Magnetic Resonance Imaging in Orthopaedics & Sports Medicine

SECOND EDITION

Magnetic Resonance Imaging in Orthopaedics & Sports Medicine

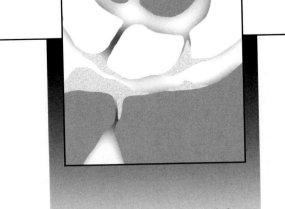

David W. Stoller, MD

Director
California Advanced Imaging

Director
Marin Radiology and National Orthopaedic Imaging Associates
San Francisco, California

Assistant Clinical Professor of Radiology
University of California at San Francisco
San Francisco, California

With 22 Contributors

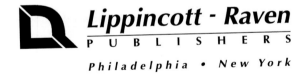

Lippincott - Raven
PUBLISHERS

Philadelphia • New York

Acquisitions Editor: James D. Ryan
Senior Developmental Editor: Delois Patterson
Project Editor: Bridget H. Meyer
Production Manager: Caren Erlichman
Production Coordinator: David Yurkovich
Designer: Doug Smock
Indexer: Maria Coughlin
Compositor: Tapsco, Inc.
Printer: Worzalla

Second Edition

Library of Congress Cataloging-in-Publication Data

Stoller, David W.
    Magnetic resonance imaging in orthopaedics & sports medicine/
David W. Stoller; with 22 contributors.—2nd ed.
        p.   cm.
    Includes bibliographical references and index.
    ISBN 0-397-51542-1
    1. Orthopedics—Diagnosis.   2. Magnetic resonance imaging.
3. Sports injuries—Diagnosis.   4. Magnetic Resonance Imaging—
atlases.   I. Title.
    [DNLM: 1. Orthopedics—atlases.   2. Orthopedics.   3. Athletic
Injuries—diagnosis—atlases.   WE   17 S875m 1997]
RD734.5.M33S75   1997
617.5′807548—dc20
DNLM/DLC
for Library of Congress   96-32807
                                                                          CIP

Care has been taken to confirm the accuracy of the information presented and to describe generally accepted practices. However, the authors, editors, and publisher are not responsible for errors or omissions or for any consequences from application of the information in this book and make no warranty, express or implied, with respect to the contents of the publication.

The authors, editors, and publisher have exerted every effort to ensure that drug selection and dosage set forth in this text are in accordance with current recommendations and practice at the time of publication. However, in view of ongoing research, changes in government regulations, and the constant flow of information relating to drug therapy and drug reactions, the reader is urged to check the package insert for each drug for any change in indications and dosage and for added warnings and precautions. This is particularly important when the recommended agent is a new or infrequently employed drug.

Some drugs and medical devices presented in this publication have Food and Drug Administration (FDA) clearance for limited use in restricted research settings. It is the responsibility of the health care provider to ascertain the FDA status of each drug or device planned for use in their clinical practice.

To my cherished son, Griffin, and my lovely wife, Marcia, for their extraordinary love and support, and to both of our families, for understanding and accommodating the sacrifices of personal time

Contributors

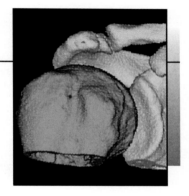

Lesley J. Anderson, MD
Orthopedic Surgeon
California Pacific Medical Center
San Francisco, California

Gordon A. Brody, MD
Chief, Hand Surgery
Sports, Orthopedic and Rehabilitation Medicine Associates
Menlo Park, California

W. Dilworth Cannon, Jr., MD
Professor of Clinical Orthopedics and Director of Sports
    Medicine
University of California at San Francisco
San Francisco, California

Richard D. Ferkel, MD
Clinical Instructor of Orthopedic Surgery
University of California, Los Angeles, Center for Health
    Science
Chief of Arthroscopy
Wadsworth VA Hospital
Los Angeles, California
Attending Surgeon and Director of Fellowship
Southern California Orthopedic Institute
Van Nuys, California

James L. Fleckenstein, MD
Associate Professor
Department of Radiology
University of Texas Southwestern Medical Center
Dallas, Texas

Russell C. Fritz, MD
Medical Director
National Orthopaedic Imaging Associates
Assistant Clinical Professor of Radiology
University of California at San Francisco
San Francisco, California

James M. Glick, MD
Associate Clinical Professor of Orthopedics
University of California at San Francisco
San Francisco, California

Steven E. Harms, MD
Director of Magnetic Resonance
University of Arkansas for Medical Science
Department of Radiology
Little Rock, Arkansas

Serena S. Hu, MD
Assistant Professor
Department of Orthopedic Surgery
University of California at San Francisco
San Francisco, California

Richard L. Jacobson, DMD, MS
Clinical Instructor of Orthodontics
UCLA School of Dentistry
Los Angeles, California

James O. Johnson, MD
Professor of Clinical Orthopedics
University of California at San Francisco
San Francisco, California

Jay A. Kaiser, MD
Medical Director
National Orthopaedic Imaging Associates
Assistant Clinical Professor of Radiology
University of California at San Francisco
San Francisco, California

Emanuel Kanal, MD
Director
MRI Department
Pittsburgh NMR Institute
Associate Professor
University of Pittsburgh
Pittsburgh, Pennsylvania

J. Bruce Kneeland, MD
Associate Professor of Radiology
Hospital of the University of Pennsylvania
Department of Radiology
Philadelphia, Pennsylvania

Thomas R. Lindquist, PhD
President
Lindquist and Associates Systems and Software
Eden Prairie, Minnesota

William J. Maloney, MD
Chief of Service
Director of Adult Reconstructive Surgery
Barnes Hospital

Associate Professor
Orthopedic Surgery
Washington University Medical Center
St. Louis, Missouri

Bruce A. Porter, MD
Medical Director
First Hill Diagnostic Imaging Center
Seattle, Washington

Thomas Schrack
MR Advanced Applications Specialist
GE Medical Systems
Waukesha, Wisconsin

Frank G. Shellock, PhD
Director
Research and Development
Future Diagnostics, Inc.
Clinical Professor of Radiology
University of Southern California
School of Medicine
Los Angeles, California

Terri M. Steinkirchner, MD
Staff Pathologist
Department of Pathology
Walnut Creek Kaiser Medical Center
Walnut Creek, California

David W. Stoller, MD
Director, California Advanced Imaging
Director, Marin Radiology and National Orthopedic Imaging
  Associates
Assistant Clinical Professor of Radiology
University of California at San Francisco
San Francisco, California

David M. Weber, PhD
MR Advanced Applications Scientist
GE Medical Systems
Echo Planar Imaging
Waukesha, Wisconsin

Eugene M. Wolf, MD
Department of Orthopedics
California Pacific Medical Center
San Francisco, California

Foreword

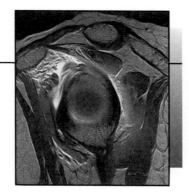

Magnetic resonance imaging is the most significant diagnostic test performed in orthopaedic and sports medicine patients. Frequently, it is the definitive examination, providing invaluable information to help the surgeon not only to understand the underlying pathology but also to make the critical decision regarding surgical intervention. In 1985, when MR imaging of the knee first became available, the clinical decision-making process was rarely influenced by its results, the direction of treatment being determined by physical examination and arthrogram. With the advent of improved and sophisticated equipment, today MR imaging is indispensable in the workup of patients with knee disorders and is fast approaching the same state of excellence for shoulder maladies. It is especially important to the professional athlete who depends on quick, accurate diagnoses to support treatment programs and to provide him or her with information that will help their return to play.

The accuracy of MR imaging for detection of meniscus and anterior cruciate tears is over 90%. In the shoulder, the diagnosis of subtle labral tears and abnormal capsular attachments, including SLAP lesions, now is made possible by these imaging techniques, thereby avoiding invasive techniques and radiation exposure. Occasionally, when further information is sought from diagnostic MR imaging, the use of intra-articular or intravenous gadolinium provides surface topographic details as well as information on vascular patterns within tissues. But the orthopaedist and radiologist should also be aware of the limitations of MR imaging, such as in the evaluation of the knee after partial meniscectomy or after meniscal repair, instances in which a Grade III signal may persist despite clinical and arthroscopic evidence of satisfactory healing.

The present compendium of musculoskeletal MR imaging is all encompassing: from the shoulder to the foot and ankle, and from bone marrow imaging to bone and soft tissue tumors. The second edition of *Magnetic Resonance Imaging in Orthopaedics and Sports Medicine* is composed of over 1,400 pages and over 3,400 images. Dr. Stoller has successfully expanded the collaboration between orthopaedic surgeons and radiologists as exemplified in numerous examples of arthroscopic, gross, and histologic correlations, in addition to enhanced clinical discussions of patient management. The beginning section provides a valuable introduction into the physics and science of MR imaging for the nonradiologist. Chapter 3, on three-dimensional MR rendering techniques, provides some interesting clinical and research concepts in volumetric analysis of internal structures, such as the menisci. Preoperative MR imaging sizing for allograft surgery is also possible. The kinematics of meniscal motion during flexion and extension as determined by MR imaging has helped to better understand knee biomechanics. The second edition also contains dedicated chapters discussing articular cartilage and muscle injuries reflecting the increased use of MR imaging for these clinical applications.

Dr. Stoller's text should become a key reference source for libraries of both radiologists and orthopaedists. It is extremely readable, and its ample illustrations help clarify points made in the text. The second edition of *Magnetic Resonance Imaging in Orthopaedics and Sports Medicine* continues to be the most comprehensive work to date on musculoskeletal imaging and should remain a classic for years to come.

W. Dilworth Cannon, Jr, MD
Professor of Clinical Orthopaedics
Director of Sports Medicine
Department of Orthopaedic Surgery
University of California at San Francisco

Preface

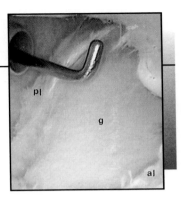

Collaborative efforts from the fields of radiology and orthopaedics have continued to define the growing indications and applications for the use of MR in orthopaedics and sports medicine. Developments such as high performance MR systems and optimized coil technology have allowed ongoing technical improvements in spatial resolution and signal to noise, as well as improving the cost effectiveness of MR studies. An understanding of both normal MR anatomy and anatomic variations of the appendicular joints has become increasingly important in having clinical applications keep pace with technological advances.

Magnetic Resonance Imaging in Orthopaedics and Sports Medicine, 2nd edition, represents a major revision of the 1993 text. More than 1500 new images have been added, the text has been significantly expanded, and four new chapters (Magnetic Resonance: Bioeffects and Safety; Principles of Echo Planar Imaging; MR Imaging of Articular Cartilage and of Cartilage Degeneration; and Magnetic Resonance Imaging of Muscle Injuries) were written. Several hundred new color arthroscopic, gross, and histologic correlative photographs have been incorporated throughout the text. Comprehensive discussions and examples of MR arthrography, fast spin-echo, fat-suppression, and echo planar techniques have also been included. MR images and concepts developed from arthroscopic correlations and numerous cadaver dissections have also been newly added.

An increased orthopaedic clinical perspective is especially evident in the chapters on the hip, the knee, the ankle and foot, the shoulder, the wrist and hand, the temporomandibular joint, the spine, and bone and soft tissue tumors. This orthopaedic contribution was made possible by the unique collective expertise of highly respected academic and orthopaedic surgeons including William J. Maloney, MD; James M. Glick, MD; W. Dilworth Cannon Jr., MD; Lesley J. Anderson, MD, Richard D. Ferkel, MD, Eugene M. Wolf, MD, Gordon A. Brody, MD, Serena S. Hu, MD, and James O. Johnston, MD.

Magnetic Resonance Imaging in Orthopaedics and Sports Medicine is a complete and current reference which addresses the growing need of radiologists, orthopaedic surgeons, and sports medicine physicians to understand and incorporate new clinical applications of bone and joint imaging into their practices.

David W. Stoller, MD

Acknowledgments

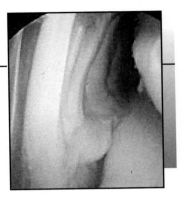

I appreciate and acknowledge the following individuals for their contributions:

J. A. Gosling, M.D., M.B., Ch.B., P. F. Harris, M.D., M.B., Ch.B., M.Sc., J. R. Humpherson, M.B., Ch.B., J. Whitmore, M.D., M.B., B.S., L.R.C.P., M.R.C.S., and P. L. T. Willan, M.B., Ch.B., F.R.C.S., for providing superior quality gross anatomic color plates from their text, *Human Anatomy*, second edition, Gower Medical Publishing.

The industrious technologist staff at California Advanced Imaging: Carolin Elquist, R.T., Kim Dick, R.T., Carol Greene, R.T., Amandra Beckford, R.T., and Ann Nelson, R.T.

Katherine Pitcoff, who served as my West Coast editor, for tirelessly preparing manuscript for presentation to Lippincott-Raven.

Jim Ryan, Medical Editor at Lippincott-Raven, Caren Erlichman, Production Manager, and Bridget Meyer, for their efforts and appreciation of the necessary quality required to bring this textbook to fruition.

Doug Smock and Dave Yurkovich for art and composition.

Chris G. Goumas, M.D., who assisted in the MR imaging of selected cadaveric joint specimens required to increase our understanding of complex appendicular joint relationships.

Kim Figone for her artistic adaptation of MR images in the cover design.

Wanda Turkle and Gordon Gee of Biomed Arts for stellar photography of text images and an unmatched professional work clinic.

Geneva C. Wright, R.T., of GE Medical Systems for supporting efforts in developing a chapter on Echo Planar Imaging.

David Frostadt of Elscint for assistance in developing color 3D CT images.

Mary Harris for assistance in typing drafts of the Preface, Foreword, and Acknowledgments.

John V. Crues III, M.D., for Figures 15-7, 15-8, 15-9, 15-10, 16-6ABC, 16-98, and 16-109

Jerrold H. Mink, M.D., for Figure 16-84

Sheila Moore, M.D., for Figures 6-72, 15-14, 16-76, and 16-101

David Seidenwurm, M.D., for Figures 16-36ABC, 16-43, 16-44, 16-71, and 16-79

Jeremy McCreary, M.D., for Figure 11-84

John Hunter, M.D., for Figure 16-37A–F

Barbara Griffiths, M.D., for Figure 7-28

Michael Schneider, M.D., for Figure 7-254

Harry K. Genant, M.D., for Figures 6-40, 14-19, 14-46, 16-23A–D, and 16-48

Clyde A. Helms, M.D., for Figure 12-6

Russell Fritz, M.D., for Figures 8-77A, 8-95, and 8-99

Frank Shellock, Ph.D., for Figures 13-19, 13-28, and 13-31, from *MRI of the Musculoskeletal System, a Teaching File,* Raven Press

Phillip Brody, M.D., for Figure 15-24

David Rubenstein, M.D., for Figure 11-109

Chris G. Goumas, M.D., for Figures 9-107, 9-137, 16-20, and 16-94

Ana Maria Magalhaes Valla Cundari, M.D., for Figure 7-251

William L. Newmeyer, M.D., for Figure 11-105D

Kevin R. Stone, M.D., for Figures 7-88B, and C, 7-120 D and F, 7-132 B and D

Contents

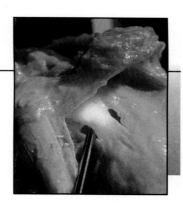

Magnetic Resonance Imaging in Orthopaedics & Sports Medicine

Magnetic Resonance Imaging in Orthopaedics & Sports Medicine, Second Edition,
edited by David W. Stoller. Lippincott-Raven Publishers, Philadelphia, © 1997.

Chapter 1

Generation and Manipulation of Magnetic Resonance Images

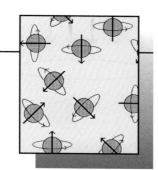

Steven E. Harms

Magnetic resonance (MR) imaging, which uses nonionizing radiation and has no demonstrated adverse biological effects, has rapidly evolved into an accepted modality for medical imaging of disease processes in the musculoskeletal system. Magnetic resonance images provide a digital representation of tissue characteristics related to spatial location and can be obtained in any tissue plane. This chapter provides an overview of MR fundamentals and addresses the factors that affect the differences in appearance (ie, contrast) among tissues in MR imaging. More detailed discussions on the fundamentals of MR imaging can be found in other sources.[1–5]

The appearance of an MR image is a function of the chemical composition of the various types of tissue. For example, soft tissues are composed of approximately 70%

water and 10% to 15% adipose, which generate all of the MR signal. At the atomic level, water and adipose are composed of hydrogen, oxygen, carbon, and phosphorus atoms. The hydrogen atom contains a proton and an orbiting electron. Understanding how an MR image is produced begins with a knowledge of magnetic fields and how these atomic components of water and fat interact with such fields.

FUNDAMENTALS OF MAGNETISM

A familiar example of magnetism is an ordinary compass needle. Like any magnet, the compass needle has a north pole and a south pole—a reflection of the dipolar nature of

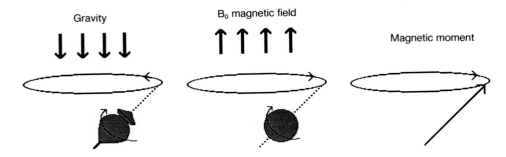

FIGURE 1-1. The hydrogen atom contains a proton that spins about an arbitrary internal axis. This spinning, positive charge produces a magnetic field, called the magnetic moment. The magnetic moment of the proton has two poles (ie, north and south) like a conventional bar magnet.

magnetism. The compass needle has a weak internal magnetic field called a magnetic moment. The earth also has an internal magnetic field, which is stronger than the magnetic field of the compass needle. In the presence of the strong magnetic field from the earth, the weak magnetic moment of the compass needle aligns with the stronger magnetic field and the needle points north. It is possible to introduce another magnetic field, such as a bar magnet, which has a magnetic field comparable in strength to the earth's magnetic field, and to twist the compass needle out of alignment with the earth's magnetic field. When the bar magnet is removed, the compass needle returns to the normal condition of pointing north in the same direction as the earth's magnetic field.

The magnetic fields associated with MR imaging are less intuitive, but follow these same principles. A spinning charged particle produces a local magnetic field. The proton

has a positive charge and spins like a top about its internal axis, as shown in Figure 1-1. The local magnetic field of the proton is called the magnetic dipole moment, and causes the proton to behave like a tiny, weak bar magnet or a weak compass needle. In the absence of any external forces, the magnetic moments of protons in tissue are oriented randomly, as shown in Figure 1-2A. If the ensemble of protons is placed in a strong, static magnetic field (B_0), their magnetic dipoles align with and against the strong field (see Fig. 1-2B). The distribution of alignments is nearly evenly divided due to the effects of thermal energy. The magnetic moments aligned with the main field are canceled by neighbors aligned against the main field. Slightly more than half of the magnetic moments align parallel to the B_0 field, however, because it takes less energy for the small magnetic moments to align with the stronger main magnetic field.

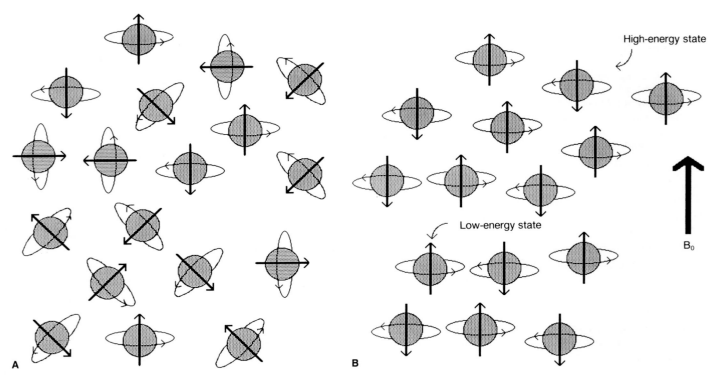

FIGURE 1-2. (**A**) A collection of protons at thermal equilibrium in the absence of a strong magnetic field. The magnetic moments produced by the spinning of the nucleus are oriented randomly. (**B**) The same collection of protons at thermal equilibrium in the presence of a strong magnetic field. The magnetic moments are aligned with or against the magnetic field B_0.

A MR signal is generated from extra magnetic moments that are aligned with B_0. At a magnetic field strength of 1.5 tesla (T), used in many clinical scanners, only approximately 8 of 2,000,000 proton magnetic moments aligned with B_0 do not have a corresponding proton magnetic moment aligned against B_0. This slight excess of protons in the lower energy state, whose individual magnetic moments add up, creates the net magnetization vector. The alignment of the magnetic moments, which occurs when the protons are placed in the B_0 field, causes the patient to acquire a slight magnetization. This process is reversible, because the magnetic moments lose alignment when the person is removed from the strong static magnetic field.

Magnetic resonance sensitivity increases as a function of magnetic field strength, because more energy is required for magnetic moments to align against the main magnetic field with increasing field strength, and a higher percentage of magnetic moments adopt the low-energy state aligned with the main B_0 field. Magnetic resonance images have low signal-to-noise ratio (SNR) compared with that of computed tomography or x-ray, because this net magnetization vector is detected from such a small percentage of the protons in the tissue.

PRECESSION AND RESONANCE

Precession and resonance are physical phenomena central to understanding MR imaging. Both result from the interaction of an object with a force. Common examples of precession include the movement of the earth and planets around the sun, the swing of a pendulum, and the rotation of a spinning top. In these cases, the precessional motion results from the effect of an orienting gravitational field on the motion of the object. The precessional motion of the magnetic dipole moment, induced by the force of a strong magnetic field, is analogous.

Resonance involves the exchange of energy between two systems. A familiar example of resonance is the vibration of two tuning forks. When energy is applied to a single tuning fork (ie, when it is struck), it resonates at a characteristic frequency. The vibration of the air produced by the first tuning fork induces resonance in a second nearby tuning fork and causes the second fork to vibrate as well. The interaction of the precessing magnetic moments with a second perturbing magnetic field is another example of resonance. In each of these examples, the motion of the object has a periodic return to the same physical location, resulting from its inherent energy (ie, momentum) or applied energy. Resonance and precession can be measured in units of numbers of cycles per second, or hertz (Hz). This unit can be scaled by a multiplier, for example, 1 million, to produce units of millions of cycles per second, or megahertz (MHz).

Precession

When a person is placed in a strong magnetic field, alignment of the magnetic moments of the protons in water and fat generates a net magnetization in the tissue. The aligned magnetic moments also precess about the main magnetic field. This precession of the magnetic moments about the main magnetic field is a cyclic process with a characteristic frequency (Fig. 1-3). A good analogy is the precession of a spinning top about the gravitational field of the earth. As the top spins, the pull of gravity is balanced by centrifugal force and the top begins to precess. As the protons spin, the attraction of the main magnetic field is balanced by centrifugal force, and the proton and its magnetic moment begin to precess. For protons in tissue, the relationship between the magnetic field strength B_0 and the precessional frequency w is given by the Larmor equation

$$w = \gamma B_0$$

where gamma is a physical constant (ie, 42.58 MHz/T) for the proton. Other MR-sensitive nuclei, such as phosphorus 31, have lower values for gamma and precess at lower frequencies.

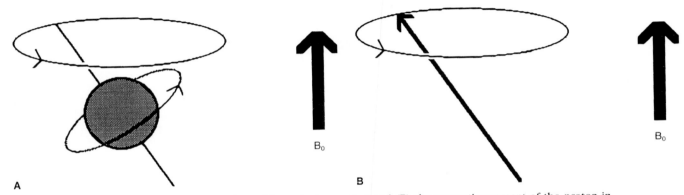

FIGURE I-3. **(A)** The precession of the spinning proton and **(B)** the magnetic moment of the proton in the presence of a strong external magnetic field.

Resonance

The net magnetism produced by precessing magnetic moments in tissue is small and cannot be measured directly with any accuracy. Instead, it is detected indirectly with a second perturbing magnetic field (B_1). A compass needle and two magnets provide a model for this process. When a compass needle is placed in a strong magnetic field (B_0), the needle aligns with the lines of magnetic flux (Fig. 1-4A). If a second perturbing magnetic field (B_1, from a second bar magnet) is placed perpendicular to the aligned compass needle, the needle realigns in a new position (see Fig. 1-4B). When the B_1 field is removed, the compass needle begins to oscillate about B_0 (see Fig. 1-4C). The resonant frequency of oscillation is governed by the strength of the aligning field (B_0), whereas the amplitude of the oscillation is determined by the strength of the perturbing field (B_1).

An analogous sequence of events is used to induce resonance in MR studies of tissue. The patient is placed in a strong magnetic field (B_0) to align the magnetic moments of water and fat protons in the tissue. Next, a perturbing magnetic field (B_1) is applied through a short (ie, 1 to 3 milliseconds) pulse of a radiofrequency (RF) wave at the Larmor frequency. RF waves have inherent perpendicular oscillating electric and magnetic field components. Therefore, a pulse of a 63.86 MHz RF wave briefly creates a magnetic field that oscillates at 63.86 MHz. The magnetic moments resonate and begin to precess about this perturbing B_1 magnetic field, and the net magnetization in tissue is realigned about a new axis away from equilibrium (Fig. 1-5). This realignment of the net magnetization vector at a new position introduces phase coherence to the individual magnetic moments in a plane perpendicular to the direction of the B_0 magnetic field. After the RF pulse is turned off and the perturbing magnetic field B_1 is removed, the displaced individual magnetic moments begin to process coherently about the B_0 field at the characteristic frequency w, given by the Larmor equation.

The resonance of the bulk magnetic moment from tissue is detected as a very small (μA) current induced in an RF antenna tuned to the Larmor frequency and located perpendicular to the B_0 field. Both the antenna used to perturb the magnetic moments and the antenna used to detect their precession must be tuned to the Larmor frequency and located perpendicular to the B_0 field.

This detection process is similar to the generation of electricity by a dynamo in a power station. In the dynamo shown in Figure 1-6, the moving water turns a turbine attached to a bar magnet. The turbine and magnet rotate at a fixed frequency and produce a magnetic field that oscillates at the same frequency (eg, the turbine and magnet rotate at 60 Hz and produce a magnetic field that oscillates at 60 Hz). If the bar magnet is near a coil of wire, the oscillating magnetic field generates electric current in the coil of wire. The electric current varies from positive to negative at a resonant frequency of 60 Hz as the bar magnet swings around near the coil of wire. This alternating current then can be stored.

Similarly, after excitation, the protons in tissue behave like tiny bar magnets rotating at the Larmor frequency. When a coil of wire (ie, the MR antenna) is located near the tissue, the rotating magnetic field caused by precession of the net magnetic moment from the tissue generates a current that

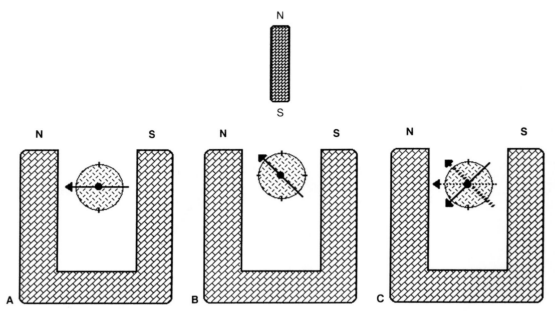

FIGURE 1-4. (**A**) Positioning a compass needle between the poles of a strong bar magnet causes it to orient itself toward the north pole of the magnet. (**B**) Reorientation of the compass needle is caused by a second perturbing magnetic field. (**C**) Induction of precession in the compass needle occurs when the second perturbing magnetic field is removed.

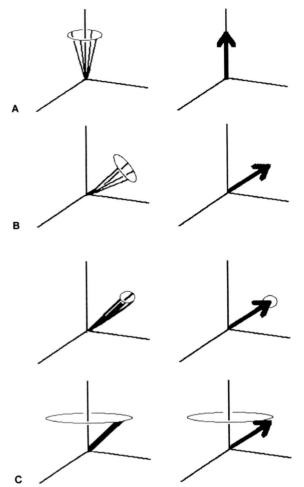

FIGURE 1-5. Note the effects of the perturbing B_1 magnetic field on the bulk magnetization vector (**A**) at the start of the B_1 pulse; (**B**) at the end of the B_1 pulse; and (**C**) some time after the pulse as the individual magnetic moments precess at their Larmor frequencies.

resonates at the Larmor frequency in the wire of the MR antenna. The amplitude of the detected signal in an MR scan is related to the size of the net magnetic moment per volume of tissue and the duration and amplitude of the applied perturbing magnetic field (B_1). The voltage induced in the antenna is digitized and stored in an MR imaging computer as a function of time.

Energy Levels

This process also can be described in quantum mechanical terms as a probability function for inducing a transition between two energy levels that correspond to the states where the magnetic moment is aligned with and against the main magnetic field. This quantum mechanical description of resonance is equally valid, but is based on a mathematical description that is difficult to visualize.

Rotating Frame of Reference

A reexamination of the precession of the net magnetization vector in tissue, as seen in Figure 1-3, shows that after excitation the precession of the bulk magnetic moment traces out a circular path. If the observer's perspective is changed (instead of viewing this precession from the side, it is viewed looking down the direction of the static magnetic field B_0), is defined as the Z axis in this new coordinate system. This is illustrated in Figure 1-7, where the intensity of the net magnetization vector is projected onto a plane that contains the X and Y axes. The vector precesses at the Larmor frequency, perhaps in a counterclockwise direction (ie, an arbitrary choice), and it can now be seen that the precession of the magnetization is a three-dimensional (3D) process with an associated amplitude (ie, length) and phase (ie, relative position in the X,Y plane). These attributes can be visualized by plotting the relative position of the net magnetization vector in the X,Y plane versus time. The result is a sine or cosine wave that resonates at the Larmor frequency. As the net magnetization vector precesses, the change in apparent position is reflected as a change in the phase of the projected vector in the X,Y plane.

If the observer also is precessing counterclockwise at the Larmor frequency, the net magnetization vector appears to be stationary. This is called the rotating frame of reference, and is commonly used in descriptions of MR scans to aid in the visualization of the effects that RF pulses, magnetic field gradient pulses, and relaxation processes have on the net magnetization vector.

Changes in the phase and Larmor frequency of a net magnetization vector relative to the position of the observer at a fixed frequency and phase can be detected. If the observer is diligent and continuously records the position of the precessing vectors, those vectors will appear to move away from the fixed reference point at some relative frequency (Fig. 1-8). However, imagine that the observer is sleepy and only opens his or her eye periodically for a brief instant to perform a measurement and recording. In this case, the precessing vectors do not appear to move continually, but adopt a new relative position in the X,Y plane each time the observer makes a measurement. The new position is recorded as phase information relative to the position of the observer. If enough observations are performed, the frequency of the precessing vectors can be determined indirectly by measuring the rate of change in the phase of the vectors and by converting this rate of change into frequency information (see Fig. 1-8).

The two methods—direct measurement of frequency and indirect determination of frequency from phase changes—yield an identical result. Every MR signal has a frequency and a phase; thus, changes in either of these two attributes can be measured via phase encoding or frequency encoding and converting into frequency information to produce a two-dimensional (2D) MR image.

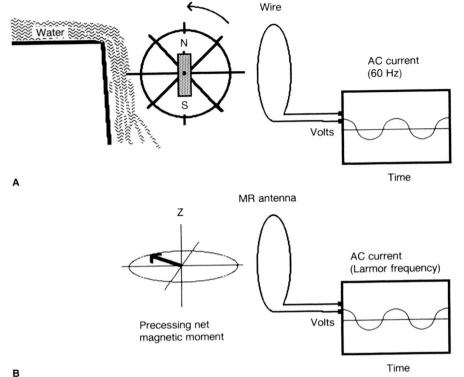

A

B

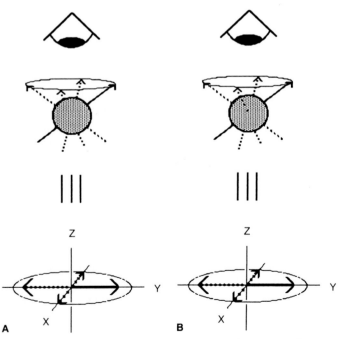

A   B

FIGURE 1-6. The dynamo model for detection of the MR signal. **(A)** A model dynamo produces current in a loop of wire through the circular motion of the bar magnet induced by the flow of water over the paddle wheels. **(B)** A model magnetic moment produces current in a loop of wire (ie, MR antenna) through precession at the Larmor frequency. The effect is analogous to the model dynamo, although the model magnetic moment rotates in a plane perpendicular to the plane of the dynamo's bar magnet.

FIGURE 1-7. A view of a precessing magnetization vector after perturbation from along the Z axis (ie, along the axis of the strong magnetic field), and a corresponding model of precession in the rotating frame of reference is continuously monitored from along the Y axis. The amplitude of the magnetization vector is zero when viewed head-on, and has maximum and minimum values when viewed from the side.

MAKING A MAGNETIC RESONANCE IMAGE

Inherently, the generation of an MR image is a four-dimensional problem that involves three spatial coordinates (ie, X, Y, Z) and one contrast dimension that reflects the signal intensity within each volume element (ie, voxel) of tissue. The spatial origin of the signal must be defined with suitable resolution in three orthogonal planes, whereas the signal intensity in the contrast dimension must be above the level of the background noise. In practice, the resolution in one spatial dimension (ie, slice dimension) may be compressed to one point to save time, producing a 2D image of a single slice. This method for generating a 2D slice-selective image is the basis for the following discussion. The benefits of true 3D volume imaging are presented later in this chapter.

Equipment

The following equipment is required to produce an MR image:

- A large homogeneous static magnetic field (B_0) to align the tissue magnetization
- Magnetic field gradient coils, which produce linear variations in the effective magnetic field as a function of spatial position in X, Y, and Z.
- An RF antenna, or RF coil, to produce a perturbing magnetic field (B_1) and to measure the MR signal

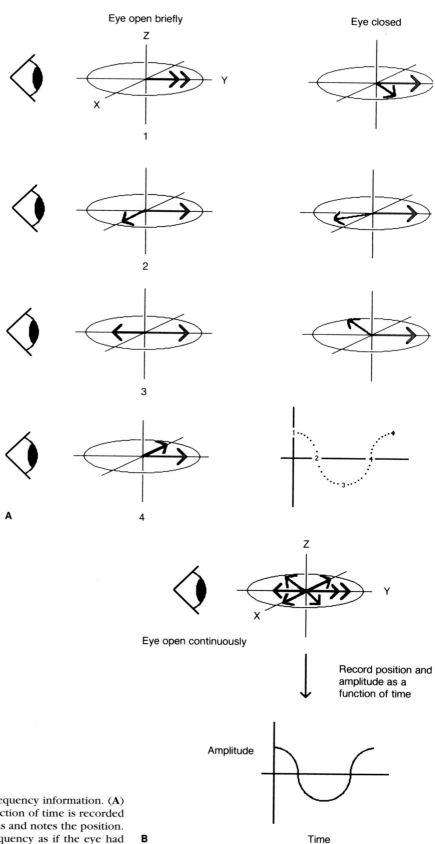

FIGURE 1-8. A model for the phase encoding of frequency information. (**A**) The amplitude of the magnetization vector as a function of time is recorded in the lower right corner each time the "eye" opens and notes the position. (**B**) This periodic sampling measures the same frequency as if the eye had been open the entire time.

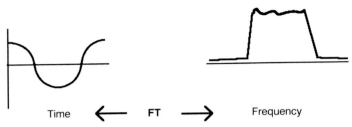

Time   ⟵   FT ⟶   Frequency

FIGURE 1-9. The 3D Fourier transform converts time to frequency information. Hence, signals measured in the time domain can be converted into frequency information used to produce MR images.

- A computer to store time domain data on frequency and phase and to convert this data to frequency information through the mathematical function called three-dimensional Fourier transform (3DFT; Fig. 1-9)
- A method to display the images through appropriate media such as film or a computer workstation.

Magnetic Field Gradient

In a perfectly homogeneous static magnetic field, all of the magnetic moments for each proton of water or fat would precess at the same Larmor frequency. However, the strength of the magnetic field can be made to vary throughout the magnet in a linear and predictable fashion, using the mag-

netic field gradient coils. All MR scanners have magnetic field gradient coils that introduce a linear change in the magnetic field B_0 oriented along three orthogonal directions: (1) left to right across the bore of the magnet, (2) up and down across the bore of the magnet; and (3) along the length of the bore of the magnet (X, Y, and Z axes in the rotating frame coordinate system).

At the exact center of the gradient coil, the linear change in magnetic field strength for all three directions is zero. This location, where each of the gradient coils induces no change in magnetic field strength, is called the isocenter of the magnet. At this point, magnetic moments always precess at the normal frequency governed by the strength of the main magnetic field. Away from isocenter, the strength of the main static magnetic field B_0 is altered by the gradient coils.

The precessional frequency of the magnetization depends on the effective strength of the total magnetic field, as calculated from the Larmor equation. Therefore, the precessional frequencies can be made to vary as a function of spatial position by applying a magnetic field gradient in the X, Y, or Z direction.

This concept of magnetic field gradient, central to all MR processes, is illustrated in Figure 1-10. If a 10-cm long container filled with water is placed in the bore of a 1.5-T

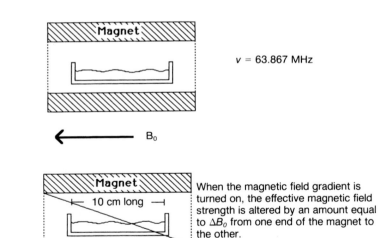

v = 63.867 MHz

A   ⟵ B_0

When the magnetic field gradient is turned on, the effective magnetic field strength is altered by an amount equal to ΔB_0 from one end of the magnet to the other.

$B_0 + \Delta B_0$ $B_0 - \Delta B_0$

B v = 63.888 MHz v = 63.846 MHz

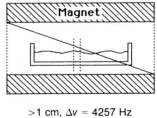

C   >1 cm, Δv = 4257 Hz

FIGURE 1-10. (A) When a 10-cm tub of water is placed in a homogeneous static magnetic field B_0, all of the water protons precess at a single frequency, w. **(B)** In the presence of a magnetic field gradient γB_0 with a strength of 1 gauss/cm applied along the Z axis, the water magnetization resonates over a frequency range of 63.888 to 63.846 MHz as a function of the spatial position in the magnet field gradient. **(C)** In the presence of a magnetic field gradient with a strength of 1 gauss/cm, the water magnetization in the central 1-cm region resonates over a frequency range of 4257 Hz. If a radio frequency pulse with a bandwidth of 4257 Hz is used as the perturbing B_1 magnetic field, only the water magnetization in the 1-cm region will be excited.

magnet, all of the protons will resonate at a frequency of 63.876000 MHz. However, in the presence of a magnetic field gradient with a strength of 10 mT/m (1 gauss/cm) applied along the Z axis (ie, the length of the magnet bore), the water protons resonate over a range of frequencies determined by the following equation:

$$(10 \text{ cm long}) \times (0.1 \text{ mT/m}) \times 42.58 \text{ MHz/T} = 42{,}580 \text{ Hz}.$$

Since the strength of the magnetic field gradient is linear as a function of position along Z, the resonant frequency is directly related to the spatial position. We use this relationship to generate MR images.

Two-Dimensional Magnetic Resonance Imaging

The generation of a 2D MR image requires three steps: (1) selection of a slice of tissue for study in a first dimension (ie, slice direction), (2) definition of the spatial position in a second dimension by measuring the rate of change in the phase of the MR signal produced by varying the amplitude of a magnetic field gradient pulse (ie, phase-encoding direction), and (3) definition of the spatial position in the third dimension by detecting the signal in the presence of a magnetic field gradient (ie, read-out direction).

Slice Selection

As shown in Figure 1-10, in the presence of a 1 gauss/cm magnetic field gradient, the water protons in a 10 cm dish resonate over a frequency range of 42,580 Hz (± 21,290 Hz), with a frequency of 63.876000 MHz at the gradient isocenter. If the RF pulse used to generate the perturbing magnetic field at 63.876000 MHz has a bandwidth of only 2129 Hz, the signal from a 5 mm section of the dish centered about the isocenter can be excited selectively when the magnetic field gradient is turned on. If the frequency of the slice-selective pulse is varied, for example to 63.878129 MHz (+2129 Hz), a 5 mm slice can be generated at a location 5 mm to the left (ie, high-frequency side) of the slice at isocenter. In this fashion, 20 contiguous 5 mm thick MR images of the entire object could be generated using frequency selective RF pulses to excite each slice.

Phase and Phase Encoding

As shown earlier, precessing magnetization has an amplitude and a relative position in the X,Y plane. In the presence of a magnetic field gradient perpendicular to the direction of the slice gradient, the magnetization vectors in different spatial locations experience different effective magnetic field strengths as a linear function of their position and, as governed by the Larmor equation, resonate at different frequencies. This condition leads to dephasing of the magnetization vectors in different parts of the slice plane. The amount of dephasing that the net magnetization vector experiences is

a function of the position in the gradient (Fig. 1-11), the strength of the applied gradient, and the length of time that the gradient pulse is on.

When the field gradient pulse is turned off, the vectors experience only the B_0 magnetic field, and then resonate at their original frequencies. However, the vectors remember the amount of dephasing they received during the time the field gradient pulse was applied (ie, phase encoding time). The strength of the applied field gradient pulse can be varied many times and the amount of dephasing that occurs with each variation can be measured for magnetization in all parts of the slice plane. The rates of change in the phase of magnetization for proximate regions of tissue are small, and a large number (128 to 256) of phase-encoding steps are required to produce adequate resolution in the time domain. These rates are converted into frequency information via 3DFT and finally into the exact spatial location from the known strength and duration of the phase encoding gradient pulse.

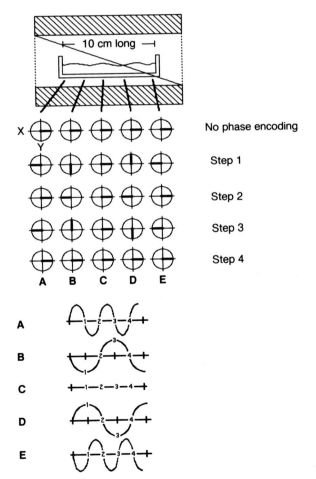

FIGURE 1-11. The phase encoding process. In the presence of a magnetic field gradient pulse, the magnetic moments temporarily precess at faster or slower speeds. This produces a shift in the phase of the detected signal. The change in phase is shown for five locations (*A through E*), following four different magnetic field gradient pulses (*1 through 4*). The resulting phase maps for A through E are shown (*bottom*).

Readout Dimension and Frequency Encoding

As shown in Figure 1-10, the relative spatial position of an object can be estimated from the resonant frequency in the presence of a magnetic field gradient. However, the resonant frequency is determined indirectly. The MR signal is measured and stored as amplitude (ie, voltage) versus time information while the readout field gradient is applied. The spatial resolution in this dimension is determined by the number of points that are sampled and the frequency bandwidth. The strength of the readout gradient and the bandwidth determine the field of view (FOV). If the frequency bandwidth in the readout dimension is 16,000 Hz, 512 points will have to be sampled to be able to distinguish signals that differ by 30 Hz.

The readout bandwidth also affects the SNR in an image. The amount of noise stored by the computer is proportional to the bandwidth. A fourfold decrease in the readout bandwidth reduces the noise by a factor of four, with a twofold improvement in image SNR. This variable bandwidth strategy is used on many commercial MR units to improve the SNR in images acquired at long echo times (TEs).

Three-Dimensional Magnetic Resonance Imaging

Conventional 2D imaging often sacrifices resolution and complete coverage in the slice dimension for speed. These trade-offs probably are acceptable in studies of the brain and body, in which the organs are large and homogeneous. However, in regions that contain fine structures, such as the knee, the volume averaging, lack of continuous slices, and thicker slices associated with 2D MR imaging can obscure pathology. 3D MR imaging can be used to generate a set of contiguous images having nearly isotropic voxels, which provide high-resolution detail of fine pathologic processes. In addition, images corresponding to any plane of tissue can be generated and viewed from a 3D data set. Hence, it is not necessary to spend time obtaining separate sets of images in all three conventional image planes. This added flexibility is advantageous for following pathologic processes such as damage to ligaments or cartilage that do not track through a single-image plane.

To date, the clinical use of 3D MR imaging has been restricted because of limitations in the performance of computers and gradients available on MR instruments. For example, a 16 bit, 128 × 128 × 256 point 3D data set requires 8 megabytes of computer memory. Storage, 3DFT, and reformatting of 3D data sets can be time-consuming on conventional MR imaging computers, making dedicated image processing workstations necessary for viewing 3D images. However, the usefulness and diagnostic importance of 3D MR imaging has spawned a new generation of MR imaging hardware to provide users with the required capabilities.

The steps involved in producing a 3D MR image are very similar to the steps used to make a 2D image. A thick-slab 3D image can be produced by exciting a large (8- to 20-cm) slice, followed by phase encoding using stepped gradient pulses in both the slice encoding and phase encoding dimensions. This method is used when a limited number of slice encoding steps are to be used. A volume 3D image can be produced by performing the initial excitation with a nonselective pulse, followed by application of a large number (128 or more) of encoding steps in the slice and phase dimensions. The data sets may be interpolated in one or more dimensions to yield true isotropic 3D images.

Image Generation

The following steps must be performed in the order presented for an MR image to be generated properly: (1) excite a slice of magnetization in the presence of a magnetic field gradient in one direction, (2) encode spatial position in the second direction (a third direction for 3D) by measuring the rate of change in the phase of the signals caused by a series of pulsed field gradients of differing amplitudes (ie, phase encoding), and (3) encode spatial position in the third direction by indirectly measuring the resonant frequency in the presence of a magnetic field gradient (ie, frequency readout).

The series of RF and gradient events for producing an MR image can be drawn schematically as a function of time. Such pulse timing diagrams for a gradient echo sequence and a spin-echo sequence are shown in Figure 1-12. The gradient echo sequence begins with the shape of a sine function [sine (x)/x] in the presence of a magnetic field gradient. The phase error introduced by the magnetic field gradient during the slice selection process is reversed when a magnetic field gradient pulse of the opposite sign and one half the area is applied after the slice selection process. Next, the appropriate phase encoding magnetic field gradient pulse is applied. This is often concomitant with the slice refocusing gradient pulse and a dephasing gradient pulse whose area is equal to one half of the area of the readout gradient pulse—applied along the readout direction during the signal acquisition period. Finally the signal is detected in the presence of the readout magnetic field gradient. A full echo generally is stored during the digitization period, although this is not required.

The data are stored in the MR imaging computer as voltage amplitude versus time. The computer performs a 3DFT to convert the time data from the readout dimension and the rate of change of the signal phase from the phase encoding dimension into frequency information. Frequency differences are proportional to the distance from the isocenter in a calibrated magnetic field gradient, and the frequency information directly corresponds to the spatial location in both directions. The resulting MR image has a resolution of 1 point in the slice direction. In the image plane, however, the resolution is represented by the following:

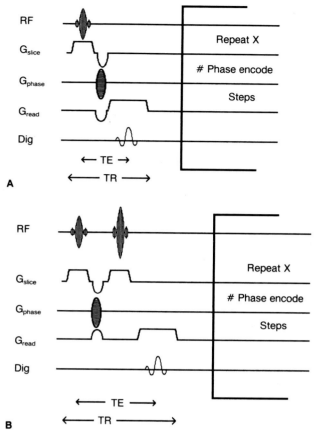

FIGURE 1-12. Timing diagrams for (**A**) a gradient echo pulse sequence and (**B**) a spin-echo pulse sequence. Time is increasing from left to right for each of the radiofrequency (RF) and gradient pulse waveforms. Dig, analog/digital converter; G_{phase}, phase-encoding gradient; G_{read}, readout or frequency gradient; G_{slice}, slice encoding gradient.

(FOV/no. of phase encoding)

× (FOV/no. of points stored during readout).

Therefore, greater resolution for smaller structures can be achieved only by increasing the number of phase encoding steps and the time required to make the image or by decreasing the FOV to alter the size of the voxels in the image. Each voxel contains signal intensity corresponding to the voltage measured during data acquisition. The enhancement or attenuation of this signal intensity using known variables produces contrast in the MR image.

PARAMETERS AFFECTING THE APPEARANCE OF MAGNETIC RESONANCE IMAGES

The appearance of an MR image is determined by many parameters. In general, these parameters can be divided into two cases: (1) those that have a fixed value governed by the physics of MR, and (2) those that can be modified by the user to alter the appearance of the image.

The goal of any MR study is to generate images of tissue anatomy in which the contrast-to-noise ratio (CNR) is sufficient to allow identification of the disease process. This is accomplished by varying the user-defined parameters to maximize differences in the values of intrinsic parameters and to emphasize differences in signal intensity between voxels containing normal and pathologic tissues.

Intrinsic Parameters

Intrinsic parameters are tissue dependent and not under operator control. Examples of intrinsic parameters are the density of water and fat within tissue, blood flow, and the rates of relaxation of the magnetic moments back to equilibrium after perturbation. Some intrinsic parameters are invariant among all tissues (eg, the strength of the magnetic field).

Proton Density

A common pathologic condition is the accumulation of edematous fluid around a tumor. The edema has a higher proportion of water than surrounding normal tissue, and hence a higher density of protons per unit volume. This increase in density of protons per unit volume can be observed using MR imaging methods that emphasize or attenuate the signal intensity in voxels based on the proton density. Typically, proton density weighted MR images are obtained using the shortest possible TE and repetition time (TR) that allows full T1 relaxation of all magnetic moments back to equilibrium.

Relaxation Times

After it is excited, the MR signal cannot be detected forever. It decays as the result of two different types of relaxation processes: (1) the return of the bulk magnetic moment to thermal equilibrium, and (2) the loss of phase coherence in the net magnetization as a result of interactions with other magnetic moments in the tissue.

The rate at which these processes return the net magnetization to equilibrium is critical, because the MR experiment must be repeated for each phase encoding step, and the amount of magnetization available for study depends on how many of the magnetic moments are realigned with the main magnetic field.

T2 AND T2* RELAXATION TIMES. After excitation, the MR signal present in the X,Y plane decays exponentially to zero over time. The time required for 63% of the signal to disappear irreversibly is called the T2 relaxation time or the transverse or spin-spin relaxation time (Fig. 1-13). This decay is caused by the many processes that produce a loss of phase coherence in the MR signal. After the RF pulse, all the magnetic moments initially precess with identical phases. However, variations in the effective magnetic field strength cause the magnetic moments to precess at different frequen-

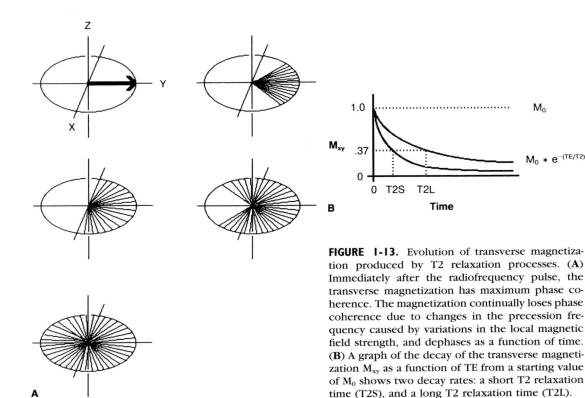

FIGURE 1-13. Evolution of transverse magnetization produced by T2 relaxation processes. **(A)** Immediately after the radiofrequency pulse, the transverse magnetization has maximum phase coherence. The magnetization continually loses phase coherence due to changes in the precession frequency caused by variations in the local magnetic field strength, and dephases as a function of time. **(B)** A graph of the decay of the transverse magnetization M_{xy} as a function of TE from a starting value of M_0 shows two decay rates: a short T2 relaxation time (T2S), and a long T2 relaxation time (T2L).

cies for short periods of time. This results in the dephasing of the vector bundle in the X,Y plane illustrated by Figure 1-13 and a decrease in the signal available for detection. Variation in the local magnetic field strength can be produced by binding to macromolecules, interactions with magnetic dipoles of other nuclei such as oxygen, and vibration of chemical bonds.

The T2* and T2 relaxation processes originate from inhomogeneities in the strength of the main magnetic field (T2*), or close interactions with other magnetic dipoles (T2). After the initial RF pulse, the individual magnetic moments precess in phase at frequencies determined by the local magnetic field strength. For a variety of reasons, however, including differences in tissue composition, the main magnetic field B_0 is not homogeneous. As the magnetic moments traverse regions of

altered magnetic field strength, they momentarily precess at higher and lower frequencies, causing dephasing of the net magnetization vector and T2* relaxation. This inhomogeneity in the main magnetic field varies slowly, and the dephasing can be reversed by application of a second RF pulse with an amplitude of π radians (ie, 180°), which flips the magnetic moments in the X,Y plane and produces a reversal of the dephasing due to static magnetic field inhomogeneity.

The RF pulse can be applied many times, and multiple echoes can be formed and acquired as shown in Figure 1-14. Eventually, the signal amplitude decays as a function of the true T2 relaxation time, which is a function of irreversible dephasing caused by random, short-duration interactions of the individual magnetic moments with neighboring magnetic moments.

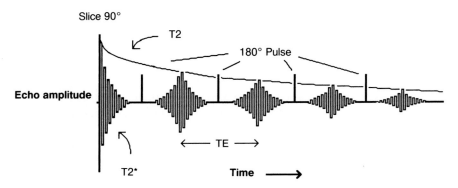

FIGURE 1-14. Evolution of transverse magnetization as a function of time in a spin-echo sequence with four echoes. After the initial slice pulse, sequential application of 180° pulses produces refocusing of T2* dephasing due to magnetic field inhomogeneities and balanced magnetic field gradient pulses. The maximum amplitude of each echo decays over a time T2, which is the time period for irreversible dephasing of transverse magnetization.

T1 RELAXATION TIME. The T1 relaxation time (ie, spin-lattice or longitudinal relaxation time) is the time required to restore 63% of the equilibrium population of magnetic moments aligned with the B_0 magnetic field following the excitation pulse. T1 relaxation is an exponential process (Fig. 1-15). In the classic picture, T1 relaxation processes involved the transfer of energy from the excited individual magnetic moments to the surrounding lattice of magnetic moments in other molecules. This transfer of energy from magnetic moments to the lattice restores the equilibrium alignment of the magnetic moments with the main magnetic field. An example of a T1 relaxation process would be the transfer of energy from an excited magnetic dipole of an individual spin to the large and small effective magnetic dipoles of groups of spins on neighboring molecules. Unlike T2 relaxation, this T1 relaxation occurs only through oscillation of local magnetic moments that occur at the Larmor frequency. These local magnetic moments originate from tumbling macromolecules and other magnetic constituents of the lattice that couple to the relaxing magnetic moment.

The T1 relaxation time for any material varies as a function of magnetic field strength, since more variations occur in the local effective magnetic field strength at lower Larmor frequencies. Therefore, T1 relaxation times tend to decrease with decreasing magnetic field strengths. At all Larmor frequencies, few paths exist to produce T1 relaxation, and the

T1 relaxation time is always longer than or equal to the T2 relaxation time. Figure 1-15 provides a pictorial representation of T1 relaxation and a graph showing the exponential recovery of aligned magnetization as a function of time after the initial RF pulse.

Extrinsic Parameters

Many types of operator-controlled parameters can alter image appearance. These include timing events, such as TR, TE, and, in inversion recovery studies, the spin inversion time. Other parameters that affect image appearance are slice thickness, digital resolution, and FOV. Image appearance also can be changed by applying more than one RF pulse prior to data collection.

TR and TE

Typically, 128 or 256 phase encoding steps are required in an MR acquisition. The TR is the amount of time between consecutive phase-encoding steps, and the TE is the time between the initial perturbing RF pulse and the center of the acquisition period. TR is generally longer than TE, except for some steady state fast scan methods, such as contrast-enhanced fast acquisition in steady state (CE-FAST) or fast imaging with steady state precession (FISP).

Slice Thickness, Field of View, and Resolution

All MR images suffer from volume averaging effects to some degree. This is most serious in the slice direction, where the effective voxel size is often 3 or 5 mm deep. Thinner slices can be obtained with 3D sequences at the expense of longer acquisition times. The size of the FOV can be modified to prevent wraparound artifacts and to increase the in-plane resolution for a fixed number of data points. When the resolution in a spatial dimension is doubled for a fixed total acquisition time, only one half as much signal is detected in each voxel and the SNR in the image is decreased by a factor of two. Scanning for twice as long does not provide twice the signal, because the SNR only increases with the square root of the number of averages (n).

Pulse Tip Angle

When the second perturbing magnetic field B_1 is applied, the individual magnetic moments precess about the new effective magnetic field. Hence, their final position is a function of the strength and duration of the perturbing field B_1. As illustrated in the rotating frame diagram in Figure 1-4, the maximum signal is detected when the B_1 magnetic field produces a displacement of $\pi/2$ radians (ie, 90°) away from the Z axis, and the bulk magnetization vector is placed in the X,Y plane. The geometric angle between the position of the net magnetization vector is placed in the X,Y plane.

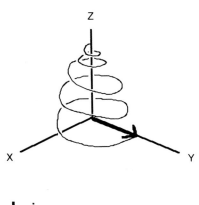

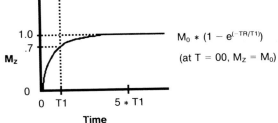

FIGURE 1-15. Contrast depends on the magnitude of the initial pulse, as seen for two tissues with a T1 of 500 and 800 msec, respectively. Restoration of longitudinal magnetization occurs as a function of time after a single $\pi/2$ radiofrequency (RF) pulse. After the $\pi/2$ RF pulse, the longitudinal magnetization is zero. The magnetization continues to precess at the Larmor frequency until it has returned to its equilibrium position with a longitudinal component M_0. The amount of longitudinal magnetization is restored as an exponential function of time.

The geometric angle between the position of the net magnetization vector and the Z axis is called the pulse tip angle. The pulse tip angle can strongly affect the contrast in an image. An example of this relationship is shown in Figure 1-16.

Signal-to-Noise Ratio and Scan Time

As discussed in the preceding sections, the SNR in an MR image is a function of many things. Invariant parameters such as the magnetic field strength influence the SNR, as do the intrinsic parameters unique to tissues such as proton density [N(H)] and T1, T2*, and T2 relaxation times. Extrinsic operator-controlled parameters affecting the SNR include the TE, TR, flip angle, FOV, and sampling bandwidth in each spatial dimension (FOV_x and FOV_y, where x = readout and y = phase encode directions), slice thickness (Δz), n, the number of points sampled in each spatial dimension (#x and #y), and noise level (N).

With a fixed field strength, flip angle, and noise level, the SNR can be calculated according to the following formula:

$$SNR \approx f(intrinsic) \cdot f(extrinsic)/N.$$

The function for the dependence of the signal strength on the intrinsic parameters in an spin-echo pulse sequence is given as the following equation:

$$f(intrinsic) \approx (N_{(H)} \cdot (1 - e^{-(TR/T1)}) \cdot (e^{-(TE/T2)}).$$

The TR is linked to T1, such that only variations in TR affect the amount of T1 weighting, or signal attenuation, in an MR image. Similarly, TE is linked to T2, and variations in the extrinsic parameter TE affect the amount of T2 weighting (ie, signal attenuation) in an image. Both T1- and T2-weighted images have lower SNRs than proton density images because contrast is produced by attenuating one signal component. These relationships between TR/T1 and TE/T2 form the basis for the following discussion of image appearance.

For any given combination of invariant and intrinsic parameters with TR and TE, the equation for the signal strength as a function of the remaining extrinsic parameters is given as the following:

$$f(extrinsic) \approx \Delta z \cdot (\sqrt{n}) \cdot (FOV_x/\#x) \cdot (FOV_y/\#y).$$

The relationship has no impact on the contrast in an image, but does have several other important consequences. For example, a twofold magnification (ie, fixed matrix size but FOV reduced by one half) reduces the SNR per voxel in the image by a factor of four. A twofold increase in resolution (ie, double the matrix size in both the phase encoding and readout dimension for a fixed FOV) reduces the SNR by $2\sqrt{2}$ but doubles the scan time (T_S), because the T_S is increased to sample twice as many phase encode steps. Sampling for twice as long (ie, n twice as large) increases the SNR by a maximum of only $\sqrt{2}$.

The total T_S for a 2D or 3D image can be defined from TR, #y, #z, and n as in the following equation:

$$T_S = TR \cdot \#y \cdot n \cdot \#z.$$

It follows from this equation that increasing the number of n, the number of phase encode steps (#y and #z; #z = 1 for a 2D image), or TR, increases the time required to complete the scan. In spin-echo imaging, signal averaging is the only way to improve the SNR without altering image resolution. The situation is more complex in fast scans, where the SNR is a function of the TR, type of pulse, and flip angle. If the Ts is held constant, an improvement in SNR can be realized only by increasing the slice thickness, increasing the FOV, or decreasing the resolution.

Contrast-to-Noise Ratio

The ability to differentiate among tissues is limited by both the inherent SNR level and the difference in signal strength (ie, contrast between adjacent voxels). For example, if the signal strength in voxel 1 is defined as S1 and in an adjacent voxel as S2, and N in the image is uniformly distributed (ie, no artifacts are present), then the CNR is given as the following equation:

$$CNR \approx \frac{|S1 - S2|}{N}.$$

This equation suggests that the contrast in an MR image can be improved by reducing the noise level or by manipulating the differential attenuation of signal in normal versus pathologic tissues using extrinsic parameters. Strategies for

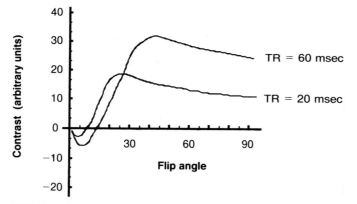

FIGURE 1-16. Tissue contrast depends on the magnitude of the initial radiofrequency (RF) pulse for a model system of two tissues with different T1 longitudinal relaxation times. As the flip angle of the RF pulse increases, the contrast between the two tissues becomes strongly dependent on the TR used between pulses. However, there is a flip angle that produces the optimum contrast for the given T1 values of 500 and 800 msec (eg, values for white matter and gray matter in the brain, respectively).

manipulating image contrast are discussed in the next section.

MANIPULATING EXTRINSIC PARAMETERS TO VARY IMAGE CONTRAST

Echo Formation

Thus far, the discussion of production of an MR image has been concerned with excitation of a slice followed by generation of a gradient echo that is detected during application of a readout gradient and contains phase information on spatial position in the phase encoding dimension. Two methods commonly are used to form the echo:

1. Refocusing of the readout gradient to form a gradient echo.
2. Simultaneous formation of a gradient echo and an RF echo using gradient reversal and an additional RF pulse.

The characteristics of the detected signal are influenced strongly by the method used to generate the echo.

Gradient Echoes

The gradient echo method collects the residual free induction decay (FID) signal still present after the initial excitation pulse. The FID disappears to zero at a time, designated T2*, that is shorter than the natural T2 relaxation time. At very short TEs, the signal attenuation from T2 and T2* are approximately equivalent, and gradient echo images provide an accurate representation of tissue signal intensity. However, at TEs longer than 10 msec, the signal intensity in gradient echo images is attenuated strongly by T2*.

Spin-Echoes

Nearly 40 years ago, Hahn[5] demonstrated that the FID signal could be regenerated by applying a second RF pulse. This second pulse reverses and refocuses the dephasing of the magnetization produced by long-lived magnetic field inhomogeneities (ie, T2* relaxation) and forms an echo at a time equal to the interval between the two RF pulses. When the amplitude of the second RF pulse produces an inversion of the signal in the X,Y plane, the echo formed during the digitization period is called a spin-echo. The second pulse has an optimum amplitude of π radians (180°) to produce the maximum intensity of the spin-echo. The signal intensity decays with time as an exponential function of the T2 relaxation time, not the T2* relaxation time (see Fig. 1-14).

It can be seen, therefore, that the contrast in an image generated from a gradient echo differs significantly from that of an image generated from a spin-echo. The contrast in a gradient echo image can be varied using ''pre-pulses'' to invert the magnetization prior to the fast scan, by increasing (or decreasing) the repetition and TEs, and by selecting

from among the different types of gradient echoes that can be acquired.

Spin-echo imaging methods collect the data after application of a 180° pulse to refocus T2* induced dephasing. The contrast in spin-echo images is a function of the T1 and T2 relaxation times and the TR and TE, with no contribution from T2*.

T1-Weighted Magnetic Resonance Imaging and TR

All MR images are T1-weighted to some degree, since the net magnetization is not restored to 100% until a period equal to 7 · (T1 relaxation time) after the initial excitation. The T1 relaxation times for water and fat in the body range from 100 to 2000 msec. The primary source of signal attenuation in a spin-echo image is the progressive saturation of the magnetic moment by the repetitive slice selection pulses. This is demonstrated in Figure 1-17 for sagittal images from a knee obtained with a 3 mm slice thickness. The signal from fat is bright, whereas image intensities from areas of muscle and fluid in a meniscal cyst are lower. At longer TR values, the amount of signal attenuation due to incomplete T1 relaxation is reduced, and the images move toward a proton density appearance. T1-weighted images also can be produced using a preliminary inversion recovery pulse and delay time. However, this method requires a sufficiently long TR interval to ensure that the magnetization has returned to equilibrium prior to the next inversion pulse.

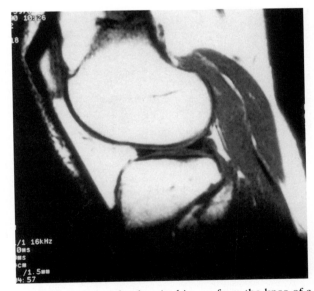

FIGURE 1-17. A T1-weighted sagittal image from the knee of a patient with a meniscal cyst. A TR of 500 msec and a TE of 15 msec have been employed using a 3-mm slice thickness and a 16-cm field of view with 256 points. The meniscus is very hypointense, the cyst and articular cartilage are hypointense, the muscle has moderate intensity, and the fat is hyperintense.

Proton Density Weighting

Images where the contrast is governed by the relative concentration of water in the tissue can be generated using long TRs (TR >2 seconds) and short TEs (TE <20 msec). These images are called proton density weighted images, and they have high SNR because the signal intensity is only slightly attenuated by T1 or T2 relaxation processes. Proton density weighted images provide improved anatomic detail, because the high SNR of these images can be used to visualize fine structures. They are usually obtained and are useful for interpretation of areas of high signal intensity observed on the T2-weighted scan in which anatomic detail is obscured. A proton density weighted image of a knee with a meniscal cyst is presented in Figure 1-18.

T2 Weighting and TE

Fluid and edema can be emphasized on MR images by using long TE times because they have longer T2 relaxation times than normal tissues. At long TEs, the exponential signal decay due to T2 relaxation attenuates the signal from fluid and edema more slowly than the signal from fat, muscle, or normal connective tissues. Therefore, fluid and edema appear bright on T2-weighted MR images acquired using long TE times and long TR times. For example, on a T2-weighted sagittal image from the same knee, the synovial fluid and

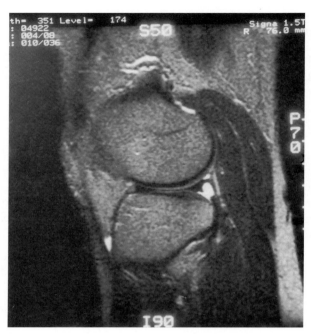

FIGURE 1-19. A T2-weighted sagittal image from the knee of a patient with a meniscal cyst. A TR of 2000 msec and a TE of 80 msec have been employed using a 3-mm slice thickness and a 16-cm field of view with 256 points. The meniscus remains hypointense, whereas the cyst is hyperintense. Fat displays moderate intensity, and muscle is hypointense. This image has a significant deficit in signal-to-noise ratio compared with that found on the T1-weighted and proton density weighted images.

region of cyst appear bright in the image, whereas regions of muscle appear dark (Fig. 1-19).

Two-Dimensional Versus Three-Dimensional Imaging

As noted earlier, true volume 3D MR imaging allows reconstruction of any image plane from the 3D data set. This is particularly useful for following small structures such as nerves, blood vessels, and cartilage. Pseudo-3D data sets can be produced from 2D studies that have been acquired radially or by contiguous slices, but this method suffers from signal attenuation where slices intersect or overlap. In addition, the resolution in the slice dimension is low and fine structures can be obscured. An example of a T1-weighted coronal image reformatted from a series of 32 contiguous sagittal slices is presented in Figure 1-20. The in-plane resolution is very low in the slice direction and the features appear smeared.

The corresponding coronal image generated from a sagittal 3D image data set is shown in Figure 1-21. Acquisition of data from a volume using nearly isotropic voxel sizes in each dimension permits observation of multiple planes without any reduction in diagnostic quality. This approach to imaging is most useful in situations in which multiple image planes or views along nonorthogonal planes are required,

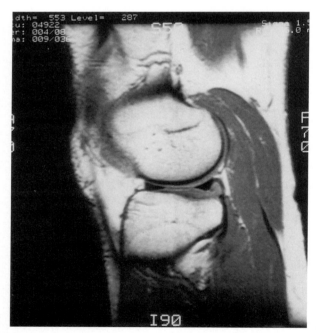

FIGURE 1-18. A proton density weighted sagittal image from the knee of a patient with a meniscal cyst. A TR of 2000 msec and a TE of 15 msec have been employed using a 3-mm slice thickness and a 16-cm field of view with 256 points. Less contrast among tissues is seen as compared with a T1-weighted image.

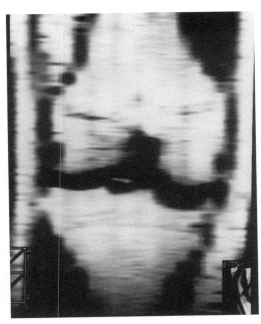

FIGURE 1-20. A coronal T1-weighted image of a knee was generated from a series of 32 contiguous sagittal 2D spin-echo images. The in-plane resolution is 32 × 128 points. A TR of 500 msec and a TE of 15 msec were used. Two-dimensional slices with the thinnest commercially available section thickness are inadequate for multiplanar reformations.

since image planes are calculated off-line on an image workstation. This method reduces total magnet time because patient preparation time used for positioning and slice definition is decreased. Finally, repeat studies are not required to sample multiple contiguous thin slices.

Manipulation of Contrast in Fast Scans

Most fast scan techniques use small RF tip angles and gradient refocusing to acquire a gradient echo. In any fast scan method the image contrast is a mixture of T1 and T2* weighting, with some dependence on the flip angle. As already noted, T2* relaxation proceeds more rapidly than conventional T2 relaxation, and fast scan sequences are more sensitive to the effects of magnetic field inhomogeneities and signal drop-out at air—tissue interfaces. Fast scan images can appear similar to either T1- or T2-weighted spin-echo scans, depending on the choice of TR, TE, type of magnetization spoiling, type of echo that is acquired, and type of RF pulse.

The simplest fast scan technique for acquiring a gradient echo is outlined in Figure 1-12*A*. These conventional fast, low-angle shot (FLASH) images are like T1-weighted spin-echo images because of the saturating effects of the repetitive low-angle RF pulse and large amplitude spoiler gradients.[6] Such FLASH or spoiled gradient recalled acquisition in the steady state (GRASS) images usually suffer from low SNR, and several excitations must be added together to produce

images with acceptable SNR. A GRASS image obtained from a knee using a 45° flip angle and eight averages is presented in Figure 1-22. The amount of magnetization available for imaging during the next phase encoding step is increased as TR is increased, and multiplanar gradient echo images have less T1 weighting and more T2* weighting.[7]

Pure proton density gradient echo images can be obtained using the 3D rotating delivery of excitation off-resonance (RODEO) technique with adiabatic RF pulses and a short TE of 2.8 msec.[8] Fast scan methods such as CE-FAST, sagittal, 3D, steady state free precession (SSFP), and time-reversed fast imaging with steady-state precession (PSIF)—which store a high-order echo generated by combinations of RF and gradient pulses—tend to be strongly T2*-weighted because the effective TE is two to three times that of the TR.[9] These types of fast scan images are useful for demonstrating fluid, which has very high intensity relative to other soft tissues. Unfortunately, these images are not truly T2-weighted, and lesions, such as bone bruises and tumors, which would be hyperintense on T2-weighted spin-echo images, may not be seen on SSFP and CE-FAST scans.

An example of a 3D SSFP image of a knee containing a meniscal cyst is presented in Figure 1-23. The regions of fluid appear to have very high intensity, but the SNR for other tissues is very low.

A combination of two RF pulses applied in rapid succession is called a composite pulse which is used in field echo

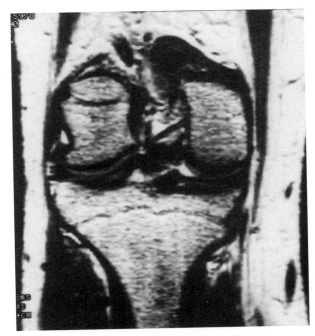

FIGURE 1-21. A coronal T1-weighted image of a knee was generated from a sagittal 3D field echo acquisition with a short TR and echo reduction (FASTER) data set. The in-plane resolution is 128 × 128 points. A TR of 18 msec and a TE of 3.2 msec were used. Reformations using thin slice 3D data produce images that are almost identical in quality to images of the original acquisition plane.

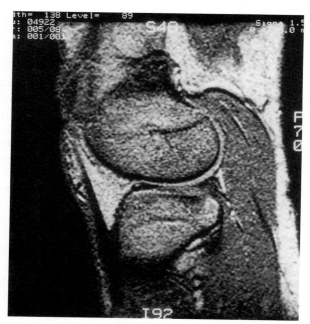

FIGURE 1-22. A sagittal spoiled gradient recalled acquisition in the steady state (GRASS) image of a knee was generated using a TR of 33 msec and a TE of 5.6 msec with a total of four averages using a 5-mm slice thickness, a 16-cm field of view, and 256 data points. This image has similar contrast to the T1-weighted spin-echo image, but has poor signal-to-noise ratio.

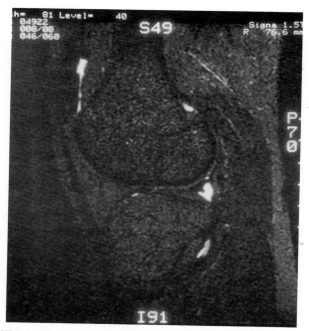

FIGURE 1-23. A sagittal 3D steady state free precession (SSFP) of a knee with a meniscal cyst. A TR of 33 msec and a TE of 9.0 msec were used. The effective TE was 66 to 99 msec. A total of two averages were used with a 1.25-mm slice thickness, a 16-cm field of view, and $128 \times 128 \times 256$ data points. Note the high-intensity fluid signal that allows easy identification of the cyst. Normal tissues are difficult to identify due to decreased signal-to-noise ratio caused by T2* losses.

acquisition with a short TR and echo reduction (FASTER) to achieve better SNR, improved T1 weighting, and fewer artifacts.[10] The second RF pulse is used to convert nonresonant magnetization into transverse magnetization, which contributes to the steady state coherence. A FASTER image of a knee is presented in Figure 1-24.

Kinematic Studies

Multiple MR images can be obtained at various defined stations of joint movement and displayed in rapid succession to provide a kinematic display that resembles joint motion. These techniques have been effectively used for the temporomandibular joint, knee, wrist, and ankle. The amount of imaging time spent at each station is critical, because multiple stations are needed for the kinematic display. A reasonable T_S per station is approximately 80 seconds, and the number of stations needed is approximately 6 to 12. Fast scans or short TR spin-echo sequences can be used.

Fat Suppression

In many cases, detection of a pathologic process is hindered by the presence of a strong signal from neighboring adipose tissue. In such cases, suppression of the fat signal offers improved conspicuity and sensitivity. Fat suppression is commonly employed for contrast-enhanced images where

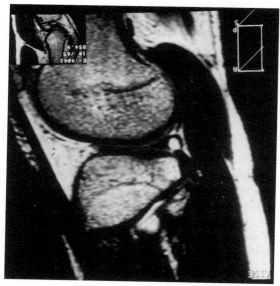

FIGURE 1-24. This field echo acquisition with a short TR and echo reduction (FASTER) image shows T1-weighted contrast similar to the T1-weighted spin-echo (see Fig. 1-17) and T1-weighted spoiled gradient recalled acquisition in the steady state (GRASS) images, except that fluids are hyperintense due to the presence of long T2 species in the steady state signal. If hyperintense fluid is not desirable, radiofrequency spoiling can be used with the FASTER sequence to make fluids appear hypointense.

the hyperintense signal from enhancing abnormalities may be masked by hyperintense fat on conventional MR images. Other common applications of fat suppression include T2-weighted images of the marrow, MR angiography of the extremities, and MR arthrography (Fig. 1-25). The various choices for fat suppression technique are summarized along with the relative merits and limitations in Table 1-1.

Subtraction is the most popular method for eliminating fat intensity in contrast-enhanced imaging. Subtraction is simple and widely available on a variety of platforms and field strengths. Subtraction has not become a popular method for musculoskeletal applications due to misregistration from movement between scans and the low SNR resulting from the subtraction.

The inversion time of inversion recovery pulse sequences can be selected so that fat recovery is at or near the null during the readout. Short tau inversion recovery (STIR) has a long history as a fat suppression method that is effective at all field strengths.[11] Conventional STIR sequences are time-consuming and have low SNR. Inversion recovery (IR) prepared fast scans suffer from blurred images due to the filling of k-space with samples that are off the fat null.

Fat presaturation employs a frequency selective 90° pulse on fat resonance in preparation for the usual pulse sequence. Fat presaturation is available on most high field MR systems. The lengthened TR associated with this method makes it most applicable to 2D methods. It is susceptible to motion artifacts and the less effective fat suppression often results in fat signal that is nearly isointense with muscle.[12]

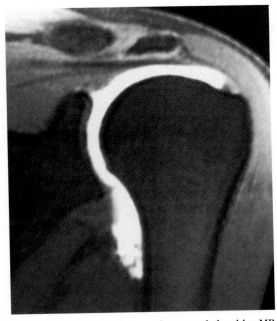

FIGURE 1-25. A 3D RODEO image of a normal shoulder MR arthrogram. A TR of 20 msec, a TE of 3.6 msec, and a slice thickness of 1.25 mm were employed. One average was obtained for a 128 × 128 × 256 data matrix and a 16-cm field of view. Fat suppression in MR arthrography avoids confusion between hyperintense joint contrast and normally hyperintense fat within the bursa space.

Another chemical shift method exploits the differences in the phases of fat and water that can occur with adjustment of the readout timing. Phase difference methods[13] can be applied at any field strength but require multiple repetitions. The trade-off is usually lower resolution or a longer scan.[13]

Image data can be gathered with phase encoding in all three spatial directions, which preserves the frequency information for spectroscopy of individual voxels. Chemical shift imaging has not achieved popularity for musculoskeletal applications due to the considerably longer scan times associated with the method.[14-16]

In 3D imaging, selective excitation of the signal from water using adiabatic techniques is possible, because no slice selection gradient is required.[12] These fat-suppressed 3D images have high SNRs without the errors associated with 2D methods. RODEO provides excellent fat suppression with rapid 3D acquisition. The off-resonance excitation of RODEO produces a very T1-weighted image along with magnetization transfer weighting. Unfortunately, the RODEO method is not widely available and performs best with a transmit-receive coil. An example of a RODEO image of a shoulder arthrogram is provided in Figure 1-25. The signal from bone and adipose have been suppressed by a factor of more than 150. The submillimeter slice thickness allows excellent visualization of fine detail in the rotator cuff.[17,18]

Recently, spatial and frequency selective excitation has become available on imaging systems. These spatial-spectral pulses can select water signal in a definable region. The pulses are inherently of long duration and favor long TR pulse sequences. The longer pulses also are more susceptible to motion artifacts.[19]

Magnetic Resonance Angiography

The signal from flowing blood can be observed selectively using magnetic resonance angiography (MRA) techniques. This is accomplished using 2D and 3D time-of-flight (TOF) methods,[20,21] in which the signal from blood is refreshed by inflow, and phase contrast[22] difference methods, in which moving spins acquire a phase shift relative to stationary spins. Different techniques can be used to enhance the signal from arterial and venous structures relative to static tissue.

In TOF methods, thin 2D or thick 3D slabs can be excited to saturate the signal from static spins. When thick slabs are used, the signal from blood flowing slowly within the slab also can be saturated. Therefore, SNR for venous structures is superior with 2D TOF MRA compared with that found with 3D methods. In an effort to reduce the saturation effects, thinner slabs may be excited and spliced together for the final angiographic display or the flip angle can be varied across the slab for data acquisition that is progressively less saturated as the blood progresses through the slab.[20,21]

TOF methods use computational postprocessing tools to find the pixels with the maximum signal intensity after conventional fast scan data has been obtained. In fast scans,

TABLE 1-1
Fat Suppression Methods

Method	Intrinsic MR Parameter Exploited	Major Features
Phase difference (Dixon)	Chemical shift	Requires multiple repetitions
Chemical shift presaturation	Chemical shift	Best suited to 2D acquisition, usually spin echo
		Favors long TR pulse sequences
		More motion artifacts due to long excitation pulses
		Incomplete fat suppression due to T1 recovery before readout
Chemical shift (time domain)	Chemical shift	4DFT acquisition is time-consuming and/or low resolution; therefore, this method has not been extensively used except for spectroscopic evaluations
RODEO	Chemical shift	Narrow frequency range can be selectively suppressed
		Optimized for high-resolution 3D acqisitions
		Single-repetition fast 3D imaging with good SNR can be performed at mid-field
Spectral-spatial selective	Chemical shift	Favors transmit-receive coils
		Long pulse length favors 2D
Inversion recovery	T1	Greater motion artifacts, available on few machines
		TI is adjusted to null the T1 corresponding to fat
		May be used as a preparation pulse for spin echo, RARE, or turbo gradient echo sequence
		When combined with fast imaging (turbo) sequence, the images are blurred due to acquisition of data off the null
Subtraction	None, simple subtraction of precontrast and postcontrast images	Can be used at any field strength
		Shows regions of contrast enhancement
		Susceptible to misregistration artifacts
		Motion limited

RODEO, rotating delivery of excitation off-resonance; TR, repetition time; 2D, two-dimensional; HDFT, four-dimensional Fourier transform; 3D, three-dimensional; SNR, signal-to-noise ratio; TI, inversion time.

blood that flows into the slice has the highest signal strength, and the reconstructed data sets yield images in which the vessels are enhanced compared with that found in normal tissue. The maximum pixel images can be enhanced by suppression of the signal from fat and by administration of gadolinium contrast agents to enhance the signal from blood.[20–23]

Phase contrast angiography exploits the change in spin magnetization phase that occurs as the nuclear spin moves in the presence of a gradient. As with time of flight techniques, phase contrast angiography can be obtained in either 2D or 3D acquisitions. 2D is considerably faster than 3D, but has significantly lower resolution.[22] Phase contrast angiography employs bipolar gradients for flow encoding in one, two, or all three flow directions (anterior-posterior, medial-lateral, or superior-inferior). The timing of the flow encoding gradients is set to correspond to a range of flow velocities. Phase contrast angiography also can be gated for optimal imaging of pulsatile flow. Recently, a series of encoding gradients have be obtained to generate flow velocity curves.

It is difficult to achieve reliable phase contrast angiograms in extremity vessels due to the high variability in vascular flow rates. For this reason, TOF techniques remain the choice of most extremity angiographic protocols.[24,25]

The 3D RODEO technique has been used to simultaneously produce both high-quality vascular images and multiple anatomic slices in a single scan.[26] This method uses TOF and improved capture of off-resonance flowing spins to enhance the SNR from vessels. The use of maximum pixel intensity ray tracing on a workstation generates the vascular images. An example of the high-quality vascular and multiple anatomic slices produced by this integrated approach is shown in Figure 1-26.

Current research into the slow movement of water and blood (ie, diffusion and perfusion) shows great promise for evaluation of hydrodynamics in the extracellular, interstitial, and intracellular spaces of tissue.[27]

Magnetic Resonance Spectroscopy

Magnetic resonance spectroscopy (MRS) generates information on tissue metabolism and has been used to study energetics and disease conditions in patients. The protons and phosphorus atoms in metabolites such as lactate, creatinine, phosphocreatinine, and adenosine triphosphate have unique magnetic environments that can be observed using MRS. The effective magnetic fields differ by only parts per million,

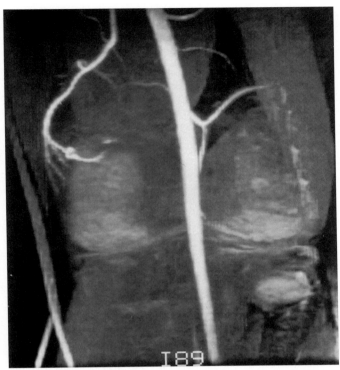

FIGURE 1-26. A maximum pixel ray casting of a 3D RODEO image of a knee with an osteosarcoma. The RODEO sequence can produce high-quality basic and angiographic images in the same scan. Even though this sequence is nonselective, high signal intensity is produced from vessels due to the acquisition of signal from frequency shifted spins.

and are small compared with the strength of the magnetic field gradients used to make MR images. In MRS, therefore, the MR signal is detected in the absence of readout gradients to provide high-resolution information on the distribution of frequencies induced by chemical differences. Levels of inorganic phosphate, phosphocreatinine, and adenosine triphosphate can be estimated using phosphorus MR imaging.[28] Spatial localization to specific volumes of tissue is achieved using slice selective gradients, phase encoding, or both.[29] With proton MRS, it is possible to detect anaerobic metabolism by means of the production of lactic acid.[30] Although MRS is a powerful tool for research studies of tissue biochemistry, clinical applications are still being developed.

New Rapid Imaging Methods

Development of a number of new techniques for obtaining faster MR imaging has been propelled by advances in both hardware and software. The three main classes of fast scanning techniques are distinguishable by the means by which they collect data for reconstruction.

"Turbo" fast scans employ short TR acquisitions in a continuous or syncopated mode, with the projections following the conventional 2DFT or 3DFT format—one line per

excitation. The image contrast is a complex function of T2 and T1, and the SNR generally is low. In most fast scan imaging methods, the major limitation on the duration of TE is the magic TE of 4.4 msec (required to generate in-phase images at 1.5 T). At multiples of this TE, the signals from water and fat are in phase because the phase evolution due to the difference in chemical shift is equal to 2π radians. The images have more signal intensity than fast scans performed using a TE of 2.2, 6.6, or 11 msec, because the signals from fat and water do not cancel each other. As already discussed, the contrast in fast scan methods can be altered in a variety of ways to generate T1-weighted, proton density weighted, T2-weighted, or other types of images. The most commonly used preparation pulse is an inversion pulse that can be used to suppress fat (STIR) or provide more T1 weighting.[31]

Instead of using the multiple echoes of a spin-echo for images of varying T2 weighting, the additional echoes can be used to generate multiple phase encoding projections during the same TR. These fast spin-echo, or rapid acquisition with relaxation enhancement (RARE) pulse sequences, are performed to reduce the scan time of long TR/ long TE acquisitions. The images from long effective TE studies tend to be sharper than single long TE acquisitions due to the filling of the peripheral reconstruction space with high SNR short TE echoes. Since the projections vary greatly in weighting and SNR, images from short effective TE acquisitions tend to be blurred compared with single-echo acquisitions. Since there is little improvement in acquisition efficiency compared with conventional short TE–short TR sequences, fast spin-echo is not typically employed for T1-weighted imaging. Because of the high-power deposition of fast spin-echo, it is practically limited to 2D acquisitions.[32]

Echo planar or spiral imaging methods employ time varying gradients during the readout to collect a greater number of projections per excitation. A low-resolution MR image can be obtained at scan times of 30 to 60 msec from a single excitation pulse.[33,34] Echo planar techniques rapidly change the gradient during the readout to generate a raster-line data collection for reconstruction space. Spiral techniques fill reconstruction space with a spiral gradient trajectory.[35] Either spin-echo or gradient echo sequences can be used but the longer readout generally dictates a more T2- or T2*-weighted image. A long readout with a narrow bandwidth results in significant chemical shift effects that can impair musculoskeletal diagnosis unless some form of fat suppression is employed.

References

1. Stark DD, Bradley WG, eds. Magnetic resonance imaging. St Louis: CV Mosby, 1988.
2. Mink JH, Reicher MA, Crues JV III, eds. Magnetic resonance imaging of the knee. New York: Raven Press, 1987.
3. Wehrli FW, Shaw D, Kneeland JB, eds. Biomedical magnetic resonance

imaging: principles, methodology, and applications. New York: VCH Publishers, 1988.

4. Matwiyoff NA. Magnetic resonance workbook. New York: Raven Press, 1989.

5. Hahn EL. Spin echoes. Phys Rev 1950;80:580.

6. Haase A. Applications to T1, T2, and chemical shift imaging. Magn Reson Med 1990;13(1):77. Snapshop Fast low-angle shot MRI.

7. Reischer MA, Lufkin RB, Smith S, et al. AJR 1986;147:363.

8. Harms SE, Flamig, Griffey RH. New MR pulse sequence: fat suppressed steady state. Radiology 1990;270:177.

9. Gyngell ML. The application of steady state free precession in rapid 2DT NMR imaging: FAST and ED fast sequences. Magn Reson Imaging 1988;6:415.

10. Harms SE, Flamig DP, Fisher CF, Fulmer JM. New method for fast MR imaging of the knee. Radiology 1989;173:743.

11 Bydder GM, Steiner RE, Blumgart LH, et al. Imaging of the liver using short T1 inversion recovery sequences. J Comput Assist Tomogr 1985;9:1084.

12. Keller PJ, Hunter WW, Schmalbrock P. Multisection fat-water imaging with chemical shift selective presaturation. Radiology 1987;164:539.

13. Dixon WT. Simple proton spectroscopic imaging. Radiology 1984;153:189.

14. Maudsley AA, Hilal SK, Perman WH, Simon HE. Spatially revolved high resolution spectroscopy by "four dimensional" NMR. J Magn Reson 1983;51:147.

15. Frahm J, Haase A, Hanickle W, Matthaei D, Bonsdorf H, Helzel T. Chemical shift selective MR imaging using a whole-body magnet. Radiology 1985;156:441.

16. Hasso A, Frahm J. Multiple chemical shift selective NMR imaging using stimulated echoes. J Magn Reson 1985;64:94.

17. Harms SE, Flamig DP, Hesley KL, et al. Fat suppressed three-dimensional MR imaging of the breast. Radiographics 1993;13:247.

18. Harms SE, Flamig DP, Hesley KL, et al. Breast MRI: rotating delivery of excitation off-resonance. Clinical experience with pathologic correlations. Radiology 1993;187:493.

19. Meyer CH, Pauly IM, Macovski A, et al. Simultaneous spatial and spectral selective excitation. Magn Reson Med 1990;15:287.

20. Keller PJ, Drayer BP, Fram EK, et al. MR angiography with two-dimensional acquisition and three-dimensional display: work in progress. Radiology 1989;173:527.

21. Laub GA, Kaiser WA: MR angiography with gradient motion refocusing. J Comput Assist Tomogr 1988;12:377.

22. Dumoulin CL Hart HR. MR angiography. Radiology 1986;161:717.

23. Harms SE, Flamig DP, Griffey RH. Clinical applications of a new fat suppressed, steady state pulse sequence for high resolution 3D applications. In: Book of abstracts. vol 1. New York: Society of Magnetic Resonance in Medicine, 1990:187.

24. Nishimura DG. Time of flight MR angiography. Magn Reson Med 1990;14:194.

25. Steinberg FL, Yucel EK, Dumoulin CL, Souza SP. Peripheral vascular and abdominal applications of MR flow imaging techniques. Magn Reson Med 1990;14:315.

26. Harms SE, Flamig DP, Siemers PT, Glastad KA, Pierce B. Zero scan time vascular MR imaging. Radiology 1990;144:177.

27. LeBihan D, Breton E, Lallemand D, Grenier P, Cabanis E, Laval-Jeantet M. MR imaging of intravoxel incoherent motors: application to diffusion and perfusion in neurologic disorders. Radiology 1989;161:401.

28. Luyten RP, Bruntink G, Sloff FM, et al. Broadband proton decoupling in human 31P NMR spectroscopy. NMR Biomed 1989;1:177.

29. Van Vaals JJ, Bergman AH, den Boef JH, et al. A single shot method for water suppressed localization and editing of spectra, images, and spectroscopic images. Mag Reson Med 1990;144:177.

30. Griffey RH. Tumor characterization using unconventional MR modalities. Invest Radiol 1990;16:451.

31 Edelman RR, Wallner B, Singer A, Atkinson DJ, Saini S. Segmented turbo FLASH: method for breath-hold MR imaging of the liver with flexible contrast. Radiology 1990;177:515.

32. Hennig J, Nauerth A, Friedburg H. RARE imaging: a fast imaging method for clinical MR. Magn Reson Med 1986;3:823.

33. Mansfield P. Multi planar image formation using NMR spin echoes. J Physiol Chem 1977;10:L55.

34. Farzaneh F, Riederer SJ, Pelc NJ. Analysis of T2 limitations and off-resonance effects on spatial resolution and artifacts in echo planar imaging. Magn Reson Med 1990;14:123.

35. Meyer CH, Hu BS, Nishimura DG, et al. Fast spiral coronary artery imaging. Magn Reson Med 1992;28:202.

Magnetic Resonance Imaging in Orthopaedics & Sports Medicine, Second Edition,
edited by David W. Stoller. Lippincott-Raven Publishers, Philadelphia, © 1997.

Chapter 2

Magnetic Resonance: Bioeffects and Safety

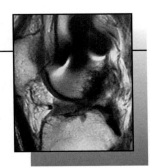

Frank G. Shellock
Emanuel Kanal

During the performance of magnetic resonance (MR) imaging, the patient is exposed to three different forms of electromagnetic radiation: a static magnetic field, gradient magnetic fields, and radiofrequency (RF) electromagnetic fields. Each of these may cause significant bioeffects if applied at sufficiently high exposure levels. Numerous investigations have been conducted to identify potentially adverse bioeffects of MR imaging.[1–83] Although none has identified the presence of any significant or unexpected hazards, the data are not comprehensive enough to assume absolute safety.

In addition to bioeffects related to exposure to the electromagnetic fields used for MR studies, there are several areas of health concern for both the patient and the health-care practitioner with respect to the use of clinical MR imaging. Therefore, this discussion of the bioeffects of static, gradient, and RF electromagnetic fields is supplemented by an overview of other safety considerations and patient management aspects related to this imaging technique.

BIOEFFECTS OF STATIC MAGNETIC FIELDS

General Bioeffects of Static Magnetic Fields

There are few data concerning the effects of high-intensity static magnetic fields on humans. Some of the original investigations on human subjects exposed to static magnetic fields were performed by Vyalov[84,85], who studied workers involved in the permanent magnet industry. These subjects, exposed to static magnetic fields ranging from 0.0015 to 0.35 T, reported feelings of headache, chest pain, fatigue, vertigo, loss of appetite, insomnia, itching, and other, more nonspecific ailments.[84,85] Exposure to other potentially hazardous environmental working conditions (such as elevated room temperature, airborne metallic dust, or chemicals) may have been partially responsible for the reported symptoms in these study subjects. Because this investigation lacked an appropriate control group, it is difficult to ascertain if there was a definite correlation between exposure to the static magnetic field and reported abnormalities. Subsequent studies performed with more scientific rigor have not substantiated many of the above findings.[86–89]

Temperature Effects

There are conflicting statements in the literature regarding the effect of static magnetic fields on body and skin temperatures of mammals. Some reports have indicated that static magnetic fields either increase or both increase and decrease tissue temperature, depending on the orientation of the organism in the static magnetic field.[19,66] Other articles state that static magnetic fields have no effect on skin and body temperatures of mammals.[55,61,88,90]

None of the investigators who identified a static magnetic field effect on temperatures proposed a plausible mechanism for this response, nor has this work been substantiated. In addition, studies that reported static-magnetic-field–induced skin or body temperature changes used either laboratory animals that are known to have labile temperatures or instrumentation that may have been affected by the static magnetic fields.[19,66] An investigation in humans indicated that exposure to a 1.5-T static magnetic field does not alter skin and body temperatures.[90] This study was performed using a special fluoroptic thermometry system demonstrated to be unperturbed by high-intensity static magnetic fields. Therefore, skin and body temperatures of human subjects are believed to be unaffected by exposure to static magnetic fields of up to 1.5 T.[55,61]

Electric Induction and Cardiac Effects

Induced biopotentials, sometimes observed during exposure to static magnetic fields, are caused by blood, a conductive fluid, flowing through a magnetic field. The induced biopotential is exhibited as an augmentation of T-wave amplitude as well as by other, nonspecific, waveform changes that are apparent on the electrocardiogram and have been observed at static magnetic field strengths as low as 0.1 T.[86,91,92] The increase in T-wave amplitude is directly related to the intensity of the static magnetic field. In other words, at low static magnetic field strengths the effects are not as predominant as those at higher field strengths. The most marked effect on the T wave is thought to be caused when the blood flows through the thoracic aortic arch. This T-wave amplitude change can be significant enough to falsely trigger the RF excitation during a cardiac-gated MR examination. Other potions of the electrocardiogram may also be altered by the static magnetic field and this varies with the placement of the recording electrodes. To facilitate cardiac gating studies, alternative lead positions can be used to attenuate the static-magnetic-field–induced electrocardiographic changes.[93] After exposure to the static magnetic field is terminated, these electrocardiographic voltage abnormalities revert to normal.

Because there are no circulatory alterations that appear to coincide with these electrocardiographic changes, no biologic risks are believed to be associated with the magnetohydrodynamic effect that occurs in conjunction with static magnetic field strengths of up to 2.0 T.[86,91,92]

Neurologic Effects

In theory, electrical impulse conduction in nerve tissue may be affected by exposure to static magnetic fields. However, this area in the bioeffects literature contains contradictory information. Some studies have reported remarkable effects on both the function and structure of those portions of the central nervous system that were associated with exposure to static magnetic fields, whereas others have failed to show any significant changes.[14,20,34,68,69,76–79,94–99] Further investigations of potential unwanted bioeffects are needed because of the relative lack of clinical studies in this field that are directly applicable to MR imaging. Currently, exposure to static magnetic fields of up to 2.0 T does not appear to significantly influence the bioelectric properties of neurons in humans.[97–99]

In summary, there is no conclusive evidence of irreversible or hazardous biologic effects related to acute, short-term exposures of humans to static magnetic fields of strengths up to 2.0 T. However, as of 1996, there were several 3.0- and 4.0-T whole-body MR systems operating at various research sites around the world. A preliminary study has indicated that workers and volunteer subjects exposed to a 4.0-T MR system have experienced vertigo, nausea, headaches, a metallic taste in their mouths, and magnetophosphenes (which are visual flashes).[50] Therefore, considerable research is required to study the mechanisms responsible for these bioeffects and to determine possible means, if any, to counterbalance them.

CRYOGEN CONSIDERATIONS

All superconductive MR systems in clinical use today use liquid helium. Liquid helium, which maintains the magnet coils in their superconductive state, will achieve the gaseous state ("boil off") at approximately −268.93°C (4.22 K).[99] If the temperature within the cryostat precipitously rises, the helium enters the gaseous state. In this situation, the marked increase in volume of the gaseous versus the liquid cryogen (with gas–liquid volume ratios of 760:1 for helium and 695:1 for nitrogen) will dramatically increase the pressure within the cryostat.[99] A pressure-sensitive carbon "pop-off" valve will give way, sometimes with a loud popping noise, followed by the rapid (and loud) egress of gaseous helium as it escapes from the cryostat. In normal situations, this gas should be vented out of the imaging room and into the external atmosphere. It is possible, however, that during this venting some helium gas might accidentally be released into the ambient atmosphere of the imaging room.

Gaseous helium is considerably lighter than air. If any helium gas is inadvertently released into the imaging room, the dimensions of the room, its ventilation capacity, and the total amount of gas released will determine whether the helium gas will reach the patient or health-care practitioner, who is in the lower part of the room.[99] Helium vapor looks like steam and is odorless and tasteless, but it may be extremely cold. Asphyxiation and frostbite are possible if a person is exposed to helium vapor for a long time. In a system quench, a considerable quantity of helium gas may be released into the imaging room. The resulting pressure differential might secondarily cause difficulty in opening the room door. In this circumstance, the first response should be to evacuate the area until the offending helium vapor is adequately removed from the imaging room environment and safely redirected to an outside environment away from patients, pedestrians, and temperature-sensitive material.[99]

With better cryostat design and insulation, many of the newer superconductive magnets use only liquid helium. However, many magnets in clinical systems use liquid nitrogen as well. Liquid nitrogen within the cryostat acts as a buffer between the liquid helium and the outside atmosphere, boiling off at 77.3 K. In the event of an accidental release of liquid nitrogen into the ambient atmosphere of the imaging room, there is a potential for frostbite, similar to that encountered with gaseous helium release. Gaseous nitrogen is roughly the same density as air and is certainly much less buoyant than gaseous helium. In the event of an inadvertent venting of nitrogen gas into the imaging room the gas could easily settle near floor level; the amount of nitrogen gas within the room would continue to increase until venting ceased. The total concentration of nitrogen gas contained within the room would be determined on the basis of the total amount of the gas released into the room, the dimensions of the room, and its ventilation capacity (the existence and size of other routes of egress such as doors, windows, ventilation ducts, and fans). A pure-nitrogen environment is exceptionally hazardous, and unconsciousness generally results within 5 to 10 seconds after exposure.[99] It is imperative that all patients and health-care personnel evacuate the area as soon as it is recognized that nitrogen gas is being released into the imaging room, and no one should return until appropriate corrective measures have been taken to clear the gas.[99]

Dewar (cryogen storage containers) storage should be conducted in a well-ventilated area in case normal boil-off rates increase the concentration of inert gas within the storage room to a dangerous level (J. E. Gray, PhD, oral communication, September 1989). At least one reported death has occurred in an industrial setting during the shipment of cryogens (J. E. Gray, PhD, oral communication, August 1989), although to our knowledge no such fatality has occurred in the medical community. There has been one report of a sudden, unexplained loss of consciousness in an otherwise healthy technologist (with no prior or subsequent similar episodes) who was passing through a cryogen storage area where multiple dewars were located (A. Aisen, PhD, oral communication, May 1989). Although there is no verification of a change in the ambient atmospheric oxygen concentration to confirm a relation to the cryogens per se, the history is strongly suggestive of such a relation.

Cryogens present a potential concern in clinical MR imaging despite their overwhelmingly safe record of use in their more than 13 years of clinical service.[99] Proper handling and storage of cryogens as well as training in the appropriate response in case of a leak should be emphasized at each site. An oxygen monitor with an audible alarm, situated at an appropriate height within each imaging room, should be a mandatory minimum safety measure for all sites; automatic linking to and activation of an imaging-room ventilation fan system when the oxygen monitor registers below 18% or 19% should be considered at each magnet installation.[99]

Electrical Considerations in a Quench

In addition to the potential for cryogen release, there is also concern about the currents that may be induced in conductors (such as biologic tissues) near the rapidly changing magnetic field associated with a quench.[99] In one study, both physiologic monitoring of a pig and monitoring of the environment were performed during an intentional quench from 1.76 T. In this study there seemed to be no significant effect on the blood pressure, pulse, temperature, and electroencephalographic and electrocardiographic measurements on the pig during or immediately after the quench.[100] Although a single observation does not prove safety for humans undergoing exposure to a quench, the data do suggest that the experience would be similar and that there would be no deleterious electrical effects on humans undergoing a similar experience and exposure.

BIOEFFECTS OF GRADIENT MAGNETIC FIELDS

MR imaging exposes the human body to rapid variations of magnetic fields produced by the transient application of magnetic field gradients during the imaging sequence. Gradient magnetic fields can induce electrical fields and currents in conductive media (including biologic tissue) according to Faraday's law of induction. The potential for interaction between gradient magnetic fields and biologic tissue is inherently dependent on the fundamental field frequency, the maximum flux density, the average flux density, the presence of harmonic frequencies, the waveform characteristics of the signal, the polarity of the signal, current distribution in the body, and the electrical properties and sensitivity of the particular cell membrane.[97-99]

For animals and human subjects, the induced current is proportional to the conductivity of the biologic tissue and the rate of change of the magnetic flux density.[98,99,101,102] In theory, the largest current densities will be produced in peripheral tissues (ie, at the greatest radius) and will linearly diminish toward the body's center[98,99,101,102] The current density will be enhanced at higher frequencies and magnetic flux densities and will be further accentuated by a larger tissue radius with a greater tissue conductivity. Current paths are affected by differences in tissue types, such that tissues with low conductivity (eg, adipose and bone) will change the pattern of the induced current.

Bioeffects of induced currents can be due either to the power deposited by the induced currents (thermal effects) or to direct effects of the current (nonthermal effects). Thermal effects due to switched gradients used in MR imaging are negligible and are not believed to be clinically significant.[96,98,99]

Possible nonthermal effects of induced currents are stimulation of nerve or muscle cells, induction of ventricular fibrillation, increased brain mannitol space, epileptogenic potential, stimulation of visual flash sensations, and altered bone healing.[98,99,101-104] The threshold currents required for nerve stimulation and ventricular fibrillation are known to be much higher than the estimated current densities that are induced under routine clinical MR conditions.[96-99,101]

The production of magnetophosphenes is considered to be one of the most sensitive physiologic responses to gradient magnetic fields.[96-99] Magnetophosphenes are thought to be caused by electrical stimulation of the retina and are completely reversible, with no associated effects on health.[96-99] They have been elicited by current densities of roughly 17 $\mu A/cm^2$. In contrast, currents required for the induction of nerve action potentials are roughly 3000

$\mu A/cm^2$, and those required for ventricular fibrillation induction of healthy cardiac tissue are calculated to be 100 to 1000 $\mu A/cm^2$.[96] Although to our knowledge there have been no reported cases of magnetophosphenes for fields of 1.95 T or less, magnetophosphenes have been reported in volunteers working in and around a 4.0-T research system.[50] In addition, a metallic taste and symptoms of vertigo seem also to be reproducible and associated with rapid motion within the static magnetic field of these 4.0-T systems.[50]

Time-varying, extremely low-frequency magnetic fields have been demonstrated to be associated with multiple effects, including clustering and altered orientation of fibroblasts, as well as increased mitotic activity of fibroblast growth, altered DNA synthesis, and reduced fentanyl-induced anesthesia.[49,64,99] Possible effects in multiple other organisms, including humans, have also been mentioned.[99] Although no studies have conclusively demonstrated carcinogenic effects from exposure to time-varying magnetic fields of various intensities and durations, several reports suggest that an association between the two is still plausible.[105-107]

BIOEFFECTS OF RF ELECTROMAGNETIC FIELDS

General Bioeffects of RF Electromagnetic Fields

RF radiation is capable of generating heat in tissues as a result of resistive losses. Therefore, the main bioeffects associated with exposure to RF radiation are related to the thermogenic qualities of this electromagnetic field.[96-99,108-116] Exposure to RF radiation may also cause nonthermal, field-specific alterations in biologic systems without a significant increase in temperature.[108-114] This topic is controversial because of assertions concerning the role of electromagnetic fields in producing cancer and developmental abnormalities and the ramifications of these effects.[108-114] A report from the United States Environmental Protection Agency claimed that the existing evidence on this issue is sufficient to demonstrate a relation between low-level electromagnetic field exposures and the development of cancer.[107] To date, there have been no specific studies performed to study potential nonthermal bioeffects of MR imaging. A thorough review of this topic, particularly as it pertains to MR, has been published by Beers.[113]

In studying RF power deposition concerns, investigators have typically quantified exposure to RF radiation by means of determining the specific absorption rate (SAR).[108-112, 116-119] SAR is the mass normalized rate at which RF power is coupled to biologic tissue and is expressed in watts per kilogram. Measurements or estimates of SAR are not trivial, particularly in human subjects, and there are several methods of determining this parameter for RF energy dosimetry.[108-112,119] The SAR that is produced during MR scanning is a complex function of numerous variables including the frequency (which, in turn, is determined by the strength of the static magnetic field), the type of RF pulse (90° or 180°), the repetition time, the pulse width, the type of RF coil used, the volume of tissue within the coil, the resistivity of the tissue, and the configuration of the anatomic region imaged.[96–99] The actual increase in tissue temperature caused by exposure to RF radiation is dependent on the subject's thermoregulatory system (involving skin blood flow, skin surface area, sweat rate, and other factors).[97–99]

The efficiency and absorption pattern of RF energy are mainly determined by the physical dimensions of the tissue in relation to the incident wavelength.[108–112] Therefore, if the tissue is large relative to the wavelength, energy is predominantly absorbed on the surface; if it is small relative to the wavelength, there is little absorption of RF power.[108–112] Because of the relation between RF energy and physical dimensions just described, studies designed to investigate the effects of exposure to RF radiation during MR imaging in the clinical setting require tissue volumes and anatomic shapes comparable to those of human subjects. In addition, laboratory animals do not accurately mimic or simulate the thermoregulatory system or responses of humans. For these reasons, results obtained in laboratory animal experiments cannot simply be "scaled" or extrapolated to human subjects.[110–112,119]

MR Imaging and Exposure to RF Radiation

Before the studies performed with MR imaging, few quantitative data had been available on the thermoregulatory responses of humans exposed to RF radiation. The few studies that existed did not directly apply to MR because these investigations either examined thermal sensations or therapeutic applications of diathermy, usually involving only localized regions of the body.[108,109,110,114]

Several studies of RF power absorption during MR scanning have been performed and have yielded useful information about tissue heating in human subjects.[28,58–60,62,63,65] During MR imaging, tissue heating results primarily from magnetic induction with a negligible contribution from the electric fields, so that ohmic heating is greatest at the surface of the body and approaches zero at the center of the body. Predictive calculations and measurements obtained in phantoms and human subjects exposed to MR scanning support this pattern of temperature distribution.[58–60,115,116]

Although one study reported that MR imaging produced significant temperature rises in internal organs,[65] this study was conducted on anesthetized dogs and is unlikely to be applicable to conscious adult human subjects because of factors related to the physical dimensions and dissimilar thermoregulatory systems of these two species. However, these data may have important implications for the use of MR in pediatric patients because this patient population is typically sedated or anesthetized for MR examinations.

An investigation using fluoroptic thermometry probes that are unperturbed by electromagnetic fields[117] demonstrated that human subjects exposed to MR imaging at SAR levels up to 4.0 W/kg (ten times higher than the level currently recommended by the United States Food and Drug Administration [FDA]) have no statistically significant increases in body temperature and have elevations in skin temperatures that are not believed to be clinically hazardous.[62] These results imply that the suggested exposure level of 0.4 W/kg for RF radiation during MR imaging is too conservative for persons with normal thermoregulatory function.[62] Additional studies are needed, however, to assess the physiologic responses of patients with conditions that may impair thermoregulatory function before they are subjected to MR procedures that require high SARs. These patients include elderly persons; patients with underlying conditions such as fever, diabetes, cardiovascular disease, or obesity; and patients taking medications that affect thermoregulation, such as calcium-channel blocking agents, beta-adrenergic blocking agents, diuretic agents, and vasodilators.

Temperature-Sensitive Organs

Some human organs that have reduced capabilities for heat dissipation, such as the testis and eye, are particularly sensitive to elevated temperatures. Therefore, these organs are primary sites of potential harmful effects if RF radiation exposures during MR are excessive.

Testes

Laboratory investigations have demonstrated detrimental effects on testicular function (including reduction or cessation of spermatogenesis, impaired sperm motility, and degeneration of seminiferous tubules) caused by RF radiation-induced heating from exposures sufficient enough to raise scrotal or testicular tissue temperatures up to 38°C to 42°C.[118] In one study, scrotal skin temperature (which is an index of intratesticular temperature) was measured in volunteer subjects undergoing MR imaging at a whole body averaged SAR of 1.1 W/kg.[63] The greatest change in scrotal skin temperature was 2.1°C and the highest scrotal skin temperature recorded was 34.2°C.[63] These temperature changes were below the threshold known to impair testicular function. However, excessive heating of the scrotum during MR imaging in patients who are already oligospermic could exacerbate certain preexisting disorders associated with increased scrotal or testicular temperatures (acute febrile illness and varicocele, for example) and lead to possible temporary or permanent sterility.[63] Additional studies designed to investigate these issues are needed, particularly if patients are scanned at whole body averaged SARs higher than those previously evaluated.

Eye

Dissipation of heat from the eye is a slow and inefficient process because of its relative lack of vascularization. Acute near-field exposures of RF radiation, if of sufficient intensity and duration, to the eyes or heads of laboratory animals have been demonstrated to be cataractogenic as a result of the thermal disruption of ocular tissues.[108,110] However, an investigation conducted by Sacks and colleagues[53] revealed that MR scanning at exposures that far exceeded typical clinical imaging levels produced no discernible effects on the eyes of rats. However, it may not be acceptable to extrapolate these data to human subjects considering the coupling of RF radiation to the anatomy and tissue volume of the laboratory rat eyes compared with those of humans.

Corneal temperatures have been measured in patients undergoing MR imaging of the brain using a send–receive head coil at local SARs up to 3.1 W/kg.[59] The largest corneal temperature change was 1.8°C and the highest temperature measured was 34.4°C. Because the temperature threshold for RF radiation-induced cataractogenesis in animal models has been demonstrated to be between 41°C to 55°C for acute, near-field exposures; it does not appear that clinical MR imaging using a head coil has the potential to cause thermal damage in ocular tissue.[59] The effect of MR at higher SARs and the long-term effects of MR on ocular tissues remain to be determined.

RF Radiation and "Hot Spots"

Theoretically, RF radiation "hot spots" caused by an uneven distribution of RF power may arise whenever current concentrations are produced in association with restrictive conductive patterns. Some have suggested that RF radiation hot spots may generate thermal hot spots under certain conditions during MR imaging. Because RF radiation is absorbed mainly by peripheral tissues, thermography has been used to study the heating pattern associated with MR imaging at high whole-body SARs.[57] This study demonstrated no evidence of surface thermal hot spots related to MR imaging in human subjects. The thermoregulatory system apparently responds to the heat challenge by distributing the thermal load, producing a "smearing" effect of the surface temperatures. Nonetheless, there is a possibility that internal thermal hot spots may develop from MR imaging.[59]

UNITED STATES FDA GUIDELINES FOR MR DEVICES

In 1988, MR diagnostic devices were reclassified from class III, for which premarket approval is required, to class II, which is regulated by performance standards as long as the device(s) are within the scope of the defined limits described below.[120] Subsequent to this reclassification, new devices had only to demonstrate that they were "substantially equivalent" to any class II device that was brought to market using the premarket notification process (510[k]) or to any of the devices described by the 13 MR-system manufacturers that had petitioned the FDA for the reclassification.

Four areas relating to the use of MR systems have been identified for which safety guidelines have been issued by the FDA. These include the static magnetic field, the gradient magnetic fields, the RF power of the examination, and the acoustic considerations. The following guidelines are excerpted from the FDA "Safety Parameter Action Levels"[120]:

Static magnetic field. Static magnetic field strengths not exceeding 2.0 T are below the level of concern for the static magnetic field. Should the static magnetic field strength exceed 2.0 T, additional evidence of safety must be provided by the sponsor.

Gradient magnetic field. Limit patient exposure to time-varying magnetic fields with strengths less than those required to produce peripheral nerve stimulation or other effects. There are three alternatives:

- Demonstrate that the maximum rate of change of magnetic field (dB/dt) of the system is 6 T/s or less.
- Demonstrate that for axial gradients, dB/dt < 20 T/sec for μs ≥ 120 msec, or dB/dt < (2,400/p) T/sec for 12 msec < μs < 120 psec, or dB/dt < 200 T/sec for μs ≤ 12 psec, where μs equals the width (in fractions of a second) of a rectangular pulse or the half period of a sinusoidal dB/dt pulse. For transverse gradients, dB/dt is considered to be below the level of concern when it is less than three times the above limits for axial gradients.
- Demonstrate with valid scientific evidence that the dB/dt for the system is not sufficient to cause peripheral nerve stimulation by an adequate margin of safety (at least a factor of three).

The parameter dB/dt must be lower than either of the two levels of concern by presentation of valid scientific measurement or quantitative evidence sufficient to demonstrate that the dB/dt is of no concern.

RF power deposition. Options to control the risk of systemic thermal overload and local thermal injury caused by RF energy absorption are as follows:

- If the SAR is 0.4 W/kg or less for the whole body and 8.0 W/kg or less spatial peak in any 1 g of tissue, and if the SAR is 3.2 W/kg or less averaged over the head, then it is below the level of concern.
- If exposure to RF magnetic fields is insufficient to produce a core temperature increase of 1°C and localized heating to no greater than 38°C in the head, 39°C in the trunk, and 40°C in the extremities, then it is considered to be below the level of concern.

The parameter of RF heating must be below either of the two levels of concern by presentation of valid scientific measurement or calculational evidence sufficient to demonstrate that RF heating effects are of no concern.

Acoustic noise levels. Acoustic noise levels associated with the device must be shown to be below the level of concern established by pertinent federal regulatory or other recognized standards-setting organizations. If the acoustic noise is not below the level of concern, the sponsor must recommend steps to reduce or alleviate the noise perceived by the patient.

MR IMAGING AND ACOUSTIC NOISE

The acoustic noise produced during MR examination represents a potential risk to patients. Acoustic noise is associated with the activation and deactivation of electrical current that induces vibrations of the gradient coils.[121] This repetitive sound is enhanced by higher-gradient duty cycles and sharper pulse transitions. Acoustic noise is thus likely to increase with decreases in section thicknesses, decreased fields of view, repetition times, and echo times.

Gradient magnetic field–related noise levels measured on several commercial MR scanners were in the range of 65 to 95 dB, which is considered to be within the recommended safety guidelines set forth by the FDA.[120] However, there have been reports that acoustic noise generated during MR scanning has caused patient annoyance, interference with verbal communication, and reversible hearing loss in patients who did not wear ear protection.[9,122] One study of patients undergoing MR imaging without earplugs resulted in temporary hearing loss in 43% of the subjects.[9] Furthermore, it is possible that significant gradient coil–induced noise may produce permanent hearing impairment in certain patients who are particularly susceptible to the damaging effects of relatively loud noises.[9,122]

The safest and least expensive means of preventing problems associated with acoustic noise during clinical MR imaging is to encourage the routine use of disposable earplugs.[9,122] The use of hearing protection has been demonstrated to successfully avoid any temporary hearing loss that may be associated with clinical MR examinations.[9,122] MR compatible headphones that significantly muffle acoustic noise are also commercially available.

An acceptable alternative strategy for reducing sound levels during MR studies is to use an "antinoise" or destructive interference technique that not only effectively reduces noise but also permits better patient–staff communication.[123] This technique requires a real-time Fourier analysis of the noise emitted from the MR system.[123] A signal, possessing the same physical characteristics but the opposite phase from the sound generated by the MR system, is then produced. The two opposite-phase signals are then combined, resulting in a cancellation of the repetitive noise while allowing other sounds such as music and voice to be transmitted to the patient.[123] A recent investigation demonstrated no significant degradation of image quality when MR imaging is performed with systems that use this antinoise method.[123] Although this technique has not yet found widespread clinical application, it has considerable potential for minimizing acoustic noise and its associated problems.

INVESTIGATIONS OF MR IMAGING BIOLOGIC EFFECTS

Investigations performed to specifically study the potential bioeffects of MR imaging are summarized in Table 2-1.[1–83] The results of this MR-related bioeffects research have been predominantly negative, supporting the widely held view that no significant health risks are associated with the use of this imaging modality. Experiments that yielded positive results identified possible nonspecific biologic responses, determined short-term biologic changes that were not considered to be deleterious, or found bioeffects that require further substantiation.

In these studies, the dosimetric aspects of the exposure(s) to static, gradient, or RF electromagnetic fields varied and included some that exceeded clinical exposures, simulated clinical exposures, or involved low-level chronic exposures. In some cases, the effects of only one of the electromagnetic fields used for MR imaging was evaluated. In theory the combination of static, gradient, and RF electromagnetic fields may produce some unusual or unpredictable bioeffects that are unique to MR imaging.

"Window" effects are often present with respect to biologic changes that occur in response to electromagnetic radiation. Window effects are those biologic changes associated with a specific spectrum of electromagnetic radiation that are not observed at levels below or above this range.[108,119] Both field strength and frequency windows have been reported.[108,119] Virtually all of the experiments conducted to date on MR biologic effects have been performed at specific windows and the results cannot be assumed to apply to all of the various field strengths or frequencies used for clinical MR imaging.

A variety of biologic systems were also used for these experiments. As previously mentioned, because the coupling of electromagnetic radiation to biologic tissues is highly dependent on organism or subject size, anatomic factors, duration of exposure, sensitivity of the involved tissues, and other variables, studies performed on laboratory preparations may not be extrapolated or directly applicable to human subjects nor to the clinical use of MR. Therefore, a cautionary approach to the interpretation of the results of these studies is advisable.

ELECTRICALLY, MAGNETICALLY, OR MECHANICALLY ACTIVATED IMPLANTS AND DEVICES

The FDA requires labeling of MR systems to indicate that the device is contraindicated for patients who have electrically, magnetically, or mechanically activated implants because electromagnetic fields produced by the MR system may interfere with the operation of these devices.[120] Therefore, patients with internal cardiac pacemakers, implantable cardiac defibrillators, cochlear implants, neurostimulators, bone-growth stimulators, implantable electronic drug infusion pumps, and other similar devices that could be adversely affected by the electromagnetic fields used for MR undergo examination with this imaging technique.[122,124–127] Ex vivo testing of certain of these implants and devices, however, may indicate that they are, in fact, MR-compatible.

text continues on page 39

TABLE 2-1
Summary of Studies on Bioeffects of MR Imaging

Study Description	Results	Reference
2.0 T • Clinical imaging conditions • Rats Studied effect of MRI on blood–brain barrier permeability	"no MRI-induced difference was detected"	Adzamil et al[1]
1.5 T • Exposure to RF radiation in excess of clinical imaging conditions • Sheep • Studied RF radiation–induced heating	"For exposure periods in excess of standard clinical imaging protocols the temperature increase was insufficient to cause adverse thermal effects."	Barber et al[2]
0.5 and 1.5 T • Clinical imaging conditions • Human subjects • Studied effect of MRI on electroencephalogram and evaluated neuropsychological status	"no measurable influence of MRI on cognitive functions"	Bartels et al[3]
0.04 T • Clinical imaging conditions • Human subjects • Studied effects of MRI on cognition	"MRI did not cause any cognitive deterioration"	Besson et al[4]
1.6 T • Quenched magnet • Pigs • Studied effect of quenching magnet	"our findings, which in the circumstances of this experiment, suggested that the risk are small"	Bore et al[5]
MRI gradient-induced electric fields • Dogs • Studied bioeffects at high MRI gradient-induced fields	"as the strength of MRI gradient-induced fields increases, biological effects in order of increasing field and severity include stimulation of peripheral nerves, nerves of respiration and finally, the heart"	Bourland et al[6]
0.38 T • Static magnetic field only • Deoxygenated erythrocytes • Studied orientation of sickle erythrocytes	"further studies are needed to assess possible hazards of MRI of sickle cell disease"	Brody et al[7]
0.35 and 1.5 T • Clinical imaging conditions • Human subjects with sickle cell disease • Studied effects of MRI on patients with sickle cell disease	"no change in sickle cell blood flow during MR imaging in vivo"	Brody et al[8]
0.35 T • Clinical imaging conditions • Human subjects • Studied effects of noise during MRI on hearing	"noise generated by MR imaging may cause temporary hearing loss, and earplugs can prevent this"	Brummett et al[9]

(Continued)

TABLE 2-1
(Continued)

Study Description	Results	Reference
Varying Gradient Fields • Human subjects • Studied neural stimulation threshold with varying oscillations and gradient-field strengths	"the threshold decreases with the number of oscillations and increases with frequency. The repeatable threshold of 63 T/s (1270 Hz) remains constant from 32 oscillations (25.6 ms) to 128 oscillations (102.4 ms)"	Budinger et al[10]
0.15 T • Simulated imaging conditions • HL60 promyelocytic cells • Studied effect of MRI on Ca^{2+}	"results demonstrate that time-varying magnetic fields associated with MRI procedures increase Ca^{2+}"	Carson et al[11]
Gradient Magnetic Fields up to 66 T/s in Dogs and 61 T/s in Humans • Dogs and human subjects • Studied physiologic responses to large-amplitude time-varying magnetic fields	Dogs: "no motion, twitch, or ECG abnormalities" Humans: brief minimal muscular twitches observed on various parts of the body, due to magnetic stimulation	Cohen et al[12]
0.5 and 1.0 T • Simulated imaging conditions • Cultured human blood cells • Studied effects of static magnetic fields and line-scan imaging on human blood cells	"neither treatment had any significant effect on any of the parameters measured"	Cooke and Morris[13]
4.7 T • Exposures to static and RF electromagnetic fields only • Isolated rabbit hearts • Studied effects on cardiac excitability and vulnerability	No measurable effect on strength interval relation or ventricular vulnerability	Doherty et al[14]
Gradient Magnetic Fields Only • Sinusoidal gradients at frequency of 1.25 kHz with amplitudes up to 40 mT/min for z coil and 25 mT/min for x coil • Human subjects • Studied physiologic effects and physiologic responses	Observed peripheral muscle stimulation; no extrasystoles or arrhythmias	Fischer[15]
0.3, 0.5 and 1.5 T • Simulated imaging conditions • Separate static/RF and gradient fields • Rats • Studied blood–brain barrier permeability	"increased brain mannitol associated with gradient fluid flux may reflect increase blood–brain barrier permeability or blood volume in brain"	Garber et al[16]
2.2–2.7 T • Simulated imaging conditions • Mouse cells • Studied oncogenic and genotoxic effects of MRI	"data clearly mitigate against an association between exposure to MR imaging modalities and both carcinogenic and genotoxic effects"	Geard et al[17]

(Continued)

TABLE 2-1
(*Continued*)

Study Description	Results	Reference
60 T/s • Gradient magnetic fields only • Human subjects • Studied effects of gradient magnetic fields on cardiac and respiratory functions	"no changes were observed"	Gore et al[18]
0.1–1.5 T • Static magnetic field only • Human subjects • Studied effects of static magnetic fields on temperature	Temperatures increased or decreased depending on field strength of magnet	Gremmel et al[19]
2.11 T • Static magnetic field only • Isolated rat hearts • Studied effect of static magnetic field on cardiac muscle contraction	"static magnetic fields used in NMR imaging do not constitute any hazard in terms of cardiac contractility"	Gulch and Lutz[20]
2.0 T • RF of 90 MHz • Simulated imaging conditions • Phantom and Caphuchin monkeys • Studied temperature changes in phantom and monkey brain during high-RF-power exposures	"blood flowing through the brain used the body as a heat sink"	Hammer et al[21]
0.35 T • Simulated imaging conditions • Mice • Studied teratogenic effects of MRI	"prolonged midgestional exposure failed to reveal any overt embryotoxicity or teratogenicity" "slight but significant reduction in fetal crown–rump length after prolonged exposure justifies further study of higher MRI energy levels"	Heinrichs et al[22]
1.5 T • Static magnetic field only • Human subjects • Studied effect of static magnetic field on somatosensory evoked potentials	"short-term exposure to 1.5 T static magnetic field does not effect SEPs in human subjects"	Hong and Shellock[23]
0.15 T • Simulated imaging conditions • Rats • Studied effects on cognitive processes	"MRI procedure has no significant effect on spatial memory processes in rats"	Innis et al[24]
2.0 T • Static magnetic field only • Human subjects • Studied effect of static magnetic field on cardiac rhythm	Cardiac cycle length was significantly increased, but this increase is probably harmless in normal subjects; safety in patients with dysrrhythmia remains to be determined	Jehenson et al[25]
1.5 T • Simulated imaging conditions • Frog embryo • Studied effect of MRI on embryogenesis	"no adverse effects of MRI components on development of this vertebrate (*Xenopus laevis*)"	Kay et al[26]

(*Continued*)

TABLE 2-1
(Continued)

Study Description	Results	Reference
2.3, 4.7, and 10 T • Static magnetic fields only • Physiologic solutions (2.3 and 4.7 T) and mathematic modeling (10 T) • Studied hydrostatic pressure and electrical potentials across vessels in presence of static magnetic fields	"A 10-T magnetic field changes vascular pressure in a model of the human vasculature by less than 0.2%"	Keltner et al[27]
1.5 T • Clinical imaging conditions • Human subjects • Studied physiologic changes during high-field-strength MRI	"temperature changes and other physiologic changes . . . were small and of no clinical concern"	Kido et al[28]
1.5 T • Simulated imaging conditions • Rats • Studied effects of MRI on receptor-mediated activation of pineal gland indole biosynthesis	"strong magnetic fields and/or radiofrequency pulsing used in MRI inhibited beta-adrenergic activation of the gland"	LaPorte et al[29]
3.5–12 kT/s • Gradient magnetic fields only • Mice • Studied effect of gradient magnetic fields on pregnancy and postnatal development	"no significant difference between the litter numbers and growth rates of the exposed litters compared with controls"	McRobbie and Foster[30]
Various Strong Magnetic Fields • Gradient magnetic fields only • Anesthetized rats • Studied cardiac response to gradient magnetic fields	"the types of pulsed magnetic fields used in the present study did not affect the cardiac cycle of anesthetized rats"	McRobbie and Foster[31]
1.89 T • Simulated imaging sequence • Rats • Studied taste aversion in rats to evaluate possible toxic effects of MRI	"rats exposed to MRI did not display any aversion to the saccharin solution"	Messmer et al[32]
1.89 T • Simulated imaging sequence • Mouse spleen cells • Studied possible interaction between ionizing radiation and MRI on damage to normal tissue	"for the normal tissues studied, MR imaging neither increases radiation damage nor inhibits repair"	Montour et al[33]
0–2.0 T • Clinical imaging conditions • Human subjects • Studied extent of changes in brain stem evoked potentials with MRI	"routine MRI examinations do not produce pathological changes in auditory evoked potentials"	Muller and Hotz[34]
1.5 T • Simulated imaging conditions • Human subjects • Studied effect of MRI on somatosensory and brain stem auditory evoked potentials	"it may be assumed that MRI causes no lasting changes"	Niemann et al[35]

(Continued)

TABLE 2-1
(Continued)

Study Description	Results	Reference
0.75 T • Static magnetic field only • Hamster cells • Studied effect of static magnetic field on DNA synthesis and survival of mammalian cells irradiated with fast neutrons	"presence of the magnetic field either during or subsequent to fast-neutron irradiation does not effect the neutron-induced radiation damage or its repair"	Ngo et al[36]
1.89 T • Static magnetic field only • Mice • Studied effects of long-term exposure to a static magnetic field	"no consistent differences found in gross and microscopic morphology, hematocrit and WBCs, plasma creatine phosphokinase, lactic dehydrogenase, cholesterol, triglyceride, or protein concentrations in magnet groups compared to two control groups"	Osbakken et al[37]
0.15 T • Simulated imaging conditions • Rats • Studied effects of MRI on behavior of rats	"results fail to provide any evidence for short or long term behavioral changes in animals exposed to MRI"	Ossenkopp et al[38]
0.15 T • Simulated imaging conditions • Rats • Studied effect of MRI on murine opiate analgesia levels	"NMRI procedures alter both day and night time responses to morphine"	Ossenkopp et al[39]
1.0 T • Static magnetic field only • Mice • Studied effect of static magnetic field on in vivo bone growth	"results suggest that exposure to intense magnetic fields does not alter physiological mechanisms of bone mineralization"	Papatheofanis and Papatheofanis[40]
2.35 T • Static and gradient magnetic fields only • Nematodes • Studied toxic effects of static and gradient magnetic fields	"static magnetic fields have no effect on fitness of test animals"; "time-varying magnetic fields cause inhibition of growth and maturation"; "combination of pulsed magnetic field gradients in a static uniform magnetic field also has a detrimental effect on the fitness of the test animals"	Peeling et al[41]
2.35 T • Simulated imaging conditions • Mice • Studied the effect of MRI on tumor development	"immune response may be enhanced following MRI exposure, as indicated by the longer latency and smaller sizes of tumors in animals receiving MRI exposure"	Prasad et al[42]
4.5 T • Simulated imaging conditions • Mice • Studied the effects of high-field-strength MR imaging on mouse testes and epididymes	"little, if any, damage to male reproductive tissues from . . . high intensity MRI exposure"	Prasad et al[43]

(Continued)

TABLE 2-1
(Continued)

Study Description	Results	Reference
0.7 T • Simulated imaging conditions • Mouse bone marrow cells • Studied the cytogenic effects of MRI	"NMR exposure causes no adverse cytogenic effects"	Prasad et al[44]
0.15 T • Simulated imaging conditions • Mice • Studied effects of MRI on immune system	"MR exposure has no adverse effect on the immune system, as evidenced by natural killer cell activity"	Prasad et al[45]
2.35 T • Simulated imaging conditions • Human peripheral blood mononuclear cells • Studied effect of MRI on natural killer cell toxicity of peripheral blood mononuclear cells with and without interleukin-2	"in neither case was cytotoxicity affected by prior exposure to MR imaging"	Prasad et al[46]
0.15 and 4.0 T • Simulated imaging conditions • Fertilized frog eggs • Studied effect of MRI on developing embryos	"no adverse effect early development"	Prasad et al[47]
0.7 T • Simulated imaging conditions • Frog spermatazoa, fertilized eggs, and embryos • Studied effects of MRI on development	"NMR exposure, at the dose used does not cause detectable adverse effects in this amphibian"	Prasad et al[48]
0.15 T • Exposed separately to static, gradient, and RF electromagnetic fields • Mice • Studied separate effects of static, gradient, and RF electromagnetic fields on morphine-induced analgesia	"time-varying, and to a lesser extent the RF, fields associated with the MRI procedure inhibit morphine-induced analgesia in mice"	Prato et al[49]
4.7 T • Clinical imaging conditions • Human subjects • Studied bioeffects of 4.7-T scanner	"mild vertigo"; "headaches, nausea"; "magnetophosphenes"; "metallic taste in mouth"	Redington et al[50]
0.04 T • Clinical imaging conditions • Human subjects • Follow-up study	"average follow-up time was 6 months. . . . none of the 35 deaths recorded was unexpected"; "using the magnetic field and radiofrequency levels currently in operation. . . . we believe NMRI to be a safe, non-invasive method of whole-body imaging"	Reid et al[51]

(Continued)

TABLE 2-1
(Continued)

Study Description	Results	Reference
4.0 T • RF of 8–170 MHz • No gradient magnetic fields • Human subjects • Studied response of human auditory system to RF pulses	"in accordance with the used RF modulation envelope three distinct chirps per sequence could be resolved"; "RF induced auditory noise is usually completely masked by noise from simultaneously switched gradient fields"	Roschmann et al[52]
2.7 T • Simulated imaging conditions • Rats • Studied effects of MRI on ocular tissues	"there were no discernible effects on the rat eye"	Sacks et al[13]
0.35 T • Simulated imaging conditions • Hamster ovary cells • Studied effects of MRI on observable mutations and cytotoxicity	"NMR imaging caused no detectable genetic damage and does not affect cell viability"	Schwartz and Crooks[54]
1.5 T • Static magnetic field only • Human subjects • Studied effect of static magnetic field on body temperature	"no effect on body temperature of normal human subjects"	Shellock et al[55]
1.5 T • Clinical imaging conditions • Human subjects • Studied changes in temperature, heart rate, and blood pressure associated with MRI	"MR imaging . . . not associated with any temperature or hemodynamic related deleterious effects"	Shellock and Crues[56]
1.5 T • Clinical imaging conditions • Human subjects • Studied thermal effects of MRI of the spine	"no surface 'hot spots' "; "temperature effects were well below known thresholds for adverse effects"	Shellock et al[57]
1.5 T • Clinical imaging conditions • Human subjects • Studied possible hypothalamic heating produced by MRI of the head	"there was probably no direct hypothalamic heating produced by clinical MRI of the head"	Shellock et al[58]
1.5 T • Clinical imaging conditions • Human subjects • Studied effect of MRI on corneal temperatures	"MR imaging . . . causes relatively minor increases in corneal temperature that do not appear to pose any thermal hazard to ocular tissue"	Shellock and Crues[59]
1.5 T • Clinical imaging conditions • Human subjects • Studied temperature changes associated with MRI of the brain	"no significant increases in average body temperature" "observed elevations in skin temperatures were physiologically inconsequential"	Shellock and Crues[60]

(Continued)

TABLE 2-1
(Continued)

Study Description	Results	Reference
1.5 T • Static magnetic field only • Human subjects • Studied effects of static magnetic field on body and skin temperatures	"there were no statistically significant changes in body or any of the skin temperatures recorded"	Shellock et al[61]
1.5 T • Clinical imaging conditions • Human subjects • Studied effect of MRI performed at high SAR levels	"recommended exposure to RF radiation during MR imaging of the body for patients with normal thermoregulatory function may be too conservative"	Shellock et al[62]
1.5 T • Clinical imaging conditions • Human subjects • Studied effect of MRI on scrotal skin temperature	"absolute temperature is below threshold known to affect testicular function"	Shellock et al[63]
0.15 T • Simulated imaging conditions • Anesthetized rats • Studied effect of MRI on permeability of blood–brain barrier	"these findings raise the possibility that exposure to clinical MRI procedures may also temporarily alter the central blood–brain permeability in human subjects"	Shivers et al[64]
1.5 T • Simulated imaging conditions • Anesthetized dogs • Studied effect of MRI performed at high SAR levels	"these findings argue for continued caution in the design and operation of imagers capable of high specific absorption rates"	Shuman et al[65]
0.4 to 8.0 T • Static magnetic field only • Mice • Studied effect of static magnetic field on temperature	"observed a field-induced increase in temperature"	Sperber et al[66]
0.4 to 1.0 T • Static magnetic field only • Human subjects • Studied the effects of static magnetic fields on tissue perfusion	"neither at the skin of the thumb nor at the forearm were the changes in local flood flow attributable to the magnetic fields applied"	Stick et al[67]
0.4 T • Static magnetic field only • Human subjects • Studied magnetic-field–induced changes in auditory evoked potentials	"strong steady magnetic fields induce changes in human auditory evoked potentials"	Stojan et al[68]
0.15 T • Clinical imaging conditions • Human subjects • Studied effect of MRI on cognitive functions	"no significant effect upon cognitive functions assessed"	Sweetland et al[69]

(Continued)

TABLE 2-1
(Continued)

Study Description	Results	Reference
0.6 T/s • Gradient magnetic field only • Mice • Studied effect of gradient magnetic fields on the analgesic properties of specific opiate antagonists	"results indicate that the time-varying fields associated with MRI have significant inhibitory effects on analgesic effects of specific myopiate-directed ligands"	Tesky et al[70]
0.15 T • Simulated imaging conditions • Rats • Studied effects of MRI on survivability and long-term stress reactivity levels	results fail to provide any evidence for changes in survivability and long-term reactivity levels in rats exposed to MRI"	Teskey et al[71]
0.01 and 1.0 T • Simulated imaging conditions and static magnetic field only • *Escherichia coli* • Studied effect of MRI and static magnetic field on various properties of *E coli*	"no mutations or lethal effects observed"	Thomas and Morris[72]
1.5 T • Simulated imaging conditions • Mice • Studied potential effects of MRI fields on eye development	"these data suggest a potential for MRI teratogenicity in a strain of mouse predisposed to eye malformations"	Tyndall and Sulik[73]
1.5 T • Simulated imaging conditions • C57BL/6J mouse • Studied combined effects of MRI and x-irradiation on the developing eye of the mouse	"MRI techniques employed for this investigation did not enhance teratogenicity of x-irradiation on eye malformations produced in the 657BL/6J mouse"	Tyndall[74]
0.35 and 1.5 T • Clinical imaging conditions • Human subjects • Studied effects of MRI on temperature	"no significant changes in central or peripheral temperatures resulting from the application of static or dynamic or radiofrequency"	Vogl et al[75]
0.35 T • Static magnetic field only • Human subjects • Studied effect of static magnetic field on auditory evoked potentials	"magnetically induced shift may be explained by changes in electric capacities of the magnetically exposed biological system"	Von Klitzing[76]
0.2 T • Static magnetic field only • Human subjects • Studied effect of static magnetic field on power intensity of electroencephalogram	"the increased control values following on inverted magnetic flux vector point to a reversible alteration of brain function induced by a static magnetic field"	Von Klitzing[77]

(Continued)

TABLE 2-1
(Continued)

Study Description	Results	Reference
0.2 T • Static magnetic field only • Human subjects • Studied encephalomagnetic fields during exposure to static magnetic field	"exposure to static magnetic fields as used in NMR equipment generates a new encephalomagnetic field in human brain"	Von Klitzing[78]
1.5 and 4.0 T • Static magnetic fields only • Rats • Studied effect of magnetic field on behavior	"at 4 T . . . in 97% of the trials the rats would not enter the magnet"	Weiss et al[79]
0.16 T • Static and gradient magnetic fields only • Anesthetized rats and guinea pigs • Studied effects of static and gradient magnetic fields on cardiac function of rats and guinea pigs	"no change in blood pressure, heart rate, or ECG"	Willis and Brooks[80]
0.3 T • Static magnetic field only • Mouse sperm cell • Studied effect of static magnetic field on spermatogenesis	"acute and subacute exposure to static magnetic fields associated with diagnostic MR imaging devices is unlikely to have any significant adverse effect on spermatogesis"	Withers et al[81]
0.35 T • Simulated imaging conditions • Hamster ovary cells • Studied effect of MRI on DNA and chromosomes	"the conditions used for NMR imaging do not cause genetic damage which is detectable by any of these methods"	Wolff et al[82]
Varying Gradient Fields • Human subjects • Studied the effects of time-varying gradient fields on peripheral nerve stimulation using trapezoidal and sinusoidal pulse trains	"the thresholds of trapezoidal pulses were higher than those of sinusoidal pulses by 11% and 30% respectively, at equivalent power level"	Yamagata et al[83]

ECG, *electrocardiogram;* MRI, *magnetic resonance imaging;* NMR, *nuclear magnetic resonance;* SEPs, *somatosensory evoked potentials;* WBCs, *white blood cells.*

Risks associated with scanning patients with cardiac pacemakers are related to the possibility of movement, reed switch closures or damage, programming changes, inhibition, reversion to an asynchronous mode of operation, electromagnetic interference, and induced currents in lead wires.[122,124,125,127] There have been anecdotal reports of a patient with a pacemaker who was scanned by MR without incident, and of another, who was not pacemaker dependent, who underwent MR imaging by having his pacemaker disabled during the procedure.[126] Although the procedure was performed with no apparent discomfort for the patient nor damage to the pacemaker, it is inadvisable to perform this type of maneuver on patients with pacemakers routinely be-

cause of the potential hazards mentioned above. There has been an MR-related death of a patient with a pacemaker.[99]

Of particular concern is the possibility that the pacemaker lead wire(s) or other similar intracardiac wire configuration could act as an antenna in which the gradient or RF electromagnetic fields may induce sufficient current to cause fibrillation, a burn, or other dangerous events.[99,122,124,125,127] Because of this theoretically deleterious and unpredicted effect, patients with residual external pacing wires, temporary pacing wires, Swan-Ganz (catheter balloon-tipped pulmonary artery) thermodilution catheters, or other types of internally or externally positioned conductive wire or similar device should not undergo MR imaging.[99,122,128]

Cochlear implants either have a relatively high-field strength cobalt samarium magnet, used in conjunction with an external magnet, to align and retain an RF transmitter coil on the patient's head or are electronically activated.[129] MR imaging is strictly contraindicated in patients with these implants because of the possibility of injuring the patient or damaging or altering the operation of the cochlear implant.

Implants that involve magnets (eg, dental implants, magnetic sphincters, magnetic stoma plugs, magnetic ocular implants, and other similar devices) may become demagnetized during MR imaging, and surgery may be required to replace the damaged implant. If possible, therefore, these implants should be removed from the patient before MR imaging.[129–131]Otherwise, MR imaging should not be performed on a patient with a magnetically activated implant or device. A patient with any other similar electrically, magnetically, or mechanically activated implant or device should be excluded from examination by MR unless the particular implant or device has been previously demonstrated to be unaffected by the magnetic and electromagnetic fields used.[122]

PATIENTS WITH METALLIC IMPLANTS AND FOREIGN BODIES

Because of the possibility of movement or dislodgment, MR imaging is contraindicated in patients who have ferromagnetic implants, materials, or foreign bodies.[97–99] Other problems that may be encountered when imaging these patients include the induction of electrical current in the object, excessive heating of the object, and the misinterpretation of an artifact produced by the presence of the object as an abnormality.[97,99,132–135] These latter potential hazards, however, are encountered infrequently or are insignificant in comparison with the possibility of movement or dislodgment of a ferromagnetic implant or foreign body caused by the magnetic fields of the MR system.

Numerous investigations have evaluated the ferromagnetic qualities of a variety of metallic implants, materials, or foreign bodies by measuring deflection forces or movements associated with the static magnetic fields used by MR scanners.[100,135–153] These studies were conducted to determine the relative risk of performing MR imaging on a patient with a metallic object with respect to whether or not the magnetic attraction was strong enough to produce movement or dislodgment (Table 2-2).

A variety of factors require consideration when the relative risk of performing an MR procedure in a patient with a ferromagnetic implant, material, device, or foreign body is evaluated. These factors include the strength of the static and gradient magnetic fields, the relative degree of ferromagnetism of the object, the mass of the object, the geometry of the object, the location and orientation of the object in situ, and the length of time the object has been in place.[98,99] Each of these should be considered before allowing a patient

with a ferromagnetic object to enter the electromagnetic environment of the MR system.

Aneurysm and Hemostatic Clips

Of the different aneurysm and vascular clips studied and reported in the literature, many of the aneurysm clips and none of the vascular clips were found to be ferromagnetic. Therefore, only patients who definitely have nonferromagnetic aneurysm clips should be exposed to the magnetic fields used for MR imaging, Any patient with one of the previously tested hemostatic clips may safely undergo MR examination.

Carotid Artery Vascular Clamps

Each of the carotid artery vascular clamps evaluated for ferromagnetism exhibited deflection forces. However, only the Poppen-Blalock clamp (Codman, Randolph, MA) was considered to be contraindicated for patients undergoing MR because of the significant ferromagnetism shown by this object. Other carotid artery vascular clamps are believed to be safe for MR imaging because of the minimal deflection forces relative to their use in an in vivo application (ie, the deflection forces are insignificant and, therefore, there is little possibility of significant movement or dislodgment of the implant).

Dental Devices and Materials

Various dental devices and materials have been tested for ferromagnetism. Although many demonstrated deflection forces, only a few pose a possible risk to patients undergoing MR because they are magnetically activated devices.

Heart Valves

Many commercially available heart valve prostheses have been tested for ferromagnetism. The majority displayed measurable deflection forces, however, the deflection forces were relatively insignificant compared with the force exerted by the beating heart. Therefore, patients with these heart valve prostheses may safely undergo MR imaging.

Intravascular Coils, Filters, and Stents

Fewer than half of the different intravascular coils, filters, and stents tested were ferromagnetic.[145,152] These ferromagnetic devices are usually attached firmly into the vessel wall 4 to 6 weeks after introduction.[152] Therefore, it is unlikely that any of them would become dislodged by attraction from

TABLE 2-2
Metallic Implants, Materials, and Foreign Bodies That Are Potential Risks
for Patients Undergoing MR Procedures

Aneurysm Clips

Drake (DR14, DR 24), Edward Weck (Triangle Park, NJ)
Drake (DR16), Edward Weck
Drake (301 SS), Edward Weck
Downs multi-positional (17-7PH)
Heifetz (17-7PH), Edward Weck
Housepian
Kapp (405 SS), V. Mueller
Kapp curved (404 SS), V. Mueller
Kapp straight (404 SS), V. Mueller
Mayfield (301 SS), Codman (Randolph, MA)
Mayfield (304 SS), Codman
McFadden (301 SS), Codman
Pivot (17-7PH), V. Mueller
Scoville (EN58J), Downs Surgical (Decatur, GA)
Sundt-Kees (301-SS), Downs Surgical
Sundt-Kees Multi-Angle (17-7PH), Downs Surgical
Vari-Angle (17-7PH), Codman
Vari-Angle Micro (17-7PM SS), Codman
Vari-Angle Spring (17-7PM SS), Codman

Cartoid Artery Vascular Clamp

Poppen-Blaylock (SS), Codman

Dental Devices and Materials

Palladium-clad magnet,* Parkell Products (Farmingdale, NY)
Titanium-clad magnet,* Parkell Products
SS-clad magnet,* Parkell Products

Intravascular Coils, Stents, and Filters

Gianturco embolization coil,† Cook (Bloomington, IN)
Gianturco bird nest IVC filter,† Cook
Gianturco zig-zag stent,† Cook
Gunther IVC filter,† Cook
New retrievable IVC filter,† Thomas Jefferson University (Philadelphia, PA)
Palmaz endovascular stent,† Ethicon (Sommerville, NJ)

Ocular Implants

Fatio eyelid spring/wire*
Retinal tack (SS martensitic), Western European

Otologic Implants

Cochlear implant (3M/House)
Cochlear implant (3M/Vienna)
Cochlear implant, Nucleus Mini 22-channel, Cochlear (Englewood, CO)
McGee piston stapes prothesis, (platinum and 17 chromium–4 nickel SS), Richards Medical (Memphis, TN)

Pellets, Bullets, and Schrapnel

BBs, Daisy
BBs Crosman
Bullet, 7.62 × 39 mm (copper, steel), Norinco
Bullet, 0.380 inch (copper, nickel, lead), Geco
Bullet, 0.45 inch (steel, lead), North America Ordinance
Bullet, 9 mm, (copper, lead), Norma

Penile Implant

OmniPhase,* Dacomed (Minneapolis, MN)

(Continued)

TABLE 2-2
(Continued)

Other Foreign Bodies

Cerebral ventricular shunt tube, connector (type unknown)
Swan-Ganz Catheter, Thermodilution,‡ American Edwards (Irvine, CA)
Tissue expander with magnetic port,* McGhan Medical (Santa Barbara, CA)

Manufacturer information is provided if given in previously published report or if otherwise known.

SS, stainless steel.

* The potential for these metallic implants or devices to produce significant injury to the patient is minimal. However, MR imaging in a patient with one of these devices may be uncomfortable for the patient or may result in damage to the implant.

† Ferromagnetic coils, filters, and stents typically become firmly incorporated into the vessel wall several weeks after placement, and therefore it is unlikely that they will become dislodged by magnetic forces after a suitable period of time, approximately 6 to 8 weeks, has passed.

‡ Although there is no magnetic deflection associated with the Swan-Ganz thermodilution catheter, there has been a report of a catheter "melting" in a patient undergoing MR imaging. Therefore, this catheter is considered a contraindication for MR imaging.

ſ The relative risks of performing MR imaging in patients with pellets, bullets, or schrapnel are related to whether the foreign bodies are positioned near a vital structure.

magnetic forces presently used for MR imaging. However, patients with intravascular coils, filters, or stents that might not be properly positioned or held firmly in place should not undergo MR imaging.

Ocular Implants

Various ocular implants have been evaluated for ferromagnetism. Of these, the Fatio eyelid spring and retinal tack made from martensitic stainless steel displayed measurable deflection forces. Although it is unlikely that the associated deflection forces would cause movement or dislodgment of an implant, it is possible that a patient with one of these implants would be uncomfortable or sustain a minor injury during MR imaging.

Orthopaedic Implants, Materials, and Devices

Most orthopaedic implants, materials, and devices tested for ferromagnetism have been demonstrated to be made from nonferromagnetic materials. Therefore, patients with these particular orthopaedic implants, materials, and devices may be imaged safely by MR. The Perfix interference screw (Instrument Makar, Okemos, MI) used for reconstruction of the anterior cruciate ligament is composed of ferromagnetic material but does not pose a hazard to the patient undergoing MR imaging because of the significant force that holds it in place in vivo. However, the resulting imaging artifact precludes diagnostic assessment of the knee using MR imaging.

Otologic Implants

MR imaging is contraindicated in patients with the cochlear implants so far evaluated for ferromagnetism. Besides being attracted by static magnetic fields, these implants are also electronically or magnetically activated. Only one of the tested otologic implants had associated deflection forces. This implant, the McGee piston stapes prosthesis composed of platinum and 17 chromium–4 nickel stainless steel (Richards Medical, Memphis, TN), was made on a limited basis in mid-1987 and was recalled by the manufacturer. Patients with this otologic implant were issued warning cards that instructed them to not be examined by MR imaging.

Pellets, Bullets, and Shrapnel

Most of the pellets and bullets that have been tested for ferromagnetism are composed of nonferromagnetic materials.[143,145] Typically, ammunition found to be ferromagnetic came from foreign countries or was used by the military. Shrapnel usually contains various amounts of steel and therefore presents a potential hazard for MR imaging. Furthermore, because pellets, bullets, and shrapnel may be contaminated with ferromagnetic materials, these objects represent relative contraindications for MR examination. Patients with these foreign bodies should be evaluated on an individual basis, with respect to whether the object is positioned near a vital neural, vascular, or soft-tissue structure. This may be assessed by taking a careful history and using plain-film radiography to determine the location of the foreign body.

Penile Implants and Artificial Sphincters

One of the penile implants tested for ferromagnetism displayed significant deflection forces. Although it is unlikely that this implant, the Omniphase (Dacomed, Minneapolis, MN), would cause serious injury to a patient undergoing MR imaging, it would undoubtedly be uncomfortable for the patient. Therefore, this implant is regarded as a relative contraindication for MR imaging. Artificial sphincters that have been tested are made from nonferromagnetic materials. However, at least one artificial sphincter currently undergoing clinical trials has a magnetic component and, therefore, patients with this device should not undergo MR imaging.

Vascular Access Ports

Of the various vascular access ports tested for ferromagnetism, two showed measurable deflection forces, but the forces were felt to be insignificant relative to the in vivo application of these implants.[142] Therefore, it is considered safe to perform MR imaging in a patient who may have one of these previously tested vascular access ports. The exception to this is any vascular access port that is programmable or electronically activated. Patients with this type of vascular access port should not undergo MR imaging.

Other Metallic Implants

Various types of other metallic implants, materials, and foreign bodies have also been tested for ferromagnetism. Of these, the cerebral ventricular shunt tube connector (type unknown) and tissue expander that is magnetically activated exhibited deflection forces that may pose a risk to patients during an MR examination. An O-ring washer used as a vascular marker also showed ferromagnetism, but the deflection force was determined to be minimal relative to the in vivo use of this device.

Each of the contraceptive diaphragms tested for ferromagnetism displayed significant deflection forces. However, we have performed MR studies on patients with these devices who did not complain of any sensation related to movement of these objects. Therefore, scanning patients with diaphragms is not believed to be considered to be physically hazardous to patients.

General Guidelines

According to the *Policies, Guidelines, and Recommendations for MR Imaging Safety and Patient Management* information issued by the Society for Magnetic Resonance Imaging Safety Committee,[122] patients with electrically, magnetically, or mechanically activated or electrically conductive devices should be excluded from MR scanning unless the particular device has been previously shown (usually by ex vivo testing procedures) to be unaffected by the electromagnetic fields used for clinical MR imaging and there is no possibility of injuring the patient. During the screening process for MR imaging, patients with these devices should be identified before the examination and before exposure to electromagnetic fields. If the device is as yet untested for MR compatibility, the patient should not be allowed to undergo MR imaging.

Screening Patients With Metallic Foreign Bodies

Patients who have had metallic foreign bodies such as slivers, bullets, shrapnel, or other types of metallic fragments should be screened before undergoing MR examination. The relative risk of scanning these patients depends on the ferromagnetic properties of the object, the shape and dimensions of the object, and the strength of the static and gradient magnetic fields of the MR system. Also important is the strength with which the object is fixed within the tissue and whether or not it is positioned in or adjacent to a vital neural, vascular, or soft-tissue structure.

A patient with an intraocular metallic foreign body is at a particular risk for significant eye injury from the static magnetic field of an MR system. In one reported case, a patient had an occult intraocular metal fragment (2.0×3.5 mm) that dislodged during MR imaging on a 0.35-T scanner, resulting in a vitreous hemorrhage that caused blindness.[154] This incident emphasizes the importance of adequate screening of patients with suspected intraocular metallic foreign bodies before MR imaging.

Research has demonstrated that small intraocular metallic fragments (as small as $0.1 \times 0.1 \times 0.1$ mm) can be detected using standard plain-film radiographs.[155] Although thin-slice (≤ 3 mm) computed tomography has been demonstrated to detect metallic foreign bodies as small as 0.15 mm, it is unlikely that a metallic fragment of this size would be dislodged during MR imaging, even with a static magnetic field up to 2.0 T.[155] Metallic fragments of various sizes and dimensions, ranging from $0.1 \times 0.1 \times 0.1$ mm to $3.0 \times 1.0 \times 1.0$ mm, have been examined to determine if they were moved or dislodged from the eyes of laboratory animals during exposure to a 2.0-T MR system.[155] Only the largest fragment ($3.0 \times 1.0 \times 1.0$ mm) rotated, but even it did not cause any discernible damage to the ocular tissue.[155] Therefore, the use of plain-film radiography may be an acceptable technique for identifying or excluding an intraocular metallic foreign body that represents a potential hazard to the patient undergoing MR imaging.[122] Patients with a high suspicion of having an intraocular metallic foreign body (for example, a metal worker exposed to metallic slivers with a history of an eye injury) should have plain-film radiographs of the orbits to rule out the presence of a metallic fragments before exposure to the static magnetic field. If a patient with a suspected ferromagnetic intraocular foreign body has no symptoms and a plain-film series of the orbits does not demonstrate a radiopaque foreign body, the risk of performing MR examination is minimal.[122] Using plain-film radiography to search for metallic foreign bodies is a sensitive and relatively inexpensive means of identifying patients who are unsuitable for MR, and can also be used to screen out patients who may have metal fragments in other potentially hazardous sites of the body.[122]

Each MR imaging site should establish a standardized policy for screening patients with suspected foreign bodies. The policy should include guidelines as to which patients require work-up by radiographic procedures, the specific procedure to be performed (including the number and types of views and patient position), and each case should be considered on an individual basis. These precautions should be taken for all patients referred for MR examination in any type of MR system, regardless of the field strength, magnet type, and the presence or absence of magnetic shielding.[122]

MR IMAGING DURING PREGNANCY

Although MR imaging is not believed to be hazardous to the fetus, only a few investigations have examined the teratogenic potential of this imaging modality. By comparison, literally thousands of studies have been performed to examine the possible hazards of ultrasound during pregnancy and controversy still exists concerning the safe use of this non-ionizing-radiation imaging technique.

Most of the earliest studies conducted to determine possible unwanted bioeffects during pregnancy showed negative results.[17,22,26,31,41,47,82] More recently, one study examined the effects of MR imaging on mice exposed during mid-gestation.[22] No gross embryotoxic effects were observed, however, there was a reduction in crown-rump length.[22] In another study performed by Tyndall and Sulik,[74] exposure to the electromagnetic fields used for a simulated clinical MR examination caused eye malformations in a genetically prone mouse strain. Therefore, it appears that the electromagnetic fields used for MR have the ability to produce developmental abnormalities.

A variety of mechanisms exist that could produce deleterious bioeffects with respect to the developing fetus and the use of electromagnetic fields during MR imaging.[86,88,89,103,108,109,118] In addition, it is well known that cells undergoing division, as in the case of the developing fetus during the first trimester, are highly susceptible to damage from different types of physical agents. Therefore, because of the limited data available at the present time, a cautionary approach is recommended for the use of MR imaging in pregnant patients.

The current guidelines of the FDA requires labeling of MR devices to indicate that the safety of MR imaging when used to image the fetus and the infant "has not been established."[120] In Great Britain, the acceptable limits of exposure for clinical MR imaging recommended by the National Radiological Protection Board in 1983 specify that "it might be prudent to exclude pregnant women during the first 3 months of pregnancy."[120]

According to the Safety Committee of the Society for Magnetic Resonance Imaging[122] (information also adopted recently by the American College of Radiology), MR examination is indicated for use in pregnant women if other non-ionizing forms of diagnostic imaging are inadequate or if the examination provides important information that would otherwise require exposure to ionizing radiation (such as x-ray exposure or computed tomography). It is recommended that pregnant patients be informed that, to date, there has been no indication that the use of clinical MR scanning during pregnancy has produced deleterious effects. However, as noted by the FDA, the safety of MR examination during pregnancy has not been proved.[120] Patients who are pregnant, or who suspect they may be pregnant, must be identified before undergoing MR imaging to assess the risks versus the benefits of the examination.

Another concern related to MR imaging in the pregnant patient is that during the first trimester of pregnancy the rate of spontaneous abortions is very high (over 30%) in the general population. Potential medico-legal implications relative to spontaneous abortions require that particular care be exercised in the use of MR imaging during this period.

CLAUSTROPHOBIA, ANXIETY, AND PANIC DISORDERS

Claustrophobia, and a variety of other psychological reactions including anxiety and panic disorders, may be encountered in as many as 5% to 10% of patients undergoing MR imaging. These sensations originate from several factors, including the restrictive dimensions of the interior of the scanner, the duration of the examination, the gradient-induced noises, and the ambient conditions within the bore of the scanner.[156–164]

Fortunately, adverse psychological responses to MR imaging are usually transient. However, there has been a report of two patients with no history of claustrophobia who tolerated MR with great difficulty and had persistent claustrophobia that required long-term psychiatric treatment.[157] Because adverse psychological responses to MR imaging typically delay or require cancellation of the examination, the following techniques have been developed and may be used to avert these problems.[122,156–164]

- Brief the patient concerning the specific aspects of the MR examination including the level of gradient-induced noise to expect, the internal dimensions of the scanner, and the length of the examination.
- Allow an appropriately screened relative or friend to remain with the patient during the procedure.
- Use headphones with calming music to decrease the repetitive noise created by the gradient coils.
- Maintain physical or verbal contact with the patient throughout the examination.
- Place the patient in a prone position with the chin supported by a pillow. In this position, the patient is able to visualize the opening of the bore, which helps to alleviate the "closed-in" feeling. An alternative method to reduce claustrophobia is to place the subject feet-first instead of head-first into the scanner.

- Scanner-mounted mirrors and mirror or prism glasses within the scanner allow the patient to see out.
- A large light at either end of the scanner decreases the anxiety of being in a long dark enclosure.
- A blindfold helps to mask the close surroundings from the patient.
- Relaxation techniques, such as controlled breathing and mental imagery, are also useful.[165] Also, several case reports have shown hypnotherapy to be successful in reducing MR-related claustrophobia and anxiety.
- Use psychological desensitization techniques before the MR examination.

Several investigators have recently attempted to compare the effectiveness of these techniques in reducing MR-induced anxiety or claustrophobia.[158,159,162] One such study demonstrated that providing detailed information about the MR procedure, in addition to relaxation exercises, successfully reduced the anxiety level of a group of patients both before and during MR examination. Similar reduction in anxiety could not be shown in patients provided with only information or stress-reduction counseling. Relaxation methods have also been shown to significantly decrease anxiety during other medical procedures. Some MR systems using a vertical magnetic field offer a more open design that might reduce the frequency of psychological problems associated with MR imaging procedures.

MONITORING PHYSIOLOGIC PARAMETERS DURING MR IMAGING

Because the typical MR system is constructed such that the patient is placed inside a cylindrical structure, routine observations and vital signs monitoring is not a trivial task. Conventional monitoring equipment was not designed to operate in the MR environment where static, gradient, and RF electromagnetic fields can adversely affect the operation of these devices. Fortunately, MR-compatible monitors have been developed and are commonly used in in-patient and out-patient MR centers.[166-174]

Physiologic monitoring is required for the safe use of MR examination in patients who are sedated, anesthetized, comatose, critically ill, or unable to communicate with the MR system operator. These patients should be routinely monitored during MR examination and, considering the current availability of MR-compatible monitors, there is no reason to exclude these types of patients from MR imaging. Every physiologic parameter that can be obtained under normal circumstances in the intensive care unit or operating room can be monitored during MR imaging, including heart rate, systemic blood pressure, intracardiac pressure, end-tidal carbon dioxide tension, oxygen saturation, respiratory rate, skin blood flow, and temperature.[167-174] Table 2-3 lists examples of MR-compatible monitors that have been successfully tested and operated at field strengths of up to 1.5 T. In addition, there are now MR-compatible ventilators for patients who require ventilatory support.

Monitors that contain ferromagnetic components (such as transformers or outer casings) can be strongly attracted by mid- and high-field MR systems, posing a serious hazard to patients and possible damage to the MR system. Because the intensity of the standard static magnetic field falls off as the third power of the distance from the magnet, simply placing the monitor a suitable distance from the MR system is sufficient to protect the operation of the device and to help prevent it from becoming a potential projectile.[171,174] If monitoring equipment is not permanently fixed in position, instructions should be given to all appropriate personnel regarding the hazards of moving this equipment too close to the MR system.[171,174]

In addition to being influenced by the static magnetic field, monitors may be adversely affected by electromagnetic interference from the gradient and RF pulses from the MR system.[171,174] In these instances, increasing the length of the patient-monitor interface and positioning the equipment outside the RF-shielded room (in the control room, for example) will enable the monitor to operate properly. It is usually necessary to position all monitors with cathode ray tubes at a location in the magnetic fringe field such that the display is not bent or distorted.

Some monitors emit spurious electromagnetic noise that can result in moderate to severe imaging artifacts.[171,174] These monitors can be modified to work during MR scanning by adding RF-shielded cables, using fiberoptic transmission of the signals (which is becoming increasingly the method of choice in the MR environment), or using a special outer casing. Also, special filters may be added to the monitor to inhibit electromagnetic noise. Of further concern is the fact that some monitoring equipment can be potentially harmful to patients if special precautions are not followed.[171,174,175-177] A primary source of adverse MR system and physiologic monitor interactions has been the interface that is used between the patient and the equipment, because this usually requires a conductive cable or other device. The presence of conductive material in the immediate MR system area is a safety concern because of the potential for monitor-related burns. There has been one report of an accident involving an anesthetized patient who sustained a third-degree burn on the finger in association with use of a pulse oximeter during MR imaging.[176] Investigation of this incident revealed that the cable leading from the pulse oximeter to the finger probe may have been looped during MR imaging and the gradient or RF magnetic fields induced sufficient current to heat the finger probe excessively, resulting in the finger burn.[176] This problem may also occur with the use of electrocardiographic lead wires or any other cable that may be looped or may form a conductive loop that contacts the patient.

The following recommendations help to prevent potential monitor-related accidents from occurring:

- Monitoring equipment should be used only by trained personnel.

TABLE 2-3
Examples of MR-compatible Monitors and Ventilators

Device and Manufacturer	Function
MRI Fiber-optic Pulse Oximeter Nonin Medical Plymouth, MN	Oxygen saturation, heart rate
MR-Compatible Pulse Oximeter Patient Monitoring System Magnetic Resonance Equipment Bay Shore, NY	Oxygen saturation, heart rate
MR-Compatible Pulse Oximeter In Vivo Research, Inc. Orlando, FL	Oxygen saturation, heart rate
Omega 1400 In Vivo Research Orlando, FL	Blood pressure, heart rate
Omni-Trak 3100 MRI Vital Signs Monitor In Vivo Research Orlando, FL	Heart rate, electrocardiogram, oxygen saturation, respiratory rate, blood pressure
Laserflow Blood Perfusion Monitor Vasomed St. Paul, MN	Cutaneous blood flow
Medpacific LD 5000 Laser-Doppler Perfusion Monitor Medpacific Seattle, WA	Cutaneous blood flow
Respiratory Rate Monitor, Models 515 and 525 Biochemical International Waukesha, WI	Respiratory rate, apnea monitoring
MicroSpan Capnometer 8800 Biochem International Waukesha, WI	Respiratory rate, end-tidal carbon dioxide tension, apnea monitoring
Aneuroid Chest Bellows Coulborun Instruments Allentown, Pennsylvania	Respiratory rate
Datex CO_2 Monitor Puritan-Bennett Corporation Los Angeles, CA	Percentage carbon dioxide
Wenger Precordial Stethescope Anesthesia Medical Supplies Santa Fe Springs, CA	Heart sounds
Fluoroptic Thermometry System, Model 3000 Luxtron Santa Clara, CA	Temperature
Omni-Vent, Series D Columbia Medical Marketing Topeka, KS	Ventilation
Ventilator models 225 and 2500 Monaghan Medical Plattsburgh, PA	Ventilation
Anesthesia Ventilator Ohio Medical Madison, WI	Ventilation
Infant Ventilator MVP-10 Bio-Med Devices Madison, CN	Ventilation

(Continued)

TABLE 2-3
(Continued)

Device and Manufacturer	Function
Ventilator model 900C Siemens-Elema Iselin, NJ	Ventilation

These devices may require modifications to make them MR-compatible, and none of them should be positioned closer than 2.5 m from the entrance of the bore of a 1.5-T MR system. In addition monitors with metallic cables, leads, or probes may cause mild to moderate imaging artifacts if placed near the imaging area of interest. Consult manufacturers to determine compatibility with specific MR systems.

- All cables and lead wires from monitoring devices that come into contact with the patient (the monitor–patient interface) should be positioned so that no conductive loops are formed.
- Monitoring devices that do not appear to operate properly during MR scanning should be immediately removed from the patient and the magnetic environment.

Techniques for Monitoring Physiologic Parameters

Blood Pressure

Noninvasive blood-pressure monitors typically use the oscillometric technique for measuring blood pressure, using a pressure transducer connected to a pressure cuff by a pneumatically filled hose. Some monitors (such as the Omega 1400, In Vivo Research, Orlando, FL) have adjustable audible and visual alarms as well as a strip-chart recorder.

Occasionally, inflation of the cuff disturbs lightly sedated patients, especially children, and thus may cause them to move and distort the MR image. For this reason, the noninvasive blood pressure monitor may not represent the optimal instrument for obtaining vital signs in all patient groups. Direct pressure monitoring of systemic or intracardiac pressures, if necessary, can be accomplished using a fiberoptic pressure transducer made entirely of plastic.

Respiratory Rate, Oxygenation, and Gas Exchange

Monitoring respiratory parameters during MR imaging of sedated or anesthetized patients is particularly important because the medications used for these procedures may produce complications of respiratory depression. Therefore, as a standard of care, a pulse oximeter, capnograph, or capnometer should always be used to monitor patients who are sedated or anesthetized during MR imaging.

The respiratory monitors used successfully on sedated pediatric or adult patients (such as model 515 Respiration Monitor and model 8800 Capnometer, Biochem International, Waukesha, WI) are relatively inexpensive and can be modified for use during MR imaging by simply lengthening the plastic tubing interface to the patient so that the monitors can be placed at least 2.5 m from the unshielded MR imager.

Pulse oximeters are used to record oxygen saturation and heart rate. Commercially available, modified pulse oximeters using hard wire cables have been used to monitor sedated and anesthetized patients during the MR imaging study and the recovery period with moderate success. These pulse oximeters tend to work intermittently during MR imaging because of interference from the gradient or RF electromagnetic fields. In certain instances, patients have been burned, presumably as a result of excessive current being induced in inappropriately looped conductive cables attached to the patient probes of the pulse oximeters.[175–177]

Newly developed portable fiberoptic pulse oximeters are now available for use during MR procedures[178] (see Table 2-3). When fiberoptic technology is used to obtain and transmit physiologic signals from patients undergoing MR imaging, there is no associated MR-related electromagnetic interference. It is physically impossible for a patient to be burned using a fiberoptic monitor during MR imaging because there are no conductive pathways formed by any metallic materials.

Cutaneous Blood Flow

Cutaneous blood flow can be monitored during MR imaging by means of the laser Doppler velocimetry technique. This noninvasive measurement technique uses laser light that is delivered to and detected from the region of interest by flexible, graded-index fiberoptic light wires. The Doppler broadening of laser light scattered by moving red blood cells within the tissue is analyzed in real time by an analogue processor that indicates instantaneous blood velocity and the effective blood volume and flow. The small circular probe can be attached to any available skin surface. Areas with a relatively high cutaneous blood flow (such as the hand, finger, foot, toe, or ear) yield the best results.

Hard-copy tracings obtained by laser Doppler velocimetry can be used to determine the patient's heart rate, respiratory rate, and cutaneous blood flow. An audible signal may be activated to permit the operator to hear blood flow changes during monitoring. This technique of continuous physiologic monitoring is particularly useful when there is concern about disturbing a sedated patient because it is easily tolerated.

Heart Rate

Monitoring the electrocardiogram during MR imaging is typically required for cardiac imaging, for gating to reduce imaging artifacts from the physiologic motion of cerebral spinal fluid in the brain and spine, and for determining the patient's heart rate. Artifacts caused by the static, gradient, and RF electromagnetic fields may severely distort the morphology of the electrocardiogram, making determination of cardiac rhythm during MR imaging extremely difficult and unreliable. Although sophisticated filtering techniques can be used to attenuate the artifacts from the gradient and RF fields, the static magnetic field produces T-wave augmentation, as previously mentioned, and other nonspecific waveform changes that are in direct proportion to the strength of the field and that cannot be easily counterbalanced.

In some instances, static magnetic field-induced augmented T waves have a higher amplitude than the R waves, resulting in false triggering and an inaccurate determination of the number of beats per minute. Electrocardiogram artifacts can be minimized during MR imaging by using special filters, by using electrocardiogram electrodes with minimal metal, by selecting lead wires with minimal metal, by twisting or braiding the lead wires, and by using special lead placements.[173]

The pulse oximeters described above may also be used to accurately record heart rate during MR examinations. These devices have probes that may be attached to the finger, toe, or ear lobe of the patient.

SAFETY CONSIDERATIONS FOR USE OF GADOLINIUM-BASED AGENTS

Although the first intravenous MR imaging contrast agent was only introduced into the clinical arena in mid-1988, less than 5 years later there are now three different contrast agents available for use. Throughout the United States, roughly one third of all MR imaging studies use contrast agents. Therefore, it is important to be familiar with the safety aspects of these medications commonly used in the clinical MR environment.[179–181]

The three MR imaging contrast agents approved for intravenous administration by the FDA are Magnevist (gadopentetate dimeglumine injection, Berlex Laboratories, Wayne, NJ), Omniscan (gadodiamide injection, Nycomed Salutar, Oslo, Norway), and ProHance (gadoteridol injection, Bracco Diagnostics, Princeton, NJ). Another agent, approved internationally, is Dotarem (gadoterate meglumine, Gd-DOTA, Guebet Laboratories, Aulnay-sous-Bois, France).

All of these contrast agents are based on the element gadolinium and have similar mechanisms of action, biodistri-

bution, and halflives.[180–183] Drug equilibration and physiologic biodistribution for each of the MR contrast agents is in the extracellular fluid space, with biologic elimination halflives of roughly 1.5 hours for each of these drugs.[180]

Gadolinium-based MR contrast agents are paramagnetic substances that develop a magnetic moment when placed in a magnetic field. The relatively large magnetic moment produced by a paramagnetic agent results in a relatively large local magnetic field that can enhance the relaxation rates of water protons in the vicinity of the MR imaging contrast agent. When placed in a magnetic field, gadolinium-based MR contrast agents decrease the T1 and T2 relaxation times in tissues in which they accumulate, although at doses used in the clinical setting, it is mainly the T1 relaxation time that is affected. The purpose is to improve contrast between two adjacent tissue compartments to make an abnormality, if one exists, more conspicuous.[180]

Free gadolinium ion is toxic, with a markedly prolonged biologic halflife of several weeks. The predominant uptake and excretion of gadolinium is by the kidneys and liver. Chelation of the gadolinium ion restricts it and markedly decreases its toxicity and alters its pharmacokinetics.[180] In fact, this chelation also decreases the ability of the gadolinium ion to accomplish its task of T1 shortening. Therefore, the goal of MR contrast-agent design and development is to decrease toxicity sufficiently without overly decreasing T1 relaxivity.

As noted above, the chelating process also alters the pharmacokinetic characteristics of the agent. For example, chelation of gadolinium ions allows an approximately 500-fold increase in the rate of renal excretion of the substance.[184,185] In each case, the chelating substance is what makes these various MR contrast agents differ from one another. The chelating agent for Magnevist is the DTPA molecule; for Omniscan it is DTPA-BMA; and for ProHance it is HP-DO3A. Magnevist has a linear structure and is an ionic compound; Omniscan has a linear structure and is nonionic; ProHance is also nonionic and possesses a macrocyclic ring structure.

Despite marked differences in their chelating molecules, their ionic versus nonionic nature, and their linear versus ring-like molecular structure, these agents appear to have remarkably similar effectiveness and safety profiles. Some differences do exist, however, both theoretically as well as on paper, as discussed below (see the section ''Adverse Effects of Specific MR Contrast Agents,'' later in this chapter). Multiple studies have documented the high safety index of MR contrast agents, especially when compared with iodinated contrast media used for computed tomography.[181,186–202] However, from a safety profile standpoint, it is inappropriate to compare ionic and nonionic MR contrast agents to ionic and nonionic computed-tomography contrast agents because of the drastically different osmotic loads associated with each of these drugs.

''The 50% lethal dose'' (LD_{50}) is the term used to denote the dose of an agent that, when administered to test animals, results in acute death of half of the population of the recipients. The LD$_{50}$ for MR contrast agents, as studied in rodents, is high. It is highest for Omniscan (>30 mmol/kg), next highest for ProHance (12 mmol/kg), and the lowest for Magnevist (6 to 7 mmol/kg). In all cases, the LD$_{50}$ is significantly in excess of the typical diagnostic dose of 0.1 mmol/kg (roughly 300, 120, and 60 times, respectively).[180,203] There are also data to suggest that there are fewer acute cardiodepressive effects from the nonionic drugs (ProHance was used in one study) than the ionic agent (Magnevist), when injected rapidly and into a central vein.[204] This may have limited clinical applicability, however, because MR contrast agents are typically injected into peripheral veins, with only small total volumes being administered.[180]

General Adverse Events of MR Contrast Agents

The total incidence of adverse reactions of all types for each of the MR imaging contrast agents ranges from approximately 2% to 4%.[181,196,205] The most common reactions are nausea, emesis, hives, headaches, and local injection site symptoms such as irritation, focal burning, or a cool sensation. With the use of Magnevist, transient elevations in serum bilirubin have been reported in 3% to 4% of patients, and with the use of both Magnevist and Omniscan, a transient elevation in iron that seems to reverse spontaneously within 24 to 48 hours has been reported in 15% to 30% of patients.[181,206] No such alterations in blood chemistry have been reported with the use of ProHance. Of special note is that here are no known contraindications for Magnevist, Ominiscan, and Prohance.

The MR contrast agent that has had FDA approval the longest and, therefore, the one for which there is the most clinical experience and information, is Magnevist. Approximately 5.7 million doses have been administered worldwide since its approval in June 1988. This figure compares with approximately 150,000 total administered doses of ProHance since its FDA approval in November 1992 and approximately 100,000 doses of Omniscan since its FDA approval in January 1993.

There have been rare reported incidents of laryngospasm or anaphylactoid reactions (requiring interventional therapy such as epinephrine) associated with the administration of each of these agents (Reich, L., PhD, Mycomed, oral communication, June 1993).[205–214] Therefore, it is advisable to establish a prolonged observation period of all patients with a history of allergy or drug reaction. The package insert for Magnevist states:

> The possibility of a reaction, including serious, fatal, anaphylactoid, or cardiovascular reactions or other idiosyncratic reactions should always be considered especially in those with a known clinical history of asthma or other allergic respiratory disorders.

Delayed reactions of hypertension, vasovagal responses, and syncope have also been reported with the use of MR contrast agents. Accordingly, the product inserts for these drugs advise that all patients should be observed for several hours after drug administration.

Adverse Effects of Specific MR Contrast Agents

The specific adverse events associated with the use of MR contrast agents vary to a minor degree.[205–219] It should be noted that the incidence of the vast majority of these events is less than 1%. To understand better the nature of these adverse events, definition of some commonly used, and misused, terms is warranted. An anaphylactoid reaction is one that involves respiratory, cardiovascular, cutaneous (and possibly gastrointestinal or genitourinary) manifestations.[215] This is not to say that all events that have such symptoms are by definition anaphylactoid. However, it does become more difficult to make the diagnosis of anaphylaxis in the absence of such symptoms, especially the classic triad of upper airway obstructive symptomatology, decreased blood pressure (or other similar severe cardiovascular symptoms), and cutaneous manifestations, such as urticaria.

As defined by the FDA, a ''serious reaction'' is one in which an adverse reaction to a drug proves fatal or life-threatening, is permanently disabling, requires in-patient hospitalization, or is an overdose (FDA docket 85D-0249). A ''life-threatening reaction,'' in FDA terminology, is one in which the initial reporter (the person initially reporting the incident) believes that the patient was at immediate risk of death from the event. Given these definitions, it is possible to understand how the interpretation of an adverse event may differ from that designated by the FDA.

Magnevist

As of June 1993, there were 13 anaphylactoid reactions with Magnevist, an estimated anaphylactoid reaction rate of 1:450,000 (L. Gifford, MD, Berlex Laboratories, oral communication, June 1993). One of the patients who had an anaphylactoid reaction died and another suffered brain damage (at the time of this writing that patient is still in a coma) subsequent to administration of Magnevist. In each case there was a history of respiratory difficulty or allergic respiratory problem, such as asthma. As previously mentioned, the current package insert for Magnevist warns that caution should be exercised when administering this agent to patients with known allergic respiratory disease.

The total reported incidence of adverse reactions to Magnevist of any kind is 2.4%, based on a retrospective review of 15,496 patients (L. Gifford, MD, Berlex Laboratories, written communication, June 1993). Of these cases, only two reactions were labeled ''serious'' by FDA standards. In one, a patient being evaluated for metastatic disease died of herniation from an intracranial tumor within 24 hours of the contrast enhanced MR study. Because of the design of the present review process, this temporal association is sufficient to have the case reported as "associated" with Magnevist administration, irrespective of any perceived or real causal relation. The second serious reaction in this series of patients occurred in an patient who was undergoing evaluation for vertigo and who had an acute progression of vertigo after the administration of Magnevist. Seizures after administration of this drug have been reported.[219] In at least one case, the Magnevist injection was believed to induce a seizure in a patient with a history of grand mal seizures (the product insert information for Magnevist has more detailed information on seizures if needed).

Mild elevations in serum chemistries associated with the use of Magnevist suggest that there may be a component of mild hemolysis in some unknown manner associated with the use of this drug. However, this association is not definite and there is no evidence demonstrating increased hemolysis as a result of Magnevist administration in patients with hemolytic anemias. The FDA has expressed concern (in the package insert) regarding the use of Magnevist as well as the other gadolinium-based agents in patients with sickle cell anemia. According to the package insert information for MR contrast agents, the enhancement of magnetic moment by Magnevist, Omniscan, or ProHance may possibly potentiate sickle erythrocyte alignment. This information was based on in vitro studies that showed that deoxygenated sickle erythrocytes align perpendicular to a magnetic field and, therefore, vasoocclusive complications may result, in vivo. However, there have been no studies performed to assess the effect of the use of these MR contrast agents in patients with sickle cell anemia and other forms of hemoglobinopathies. In addition, there has been no report of sickle crisis precipitated by the administration of any of these drugs.

Of the three MR contrast agents, Magnevist has the highest of the osmolalities, measuring 1960 mmol/kg of water, or roughly six to seven times that of plasma (approximately 285 mmol/kg of water).[220] Doses greater than and sometimes double those used in the United States (doses of up to 0.3 mmol/kg) have already been investigated in the clinical setting[206,221-223] and have been used for some time in Europe with no apparent significant deleterious effects.[224]

Because the osmolality of Magnevist is approximately six to seven times the osmolality of plasma, one might expect local irritative reactions as a possible adverse response with the use of this relatively hyperosmolar substance. Indeed, there has been at least one incident of possible phlebitis that required hospitalization and that was related temporally to the administration of an intravenous dose of Magnevist (J. LaFlore, MD, Berlex Laboratories, oral communication, 1990). The mechanism or mechanisms behind this reaction are still unclear, although objective studies have demonstrated that tissue sloughing can occur as a result of extravasation of gadolinium dimeglumine.[216,217]

There have also been several cases of erythema, swelling, and pain at or proximal to the site of administration that were of delayed onset, typically appearing 1 to 4 days after the intravenous administration of the gadolinium-DTPA. The symptoms typically progressed for several days, plateaued, and then resolved over several more days.[218] Nevertheless, severe adverse local reactions to even considerable quantities (>10 cc) of Magnevist extravasation seem to be rare, at best.

Of note, Magnevist is the only one of the three MR contrast agents approved in the United states that has a package insert that recommends a slow, intravenous administration at a rate not to exceed 10 mL/min. The FDA has approved rapid bolus intravenous administration of Omniscan and ProHance. Studies that have used rapid intravenous administration of Magnevist indicate that there is no significant difference in the incidence of adverse effects compared with the slow, intravenous administration of this drug.[194,206,218]

Omniscan

Because Omniscan is the MR contrast agent most recently approved by the FDA, there are relatively few data available related to the safety aspects of this drug. Of the estimated 100,000 doses that have been distributed, there have been 28 reports of adverse reactions of any type, of which 20 were nausea and emesis. There was a single case of laryngospasm that was successfully treated with epinephrine, as well as a single case of seizures (in a patient with a history of seizure disorders) after Omniscan administration. There have been no reports of patient hospitalizations or permanent disabilities related to the use of Omniscan (L. Reich, PhD, Mycomed, written communication, July 1993).

Omniscan has an osmolality value of 789 mmol/kg of water.[220] The manufacturer of Omniscan is in the process of applying for approval of higher total dose administration for specific situations in which this might be of clinical significance and benefit (Reich L., PhD, Sanofi Winthrop Pharmaceuticals, oral communication, June 1993).

ProHance

ProHance was approved for use 2 months before the release of Omniscan, and there is also a relative lack of postmarket safety data concerning this MR contrast agent. Of the estimated 150,000 doses administered, there have been no deaths associated with the use of ProHance. Ten anaphylactoid reactions have occurred in association with the use of this MR contrast agent, of which five required hospitalization, or ended in permanent disabilities (R. Rogan, MD, Bracco Diagnostics, written communication, June 1993).

For specific clinical indications, ProHance has FDA approval (the only one of the three MR contrast agents) for administration up to a total dose of 0.3 mmol/kg, three times the standard dose for each of the other two FDA-approved MR contrast agents. The relatively low (630 mmol/kg) water osmolality[42] of ProHance may be one of the major factors that permits higher doses of this MR contrast agent to be used without significant deleterious effects on the patient. However, this possibility is pure speculation. Here, too, total adverse effects of any type seem to total less than 4%, with nausea and taste disturbance each having an incidence of roughly 1.4% and all other adverse reactions being less than 1% each (A. Y. Olukotun, MD, and R. Rogan, MD, Bracco Diagnostics, written communication, June 1993).

With emphasis on osmolality, ProHance was compared with Magnevist in an investigation into the effect of extravasation in the rat model.[39] The findings indicated that extravasation of Magnevist was associated with more necrosis, hemorrhage, and edema than was ProHance, although the authors of this report cautioned about extrapolating the results of their study to contrast agent extravasation in human subjects.

Administration of MR Contrast Agents in Renal Failure

As previously indicated, toxicity may result from the dissociation of the gadolinium ion from its chelate. After intravenous administration of gadolinium-based contrast agents, some displacement of gadolinium will result from competition for the chelating molecule, such as DTPA, by intravascular copper and zinc, normally found in small amounts within the bloodstream, resulting in the release of free gadolinium ion (Gd^{3+}). Although gadolinium is a highly toxic substance, the total concentration of the released free gadolinium is very low and is cleared very rapidly, allowing a low concentration of free ion to be maintained. In fact, in patients with normal renal function, the rate of dissociation is lower than that of clearance, thus preventing any accumulation phenomenon from occurring.[185] It is also believed that macrocyclic molecules tend to bind the gadolinium more tightly than do linear ones.[183,225]

As additional copper and zinc ions are leaked into the intravascular space in an attempt to reestablish their concentration equilibrium, more gadolinium is displaced from its chelate. This cycle continues until the kidneys clear all of the gadolinium-chelate from the body by glomerular filtration. In renal failure, therefore, there is a potential concern for the accumulation of free gadolinium ion, as there is in any patient with a decreased rate of renal clearance.

The safety of administering MR contrast agents to patients with impaired renal function, or even overt renal failure, has not been clearly established, although several studies suggest that they should be well tolerated.[190,206,226–230] Although there is a concern that decreasing the rate of clearance of the gadolinium chelate might increase the concentration of free gadolinium within the body, data suggest that, for a given level of renal function, administration of lower volume doses may be safer than administering standard doses of iodine-based contrast agents to the same patient.[226] Similarly, the safety of administering an MR contrast agent to patients with elevated levels of copper (such as patients with Wil-

son's disease) or zinc has not been firmly established, and will likely depend on factors such as the glomerular filtration rate and renal clearance rates, as well as the blood copper levels.[185] It has also been shown that Magnevist is dialyzable, with more than 95% of the administered dose being removed by the third dialysis treatment.[28,52]

Chronic and Repeated Administration of MR Contrast Agents

There is concern related to the total storage or accumulation of MR contrast agents, or even free gadolinium ion, after multiple doses are administered throughout a patient's lifetime. The amount of detectable drug still in the liver, kidneys, and bone days after administration seems to be higher for Omniscan than for Magnevist,[181] and both seem to be higher than the level for ProHance.[183,225] Currently, there are no data available regarding the safety of long-term cumulative exposure to low doses of free gadolinium ion. Therefore, there may be a clinical limitation on the number of times a patient can be safely scanned with gadolinium-based contrast drugs. To date, this question remains unanswered and is a topic that warrants further investigation.

Use of MR Contrast Agents During Pregnancy and Lactation

Magnevist has been shown to cross the placenta and appear in the fetal bladder only moments after intravenous administration. It is assumed that the other MR contrast agents behave in a similar fashion and cross the blood–placenta barrier easily. From the fetal bladder, the contrast agent is excreted into the amniotic fluid, swallowed by the fetus, and subsequently filtered and excreted in the urine of the fetus again, with the entire cycle being repeated innumerable times.

There are no data available to assess the rate of clearance of MR contrast agents from the amniotic fluid cycle. Therefore, it is our opinion that there is no information to support the safety of the use of MR contrast agents in pregnant women. Our conservative approach is to recommend against the administration of any of the MR contrast agents to a pregnant patient until more data become available. Pregnant patients should only receive these drugs if the potential benefit justifies the potential risk to the fetus. In any case, if it is deemed necessary to administer MR contrast agents to a pregnant patient to facilitate MR imaging, written informed consent that specifically stipulates that the risk associated with the use these drugs during pregnancy is presently unknown should be provided.

Magnevist has been shown to be excreted in very low concentrations (0.011% of the total dose) in human breast milk over approximately 33 hours.[231,232] The concentration of the contrast agent in breast milk peaks at approximately 4.75 hours and decreases to less than a fifth of this level (<1 μmol/L) 22 hours after the injection.[231,232] For this reason, and as an extra precaution to ensure that the nursing child does not receive the drug in any notable quantity by mouth, we recommend that nursing mothers express their breasts and not breast feed for 36 to 48 hours after the administration of an MR contrast agent. However, it should be noted that the LD_{50} of gadolinium chloride or gadolinium acetate (which easily release free gadolinium ions) when given intravenously is approximately 1000 times lower if taken orally because of the very low absorption of gadolinium from the gastrointestinal tract.[233] This finding supports other data that have demonstrated that 99.2% of orally administered Magnevist was fecally excreted and not absorbed.[234]

References

1. Adzamli IK, Jolesz FA, Blau M. An assessment of blood-brain barrier integrity under MRI conditions: brain uptake of radiolabeled Gd-DTPA and In-DTPA-IgG. J Nucl Med 1989;30:839.
2. Barber BJ, Schaefer DJ, Gordon CJ, et al. Thermal effects of MR imaging: worst-case studies in sheep. AJR Am J Roentgenol 1990;155:1105.
3. Bartels MV, Mann K, Matejcek M, et al. Magnetresonanztomographie und Sicherheit: Elektroenzephalographische und neuropsychologische Befunde vor und nach MR-Untersuchungen des Gehirns. Fortschr Res Rontgenstr 1986;145:383.
4. Besson J, Foreman EI, Eastwood LM, et al. Cognitive evaluation following NMR imaging of the brain. J Neurol Neurosurg Psychiatry 1984;47:314.
5. Bore PJ, Galloway GJ, Styles P, et al. Are quenches dangerous? Magn Reson Imaging 1986;3:112.
6. Bourland JD, Nyenhuis JA, Mouchawar GA, et al. Physiologic indicators of high MRI gradient-induced fields. In: Book of Abstracts, Society of Magnetic Resonance in Medicine 1990:1276.
7. Brody AS, Sorette MP, Gooding CA, et al. Induced alignment of flowing sickle erythrocytes in a magnetic field: a preliminary report. Invest Radiol 1985;20:560.
8. Brody AS, Embury SH, Mentzer WC, et al. Preservation of sickle cell blood flow patterns during MR imaging: an in vivo study. AJR Am J Roentgenol 1988;151:139.
9. Brummett RE, Talbot JM, Charuhas P. Potential hearing loss resulting from MR imaging. Radiology 1988;169:539.
10. Budinger TF, Fischer H, Hentschel D, et al. Physiological effects of fast oscillating magnetic field gradients. J Comput Assist Tomogr 1991;15:909.
11. Carson JJL, Prato FS, Drost DJ, et al. Time-varying fields increase cytosolic free Ca2+ in HL-60 cells. Am J Physiol 1990;259:C687.
12. Cohen MS, Weisskoff R, Rzedzian R, et al. Sensory stimulation by time-varying magnetic fields. Magn Reson Med 1990;14:409.
13. Cooke P, Morris PG. The effects of NMR exposure on living organisms: II. a genetic study of human lymphocytes. Br J Radiol 1981;54:622.
14. Doherty JU, Whitman GJR, Robinson MD, et al. Changes in cardiac excitability and vulnerability in NMR fields. Invest Radiol 1985;20:129.
15. Fischer H. Physiological effects of fast oscillating magnetic field gradients. Radiology 1989;173:382.
16. Garber HJ, Oldendorf WH, Braun LD, et al. MRI gradient fields increase brain mannitol space. Magn Reson Imaging 1989;7:605.
17. Geard CR, Osmak RS, Hall EJ, et al. Magnetic resonance and ionizing radiation: a comparative evaluation in vitro of oncongenic and genotoxic potential. Radiology 1984;152:199.
18. Gore JC, McDonnell MJ, Pennock JM, et al. An assessment of the safety of rapidly changing magnetic fields in the rabbit: implications for NMR imaging. Magn Reson Imaging 1982;1:191.
19. Gremmel H, Wendhausen H, Wunsch F. Biologische Effekte statischef Magnetfelder bei NMR-Tomographie am Menschen. Wiss, Radiologische, Klinik, Christian-Albrechts-Universitat zu Kiel, 1983.
20. Gulch RW, and Lutz O. Influence of strong static magnetic fields on heart muscle contraction. Physics Med Biol 1986;31:763.
21. Hammer BE, Wadon S, Mirer SD, et al. In vivo measurement of RF heating in Capuchin monkey brain, In: Book of Abstracts, Society of Magnetic Resonance in Medicine 1991:1278.
22. Heinrichs WL, Fong P, Flannery M, et al. Midgestational exposure of pregnant balb/c mice to magnetic resonance imaging. Magn Reson Imaging 1988;6:305.
23. Hong CZ, Shellock FG. Short-term exposure to a 1.5 Tesla static magnetic field does not effect somato-sensory evoked potentials in man. Magn Reson Imaging 1989;8:65.
24. Innis NK, Ossenkopp KP, Prato FS, et al. Behavioral effects of exposure to nuclear magnetic resonance imaging: II. spatial memory tests. Magn Reson Imaging 1986;4:281.
25. Jehenson P, Duboc D, Lavergne T, et al. Change in human cardiac rhythm by a 2 Tesla static magnetic field. Radiology 1988;166:227.
26. Kay HH, Herfkens RJ, Kay BK. Effect of magnetic resonance imaging on *Xenopus laevis* embryogenesis. Magn Reson Imaging 1988;6:501.
27. Keltner JR, Roos MS, Brakeman PR, et al. Magnetohydrodynamics of blood flow. Magn Reson Med 1990;16:139.
28. Kido DK, Morris TW, Erickson JL, et al. Physiologic changes during high field strength MR imaging. Am J Neuroradiol 1987;8:263.
29. LaPorte R, Kus L, Wisniewski RA, et al. Magnetic resonance imaging (MRI) effects on rat pineal neuroendocrine function. Brain Res 1990;506:294.
30. McRobbie D, Foster MA. Cardiac response to pulsed magnetic fields with regard to safety in NMR imaging. Physics Med Biol 1985;30:695.
31. McRobbie D, Foster MA. Pulsed magnetic field exposure during pregnancy and implications for NMR foetal imaging: a study with mice. Magn Reson Imaging 1985;3:231.
32. Messmer JM, Porter JH, Fatouros P, et al. Exposure to magnetic resonance imaging does not produce taste aversion in rats. Physiol Behav 1987;40:259.
33. Montour JL, Fatouros PP, Prasad UR. Effect of MR imaging on spleen colony formation following gamma radiation. Radiology 1988;168:259.
34. Muller S, Hotz M. Human brainstem auditory evoked potentials (BAEP) before and after MR examinations. Magn Reson Med 1990;16:476.
35. Niemann G, Schroth G, Klose U, et al. Influence of magnetic resonance imaging on somatosensory potential in man. J Neurol 1988;235:462.
36. Ngo FQH, Blue JW, Roberts WK. The effects of a static magnetic field on DNA synthesis and survival of mammalian cells irradiated with fast neutrons. Magn Reson Med 1987;5:307.
37. Osbakken M, Griffith J, Taczanowsky P. A gross morphologic, histologic, hematologic, and blood chemistry study of adult and neonatal mice chronically exposed to high magnetic fields. Magn Reson Med 1986;3:502.
38. Ossenkopp KP, Kavaliers M, Prato FS, et al. Exposure to nuclear magnetic imaging procedure attenuates morphine-induced analgesia in mice. Life Sci 1985;37:1507.
39. Ossenkopp KP, Innis NK, Prato FS, et al. Behavioral effects of exposure to nuclear magnetic resonance imaging: I. open-field behavior and passive avoidance learning in rats. Magn Reson Imaging 1986;4:275.
40. Papatheofanis FJ, Papatheofanis BJ. Short-term effect of exposure to

intense magnetic fields on hematologic indices of bone metabolism. Invest Radiol 1989;24:221.

41. Peeling J, Lewis JS, Samoiloff MR, et al. Biological effects of magnetic fields on the nemtode Panagrellus redivivus. Magn Reson Imaging 1988;6:655.

42. Prasad N, Kosnik LT, Taber KH, et al. Delayed tumor onset following MR imaging exposure. In: Book of Abstracts, Society of Magnetic Resonance in Medicine 1990:275.

43. Prasad N, Prasad R, Bushong SC, et al. Effects of 4.5 T MRI exposure on mouse testes and epididymes. In: Book of Abstracts, Society of Magnetic Resonance in Medicine 1990:606.

44. Prasad N, Bushong SC, Thornby JI, et al. Effect of nuclear resonance on chromosomes of mouse bone marrow cells. Magn Reson Imaging 1984;2:37.

45. Prasad N, Lotzova E, Thornby JI, et al. Effects of MR imaging on murine natural killer cell cytotoxicity. AJR Am J Roentgenol 1987;148:415.

46. Prasad N, Lotzova E, Thornby JI, et al. The effect of 2.35-T MR imaging on natural killer cell cytotoxicity with and without interleukin-2. Radiology 1990;175:251.

47. Prasad N, Wright DA, Ford JJ, et al. Safety of 4-T MR imaging: A study of effects of developing frog embryos. Radiology 1990;174:251.

48. Prasad N, Wright DA, Forster JD. Effect of nuclear magnetic resonance on early stages of amphibian development. Magn Reson Imaging 1982;1:35.

49. Prato FS, Ossenkopp KP, Kavaliers M, et al. Attenuation of morphine-induced analgesia in mice by exposure to magnetic resoance imaging: separate effects of the static, radiofrequency and time-varying magnetic fields. Magn Reson Imaging 1987;5:9.

50. Redington RW, Dumoulin CL, Schenck JL, et al. MR imaging and bio-effects in a whole body 4.0 Tesla imaging system. In: Book of Abstracts, Society of Magnetic Resonance Imaging 1988;1:20.

51. Reid A, Smith FW, Hutchison JMS. Nuclear magnetic resonance imaging and its safety implications: follow-up of 181 patients. Br J Radiol 1982;55:784.

52. Roschmann P. Human auditory system response to pulsed radiofrequency energy in RF coils for magnetic resonance at 2.4 to 170 MHz. Magn Reson Med 1991;21:197.

53. Sacks E, Worgul BV, Merriam GR, et al. The effects of nuclear magnetic resonance imaging on ocular tissues. Arch Ophthalmol 1986;104:890.

54. Schwartz JL, Crooks LE. NMR imaging produces no observable mutations or cytotoxicity in mammalian cells. AJR Am J Roentgenol 1982;139:583.

55. Shellock FG, Schaefer DJ, Gordon CJ. Effect of a 1.5 T static magnetic field on body temperature of man. Magn Reson Med 1986;3:644.

56. Shellock FG, Crues JV. Temperature, heart rate, and blood pressure changes associated with clinical MR imaging at 1.5 T. Radiology 1987;163:259.

57. Shellock FG, Schaefer DJ, Grundfest W, et al. Thermal effects of high-field (1.5 Tesla) magnetic resonance imaging of the spine: clinical experience above a specific absorption rate of 0.4 W/kg. Acta Radiol Suppl 1986;369:514.

58. Shellock FG, Gordon CJ, Schaefer DJ. Thermoregulatory responses to clinical magnetic resonance imaging of the head at 1.5 Tesla: lack of evidence for direct effects on the hypothalamus. Acta Radiol Suppl 1986;369:512.

59. Shellock FG, Crues JV. Corneal temperature changes associated with high-field MR imaging using a head coil. Radiology 1986;167:809.

60. Shellock FG, Crues JV. Temperature changes caused by clinical MR imaging of the brain at 1.5 Tesla using a head coil. Am J Neuroradiol 1988;9:287.

61. Shellock FG, Schaefer DJ, Crues JV. Effect of a 1.5 Tesla static magnetic field on body and skin temperatures of man. Magn Reson Med 1989;11:371.

62. Shellock FG, Schaefer DJ, Crues JV. Alterations in body and skin temperatures caused by MR imaging: is the recommended exposure for radiofrequency radiation too conservative? Br J Radiol 1989; 62:904.

63. Shellock FG, Rothman B, Sarti D. Heating of the scrotum by high-field-strength MR imaging. AJR Am J Roentgenol 1990;154:1229.

64. Shivers RR, Kavaliers M, Teskey GC, et al. Magnetic resonance imaging temporarily alters blood-brain barrier permeability in the rat. Neurosci Lett 1987;76:25.

65. Shuman WP, Haynor DR, Guy AW, et al. Superficial and deep-tissue increases in anesthetized dogs during exposure to high specific absorption rates in a 1.5-T MR imager. Radiology 1988;167:551.

66. Sperber D, Oldenbourg R, Dransfeld K. Magnetic field induced temperature change in mice. Naturwissenschaften 1984;71:100.

67. Stick VC, Hinkelmann ZK, Eggert P, et al. Beeinflussen starke statische magnetfelder in der NMR-Tomographie die gewebedurchblutung? [Strong static magnetic fields of NMR: do they affect tissue perfusion?] Fortschr Rontgenstr 1991;154:326.

68. Stojan L, Sperber D, Dransfeld K. Magnetic-field-induced changes in the human auditory evoked potentials. Naturwissenschaften 1988;75:622.

69. Sweetland J, Kertesz A, Prato FS, et al. The effect of magnetic resonance imaging on human congnition. Magn Reson Imaging 1987; 5:129.

70. Teskey GC, Prato FS, Ossenkopp KP, et al. Exposure to time varying magnetic fields associated with magnetic resonance imaging reduces fentanyl-induced analgesia in mice. Bioelectromagnetics 1988;9:167.

71. Teskey GC, Ossenkopp KP, Prato FS, et al. Survivability and long-term stress reactivity levels following repeated exposure to nuclear magnetic resonance imaging procedures in rats. Physiol Chem Physics Med NMR 1987;19:43.

72. Thomas A, Morris PG. The effects of NMR exposure on living organisms: I. a microbial assay. Br J Radiol 1981;54:615.

73. Tyndall DA, Sulik KK. Effects of magnetic resonance imaging on eye development in the C57BL/6J mouse. Teratology 1991;43:263.

74. Tyndall DA. MRI effects on the tertogenicity of X-irradiation in the C57BL/6J mouse. Magn Reson Imaging 1990;8:423.

75. Vogl T, Krimmel K, Fuchs A, et al. Influence of magnetic resonance imaging on human body core and intravascular temperature. Med Physics 1988;15:562.

76. Von Klitzing L. Do static magnetic fields of NMR influence biological signals. Clin Physics Physiol Measurement (Bristol) 1986;7:157.

77. Von Klitzing L. Static magnetic fields increase the power intensity of EEG of man. Brain Res 1989;483:201.

78. Von Klitzing L. A new encephalomagnetic effect in human brain generated by static magnetic fields. Brain Res 1991;540:295.

79. Weiss J, Herrick RC, Taber KH, et al. Bio-effects of high magnetic fields: a study using a simple animal model. Magn Reson Imaging 1990;8(suppl 1):166.

80. Willis RJ, Brooks WM. Potential hazards of NMR imaging. No evidence of the possible effects of static and changing magnetic fields on cardiac function of the rat and guinea pig. Magn Reson Imaging 1984;2:89.

81. Withers HR, Mason KA, Davis CA. MR effect on murine spermatogenesis. Radiology 1985;156:741.

82. Wolff S, Crooks LE, Brown P, et al. Tests for DNA and chromosomal damage induced by nuclear magnetic resonance imaging. Radiology 1980;136:707.

83. Yamagata H, Kuhara S, Eso Y, et al. Evaluation of dB/dt thresholds for nerve stimulation elicited by trapezoidal and sinusoidal gradient fields in echo-planar imaging. In: Book of Abstracts, Society of Magnetic Resonance in Medicine 1991:1277.

84. Vyalov AM. Magnetic fields as a factor in the industrial enviroment. Vestn Akad Med Nauk 1967;8:72.

85. Vyalov AM. Clinico-hygenic and experimental data on the effect of magnetic fields under industrial conditions. In: Kholodov Y, ed. Influence of magnetic fields on biological objects. Moscow: 1971. Joint Publications Research Service 1974;63-38:20.

86. Barnothy MF. Biological effects of magnetic fields, Vols 1 and 2. New York: Plenum Press, 1964, 1969.

87. Persson BR, Stahlberg F. Health and safety of clinical NMR examinations. Boca Raton, FL: CRC Press, 1989.

88. Tenforde TS. Magnetic field effects on biological systems. New York: Plenum Press, 1979.

89. Michaelson SM, Lin JV. Biological effects and health implications of radiofrequency radiation. New York: Plenum Press, 1987.

90. Tenforde TS. Thermoregulation in rodents exposed to high-intensity stationary magnetic fields. Bioelectromagnetics 1986;7:341.

91. Beischer DE, Knepton J. Influence of strong magnetic fields on the electrocardiogram of squirrel monkey (*Saimiri sciures*). Aerospace Med 1964;35:939.

92. Tenforde TS, Gaffey CT, Moyer BR, et al. Cardiovascular alterations in Macaca monkeys exposed to stationary magnetic fields. Experimental observations and theoretical analysis. Bioelectromagnetics 1983; 4:1.

93. Dimick RM, Hedlund LW, Herfkens RJ, et al. Optimizing electrocardiographic electrode placement for cardiac-gated magnetic resonance imaging. Invest Radiol 1987;22:17.

94. Abdullakhozhaeva MS, Razykov SR. Structural changes in central nervous system under the influence of a permanent magnetic field. Bull Exp Biol Med 1986;102:1585.

95. Hong CZ. Static magnetic field influence on human nerve function. Arch Phys Med Rehabil 1987;68:162.

96. Budinger TF. Nuclear magnetic resonance (NMR) in vivo studies: Known thresholds for health effects. J Comput Assist Tomogr 1981;5:800.

97. Shellock FG, Crues JV. MRI: Safety considerations in magnetic resonance imaging. MRI Decisions 1988;2:25.

98. Shellock FG. Biological effects and safety aspects of magnetic resonance imaging. Magnetic Resonance Quarterly 1989;5:243.

99. Kanal E, Talagala L, Shellock FG. Safety considerations in MR imaging. Radiology 1990;176:593.

100. Davis PL, Crooks L, Arakawa M, et al. Potential hazards in NMR imaging: Heating effects of changing magnetic fields and RF fields on small metallic implants. AJR Am J Roentgenol 1981;137:857.

101. Reilly JP. Peripheral nerve stimulation by induced electric currents: exposure to time-varying magnetic fields. Med Biol Engineering Computing 1989;27:101.

102. Bernhardt J. The direct influence of electromagnetic fields on nerve and muscle and muscle cells of man within the frequency range of 1 Hz to 30 MHz. Radiation Environ Physics 1979;16:309.

103. Adey WR. Tissue interactions with nonionizing electromagnetic fields. Physiol Rev 1981;61:435.

104. Watson AB, Wright JS, Loughman L. Electrical thresholds for ventricular fibrillation in man. Med J Australia 1973;1:1179.

105. Modan B. Exposure to electromagnetic fields and brain malignancy: a newly discovered menace? Am J Industrial Med 1988;13:625.

106. Brown HD, Chattopadhyay SK. Electromagnetic-field exposure and cancer. Cancer Biochemistry Biophysics 1988;9:295.

107. Pool R. Electromagnetic fields: the biological evidence. Science 1990;249:1378.

108. NCRP Report No. 86. Biological effects and exposure criteria for radiofrequency electromagnetic fields. Bethesda, MD: National Council on Radiation Protection and Measurements, 1986.

109. Erwin DN. Mechanisms of biological effects of radiofrequency electromagnetic fields: an overview. Aviation Space Environ Med 1988;59(suppl 11):A21.

110. Gordon CJ. Thermal physiology. In: Biological effects of radiofrequency radiation, EPA 600/8-830-026A. Washington, DC: United States Environmental Protection Agency, 4-1.

111. Gordon CJ. Normalizing the thermal effects of radiofrequency radiation: body mass versus total body surface area. Bioelectromagnetics 1987;8:111.

112. Gordon CJ. Effect of radiofrequency radiation exposure on thermoregulation. ISI Atlas of Science, Plants and Animals 1988;1:245.

113. Beers J. Biological effects of weak electromagnetic fields from 0 Hz to 200 MHz: a survey of the literature with special emphasis on possible magnetic resonance effects. Magn Reson Imaging 1989;7:309.

114. Coulter JS, Osbourne SL. Short wave diathermy in heating of human tissues. Arch Phys Ther 1936;17:679.

115. Bottomley PA, Edelstein WA. Power disposition in whole body NMR imaging. Med Physics 1981;8:510.

116. Bottomley PA, Redington RW, Edelstein WA, et al. Estimating radiofrequency power disposition in body NMR imaging. Magn Reson Med 1985;2:336.

117. Wickersheim KA, Sun MH. Fluoroptic thermometry. Medical Electronics February 1987:84.

118. Berman E. Reproductive effects. In: Biological effects of radiofrequency radiation, EPA 600/8-83-026A. Washington, DC: Environmental Protection Agency, 1984.

119. Michaelson SM, Lin JC. Biological effects and health implications of radiofrequency radiation. New York: Plenum Press, 1987.

120. United States Food and Drug Administration. Magnetic resonance diagnostic device: panel recommendation and report on petitions for MR reclassification. Federal Register 1988;53:7575.

121. Hurwitz R, Lane SR, Bell RA, et al. Acoustic analysis of gradient-coil noise in MR imaging. Radiology 1989;173:545.

122. Shellock FG, Kanal E. Policies, guidelines, and recommendations for MR imaging safety and patient management. J Magn Reson Imaging 1991;1:97.

123. Goldman AM, Grossman WE, Friedlander PC. Reduction of sound levels with antinoise in MR imaging. Radiology 1989;173:549.

124. Hayes DL, Holmes DR, Gray JE. Effect of a 1.5 Tesla nuclear magnetic resonance imaging scanner on implanted permanent pacemakers. J Am Coll Cardiol 1987;10:782.

125. Gangarosa RE, Minnis JE, Nobbe J, et al. Operational safety issues in MRI. Magn Reson Imaging 1987;5:287.

126. Alagona P, Toole JC, Maniscalco BS, et al. Nuclear magnetic resonance imaging in a patient with a DDD pacemaker. PACE Pacing Clin Electrophysiol 1989;12:619.

127. Edelman RR, Shellock FG, Ahladis J. Practical MRI for the technologist and imaging specialist, In: Edelman RR, Hesselink J, eds. Clinical magnetic resonance imaging. Philadelphia: WB Saunders, 1990.

128. ECRI. A new MRI complication? Health Devices Alert May 27, 1988:1.

129. Dormer KJ, Richard GJ, Hough JVD, et al. The use of rare-earth magnet couplers in cochlear implants. Laryngoscope 1981;91:1812.

130. Shellock FG. Ex vivo assessment of deflection forces and artifacts associated with high-field MRI of 'mini-magnet' dental prostheses. Magn Reson Imaging 1989;7(suppl 1):IT-03.

131. Liang MD, Narayanan K, Kanal E. Magnetic ports in tissue expanders: a caution for MRI. Magn Reson Imaging 1989;7:541.

132. Lund G, Nelson JD, Wirtschafter JD, et al. Tatooing of eyelids: magnetic imaging artifacts. Opthalmic Surg 1986;17:550.

133. Sacco DA, Steiger DA, Bellon EM, et al. Artifacts caused by cosmetics in MR imaging of the head. AJR Am J Roentgenol 1987;148:1001.

134. Jackson JG, Acker JD. Permanent eyeliner and MR imaging. AJR Am J Roentgenol 1987;149:1080.

135. Pusey E, Lufkin RB, Brown RKJ, et al. Magnetic resonance imaging artifacts: mechanism and clinical significance. Radiographics 1986;6:891.

136. Buchli R, Boesiger P, Meier D. Heating effects of metallic implants by MRI examinations. Magn Reson Med 1988;7:255.

137. Shellock FG, Crues JV. High-field MR imaging of metallic biomedical implants: an in vitro evaluation of deflection forces and temperature changes induced in large prostheses. Radiology 1987;165:150.

138. Shellock FG, Crues JV. High-field MR imaging of metallic biomedical implants: an ex vivo evaluation of deflection forces. AJR Am J Roentgenol 1988;151:389.

139. Dujovny M, Kossovsky N, Kossowsky R, et al. Aneurysm clip motion

during magnetic resonance imaging: in vivo experimental study with metallurgical factor analysis. Neurosurgery 1985; 17:543.

140. Shellock FG, Schatz CJ, Shelton C. et al. Ex vivo evaluation of 9 different ocular and middle-ear implants exposed to a 1.5 Tesla MR scanner. Radiology 1990; 177:271.

141. Shellock FG, Schatz CJ. High-field strength MRI and otologic implants. Am J Neuroradiol 1991; 12:279.

142. Shellock FG, Meeks T. Ex vivo evaluation of ferromagnetism and artifacts for implantable vascular access ports exposed to a 1.5 T MR scanner. J Magn Reson Imaging 1991; 1:243.

143. Teitelbaum GP, Yee CA, Van Horn DD, et al. Metallic ballistic fragments: MR imaging safety and artifacts. Radiology 1990; 175:855.

144. Shellock FG. MR imaging of metallic implants and materials: A compilation of the literature. AJR Am J Roentgenol 1988; 151:811.

145. Shellock FG, Curtis JS. MR imaging and biomedical implants, materials, and devices: an updated review. Radiology 1991; 180:541.

146. Holtas S, Olsson M, Romner B, et al. Comparison of MR imaging and CT in patients with intracranial aneurysm clips. Am J Neuroradiol 1988; 9:891.

147. Huttenbrink KB, Grobe-Nobis W. Experimentelle Untersuchungen und theoretische Betrachtungen uber das Verhalten von Stapes-Metall-Prothesen im Magnetfeld eines Kernspintomographen. [Experiments and theoretical considerations on behaviour of metallic stapedectomy-protheses in nuclear magnetic resonance imaging.] Laryngologicie Rhinologie Otologie 1987; 66:127.

148. Becker R, Norfray JF, Teitelbaum GP, et al. MR imaging in patients with intracranial aneurysm clips. Am J Neuroradiol 1988; 9:885.

149. Randall PA, Kohman LJ, Scalzetti EM, et al. Magnetic resonance imaging of prosthetic cardiac valves in vitro and in vivo. Am J Cardiol 1988; 62:973.

150. Romner B, Olsson M, Ljunggren B, et al. Magnetic resonance imaging and aneurysm clips. J Neurosurg 1989; 70:426.

151. Augustiny N, von Schulthess GK, Meier D, et al. MR imaging of large nonferromagnetic metallic implants at 1.5 T. J Comput Assist Tomogr 1987; 11:678.

152. Teitelbaum GP, Bradley WG, Klein BD. MR imaging artifacts ferromagnetism, and magnetic torque of intravascular filters, stents, and coils. Radiology 1988; 166:657.

153. Yuh WTC, Hanigan MT, Nerad JA, et al. Extrusion of a magnetic eye implant after MR examination: a potential hazard to the enucleated eye. In: Book of Abstracts, American Society of Neuroradiology 1991:97.

154. Kelly WM, Pagle PG, Pearson A, et al. Ferromagnetism of intraocular foreign body causes unilateral blindness after MR study. Am J Neuroradiol 1986; 7:243.

155. Williams S, Char DH, Dillon WP, et al. Ferrous intraocular foreign bodies and magnetic resonance imaging. Am J Ophthalmol 1988; 105:398.

156. Flaherty JA, Hoskinson K. Emotional distress during magnetic resonance imaging. New Engl J Med 1989; 320:467.

157. Fishbain DA, Goldberg M, Labbe E, et al. Long-term claustrophobia following magnetic resonance imaging. Am J Psychiatry 1988; 145:1038.

158. Quirk ME, Letendre AJ, Ciottone RA, et al. Anxiety in patients undergoing MR imaging. Radiology 1989; 170:463.

159. Quirk ME, Letendre AJ, Ciottone RA, et al. Evaluation of three psychological interventions to reduce anxiety during MR imaging. Radiology 1989; 173:759.

160. Hricak H, Amparo EG. Body MRI: alleviation of claustrophobia by prone positioning. Radiology 1984; 152:819.

161. Weinreb JC, Maravilla KR, Peshock R, et al. Magnetic resonance imaging: Improving patient tolerance and safety. AJR Am J Roentgenol 1984; 143:1285.

162. Klonoff EA, Janata JW, Kaufman B. The use of systematic desentization to overcome resistance to magnetic resonance imaging (MRI) scanning. J Behav Ther Exp Psychiatry 1986; 17:189.

163. Granet RB, Gelber LJ. Claustrophobia during MR imaging. New Jersey Med 1990; 87:479.

164. Phelps LA. MRI and Claustrophobia. Am Fam Physician 1990; 42:930.

165. McGuinness TP. Hypnosis in the treatment of phobias: A review of the literature. Am J Clin Hypnosis 1984; 26:261.

166. Karlik SJ, Heatherley T, Pavan F, et al. Patient anesthesia and monitoring at a 1.5 T MRI installation. Magn Reson Med 1988; 7:210.

167. Barnett GH, Ropper AH, Johnson KA. Physiological support and monitoring of critically ill patients during magnetic resonance imaging. J Neurosurg 1988; 68:244.

168. Dunn V, Coffman CE, McGowan JE, et al. Mechanical ventilation during magnetic resonance imaging. Magn Reson Imaging 1985; 3:169.

169. McArdle CB, Nicholas DA, Richardson CJ, et al. Monitoring of the neonate undergoing MR imaging: Technical considerations. Radiology 1986; 159:223.

170. Roth JL, Nugent M, Gray JE, et al. Patient monitoring during magnetic resonance imaging. Anesthesiology 1985; 62:80.

171. Shellock FG. Monitoring during MRI. An evaluation of the effect of high-field MRI on various patient monitors. Medical Electronics September 1986:93.

172. Shellock FG. Monitoring sedated patients during MRI. Radiology 1990; 177:586. Letter.

173. Wendt RE, Rokey R, Vick GW. et al. Electrocardiographic gating and monitoring during NMR imaging. Magn Reson Imaging 1988; 6:89.

174. Holshouser BA, Hinshaw DB, Shellock FG. Sedation, anesthesia, and physiologic monitoring during MRI. In: Hasso AN, Stark DD, eds. Categorical course syllabus, spine and body magnetic resonance imaging. American Roentgen Ray Society, May 1991.

175. Kanal E, Applegate GR. Thermal injuries/incidents associated with MR imaging devices in the US: A compilation and review of the presently available data. In: Book of Abstracts, Society for Magnetic Resonance Imaging 1990:274.

176. Shellock FG, Slimp G. Severe burn of the finger caused by using a pulse oximeter during MRI. AJR Am J Roentgenol 1989; 153:1105.

177. Kanal E, Shellock FG. Burns associated with clinical MR examinations. Radiology 1990; 175:585.

178. Shellock FG, Myers SM, Kimble K. Monitoring heart rate and oxygen saturation during MRI with a fiber-optic pulse oximeter. AJR Am J Roentgenol 1992; 158:663.

179. Runge V. Clinical application of magnetic resonance contrast media in the head. In: Runge V, ed. Contrast media in magnetic resonance imaging: a clinical approach. Philadelphia: JB Lippincott, 1992.

180. Oksendal A, Hals P. Biodistribution and toxicity of MR imaging contrast media. J Magn Reson Imaging 1993; 3:157.

181. Harpur E, Worah D, Hals P, Holtz E, Furuhama K, Nomura H. Preclinical safety assessment and pharmacokinetics of gadodiamide injection, a new magnetic resonance imaging contrast agent. Invest Radiol 1993; 28:S280-S43.

182. Tweedle M, Eaton S, Eckelman W, et al. Comparative chemical structure and pharmacokinetics of MRI contrast agents. Invest Radiol 1988; 23(suppl 1):S236.

183. Tweedle M. Physiochemical properties of gadoteridol and other magnetic resonance contrast agents. Invest Radiol 1992; 27(suppl 1):S2.

184. Chang C. Magnetic resonance imaging contrast agents. Design and physiochemical properties of gadodiamide. Invest Radiol 1993; 28 (suppl 1):S21.

185. Cacheris W, Quay S, Rocklage S. The relationship between thermodynamics and the toxicity of gadolinium complexes. Magn Reson Imaging 1990; 8:467.

186. Felix R, Schorner W. Intravenous contrast media in MRI: clinical experience with gadolinium-DTPA over four years. Second European Congress of NMR in Medicine in Biology. Berlin: 1988.

187. Niendorf H, Ezumi K. Magnevist (Gd-DTPA): Tolerance and safety after 4 years of clinical trials in more than 7000 patients. Second European Congress of NMR in Medicine in Biology. Berlin: 1988.

188. Niendorf H, Valk J, Reiser M. First use of Gd-DTPA in pediatric MRI. Second European Congress of NRM in Medicine in Biology. Berlin: 1988.

189. Ball WJ, Nadel S, Zimmerman R, et al. Phase III multicenter clinical investigation to determine the safety and efficacy of gadoteridol in children suspected of having neurologic disease. Radiology 1993; 186:769.

190. Niendorf H, Haustein J, Cornelius I, Alhassan A, Claus W. Safety of Gadolinium-DTPA: extended clinical experience. Magn Reson Med 1991;22:222.

191. Sullivan M,. Goldstein H, Sansone K, Stoner S, Holyoak W, Wiggins J. Hemodynamic effects of Gd-DTPA administered via rapid bolus or slow infusion: a study in dogs. Am J Neuroradiol 1990;11:537.

192. Goldstein H, Kashanian F, Blumetti R, Holyoak W, Hugo F, Blumenfield D. Safety assessment of gadopentetate dimeglumine in US clinical trials. Radiology 1990;174:17.

193. Hajek P, Sartoris D, Gylys-Morin V, et al. The effect of intra-articular gadolinium-DTPA on synovial membrane and cartilage. Invest Radiol 1990;25:179.

194. Kashanian F, Goldstein H, Blumetti R, Holyoak W, Hugo F, Dolker M. Rapid bolus injection of gadopentetate dimeglumine: absence of side effects in normal volunteers. Am J Neuroradiol 1990;11:853.

195. Brasch R. Safety profile of gadopentetate dimeglumine. MRI Decisions 1989;3:13.

196. McLachlan S, Lucas M, DeSimone D, et al. Worldwide safety experience with gadoteridol injection (ProHance). In: Book of Abstracts, Society of Magnetic Resonance in Medicine 1992:1426.

197. Berlex. A two year report on the safety and efficacy of Magnevist (gadopentetate dimeglumine) injection. Wayne, NJ: Berlex Laboratories, 1990.

198. DeSimone D, Morris M, Rhoda C, et al. Evaluation of the safety and efficacy of gadoteridol injection (a low osmolal MR contrast agent): clinical trials report. Invest Radiol 1991;26(suppl 1):S212.

199. Carvlin M, DeSimone D, Meeks M. Phase II clinical trial of gadoteridol injection, a low osmolal magnetic resonance imaging contrast agent. Invest Radiol 1992;27(suppl 1):S16.

200. Runge V, Bradley W, Brant-Zawadski M, et al. Clinical safety and efficacy of gadoteridol: a study in 411 patients with suspected intracranial and spinal disease. Radiology 1991;181:701.

201. McLachlan S, Eaton S, DeSimone D.. Pharmacokinetic behavior of gadoteridol injection. Invest Radiol 1992;27(suppl 1):S12.

202. Soltys R. Summary of preclinical safety evaluation of gadoteridol injection. Invest Radiol 1992;27(suppl 1):S7.

203. Weinmann HJ, Gries H, Speck U. Gd-DTPA and low osmolar Gd chelates. In: Runge V, ed. Enhanced magnetic resonance imaging. St. Louis: CV Mosby, 1989.

204. Muhler A, Saeed M, Brasch R, Higgins C. Hemodynamic effects of bolus injection of gadodiamide injection and gadopentetate dimeglumine as contrast media at MR imaging in rats. Radiology 1992;183:523.

205. LaFlore J. Goldstein H, Rogan R, Keelan T, Ewell A. A prospective evaluation of adverse experiences following the administration of Magnevist (gadopentetate dimeglumine) injection. In: Book of Abstracts, Society of Magnetic Resonance in Medicine, 1989:1067.

206. Niendorf H, Dinger J, Haustein J, Cornelius I, Alhassan A, Claub W. Tolerance data of Gd-DTPA: a review. Eur J Radiol 1991;13:15.

207. Takebayashi S, Sugiyama M, Nagase M, Matsubara S. Severe adverse reaction to IV gadopentetate dimeglumine. AJR Am J Roentgenol 1990;14:912.

208. Shellock FG, Hahn P, Mink JH, Itskovich E. Adverse reaction to intravenous gadoteridol. Radiology 1993;189:1.

209. Salonen O. Case of anaphylaxis and four cases of allergic reaction following Gd-DTPA administration. J Comput Assist Tomogr 1990;14:912.

210. Tishler S, Hoffman JC. Anaphylactoid reactions to IV gadopentetate dimeglumine. Am J Neuroradiol 1990;11:1167.

211. Weiss K. Severe anaphylactoid reaction after IV Gd-DTPA. Magn Reson Imaging 1990;8:817.

212. Tardy B, Guy C, Barral G. Page Y, Ollagnier M, Bertrand C. Anaphylactic shock induced by intravenous gadopentetate dimeglumine. Lancet 1992;339:494.

213. Omohundro J, Elderbrook M, Ringer T. Laryngospasm after administration of gadopentetate dimeglumine. J Magn Reson Imaging 1992;1:729.

214. Chan C, Bosanko C, Wang A. Pruritis and paresthesia after IV administration of Gd-DTPA. Am J Neuroradiol 1989;10:S53.

215. American College of Radiology: Manual on iodinated contrast media. 1991.

216. McAlister W, McAlister V, Kissane J. The effect of Gd-dimeglumine on subcutaneous tissues: a study with rats. Am J Neuroradiol 1990;11:325.

217. Cohan R, Elder R, A, et al. Extravascular toxicity of two magnetic resonance contrast agents: preliminary experience in the rat. Invest Radiol 1991;26:224.

218. Kanal E, Applegate G, Gillen C. Review of adverse reactions, including anaphylaxis, in 5260 cases receiving Gadolinium-DTPA by bolus injection. Radiology 1990;177:159.

219. Harbury O. Generalized seizure after IV gadopentetate dimeglumine. Am J Neuroradiol 1991;12:666.

220. Watson A, Rocklage S, Carvlin M. Contrast media: In: Stark D, Bradley W, eds. Magnetic resonance imaging. St. Louis: CV Mosby, 1991.

221. Niendorf H, Haustein J, Louton T, Beck W, Laniado M. Safety and tolerance after intravenous administration of 0.3 mmol/kg Gd-DTPA. Invest Radiol 1991;26(suppl 1):S221.

222. Niendorf H, Laniado M, Semmler W, Schomer W, Felix R. Dose administration of gadolinium-DTPA in MR imaging of intracranial tumors. Am J Neuroradiol 1987;8:803.

223. Haustein J, Bauer W, Hibertz T, et al. Double dosing of Gd-DTPA in MRI of intracranial tumors. In: Book of Abstracts, Society of Magnetic Resonance in Medicine, 1990:258.

224. Leander P, Allard M, Caille J, Golman K. Early effect of gadopentetate and iodinated contrast media on rabbit kidneys. Invest Radiol 1992;27:922.

225. Wedeking P, Kumar K. Tweedle M. Dissociation of gadolinium chelates in mice: relationship to chemical characteristics. Magn Reson Imaging 1992;10:641.

226. Haustein J, Niendorf H, Louton T. Renal tolerance of Gd-DTPA: a retrospective evaluation of 1,171 patients. Magn Reson Imaging 1990;8(suppl 1):43.

227. Frank J, Choyke P, Girton M, Morrison P, Diggs R, Skinner M. Gadopentetate dimeglumine clearance in renal insufficiency in rabbits. Invest Radiol 1990;25:1212.

228. Haustein J, Niendorf H, Krestin G, et al. Renal tolerance of Gadolinium-DTPA/Dimeglumine in patients with chronic renal failure. Invest Radiol 1992;27:153.

229. Runge V, Rocklage S, Niendorf H, et al. Gadolinium chelates. Society of Magnetic Resonance in Medicine Workshop on Contrast Enhanced Magnetic Resonance. Berkeley, CA: 1991:229. Discussion.

230. Lackner K, Krahe T, Gotz R, Haustein J. The dialysability of Gd-DTPA. In: Bydder G, Felix R, Bucheler E, ed. Contrast media in MRI. Bussum: Medicom Europe, 1990:321.

231. Schmiedl U, Maravilla K, Gerlach R, Dowling C. Excretion of gadopentetate dimeglumine in human breast milk. AJR Am J Roentgenol 1990;154:1305.

232. Rofsky N, Weinreb J, Litt A. Quantitative analysis of gadopentetate dimeglumine excreted in breast milk. J Magn Reson Imaging 1993;3:131.

233. Nell G, Rummel W. Pharmacology of intestinal permeation: In: Csaky T, ed. Handbook of experimental pharmacology, vol 70, part II. Berlin: Springer-Verlag, 1984:489.

234. Weinmann H, Brasch R, Press W, Wesbey G. Characteristics of gadolinium-DTPA complex: a potential NMR contrast agent. AJR Am J Roentgenol 1984;142:619.

Magnetic Resonance Imaging in Orthopaedics & Sports Medicine, Second Edition,
edited by David W. Stoller. Lippincott-Raven Publishers, Philadelphia, © 1997.

Chapter 3

Three-Dimensional Magnetic Resonance Rendering Technique

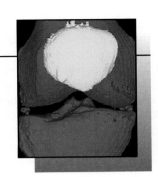

Thomas R. Lindquist
Thomas Schrack
David W. Stoller

Although radiologists are skilled at interpreting original cross-sectional images, situations exist in which the complexity of an anatomic region or the need to improve communication with other physicians warrants computer-based medical three-dimensional (3D) imaging. 3D rendering is a technique for producing images that ideally approach the clarity and style of a medical artist's illustration. In a medical illustration, the artist has the freedom to select what to depict, what vantage point to use, how to shade and color structures of interest, and how to use cutaway views or transparency to best effect. In producing computer-based 3D images, computer algorithms do much of the work, and the user makes decisions to guide the process.

Unlike a typical computer-graphics task, which renders images from precise geometric descriptions of idealized objects, medical 3D rendering must faithfully extract and represent clinical features of interest that lie embedded within millions of original image data points, such as those generated by a magnetic resonance (MR) scanner. Despite formidable challenges, technical advances have already made it possible to produce clinically useful 3D renderings from MR data. This chapter reviews some of the methods for 3D processing using a commercially available computer workstation.

For readers interested in technical details, the surface-rendering algorithms used in this workstation have roots that can be found in work by Artzy and colleagues.[1] However, in its handling of multiple surfaces and volumes, the approach taken here is substantially different from other volume-rendering approaches (eg, Levoy's).[2] Surveys of the overall field of 3D medical image rendering algorithms can be found in publications by Tiede and colleagues[3] and by Stytz and colleagues.[4]

TWO-DIMENSIONAL (2D) IMAGES AND THREE-DIMENSIONAL (3D) VOLUMES

3D processing begins with either a two-dimensional (2D) or a 3D acquisition and manipulates the resultant 2D images into a 3D display. The display can be any one of numerous types, ranging from but not restricted to surface renderings and volume renderings.

Image Quality

The quality of a 3D-rendered image depends to a great extent on the quality and coverage of the original cross-sectional 2D images from which it is derived. If the original 2D images have poor spatial resolution, so will the resultant 3D image. If gaps in coverage exist between the original slices, the small structures that lie in these gaps will not be seen in the 3D image. Similarly, if the original images represent a relatively thick slab of anatomy, small details in the slice-to-slice direction will be lost, even if each original image seems sharp in its own plane. In addition, inconsistencies in the original images, caused by poor signal-to-noise ratio or drop-offs in sensitivity, generally also appear in the 3D image. In fact, the inconsistency is probably accentuated in the 3D image because numerical consistency in the image data is usually more critical to a 3D processing algorithm than to a human observer of a 2D image. The human eye easily accommodates gradual drop-offs in brightness across an image, whereas a simple threshold-based classification algorithm responds incorrectly when the inherent contrast of a structure (compared with its surroundings) is less than the nonuniformities caused by the imaging technique.

Acquisition Parameters

When 3D processing of images from an acquisition is anticipated, the choice of acquisition parameters (eg, coils, slice selections, or pulse sequences) should ensure an adequate in-plane spatial resolution and signal-to-noise ratio for the tissues of interest and also should provide sufficient self-consistency and sufficient sampling, both within each image and from image to image. If high spatial resolution is to be maintained in all three dimensions, the acquired image set should have a large number of thin, contiguous slices, as is the case when a 3D volume acquisition is performed.

The methods described in this chapter allow and can make use of multiple acquisitions from the same patient. For example, one pulse sequence that yields T1-weighted images may be performed to make a particular tissue visibly brighter than or darker than its surroundings. A second pulse sequence that yields T2-weighted images may be performed to enhance the contrast of a different tissue. As long as the two original image sets have the same geometric locations, they may be used jointly to produce combined 3D renderings that show the two (or more) tissues at once, each derived from its most favorable acquisition.

In addition to spatial resolution requirements, contrast plays an important role when 3D renderings and segmentation are planned. Most segmentation tools and algorithms, and especially automatic segmentation techniques, rely heavily on distinct contrast between tissue types. For example, if segmentation is required between synovial fluid and cartilage, then scan parameters should be optimized to provide strong contrast between the two tissues.

Data Processing

After the original images have been acquired, they may be electronically transmitted from the MR scanner to a workstation computer equipped with a suitable direct link. If a direct link is not installed, the scanner images may be saved on an archive tape that is then brought to the workstation computer for input. Figure 3-1 summarizes how the acquired data is then used as input for 3D processing. The user first selects a set of original 2D cross-sectional MR images and then defines, using tools created for the medical imaging worksta-

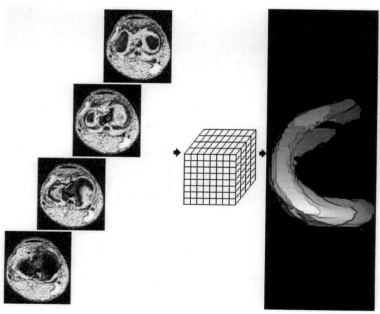

FIGURE 3-1. Original MR images (*left*) are acquired and processed into one or more 3D volumes (*middle*), which are subsequently used to render the final images (*right*).

tion, one or more 3D volumes, each representing an anatomic structure of interest. The resultant volumes are then used for interactive rendering or for batch high-resolution rendering. The final rendered images may represent single or multiple anatomic structures and may make use of options such as color or transparency to depict most suitably the features of clinical interest.

Workstation Software and Hardware Requirements and Recommendations

Although postprocessing tools normally exist on the operator's scanning console, postprocessing often interferes with routine scanning. For this reason, most postprocessing of image data, whether 2D reformatting or 3D rendering, usually requires an off-line workstation. Workstation hardware and software vary greatly from vendor to vendor, but certain requirements can be assumed.

Software

The software on the workstation should be both flexible and "user-friendly." ("User-friendly" is a relative assessment, dependent on user experience and training.) The software packaging should allow the user to create various model types for reformatting and rendering. Moreover, the performance should permit a typical data set for the postprocessing of 60 slices with a 256×256 resolution to be loaded within 1 minute. Once the model is generated and displayed, the software should allow the data to be manipulated to display the model in both an explicit and a real-time fashion.

Hardware

Workstations are available in many configurations from numerous vendors. They may be part of an MR manufacturer's product structure or be purchased from a workstation vendor directly. When they are part of the MR vendor's product structure, workstations come equipped with the software necessary for postprocessing (software packages vary greatly in cost and capabilities from vendor to vendor) and have the added benefit of the vendor's applications support and training. In general, the workstation (common brands include SUN Sparc and Silicon Graphics) should have a fast central processing unit and a minimum of 256 Mb of memory.

SEGMENTATION

The most useful 3D renderings usually include only those anatomic structures that are most relevant to the given case. Rendering additional structures tends to cover or obfuscate the area to be examined. This situation leads to the need for "segmentation," or the extraction of a desired structure (ie,

the one that is to be seen in the renderings) from other structures in the same original image set. In a few cases, segmentation may be defined entirely by the image data themselves (eg, when all pixels of a particular brightness are selected). More typically, however, segmentation is determined by geometric constraints (eg, disarticulation boundaries imposed by a user) or by connectivity requirements. Methods for segmentation are discussed later in this chapter.

Segmentation in no way precludes examination of multiple anatomic structures. Rather, it provides entirely separate representations for each structure of interest, giving the user a set of building blocks, any combination of which can be collectively rendered.

Preprocessing

The segmentation of data may be facilitated by performing one of a variety of automatic preprocessing algorithms before segmentation. One such algorithm is a smoothing filter, which reduces the noise of the original image set. Although this operation may result in a small loss in spatial resolution, the gain in smoothness of tissue values makes this type of preprocessing warranted, unless the highest possible spatial resolution is needed.

Another preprocessing algorithm, specifically developed for MR, performs an autonormalization function; that is, the algorithm derives sensitivity correction information from the original image set itself and applies that correction information to the original images. This process yields images with significantly improved consistency in brightness and contrast.

Segmentation Tools

Generating Binary Volumes

Segmentation is the processing step that generates a 3D binary volume from the original, or preprocessed, image set. The binary volume represents a particular anatomic structure of interest to the user (eg, the meniscus in a study of the knee). The binary volume contains 1 bit of information for each location (ie, voxel) in 3D space, defining whether or not that voxel is within or outside of the structure of interest.

Two independent criteria both must be satisfied for a given voxel to be considered in the structure of interest:

1. The brightness at the voxel's location, as seen in the original images, must be within a specified range of values selected by the user for that tissue. The user determines the range by viewing the original image and interactively adjusting the range of brightness. Pixels with values in the range are given a distinctive color to indicate which will be included in the resultant binary volume.

2. The voxel's location must lie within a geometric volume of interest and any disarticulation boundaries established by the

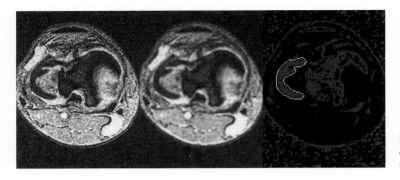

FIGURE 3-2. Original image (*left*), after preprocessing (*middle*), and after segmentation operations to extract the meniscus (*right*).

user. The user defines these boundaries by means of various manual and automatic boundary-drawing tools.

As an example of segmentation, the three images in Figure 3-2, *left* to *right*, illustrate three stages in the generation of a meniscal volume from an axial knee study. The left image shows an original image, as acquired from an MR scanner; the middle image shows the effect of preprocessing by means of a smoothing filter to reduce random noise fluctuations, even though this results in a slight loss in spatial resolution; and the image at the right shows the results of selecting a threshold range of pixel values (those in the user-selected range for the meniscus are medium gray) and defining disarticulation boundaries (in white) to limit further what will be present in the binary volume and hence in the final 3D renderings. In this case, the disarticulation contour was drawn automatically by the workstation computer in response to a single point placed by the user in the interior of the meniscus. In this example, the binary volume being defined contains only the meniscus, because other tissue that is in the same range of brightness (ie, pixel value) is not included within the disarticulation contour defined here.

Disarticulation Methods

As noted previously, the automatic-boundary–generating method is able to generate, with some limitations, the boundary between the pixels that are within the threshold range and those that are outside the threshold range. This process can be accomplished provided that there are few, if any, pixels along the boundary that are in the currently defined in-threshold range but not part of the desired tissue. Automatic boundary generation cannot be used when abutting tissues have nearly the same brightness for the pulse sequence that was used or when there is partial volume averaging of abutting tissues.

When fully automatic methods cannot be used, the user can hand-trace the desired disarticulation contour with the workstation computer's mouse. Alternatively, automatically generated contours may be edited by the user by manually tracing over the portion to be changed.

It is necessary for the user to ensure that disarticulation contours are properly set on each original slice that contains any anatomic structure to be included in a particular binary volume. To assist in this undertaking, computer tools allow the replication of disarticulation contours through several adjacent slices. For automatically generated contours, the workstation computer uses the geometric center of an existing contour to begin generating a contour on the next slice.

After the threshold range has been selected and any required disarticulation contours have been defined, the binary volume representing the desired anatomic structure is computed. The procedure used here may be repeated for as many different binary volumes as the user may eventually wish to render.

Common Segmentation Techniques

Segmentation of 3D models is the operation that enables the user to differentiate one section of anatomy from another, either by removing it from the model or by "painting" it with a color to display it in sharp contrast to another structure. Various segmentation techniques are available, and each has its own advantages and disadvantages. The user must decide which technique is most useful and best maintains the integrity of the anatomic data. Table 3-1 provides a summary of a few of the more common commonly applied techniques and their benefits and detractions.

INTERMEDIATE 3D DATA

Thus far, the concept of segmentation leading to binary volumes has been described in some detail. A binary volume is one of several intermediate 3D data structures that may be used in a workstation. Although these data structures cannot be directly viewed as 2D images, they are important because of their information content and their effect on the final images.

Processing of Binary Volumes

As already discussed, a binary volume is a concise and useful representation of the results of segmentation. It may, for example, be used as input for a program that interactively rotates, cuts, measures, renders, and displays such volumes. It may also be used as input to a 3D surface extraction program that generates yet another intermediate data structure called a "voxel surface."

The spatial resolution content of a binary volume is fundamentally limited by the spatial resolution of the original slices from which it was built and by the center-to-center distance of

TABLE 3-1
Common Segmentation Techniques

Technique	Advantage	Disadvantages
Manual		
User defines tracers or "cuts" to identify boundaries between tissues or anatomy	User maintains ultimate control in defining true boundaries	Time consuming, tedious; risk of user error; low reproducibility factor
Voxel-Value Thresholding		
The inclusion or exclusion of tissues or anatomy by virtue of their inherent voxel intensity	User-defined threshold values ensure wanted anatomy is included; requires less computer power by reducing the 3D model size	After voxels are deleted from model, they are no longer visible; requires high degree of contrast between tissues
Automatic Edge Detection		
Various algorithms to detect edges of a selected anatomy that can then be displayed or removed	Fast; requires little user input; highly reproducible	Effectiveness limited to the particular algorithm; low contrast between tissue boundaries may result in "bleeding" into unwanted tissues that then require manual segmentation
Voxel Connectivity		
Removes all voxels not directly "connected" to a selected voxel	Fast method for removing noise and "floaters"; requires user simply to "select" wanted anatomy to the exclusion to all others regardless of contrast	May require other segmentation techniques to "separate" one tissue from another
Voxel Erosion or Dilation		
Removes or adds layers of voxels along a surface; used in conjunction with other segmentation techniques such as voxel connectivity	Does not require high tissue contrast; highly reproducible; fast method for separating one tissue from another	Risk of losing small number of voxels of wanted anatomy as well as including some unwanted anatomy

the original slices. To retain even this much spatial resolution, there must be at least as many volume elements (ie, voxels) as there were total pixels in all of the original slices. In practice, because the slice-to-slice distance is usually considerably larger than the original pixel size, volumes are usually computed using some form of interpolation in at least the slice-to-slice direction. The interpolation computation not only performs slice-to-slice pixel value interpolation but also derives new disarticulation contours at the interpolated slice positions. Typically, a volume is built with voxels that are approximately cubic; that is, the voxel size in the slice-to-slice direction is chosen to be as small as its size in the original image plane. This approach yields a binary volume that, when rendered, looks less "blocky," although the resolution is not improved.

It should be noted that volumes other than binary volumes may also be generated. These volumes may contain the full resolution pixel values of the original image data (eg, 12 bits per voxel instead of 1) and are useful for volume rendering.

Isotropic Voxels and Their Benefits

In addition to high spatial resolution, it is necessary to ensure that the resolution is equal in all dimensions in the voxel. When all sides of the cube are equal, then the voxels are

said to be isotropic. Voxels that have unequal sides are anisotropic. To maintain the same high resolution on any reformatted plane outside the slice direction, the voxel must be isotropic. In practical terms, this requirement means keeping the phase and frequency steps equal, as well as the field of view and slice thickness. For example, a matrix of 256 × 256 phase and frequency steps with a 1-mm-thick slice should keep a field of view of no more than 25 cm. In this case, the voxels will maintain approximately 1-mm resolution on all three dimensions. Images with anisotropic voxels yield reformatted images of lower, poorer resolution, noted by the appearance of a "stair-step" artifact along the edges of the anatomy and an overall "fuzzing" of the image (Fig. 3-3).

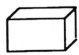

Isotropic Voxel   Anisotropic Voxels

FIGURE 3-3. Examples of isotropic (*left*) and anisotropic (*right*) voxels.

Voxel Surfaces

When a large number of high-resolution surface renderings are to be made, a surface representation such as the voxel surface data structure becomes useful. As its name implies, a voxel surface contains information on only those voxels that lie on the surface of a binary volume. A voxel surface can be generated by means of a 3D boundary detection program applied to an existing binary volume. In addition, if the user has placed a ''seed point'' on some desired anatomic point that can be selected on any original image, the boundary detection algorithm limits itself to generating only those surface elements that are connected to the user-specified seed point. This technique may be useful for excluding unwanted anatomic structures or noise.

SURFACE AND VOLUME RENDERING

The differences between surface and volume rendering are important with respect to their manipulation capabilities, computer-power requirements, and memory use. Stated in simple terms, a surface-rendered 3D model uses and displays only the voxels along the surface of the model. These models require little memory and raw computer power when compared with volume-rendered models. The 3D model is essentially an empty shell of the whole data set as it contains none of the information below the first layer of voxels. In contrast, a volume-rendered 3D model uses all the information from the data set (Fig. 3-4). Although the display of the model itself is of the surface voxels, it is not an empty shell. It can, therefore, be manipulated far more than the surface-rendered model. For example, a volume-rendered model can be segmented to view the interior structures of the anatomy. Of course, such manipulations cannot be performed on a surface rendering, because none of the interior voxel infor-

mation is present. Although the manipulation properties of a volume rendering far exceed those of the surface rendering, the volume rendering requires far more computer power and memory. To manipulate 3D volume-rendered models quickly and efficiently, a powerful workstation is recommended.

Rendering of Surfaces

The algorithms used in surface rendering normally perform hidden surface removal; that is, for each pixel in the rendered image, only the projected element of that surface closest to the viewer is retained. The rendered brightness of a surface element is normally modeled after the diffuse reflection of light from a surface. The brightest surface elements are those that are closest to the viewer and that are tipped most favorably to reflect light to the viewer, in what might be described as ''miner's-lamp illumination.'' If the selected rendering parameters make brightness decrease rapidly with the tipping angle, the surface takes on a somewhat specular appearance.

Using the segmentation methods just described, the most natural-looking surface renderings are obtained when disarticulations do not actually cut through in-threshold regions. The best mathematical estimates of actual surface orientation come from the image pixels that are immediately exterior to the in-threshold pixels; thus, these neighboring pixels should not be eliminated unless necessary. Images in Figure 3-5 (see also Fig. 3-1) show examples of surface renderings.

Rendering of Volumes

Volume-rendering techniques have been developed as an alternative to the surface rendering method. In volume rendering, rays are mathematically projected through the entire

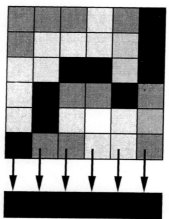
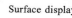
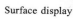
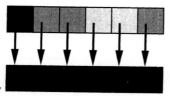

Surface display

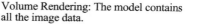

Volume Rendering: The model contains all the image data.

Surface Rendering: The model contains only the outer edge data.

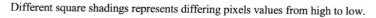
Different square shadings represents differing pixels values from high to low.

FIGURE 3-4. Differing pixel values (*various square shadings*), from high to low.

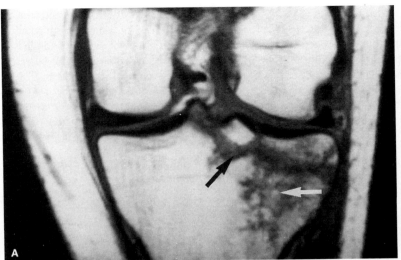

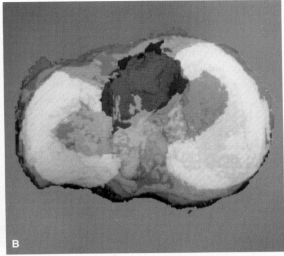

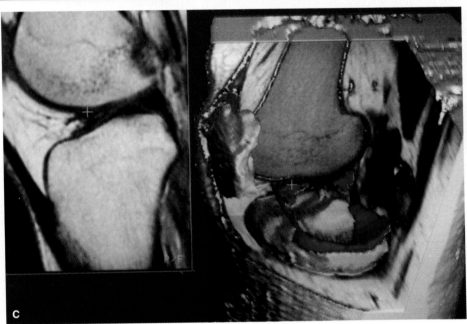

FIGURE 3-5. (A) A 3D MR T1-weighted coronal image of a lateral tibial plateau fracture (*black arrow*) involving the anterior intercondyloid fossa and tibial spine. Adjacent marrow hemorrhage (*white arrow*) is identified by diffuse low signal intensity. (B) The corresponding axial 3D rendering generated from 0.7-mm axial 3D Fourier transform images demonstrates anterior tibial plateau avulsion (*dark green*) separate from marrow edema (*light gray*) and meniscal cartilages (*transparent yellow*). (C) 3D knee rendering generated from T1-weighted sequence in another case (C, 3AA Medial Imaging Systems Divisions, St. Paul, MN at Cemax-ICON, Fremont, CA).

volume and not just its surface elements. In addition, the full resolution (eg, 12 bits per voxel) of the original slice data may be retained and used during the projection process. Color assignments may be made to different ranges in the values of the voxels. Opacity assignments may also be made to different structures.

In one type of volume rendering, opacities are assigned only to voxel surfaces. In certain other systems, all voxels have opacity, and gradients in the voxel values may be computed during the volume rendering to give surfacelike renderings. In either case, volume-rendering methods can produce quasiradiographic images, in which the brightness of a pixel in the final rendered image is related to the summed voxel values along a ray. Unlike actual radiographs, these images can be derived from any multislice modality, such as MR. These images can be generated with or without disarticulations and at any desired pose.

Another method of generating 2D images from volumes is based on a maximum- or minimum-intensity projection algorithm. These images are useful mainly in portraying vasculature, from original bright blood or dark blood images acquired using a suitable MR angiographic technique. There is no segmentation or true 3D representation of different tissues with this method; therefore, its application is limited primarily to MR angiography.

CORENDERING

In many cases, it is desirable to view one anatomic structure in the context of several nearby structures. Software is available that allows such ''corendering,'' to a limit of eight objects, any of which may be of either a surface or volumetric type. Arbitrary or standardized colors and brightnesses may be assigned to each object. In addition, any desired opacity can be assigned to any surface.

The final images are based on a rendering model in which the rendered simulated light from a deeper object is partially absorbed when passing through any intervening surface. The final color of any pixel is the net effect of all of the brightnesses and attenuations that occur along the ray that passes through that pixel.

IMAGE PRESENTATION

Since its introduction a few years ago, the laser imager has proven to be a high-quality hard-copy device well suited to multiformat presentation of gray-scale images from digital modalities such as MR. Many 3D images, however, benefit from the addition of color or motion, making it desirable to have supplemental output available, such as color hard copy, a remote color display system, or videotaping. These may be produced by ancillary devices and systems (eg, a color laser imager), which obtain color images from the primary workstation either digitally or by video.

For "true" 3D viewing, rendered images can be computed at poses that are at roughly 5° to 10° rotational increments about an axis vertical to the observer. Any two consecutive images then form a stereo pair. Stereo pairs can be displayed or filmed using a side-by-side format and viewed directly by cross-eyed stereo viewing. Another approach is to use ancillary equipment with a special display and glasses. Although the 3D effect of stereo-pair viewing can be rather dramatic, its contribution to the clinical interpretation of the rendered images is questionable. As technology continues to evolve, the use of low-cost remote workstations for interactive 3D operations is becoming feasible. In the not-too-distant future, media delivered from the radiology department to surgeons, radiation treatment planners, and other referring physicians could well include electronically transmitted data files with 3D volumes, which can then be interactively reviewed, analyzed, and discussed by means of desktop computers.

References

1. Artzy E, Frieder G, Herman GT. The theory, design, implementation, and evaluation of a three-dimensional surface detection algorithm. Comput Graphics Image Process 1981;15:1.
2. Levoy M. Display of surfaces from volume data. IEEE Comput Graphics Appl 1988;8(3):29.
3. Tiede U, et al. Investigation of medical 3D-rendering algorithms. IEEE Comput Graphics Appl 1990;10(2):41.
4. Stytz MR, Frieder G, Frieder O. Three-dimensional medical imaging: algorithms and computer systems. ACM Computing Surveys 1991; 23:421.

Magnetic Resonance Imaging in Orthopaedics & Sports Medicine, Second Edition,
edited by David W. Stoller. Lippincott-Raven Publishers, Philadelphia, © 1997.

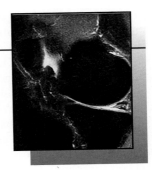

Chapter 4

Principles of Echo Planar Imaging: Implications for the Musculoskeletal System

David M. Weber

DEFINITION OF EPI: A FAMILIAR
  PERSPECTIVE
  Comparison of EPI to Spin-Echo
    Imaging
  Comparison of EPI to Fast Spin-
    Echo Imaging
    Effective TE
    *Transitioning from "ETL" to
      "Shots"*

EPI CHARACTER TRAITS
  High Sensitivity to Off-Resonance
    Artifacts
    *The Chemical Shift of Fat
    Geometric Distortion Artifact*
  Increased Magnetic Susceptibility-
    Weighted Contrast
IMPACT OF HIGH PERFORMANCE
  MR SYSTEMS ON EPI

Benchmarks of High Performance
    *Gradient Amplitude
    Gradient Slew Rate
    RF Receiver Bandwidth*
  High Performance EPI
    Technologies
  Peripheral Nerve Stimulation
  High Performance Echo Planar
    Imaging
SUMMARY

Since its first introduction in 1977 by Mansfield,[1] the concept of echo planar imaging (EPI) has fired the imagination of scientists and clinical practitioners interested in magnetic resonance (MR) imaging. EPI was introduced as a technique to reduce the MR examination to a "snapshot" acquisition, much like a conventional radiograph. This concept generated a good deal of speculation about the clinical impact of an EPI-equipped MR scanner. From completing the entire MR examination in a matter of seconds to expanding the potential applications of MR imaging into territories traditionally claimed by other modalities, the perceived potential of EPI was indeed great.

It was not until this decade, however, that the technical challenges involved in developing EPI into a clinical tool have been overcome. The early resonant gradient systems were the first to bring EPI into the clinical setting.[2-4] These

systems provided a platform for early development of a number of new MR applications such as neurofunctional, perfusion, and diffusion-weighted studies. Limitations in the gradient hardware and the software implementation, however, resulted in little impact on day-to-day clinical MR imaging.

The development of a second generation of EPI hardware, described as "nonresonant," began in response to the clinical limitations of the resonant systems.[5] The primary design goal of the nonresonant system is to apply EPI-capable gradient hardware to all types of MR acquisitions, enhancing the overall productivity of the imager. The secondary design goal of the nonresonant approach is to provide a more versatile EPI software implementation. User-selectable fields of view (FOV), image matrix, scan plane, and other scan parameters that determine image quality permit the extension of EPI applications further into mainstream clinical MR imaging.

One branch of MR applications, for example, that is not traditionally associated with echo-planar imaging is musculoskeletal imaging. Although the speed associated with snapshot EPI could be of potential use to dynamic musculoskeletal exams, the small FOV and high resolution requirements have limited this application development. The modern versatility of EPI, however, facilitates the extension of EPI

Acknowledgments. *The author acknowledges the invaluable support provided by the Ultra-Fast Imaging Program Team at General Electric Medical Systems, MRI Division, Milwaukee, WI. Particular thanks go to Tom Schrack, Rodney Bell, Joe Maier, Paul Licato, Steve Huff, Steve Chen, Fred Epstein, Fred Wirth, Tom MacFarland, Neil Hattes, Perry Frederick, and Bob Vavrek for leading the efforts in the design and implementation of this ground-breaking EPI technology.*

imaging beyond (generally lower resolution) snapshot techniques. From the perspective of speed and resolution, "multishot" EPI protocols are competitive with mainstream fast techniques, such as turbo or fast spin-echo (FSE). Additionally, EPI has its own unique contrast characteristics that may prove to be advantageous for musculoskeletal imaging.

The discussion that follows is divided into three sections. The first section is a review of the underlying principles of echo planar acquisition, identifying the similarities and differences between EPI and the more mainstream MR acquisition techniques such as spin-echo and FSE. The second section concentrates on the unique properties of EPI acquisition, or what we refer to as the "character traits" of EPI. It is these character traits that ultimately determine potential applications of EPI for musculoskeletal imaging. After these discussions, which concentrate on the generic properties of the echo planar acquisition and demonstrate these properties from images obtained on a conventional MR imaging system, similar to the many that are commercially available today, the final section of the chapter specifically addresses the impact that a higher performance MR system would have on echo planar acquisition from both an imaging performance and application perspective.

DEFINITION OF EPI: A FAMILIAR PERSPECTIVE

Comparison of EPI to Spin-Echo Imaging

The easiest way to begin the definition of EPI is to revisit conventional spin-echo acquisitions. Figure 4-1 illustrates the basic spin-echo pulse sequence (see Fig. 4-1A), the raw image data that is collected during that pulse sequence (see Fig. 4-1B), and the typical image quality that results from the completion of the scan (see Fig. 4-1C; shown is a fat-suppressed image). With an emphasis on keeping the analysis simple, the whole process can be summed up by saying that within each repetition time (TR) period, the pulse sequence is executed and one line of image data (ie, one phase encode) is collected. The pulse sequence is then repeated for a number of TR periods until all of the phase encodes are collected. The scan time for this technique can, therefore, be represented by the formula in equation 1:

$$\text{Scan time } \alpha \text{ (TR period)} \times \text{(total \# phase encodes)} \quad (1)$$

With TR periods of 2 to 3 seconds and 128 to 256 phase encodes, the scan time easily approaches 6 to 12 minutes.

In Figure 4-2, the same simple analysis is applied to EPI. Figure 4-2A is an illustration of the pulse sequence; Figure 4-2B illustrates the data collected during a single TR period; and Figure 4-2C demonstrates the resulting image quality. When Figure 4-2C is compared with Figure 4-1C, it seems that the EPI image is, in fact, very similar to the spin-echo image. The reason for this similarity is that the first half of

the EPI pulse sequence is identical to a standard spin-echo pulse sequence—a slice selective 90° to 180° excitation.

It is in the second half of the pulse sequence, however, that EPI differs significantly from a standard spin-echo acquisition. First, the readout or "frequency" gradient oscillates rapidly from positive to negative amplitude to form a train of gradient echoes. Each echo in this "echo train" is phase encoded differently by the phase encode "blips" that occur on the phase axis. Figure 4-2B illustrates how the image data, or k-space, is collected. At the beginning of the echo train, the acquisition commences from the bottom left of k-space and proceeds to sweep over and up, as indicated by the arrows. Each oscillation of the readout gradient corresponds to one line of image data and each phase encode blip corresponds to a transition from one line to the next. By the end of the echo train, the data acquisition has swept to the top of k-space.

Functionally speaking, the most prominent difference between the spin-echo acquisition and the EPI acquisition is that the EPI pulse sequence acquires *multiple* lines of image data during one TR interval. For the particular case illustrated here, with an echo train length (ETL) equal to eight, a total of eight lines of image data are acquired. As with spin-echo, however, there are still not enough lines of image data after one TR interval to complete the entire image. Therefore, the pulse sequence must be repeated in subsequent TR intervals. During the second TR interval, another group of ETL phase encodes is collected in a pattern that it interleaved with the first set. This interleaved pattern is repeated in multiple TR intervals until the entire set of phase encodes is collected. The scan time equation (equation 2) for EPI is:

$$\text{Scan time } \alpha \text{ (TR period)} \times \text{(total \# phase encodes)/ETL}$$
$$= \text{(TR period)} \times \text{(\# shots)} \quad (2)$$

As with spin-echo acquisitions, the scan time for EPI is proportional to the TR period multiplied by the number of phase encodes. Unlike spin-echo imaging, however, it is inversely proportional or *reduced* by the ETL.

Comparison of EPI to Fast Spin-Echo Imaging

For those familiar with FSE or rapid acquisition with relaxation enhancement (RARE) techniques,[6] this EPI analysis should be familiar. EPI has many similarities to FSE: both techniques collect multiple lines of image data during each TR interval and both have an associated ETL, which is an approximate measure of the extent to which the acquisition will be faster than a conventional spin-echo technique.

Effective TE

Since EPI is an echo train imaging technique like FSE, the concept of "effective TE" also comes into play. Like FSE, the echo time (TE) that is prescribed for a particular

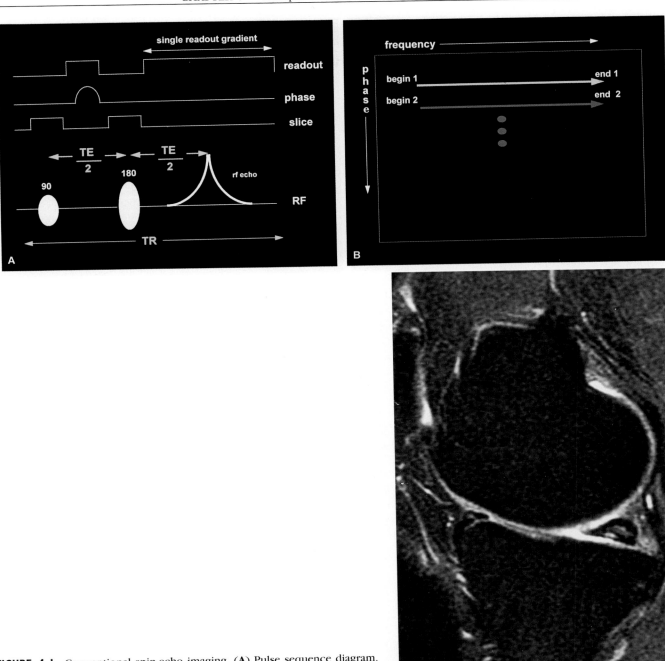

FIGURE 4-1. Conventional spin-echo imaging. (**A**) Pulse sequence diagram. (**B**) Raw data, or, "k-space." (**C**) Typical T2-weighted image. Within each TR period, the pulse sequence is executed and one line of image data (ie, one phase encode) is collected.

acquisition is the true TE for only the central most phase encodes of the image data. As illustrated in Figure 4-2B, the EPI echo train commences data collection in the bottom half of k-space and proceeds sequentially through phase encode values, crossing the center of k-space and then continuing on to the upper half of k-space. Figure 4-2B depicts the EPI acquisition beginning its traversal of k-space at the bottom most phase encode value, resulting in the collection of the

center phase encode values exactly halfway through the echo train (TE$_{eff}$/2, see Fig. 4-2A). If this type of acquisition is used, the minimum effective TE is equal to the time duration of the echo train.

In order to achieve effective TEs shorter than the duration of the echo train, the EPI acquisition could employ a partial-Fourier scheme, as depicted in Figure 4-3. Here, the echo train commences acquisition at a phase encode value closer

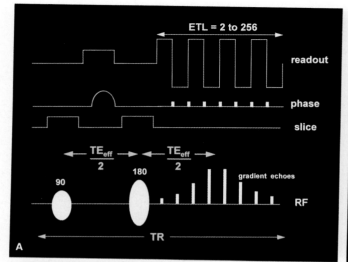

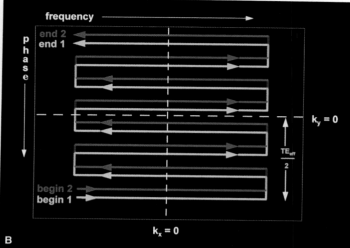

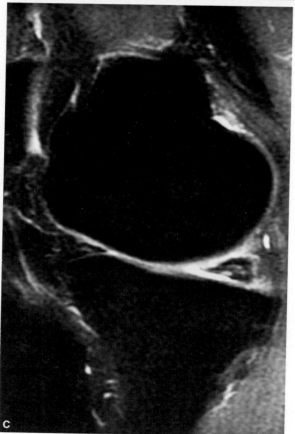

FIGURE 4-2. Echo planar imaging. (**A**) Pulse sequence diagram. (**B**) Raw data, or "k-space." (**C**) Typical T2-weighted image. Within each TR period, multiple lines of image data are collected.

to the center of k-space. The bottom half of k-space is, therefore, only partially collected and partial-Fourier processing methods are employed to properly reconstruct the image data. The minimum effective TE is achieved by minimizing the number of phase encodes collected in the bottom half of k-space (partial-Fourier methods require that some nonzero minimum number be collected). Assuming that 5% to 15% of the bottom half of k-space is collected, then the center of k-space is traversed 5% to 15% of the way into

the echo train ($TE_{eff}/2$). The effective TE would, therefore, be in the range of 10% to 30% of the echo train duration.

Transitioning from "ETL" to "Shots"

One minor difference between FSE and EPI is simply in the terminology that we use to describe the acquisition. During an FSE protocol selection, we actually choose an ETL and describe the protocol based on this ETL selection. For

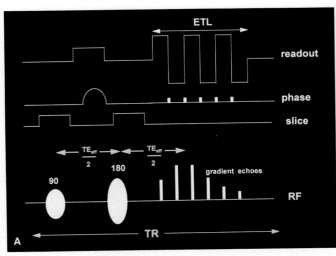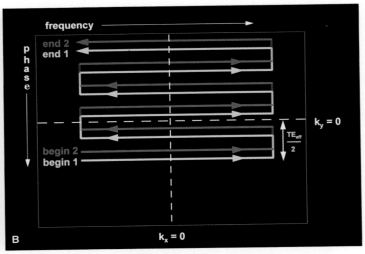

FIGURE 4-3. Partial Fourier EPI. **(A)** Pulse sequence diagram. **(B)** Raw data, or "k-space." The acquisition commences at a phase encode value closer to the center of k-space. The bottom half of k-space is only partially collected, and partial Fourier processing methods are employed to reconstruct the image data. The minimum effective TE is achieved by minimizing the number of phase encodes collected in the bottom half of k-space.

example, an image may be acquired ". . . using an 8 ETL fast spin-echo protocol. . . ." During an EPI protocol selection, however, instead of selecting an ETL, we choose the number of "shots." The number of shots is just another term for the number of TR periods that are used to complete the acquisition. If the case illustrated in Figure 4-2 is a 256 phase encode acquisition, for example, a total of 32 shots, or TR periods, is needed to complete the image acquisition. The terminology would indicate that the image was acquired ". . . using a 32 shot EPI protocol. . . ." By prescribing the number of shots and the total number of phase encodes in the image, the ETL is calculated automatically by the relationship shown in equation 3:

$$\# \text{ shots} = (\text{total } \# \text{ phase encodes collected})/\text{ETL} \qquad (3)$$

where "total # phase encodes collected" takes into account the potential partial-Fourier acquisition described earlier. A 256 phase encode image, for example, with only 10% of the bottom half of k-space acquired, would call for the collection of only 141 phase encodes. EPI protocols that use more than one shot to complete the image acquisition are referred to as multishot EPI protocols. Those that use only one shot to acquire the image are referred to as "single-shot" or snapshot EPI protocols.

Obviously, the acquisition is completed much faster with a single-shot protocol than a multishot protocol. Multishot protocols are needed because with EPI, as with all other types of MR acquisitions, there is a trade-off between image quality and scan time. Figure 4-4 compares a multishot EPI protocol and a single-shot EPI protocol. Both protocols acquired 18 image locations in the knee. The multishot protocol (8 shots in this case) was completed in approximately 2 minutes (see Fig. 4-4A), whereas the single-shot protocol was completed in only 5 seconds (see Fig. 4-4B). On the

other hand, the multishot image appears sharper, has a higher pixel resolution, and is less "distorted" or "misshapen" than the single-shot image. This distortion artifact in the single-shot image is a very common EPI artifact, as discussed in detail later.

EPI CHARACTER TRAITS

Let's return for a moment to the comparison of EPI and FSE. We have already pointed out a number of similarities between EPI and FSE and have discussed one minor difference in terminology between the two. There is, however, a more significant difference between EPI and FSE that makes EPI unique in its own right. This difference is illustrated in Figure 4-5. Looking at this block diagram of the FSE and the EPI acquisitions, it can be seen that during the FSE echo train, there is a 180° radiofrequency (RF) refocusing pulse associated with each echo. That is, each line of image data that is collected is preceded by its own RF refocusing pulse. The EPI echo train, on the other hand, does not contain *any* RF refocusing pulses. Each line of image data is collected by simply reversing the polarity of the readout gradient to form another gradient echo.

This lack of RF refocusing pulses in EPI is responsible for virtually all of the unique behavior of EPI. The two primary implications of excluding the RF refocusing pulses during the echo train are (1) a high sensitivity to off-resonance artifacts, and (2) increased magnetic susceptibility-weighted contrast. Each of these EPI character traits is discussed later, with an emphasis on their effect, direct or indirect, on the potential for EPI in musculoskeletal imaging.

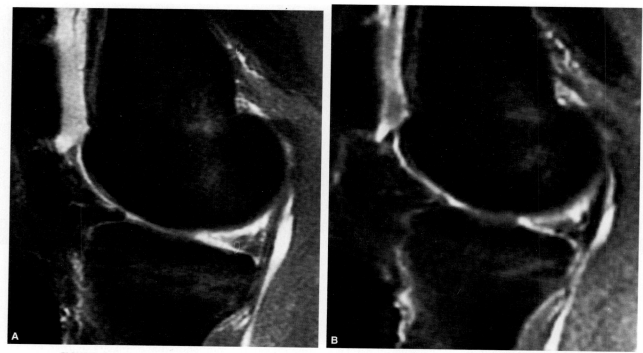

FIGURE 4-4. A comparison between images acquired with (**A**) a multishot EPI protocol and (**B**) a single-shot EPI protocol. Both protocols imaged 18 image locations in the knee. The multishot protocol (eight shots) was completed in approximately 2 minutes, whereas the single-shot protocol was completed in only 5 seconds.

High Sensitivity to Off-Resonance Artifacts

The primary negative effect of excluding RF refocusing pulses from the EPI echo train is that EPI is rendered very sensitive to off-resonance artifacts. After the initial RF excitation, a ''spin'' that is precessing off-resonance will gradually begin *accumulating* a phase error. That is, more and more phase error will be built up through the course of the echo train since there are no RF refocusing pulses to correct the phase error buildup.

In addition to this gradual phase error accumulation, the phase encode gradient pulses also cause the spins to accumulate an increasing amount of phase during the echo train. This phase encode buildup is controlled and predictable, and provides information about the position of the spin along the phase encode direction. However, when EPI raw data is submitted to the MR reconstruction process, there is no way of distinguishing the phase error buildup from the phase encode buildup. In fact, whatever phase is seen is treated as if it were caused by the phase encode gradient. The result is that off-resonance spins that have accumulated phase error are mispositioned in the phase encode direction.

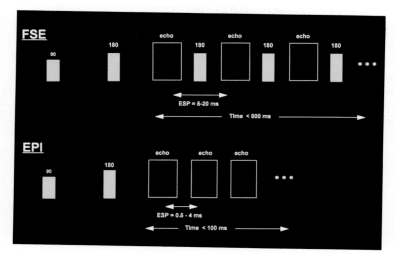

FIGURE 4-5. Block diagram comparison of FSE and EPI acquisitions. EPI is very similar to FSE, but it does not employ RF refocussing pulses during the echo train.

The Chemical Shift of Fat

An example of a common off-resonance artifact in EPI imaging is the chemical shift of fat. Since fat precesses at 220 Hz off-resonance (at 1.5 tesla), the fat signal accumulates phase error during the echo train and ends up mispositioned or shifted in the phase encode direction. Although this fundamental process also causes a chemical shift of fat in conventional imaging, the EPI chemical shift is (1) in the phase encode direction rather than the frequency direction, and (2) much larger than the shift in conventional imaging. For a given FOV and spatial resolution, the magnitude of the chemical shift of fat (in pixels) is given by the formula in equation 4:

$$\text{Shift (pixels)} = (220 \text{ Hz}) \times (\text{echo train duration}) \quad (4)$$

It is, therefore, proportional to both the off-resonance frequency shift (220 Hz for fat) and the amount of time the spins are given to accumulate phase error (the echo train duration). Although echo trains vary in duration from protocol to protocol, they are usually on the order of 100 msec, resulting in chemical shifts for fat of approximately 22 pixels!

Figure 4-6 is a comparison of an EPI image acquired without any type of fat suppression (see Fig. 4-6A) versus the same EPI acquisition with fat suppression (see Fig. 4-6B). The bone marrow and subcutaneous fat signal in Figure 4-6A are shifted approximately one fourth of the FOV, resulting in a significant artifact. The artifact is completely eliminated in Figure 4-6B. Fat suppression techniques are, therefore, a requirement for all types of EPI.

A common fat suppression technique is frequency-selective saturation, or "chemsat." The strategy of chemsat is to selectively excite the narrow bandwidth of frequencies around fat and then dephase or spoil this signal prior to the imaging pulse sequence. Therefore, when the imaging sequence commences, exciting a wider bandwidth of frequencies, there is little or no contribution from fat. One shortcoming of this technique is its sensitivity to RF or B_1 inhomogeneity. Inhomogeneities in the RF field within the imaging FOV can cause insufficient excitation of fat (ie, flip angle not equal to 90°) and, hence, incomplete dephasing of the fat signal.

An alternative fat suppression technique is "spectral-spatial" excitation.[7,8] As the name implies, this technique involves an RF excitation pulse that is not only spectrally, or frequency selective,

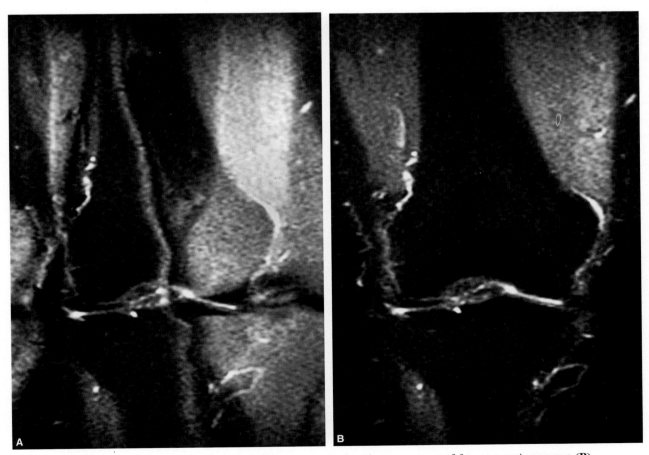

FIGURE 4-6. Comparison of (**A**) an EPI image acquired without any type of fat suppression versus (**B**) the same EPI acquisition with fat suppression. The subcutaneous fat signal in image (**A**) is shifted approximately one fourth of the field of view.

but is also spatially selective. The strategy behind spectral-spatial excitation for fat suppression is to replace the wide bandwidth spatially selective excitation that is used in the imaging pulse sequence with a narrow bandwidth spatially selective excitation centered on water. In other words, the slice selective excitation at the beginning of the imaging sequence excites only the water signal, leaving the fat signal untouched. The advantage of this technique over the chemsat technique is that the fat suppression is less sensitive to RF inhomogeneity. With this technique, unlike with chemsat, inhomogeneities causing insufficient flip angles result only in variations of the water signal as opposed to varying contributions of fat. Figure 4-7 compares EPI with chemsat fat suppression (see Fig. 4-7*A*) with spectral-spatial fat suppression (see Fig. 4-7*B*). In addition to improved fat suppression in the extraskeletal regions, bone marrow suppression is considerably improved, rendering the bone virtually black in the spectral-spatial image (see Fig. 4-7*B*). All of the following EPI images were obtained using the spectral-spatial fat suppression technique.

Geometric Distortion Artifact

There is another type of off-resonance artifact in EPI that is more difficult to deal with than the chemical shift of fat. This is the artifact that results from off-resonance *water*

protons. In regions of the FOV where the magnetic field is homogeneous, the water signal is, of course, on resonance. There are regions, however, particularly in the vicinity of tissue-to-air or tissue-to-bone interfaces, where differences in magnetic susceptibility cause inhomogeneities in the magnetic field. These inhomogeneities result in water protons precessing off-resonance. The frequency shift of these off-resonance spins varies from region to region and from patient to patient, and behaves exactly the same way as off-resonance fat, resulting in mispositioning in the phase encode direction. Figure 4-8 is a good illustration of this type of off-resonance artifact. Although difficult to recognize, this is a sagittal single-shot EPI image of the knee with 14 × 14 cm FOV and a 256 × 192 image matrix acquired on a conventional MR scanner (10 millitesla per meter [mT/m] gradient amplitude, 17 tesla per meter per second [T/m/sec] gradient slew rate). The ETL for this acquisition was 104 and the time between each echo (the "echo spacing") was approximately 6 msec, resulting in an echo train duration of about 624 msec.

The long echo train duration is responsible for the very long effective TE of 160 milliseconds, eliminating virtually all signal except the articular cartilage (~10% of the bottom half of k-space was collected in this partial-Fourier acquisi-

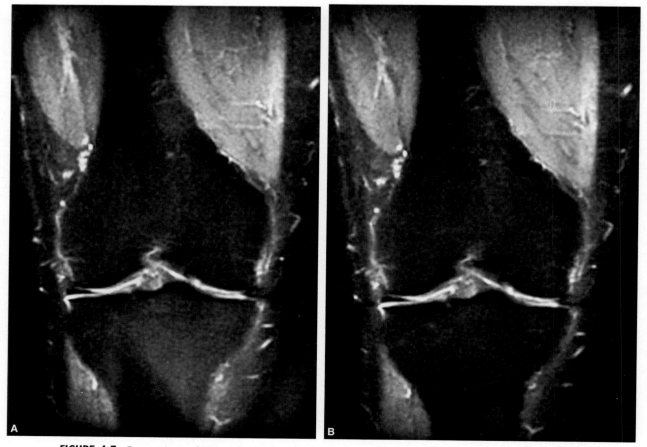

FIGURE 4-7. Comparison of EPI with (**A**) chemsat fat suppression and (**B**) spectral-spatial fat suppression. In addition to the improved fat suppression in the extraskeletal regions, bone marrow suppression is considerably improved, rendering the bone virtually black in the spectral-spatial image (**B**).

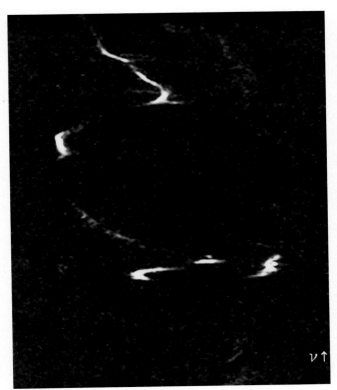

FIGURE 4-8. Single-shot EPI image of the knee with 14×14 cm FOV and a 256×192 image matrix acquired on a conventional MR scanner (10 mT/m gradient amplitude, 17 T/m/second gradient slew rate). The echo train length for this acquisition was 104, and the total echo train duration was 624 msec. This resulted in severe geometric distortion and significant signal loss.

tion). In addition to the long effective TE, the long echo train duration allows off-resonance water signals to accumulate significant phase errors. The result is an extreme geometric distortion of the articular cartilage signal along the phase encode direction.

Unlike the fat artifact, it is not possible to simply apply a water suppression scheme to remove this artifact. After all, it is the water that we wish to image. Therefore, as shown in equation 4 for fat, the only other way to reduce these artifacts is to reduce the echo train duration. One way to reduce the echo train duration is to perform the EPI acquisition on a higher performance MR imaging system with enhanced hardware. The enhanced system would be able to collect each echo in the echo train considerably faster, reducing the total time duration of the echo train. With conventional MR imaging systems, however, such as the one on which Figure 4-8 was acquired, another way to reduce the echo train time is to reduce the number of echoes in the echo train. With the single-shot protocol, this reduction in ETL would necessarily reduce the spatial resolution of the image. Figure 4-9 is an example of a 64×48 matrix single-shot image with the same FOV as the image in Figure 4-8. The ETL for this acquisition was reduced to 32, and the echo spacing was reduced to about 3 msec, resulting in a total echo train duration of 96 milliseconds. Although the

resolution is significantly reduced, the geometric distortion and the effective TE ($TE_{eff} = 31$ msec, 30% partial-Fourier acquisition) are also reduced. Conventional MR systems are, therefore, capable of single-shot imaging without significant distortion artifacts, but at the cost of image resolution.

Considering the high resolution requirements of musculoskeletal examinations, another tactic on a conventional MR system that would maintain the same resolution as Figure 4-8 and still reduce the geometric distortion is to use a multishot protocol. By employing multiple shots, the ETL of each shot is reduced, as is the echo train duration, and, consequently, the geometric distortion. Figure 4-10 illustrates the reduction of the geometric distortion (and effective TE) as the number of shots is increased from 1 (see Fig. 4-10A), to 2 (see Fig. 4-10B), to 4 (see Fig. 4-10C), to 8 (see Fig. 4-10D), and, finally, to 16 shots (see Fig. 4-10E). After two shots, the geometric distortions are moderately reduced. After 4 shots, they are reduced further; by 8 and 16 shots, the image is nearly identical to a conventional spin-echo image. The price of this improved image quality is, of course, scan time. Whereas the single-shot image in Figure 4-10A was completed in 0.6 seconds, the 2-shot to 16-shot images in Figures 10B through 10E took 6, 12, 24, and 48 seconds, respectively, to complete.

It can be seen, therefore, that EPI protocols are feasible

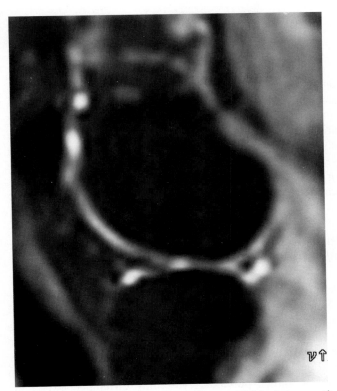

FIGURE 4-9. Single-shot image with the same field of view as the image in Figure 4-8. Using a 64×64 matrix, the echo train length for this acquisition was reduced to 32 and the echo train duration was reduced to 96 msec. Although the resolution is significantly reduced, the geometric distortion (and the effective TE [31 msec, 30% partial Fourier acquisition]) is also reduced.

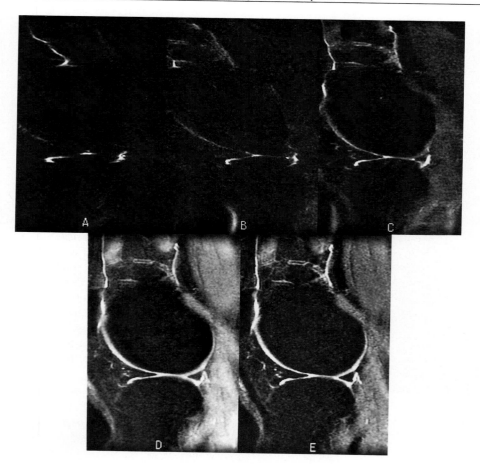

FIGURE 4-10. Demonstration of the reduction of geometric distortion as the number of shots is increased from 1 to 16 (**A** through **E**). After 2 shots (**B**) the geometric distortions are moderately reduced. After 4 shots (**C**) they are reduced further, and by 8 (**D**) and 16 shots (**E**) the image is nearly identical to a conventional spin-echo image.

on a conventional MR imaging system. In order to compensate for EPI's high sensitivity to off-resonance distortions, multishot EPI protocols must be employed. Eight to 16 shots are usually sufficient to achieve image quality similar to conventional imaging methods. However, in regions with very low inherent homogeneity, such as near bowel, lung, or other tissue-to-air interfaces, additional shots may be required to achieve acceptable image quality.

Increased Magnetic Susceptibility-Weighted Contrast

Another effect of excluding RF refocusing pulses from the EPI echo train is an increase in the magnetic susceptibility-weighted image contrast. The contrast of an EPI image is determined, in part, by the RF excitation scheme prior to the echo train but, also, in part, by the echo train itself.

Figure 4-11*A* depicts an EPI pulse sequence similar to the one shown previously (the only difference is that the phase encode and slice select gradient pulses have been removed for clarity). This is referred to as a "spin-echo EPI" pulse sequence. The reference to "spin-echo" comes from the first half of the pulse sequence in which a 90° to 180° excitation scheme is performed. The 90° and 180° RF pulses

are separated by time τ, and they set up an RF echo or spin-echo at an equal time, τ, after the 180° pulse (during the echo train). As in a classic spin-echo acquisition, after the initial 90° excitation the MR signal decays at a rate determined by T2. Therefore, the magnitude of the peak of the RF echo is governed by T2. In addition to this behavior, the rate at which the RF echo is formed and subsequently decays is determined by T2*. A longer T2* results in a broader echo formation and a shorter T2* produces narrower echoes.

Although not shown in this diagram, the phase encode pulses would be set up to sweep through the center of k-space at a time corresponding to the peak of the RF echo. Since the RF or "spin" echo corresponds to the center of k-space, the image is dominated by spin-echo–like, or T2-weighted contrast.

Figure 4-11*B* depicts an EPI pulse sequence with a modified RF excitation scheme. The 180° refocussing pulse prior to the echo train has been removed, leaving only the 90° excitation pulse. This pulse sequence, referred to as "gradient echo EPI," forms no RF echo during the echo train. The MR signal decays continuously throughout the echo train at a rate determined by T2*. The phase encode pulses (if added) would sweep through the center of k-space at the prescribed effective echo time, TE_{eff}, yet there would be no RF echo with which to coincide. The resulting image would be dominated by T2*-weighted contrast.

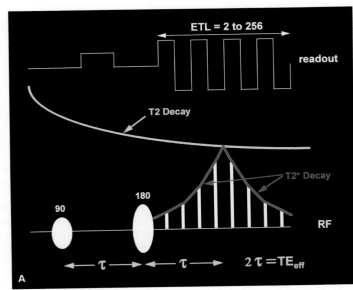
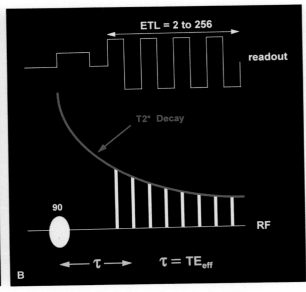

FIGURE 4-11. Illustration of image contrast parameters in the EPI pulse sequence. (**A**) Spin-echo EPI. From the time of the 90° excitation, the MR signal decays at a rate determined by T2. Therefore, the magnitude of the peak of the RF echo is governed by T2, and the resulting image is dominated by T2 contrast. In addition to this behavior, the rate at which the RF echo is formed and subsequently decays is determined by T2*. The image contrast, therefore, is partially influenced by T2* effects (ie, magnetic susceptibility). (**B**) Gradient echo EPI. The MR signal decays continuously throughout the echo train at a rate determined by T2*. The resulting image is heavily T2*-weighted.

As can be seen, variations in the initial RF excitation scheme can produce an EPI image dominated by either T2-weighted image contrast or T2*-weighted image contrast. In addition, the EPI echo train itself influences image contrast. As shown in Figure 4-11A (the spin-echo EPI diagram), the rate at which the RF echo is formed (and later decays) is governed by T2*, not T2. Even though the echoes corresponding to the central most phase encodes are arranged to coincide with the T2-governed RF echo peak, the remaining echoes in the echo train (corresponding to noncentral phase encode values) are collected during the rise and fall of the RF echo. Subsequently, these echoes offer significant T2* contributions to the image. Relative to conventional spin-echo imaging, where all phase encoded echoes coincide with a separate RF echo, spin-echo EPI has increased T2* contributions to the image contrast.

A similar comparison can be made between gradient echo EPI and conventional gradient echo imaging. Although no RF echo is formed in either case, each phase encoded echo in conventional gradient echo imaging has a common TE that determines the extent of the T2* contribution. In gradient echo EPI, however, each phase encoded echo has a different TE, ranging from the prescribed TE_{eff} to $TE_{eff} \pm$ some fraction of the echo train duration, depending on where the TE_{eff} resides within the echo train. In most cases, the TE_{eff} resides in the early echoes of the echo train, leaving the remaining echoes (and the majority of the noncentral phase encodes) at longer TEs. The result is a larger T2* contribution to image contrast in gradient echo EPI than in conventional gradient echo imaging.

Figure 4-12 summarizes the T2* image contrast behavior of EPI relative to other imaging pulse sequences, including gradient echo, spin-echo, and FSE. In order of decreasing T2* contribution (for equivalent TE or TE_{eff}), this list reads as (1) gradient echo EPI, (2) conventional gradient echo, (3) spin-echo EPI, (4) conventional spin-echo, and (5) FSE. Although not discussed here, the comparative T2*-weighted behavior of spin-echo and FSE has been addressed by other authors.[9,10] In short, the proximity of the 180° RF pulses in the FSE echo train produces a lengthening of the apparent T2 and T2*. This effect is most evident in the bright fat signal seen with FSE, although it also contributes to the brighter signal from edematous or hemorrhagic tissue when using FSE.

Considering the relative relationship of each pulse sequence on the T2* scale, Figure 4-12 also depicts the expected image contrast behavior for musculoskeletal imaging. The image contrast of marrow disease and articular cartilage, for example, should increase as the T2* weighting decreases. On the other hand, the image contrast of the meniscus should increase as T2* weighting increases. The images displayed in Figures 4-13 and 4-14 support these expectations. Figure 4-13 is a series of sagittal knee images in a subject with bone marrow edema. Images in Figures 4-13A through 4-13E were acquired with gradient echo EPI, conventional gradient echo, spin-echo EPI, conventional spin-echo, and FSE, respectively. All acquisitions were fat-suppressed. Consistent with the expected behavior for marrow disease, the image contrast monotonically increases as the T2* weighting decreases. Figure 4-14 displays a similar progres-

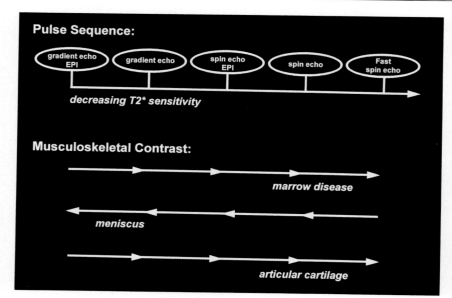

FIGURE 4-12. Summary of the T2* image contrast behavior of EPI relative to other pulse sequences. Gradient echo EPI is the most sensitive to T2* effects and FSE is least sensitive to T2* effects. The expected image contrast behavior for musculoskeletal anatomy is also depicted. The image contrast of marrow disease and articular cartilage increase as the T2* weighting decreases, and the image contrast of the meniscus increases as T2* weighting increases.

sion of images from a subject with a meniscal tear. Images in Figure 4-14*A* through 4-14*D* represent gradient echo EPI, spin-echo EPI, conventional spin-echo, and FSE, respectively. Conventional gradient echo imaging was not performed in this case. Although monotonic variation of the meniscal signal was not observed, the meniscal signal is generally brighter on the EPI acquisitions than on the spin-echo or FSE images.

One implication of these preliminary results is that spin-echo EPI, from a contrast perspective, may represent a favorable compromise between gradient echo and spin-echo (or FSE) imaging. For example, imaging protocols that call for

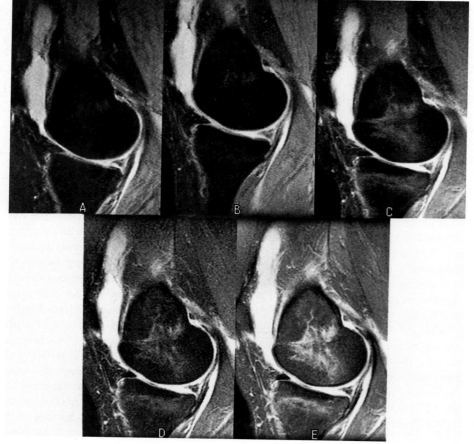

FIGURE 4-13. Fat-suppressed sagittal knee images of a subject with bone marrow edema. (**A**) Gradient echo EPI. (**B**) Conventional gradient echo. (**C**) Spin-echo EPI. (**D**) Conventional spin-echo. (**E**) Fast spin-echo. Contrast monotonically increases as the T2* weighting decreases.

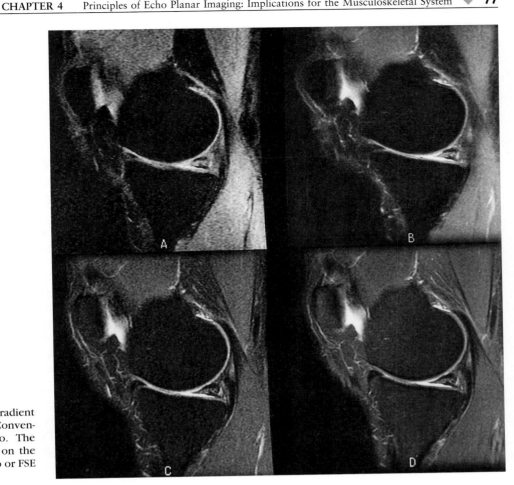

FIGURE 4-14. Meniscal tear. (**A**) Gradient echo EPI. (**B**) Spin-echo EPI. (**C**) Conventional spin-echo. (**D**) Fast spin-echo. The meniscal signal is generally brighter on the EPI acquisitions than on the spin-echo or FSE images.

gradient echo techniques to demonstrate meniscus and FSE techniques to demonstrate marrow disease could potentially be streamlined to require only a single spin-echo EPI acquisition.

IMPACT OF HIGH PERFORMANCE MR SYSTEMS ON EPI

Up to this point, discussion has concentrated on introducing and demonstrating two fundamental characteristics of EPI and demonstrating these principles on conventional MR imaging systems. Now, however, we address the effect of using a high performance MR system on the potential musculoskeletal applications of EPI.

The simple answer to this question is that EPI will be affected in the same way that all other MR pulse sequences are affected by higher performance hardware. The minimum TEs and TRs will decrease, the minimum attainable slice thickness and FOV will decrease, and the maximum resolution and maximum number of slices per TR will increase. In short, the overall efficiency of the acquisition will improve. In terms of EPI performance, however, the improvement that will have the greatest impact on clinical applica-

tions is that viable ETLs will increase on a higher performance MR system. This, not surprisingly, is the same improvement that FSE will realize on a higher performance MR system. EPI protocols that produced good image quality with eight shots on a conventional MR imaging system should be expected to produce equivalent image quality in four, two, or possibly even one shot on a higher performance imaging system.

Benchmarks of High Performance

Single-shot EPI imaging with image matrices of 128^2 to 256^2 obviously require echo trains of significant length. In order to avoid large off-resonance artifacts, these long echo trains must be completed in a reasonably short amount of time. The severe off-resonance artifacts shown in Figure 4-8, a single-shot image, were the result of an extremely long echo train duration. The time between each echo in this echo train (referred to as echo spacing) was approximately 6 msec. In order to reduce the total echo train duration to a point where the off-resonance artifacts are acceptable, the echo spacing must be reduced to approximately 500 to 800 μsec, a factor of approximately 8 to 12 for improvement in speed.

Improvements in speed can be achieved by (1) increasing the gradient slew rate, (2) increasing the gradient amplitude, and (3) increasing the maximum receiver bandwidth. Each of these modifications plays an important role in speeding up the EPI acquisition.

Gradient Amplitude

Figure 4-15 is an illustration of a typical MR gradient waveform. The gradient amplitude initially rises (usually linearly) from zero, to reach a constant "flat top." The maximum gradient amplitude of the MR imager is measured either in millitesla per meter or gauss per centimeter (G/cm) and defines how high the flat top can be. The relationship between these units of measure is given by the following formula.

$$10 \text{ mT/m} = 1 \text{ g/cm} \tag{5}$$

If the gradient waveform in Figure 4-15 is a readout gradient, the height of the flat top would influence the size of the FOV. The higher the flat top, or the maximum gradient amplitude, the smaller the FOV. If the gradient waveform is a slice select gradient, the maximum amplitude would influence the minimum attainable slice thickness. The higher the amplitude, the thinner the slice. In general, the maximum gradient amplitude of an MR system relates to maximum image spatial resolution. The maximum gradient amplitude requirements for good quality single-shot EPI are in the vicinity of 20 to 25 mT/m.

Gradient Slew Rate

The gradient slew rate specification characterizes the speed of the gradient system. As can be seen in Figure 4-15, the slew rate is actually the slope of the linear "ramp" section of the gradient waveform. The slew rate is defined as follows:

$$\text{Slew rate} = \text{maximum gradient amplitude/}$$
$$\text{rise time to maximum amplitude} \tag{6}$$

Gradient slew rate is typically measured in tesla per meter per second. With conventional MR imaging acquisitions, the maximum slew rate of the system influences the minimum attainable TE and TR. For FSE and EPI pulse sequences, the maximum slew rate influences echo spacing. The slew rate requirements for single-shot EPI are in the range of 80 to 150 T/m/sec.

RF Receiver Bandwidth

In addition to the characteristics of the gradient system, another important component of high performance EPI is the RF receiver. The RF receiver bandwidth specification describes how fast the MR signal can be digitized. The higher the receiver bandwidth, the faster the digitization. With a gradient system that has faster slew rates and higher gradient amplitudes, the time allotted for acquisition of the MR signal decreases, and the MR imager is required to collect its 128, 256, or 512 data samples in a shorter amount of time. This means that the time allotted to each data point, Δt, decreases (see Fig. 4-1). The RF receiver bandwidth is defined as follows:

$$\text{Bandwidth} = 1/\Delta t \tag{7}$$

Therefore, as Δt decreases, the RF receiver bandwidth increases. An increased or "wider" receiver bandwidth is an essential component of single-shot EPI. Receiver bandwidths on the order of 200 kHz to 1 MHz are routinely used for single-shot echo planar acquisitions.

High Performance EPI Technologies

The first whole-body clinical EPI imagers[2–4] used an oscillating sinusoidal readout gradient that peaked at 25 mT/m (Fig. 4-16A). Since sinusoidal readout gradients were used, the "slew rate" of the acquisition varied continuously but averaged about 80 T/m/sec. At these gradient performance levels, EPI echoes were collected at the rate of 1 every 500 μsec

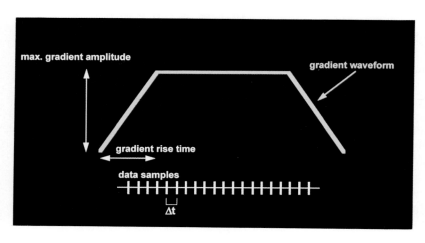

FIGURE 4-15. Typical MR gradient waveform.

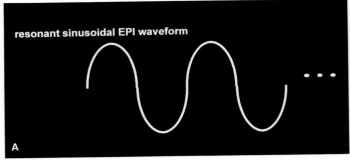 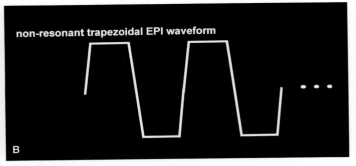

FIGURE 4-16. Illustration of (**A**) a sinusoidal EPI readout gradient from early "resonant" high performance gradient systems and (**B**) a trapezoidal EPI readout gradient from nonresonant high performance gradient system. Both systems are capable of performing high quality single-shot EPI. Nonresonant technology, however, expands the versatility of the gradient system, facilitating a variety of EPI imaging protocols and a allowing the application of the high performance gradients to non-EPI imaging.

for a single-shot protocol with 3-mm spatial resolution. Although fast enough for good quality single-shot EPI, these "resonant" gradient systems had limited application to other MR imaging pulse sequences since sinusoidal gradient shapes could not easily be utilized outside of the echo planar pulse sequence.

In order to address the limited versatility of resonant EPI systems, nonresonant gradient technologies were developed.[5] Nonresonant systems are not only capable of the speed necessary to perform single-shot EPI protocols, but they can also maintain the versatility to apply this speed to other types of MR pulse sequences. The readout gradient echo train consists of an oscillating trapezoidal gradient (see Fig. 4-16B) rather than the sinusoidal readout gradients used by the resonant systems. The nonresonant system used to produce the examples that follow operates at a maximum gradient amplitude of 23 mT/m and a gradient slew rate of 120 T/m/sec. Using the same 3-mm resolution protocol as the resonant systems, this nonresonant system is capable of collecting an EPI echo every 580 μsec. In addition to the 3-mm resolution protocol, the nonresonant system is capable of supporting a continuum of protocols spanning low to high resolution.

Peripheral Nerve Stimulation

In order to obtain the very short echo train durations required for high resolution EPI imaging, the gradient magnetic fields must switch from peak positive to peak negative amplitude very rapidly (ie, they must be able to slew rapidly). The speed at which the magnetic field changes within the bore of the magnet is characterized by the quantity dB/dt. This is a measurement of the change in the magnetic field (B) over time (often given in tesla per second (T/sec). For example, the maximum dB/dt for a conventional MR imaging system is approximately 10 T/sec. Higher performance EPI systems operate at maximum dB/dt levels of 45 to 60 T/sec. As the dB/dt level increases, the possibility of stimulating the peripheral nerves along the surface of the skin increases.[11] Although not considered to be a safety issue, peripheral nerve stimulation (PNS) may raise issues of patient comfort. The point at which the mean PNS threshold (ie, where 50% of a population experience PNS) is reached is a function of the dB/dt and the gradient ramp time. This threshold is depicted in Figure 4-17A.[11] The ramp time is simply the time during which the patient is exposed to the changing magnetic field, or, for EPI, the time required to switch from negative to positive gradient amplitude (see Fig. 4-17B). Note that as ramp times become shorter in duration, higher dB/dt levels are possible without increasing the potential for PNS.

PNS has been described as a light "touching" sensation felt on the surface of the skin. The areas of the body where these sensations are felt vary along the x, y, and z gradients. However, some of the more common sites include the bridge of the nose, the arms, the chest, and the upper abdomen. Clasping the hands together increases the possibility of PNS, and leaving the hands unclasped during EPI scans reduces the possibility of PNS by approximately 45%.[12]

High Performance Echo Planar Imaging

As discussed above, an MR imaging system equipped with the proper gradient and RF receiver hardware is capable of performing EPI protocols with very long ETLs. The ETL can, in fact, be long enough to collect all of the phase encodes in a single TR period, providing a single-shot acquisition. The image illustrated in Figure 4-8 is a single-shot protocol acquired on a conventional imaging system. Figure 4-18 illustrates the results of repeating the same protocol on a high performance imaging system. This is a single-shot image with a 14 × 14 cm FOV and a 256 × 192 image matrix acquired in about one quarter of a second. The echo train duration was 226 msec, compared with 624 msec for the image in Figure 4-8. Although distortions are apparent, the image does not suffer from the severe distortions and signal loss of the previous single-shot image.

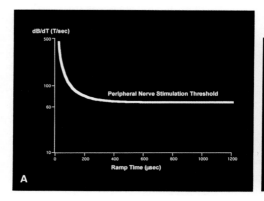

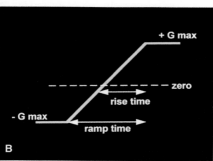

FIGURE 4-17. (**A**) Illustration of mean peripheral nerve stimulation threshold in T/second verses ramp time in milliseconds. (**B**) Illustration of gradient "ramp time" verses "rise time." The probability of peripheral nerve stimulation increases as the ramp time increases.

The distortion present in Figure 4-18 can be reduced by using the same strategies that were used on the conventional imaging system, that is, reducing the resolution of the single-shot protocol or increasing the number of shots. The images in Figure 4-19 show the results of implementing each of these alternatives. Figure 4-19A is a lower resolution single-shot image (24 × 24 cm FOV, 256 × 192 matrix, echo train duration = 140 msec). Although the distortion in the anterior aspect of the tibia is markedly reduced, it is at the cost of image resolution. Figure 4-19B is a two-shot protocol with resolution equivalent

to Figure 4-18 (14 × 14 cm FOV, 256 × 192 matrix) but with an echo train duration of 113 msec. The reduction in distortions here are at the cost of scan time (a 2-second acquisition verses ¼ second).

As discussed earlier, multishot protocols provide image contrast benefits and may expand the musculoskeletal applications of EPI. The scan time of these multishot EPI protocols can potentially be reduced on a high performance imaging system by reducing the number of shots. The applicability of single-shot EPI on high performance systems, however, remains an open issue. Single-shot techniques offer the ability to capture an image of structure while it is in motion. Multishot techniques (even two-shot protocols) suffer severe motion artifacts under these conditions. Single-shot EPI techniques, therefore, offer the capability to perform dynamic musculoskeletal examinations.

As seen in Figures 4-18 and 4-19, however, single-shot EPI musculoskeletal imaging is limited by both acceptable levels of geometric distortion and/or image resolution. The efficacy of dynamic musculoskeletal EPI ultimately depends on the minimum requirements for both of these effects; minimum requirements that, for the most part, have yet to be established. It is clear, however, that with today's state-of-the-art high performance imagers, single-shot EPI will not produce the image quality that is routinely achieved with non-EPI methods such as FSE. The question remains, therefore, of whether applications exist in which the dynamic advantages of single-shot EPI outweigh the reductions in image quality.

SUMMARY

With this review of the basic principles and imaging characteristics of EPI on both conventional and higher performance MR imaging systems, we hope to have stripped away some of the myths and misconceptions of EPI and to place it in its proper role among the family of MR acquisition techniques. As with FSE, EPI employs an echo train that collects multiple phase encode values

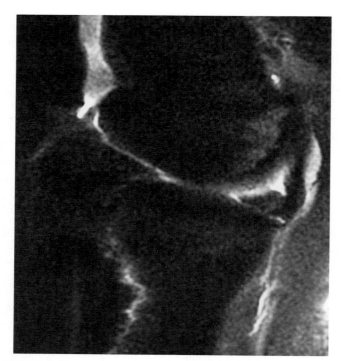

FIGURE 4-18. Single-shot image with a 14 × 14 cm FOV and a 256 × 192 image matrix acquired in about one quarter of a second on a high performance imaging system. The echo train duration was 226 msec compared with 624 msec for the image in Figure 4-8. Although some distortion is apparent, the image does not suffer from severe distortions and signal loss.

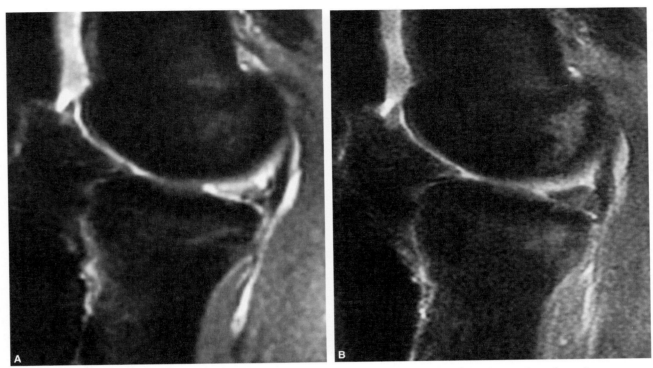

FIGURE 4-19. **(A)** Lower resolution single-shot image (24 × 24 cm FOV, 256 × 192 matrix, echo train duration = 140 msec). Distortion in the anterior aspect of the tibia is markedly reduced when compared with Figure 4-8. **(B)** Two-shot protocol with equivalent resolution to Figure 4-18 (14 × 14 cm FOV, 256 × 192 matrix) but with an echo train duration of 113 msec.

during each TR interval, and the length of this echo train provides an approximate measure of the speed advantage of EPI relative to conventional spin-echo imaging.

From the perspective of clinical applications, the most important characteristics of EPI are its high sensitivity to off-resonance artifacts and its increased T2* contrast. The sensitivity to off-resonance artifacts requires the use of both fat-suppression techniques and multishot protocols on conventional MR systems, and on high performance systems, depending on the resolution required. Increased T2* contrast may play an important role in establishing EPI as a favorable compromise between spin-echo and gradient echo techniques. Like FSE, EPI can be performed on both a conventional MR imaging system and higher performance imaging systems. The impact of a high performance MR system on EPI applications is really the same as its impact on all other types of MR acquisition techniques: imaging efficiency increases. For EPI, this translates to the ability to perform considerably longer echo trains. Protocols that required 16 shots on a conventional system may require only 8 or 4 shots on a higher performance system. High performance systems also open the door to performing single-shot EPI protocols with the potential for exploring dynamic musculoskeletal applications

References

1. Mansfield P. Multi-planar image formation using NMR spin-echoes. J Phys Chem 1977;10:L55.
2. Rzedzian R. A method for instant whole-body MR imaging at 2.0 tesla and system design considerations in its implementation. Proc SMRM 1987:229.
3. Rzedzian R. U.S. Patent #4628264, Advanced NMR Systems, Wobern Mass, 1986.
4. Cohen M, et al. Ultra-fast imaging. Magn Reson Imaging 1991;9:1.
5. Weber DM. Non-resonant EPI gradients will enhance conventional MRI. MR 1993;Sept/Oct:29.
6. Hennig J, et al. RARE imaging: a fast method for clinical MRI. Magn Reson Med 1986;3:823.
7. Meyer CH, Pauly JM. U.S. Patent #4999580.
8. Meyer CH, et al. Simultaneous spatial and spectral selective excitation. Magn Reson Med 1990;15:287.
9. Jones KM, et al. Evaluation of brain hemorrhage: comparison of fast spin-echo and conventional dual spin-echo images. Radiology 1992;182:53.
10. Jolesz FA. Fast spin-echo technique extends versatility of MR. Diagn Imaging 1992:78.
11. Reilly JP. Peripheral nerve stimulation by induced electric currents: exposure to time-varying magnetic fields. Med Biol Eng Comput 1989;27:101.
12. Schaefer DJ, et al. Determination of gradient induced, human peripheral nerve stimulation thresholds for trapezoidal pulse trains. Proc SMRM 1994:101.

Magnetic Resonance Imaging in Orthopaedics & Sports Medicine, Second Edition,
edited by David W. Stoller. Lippincott-Raven Publishers, Philadelphia, © 1997.

Chapter 5

MR Imaging
of Articular Cartilage
and of Cartilage Degeneration

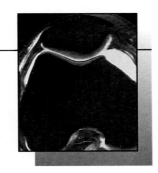

J. Bruce Kneeland

STRUCTURE OF NORMAL ARTICULAR CARTILAGE
MR IMAGING OF NORMAL ARTICULAR CARTILAGE
MR IMAGING OF CARTILAGE DEGENERATION
   Standard Protocols and Techniques
   "Exotic" Techniques
SUMMARY

Articular cartilage is a remarkable form of connective tissue that provides the joints with both the friction and lubrication that make normal motion possible. It also serves to absorb mechanical shock and to distribute the load over the underlying bone. Under ideal circumstances, articular cartilage will function over the lifetime of the joint. However, it can be damaged by trauma, osteoarthritis (OA), and inflammatory disorders.

Although the MR imaging of cartilage has been carefully studied, there is considerable disagreement with regard to the MR appearance of normal cartilage, the best technique for imaging cartilage abnormalities, and the accuracy of these techniques in the detection of abnormalities. Cartilage has proven exceedingly difficult to evaluate accurately with MR imaging. In part this is due to the limits of resolution, since articular cartilage is a thin layer of material relative to the size of the voxels that are typically used for MR imaging, and it generally lies on curved surfaces. These difficulties can be addressed by (1) using three-dimensional (3D) gradient echo acquisition techniques, which permit much thinner sections for the same gradient strength; and (2) using higher performance gradients, which are currently becoming available from equipment manufacturers and which permit both thinner sections and smaller fields of view (Fig. 5-1). Resolution alone, however, is probably not the entire explanation for the problems associated with MR imaging of cartilage, since there has been considerable difficulty noted in imaging the cartilage of the patella, which is not only the thickest in

the body, but which resides on a relatively flat surface and, because of its superficial location, is amenable to higher resolution than is used for routine MR studies of the whole knee.

This chapter provides a review of the disagreements surrounding the imaging of cartilage and a discussion of some of the more exotic techniques that may assist in its evaluation.

STRUCTURE OF NORMAL ARTICULAR CARTILAGE

The structure of normal articular cartilage has been carefully studied.[1] Articular cartilage consists of a small population of specialized cells, called chondrocytes, and a large extracellular matrix (ECM). The primary components of the ECM are water and the macromolecules collagen and proteoglycan. The structure of cartilage varies throughout its depth, and consists of four histologic zones or layers. The most superficial zone has thin collagen fibers with long axes oriented parallel to the articular surface. The proteoglycan content is at its minimum in this zone. The middle zone has thicker collagen fibers with a more random orientation. The deep zone contains the lowest water content and the highest proteoglycan concentration. Collagen fibers in this zone are oriented perpendicular to the surface of the cartilage. The deepest layer is the zone of calcified cartilage, which contains an abundance of hydroxyapatite salts.

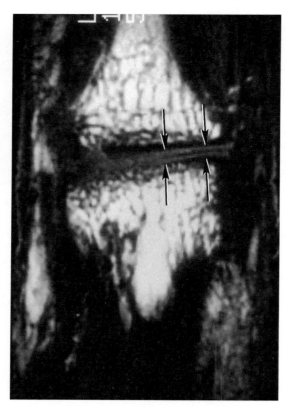

FIGURE 5-1. Coronal image of distal interphalangeal joint of an asymptomatic subject (the author) obtained with a 3-cm field of view and a 1.5-mm section thickness using dedicated gradient and radiofrequency coils. The articular cartilage is indicated between the arrows.

The ECM is further subdivided into pericellular, territorial, and interterritorial regions, depending on proximity to chondrocytes. These regions differ in proteoglycan content and the content, fibril diameter, and organization of collagen; but they are too small to be resolved by current MR techniques.

Chondrocytes are responsible for the maintenance of articular cartilage. They occupy less than 10% of the total volume of the cartilage, however, and the chemical composition, physical properties, and MR appearance of cartilage is primarily determined by the ECM.

Water is the most abundant component of articular cartilage, with concentrations ranging from 80% on the surface to 65% in the deep zone. About 30% of the water is bound to collagen molecules. Most of the remainder is located within the spaces between the macromolecules. These spaces ("pores") are very small and provide considerable resistance to the passage of the water, giving cartilage a good deal of its resistance to joint loading. The affinity of cartilage for water arises primarily from the presence of proteoglycans. Its negative charges serve to attract free-floating positive ions in solution, such as Na^+, which, in turn, attract water molecules through osmotic pressure (this phenomenon is an example of the "Donnan" equilibrium).

Proteoglycans are complex macromolecules that consist of protein and polysaccharides. The most common (80% to 90%) of the proteoglycans, which is called aggrecan, consists of a protein core with a long extended domain to which are attached many glycosaminoglycan side chains. The aggrecan molecules are, in turn, attached to hyaluronate—a long, linear polysaccharide. The resulting structure is frequently described as having a "lamp-brush" appearance. A large number of carboxyl and sulfate residues are present on the glycosaminoglycan side chains, which are ionized under physiological conditions to give COO^- and SO_4^- anions which, as noted above, serve to attract positive counter-ions and water molecules. In addition, these negative charges provide a strong electrostatic repulsive force between the proteoglycans. These two forces are responsible for the swelling pressure of cartilage. The configuration of the proteoglycan macromolecules also contributes to the previously mentioned resistance of the matrix to the passage of water molecules and consequently affects the mechanical properties of cartilage as well. There are several other types of proteoglycans that contribute only a small fraction to the proteoglycan mass. They are, however, believed to be functionally important.

Collagens are proteins with a characteristic triple helical structure. Although many different types of collagen are found in cartilage, the most common type (90% to 95%) is known as type II collagen. Collagen molecules aggregate into fibers that are 10 to 100 nm in diameter. The major role of type II collagen fibers is to provide the tensile force that opposes the hydrophilic tendency of the proteoglycans to expand the cartilage and to immobilize the proteoglycans. Other types of collagens have a variety of structures, although many of them are similar to that of type II collagen. The function of these other collagens is less well understood, but at least some of them are involved in cross-linking the type II collagen molecules. Although there are many other molecules present in the ECM in low concentrations, their functions are generally not understood.

MR IMAGING OF NORMAL ARTICULAR CARTILAGE

Although early studies of the MR appearance of cartilage, such as that by Yulish and colleagues,[2] demonstrated a rather homogeneous appearance, subsequent investigations described the presence of layers. In one of the earliest reviews, Lehner and associates[3] studied the appearance of bovine cartilage specimens and noted the presence of two layers: (1) a superficial zone, with lower signal on heavily T1-weighted inversion recovery sequences and higher signal on T2-weighted spin-echo images; and (2) a deeper layer, with brighter signal on the inversion recovery images and lower signal on the T2-weighted images. The differences in the MR appearance of the two layers was attributed to differences in water concentration.

Using higher resolution in a subsequent investigation,

Modl and colleagues[4] depicted three layers in specimens of human articular cartilage evaluated with T2-weighted spin-echo images. They described a thin, low signal superficial layer; a higher signal middle layer; and a low signal deep layer. In a subsequent unpublished work, the same investigators noted that on more T1-weighted images the low signal deep layer was less thick, and that the apparent thickness of this layer increased with increasing degrees of T2 weighting. Correlation of the MR images with histologic sections of the cartilage showed a rough qualitative correlation between the zones seen with MR imaging and those seen histologically, but the authors failed to establish a precise quantitative correlation between the thicknesses of the layers demonstrated with the two techniques. For these reasons, the exact origin of the layers seen on MR scans is still uncertain, but it is thought likely that they are related to zonal differences in the thickness and orientation of the collagen fibers and that these fibers affect the water protons through the mechanism of static susceptibility (ie, the effect of the fibers on the static magnetic field).

Figure 5-2 illustrates the appearance of patellar cartilage using spin-echo and 3D gradient echo sequences. On T1-weighted images, the cartilage appears relatively homogeneous, although the layers may be seen faintly. On intermediate and T2-weighted spin-echo images, two layers are clearly delineated: a thin, low signal superficial layer as well as an equally thin, brighter layer just deep to the superficial low signal layer. Deep to these two layers lies a much thicker layer that occupies most of the thickness of the cartilage and that becomes progressively darker with increasing T2 weighting. At significantly higher resolution, the presence of vertical, low signal striations within this lower signal, deep layer cartilage can be seen. (Erickson SJ, personal communication). This MR finding has been attributed to the radially oriented collagen fibers in the deep layer of the cartilage, although this has not been confirmed histologically.

Rubenstein and colleagues[5] described a somewhat different pattern of signal intensities on MR images of bovine cartilage specimens obtained with spin-echo sequences. They report a high signal superficial layer, a low signal middle layer, and a moderately bright deep layer. In this study, the apparent thickness of the high signal superficial layer was noted to decrease with increased T2 weighting. The reason for the discrepancy between their results and those of Modl's group is unclear, although the resolution of the images in Rubenstein's study was considerably less than that in Modl's and a thin superficial layer might have been missed.

Rubenstein and coworkers also noted an apparent loss of layered structure when the orientation of the cartilage was such that the ''magic-angle'' effect was present. This led to the conclusion that interaction between collagen and water was responsible for the MR appearance of the layers, and that the mechanism was that of a ''dipole–dipole'' interaction between the free water protons and those bound to the mac-

romolecules. It should be noted, however, that if collagen fibers are assumed to have a roughly cylindrical shape, then a similar null point would be generated at the same angle on the basis of susceptibility and hence that mechanism cannot be excluded (Leigh JS, personal communication).

Recht and associates[6] demonstrated a pattern of layers similar to that shown by Modl in the cartilage of human cadaveric knee specimens using spin-echo images (see Fig. 3 of that article), although they did not specifically comment on this finding in the text of their article. Using 3D gradient echo sequences, however, they noted a variety of different patterns with the different gradient echo sequences. Spoiled gradient echo sequences, felt to be the best for assessment of cartilage, produced a completely different pattern of layers with a thick, high signal superficial layer; a thin, low signal middle layer; and a thick, high signal deep layer (see Fig. 5-2). The thickness of these layers did not correspond to those seen with spin-echo sequences.

A 3D spoiled gradient echo sequence of the patellar cartilage is shown in Figure 5-2E. A thin, low signal intensity line is faintly visualized within the cartilage, sandwiched between brighter and much thicker deep and superficial layers. This line may correspond to the line described by Recht and colleagues. In this particular case, it appears to lie at the superior margin of the relatively darker deeper layer seen on intermediate and T2-weighted spin-echo images.

A pattern of signal intensity qualitatively similar to that seen by Modl was noted by Paul and coworkers,[7] using relatively T1-weighted and ''intermediate'' spin- and gradient-echo sequences in asymptomatic human subjects. This group of investigators, however, explained the signal differences on the basis of different zonal concentrations of proteoglycan. The ''bell-shaped'' pattern of proteoglycan concentrations cited in the literature, however, differs from the more widely accepted scheme of signal intensities described earlier.

Other authors have reported still different patterns of signal intensity, depending on the imaging sequence used. Hayes and coworkers[8] noted a thin, high signal, superficial layer and a low signal deep layer on T1-weighted spin-echo images. Fry and coworkers[9] demonstrated a thin, low signal superficial layer and a high signal deep layer using a T1-weighted gradient echo sequence.

The structural basis for the appearance of the MR images, and the reasons that they differ from one another are as yet unknown.

MR IMAGING OF CARTILAGE DEGENERATION

Standard Protocols and Techniques

Osteoarthritis, or osteoarthrosis, is the term used for a disorder of uncertain etiology that is characterized by focal cartilage erosions and fissures, progressive cartilage loss, bony sclerosis, cyst, and osteophyte formation. The earliest

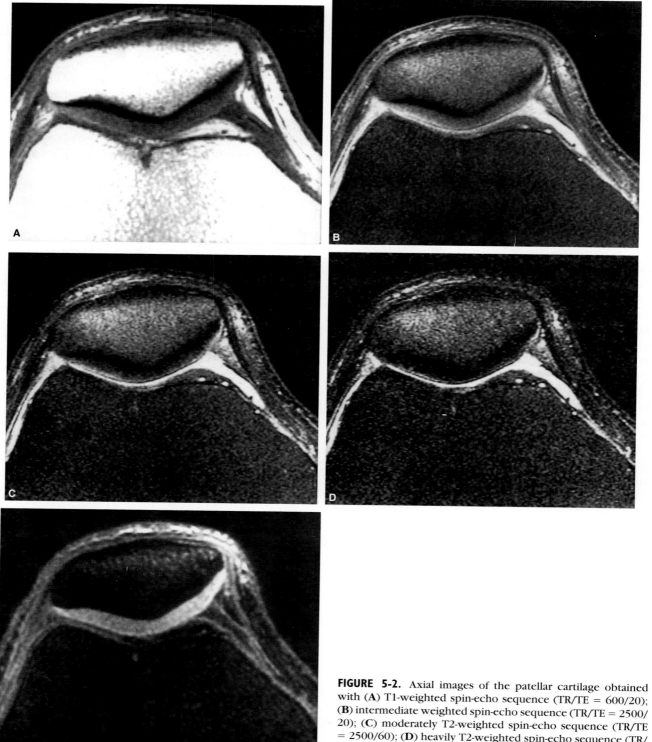

FIGURE 5-2. Axial images of the patellar cartilage obtained with (**A**) T1-weighted spin-echo sequence (TR/TE = 600/20); (**B**) intermediate weighted spin-echo sequence (TR/TE = 2500/20); (**C**) moderately T2-weighted spin-echo sequence (TR/TE = 2500/60); (**D**) heavily T2-weighted spin-echo sequence (TR/TE = 2500/100); and (**E**) a fat-suppressed, 3D, spoiled gradient echo sequence (TR/TE/flip angle = 50/11/60°).

changes of OA probably arise in the cartilage and consist of a partial breakdown in the proteoglycan matrix with a decrease in total content. The total concentration of collagen remains unaltered in the earliest stages, although there are generally changes in the size and arrangement of fibers. There is a also a small increase in the total water content. All of these changes in the macromolecular matrix lead to an alteration in the mechanical properties of cartilage, with the result that it can no longer serve as an effective load-bearing material. Mechanical failure, in turn, makes the cartilage more susceptible to damage.[10]

Until recently, therapy in the early stages of the disease has been ineffective at halting or reversing its course and has largely been directed toward symptomatic relief. In its later stages, joint surface replacement (arthroplasty) is the only effective treatment. Novel techniques for the treatment of OA, such as chondroprotective drugs and repopulation of cartilage defects by chondrocyte precursor cells with subsequent regeneration of the cartilage,[11-13] have led to a demand for more accurate noninvasive assessment of cartilage.

MR imaging can be used for diagnosis of osteoarthritic changes, although most studies have focused on the focal osteoarthritic changes seen in the patellar cartilage called "chondromalacia patellae." (The term chondromalacia patellae is somewhat of a misnomer, having been used originally to describe a softening of the cartilage, but it since has been generalized to include all degrees of degeneration of the patellar cartilage as well as a number of unrelated pain syndromes arising in the retropatellar region.) More than a half dozen different pathologic–arthroscopic classification schemes for chondromalacia patellae have been described in the orthopedic literature, including two widely cited schemes by Outerbridge[14] and Shahriaree.[15] Most schemes describe an early grades with softening or blistering of the cartilage, followed by higher grades with irregularity of the surface of the cartilage, shallow and then deep erosions and fissures, and ultimately full-thickness loss of cartilage and eburnation of the underlying bone.

Detection of early grades of abnormality, in which there are changes in the structure of the cartilage but no erosions or clefts, remains problematic with MR imaging. Early studies described the presence of low signal foci within cartilage that had undergone early changes of OA on T1-weighted spin-echo images[2] and on intermediate weighted spin-echo images obtained with fat suppression.[16] A subsequent publication described the presence of foci of bright signal on T2-weighted images in regions of early OA[17] (Fig. 5-3). A focus of low signal was also reported in a single case of early cartilage degeneration using a fat-suppressed 3D spoiled gradient echo sequence.[6] Other studies, however, failed to demonstrate any consistent changes in the MR signal intensity, regardless of pulse sequence, in cartilage containing early changes of OA.[8,18] Without considering the accuracy (or lack thereof) of these findings, it is important to remember one particular pitfall, that is, pulsation artifact from the popliteal artery can produce an apparent focus of bright signal in the cartilage (Fig. 5-4).

Higher grades of injury—such as fibrillation, erosions, and clefts—produce alteration in the morphology of the cartilage, which can be seen on MR scans as surface irregularities and focal defects in occupied by joint fluid (Figs. 5-5 through 5-8). Numerous studies have been performed in the attempt to identify the optimum pulse sequences for the detection of these cartilage abnormalities and to assess the accuracy of these sequences.[6,19] Fat suppression is generally an important component in the more accurate sequences and improves the accuracy of almost any sequence.[20] The highest reported accuracy (95%) for any technique for the detection of cartilage abnormalities is a 3D, fat-suppressed, spoiled gradient echo sequence proposed by Recht and colleagues.[6] Similar findings were reported by Disler and coworkers.[21] In our experience, however, the accuracy of this sequence

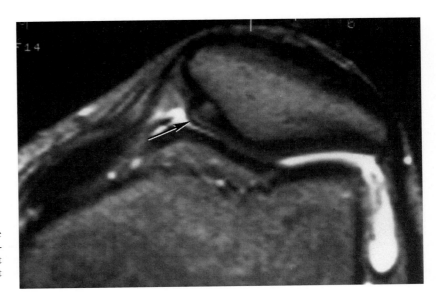

FIGURE 5-3. Axial T2-weighted spin-echo image through the patellofemoral space with a focus of increased signal and local swelling on the medial facet (*arrow*) that at arthroscopy was found to represent softening and blistering of the cartilage.

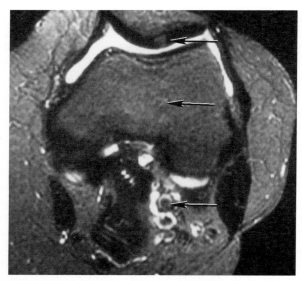

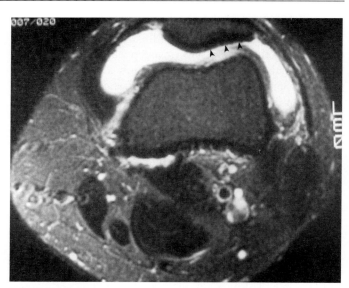

FIGURE 5-4. Axial T2-weighted spin-echo image through the knee demonstrating an apparent focus of bright signal in the patellar cartilage that represents pulsation artifact from the popliteal artery (*arrows*).

FIGURE 5-5. Axial T2-weighted spin-echo image through the knee illustrates a mild superficial irregularity of the patellar cartilage (*arrowheads*) that was found to represent fibrillation of the cartilage at arthroscopy.

is considerably lower in clinical practice and we prefer the use of fat-suppressed T2-weighted fast spin-echo sequences to detect the morphologic changes of osteoarthritic cartilage (see Fig. 5-8). We have found that this sequence provides excellent contrast between the low signal cartilage and the high signal joint fluid and that the frequently present high signal in the underlying bone often serves as a useful indicator of injury to the overlying cartilage (see Figs. 5-7 and 5-8). Thinner sections (1 to 2 mm) can now be obtained with two-dimensional (2D) fast spin-echo sequences on the higher performance gradient subsystems currently becoming commercially available. These thinner sections will most likely increase the accuracy of the 2D techniques, assuming the radiofrequency coils provide sufficient signal-to-noise ratio to support them.

The 3D gradient echo sequences can also be used to calculate the volume of articular cartilage with reasonably high accuracy.[22] This technique may make it possible to follow a progression of diffuse cartilage loss.

Although MR arthrography can also been used to detect cartilage defects (Fig. 5-9),[19,23–25] results of studies on the usefulness of intraarticular contrast are mixed, with some investigators noting a significant increase in accuracy for the detection of cartilaginous defects[24,25] and others have noting little or no improvement.[19,23] Since a variety of MR techniques were used in these studies, both before and after the intraarticular injection of contrast, comparison among them is difficult.

In view of the uncertainties surrounding the comparative accuracies of arthrographic and nonarthrographic tech-

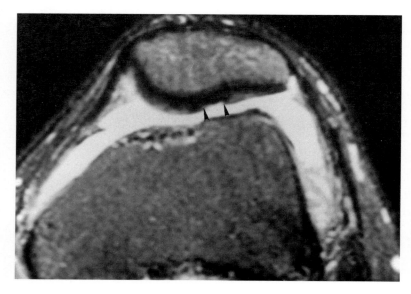

FIGURE 5-6. Axial T2-weighted spin-echo image through the knee illustrates a superficial defect of the cartilage (*arrowheads*) that represented a shallow erosion at arthroscopy.

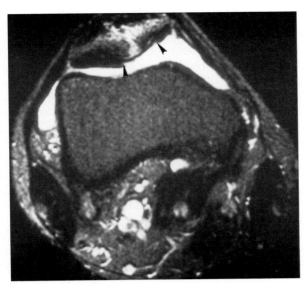

FIGURE 5-7. Axial T2-weighted spin-echo image through the knee illustrates a deep defect of the cartilage (*arrowheads*) that represented a deep erosion at arthroscopy.

niques, and considering the greater patient morbidity and logistical difficulties associated with the performance of MR arthrographic studies, MR arthrography is not routinely practiced for the detection of cartilaginous defects.

"Exotic" Techniques

In an effort to improve the accuracy of MR imaging for the evaluation of osteoarthritic changes in cartilage, particularly in their early stages, a number of more "exotic" techniques have been attempted, including magnetization transfer

weighted imaging, diffusion weighted imaging, and T1ρ and [23]Na imaging.

Magnetization transfer contrast (MTC) imaging, also called "saturation transfer" imaging, relies on the transfer of magnetization between the protons that are bound to macromolecules and the "mobile" protons in the free water molecules.[26] MR imaging only detects the nuclear magnetic resonance signal from mobile protons. However, even though bound protons are not directly observable, they can, if excited, transfer some of this excitation to the mobile protons and alter the magnitude of the detected signal. The efficiency of this transfer depends upon the concentration of the macromolecules as well as the interaction between the macromolecules and water.

MTC imaging has been used in two different techniques for the identification of early osteoarthritic injury to cartilage. In one, MTC imaging is used to increase the contrast between cartilage and joint fluid,[27] and in the other it is used as a direct probe.[28] The attempt to increase contrast between cartilage and joint fluid by use of MTC by takes advantage of the fact that joint fluid, with its usual small concentration of protein, demonstrates only a small degree of magnetization transfer whereas cartilage, with its much higher concentration of macromolecules, demonstrates a much larger effect. This technique relies on subtraction of pre- and post-MTC images, and for this reason is both time-consuming and dependent on a precise spatial registration of the two sets of images. In addition, in studying this technique Peterfy and colleagues[27] found that routine fat-suppressed gradient echo imaging provided superior contrast.

The rationale for the use of MTC imaging as a direct probe of cartilage structure is based on the theory that an alteration of the interaction between the bound protons on macromolecules and the mobile protons in free water would

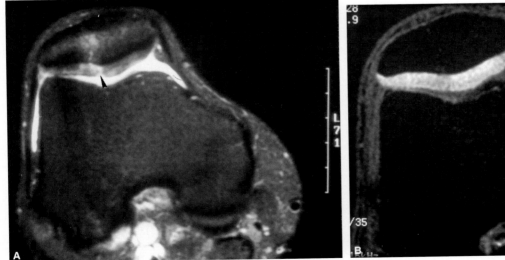

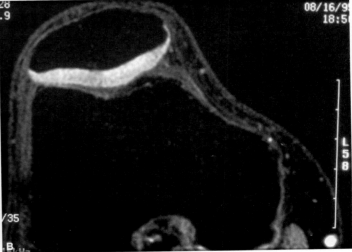

FIGURE 5-8. Axial T2-weighted fast spin-echo (**A**) and 3D spoiled gradient echo (**B**) images through the patellofemoral joint illustrate the presence of a cartilage defect (*arrowhead*) that is seen on the spin-echo but not on the gradient echo sequence. (Courtesy of David Rubin, MD, Pittsburgh)

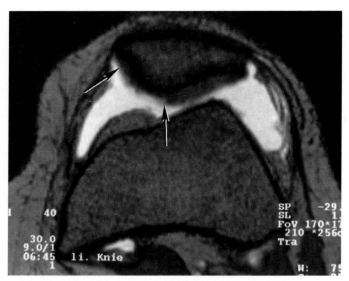

FIGURE 5-9. Axial spoiled 3D gradient echo image through the patellofemoral joint obtained following the intraarticular injection of dilute solution of a gadolinium chelate. There is an extensive defect of the cartilage on the medial facet and medial ridge (*arrows*).

occur with the breakdown of the macromolecular matrix that is observed in early OA. Vahlensieck and coworkers[28] studied the use of MTC MR imaging in the evaluation of OA in a small number of knee specimens. They found a reduction in magnetization transfer in areas of collagen loss, although they also noted that the MTC images were less sensitive than T2-weighted spin-echo images for the detection of OA in general. These findings were attributed to the fact that the majority of magnetization transfer occurs between collagen and water rather than between proteoglycans and water, and to the fact that significant injury to the proteoglycan matrix usually precedes injury to the collagen matrix.[29] These findings suggest that MTC imaging can be of only limited value for the evaluation of early osteoarthritic changes in cartilage. However, in a recent article Gray and colleagues[30] reported evidence of magnetization transfer between proteoglycans and water, and further demonstrated that although the absolute magnitude of the magnetization transfer is greater with collagen than with the proteoglycans, the relative changes in magnetization transfer that result from the breakdown of proteoglycans might well be more pronounced with the breakdown of collagen in the physiological concentration range. Thus the efficacy of MTC imaging for the detection of the early changes of OA in cartilage remains an open question.

In diffusion weighted sequences, signal intensity is heavily influenced by the speed at which the water molecules diffuse.[31] In normal cartilage, the macromolecular matrix slows the diffusion of water considerably in comparison with pure water. As this matrix breaks down in the early stages of OA, water molecules diffuse more rapidly. Therefore, it should be possible to detect the presence of this breakdown of the matrix by the detection of regions with an increased

rate of diffusion. Burstein and colleagues[32] have demonstrated an increase in diffusion rates in samples of bovine cartilage that were treated with enzymes to breakdown the macromolecular matrix. There are, however, several practical problems in implementing their techniques in the clinical setting, in particular the degree of immobilization required. Immobilization is important because (1) precise registration between the two sequences is required since this technique is usually implemented as a subtraction technique between sequences obtained with and without diffusion weighting gradients, and (2) involuntary bulk motion of the extremity that is of the same magnitude as the distance that water diffuses during the data acquisition period will make an artifactual contribution to the diffusion that is measured. Faster versions of diffusion weighted imaging, using echo planar and gradient echo techniques, minimize these two difficulties,[31] but it is very difficult to obtain the small fields of view that are necessary to image cartilage with these techniques due to the tremendous demands placed on the gradient system. Although dedicated gradient coils should make this technique more feasible, it is unclear at this time whether it can be successfully implemented and, if so, whether it will prove more sensitive than other available techniques for the detection of the early changes of OA in cartilage.

T1ρ imaging is a method of generating tissue contrast that depends on frequency motions of molecules that are lower than those that determine T1 time but faster than the static component that heavily influences T2 time.[33] The application of this technique to the study of cartilage is based on the idea that the motion of the macromolecular matrix takes place at considerably lower frequencies than those that are normally present in proteins in solution. In addition, it has been suggested that the breakdown of the macromolecular matrix is associated with a change in T1ρ. To date, only the technical feasibility of performing T1ρ imaging of cartilage has been demonstrated, and it is unknown whether the technique will prove useful for the evaluation of the early changes of OA.

A third technique of potential interest in the cartilage evaluation is the imaging of sodium (^{23}Na) ions. Sodium ions are of considerable interest because they are "bound" to the negative charges of the proteoglycans. Lesperance and colleagues[34] have used Na imaging to estimate the total quantity of proteoglycans (the "fixed charge density") present in cartilage. It is also possible to directly image only the ^{23}Na that is bound to the proteoglycans by using "multiple quantum filtering" techniques. The rationale for the use of Na imaging is based on the expectation that as the macromolecular matrix of proteoglycans becomes disrupted in early OA, the signal from the bound ^{23}Na decreases. Preliminary work with cartilage treated with enzymes to breakdown the proteoglycan matrix has demonstrated that there is a marked decrease in the signal from the bound ^{23}Na. There are formidable obstacles to the implementation of this technique in the clinical setting, however. In particular, the low signal-to-noise ratio of sodium in comparison to protons and the consequent difficulty in obtaining images with sufficient resolution to display cartilage. Thus it is unknown whether this technique will prove practical or, if so, whether it will prove more sensitive than other techniques for the breakdown of the proteoglycan matrix.

SUMMARY

The MR imaging of cartilage remains a controversial topic. There is considerable disagreement on the MR appearance of normal cartilage and the accuracy of MR imaging for the detection of the early changes of osteoarthritis. The study of cartilage may be amenable to the application of more sophisticated or exotic techniques because of its relatively simple structure. Indeed, cartilage may be the first tissue for which MR imaging will see its full potential as a biophysical probe of molecular structure and function.

References

1. Mankin HJ, et al. Form and function of articular cartilage. In: Simon SR, ed. Orthopedic basic science. American Academy Orthopedic Surgery, 1994:3.
2. Yulish BS, et al. Chondromalacia patellae: assessment with MR imaging. Radiology 1987;164:763.
3. Lehner KB, et al. Structure, function, and degeneration of bovine hyaline cartilage: assessment with MR imaging in vitro. Radiology 1989;170:495.
4. Modl JM, et al. Articular cartilage: correlation of histologic zones with signal intensity at MR imaging. Radiology 1991;181:853.
5. Rubenstein JD, et al. Effects of collagen orientation on the MR imaging characteristics of bovine articular cartilage. Radiology 1993;188:219.
6. Recht MP, et al. Abnormalities of articular cartilage in the knee: analysis of available MR techniques. Radiology 1993;187:473.
7. Paul PK, et al. Variation in MR signal intensity across normal human knee cartilage. J Magn Reson Imaging 1993;3:569.
8. Hayes CW, Sawyer RW, Conway WF. Patellar cartilage lesions: in vitro detection and staging with MR imaging and pathologic correlation. Radiology 1990;176:479.
9. Fry ME, et al. High-resolution magnetic resonance imaging of the interphalangeal joints of the hand. Skeletal Radiol 1991;20:273.
10. Mankin HJ, Brandt KD. Biochemistry and metabolism of articular cartilage in osteoarthritis. In: Moskowitz RW, ed. Osteoarthritis: diagnosis and medical/surgical management. Philadelphia: WB Saunders, 1992:109.
11. Howell DS, Altman RD. Cartilage repair and conservation in osteoarthritis. Rheum Dis Clin North Am 1993;19:713.
12. Buckwalter JA, Mow VC, Ratcliffe A. Restoration of injured or degenerated articular cartilage. J Am Acad Orthop Surg 1994;2:192.
13. Brittberg M, et al. Treatment of deep cartilage defects in the knee with autologous chondrocyte transplantation. N Eng J Med 1994;331:889.
14. Outerbridge RE. The etiology of chondromalacia patellae. Clin Orthop 1975;110:177.
15. Shahriaree H. Chondromalacia. Contemp Orthop 1985;11:27.
16. Konig H, et al. Cartilage disorders: comparison of spin-echo, CHESS, and FLASH sequence MR images. Radiology 1987;164:753.
17. McCauley TR, et al. Chondromalacia patellae: diagnosis with MR imaging. AJR 1992;158:101.
18. Adam G, et al. Experimental hyaline cartilage lesions: two-dimensional spin-echo versus three-dimensional gradient-echo MR imaging. J Magn Reson Imaging 1991;1:665.
19. Gagliardi JA, et al. Detection and staging of chondromalacia patellae: relative efficacies of conventional MR imaging, MR arthrography, and CT arthrography. AJR 1994;163:629.
20. Rose PM, et al. Chondromalacia patellae: fat-suppressed MR imaging. Radiology 1994;193:437.
21. Disler DG, et al. Detection of knee hyaline cartilage defects using fat-suppressed three-dimensional spoiled gradient echo MR imaging: comparison with standard MR imaging and correlation with arthroscopy. AJR 1995;165:377.
22. Peterfy CG, et al. Quantification of the volume of articular cartilage in the metacarpophalangeal joints of the hand: accuracy and precision of three-dimensional MR imaging. AJR 1995;165:371.
23. Chandnani V, et al. Knee hyaline cartilage evaluated with MR imaging: a cadaveric study involving multiple imaging sequences and intraarticular injection of gadolinium and saline solution. Radiology 1991;178:557.
24. Gylys-Morin VM, et al. Articular defects: detectability in cadaver knees with MR. AJR 1987;148:1153.
25. Kramer J, et al. Postcontrast MR arthrography in assessment of cartilage lesions. J Comput Assist Tomogr 1994;18:218.
26. Wolff SD, et al. Magnetization transfer contrast: MR imaging of the knee. Radiology 1991;179:623.
27. Peterfy CG, et al. MR imaging of the arthritis knee: improved discrimination of cartilage, synovium, and effusion with pulse saturation transfer and fat-suppressed T1-weighted sequences. Radiology 1994;191:423.
28. Vahlensieck M, et al. Magnetization transfer contrast (MTC) and MTC-subtraction: enhancement of cartilage lesions and intracartilaginous degeneration in vitro. Skeletal Radiol 1994;23:535.
29. Kim DK, et al. Analysis of water-macromolecule proton magnetization transfer in articular cartilage. Magn Reson Med 1993;29:211.
30. Gray ML, et al. Magnetization transfer in cartilage and its constituent macromolecules. Magn Reson Med 1995;34:319.
31. LeBihan D. Molecular diffusion nuclear magnetic resonance imaging. Magn Reson Q 1991;7:1.
32. Burstein D, et al. Diffusion of small solutes in cartilage as measured by nuclear magnetic resonance (NMR) spectroscopy and imaging. J Orthop Res 1993;11:465.
33. Sepponen RE, et al. A method for $T1\rho$ imaging. J Comput Assist Tomogr 1985;9:1007.
34. Lesperance LM, Gray ML, Burstein D. Determination of fixed charge density in cartilage using nuclear magnetic resonance. J Orthop Res 1992;10:1.

Magnetic Resonance Imaging in Orthopaedics & Sports Medicine, Second Edition,
edited by David W. Stoller. Lippincott-Raven Publishers, Philadelphia, © 1997.

Chapter 6

The Hip

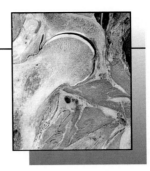

David W. Stoller
William J. Maloney
James M. Glick

The hip—consisting of the acetabulum, femoral articulation, supporting soft tissue, muscle, and cartilage structures—is a functionally and structurally complex joint. Disease processes involving the hip joint include trauma, osteonecrosis, arthritis, infection, and neoplasia—conditions that are frequently not detected by conventional radiographic techniques until they have reached an advanced clinical stage. The various imaging modalities have different strengths and weaknesses in facilitating diagnosis. Plain films, for example, are limited in assessment of soft tissues and articular structures. Contrast arthrography is useful in evaluation of the joint spaces and for sampling of synovial fluid in cases of infection; and computed tomography (CT), by reformatting axial scans with sufficient bone detail to generate sagittal and coronal images, provides a multiplanar three-dimensional (3D) perspective on hip disease.[1]

Magnetic resonance (MR) imaging has also been successfully used to evaluate pathologic processes in the hip.[2,3] The excellent spatial and contrast resolution provided by MR imaging facilitates early detection and evaluation of femoral head osteonecrosis, definition of hyaline articular cartilage damage in arthritis, identification of joint effusions,

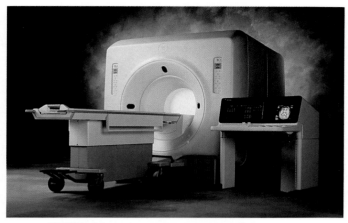

FIGURE 6-1. Body coil for MR imaging of the hip.

and characterization of osseous and soft tissue tumors about the hip. With direct, noninvasive MR imaging of bone marrow, fractures and infiltrative diseases can be identified earlier than with radiographic studies. In addition, the cartilaginous epiphysis in an infant or child, which is not visible on routine radiographs, can be demonstrated on MR images. The use of surface coils, including pelvic phased array coils, produces more anatomic detail in imaging of the hip joint capsule and acetabular labrum.

IMAGING PROTOCOLS FOR THE HIP

With the body coil used in most MR examinations of the hip, and with a large (32 to 40 cm) field of view (FOV), both hips are seen and can be compared (Fig. 6-1). Phased array torso coils improve the signal-to-noise ratio while still providing visualization of both hips (Fig. 6-2).

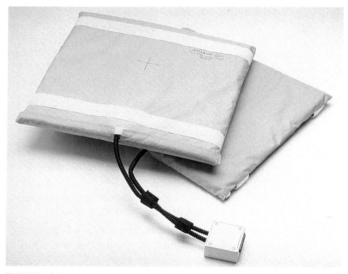

FIGURE 6-2. Torso phased array coils used to evaluate the hips. Signal-to-noise is optimized for improved image quality when using smaller FOVs.

T1-weighted images can be acquired in the axial, sagittal, or coronal planes. Examinations are performed with a 512 × 256 or 256 × 256 acquisition matrix, using 1 or 2 excitations (NEX). Thin (3 to 4 mm) sections are obtained either contiguously or with a minimal interslice gap. Three-millimeter sections are preferred in pediatric patients, or when precise assessments are required to display articular cartilage surfaces and the labrum. Three-dimensional Fourier transform volume images allow acquisition of slices as thin as 1 mm. Preliminary work with 3D fast spin-echo and echo planar imaging techniques has shown potential both in generating thin section T2-weighted images and in increasing the speed of the MR examination of the hips.

Conventional T2-weighted images or fat-suppressed T2-weighted fast spin-echo images are acquired in the axial plane to evaluate arthritis, infection, and neoplasia. Short TI inversion recovery (STIR) and fast spin-echo STIR sequences are useful in identifying hip effusions, bone marrow pathology, osseous trauma, and muscle hemorrhage and edema.[4–6] Coronal T2* surface coil imaging is useful in identifying capsular and labral abnormalities at fields of view of 16 to 20 cm.

When imaging only one hip in the sagittal plane, smaller FOVs (20 to 24 cm) should be used to obtain high spatial resolution (Fig. 6-3). Signal-to-noise ratio may be a limiting factor, however. With a shoulder surface coil (Fig. 6-4)

text continues on page 97

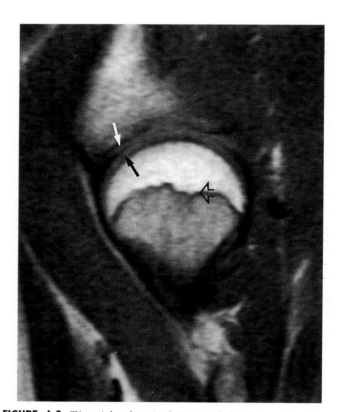

FIGURE 6-3. T1-weighted sagittal image of the femoral head in a 12-year-old child shows separation of hyaline articular cartilage in the acetabulum (*white arrow*) and femoral head (*black arrow*). The open physis, demonstrating low signal intensity, is transversely oriented (*open arrow*) (TR, 600 msec; TE, 20 msec).

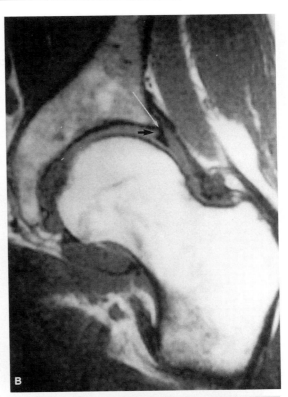

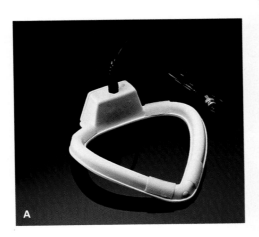

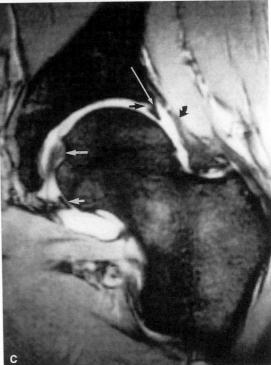

FIGURE 6-4. Capsular anatomy. (**A**) Shoulder surface coil is used to image the hip joint. (**B**) A T1-weighted coronal image obtained with the surface coil displays low signal intensity labrum (*white arrow*) and intermediate signal intensity articular cartilage (*black arrow*). The lateral extent of the articular cartilage should not be mistaken for a partial lateral tear (TR, 500 msec; TE, 20 msec). (**C**) A coronal T2*-weighted image obtained with the surface coil identifies capsular structures in contrast to the bright signal intensity joint fluid. The acetabular labrum (*long white arrow*) and cartilage (*straight black arrow*), ligamentum teres (*medium white arrow*), transverse ligament (*short white arrow*), and iliofemoral ligament (*curved black arrow*) are noted (TR, 400 msec; TE, 15 msec; flip angle, 20°).

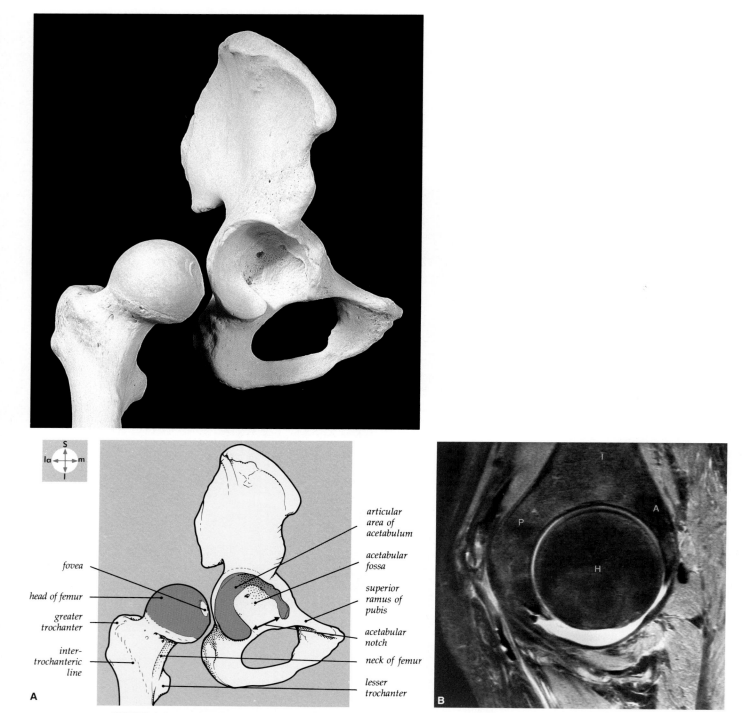

FIGURE 6-5. (**A**) Articular surfaces of the hip joint are comprised of the acetabulum of the hip bone and the head of the femur. (**B**) Sagittal MR arthrogram of the hip demonstrating capsular distention and the articular relationship of the femoral head (H) to the anterior (A) and posterior (P) aspects of the acetabulum and ilium (I). Fat-suppressed T2-weighted fast spin-echo image.

placed anterolateral to the hip joint, FOVs as small as 16 to 20 cm can be used. These images are obtained with T1-weighted or T2*-weighted contrast to display capsular and ligamentous anatomy. This technique is particularly useful in separating femoral head from acetabular articular cartilage and for demonstrating intraarticular loose bodies.[7]

ANATOMY OF THE HIP

Gross and Arthroscopic Anatomy

The femoral head represents a multiaxial, synovial ball-and-socket joint (Fig. 6-5). The acetabulum, which provides bony coverage of 40% of the femoral head (Fig. 6-6), has a horseshoe-shaped lunate surface (Fig. 6-7). The acetabular fossa lies in the inferomedial portion of the acetabulum. This region is occupied by the pulvinar (fat pad) and round ligament (ligamentum teres) (Fig. 6-8). A recently described stellate crease (Fig. 6-9) or bare area exists above the antero-superior margin of the acetabular fossa within the articular area of the acetabulum.

The dense fibrocartilaginous labrum of the acetabulum increases the depth of the acetabulum (Figs. 6-10 and 6-11). In some patients the labrum is intraarticular in location, and in these patients, this may be a predisposing factor for the development of osteoarthritis. Arthroscopically, three distinct gutters can be identified peripheral to the labrum. These include a perilabral sulcus, and the anterior and posterior synovial gutters, which are the margins of the hip joint.[8] The innominate, or hip, bone includes the ilium, ischium, and pubic bones. At birth, the triradiate or Y cartilage, located at the center of the acetabulum, separates the ilium, ischium, and pubis.[9,10] The fovea capitis, a small depression on the medial femoral head, is the site of attachment of the ligamentum teres originating in the acetabular fossa (Fig. 6-12). The ligamentum teres demonstrates a banded, pyramidal morphology (Figs. 6-8 and 6-13). The transverse acetabular ligament bridges the notch at the inferolateral acetabulum and, together with the acetabular labrum, forms a complete ring around the acetabulum (see Fig. 6-13). The femoral head, covered by articular cartilage, forms two thirds of a sphere proximal to its transition into the femoral neck (Fig.

text continues on page 104

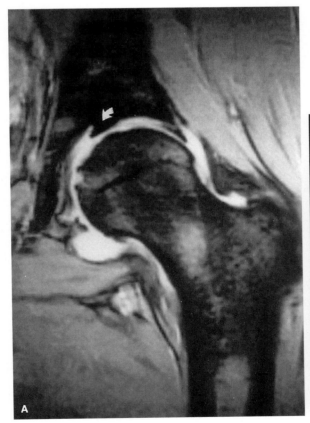
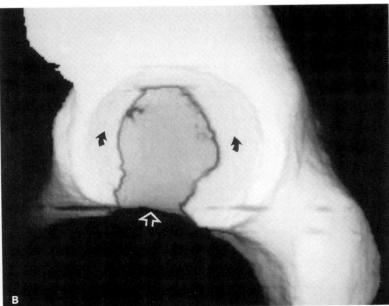

FIGURE 6-6. A normal cortical articular ridge of the acetabulum (*arrow*) is seen on (**A**) T2*-weighted coronal and (**B**) 3D CT images. This bony ridge should not be mistaken for osseous pathology. The acetabular notch (*open arrow*) is shown on 3D CT rendering. (**A:** TR, 400 msec; TE, 20 msec; flip angle, 25°).

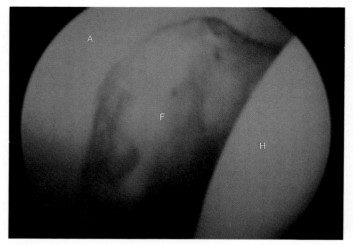

FIGURE 6-7. Anterior view of the lunate surface of the acetabulum (A), the acetabular fossa (F), and the femoral head (H).

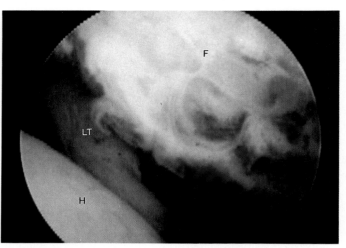

FIGURE 6-8. The ligamentum teres (LT) is shown coursing toward its insertion into the fovea of the femoral head (H). There is tissue deep in the acetabular fossa (F). Arthroscopic view with anterior down and posterior up.

FIGURE 6-9. The stellate crease (*arrows*) is shown above the acetabular fossa (F) and within the lunate surface of the acetabulum. The stellate crease represents a bare area deficient in hyaline cartilage and not degeneration. Arthroscopically, this bare area may appear as an indentation. The femoral head (H) is indicated. Anterior is down and posterior is up.

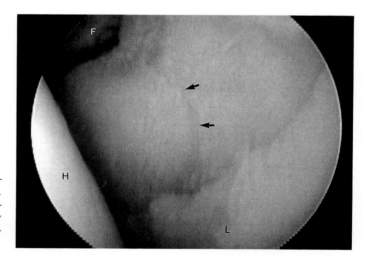

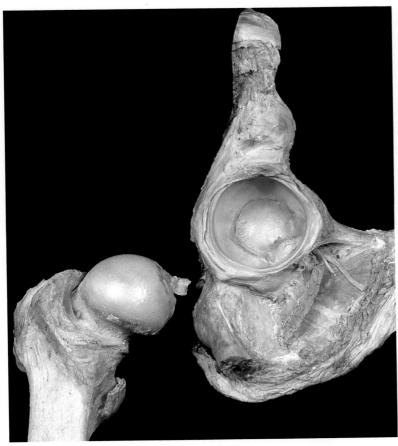

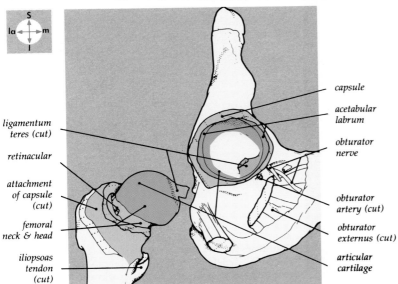

ligamentum
teres (cut)

retinacular

attachment
of capsule
(cut)

femoral
neck & head

iliopsoas
tendon
(cut)

capsule

acetabular
labrum

obturator
nerve

obturator
artery (cut)

obturator
externus (cut)

articular
cartilage

FIGURE 6-10. Internal features are revealed by disarticulation of the joint after cutting the ligamentum teres and joint capsule.

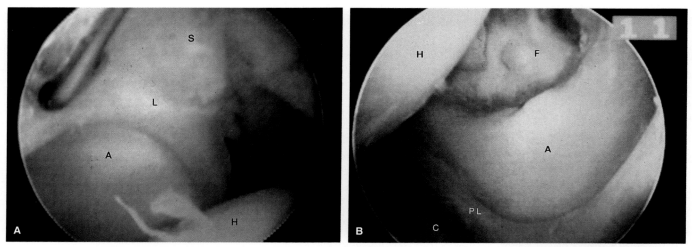

FIGURE 6-11. **(A)** A probe shown on the acetabular labrum (L). The articular area of the acetabulum (A), synovium (S) and femoral head (H) are indicated as seen on an anterior-to-posterior view. **(B)** The posterior labrum (PL) is shown overlying the articular cartilage (A) of the acetabular perimeter. The capsule (C), femoral head (H), and acetabular fossa (F) are demonstrated. Anterior is down and posterior is up.

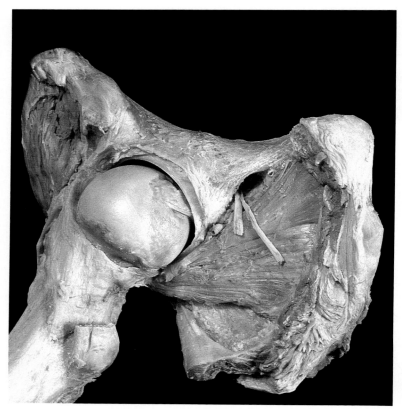

FIGURE 6-12. **(A)** The joint capsule has been opened anteriorly and reflected to show the interior of the joint. The femur has been abducted and externally rotated. *continued*

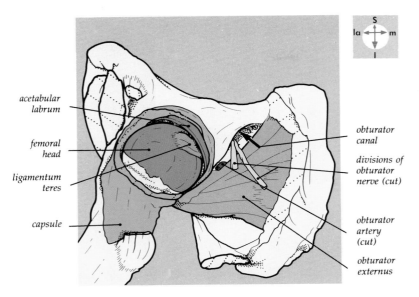

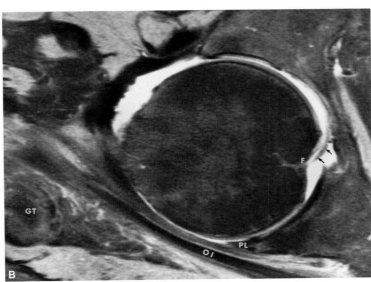

FIGURE 6-12A. *Continued.*

FIGURE 6-12. *Continued.* **(B)** Axial MR arthrogram identifying the fovea (F), ligamentum teres (*arrows*), posterior labrum (PL), obturator internus tendon (OI), and greater trochanter (GT). Fat-suppressed T2-weighted fast spin-echo image.

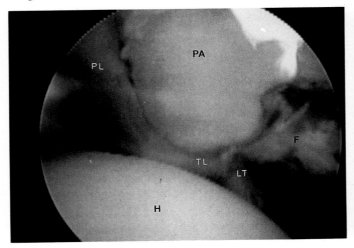

FIGURE 6-13. The transverse ligament (TL) does not need to be continuous with the labrum in completing a ring around the acetabulum. The posterior labrum (PL), ligamentum teres (LT), femoral head (H), posterior acetabulum (PA) and acetabular fossa (F) are identified.

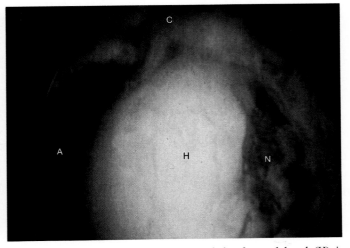

FIGURE 6-14. The articular cartilage of the femoral head (H) is shown. The acetabulum (A), capsule (C), and femoral neck (N) are labeled.

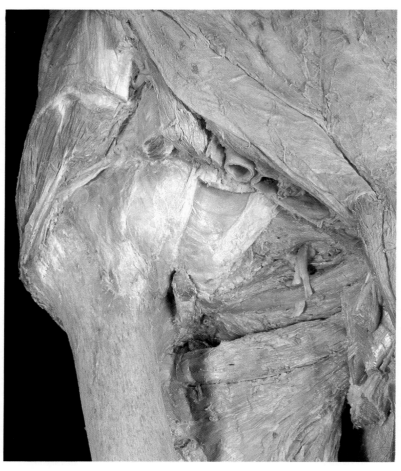

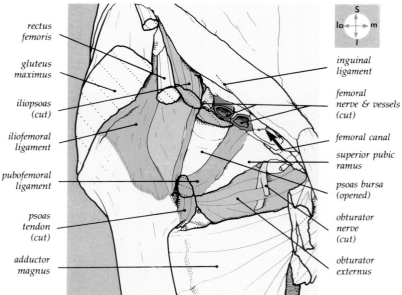

rectus
femoris

gluteus
maximus

iliopsoas
(cut)

iliofemoral
ligament

pubofemoral
ligament

psoas
tendon
(cut)

adductor
magnus

inguinal
ligament

femoral
nerve & vessels
(cut)

femoral canal

superior pubic
ramus

psoas bursa
(opened)

obturator
nerve
(cut)

obturator
externus

FIGURE 6-15. Anterior surface of the joint capsule, associated ligaments, and adjacent structures.

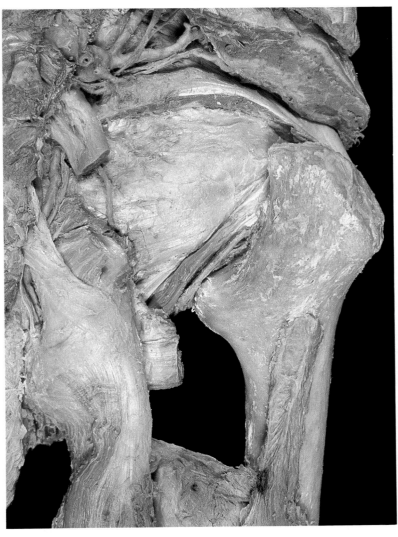

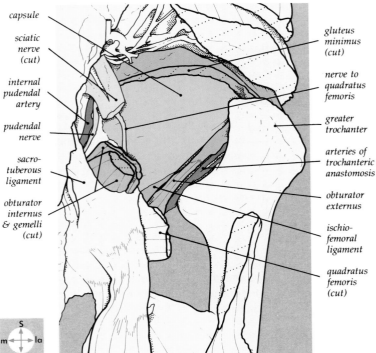

capsule

sciatic
nerve
(cut)

internal
pudendal
artery

pudendal
nerve

sacro-
tuberous
ligament

obturator
internus
& gemelli
(cut)

gluteus
minimus
(cut)

nerve to
quadratus
femoris

greater
trochanter

arteries of
trochanteric
anastomosis

obturator
externus

ischio-
femoral
ligament

quadratus
femoris
(cut)

FIGURE 6-16. Posterior surface of the joint capsule and the ischiofemoral ligament.

6-14). There is no articular cartilage surface over the fovea capitis. The insertion of the ligamentum teres into the fovea fills what has been referred to as a "bare area."[8] The femoral head articular cartilage surface measures 3 mm in its thickest regions posteriorly and superiorly, thinning to 0.5 mm along its peripheral and inferior margins.

The inelastic fibrous capsule of the hip joint is reinforced by the iliofemoral, pubofemoral, and ischiofemoral ligaments (thickenings of the hip capsule) (Figs. 6-15 and 6-16). The iliofemoral ligament, or ligament of Bigelow, is the strongest and thickest of the capsular ligaments and has an inverted Y shape anteriorly. The pubofemoral and ischiofemoral ligaments are less substantial. Deep circular fibers form the ischiofemoral ligament from the zona orbicularis (Fig. 6-17). Arthroscopically, the zona orbicularis may be mistaken for the acetabular labrum.[8] Twisting and shortening of the capsule limits full hip extension. The main hip abductors, the gluteus minimus and gluteus medius, insert on the greater trochanter. The iliopsoas tendon, a major hip flexor, passes anterior to the hip joint and attaches to the lesser trochanter (Fig. 6-18).

The calcar femorale refers to the weight-bearing bone in the femur, radiating from the inferomedial femoral cortex toward the greater trochanter. Weight-bearing stress trabeculae form the boundaries of Ward's triangle in the femoral neck and head. On conventional radiography, Ward's triangle appears as a region of decreased bone density distal to the intersection of femoral neck weight-bearing trabeculae.

The secondary ossification centers of the femoral head, the greater and lesser trochanters, appear at 4 to 7 months of fetal development. In the adult, the mean femoral neck shaft angle is 125°, and femoral anteversion averages 14°. The neck shaft and femoral anteversion angles decrease during skeletal maturation. The intertrochanteric line between the greater and lesser trochanters is the attachment site of

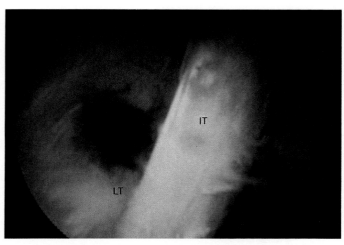

FIGURE 6-18. Arthroscopic view of the iliopsoas tendon (IT) relative to its lesser trochanter (LT) insertion. The iliopsoas flexes, laterally rotates, and adducts the thigh.

the iliofemoral ligament. Therefore, it can be seen that 95% of the femoral neck is intracapsular. This has implications for the hip joint in cases of osteomyelitis of the proximal femoral metaphysis. Since this area is intraarticular, the hip joint may become secondarily infected.

The medial and lateral circumflex arteries provide most of the blood supply to the femoral head and proximal femur through anastomotic rings at the base of the femoral neck and head. Fractures involving the femoral neck can damage the blood supply to the femoral head leading to osteonecrosis. The lateral part of the extracapsular arterial ring provides most of the blood supply to the femoral head. The obturator artery provides a variable vascular supply to the femoral head through the ligamentum teres.

Normal Magnetic Resonance Appearance of the Hip

Axial Images

The axial plane displays the relationship between the femoral head and the acetabulum with supporting musculature on cross-sectional gross images (Fig. 6-19) and MR scans (Fig. 6-20). Axial images made at the level of the acetabular roof may show a partial volume effect with the femoral head. Signal intensity inhomogeneity within the acetabulum is secondary to a greater distribution of red (hematopoietic) marrow stores. The hip musculature demonstrates intermediate signal intensity on T1-weighted images. The gluteal muscles—the gluteus medius laterally, the gluteus minimus deep, and the gluteus maximus posteriorly—can be differentiated from one another by high signal intensity fat along fascial divisions. The tensor fasciae latae muscle

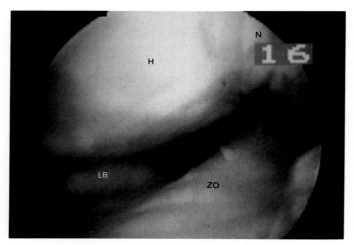

FIGURE 6-17. The zona orbicularis (ZO), femoral head (H) and neck (N), and associated loose body (LB) are demonstrated. The zona orbicularis is a capsular condensation, which should not be mistaken for the acetabular labrum.

text continues on page 111

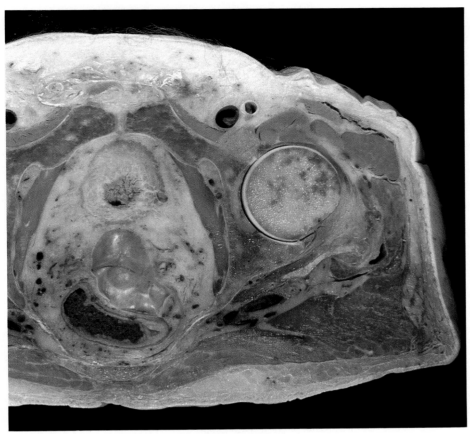

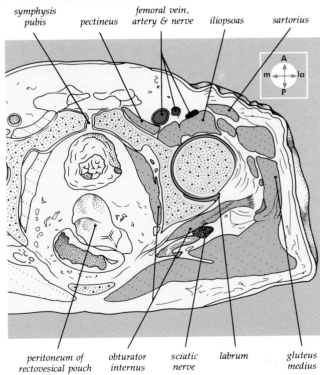

FIGURE 6-19. A transverse section through the hip joint shows its anatomic relations.

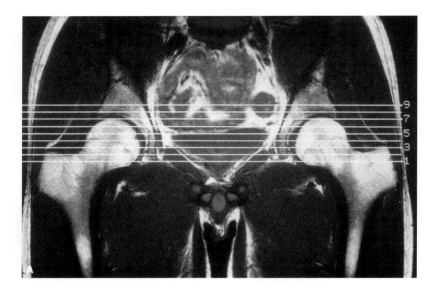

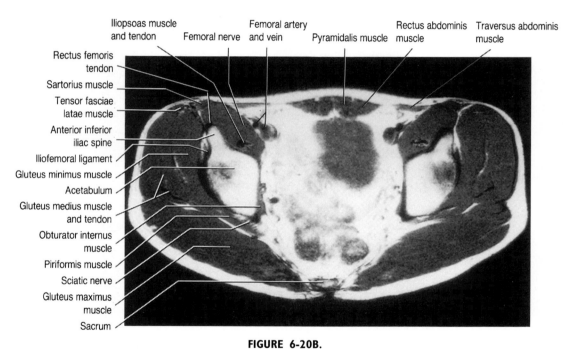

Iliopsoas muscle and tendon
Femoral nerve
Femoral artery and vein
Pyramidalis muscle
Rectus abdominis muscle
Traversus abdominis muscle

Rectus femoris tendon
Sartorius muscle
Tensor fasciae latae muscle
Anterior inferior iliac spine
Iliofemoral ligament
Gluteus minimus muscle
Acetabulum
Gluteus medius muscle and tendon
Obturator internus muscle
Piriformis muscle
Sciatic nerve
Gluteus maximus muscle
Sacrum

FIGURE 6-20B.

FIGURE 6-20. Normal axial MR anatomy. (**A**) Coronal localizer used to graphically prescribe axial T1-weighted image locations from superior to inferior (**B** through **J**, respectively). *continued*

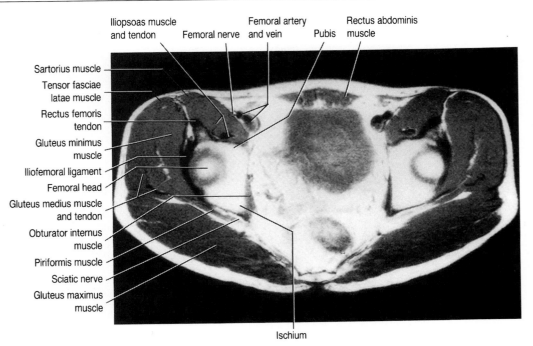

Iliopsoas muscle and tendon

Femoral nerve

Femoral artery and vein

Pubis

Rectus abdominis muscle

Sartorius muscle

Tensor fasciae latae muscle

Rectus femoris tendon

Gluteus minimus muscle

Iliofemoral ligament

Femoral head

Gluteus medius muscle and tendon

Obturator internus muscle

Piriformis muscle

Sciatic nerve

Gluteus maximus muscle

Ischium

FIGURE 6-20C.

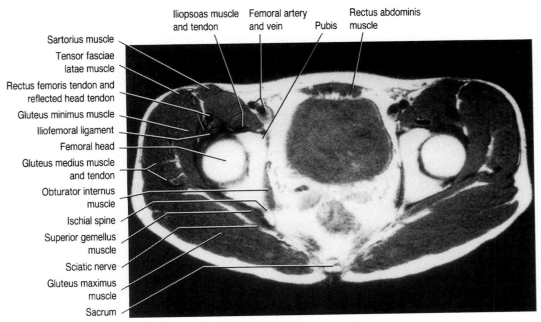

Iliopsoas muscle and tendon

Femoral artery and vein

Pubis

Rectus abdominis muscle

Sartorius muscle

Tensor fasciae latae muscle

Rectus femoris tendon and reflected head tendon

Gluteus minimus muscle

Iliofemoral ligament

Femoral head

Gluteus medius muscle and tendon

Obturator internus muscle

Ischial spine

Superior gemellus muscle

Sciatic nerve

Gluteus maximus muscle

Sacrum

FIGURE 6-20D.

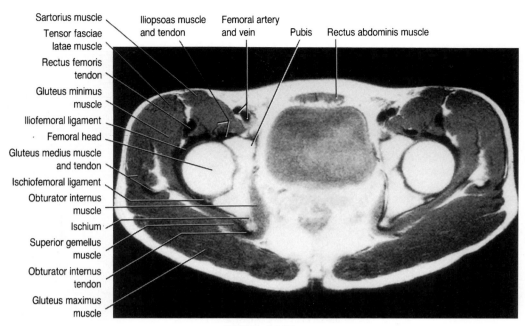

Sartorius muscle
Tensor fasciae latae muscle
Rectus femoris tendon
Gluteus minimus muscle
Iliofemoral ligament
Femoral head
Gluteus medius muscle and tendon
Ischiofemoral ligament
Obturator internus muscle
Ischium
Superior gemellus muscle
Obturator internus tendon
Gluteus maximus muscle

Iliopsoas muscle and tendon
Femoral artery and vein
Pubis
Rectus abdominis muscle

FIGURE 6-20E.

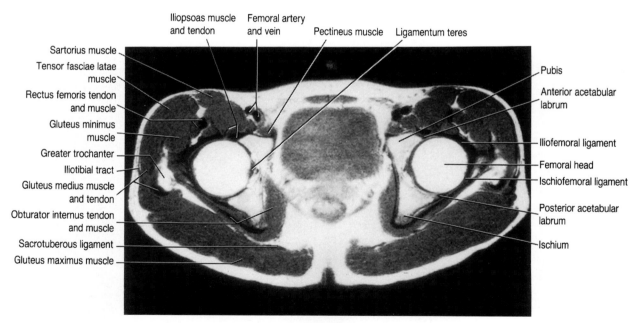

Sartorius muscle
Tensor fasciae latae muscle
Rectus femoris tendon and muscle
Gluteus minimus muscle
Greater trochanter
Iliotibial tract
Gluteus medius muscle and tendon
Obturator internus tendon and muscle
Sacrotuberous ligament
Gluteus maximus muscle

Iliopsoas muscle and tendon
Femoral artery and vein
Pectineus muscle
Ligamentum teres

Pubis
Anterior acetabular labrum
Iliofemoral ligament
Femoral head
Ischiofemoral ligament
Posterior acetabular labrum
Ischium

FIGURE 6-20F.

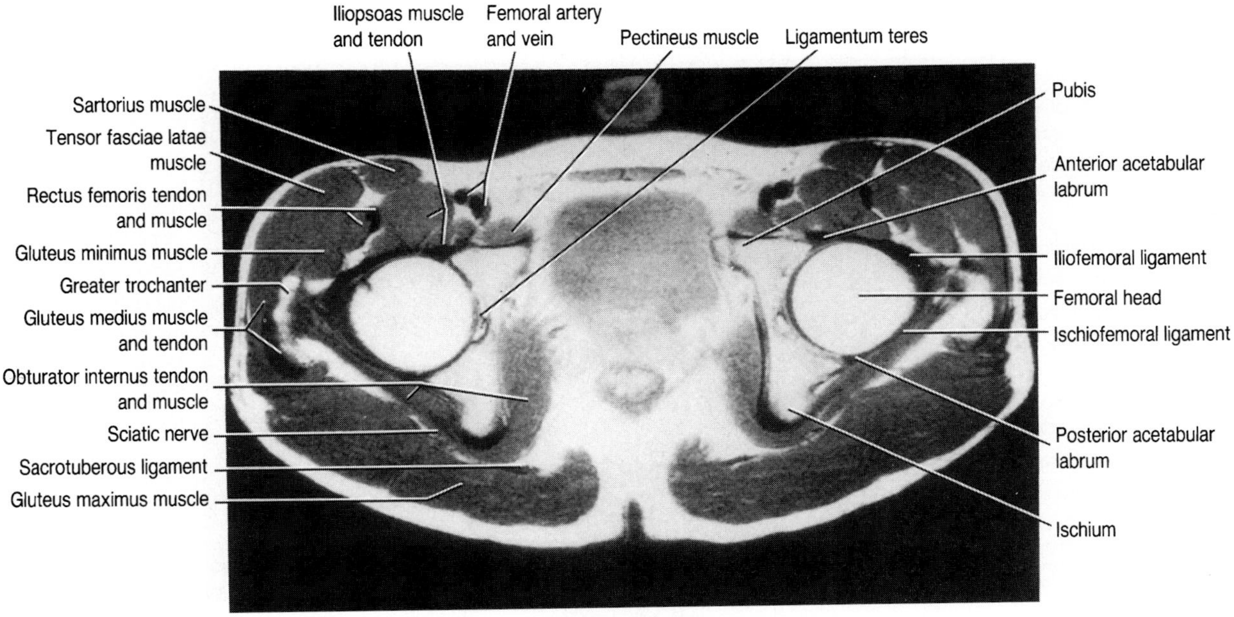

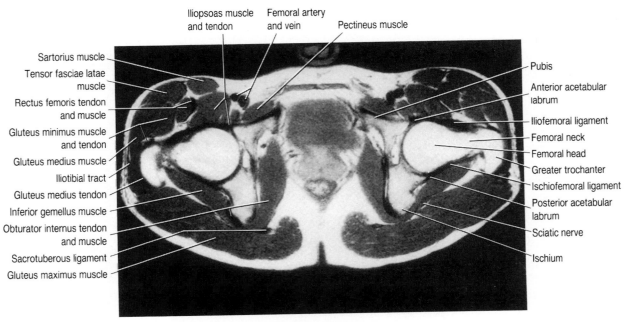

FIGURE 6-20G.

FIGURE 6-20H.

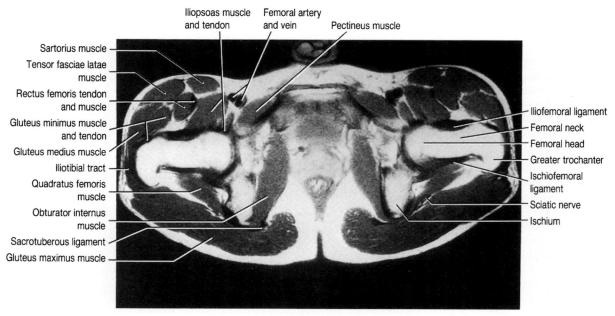

FIGURE 6-20I.

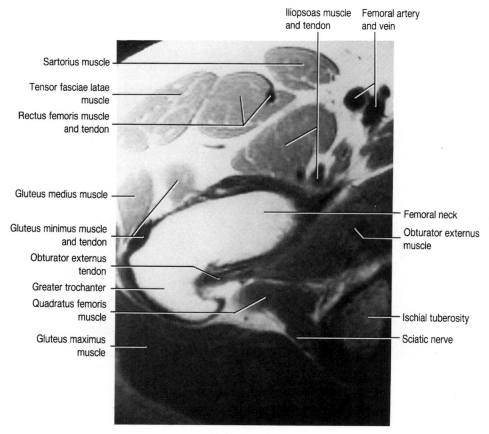

FIGURE 6-20J.

is seen anterior to the gluteus medius and is bordered anteriorly by subcutaneous fat. The iliopsoas muscle group is anterior to the femoral head in a 12-o'clock position. The sartorius muscle is the most anterior, and the rectus femoris is positioned between the more lateral tensor fasciae latae and the medial iliopsoas. The obturator internus muscle is visualized medial to the anterior and posterior acetabular columns.

The sciatic nerve, located directly posterior to the posterior column of the acetabulum, demonstrates intermediate signal intensity. It exits the pelvis through the greater sciatic foramen (the greater sciatic foramen is bordered by the ilium, the rim of the greater sciatic notch, the sacrotuberous ligament, and the sacrospinous ligament) inferior to the piriformis muscle. Entrapment of the sciatic nerve at this location may be associated with the piriformis syndrome. Asymptomatic hypertrophy of the piriformis muscle in this syndrome is best appreciated on axial images. The piriformis originates from the anterior sacrum and greater sciatic notch, and inserts on the upper border of the greater trochanter. The piriformis divides the greater sciatic foramen into superior and inferior portions. The external iliac vessels, which are of low signal intensity, are medial to the iliopsoas muscle and anterior to the anterior acetabular column. The low signal intensity tendon of the rectus femoris blends with the low signal intensity cortex of the anterior inferior iliac spine. The tendon of the reflected head of the rectus femoris muscle is anterolateral to the iliofemoral ligament and follows the contours of the lateral acetabulum. At the level of the femoral head, the more distal femoral artery and vein are visualized. The femoral head articular cartilage demonstrates intermediate signal intensity, and the anterior and posterior fibrocartilaginous acetabular labrum may also be identified at this level. The acetabular labrum is triangular, with the apex oriented laterally.

At the level of the greater trochanter and femoral neck, the obturator internus is identified medial to the pubis and ischium. The iliofemoral ligament is of low signal intensity and blends with the dark (ie, low signal intensity) cortex of the anterior femoral neck. The sciatic nerve, lateral to the ischial tuberosity, is encased in fat between the quadratus femoris muscle anteriorly and the gluteus maximus muscle posteriorly. The iliotibial tract can be seen peripherally as a thin, low signal intensity band surrounded by high signal intensity fat on the medial and lateral surfaces. The low signal intensity obturator vessels are encased in high signal intensity fat and can be identified posterolateral to the pubic bone, between the pectineus and obturator internus muscles. The adductor muscles anteromedially, the obturator externus and the quadratus femoris muscles medially, the ischial tuberosity attachment of the long head of the biceps femoris, and the semitendinosus tendons posteriorly, can be visualized at the level of the proximal femur. The ischiofemoral ligament is also identified anterior to the quadratus femoris,

medial to the ischium, and applied to the posterior hip capsule. The sacrotuberous ligament is seen posteromedial to the ischium.

Sagittal Images

The gluteus medius muscle and the tendon attachment to the greater trochanter are demonstrated on lateral sagittal images (Fig. 6-21). The tendon of the obturator externus is anterior and inferior to the greater trochanter. The piriformis tendon is situated between the iliofemoral ligament anteriorly and the gluteus medius tendon posteriorly. On lateral sagittal images, the ilium, the anterior inferior iliac spine, the acetabular roof, and the femoral head are seen on the same sagittal section. The iliofemoral ligament extends inferiorly, directly anterior to the anterior acetabular labrum. The iliopsoas muscle and tendon course obliquely anterior to the iliofemoral ligament, anterior to the femoral head. The ischiofemoral ligament is closely applied to the surface of the posterior femoral head, anterior to the inferior gemellus muscle and obturator internus tendon. The femoral physeal scar is seen as a horizontal band of low signal intensity, in an anterior to posterior orientation. In the sagittal plane, the intermediate signal intensity hyaline cartilage of the femoral head and acetabulum can be separately defined, and the posterior gluteal and anterior rectus femoris muscles are displayed in the long axis.

Distally, the vastus musculature is seen anterior to the proximal femoral diaphysis, and the biceps femoris is viewed posteriorly. The sciatic nerve can be followed longitudinally between the anterior quadratus femoris and the posterior gluteus maximus. The low signal intensity attachment of the sartorius to the anterosuperior iliac spine is shown anteriorly on sagittal images. The low signal intensity iliopsoas tendon spans the hip joint anteriorly, crossing to its insertion on the lesser trochanter. The adductor muscle group is displayed inferior to and medial to the iliopsoas tendon and the pectineus muscle.

On medial sagittal images, the acetabulum encompasses 75% of the femoral head, and the low signal intensity transverse acetabular ligament bridges the uncovered anterior inferior gap. On extreme medial images through the hip joint, the ligamentum teres may be seen within the acetabular fossa. At this level, the ischial tuberosity can be seen posterior and inferior to the acetabular fossa.

Coronal Images

The coronal plane is used in the evaluation of the acetabular labrum, the hip joint space, and the subchondral acetabular and femoral marrow, as seen on coronal gross (Fig. 6-22) and MR (Fig. 6-23) sections. Acetabular and femoral head articular cartilage may be more difficult to separate on coronal images than on sagittal images. The fibrocartilaginous limbus, or acetabular labrum, is visualized as a low

text continues on page 121

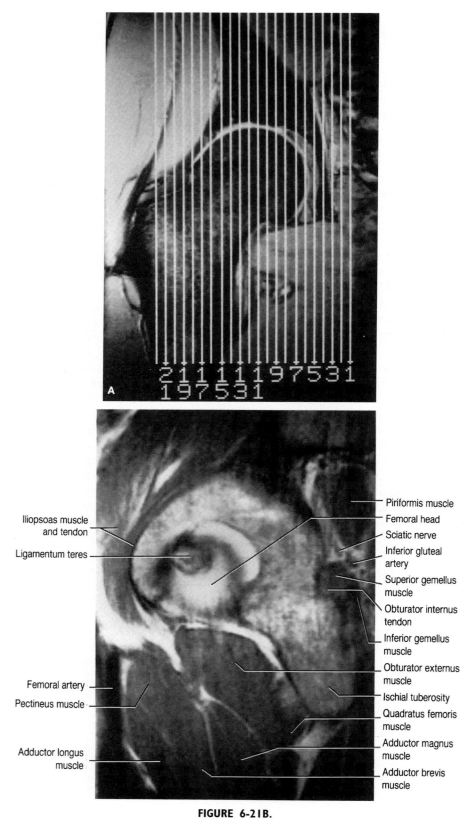

FIGURE 6-21B.

FIGURE 6-21. Normal sagittal MR anatomy. (**A**) T2*-weighted coronal localizer used to graphically prescribe sagittal T1-weighted image locations from medial to lateral (**B** through **O**, respectively).

continued

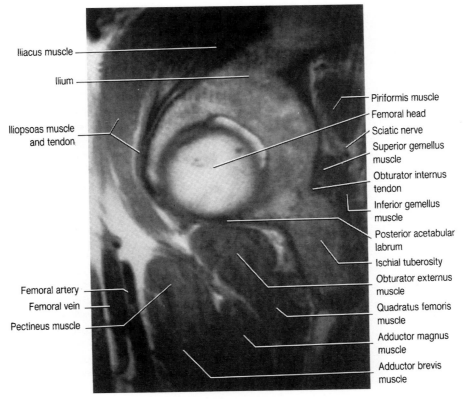

Iliacus muscle
Ilium
Iliopsoas muscle and tendon
Femoral artery
Femoral vein
Pectineus muscle

Piriformis muscle
Femoral head
Sciatic nerve
Superior gemellus muscle
Obturator internus tendon
Inferior gemellus muscle
Posterior acetabular labrum
Ischial tuberosity
Obturator externus muscle
Quadratus femoris muscle
Adductor magnus muscle
Adductor brevis muscle

FIGURE 6-21C.

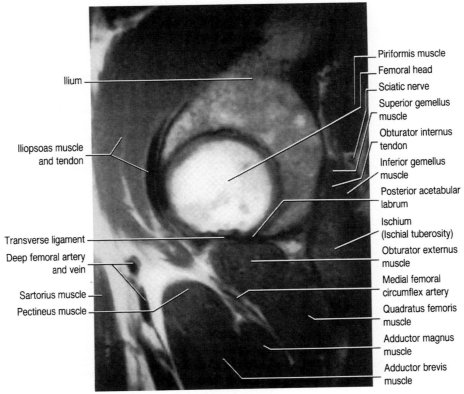

Ilium
Iliopsoas muscle and tendon
Transverse ligament
Deep femoral artery and vein
Sartorius muscle
Pectineus muscle

Piriformis muscle
Femoral head
Sciatic nerve
Superior gemellus muscle
Obturator internus tendon
Inferior gemellus muscle
Posterior acetabular labrum
Ischium (Ischial tuberosity)
Obturator externus muscle
Medial femoral circumflex artery
Quadratus femoris muscle
Adductor magnus muscle
Adductor brevis muscle

FIGURE 6-21D.

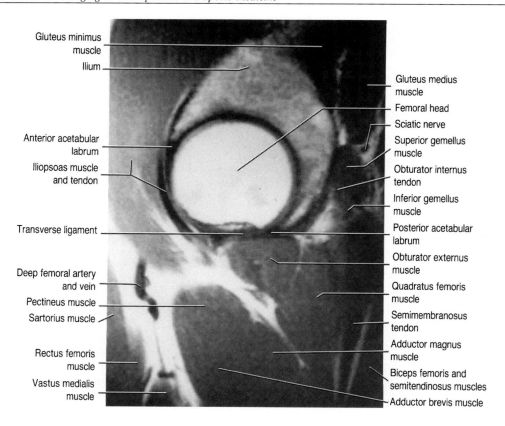

Gluteus minimus muscle

Ilium

Anterior acetabular labrum

Iliopsoas muscle and tendon

Transverse ligament

Deep femoral artery and vein

Pectineus muscle

Sartorius muscle

Rectus femoris muscle

Vastus medialis muscle

Gluteus medius muscle

Femoral head

Sciatic nerve

Superior gemellus muscle

Obturator internus tendon

Inferior gemellus muscle

Posterior acetabular labrum

Obturator externus muscle

Quadratus femoris muscle

Semimembranosus tendon

Adductor magnus muscle

Biceps femoris and semitendinosus muscles

Adductor brevis muscle

FIGURE 6-21E.

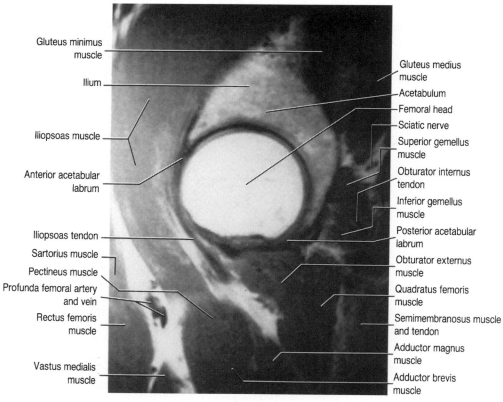

Gluteus minimus muscle

Ilium

Iliopsoas muscle

Anterior acetabular labrum

Iliopsoas tendon

Sartorius muscle

Pectineus muscle

Profunda femoral artery and vein

Rectus femoris muscle

Vastus medialis muscle

Gluteus medius muscle

Acetabulum

Femoral head

Sciatic nerve

Superior gemellus muscle

Obturator internus tendon

Inferior gemellus muscle

Posterior acetabular labrum

Obturator externus muscle

Quadratus femoris muscle

Semimembranosus muscle and tendon

Adductor magnus muscle

Adductor brevis muscle

FIGURE 6-21F.

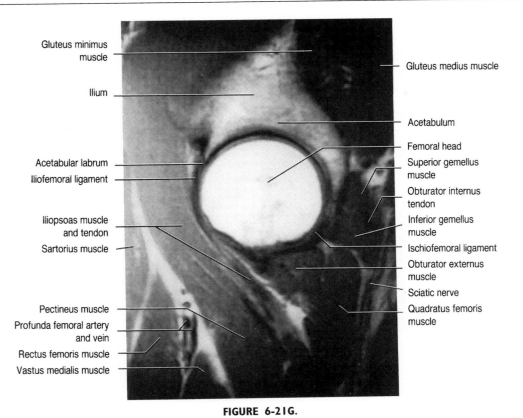

Gluteus minimus muscle

Ilium

Acetabular labrum

Iliofemoral ligament

Iliopsoas muscle and tendon

Sartorius muscle

Pectineus muscle

Profunda femoral artery and vein

Rectus femoris muscle

Vastus medialis muscle

Gluteus medius muscle

Acetabulum

Femoral head

Superior gemellus muscle

Obturator internus tendon

Inferior gemellus muscle

Ischiofemoral ligament

Obturator externus muscle

Sciatic nerve

Quadratus femoris muscle

FIGURE 6-21G.

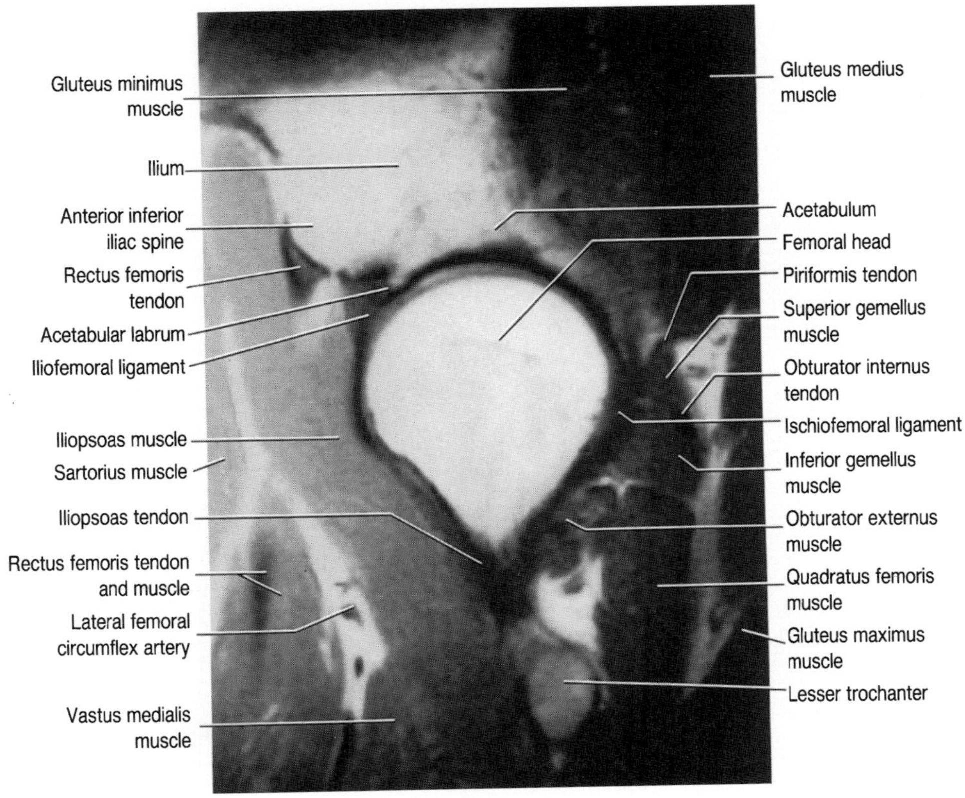

Gluteus minimus muscle

Ilium

Anterior inferior iliac spine

Rectus femoris tendon

Acetabular labrum

Iliofemoral ligament

Iliopsoas muscle

Sartorius muscle

Iliopsoas tendon

Rectus femoris tendon and muscle

Lateral femoral circumflex artery

Vastus medialis muscle

Gluteus medius muscle

Acetabulum

Femoral head

Piriformis tendon

Superior gemellus muscle

Obturator internus tendon

Ischiofemoral ligament

Inferior gemellus muscle

Obturator externus muscle

Quadratus femoris muscle

Gluteus maximus muscle

Lesser trochanter

FIGURE 6-21H.

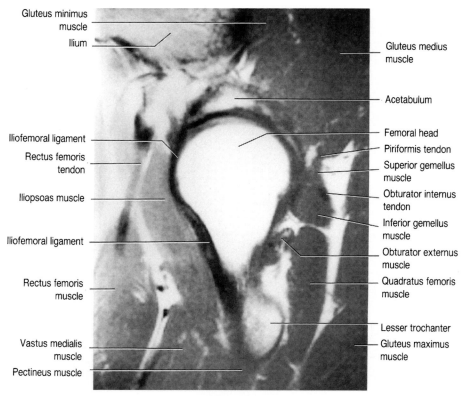

Gluteus minimus muscle

Ilium

Gluteus medius muscle

Acetabulum

Iliofemoral ligament

Rectus femoris tendon

Femoral head

Piriformis tendon

Superior gemellus muscle

Iliopsoas muscle

Obturator internus tendon

Inferior gemellus muscle

Iliofemoral ligament

Obturator externus muscle

Rectus femoris muscle

Quadratus femoris muscle

Vastus medialis muscle

Lesser trochanter

Gluteus maximus muscle

Pectineus muscle

FIGURE 6-21I.

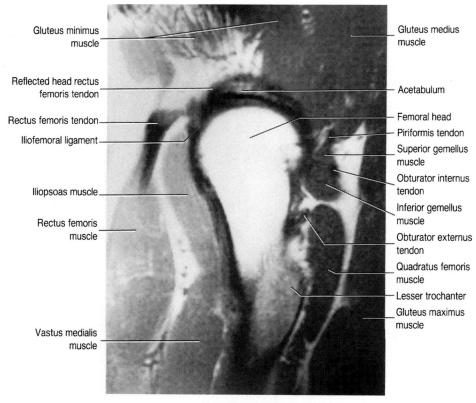

Gluteus minimus muscle

Gluteus medius muscle

Reflected head rectus femoris tendon

Acetabulum

Rectus femoris tendon

Femoral head

Iliofemoral ligament

Piriformis tendon

Superior gemellus muscle

Iliopsoas muscle

Obturator internus tendon

Inferior gemellus muscle

Rectus femoris muscle

Obturator externus tendon

Quadratus femoris muscle

Lesser trochanter

Gluteus maximus muscle

Vastus medialis muscle

FIGURE 6-21J.

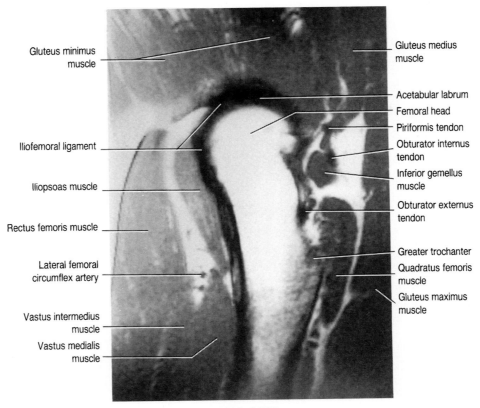

Gluteus minimus muscle

Gluteus medius muscle

Acetabular labrum

Femoral head

Piriformis tendon

Obturator internus tendon

Iliofemoral ligament

Inferior gemellus muscle

Iliopsoas muscle

Obturator externus tendon

Rectus femoris muscle

Greater trochanter

Lateral femoral circumflex artery

Quadratus femoris muscle

Gluteus maximus muscle

Vastus intermedius muscle

Vastus medialis muscle

FIGURE 6-21K.

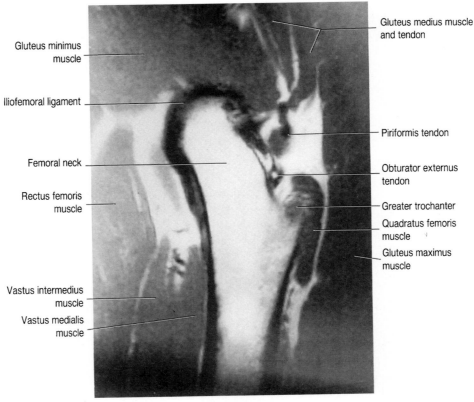

Gluteus minimus muscle

Gluteus medius muscle and tendon

Iliofemoral ligament

Piriformis tendon

Femoral neck

Obturator externus tendon

Rectus femoris muscle

Greater trochanter

Quadratus femoris muscle

Gluteus maximus muscle

Vastus intermedius muscle

Vastus medialis muscle

FIGURE 6-21L.

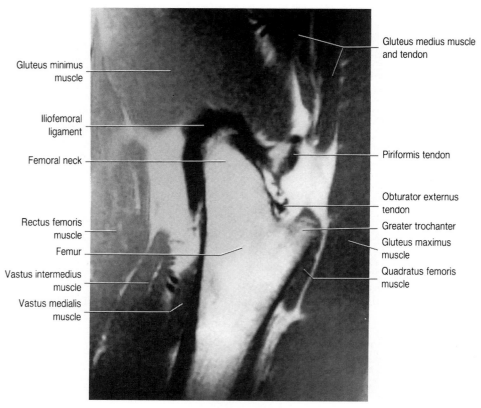

Gluteus minimus muscle

Iliofemoral ligament

Femoral neck

Rectus femoris muscle

Femur

Vastus intermedius muscle

Vastus medialis muscle

Gluteus medius muscle and tendon

Piriformis tendon

Obturator externus tendon

Greater trochanter

Gluteus maximus muscle

Quadratus femoris muscle

FIGURE 6-21M.

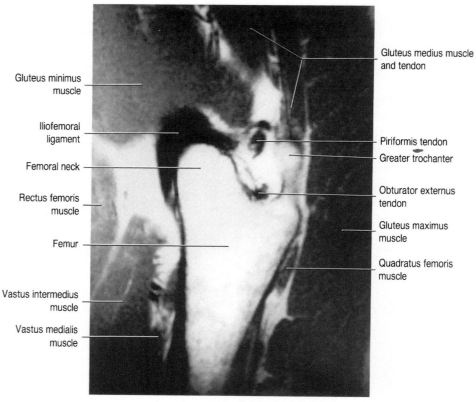

Gluteus minimus muscle

Iliofemoral ligament

Femoral neck

Rectus femoris muscle

Femur

Vastus intermedius muscle

Vastus medialis muscle

Gluteus medius muscle and tendon

Piriformis tendon

Greater trochanter

Obturator externus tendon

Gluteus maximus muscle

Quadratus femoris muscle

FIGURE 6-21N.

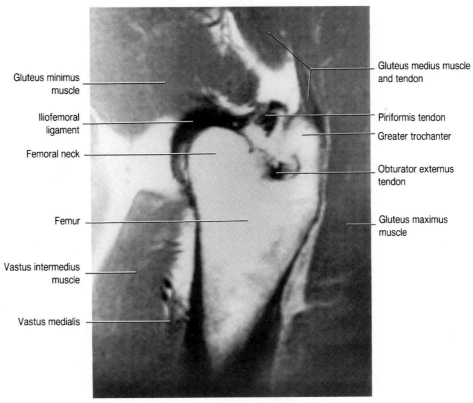

Gluteus minimus muscle

Iliofemoral ligament

Femoral neck

Femur

Vastus intermedius muscle

Vastus medialis

Gluteus medius muscle and tendon

Piriformis tendon

Greater trochanter

Obturator externus tendon

Gluteus maximus muscle

FIGURE 6-210.

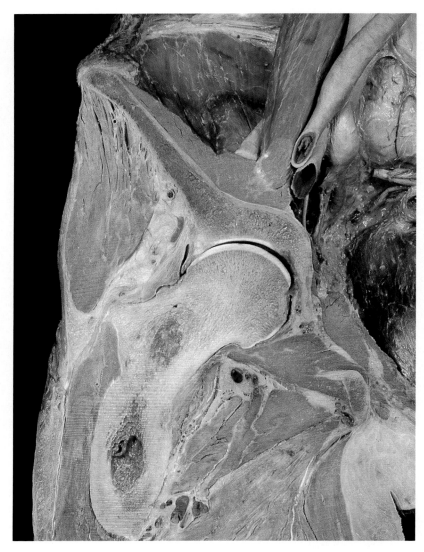

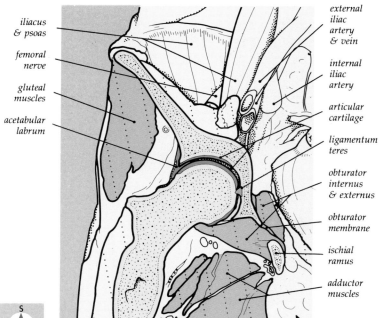

iliacus & psoas

femoral nerve

gluteal muscles

acetabular labrum

external iliac artery & vein

internal iliac artery

articular cartilage

ligamentum teres

obturator internus & externus

obturator membrane

ischial ramus

adductor muscles

FIGURE 6-22. (A) A coronal section through the hip joint shows its anatomic relations. *continued*

A

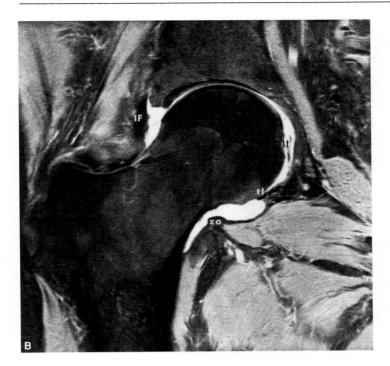

FIGURE 6-22. *Continued.* **(B)** Coronal MR arthrogram displaying hip joint and capsular anatomy. The distal insertion of the capsule is at the base of the femoral neck. The zona orbicularis (zo) is seen as an area of capsular thickening and tightening over the middle of the femoral neck. The transverse ligament (tl), iliofemoral ligament (IF) and ligamentum teres (lt) are identified. The acetabular labrum is absent. This coronal MR section cuts through the supraarticular recess, the infraarticular recess, and the recess colli (the recess at the base of the femoral neck). Fat-suppressed T2-weighted fast spin-echo image.

signal intensity triangle interposed between the superolateral aspect of the femoral head and the inferolateral aspect of the acetabulum. The joint capsule is visualized as a low signal intensity structure circumscribing the femoral neck. In the presence of fluid, the capsule distends and the lateral and medial margins become convex. Anterior coronal images demonstrate that the articular cartilage of the femoral head can be seen medially at the ligamentum teres insertion site. The reflected head of the rectus femoris is shown lateral to the proximal portion of the iliofemoral ligament.

Anteriorly, the iliopsoas muscle and tendon are in a 7-o'clock position relative to the femoral head. The low signal intensity iliofemoral ligament is present on the lateral aspect of the femoral neck, near the greater trochanter. The superior acetabular labrum is located deep to the proximal portion of the iliofemoral ligament along the lateral inferior margin of the acetabulum. The orbicular zone may be identified as a small outpouching on the medial aspect of the junction of the femoral head and neck. The intraarticular femoral fat pad is located between the medial femoral head and the acetabulum, and displays increased signal intensity on T1-weighted images. The obturator externus muscle crosses the femoral neck on posterior coronal images. Inhomogeneity of marrow signal intensity in the acetabulum, ilium, and ischium is a normal finding on T1-weighted images. This represents normal red and yellow marrow inhomogeneity.

text continues on page 127

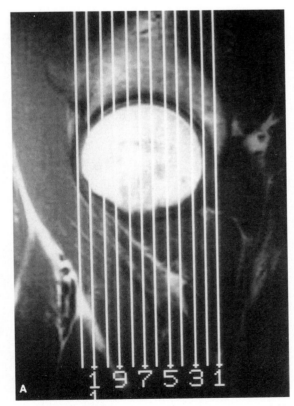

FIGURE 6-23. Normal coronal MR anatomy. **(A)** Sagittal localizer used to graphically prescribe coronal T1-weighted image location from **(B)** anterior to **(L)** posterior.   *continued*

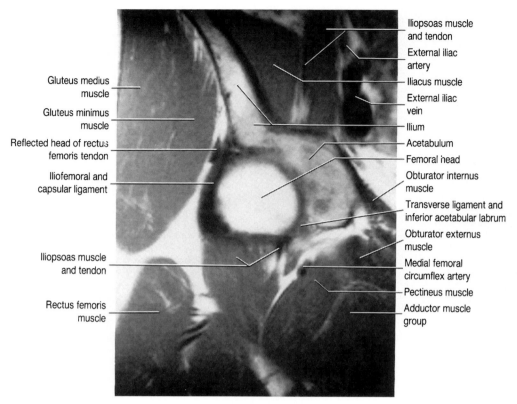

Gluteus medius muscle

Gluteus minimus muscle

Reflected head of rectus femoris tendon

Iliofemoral and capsular ligament

Iliopsoas muscle and tendon

Rectus femoris muscle

Iliopsoas muscle and tendon

External iliac artery

Iliacus muscle

External iliac vein

Ilium

Acetabulum

Femoral head

Obturator internus muscle

Transverse ligament and inferior acetabular labrum

Obturator externus muscle

Medial femoral circumflex artery

Pectineus muscle

Adductor muscle group

FIGURE 6-23B.

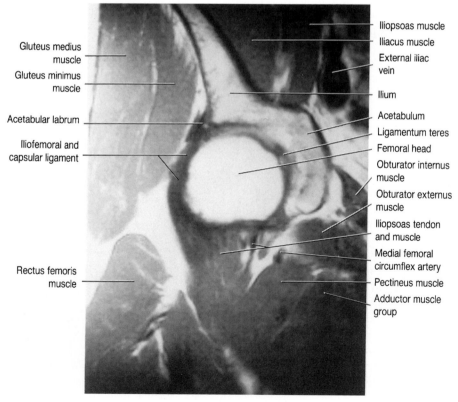

Gluteus medius muscle

Gluteus minimus muscle

Acetabular labrum

Iliofemoral and capsular ligament

Rectus femoris muscle

Iliopsoas muscle

Iliacus muscle

External iliac vein

Ilium

Acetabulum

Ligamentum teres

Femoral head

Obturator internus muscle

Obturator externus muscle

Iliopsoas tendon and muscle

Medial femoral circumflex artery

Pectineus muscle

Adductor muscle group

FIGURE 6-23C.

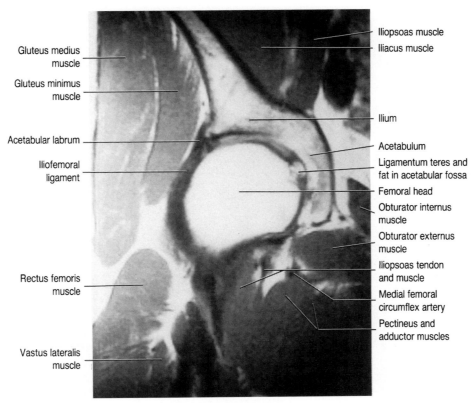

Gluteus medius muscle

Gluteus minimus muscle

Acetabular labrum

Iliofemoral ligament

Rectus femoris muscle

Vastus lateralis muscle

Iliopsoas muscle

Iliacus muscle

Ilium

Acetabulum

Ligamentum teres and fat in acetabular fossa

Femoral head

Obturator internus muscle

Obturator externus muscle

Iliopsoas tendon and muscle

Medial femoral circumflex artery

Pectineus and adductor muscles

FIGURE 6-23D.

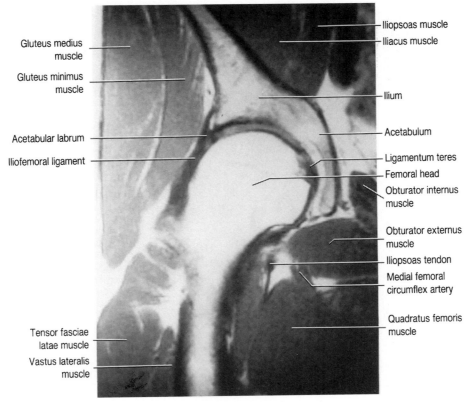

Gluteus medius muscle

Gluteus minimus muscle

Acetabular labrum

Iliofemoral ligament

Tensor fasciae latae muscle

Vastus lateralis muscle

Iliopsoas muscle

Iliacus muscle

Ilium

Acetabulum

Ligamentum teres

Femoral head

Obturator internus muscle

Obturator externus muscle

Iliopsoas tendon

Medial femoral circumflex artery

Quadratus femoris muscle

FIGURE 6-23E.

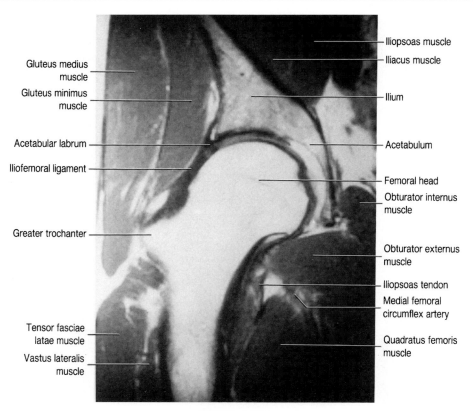

Gluteus medius muscle

Gluteus minimus muscle

Acetabular labrum

Iliofemoral ligament

Greater trochanter

Tensor fasciae latae muscle

Vastus lateralis muscle

Iliopsoas muscle

Iliacus muscle

Ilium

Acetabulum

Femoral head

Obturator internus muscle

Obturator externus muscle

Iliopsoas tendon

Medial femoral circumflex artery

Quadratus femoris muscle

FIGURE 6-23F.

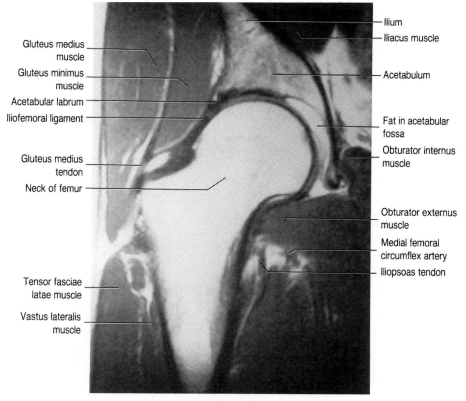

Gluteus medius muscle

Gluteus minimus muscle

Acetabular labrum

Iliofemoral ligament

Gluteus medius tendon

Neck of femur

Tensor fasciae latae muscle

Vastus lateralis muscle

Ilium

Iliacus muscle

Acetabulum

Fat in acetabular fossa

Obturator internus muscle

Obturator externus muscle

Medial femoral circumflex artery

Iliopsoas tendon

FIGURE 6-23G.

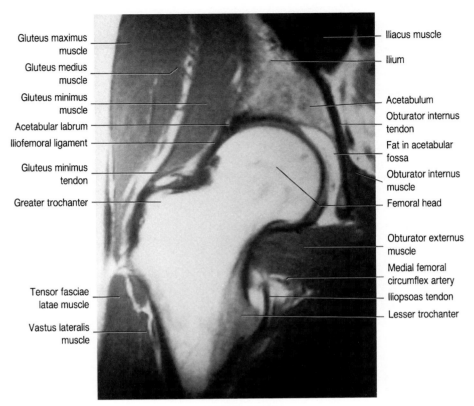

Gluteus maximus muscle
Gluteus medius muscle
Gluteus minimus muscle
Acetabular labrum
Iliofemoral ligament
Gluteus minimus tendon
Greater trochanter
Tensor fasciae latae muscle
Vastus lateralis muscle

Iliacus muscle
Ilium
Acetabulum
Obturator internus tendon
Fat in acetabular fossa
Obturator internus muscle
Femoral head
Obturator externus muscle
Medial femoral circumflex artery
Iliopsoas tendon
Lesser trochanter

FIGURE 6-23H.

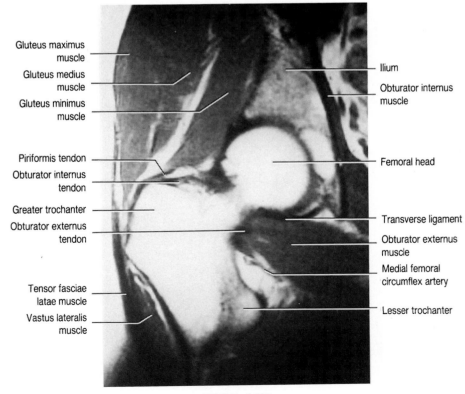

Gluteus maximus muscle
Gluteus medius muscle
Gluteus minimus muscle
Piriformis tendon
Obturator internus tendon
Greater trochanter
Obturator externus tendon
Tensor fasciae latae muscle
Vastus lateralis muscle

Ilium
Obturator internus muscle
Femoral head
Transverse ligament
Obturator externus muscle
Medial femoral circumflex artery
Lesser trochanter

FIGURE 6-23I.

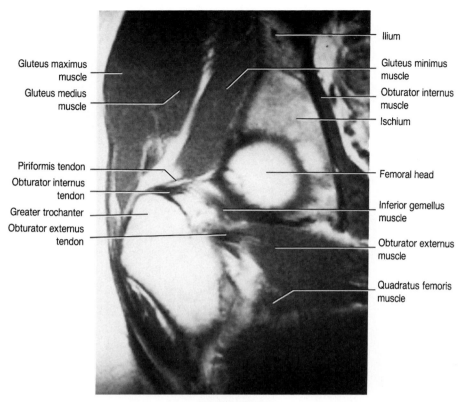

Gluteus maximus muscle

Gluteus medius muscle

Piriformis tendon

Obturator internus tendon

Greater trochanter

Obturator externus tendon

Ilium

Gluteus minimus muscle

Obturator internus muscle

Ischium

Femoral head

Inferior gemellus muscle

Obturator externus muscle

Quadratus femoris muscle

FIGURE 6-23J.

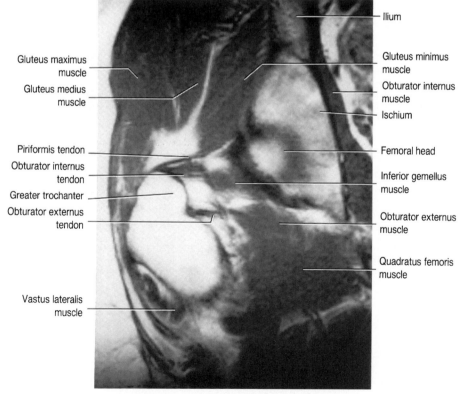

Gluteus maximus muscle

Gluteus medius muscle

Piriformis tendon

Obturator internus tendon

Greater trochanter

Obturator externus tendon

Vastus lateralis muscle

Ilium

Gluteus minimus muscle

Obturator internus muscle

Ischium

Femoral head

Inferior gemellus muscle

Obturator externus muscle

Quadratus femoris muscle

FIGURE 6-23K.

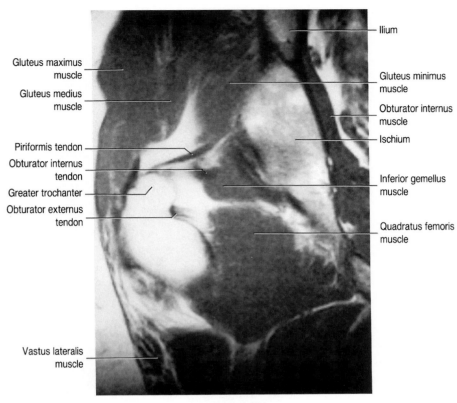

Gluteus maximus muscle

Gluteus medius muscle

Piriformis tendon

Obturator internus tendon

Greater trochanter

Obturator externus tendon

Vastus lateralis muscle

Ilium

Gluteus minimus muscle

Obturator internus muscle

Ischium

Inferior gemellus muscle

Quadratus femoris muscle

FIGURE 6-23L.

PATHOLOGY OF THE HIP

Avascular Necrosis

Avascular necrosis (AVN) of bone most commonly involves the femoral head. It is usually caused by trauma, typically occurring after a displaced femoral neck fracture and less frequently after a fracture-dislocation of the hip. Necrosis results when the vascular supply to the femoral head is disrupted at the time of injury. Nontraumatic AVN occurs in a younger population and is commonly bilateral.[11] Although the etiology is not well understood, a popular theory suggests a vascular etiology secondary to fat embolism, which leads to inflammation and focal intravascular coagulation.[12] Nontraumatic AVN is associated with several clinical conditions such as alcoholism, hypercortisolism, Gaucher's disease, obesity, hemoglobinopathies, pancreatitis, and dysbaric phenomena (Fig. 6-24). In a significant number of cases, none of the known risk factors can be identified, and the disease is considered idiopathic.[13–15]

Diagnosis and Pathology

Early diagnosis is important in improving the chances of saving the femoral head, because all prophylactic treatment procedures (discussed later in this chapter) are more successful in the initial stages of AVN. This becomes an issue when evaluating the asymptomatic hip in a patient with nontraumatic AVN on the contralateral side (Fig. 6-25). In addition to MR imaging, nuclear scintigraphy with technetium-labeled phosphate analogues, such as methylene diphosphonate (^{99m}TC-MDP), may be used for the early detection of osteonecrosis.[16] During the acute phase of the disease, decreased uptake of bone tracer is associated with vascular compromise. Increased accumulation of radiopharmaceutical tracer occurs with chronic vascular stasis in repair and in revascularization. Dynamic scanning is useful to assess regional blood flow in this setting. The specificity of marrow scanning with technetium sulfur colloid (^{99m}TC-sulfur colloid) is variable and depends on the status of the underlying disease and on the pattern of marrow composition.

The anterolateral portion of the femoral head is characteristically involved in AVN, but no specific area of the femoral head is protected or spared in this disorder.[17] The articular cartilage is intact at the initial presentation of the wedge-shaped subchondral bone infarct. An ineffective healing response with resorption of bone predominates. Partial resorption of necrotic bone and replacement with fibrous granulation tissue characterize the lack of central repair and incomplete peripheral repair of the necrotic focus. The deposition of viable bone on necrotic bone forms thickened trabeculae, which produce a mixed sclerotic and lucent or cystic radiographic appearance. Collapse of unsupported articular cartilage, secondary to subchondral fracture, leads to subsequent joint destruction.

text continues on page 130

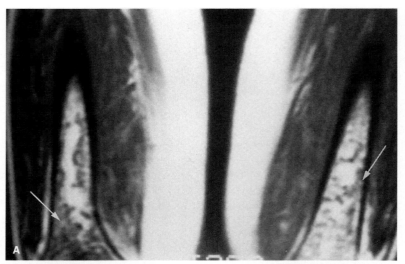

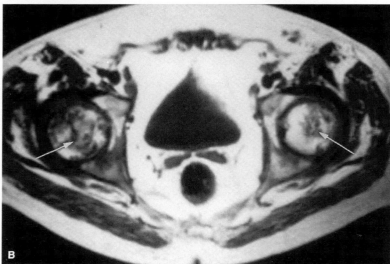

FIGURE 6-24. Diffuse osteonecrosis (*arrows*) demonstrates low signal intensity. Serpiginous areas can be seen on (**A**) T1-weighted coronal and (**B**) axial images in a patient with history of ethanol abuse (TR, 600 msec; TE, 20 msec).

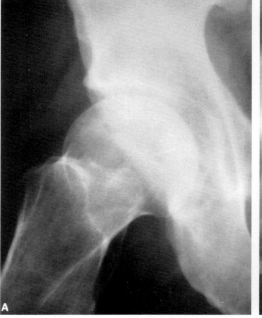

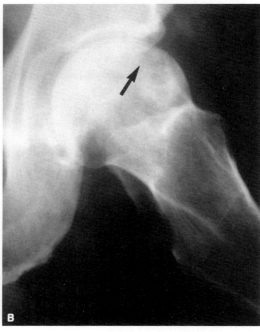

FIGURE 6-25. Avascular necrosis (AVN). Frog-lateral views are negative in the asymptomatic right hip (**A**) and show patchy sclerosis of the left femoral head (*arrow*) in the symptomatic left hip (**B**). *continued*

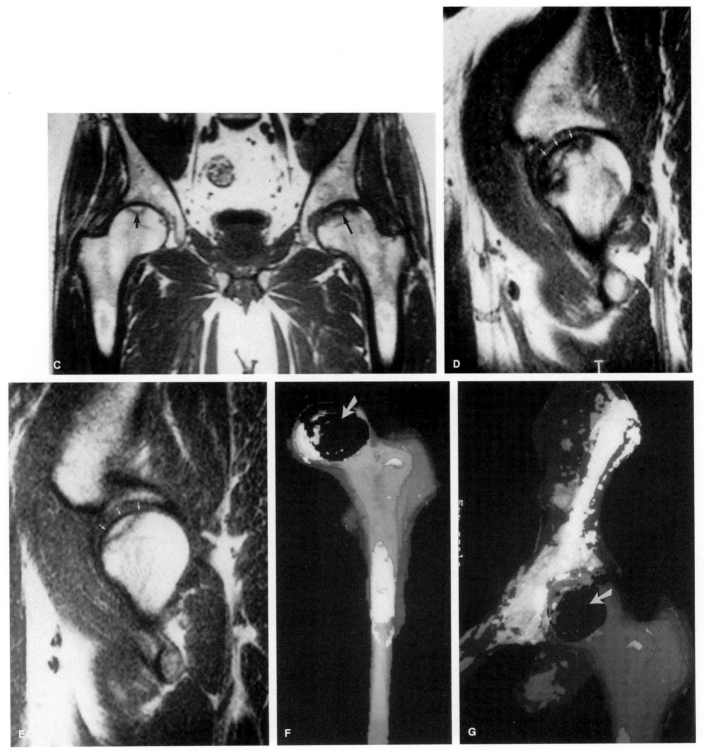

FIGURE 6-25. *Continued.* (**C**) Coronal T1-weighted image demonstrates AVN with greater than 30% involvement in the left femoral head (*long arrow*) and less than 10% involvement of the right femoral head (*short arrow*). Sagittal T1-weighted images more accurately depict early subchondral collapse with flattening (*arrows*) of the left femoral head (**D**), but show normal spherical morphology of the right femoral head (*arrows* on **E**). Three-dimensional MR rendering and mapping of the left femoral head AVN (*arrows*) with (**F**) and without (**G**) disarticulation of the femur.

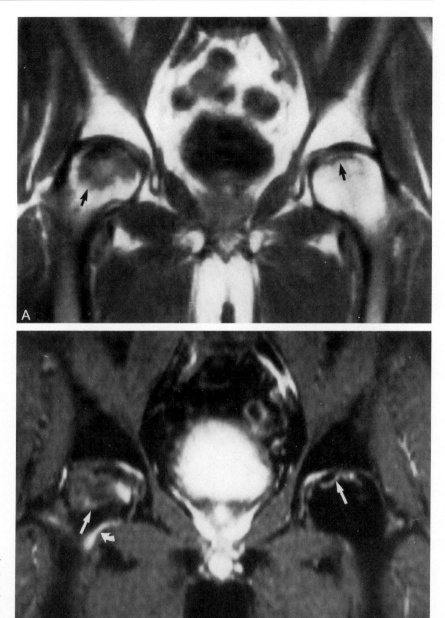

FIGURE 6-26. Avascular necrosis (AVN). **(A)** T1-weighted image shows low signal intensity bilateral osteonecrosis of the hips (*arrows*) (TR, 600 msec; TE, 20 msec). **(B)** On a short TI inversion recovery image, AVN (*straight arrows*) and associated joint effusion (*curved arrow*) demonstrate bright signal intensity (TR, 1400 msec; TI, 125 msec; TE, 40 msec).

Magnetic Resonance Imaging

In detection of AVN of the hip, MR imaging is more sensitive than CT or radionuclide bone scintigraphy.[18,19] In differentiating AVN from non-AVN disease of the femoral head, MR imaging has a specificity of 98% and a sensitivity of 97%.[20] MR imaging is also effective in assessing joint effusions, marrow conversion, edema, and articular cartilage congruity, none of which is possible with bone scintigraphy, standard radiographs, or CT.

Evaluation of patients with AVN can be accomplished with a T1-weighted axial localizer, and coronal images acquired with either a T1- and T2-weighted spin-echo se-

quence, a fat-suppressed T2-weighted fast spin-echo sequence, or a STIR (fast spin-echo STIR) sequence. Imaging in the sagittal plane may be helpful in defining early changes of cortical flattening associated with subchondral collapse (see Fig. 6-25). Short TI inversion recovery pulse sequences, which negate yellow marrow–fat signal, provide excellent contrast for the detection of marrow replacement, fluid, and necrotic tissue (Fig. 6-26).

Premature fatty marrow conversion associated with avascular necrosis can be detected using chemical-shift imaging techniques. On fat- and water-selective images, fatty and hematopoietic marrow and distribution of water within the ischemic focus can be differentiated. Gradient-echo coronal images, although not as sensitive for fluid within reparative tissue and necrosis, demonstrate associated hip joint effusions, subchondral fluid, and changes in articular cartilage contours (Figs. 6-27 through 6-29). When compared with coronal images acquired with a body coil, sagittal images acquired with a surface coil and a small FOV may provide superior anteroposterior (AP) and superoinferior localization of AVN by demonstrating joint-space narrowing, articular cartilage fracture, and the double-line sign (Fig. 6-30).[21] The characteristic double-line sign can be observed in up to 80% of lesions and cannot be attributed to a chemical-shift artifact or misrepresentation (Fig. 6-31). On T2-weighted images, the double-line sign is visualized as an inner border of high signal intensity, paralleling the low signal intensity periphery.

Staging

There are a number of staging systems for AVN,[12,22–25] but the most popular is that of Ficat and Arlet,[23] modified to include preclinical and preradiologic stages of the disease.[22] This modification is important because the disease can be present in the absence of clinical and radiologic signs.

In stage 0 disease (diagnosed on the basis of scintigraphic or MR imaging when a painful contralateral hip is being evaluated), no clinical or radiographic changes are found (Fig. 6-32). There is a double-line sign on MR image in the asymptomatic hip in this stage.

In stage I and stage II disease, the joint remains normal and the femoral head is spherical. In stage I disease, the trabeculae appear normal or slightly porotic and progress to diffuse porosis and sclerosis in stage II. In stage I, MR imaging may show a single line on T1-weighted images and a double line on T2-weighted images. The double-line sign, specific and pathognomonic for AVN, consists of concentric low and high signal intensity bands on T2-weighted images. The hyperintensity at the periphery of the necrotic focus is probably caused by hypervascular granulation tissue, a hyperemic response adjacent to thickened trabeculae.[17] Pathologic specimens from lesions in these early stages show viable bone on necrotic bone with marrow spaces infiltrated by mononuclear cells and histiocytes, explaining the radiographic changes. In stage II disease, a shell of reactive bone demarcates the area of infarct. Within this area, the trabeculae and marrow spaces are acellular.

The onset of stage III disease is marked by the loss of the spherical shape of the femoral head. The AP radiograph may appear normal, but the lateral view often reveals a crescent sign, or radiolucency, under the subchondral bone.

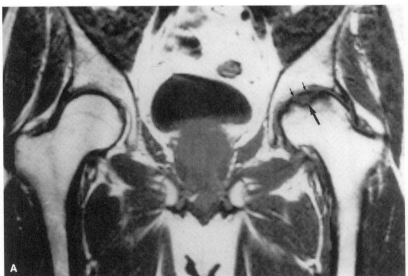
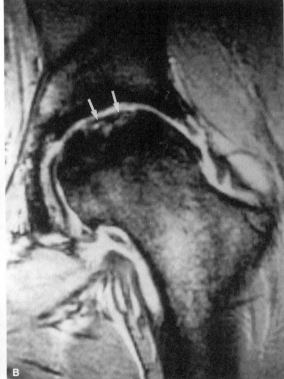

FIGURE 6-27. Avascular necrosis (AVN). **(A)** T1-weighted coronal image demonstrates a low signal intensity focus of AVN (*large arrow*). The apparent cortical outline is shown (*small arrows*). **(B)** T2*-weighted coronal image displays a subchondral fracture (*arrows*) with fluid signal intensity in the necrotic interface.

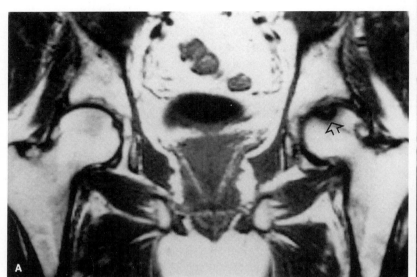
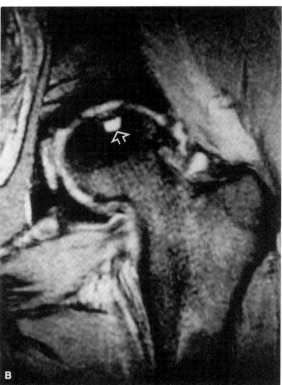

FIGURE 6-28. Avascular necrosis. Subchondral fluid in the osteonecrotic focus (*open arrows*) demonstrates (**A**) low signal intensity on a coronal T1-weighted image and (**B**) bright signal intensity on a T2*-weighted image.

This represents a fracture between the subchondral bone and the underlying femoral head. The crescent sign is the earliest indication of mechanical failure from accumulated stress fractures of nonrepaired necrotic trabeculae.[17] At this stage, there is also separation of the subchondral plate from the underlying necrotic cancellous bone. The necrotic area becomes radiodense as a result of mineral deposition in the marrow spaces. The joint space remains preserved or may actually increase in height.

In stage IV disease, the femoral head undergoes further collapse, leading to articular cartilage destruction and joint space narrowing (Fig. 6-33). Segmental collapse and subchondral fracture may result in pain and disability. Frequently this is the stage at which the patient presents for evaluation, although they may seek attention earlier. Pain in these patients may be attributed to increased intraosseous pressure and microfracture.

A recently proposed classification system incorporates components from several sources: (1) the Ficat and Arlet four-part staging classification; (2) quantification of the extent of femoral head involvement, as determined by MR imaging (<15%, 15% to 30%, or >30%); and (3) the location of the necrotic focus (medial—rarely progressive; central—prognosis of intermediate severity; or lateral—worst prognosis]).[17]

The specificity of radiographic staging of AVN is improved by the use of CT, which is also helpful in defining the associated sclerotic arc, in detecting acetabular dome and femoral head contour changes, in assessing the joint space, and in evaluating the extent of femoral head involvement.[26] Disruption of the normal pattern of bony trabeculae can be observed on CT scans in osteonecrosis of the femoral head.[27] Clumping and fusion of peripheral aspects of the femoral head asterisk may be identified prior to conventional radiographic sclerosis or subchondral fracture. These CT changes do not, however, reflect the early vascular marrow histologic processes in AVN.

Mitchell and colleagues have described an MR classification system for AVN based on qualitative assessment of alterations in the central region of MR signal intensity in the osteonecrotic focus.[16,28] In MR class A disease, the osteonecrotic lesion demonstrates signal characteristics analogous to fat: a central region of high signal intensity on short repetition time/echo time (TR/TE) settings (T1-weighted) and intermediate signal intensity on long TR/TE settings (T2-weighted) (Figs. 6-34 and 6-35). Class B hips demonstrate the signal characteristics of blood or hemorrhage: high signal intensity on both short and long TR/TE sequences (Fig. 6-36). Hips identified as class C demonstrate the signal properties of fluid: low signal intensity on short TR/TE se-

text continues on page 136

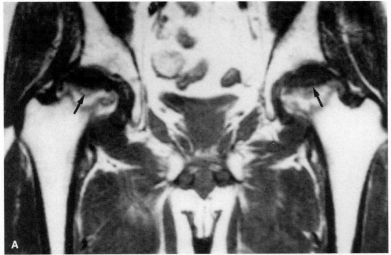

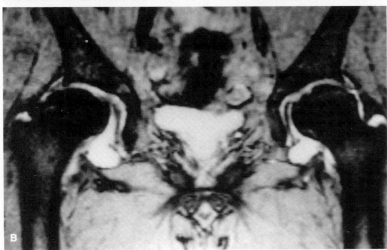

FIGURE 6-29. Bilateral avascular necrosis. (**A**) Superior delineation of the necrotic focus (*arrows*) is seen on a T1-weighted coronal image. (**B**) Spherical morphology of left femoral head is displayed on a T2*-weighted image. The right femoral head shows remodeling and flattening of its superior articular surface.

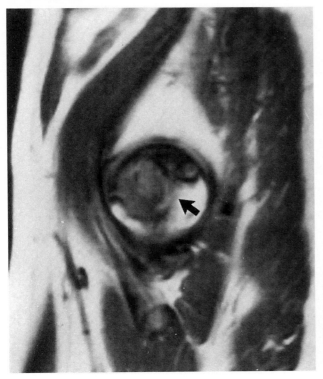

FIGURE 6-30. Femoral head AVN demonstrates low signal intensity on a T1-weighted sagittal image (*arrow*). The sagittal imaging plane displays anterior-to-posterior relationships in determining the extent of femoral head involvement (TR, 600 msec; TE, 20 msec).

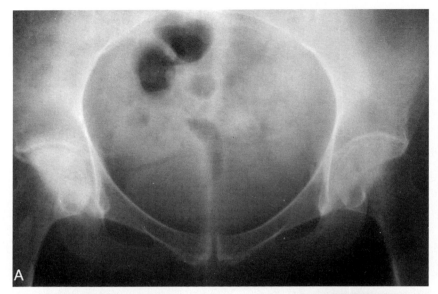

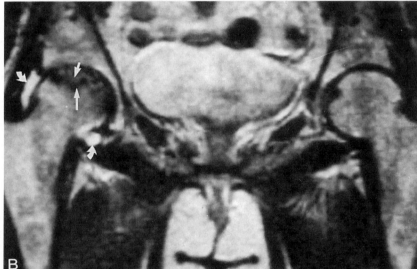

FIGURE 6-31. (**A**) AP radiograph in a patient with right hip pain is unremarkable. (**B**) A T2-weighted coronal image displays right femoral head osteonecrosis with the characteristic double-line sign. Low signal intensity periphery (*long straight arrow*) and high signal intensity inner border (*short straight arrow*) are differentiated. Bright signal intensity hip effusion is also shown (*curved arrows*) (TR, 2000 msec; TE, 60 msec).

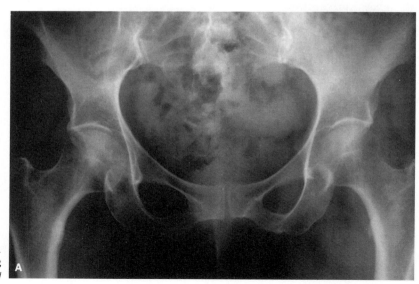

FIGURE 6-32. Avascular necrosis (AVN) in Ficat stage 0. (**A**) AP radiograph is negative in a patient presenting with unilateral hip pain. *continued*

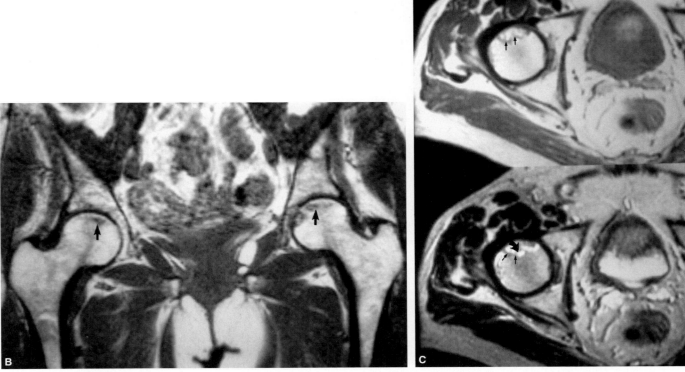

FIGURE 6-32. *Continued.* **(B)** A T1-weighted coronal image displays stage 0 disease with bilateral AVN (*arrows*) demonstrating central fat signal intensity (TR, 600 msec; TE, 20 msec). **(C)** On a T2-weighted coronal image, the double-line sign with a low signal intensity peripheral border (*straight arrows*) and a high signal intensity inner band (*curved arrow*) is seen (TR, 2000 msec; TE, 20, 80 msec).

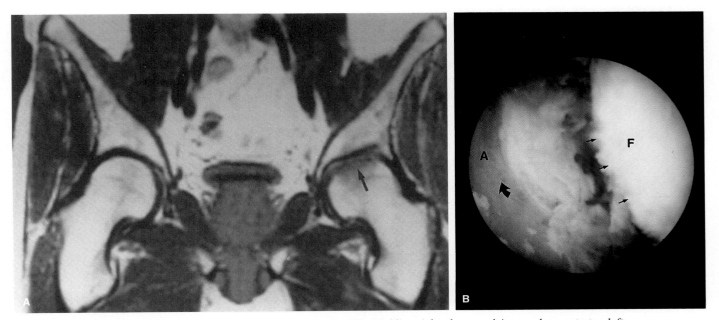

FIGURE 6-33. Avascular necrosis in Ficat stage IV. **(A)** T1-weighted coronal image demonstrates left femoral head AVN (*arrow*) with associated flattening of the superior surface of the femoral head and joint-space narrowing (TR, 600 msec; TE, 20 msec). **(B)** At arthroscopy, degenerative changes of the femoral head (*small arrows*) and denuded acetabular articular cartilage (*curved arrow*) associated with secondary narrowing of the hip joint are seen (A, acetabulum; F, femur).

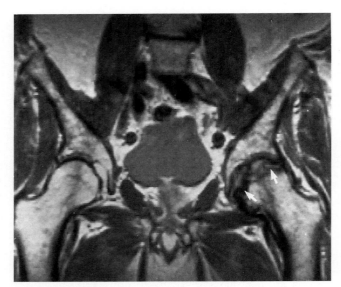

FIGURE 6-34. T1-weighted coronal image of AVN of the left femoral head shows a central focus of high signal intensity (*arrows*) (TR, 600 msec; TE, 20 msec).

quences and high signal intensity on long TR/TE sequences (Fig. 6-37). Class D hips exhibit the signal characteristics of fibrous tissue: low signal intensity on short and long TR/TE sequences (Fig. 6-38). In all four classes, there is a peripheral band of low signal intensity that outlines the central focus of AVN. This border is most visible on T1-weighted images of class A and B hips (the central focus of necrosis is bright in signal intensity) and on T2-weighted images of class C hips. Manipulation of TR/TE pulse parameters does not affect the low signal intensity border.

Treatment

The aim of treatment is to save the femoral head, not replace it, because most patients with nontraumatic AVN are relatively young. Unfortunately, surprisingly little is written

about the natural history of the disease. Some clinicians still recommend restricted activity and protected weight-bearing as initial therapy, and Steinberg and colleagues have published a retrospective study of 48 patients treated nonoperatively.[29] Their results indicate that limiting weight-bearing has no beneficial effect on the outcome. Disease was progressive in 92% of patients. A subsequent study showed disease progression in over 80% of patients, regardless of the stage of disease at presentation, and progression of the disease in all patients who presented with some collapse of the femoral head.[11]

Many clinicians recommend early surgical intervention because of the high rate of progression with nonoperative treatment. Conservative or prophylactic procedures include core decompression with or without bone grafts,[11,22,30-35] osteotomy,[14,36] and electrical stimulation.[30,37,38] The rationale for core decompression, the most commonly used of these proceeders, is to alleviate the elevated intraosseous pressure, permitting neovascularization (Fig. 6-39). Success rates reported in the literature vary dramatically—from 40% to 90%—depending on the criteria used to grade results. Smith and coworkers[39] found that core decompression was successful in 59% of Ficat stage I lesions, success being defined as no subsequent operation or radiographic evidence of progression), but recommended an alternative treatment for stage IIB or III lesions, and possibly even stage IIA lesions.[39]

Cancellous, cortical, muscle pedicle, and microvascular bone grafts have been used with core decompression. The use of a cortical graft for necrotic bone was first described by Phemister,[40] and the procedure was later modified by Bonfiglio and Voke.[30] Urbaniak and associates first used a vascularized fibular graft after coring of the femoral head.[41] Long-term follow-up results with free vascularized fibular grafting reported a decreased need for pain medication (86%) and high rate of patient satisfaction (81%).[42] Brown and colleagues used a 3D model to incorporate biomechanical variables in coring and bone grafting of a necrotic femoral head.[43] For coring, they recommended that the tract not ex-

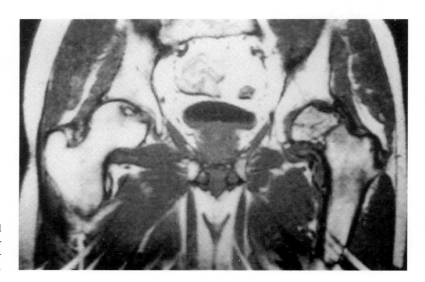

FIGURE 6-35. Avascular necrosis (AVN), class A. Bilateral AVN demonstrates fat marrow signal intensity. The sclerotic interface of the left femoral head involvement mimics a femoral neck fracture (TR, 600 msec; TE, 20 msec).

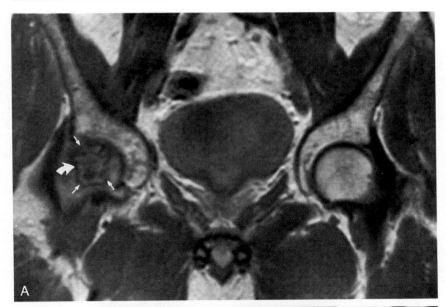

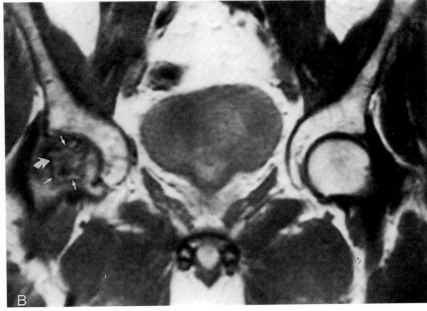

FIGURE 6-36. Right femoral head AVN (*straight arrows*) demonstrates intermediate to high signal intensity on (**A**) T1-weighted and (**B**) intermediate weighted images. The lesion is demarcated by a peripheral rim of low signal intensity (*curved arrows*).

tend near the subchondral plate. The greatest structural benefit with cortical bone-grafting was shown for grafts that penetrated deep into the superocentral or lateral aspect of the lesion with subchondral plate abutment. Increased stresses on necrotic cancellous bone occurred in central or lateral grafts that were placed proximal to the subchondral plate.[43]

A variety of proximal femoral osteotomies have been used with varying results.[15,34] The principle underlying osteotomy involves redirecting stresses from structurally compromised trabeculae. These procedures are most successful in cases with limited femoral head involvement. Patients who remain on corticosteroids or who have persistent metabolic bone disease do not benefit greatly from osteotomy. Pulsed electromagnetic fields and implantable direct current

stimulators have also been used in the treatment of AVN, also with varying results.[34,37,38]

Once the femoral head has collapsed, the success of prophylactic procedures diminishes significantly. The chance of saving the femoral head is small, and most patients go on to require femoral head replacement. In general, total hip replacement is more reliable than bipolar endoprosthesis.[44] Hip fusion is also an alternative in young patients with unilateral disease, especially the heavy, active male.

Clinical and Pathologic Correlation

Symptoms of AVN correlate well with MR classification: they are least severe in class A hips and most severe in class

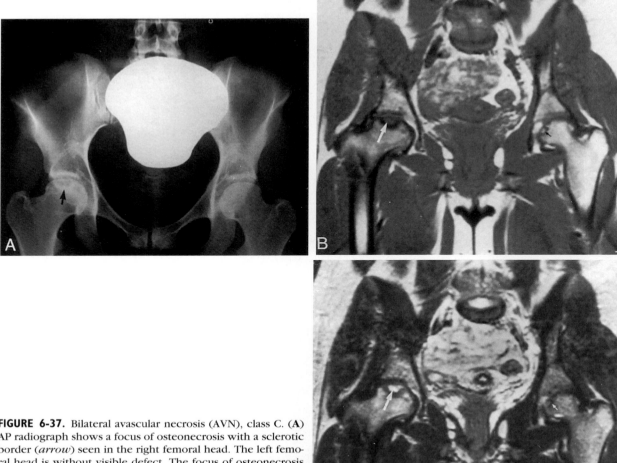

FIGURE 6-37. Bilateral avascular necrosis (AVN), class C. (**A**) AP radiograph shows a focus of osteonecrosis with a sclerotic border (*arrow*) seen in the right femoral head. The left femoral head is without visible defect. The focus of osteonecrosis (*large arrows*) demonstrates low to intermediate signal intensity on the corresponding intermediate weighted image (**B**) and high signal intensity characteristic of class C AVN on a T2-weighted image (**C**). An associated focus of AVN is seen in the contralateral hip (*small arrows*).

D hips. MR signal intensity, therefore, can be seen to follow a chronologic progression from acute (ie, class A) to chronic (ie, class D) AVN. Compared with conventional radiographic staging, approximately 50% of radiographic stage I and over 80% of stage II lesions demonstrate fat-like central signal intensity on MR scans and are classified as MR class A. Class A lesions are infrequent in more advanced radiographic stages.

MR findings can also be correlated with histologic changes (Fig. 6-40). The central region of high signal intensity corresponds to necrosis of bone and marrow, prior to the development of capillary and mesenchymal ingrowth.[45] The low signal intensity peripheral band corresponds to a sclerotic margin of reactive tissue at the interface between necrotic and viable bone. Low signal intensity on T1-weighted images and intermediate to high signal intensity on T2-weighted images can be attributed to the high water content of mesenchymal tissue and thickened trabecular bone. The double-line sign is thought to represent a hyperemic or inflammatory response causing granulation tissue inside the reactive bone interface, and is present in 80% of cases of AVN.[16] In areas of proposed vascular engorgement and inflammation, decreased signal intensity on T2-weighted images is associated with successful core decompression treatments. With intravenous gadolinium administration, enhanced and nonenhanced areas correspond to viable and necrotic bone, respectively.[46,47] In one study, perfusion, as assessed on gadolinium-enhanced T1-weighted images, and marrow composition, as measured with hydrogen-1 MR spectroscopy, was evaluated in patients with systemic lupus erythematosus (SLE) (ie, patients at risk for AVN) and control patients without AVN. Femoral head perfusion was shown to be inversely related to marrow fat content in healthy subjects and was higher in SLE patients without AVN.[48]

Beltran and colleagues have correlated collapse of the femoral head after core decompression with the extent or

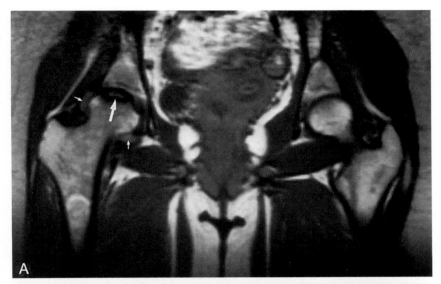

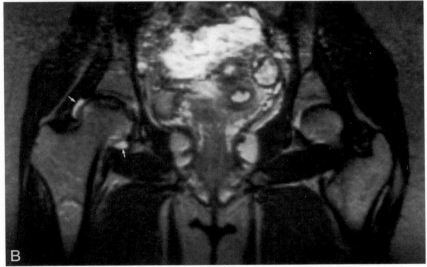

FIGURE 6-38. AVN, class D. Right femoral head osteonecrosis with a low signal intensity focus (*large arrow*) on (**A**) T1-weighted and (**B**) T2-weighted images. Associated capsular effusion demonstrates an increased signal intensity on the T1-weighted image (*small arrows*) (**A:** TR, 800 msec; TE, 20 msec; **B:** TR, 2000 msec; TE, 60 msec).

percentage of involvement of AVN as determined preoperatively by MR imaging.[49] When less than 25% of the weight-bearing surface was involved, femoral head collapse did not occur after core decompression. With 25% to 50% involvement, femoral head collapse occurred in 43% of hips. With greater than 50% involvement, femoral head collapse occurred in 87% of hips. Mean time to collapse was 6.7 months after diagnosis and treatment. Therefore, if a large area or volume of the femoral head is involved, subchondral collapse may occur with core decompression, despite the absence of subchondral fracture on conventional films. In untreated patients, Shimizu and colleagues reported a 74% rate of femoral head collapse by 32 months if the necrotic focus involved one fourth the femoral head diameter, or at least two thirds of the weight-bearing area.[50]

Joint effusions, which demonstrate low signal intensity on T1-weighted images and high signal intensity on T2-weighted images, are commonly associated with more ad-

vanced stages of AVN (Fig. 6-41).[51] It is not known whether the presence or absence of a joint effusion is of prognostic significance for the course and treatment of the disease. However, joint effusion is also associated with a bone marrow edema (BME) pattern prior to the irreversible demarcation (double-line sign) of the necrotic focus.

A second pattern of MR signal intensity, diffuse low signal intensity on T1-weighted images with increased signal intensity on T2-weighted images, has been described by Turner and colleagues.[52] The area of diffuse low signal intensity on T1-weighted images extends from the femoral head and neck into the intertrochanteric area. Although no focal findings were identified initially, AVN was subsequently demonstrated by core biopsy and focal MR morphologic patterns specific for osteonecrosis. The diffuse pattern of low signal intensity in and adjacent to the femoral head was shown to be transient in five of six patients, and may represent a BME pattern (see later in this chapter) preceding focal

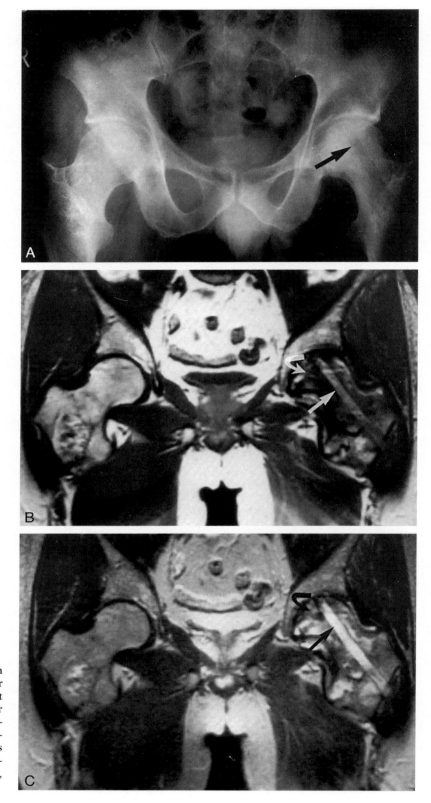

FIGURE 6-39. Core decompression. (**A**) AP radiograph allows identification of the core decompression tract for AVN (*arrow*). Unsuccessful core decompression for left femoral head AVN (*curved arrows*) with diffuse vascular edema is seen with (**B**) low signal intensity on a T1-weighted scan and (**C**) with high signal intensity on a T2-weighted scan. The core tract (*straight arrows*) displays increased signal intensity from fluid contents on the T2-weighted image (**B:** TR, 600 msec; TE, 20 msec; **C:** TR, 2000 msec; TE, 60 msec).

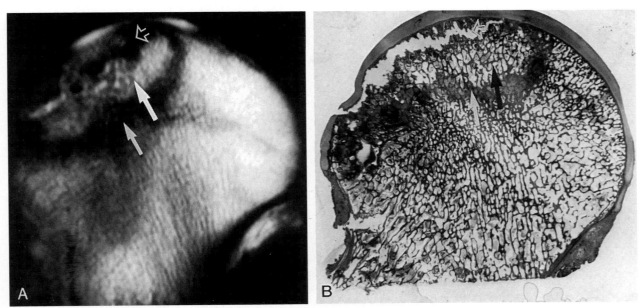

FIGURE 6-40. AVN. **(A)** A T1-weighted coronal image demonstrates high signal intensity cortical necrosis (*large arrow*), low signal intensity sclerotic peripheral interface between necrosis and viable marrow (*small arrow*), and low signal intensity subchondral fracture (*open arrow*) (TR, 600 msec; TE, 20 msec). **(B)** A macroslide of a gross specimen shows corresponding subchondral collapse (*open arrow*), reactive periphery (*white arrow*), and cortical necrosis (*black arrow*).

anterosuperior femoral head osteonecrosis. When there is also increased uptake on corresponding radionuclide bone scans, careful observation may be required to differentiate diffuse MR patterns of early AVN from transient osteoporosis of the hip. A BME pattern may represent an earlier stage of a reversible form of AVN. These changes have also been reported in the acetabular bone prior to the development of sclerosis and granulation tissue at the interface surrounding devitalized or necrotic bone (Figs. 6-42 and 6-43).

Value of Magnetic Resonance Imaging

One of the most important contributions MR imaging has made to the detection of AVN is identification of an osteonecrotic lesion in patients with normal bone scintigraphy and conventional radiography.[1,53] Since MR imaging is sensitive to changes of marrow fat signal intensity, MR findings of osteonecrosis may not be apparent for up to 5 days after the initial ischemic insult, until there is death of marrow fat cells. Marrow fat cells are more resistant to ischemia than are hematopoietic cells (which die within 6 to 12 hours) or osteocytes (which die within 12 to 48 hours). Therefore, prior to the death of fat marrow cells, (ie, before AVN is apparent on MR scans), scintigraphy may demonstrate a focus of decreased radiopharmaceutical uptake when MR findings are negative. However, as bone remodeling occurs with disease progression, bone scintigraphy may no longer be diagnostic and the osteonecrotic lesion may not be detected. This represents a severe limitation of scintigraphy compared with MR, which remains positive throughout the

course or progression of AVN or until the lesion is healed. Contrast-enhanced imaging may allow even earlier identification of changes in AVN, as discussed later.

Focal MR abnormalities, subsequent to the presentation of diffuse BME, can be observed as early as 6 to 8 weeks from the time of detection. The demonstration of marrow necrosis and acellular lacunas can differentiate osteonecrosis in its early stages from transient osteoporosis of the hip. The finding of symptomatic hip joint effusion prior to any alteration in marrow signal intensity may correspond to an elevation of intraosseous intramedullary pressures.

Genez and colleagues determined that in the early stages of AVN, histologic findings of osteonecrosis may be present in the absence of abnormal MR findings.[54] In fact, intravenous gadolinium-enhanced images appear to improve the early detection of AVN by demonstrating areas of decreased enhancement, despite normal findings on T1- and T2-weighted images. For example, using contrast-enhanced imaging, it was possible to identify early changes of AVN in 6% of 100 asymptomatic renal transplant patients at risk because of treatment with corticosteroids.[55] In another study of renal transplant recipients, followed for 22 months using serial radiographs and MR, previously untreated AVN was shown to have a benign course without progression from Ficat stage 0.[56] Jiang and Shih reported that the presence of a complete or dense physeal scar on MR scans was associated with a high risk for AVN of the femoral head.[57] Segmental or incomplete scars in AVN were uncommon. The sealed off or complete scar was shown to be a risk factor in patients

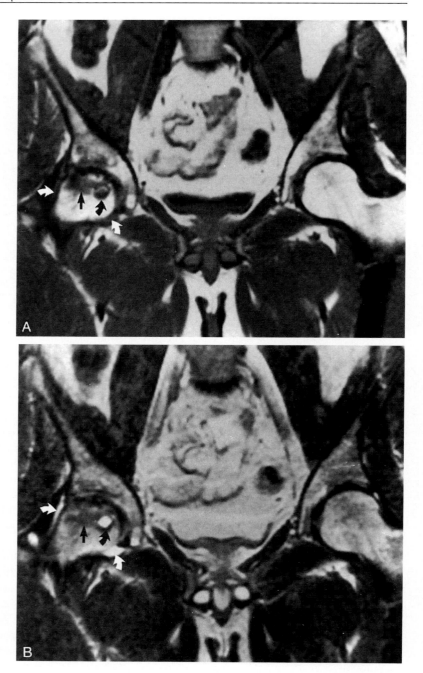

FIGURE 6-41. Advanced AVN with low signal intensity central cortical focus (*straight arrows*) on (**A**) T1-weighted and (**B**) T2-weighted images. Associated joint-space narrowing, degenerative cyst (*curved black arrows*), and effusion (*curved white arrows*) are indicated. Cyst and hip effusion demonstrate low signal intensity on T1-weighted sequences and high signal intensity on T2-weighted sequences (**A:** TR, 800 msec; TE, 20 msec; **B:** TR, 1500 msec; TE 80 msec).

with or without a history of steroid or alcohol abuse (associated lipogenic factors). Because it is possible to identify MR changes of focal osteonecrosis when radionuclide scans are negative and CT and plain film findings are normal,[58] a limited or modified MR examination could be used as a low-cost screening tool in at risk populations.

One of the advantages of chronologic or temporal staging and assessment of the percentage of marrow involvement is that the additional information may facilitate therapy choices

prior to reactive bone changes including subchondral fracture, collapse, and fragmentation. In the later stages of AVN (ie, stages 3 and 4), core decompression is frequently used to palliate pain without altering disease progression. A 3D MR rendering can be used to evaluate the volume of osteonecrotic involvement of the femoral head relative to its cross-sectional area (see Fig. 6-25). This technique can be useful for differentiating and separating the necrotic zone of involvement and for identifying its location in the femoral

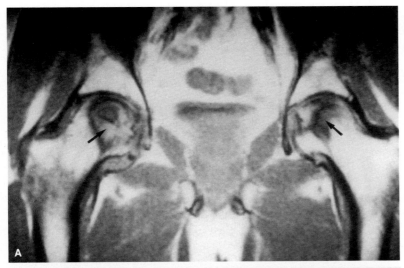

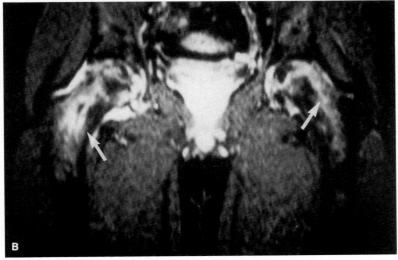

FIGURE 6-42. Avascular necrosis. Bilateral class A AVN (*arrows*) on (**A**) coronal T1-weighted and (**B**) short TI inversion recovery (STIR) images. Femoral neck edema or hyperemia (*arrows*) is best demonstrated on STIR sequence (**A:** TR, 600 msec; TE, 20 msec; **B:** TR, 1400 msec; TI, 125 msec; TE, 40 msec).

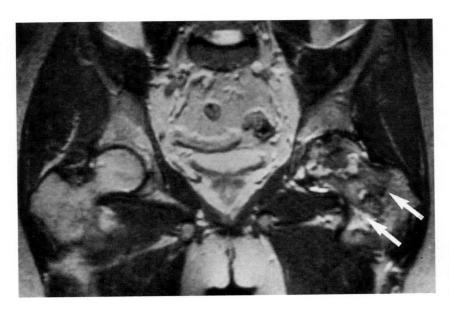

FIGURE 6-43. A T2-weighted coronal image showing a diffuse pattern of AVN in the femoral head and neck (*arrows*) with a high signal intensity area of marrow edema (TR, 2000 msec; TE, 60 msec).

head and its relationship to the weight-bearing surface. Information from quantitative assessment of femoral head volume may assist in the decision to perform a core decompression or a rotational osteotomy.

3D rendering is also best suited for displaying osteonecrotic involvement of the femoral head. Disarticulation of the femur and femoral head from the acetabulum may facilitate superior surface viewing of the femoral head and the associated necrotic focus (see Fig. 6-25). Separate disarticulation and composite volume rendering can be performed in order to display associated joint effusions. Volume transmission enables viewing of the femoral head through the acetabulum using various degrees of pelvic rotation in horizontal and vertical planes. In a quantitative approach to following early stages of AVN, weight-bearing areas of involvement are an important and reliable parameter to monitor in follow-up.[59]

Legg-Calvé-Perthes Disease

Legg-Calvé-Perthes disease is a childhood hip disorder that results in infarction of the bony epiphysis of the femoral head. Although the etiology is unclear, certain risk factors have been identified, including gender (boys are affected four times more often than girls), socioeconomic class (high incidence in low socioeconomic classes and in children with low birth weight), and inguinal hernia and genitourinary anomalies in children.[60,61]

Legg-Calvé-Perthes disease is a dynamic condition, and the results of the physical examination depend on the stage of the disease at the time of presentation. Early in the disease, the physical findings are similar to those of irritable hip syndrome. The child often has a limp with groin, thigh, or knee pain. Children aged 4 to 9 years are the most commonly affected. Children who present with knee pain must be carefully examined for hip pathology. As the disease progresses, a flexion and adduction contracture may develop, and lateral overgrowth of the femoral head cartilage may cause loss of abduction. Attempts at abduction lead to hinging and possible subluxation of the femoral head. Eventually, the hip may only move in the flexion-extension plane.

Diagnosis

Diagnosis of Legg-Calvé-Perthes disease is usually made from radiographs. Signs include widening of the inferomedial joint space, epiphyseal sclerosis, a subchondral fracture line, and a small epiphysis. Plain film findings may be negative early in the course of the disease, and scintigraphy and MR imaging may provide additional information.

Staging

The most commonly used classification systems for Legg-Calvé-Perthes disease are based on radiographic estimates of the amount of femoral head involvement. Catterall has defined four groups,[62] and Salter and Thompson have

described two groups based on such estimates.[63] In Catterall's classification,[62] group I represents involvement of the anterior aspect of the epiphysis without a metaphysical reaction, sequestrum, or subchondral fracture line. Group II shows more extensive or severe involvement of the anterior aspect of the epiphysis, with preservation of the medial and lateral segments. A sequestrum is present, as is a metaphyseal reaction anterolaterally. A subchondral fracture line is present, which does not extend to the apex of the femoral epiphysis. In group III, the entire epiphysis is dense. There is a diffuse metaphyseal reaction with femoral neck widening. A subchondral fracture line is visualized posteriorly. Group IV disease is characterized by involvement of the entire femoral head, with flattening, mushrooming, and eventual collapse. There is an extensive metaphyseal reaction and associated posterior remodeling. In Catterall's grouping of Legg-Calvé-Perthes disease, it should be possible to separate group I cases, without sequestrum or metaphyseal lesion, from cases of groups II and III, with viable bone posteriorly and medially, and from group IV cases, in which the entire epiphysis is involved, with collapse and loss of epiphyseal height. The more advanced the stage at the time of presentation, the poorer the prognosis. It is important to understand that the disease is progressive, and final radiographic staging may take up to 9 months. Green and colleagues have correlated the degree of epiphyseal extrusion with prognosis: when more than 20% of the epiphysis is extruded laterally, the prognosis is poor; when more than 50% of the femoral head is also involved, only 8% have good results.[64] Pathologically, the early stages of the disease are characterized by overgrowth of the articular cartilage medially and laterally.[65,66] Infarction within the femoral head can lead to trabecular fracture and decreased epiphyseal height.

On radiographic examination, increased bony tissue density is found in the area of infarction, representing appositional new bone and calcification of necrotic marrow. Revascularization occurs through creeping substitution of necrotic bone with fibrocartilage, causing the fragmented appearance seen on plain film radiographs during this phase of the disease. The thickened articular cartilage is repaired from subchondral bone and from within the abnormal cartilage anteriorly and laterally. Unossified cartilage that streams down from the growth plate can lead to metaphyseal cysts. In the late stages, the fibrocartilage is reossified. The last area to heal is superior and anterior.

Treatment

It is important to determine prognosis at the time of presentation, because more than 50% of patients with Legg-Calvé-Perthes disease do well with no treatment.[67] The younger the child at the time of presentation, the better the prognosis. Children who present after 8 years of age do poorly. In general, girls do not do as well and may have a more severe form of the disease. The earlier the stage of the disease at the time of presentation, the better the prognosis. Catterall has identified clinical and radiographic "head at risk" signs that he correlated with the chance of developing significant femoral head deformity.[62] Clinically, progressive loss of movement, adduction contracture, flexion with abduction, and obesity are all poor prognostic signs. Radiographically, both epiphyseal and metaphyseal signs may be associated with a poor prognosis. The epiphyseal signs are calcification lateral to the epiphysis and a lytic area laterally (Gage's sign). In the metaphysis, horizontal inclination of the growth plate and diffuse metaphyseal reaction are risk signs. Two or more of these signs correlate with a poor prognosis.[62] Lateral subluxation of the femoral head is also associated with a poor outcome.

Decisions about whether to treat a particular patient can be difficult. Catterall recommends definitive treatment for all "at risk" cases, for groups II and III disease in patients older than 7 years of age, and for group IV cases in which serious deformity has not occurred.[62] A more conservative approach, that is, observation, can be taken with group I cases and group II and III cases that are not "at risk." Arthrography may be helpful in determining incongruity of the femoral head. After healing is established radiographically, treatment is not required because the femoral head will not deteriorate further. Radiographic signs of healing are an increase in height and size of viable bone on the medial side of the epiphysis and an increase in height and quality of new bone formed laterally.

The principles of treatment involve restoring hip motion and decreasing the forces across the hip joint. To accomplish this, the femoral head must be positioned within the acetabulum. This can be achieved with physical therapy and bracing or femoral osteotomy. Neither treatment modality is clearly superior, and both have advantages and disadvantages. In the long term, approximately 86% of patients develop osteoarthritis, but most are able to function relatively well until the fifth or sixth decade of life.[68]

Magnetic Resonance Imaging

Magnetic resonance imaging is used to identify both morphologic and signal characteristics of the femoral epiphysis

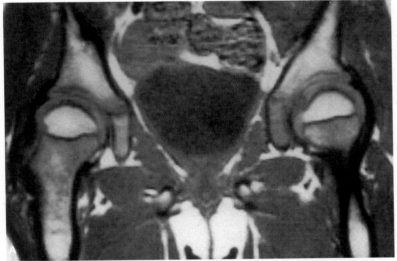
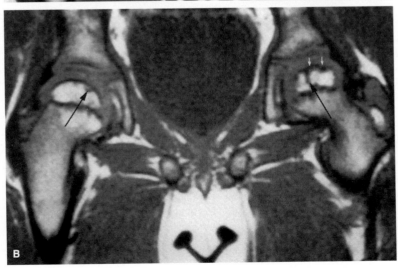

FIGURE 6-44. T1-weighted coronal images in Legg-Calvé-Perthes disease. (**A**) Normal femoral head capital epiphyses. (**B**) The earliest MR signs of Legg-Calvé-Perthes disease include peripheral irregularity of marrow-fat–containing epiphyseal ossification center (*white arrows*). Low signal intensity foci or linear segments are seen within the right and left ossification centers (*black arrows*). No subarticular collapse is present, and conventional radiographs are normal (TR, 500 msec; TE, 20 msec).

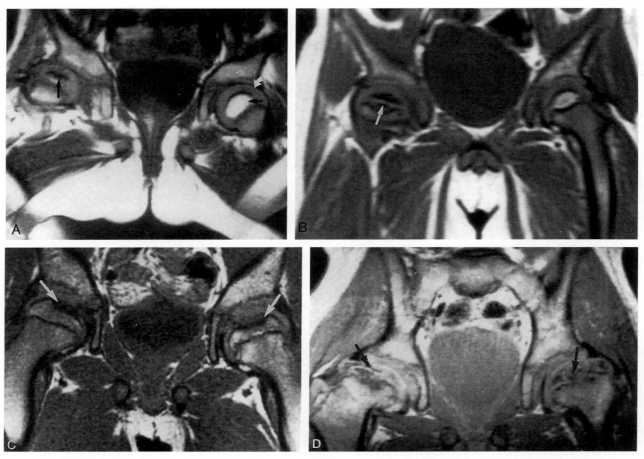

FIGURE 6-45. Coronal T1-weighted images show the spectrum of Legg-Calvé-Perthes disease from (**A, B**) early to (**C, D**) late advanced involvement. (**A**) Small, laterally displaced ossific nucleus with loss of yellow marrow signal intensity (*long black arrow*) is present early in the disease. Normal contralateral epiphyseal cartilage (*curved arrow*) and high signal intensity marrow (*short black arrow*) are seen. (**B**) Complete loss of right femoral epiphyseal marrow signal intensity (*arrow*) occurs as the disease progresses. (**C**) Bilateral low signal intensity osteonecrotic foci in the femoral epiphysis (*arrows*) becomes apparent later in the disease. Articular cartilage is thinner in the older child. (**D**) Advanced remodeling with coxa plana and coxa magna of the femoral heads (*arrows*) is indicative of late advanced involvement (TR, 600 msec; TE, 20 msec).

in the early stages of radiographically negative disease (Fig. 6-44) and in more advanced disease (Fig. 6-45). In addition to low signal intensity within the epiphyseal marrow center on T1- and T2-weighted images, associated findings include an intraarticular effusion and a small, laterally displaced ossification nucleus.[69,70]

Revascularization of the necrotic portion of the femoral epiphysis may occur after treatment of Legg-Calvé-Perthes disease with varus osteotomy. The initial low signal intensity focus is replaced with high signal intensity marrow fat. Coxa plana and coxa magna may result from later remodeling (Fig. 6-46). Before diffuse loss of signal intensity of the ossific nucleus is observed, low signal intensity irregularity occurs along the periphery of the fat-containing ossific nucleus, and linear areas of low signal intensity may transverse the femoral ossification center (see Fig. 6-44). These changes correlate with positive bone scintigraphy in stage I disease.

Since articular cartilage demonstrates increased signal intensity on T2*-weighted images (Fig. 6-47), this sequence is useful in evaluating the thickness of the articular cartilage, which may be increased in the initial stages of Legg-Calvé-Perthes disease. Fat-suppressed T2-weighted fast spin-echo or STIR (including fast spin-echo STIR) sequences are more accurate than gradient-echo techniques, however, demonstrating degenerative changes of the articular cartilage with the influx of fluid in areas of articular cartilage irregularity. The physeal cartilage may also demonstrate increased signal intensity on T2-weighted images in early stage disease.[71] Coronal or sagittal images may be used to display both acetabular and femoral head cartilage surfaces. Measurements of acetabular and femoral head articular cartilage show an increased thickness in affected hips.

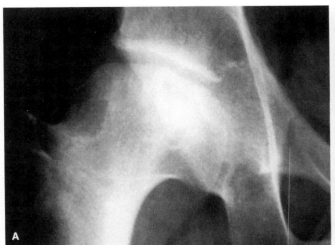

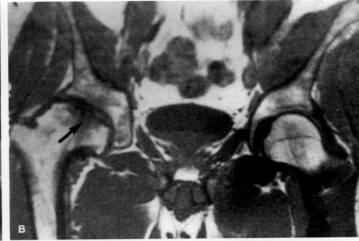

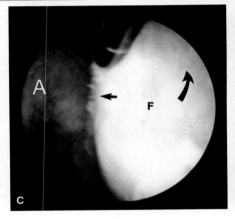

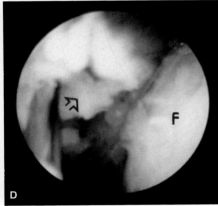

FIGURE 6-46. (A) AP radiograph of the right hip demonstrates remodeling with coxa magna and coxa plana from chronic Legg-Calvé Perthes disease. (B) T1-weighted coronal image displays low signal intensity osteonecrotic focus (*arrow*) (TR, 600 msec; TE, 20 msec). (C) The arthroscopic view shows secondary degeneration of the femoral head (F) articular cartilage (*straight arrow*). The transition from white articular cartilage to exposed yellow bone (*curved arrow*) is shown. (D) Arthroscopy also reveals intraarticular cartilage debris (*open arrow*) (A, acetabulum).

Loss of containment of the femoral head in the acetabulum was identified in a majority of cases studies by Rush and colleagues, who found hypertrophy of the synovium within the iliopsoas recess of the hip capsule in 7 of 20 cases.[72] This was visualized as a frond-like structure adjacent to the inferomedial joint space. Epiphyseal cartilage thickness also contributes to loss of containment.[71]

Ranner, in a study of 13 patients with Legg-Calvé-Perthes disease among 45 patients presenting with acute hip pain, demonstrated that MR imaging was as sensitive as isotope bone scans and allowed more precise localization of involvement than conventional radiography.[73] Although revascularization of the necrotic focus may be more accurately determined with nuclear scintigraphy, MR imaging is preferable for evaluating the position, form, and size of the femoral head and surrounding soft tissues. BME, detected on MR scans in pediatric patients with symptomatic hips, may resolve without resultant osteonecrosis. Cartilaginous physeal and metaphyseal abnormalities identified on MR imaging are common in Legg-Calvé-Perthes disease and frequently result in growth arrest. Transphyseal bone bridging and metaphyseal extension of physeal cartilage were seen in 63% and 81% of cases, respectively, and were strong predictors of abnormal growth.[71] Epiphyseal

abnormalities, seen in a majority of cases, are not associated with growth disturbances.

Slipped Capital Femoral Epiphysis

Slipped capital femoral epiphysis (SCFE) is a childhood disorder of the hip characterized by posterior inferior displacement of the proximal femoral epiphysis. Although the precise etiology is unknown, current theories indicate that obesity, trauma, and hormonal abnormalities are associated with the development of the disease.[74] Mechanically, a vertical growth plate and retroversion of the femoral neck appear to be risk factors.[75] Histologically, the slip occurs through the zone of hypertrophy in the growth plate. Agamanolis and colleagues demonstrated a generalized chondrocyte degeneration throughout the growth plate suggesting a primary pathology.[76]

The child with SCFE usually presents with pain and a limp. Often the pain is located only in the thigh or knee, leading to frequently missed diagnoses. It is important to remember that knee pain in the child can be secondary to hip disease. On physical examination, there is frequently limitation of motion, especially internal rotation and abduc-

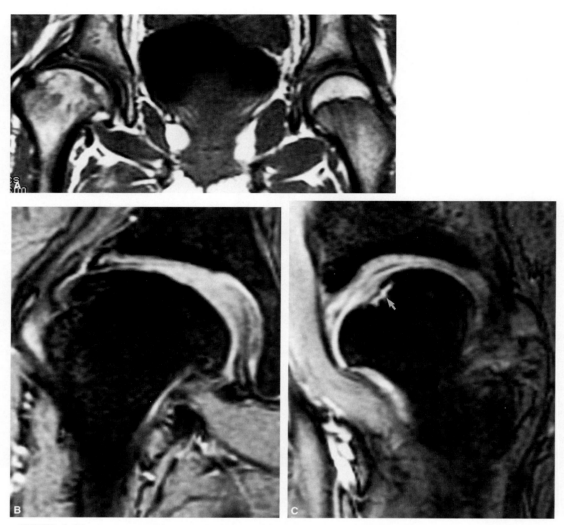

FIGURE 6-47. An 11-year old girl with chronic changes of Legg-Calvé-Perthes disease on the right. There is enlargement of the right capital epiphysis with decreased superolateral coverage, and loss of epiphyseal height on T1 coronal (**A**) and T2* coronal (**B**) images. T2* coronal image (**B**) shows flattening of the femoral head and acetabulum. Sagittal T2* image (**C**) identifies the hyperintense anterior epiphyseal involvement (*arrows*). The overlying articular cartilage appears more congruent than the necrotic focus within the capital epiphysis.

tion. As the examiner flexes the hip, it moves into external rotation and the patient often holds the leg externally rotated when standing.

Diagnosis

Initial evaluation should include both AP and frog lateral radiographs. Since the major direction of the slip is usually posterior, it is often most easily noted on a frog lateral view. Both hips should be evaluated, because slips are bilateral in 20% to 25% of cases.

Classification

Slipped capital femoral epiphysis can be classified according to the either the duration of symptoms or the degree of slippage. Acute slips may be diagnosed in patients who have had symptoms for less than 3 weeks and in whom no chronic radiographic changes are found. Symptoms lasting 3 weeks or longer indicate a chronic slip, and chronic radiographic changes include resorption of the superior femoral neck and new bone formation on the inferior femoral neck. An acute-on-chronic slip has chronic symptoms and radiographic changes with acute progression of the slip. Slips are also classified as mild, moderate, or severe based on the amount of slippage.

Treatment

The goal of treatment of SCFE is to stabilize the femoral capital epiphysis, leading to early fusion of the growth plate. For mild to moderate slips, the most common procedure is

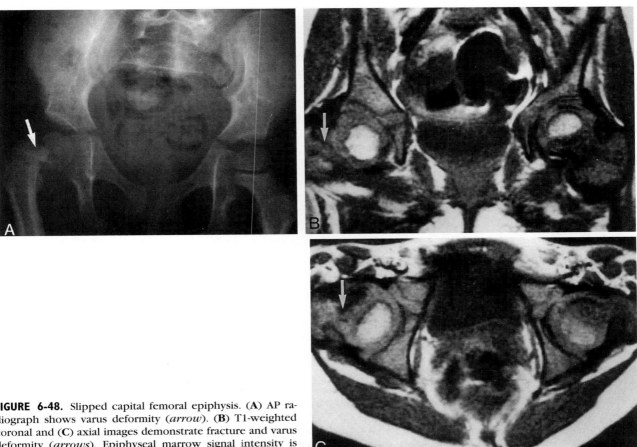

FIGURE 6-48. Slipped capital femoral epiphysis. **(A)** AP radiograph shows varus deformity (*arrow*). **(B)** T1-weighted coronal and **(C)** axial images demonstrate fracture and varus deformity (*arrows*). Epiphyseal marrow signal intensity is preserved (TR, 500 see; TE, 30 msec).

in situ pinning. Many types of hardware are used, including a variety of multiple pin techniques and single screws. With severe slips, some advocate a gentle closed reduction, open reduction, or cuneiform osteotomy.[77] The complication rate is high with internal fixation.[78] Chondrolysis can occur and has been attributed to pin penetration. Unrecognized pin penetration is a major problem. AVN, another serious complication of treatment in SCFE, may follow closed reduction, open reduction, osteotomy, or vascular damage from internal fixation. It is important to remember that this is an iatrogenic complication. Bone graft epiphysiodesis has gained popularity in some centers because of the high complication rate with internal fixation.[79] In the long term, the resultant biomechanical abnormality predisposes the patient to degenerative arthritis.[80]

Magnetic Resonance Imaging

Although MR imaging has played a limited role in the evaluation of SCFE, it is possible to display the morphology of the articular cartilage epiphysis prior to the development of bright signal intensity fat within the femoral ossification center.[73] The widened growth plate and epiphyseal slippage

are clearly demonstrated on MR images (Fig. 6-48). MR imaging may also be useful in identifying associated osteonecrosis—reported in up to 15% of children—prior to its appearance on conventional radiographs.[81] Associated incongruity of the joint surfaces and changes in the articular cartilage covering of the femoral head and acetabulum are best seen on coronal and axial plane images. The relationship of the femoral epiphysis to its containment within the acetabulum is best displayed on axial images showing anterior and posterior position relative to the acetabulum.

Developmental Dysplasia of the Hip

In developmental dysplasia of the hip (DDH), also known as infantile hip dysplasia, the left hip is affected in 40% to 60% of cases and bilateral involvement occurs in 20%. Infants at risk for DDH include those with a positive family history, breach presentation, torticollis, scoliosis, metatarsus adductus, and structural abnormalities such as underdevelopment of the anterior capsule, ligament of Bigelow, or rectus muscle.

Classification

Developmental dysplasia of the hip is classified according to the configuration of the acetabulum and the limbus.[82] A type 1 hip is characterized by positional instability. In types 2 and 3, there is subluxation and dislocation of the hip, respectively. In dislocation of the femoral epiphysis, the femoral head is uncovered by the cartilaginous acetabulum and displaced superolaterally. The hourglass configuration of the joint capsule is caused by compression between the limbus and the ligamentum teres. Constriction by the iliopsoas tendon may block attempts at reduction. Most cases of DDH present with a type 1 hip and positional instability. Failed hip reduction may be secondary to thickening of the ligamentum teres, an unfolded or blunted limbus, and severe deformity of the acetabulum or femoral head.

Diagnosis

Ortolani's and Barlow's tests are used in the early postnatal period to assess the dislocated and dislocatable hip, respectively. In Ortolani's test, hip abduction at 90° flexion with anterior pressure directs the dislocated femoral head into the acetabulum. In Barlow's test, an unstable femoral head can be dislocated by application of posterior pressure in adduction.

Radiographic diagnosis of DDH is more accurate than either of these clinical tests. Conventional radiographic assessment of the ossific nucleus relative to Hilgenreiner's line demonstrates its location in the lower medial quadrant. Shenton's line, connecting the medial border of the femoral metaphysis and the superior border of the obturator foramen, should form a smooth uninterrupted arc in the normal hip, with no subluxation or dislocation. The acetabular index (ie, the slope of the ossified acetabular roof), which is 27° to 30° at birth, is an unreliable measurement in newborns and changes with rotation of the pelvis. A 45° bilateral abduction and internal rotation view or Van Rosen view may prematurely reduce the positionally unstable hip.

Ultrasonography is often used to evaluate the cartilaginous femoral head prior to the appearance of the ossific nucleus in children up to 1 year of age. In fact, this technique may also be used in older children. Sonographic findings of increased thickness of the acetabular cartilage are reported to be an early sign of DDH.[83] Osseous dysplasia of the acetabular rim and coverage of the acetabular roof can also be assessed. CT, using a limited number of CT scans with coronal reformations and optional 3D renderings, may be a more appropriate modality for patients in plaster or with equivocal conventional radiographs.[84,85]

Magnetic Resonance Imaging

Magnetic resonance imaging can be successfully used in the evaluation of developmental hip dysplasia (Fig. 6-49).[80,85,86] The femoral epiphyseal articular cartilage displays intermediate signal intensity on T1-weighted images, and bright signal intensity on gradient-echo images. T1-weighted coronal and axial images display the exact position of the intermediate signal intensity capital epiphysis, which is particularly useful when the position of the capital epiphysis is uncertain on conventional radiographs and when serial follow-up examinations are required. MR examination can be used for children in and out of plaster casts, eliminating the need to repeatedly expose the child to ionizing radiation. MR imaging is also useful when the ossific nucleus is not yet visible on plain radiography or CT. T2-weighted images are helpful when evaluating complications associated with DDH, such as ischemic necrosis and associated effusions, which are not effectively detected with ultrasound or conventional radiography. 3D MR rendering is useful in displaying complex femoral head and acetabular spatial relationships, as well as associated dysplasia (Fig. 6-50).[87]

With MR imaging, the etiology of DDH and the failure to achieve adequate reduction can be determined without the use of invasive arthrography.[88] However, an hourglass configuration of the acetabulum or an inverted, hypertrophied limbus must be excluded. With inversion, the intermediate signal intensity limbus is often seen in the lateral aspect of the joint, with increased fat (ie, high signal intensity on T1-weighted images) noted medially. An interposed iliopsoas tendon crossing the joint space prevents reduction of the femoral head in the acetabulum and may create an hourglass configuration of the joint capsule (Fig. 6-51). Supralateral subluxation or dislocation is best identified on coronal MR images, and AP relationships and dysplasia of the acetabular wall are best demonstrated on axial plane images (Fig. 6-52). The coronal plane is the most useful for evaluating acetabular labral coverage beyond the lateral margin of the bony acetabulum relative to the femoral capital epiphysis (Fig. 6-53). This is important in determining the coverage of the femoral head and possible need for increased coverage through surgical osteotomy. Adequate coverage provided by the bony acetabulum and acetabular labrum together may direct the surgeon to more conservative management of DDH patients.

MR imaging is also useful in the long-term follow-up and postoperative evaluation of patients with DDH (Figs. 6-54 and 6-55). There is no artifact from plaster or fiberglass abduction spica casts, allowing for noninvasive eval-

text continues on page 156

FIGURE 6-50. (**A**) T1-weighted coronal image in developmental dysplasia of hip. Severe acetabular dysplasia and deformity of the femoral head (*curved black arrow*) is shown in an adult patient with untreated disease. The pseudocapsule is outlined (*white arrows*) (TR, 500 msec; TE, 20 msec). (**B**) Three-dimensional MR rendering (blue, pelvis and spine; orange, femur; red, capsule).

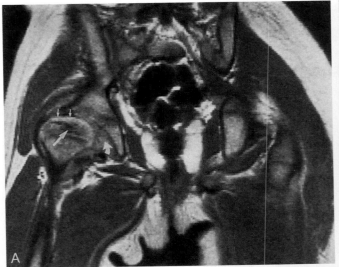

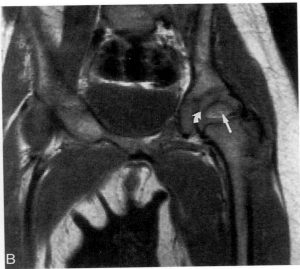

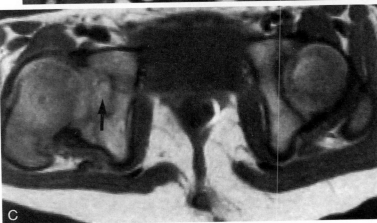

FIGURE 6-49. T1-weighted images showing developmental dysplasia of the hip (DDH). (A) Superolateral subluxation of the right femoral head and interposed soft tissue (*curved arrow*) is seen within the acetabulum. Osteonecrosis (*large straight arrow*) and flattening of the cartilaginous epiphysis (*small straight arrows*) are also present. (B) A normal left hip is shown for comparison. Note the intact intermediate signal intensity articular cartilage (*curved arrow*) and bright signal intensity yellow marrow epiphyseal center (*straight arrow*). (C) An axial image shows interposed tissue (*arrow*) that resulted in lateral subluxation. Normal anteroposterior relationships are maintained (TR, 600 msec; TE, 20 msec).

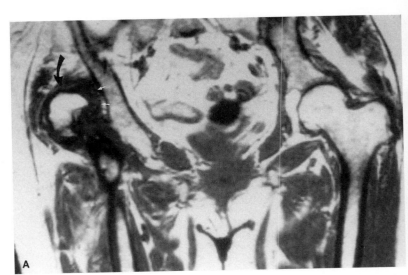

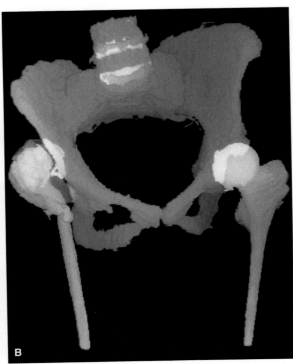

FIGURE 6-50. *Continued.*

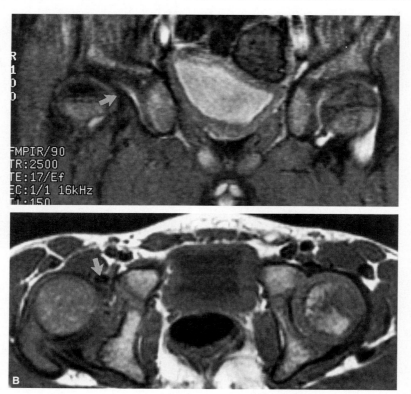

FIGURE 6-51. Interposed iliopsoas tendon (*arrow*) is seen invaginating the anterior hip capsule on the right on (**A**) fast spin-echo STIR coronal and (**B**) T1-weighted axial images. Note the associated increased medial joint space.

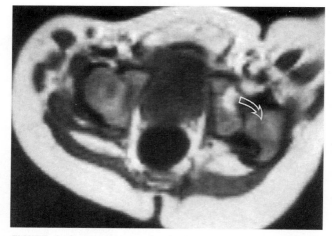

FIGURE 6-52. This T1-weighted axial image demonstrates left posterior dislocation (*arrow*) in developmental dysplasia of the hip. Associated acetabular dysplasia is shown (TR, 600 msec; TE, 20 msec).

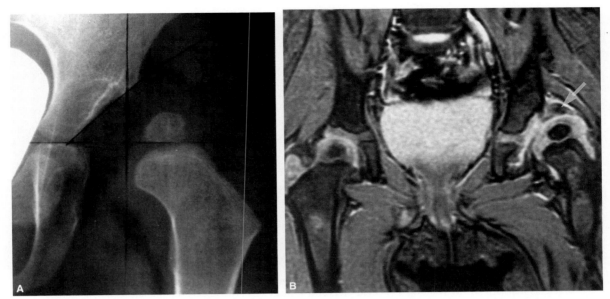

FIGURE 6-53. Coronal radiograph (**A**) shows complete lateral uncovering of the femoral capital epiphysis associated with a shallow acetabulum in developmental dysplasia of the hip. Corresponding T2* coronal MR image (**B**), however, demonstrates improved coverage by a mildly deformed but primarily everted labrum (*arrows*).

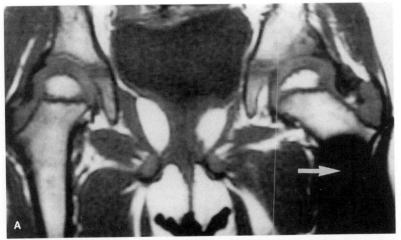

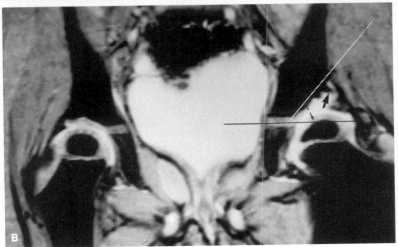

FIGURE 6-54. Coronal (**A**) T1-weighted and (**B**) T2*-weighted images in developmental dysplasia of the hip treated with varus osteotomy (*white arrow*). The acetabulum is shallow, and the labrum is inverted (*black arrows*). The acetabular index, formed by Hilgenreiner's or the Y-line through the triradiate cartilage, and the tangent through acetabular roof is abnormal (>30°) (**A:** TR, 500 msec; TE, 20 msec; **B:** TR, 400; TE, 20 msec; flip angle, 25°).

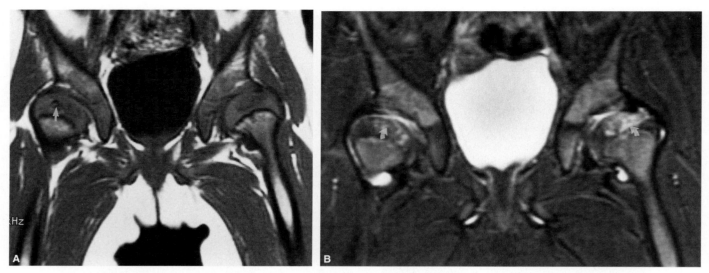

FIGURE 6-55. Ischemic necrosis complicating developmental dysplasia of the hip. The right ossific nucleus is hypointense (*arrow*) on T1-weighted coronal image (**A**). The left ossific nucleus is not visualized. Hyperintense signal inhomogeneity (*arrows*) is present within the articular cartilage of the capital epiphysis on fat-suppressed T2-weighted fast spin-echo coronal image (**B**).

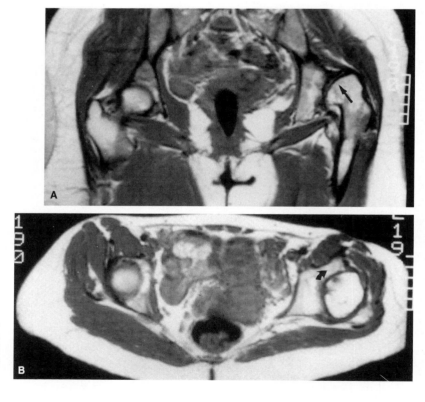

FIGURE 6-56. (**A**) Coronal and (**B**) axial T1-weighted images in an adult patient with chronic developmental dysplasia of the hip. Deformities of the acetabulum (*curved arrow*) and remodeling of the femoral head (*straight arrow*) can be seen (TR, 500 msec; TE, 15 msec).

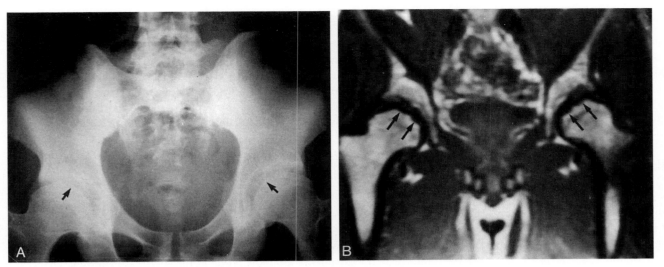

FIGURE 6-57. (A) AP radiograph and (B) T1-weighted coronal image show multiple epiphyseal dysplasia and bilateral irregularity of the femoral head (*arrows*) (TR, 800 msec; TE, 20 msec).

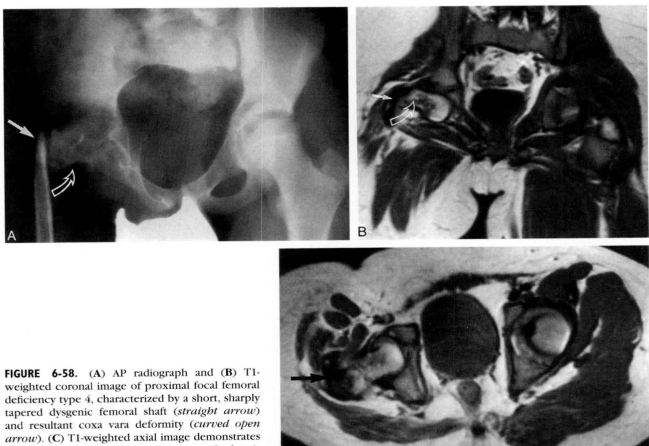

FIGURE 6-58. (A) AP radiograph and (B) T1-weighted coronal image of proximal focal femoral deficiency type 4, characterized by a short, sharply tapered dysgenic femoral shaft (*straight arrow*) and resultant coxa vara deformity (*curved open arrow*). (C) T1-weighted axial image demonstrates a region of low signal intensity pseudarthrosis (*arrow*) bridging the femoral head and neck to the ossified diaphysis (TR, 600 msec; TE, 20 msec).

uations of the femoral head. In the young, sequelae of DDH may require reconstruction of the acetabulum using a pelvic osteotomy or shelf procedure to redirect, reposition, and augment the hip socket (Fig. 6-56). Later in life, patients often develop secondary osteoarthritis requiring total hip replacement.

Miscellaneous Pediatric Hip Conditions

Multiple epiphyseal dysplasia is an autosomal dominant condition involving the epiphyseal chondrocytes of the growth plate with resultant joint incongruity and premature degenerative arthritis. MR imaging demonstrates irregularity of the femoral head and articular and cortical surfaces (Fig. 6-57). Joint-space narrowing and secondary degenerative joint disease are present by the third or fourth decade of life.

Proximal focal femoral deficiency is a term used to describe the unilateral lack of or shortening of the proximal segments of the femur. The radiographic classification system (classes A through D) is based on the presence or absence of a femoral head or acetabular dysplasia, and on the shape of the femoral segment.[89] We have used MR imaging to evaluate severe pseudoarthrosis and subtrochanteric varus deformity (Fig. 6-58). On MR examination, fibrous and osseous connections between the femoral head and shaft can be differentiated. In coxa vara, MR imaging is successful in displaying articular cartilage and epiphyseal morphology (Fig. 6-59).

Diaphyseal sclerosis, or Engelmann's disease, is characterized by long bone sclerosis involving both endosteal and cortical surfaces with relative sparing of the epiphysis and metaphysis. Bilateral symmetry and varying degrees of pain are usually associated with this condition. Although MR imaging is not indicated as the initial study of choice, its use allows the assessment of low signal intensity cortical thickening without the ionizing radiation (Fig. 6-60).

Hip Pain in the Athlete

Overuse Syndromes

Hip pain in the athlete is most commonly secondary to overuse, resulting in tendinitis, bursitis, or muscle strain. Runners are most prone to these types of injuries, which are often associated with repetitive drills or a change in the intensity or duration of a workout schedule. Muscle edema involving the adductor muscle groups can be demonstrated without tears in marathon and ultramarathon runners (Fig. 6-61). The antagonist muscle groups are most susceptible to injury. Although the injury can occur anywhere within the muscle, the origin or insertion of the muscle is most likely to be affected. In the adductors, the resulting tendinitis and periostitis cause the so-called pulled groin. Similarly, the pulled hamstring usually is a result of periostitis–tendinitis at the ischial tuberosity where the hamstring muscles originate.

In evaluating the athlete with hip pain, a careful history is critical. The physician needs a detailed account of the training habits of the athlete and any recent modifications to that regimen. On physical examination, pain can often be elicited with deep palpation in the area of the musculotendi-

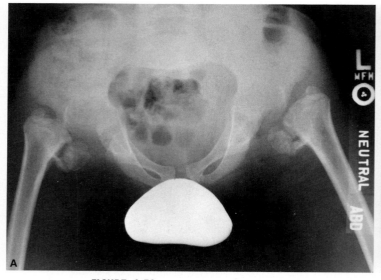
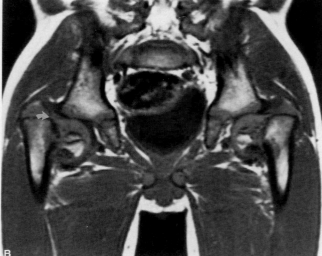

FIGURE 6-59. **(A)** Coxa vara with multiple epiphyseal dysplasia. T1- **(B)** and fat-suppressed T2-weighted fast spin-echo images document the cartilaginous continuity (*curved arrow*) between the capital epiphysis and femur.

continued

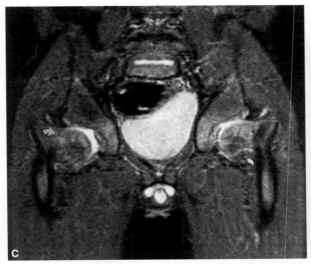

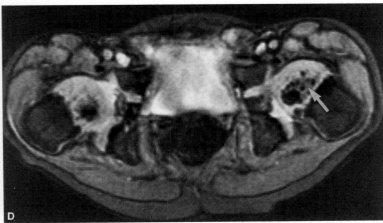

FIGURE 6-59. *Continued.* (**C**) Coronal images document the cartilaginous continuity (*curved arrow*) between the capital epiphysis and femur. Irregular and punctate morphology of the ossific nucleus (*arrow*) is appreciated on T2* axial image (**D**).

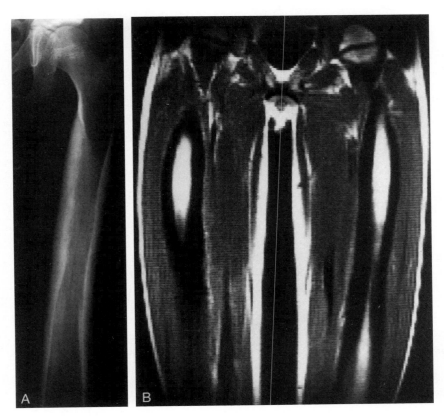

FIGURE 6-60. (**A**) AP radiograph of the femur shows diaphyseal sclerosis characteristic of Engelmann's disease. (**B**) The corresponding T1-weighted coronal MR image demonstrates low signal intensity cortical thickening (TR, 500 msec; TE, 40 msec).

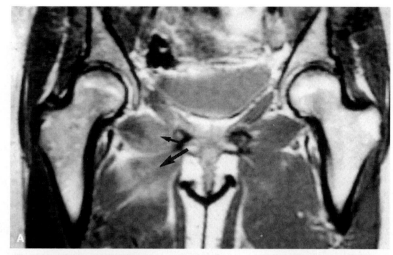

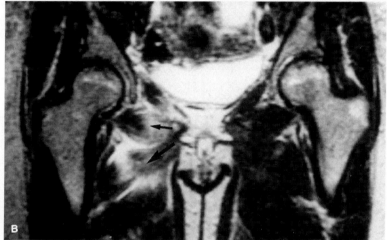

FIGURE 6-61. After a 160-km (100-mile) run, an ultramarathon runner presented with a grade 1 muscle strain. Coronal (**A**) intermediate weighted and (**B**) T2-weighted images display increased signal intensity edema and hemorrhage involving the obturator externus (*small arrow*) and adductor brevis (*large arrow*) muscles. Normal muscle size and morphology were preserved (TR, 2000 msec; TE, 20, 80 msec).

nous junction or the muscle itself. In addition, pain with resistive muscle contraction can localize the traumatized muscle group.

MUSCLE STRAINS. Muscle strains can be graded using a system similar to that used for ligament injuries. A grade 1 strain may simply result in a muscle spasm or cramp. In grade 2 strains, which result from true overuse, discomfort occurs during sporting activity or training but usually resolves with rest. The grade 3 strain is a true muscle tear that can occur within the muscle, at the muscle-tendon junction, or at the origin or insertion of the muscle.

Muscle tears and avulsions demonstrate high signal intensity in areas of edema or hemorrhage on conventional T2, fat-suppressed T2-weighted fast spin-echo, and STIR sequences.[90–92] Axial plane imaging is useful for the demonstration of associated muscle retraction and atrophy, which demonstrate high signal intensity on T1-weighted images. Coronal or sagittal images provide a longitudinal display of the entire muscle group on a single image. A comparison with the contralateral extremity is important in evaluating relative symme-

try of muscle groups. In a grade 1 muscle strain, MR findings include edema, hemorrhage, or both, with preservation of muscle morphology (Fig. 6-62). In a grade 2 muscle strain or tear, hemorrhage with tearing and disruption of up to 50% of the muscle fibers occurs (Figs. 6-63 and 6-64). Subacute hemorrhage, of bright signal intensity on T1-weighted images, is commonly seen in grade 2 injuries (Fig. 6-65). There is a complete tearing with or without muscle retraction in grade 3 muscle tears (Fig. 6-66).

Rectus femoris muscle strains are frequently seen in sprinting or kicking sports such as soccer. Hasselman and coworkers[93,94] have described three chronic strain injuries involving the mid-muscle belly of the rectus femoris. The most common rectus femoris injury involves minimally disruptive trauma with pain at the site of injury. Partial or complete disruption of the muscle tendon unit is frequently associated with rupture of distal muscle fibers from the posterior tendon insertion, with associated proximal muscle retraction.[93,94] Another type of acute strain occurs in the mid-muscle belly with disruption of the muscle tendon junction of the deep intramuscular tendon of the indirect head, with

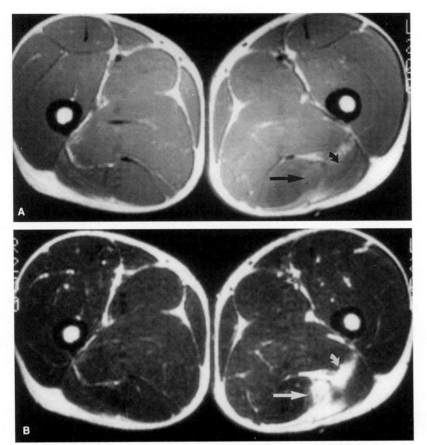

FIGURE 6-62. A grade 1 muscle strain caused edema and hemorrhage in the lateral aspect of the semitendinosus muscle (*straight arrow*) and medial aspect of the biceps femoris muscle (*curved arrow*) in a professional sprinter who presented with acute thigh pain. **(A)** Normal muscle morphology is shown on an intermediate weighted image, whereas **(B)** edema and hemorrhage are demonstrated on the T2-weighted image (TR, 2000; TE, 20, 80 msec).

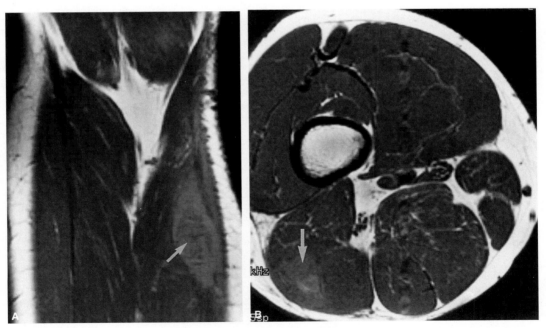

FIGURE 6-63. Grade 1 to 2 muscle strain with focal hemorrhage and disruption of the lateral biceps femoris (*long head*) muscle fibers. Hemorrhage (*arrow*) is intermediate in signal intensity on T1-weighted **(A)** coronal and **(B)** axial images.

continued

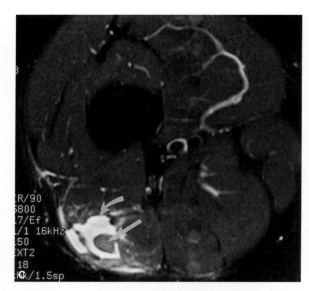

FIGURE 6-63. *Continued.* A more organized central component of the hematoma is hypointense (*straight arrow*) with surrounding hyperintensity (*curved arrow*) on fast spin-echo STIR image (**C**).

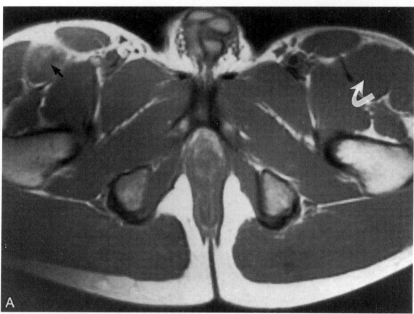

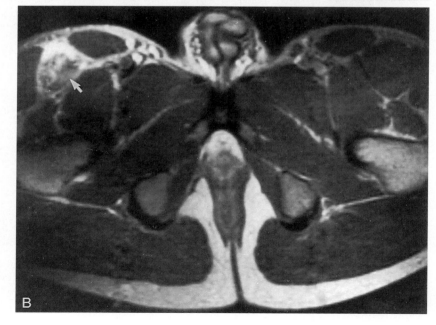

FIGURE 6-64. A grade 2 muscle tear of the right rectus femoris muscle with atrophy and edema (*arrows*) is shown on (**A**) intermediate weighted and (**B**) T2-weighted axial images. Edematous muscle fibers display increased signal intensity on the T2-weighted image. A normal size left rectus femoris muscle is shown for comparison (*curved arrow*) (TR, 2000 msec; TE, 20, 80 msec).

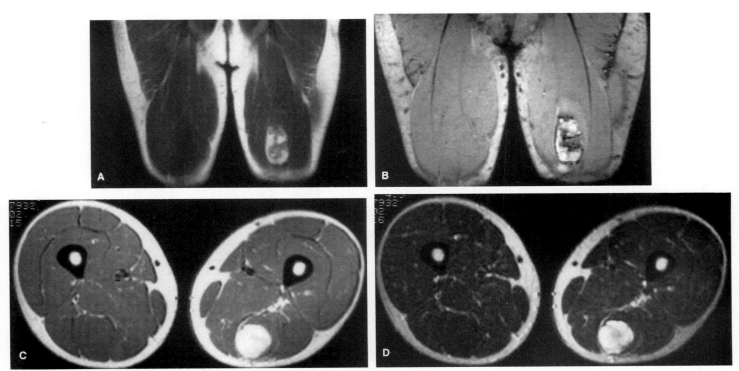

FIGURE 6-65. A grade 2 semitendinosus muscle tear is indicated by hemorrhage seen on coronal (**A**) T1-weighted and (**B**) T2*-weighted images. A subacute hemorrhage, of bright intensity on the T1-weighted image, shows focal areas of hemosiderin on the T2*-weighted image (**A:** TR, 600 msec; TE, 20 msec; **B:** TR, 500 msec; TE, 20 msec; flip angle, 25°). Axial (**C**) intermediate weighted and (**D**) T2-weighted images show semitendinosus hemorrhage involving disruption of approximately 50% of the muscle fibers (**C, D:** TR, 2000 msec; TE, 20, 80 msec).

distal retraction of muscle fibers. This injury is associated with local hemorrhage and edema. A chronic pseudocyst within the deep intramuscular tendon of the indirect head of the rectus may develop as the hematoma organizes.

Fibrous encasement of the deep tendon, with scar tissue formation, is hypointense on T2-weighted images (Fig. 6-67) and may be mistaken for a soft tissue neoplasm. In fibrous encasement, T2-weighted images display a small low signal intensity lesion with a surrounding hyperemic rim deep within the mid-muscle belly. A tumor, however, would not present with the typical cylindrical shape corresponding to the tendon of the indirect head of the rectus femoris. Gradient-echo images may demonstrate susceptibility artifact in the area of hemorrhage. If the differential diagnosis includes a neoplastic process such as a malignant fibrous histiocytoma or a synovial sarcoma, intravenous gadolinium should be administered.

Hamstring muscle injuries (semimembranosus, semitendinosus, and biceps femoris) have a variable appearance over time that can be characterized using MR imaging.[95] Distinctive findings are seen in acute, subacute, and chronic injuries. Conjoined tendon (the hamstring muscle originates in a conjoined tendon from the posterolateral aspect of the ischial tuberosity) injuries, with associated muscle edema,

hemorrhage, and partial tearing of the musculotendinous junction are seen in acute trauma. Proximal injuries, the most frequent to affect the hamstring muscle group, demonstrate an abnormal increased signal intensity that is contained by muscle fascia. Increased signal intensity on T2-weighted images or STIR sequences is secondary to hemorrhage or edema. Musculotendinous junction injuries with edema or hemorrhage may display a feather-like area of high signal intensity on T2, fat-suppressed T2-weighted fast spin-echo, or STIR images. Subacute injuries may demonstrate increased signal intensity on T1-weighted images. Exertional muscle injuries show a more diffuse pattern of hyperintensity on T2 or STIR sequences. A subacute ischial avulsion may be mistaken for osteomyelitis or neoplasia with an aggressive pattern on corresponding radiographs. MR imaging may show associated edema on fat-suppressed or STIR images. Chronic injuries frequently demonstrate atrophy and fatty replacement of muscles.

Treatment of a grade 2 strains centers on identifying the offending activity. The injury usually responds to cutting back or altering the training schedule. Cycling or swimming can be temporarily substituted for running to maintain aerobic conditioning. Physiotherapy is beneficial in decreasing muscle spasm and ultimately in regaining flexibility and

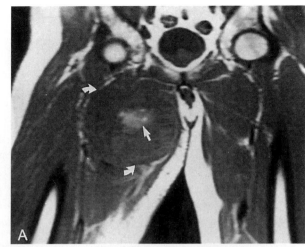

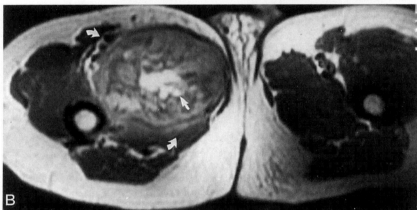

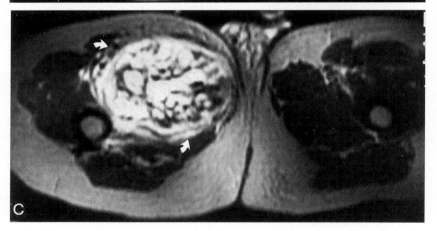

FIGURE 6-66. (A) T1-weighted image displays a complete grade 3 rupture of the adductor magnus muscle (*curved arrow*) with central subacute hemorrhagic component demonstrating bright signal intensity (TR, 600 msec; TE, 20 msec). Axial (B) intermediate weighted and (C) T2-weighted images demonstrate increasing signal intensity within the edematous muscle fibers (*curved arrows*). The central hemorrhagic component (*straight arrow*) seen on the intermediate weighted scan becomes isointense with surrounding edema on T2-weighted image (B, C: TR, 2000 msec; TE, 20, 80 msec).

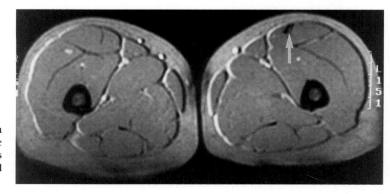

FIGURE 6-67. Focal low signal intensity sequela from trauma to the deep intramuscular tendon of the indirect head of the rectus femoris muscle (*arrow*). The hypointensity represents fibrous (scar) encasement of the deep tendon. Fat-suppressed T2-weighted fast spin-echo axial image.

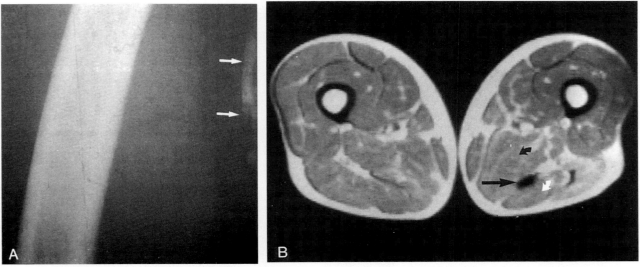

FIGURE 6-68. (A) A lateral radiograph of the thigh shows myositis ossificans demonstrating linear calcification (*arrows*). (B) T1-weighted axial image shows low signal intensity calcific deposition (*straight arrow*) in the fascial plane between the semitendinosus muscle (*curved white arrow*) and the semimembranosus muscle (*curved black arrow*) (TR, 800 msec; TE, 20 msec).

strength. Grade 3 strains are more difficult to treat and usually require a period of 6 to 8 weeks of rest. Return to full activity is allowed when pain has resolved and muscle strength has returned. This can be effectively judged by using Cybex testing.

Although conventional radiography should remain the initial diagnostic examination for excluding posttraumatic myositis ossificans secondary to muscle trauma, MR scans have shown small areas of calcification or ossification as signal void, or low signal intensity on T1- and T2-weighted images (Fig. 6-68).

Intramuscular hemorrhage may occur spontaneously or with minimal trauma in patients on anticoagulants (Fig. 6-69). On MR examination of the diabetic patient, intramus-

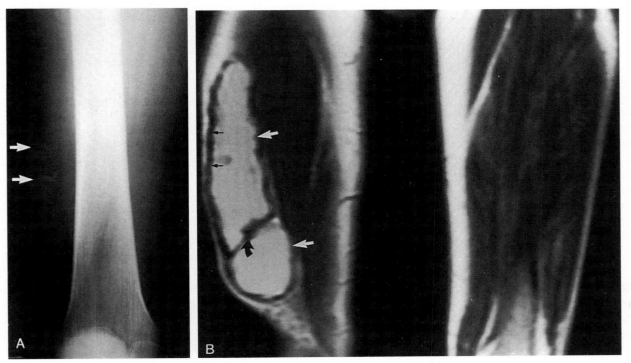

FIGURE 6-69. (A) AP radiograph of anterior thigh hemorrhage shows focal soft tissue calcific deposition (*arrows*). (B) T1-weighted coronal image displays a high signal intensity subacute hemorrhage in the region of the vastus lateralis muscle (*white arrows*). The low signal intensity hemosiderin periphery (*small black arrows*) and internal septations (*curved arrow*) are shown (TR, 800 msec; TE, 20 msec).

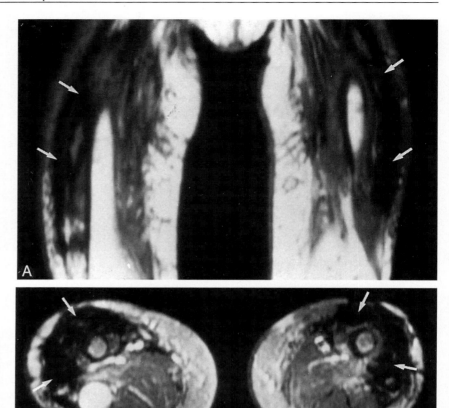

FIGURE 6-70. Chronic intramuscular hemorrhage was caused by repeated injections of insulin in this diabetic patient. Low signal intensity paramagnetic hemosiderin deposition (*short arrows*) in vastus lateralis and intermedius muscles can be seen on T1-weighted (**A**) coronal and (**B**) axial images. High signal intensity focal subacute hemorrhage is shown within the long head of the biceps femoris muscle (*long arrow*) on the axial image (TR, 600 msec; TE, 20 msec).

cular hemosiderin deposits in sites of insulin injections can also be identified (Fig. 6-70).

Muscle and soft tissue inflammation may appear similar to a grade 1 muscle strain (Fig. 6-71). Acute fasciitis is detected as a diffuse increase in signal intensity conforming to the involved muscle group (Fig. 6-72). Corresponding gallium scintigraphy and CT may be negative. Soft tissue edema in infection demonstrates low signal intensity on T1-weighted images and increased signal intensity on T2-weighted images. If soft tissue infection is suspected, MR evaluation may be the examination of choice.

BURSITIS. The two main bursal groups that can become inflamed and cause hip pain in the athlete are (1) the trochanteric bursa, which is actually three discrete bursae, and (2) the deep gluteal or ischiogluteal bursa. In addition, the iliopsoas bursa, which lies deep to the iliopsoas muscle, can occasionally cause hip pain.

The trochanteric bursa becomes inflamed with repetitive irritation of the tensor fascia latae sliding over the greater trochanter (Fig. 6-73). This condition is common in runners and those who play racquet sports, causing pain in the lateral aspect of the thigh. Inflammation of the deep gluteal bursa causes pain deep in the buttock and can be confused with referred pain from the lower back. In both cases, it is important to differentiate between bursitis and lumbar disease. Treatment consists of activity modification, physical therapy, and nonsteroidal antiinflammatory medications. Occasionally, local steroid injection and, less commonly, surgical intervention play a role.

Iliopsoas bursitis may be accompanied by a snapping sensation caused by the psoas tendon passing over the iliopectineal eminence on the pubis.[96] Treatment is initially conservative, but if pain and snapping persist, the prominence on the iliopectineal eminence can be resected along with a partial release of the iliopsoas tendon. The snapping hip syndrome has also been associated with iliotibial band syndrome (external snapping hip syndrome) with irritation of the greater trochanteric bursa by the iliotibial band.[97] Rare cases of snapping hip syndrome have also been caused by snapping of the iliofemoral ligaments over the femoral head and the long head of the biceps femoris over the ischial tuberosity. Intraarticular loose bodies and labral tears are unusual, but should be considered in the differential diagnosis of snapping hip syndrome.[98]

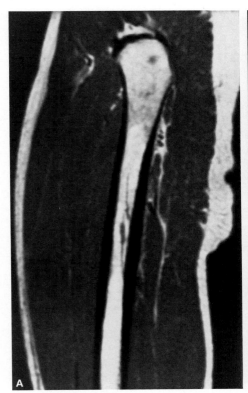
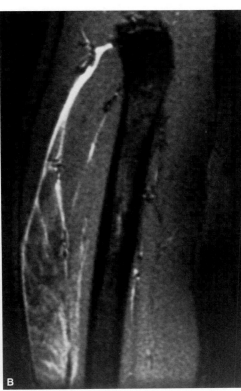

FIGURE 6-71. The feather-like distribution of muscle edema in a grade 1 muscle strain of the vastus lateralis muscle is not apparent on the T1-weighted sagittal image (**A**), However, is hyperintense on the fast spin-echo STIR image (**B**). Soft tissue inflammation may also have a similar presentation.

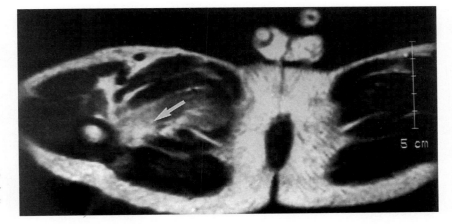

FIGURE 6-72. High signal intensity edema (*arrow*) along the muscle fascial plane is seen on this T2-weighted axial image in a 3-year-old boy with acute fasciitis (TR, 200 msec; TE, 60 msec).

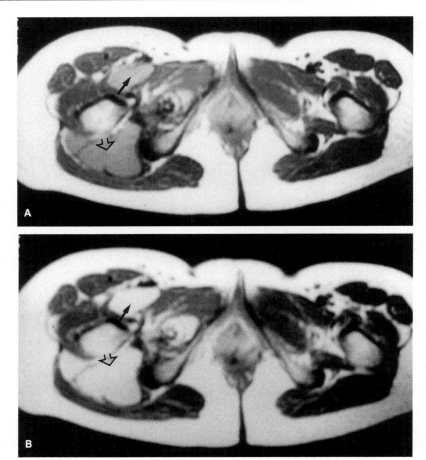

FIGURE 6-73. Trochanteric bursitis. Axial **(A)** intermediate weighted and **(B)** T2-weighted images display inflammation with synovial fluid distention in the trochanteric and ischiotrochanteric bursa in a patient with rheumatoid arthritis (*open arrow*). There is associated involvement of the iliopsoas bursa (*black arrow*). No hip effusion is present (TR, 2000 msec; TE, 20, 80 msec).

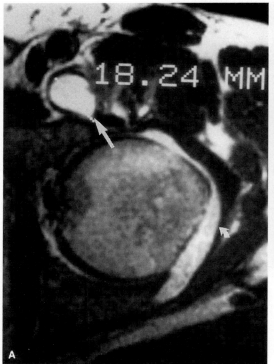

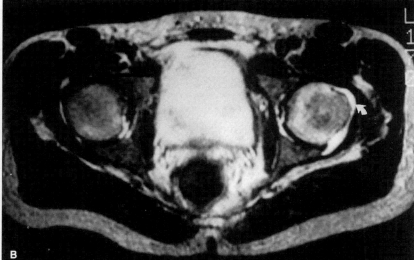

FIGURE 6-74. T2-weighted images of iliopsoas bursitis. **(A)** High signal intensity iliopsoas bursal distention can be seen medial to the iliopsoas tendon (*arrow*). Associated joint effusion is indicated (*curved arrow*). **(B)** Three months later, complete resolution of bursal fluid with no interval change in joint effusion (*curved arrow*). The initial complaint of bursitis with hip clicking in internal and external rotation was also resolved.

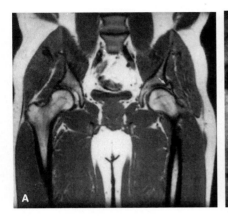
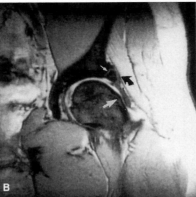

FIGURE 6-75. An old acetabular margin anterior inferior iliac spine avulsion fracture (*small white arrow*) is shown at the attachment of the reflected head of the rectus femoris (*curved black arrow*) on (**A**) a T1-weighted image obtained with a body coil and on (**B**) a T2*-weighted image obtained with a surface coil. Remodeling of the opposing surface of the femoral head has taken place (*large white arrow*) (**A:** TR 600 msec; TE, 20 msec; **B:** TR, 400 msec; TE, 20 msec; flip angle, 25°).

Axial MR images with T2 weighting are useful in demonstrating iliopsoas bursal collections adjacent to the iliopsoas tendon in patients presenting with clicking of the hip during range-of-motion activities with internal and external rotation (Fig. 6-74). Identification of bursal fluid correlates with snapping or clicking of the hip on clinical examination. Bursal fluid should not be mistaken for a malignant soft tissue neoplasm such as synovial sarcoma, which has similar imaging characteristics (ie, low signal intensity on T1-weighted and bright signal intensity on T2-weighted images).

Avulsion Fracture

The three bony structures in the hip region prone to avulsion injury are (1) the anterior superior iliac spine, (2) the anterior inferior iliac spine, and (3) the ischial tuberosity. Avulsion injuries, which are becoming more common, frequently occur in adolescents or young adults participating in athletics. It is important to evaluate the contralateral side as well as the injured side in these injuries, because they occur through secondary centers of ossification and because what appears to be a fracture may simply be an anatomic variant. Axial T2-weighted, T2*-weighted, or STIR images are usually necessary to identify areas of edema or hemorrhage associated with these fractures. When imaging with fat marrow signal, which is bright on T1-weighted images, or cortical signal intensity which demonstrates low signal intensity on T1-weighted images, avulsed bone appears dark on either gradient-echo or STIR images and may be indistinguishable from adjacent tendons or ligaments on these pulse sequences. MR evaluation of avulsion fractures should follow an initial evaluation with conventional film radiography or bone scintigraphy.

The anterior superior iliac spine is injured secondary to overpull of the sartorius muscle. This occurs with the hip in extension and the knee flexed, and thus can be seen in kicking athletes such as soccer players. Avulsion of the anterior inferior iliac spine is less common than injury to the anterior superior iliac spine and occurs as a result of overpull of the straight head of the rectus (Fig. 6-75). The mechanism of injury and the type of athlete at risk are similar in both injuries, and both are treated in the same manner. A few days of bed rest for pain relief, followed by protected weight-bearing until comfort is achieved, is adequate.[99]

Avulsion fracture of the ischial tuberosity results from overpull of the hamstring muscles. This occurs with the hip flexed and the knee in extension. During physical examination, this maneuver elicits pain, as does rectal examination. Gymnasts are prone to this injury, and Milch describes seeing it in a dancer doing splits.[100] Treatment is a short period of bed rest followed by protected weight-bearing. Although the fracture invariably heals, exuberant callus formation can occur causing chronic pain.[101] This callus formation may be confused with malignancy, leading to biopsy. Excision may be required for pain relief. Avulsion injuries of the iliac crest or lesser and greater trochanters are relatively rare.[98]

Heterotopic Ossification

Heterotopic ossification occurs secondary to trauma or surgery, or in patients who have sustained burns or paralysis. Patients with ankylosing spondylitis and diffuse idiopathic skeletal hyperostosis are also at risk for heterotopic bone formation. Large areas of bone marrow containing mature heterotopic ossification demonstrate fat marrow signal intensity on T1-weighted images (Fig. 6-76). Capsular trauma may produce bone formations that resemble an avulsion-type injury (Figs. 6-77 and 6-78).

Fractures of the Femur and Acetabulum

Fractures about the hip may be associated with significant morbidity, especially when diagnosis and treatment are delayed.[102–104] Femoral fractures are classified as either intracapsular or extracapsular. Intracapsular femoral neck fractures are subcapital, transcervical, or basicervical in location.

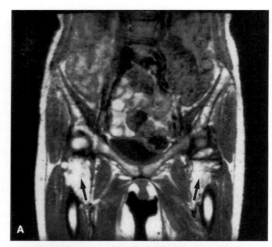

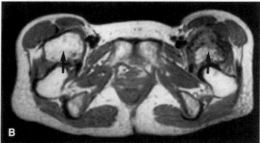

FIGURE 6-76. T1-weighted (**A**) coronal and (**B**) axial images of massive mature heterotopic bone (*arrows*) located anterior to the hip joints and extending to the level of the lesser trochanters in a patient with Guillain-Barré paralysis (TR, 600 msec; TE, 20 msec).

The incidence of posttraumatic osteonecrosis increases as the fracture site nears the femoral head, culminating in a 30% incidence for fractures in closest proximity to the femoral head. The less common capital fracture is an intracapsular fracture of the femoral head. Extracapsular fractures are intertrochanteric or subtrochanteric.

Stress fractures of the hip most frequently involve the femoral neck. They occur in two patient populations: the young adult, in whom stress fractures result from overuse and repeated stress to normal bone (eg, military recruits and runners); and osteoporosis patients (especially women), in whom the fractures are more appropriately termed insufficiency fractures and may occur with normal activity or a seemingly insignificant increase in activity.[105,106]

Patients usually present with groin pain aggravated by weight-bearing. Passive movement is often painful, especially rotation. Radiographic findings are often normal, and symptoms can be subtle. A careful history and a high index of suspicion are necessary to avoid missing the injury.

Classification and Treatment

Blickenstaff and Morris have classified stress fractures into three types.[107,108] In type I fractures, plain radiographs reveal endosteal or periosteal callus without a definite fracture line. In type II fractures, a fracture line is clearly seen, and type III fractures are displaced. Treatment may be based on the fracture type. For type I fractures, some physicians

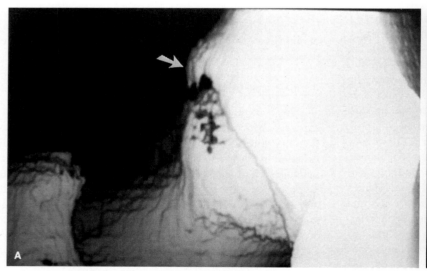

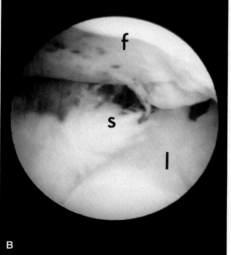

FIGURE 6-77. (**A**) Three-dimensional CT rendering of posterior capsule trauma (*arrow*) with heterotopic ossification shown in posterior view of the left hip. (**B**) An arthroscopic view shows the hyperplastic synovium (s) located deep to the capsular ossification (f, femur; l, labrum).

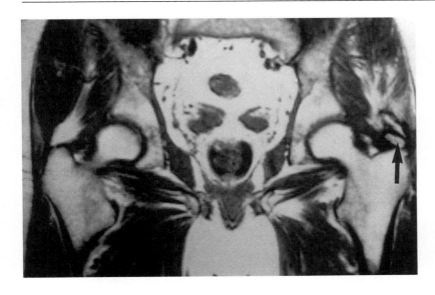

FIGURE 6-78. Heterotopic bone formation (*arrow*) after capsular trauma to the left hip. On T1-weighted coronal image, mature ossifications demonstrate fat marrow signal intensity (TR, 600 msec; TE, 20 msec).

recommend bed rest until the patient is pain free, followed by progressive weight-bearing. DeLee,[109] however, recommends prophylactic pinning for type I fractures, especially if the callus is on the lateral or tension side of the femoral neck. Type II and III fractures are treated with internal fixation. The complication rate with internal fixation of type III fractures is high and includes nonunion, malunion, and avascular necrosis.

Diagnosis and Magnetic Resonance Imaging

In general, fractures of the acetabulum are best assessed with thin section CT and subsequent image reformation and 3D rendering (Fig. 6-79). 3D reconstruction can be used to classify injuries of a single structural component (elementary fractures) and associated fractures representing combinations of elementary fracture types.[110] The posterior wall fracture is the most common acetabular fracture type. This is also referred to as a posterior lip or posterior rim fracture. A transverse fracture extends across both anterior (iliopubic) and posterior (ilioischial) acetabular columns. An anterior column fracture is usually seen in association with a posterior column or transverse fracture. In posterior column fracture, hip abduction is part of the mechanism of injury, in addition to the indirect forces acting through the femur in the position of hip flexion (this is the mechanism of posterior wall fractures). A transverse and posterior wall fracture represents the most common type of associated or complex acetabular fracture. Fracture of both the anterior and posterior columns is the most complex of acetabular fractures and is associated with comminution, rotation, and displacement. A T-shaped fracture is a transverse fracture with a vertical component that extends through the medial aspect of the acetabulum and divides the ischiopubic ramus. An anterior column fracture, in association with a transverse fracture, produces an anterior column and posterior hemitransverse

fracture. A combination of posterior column fracture and posterior wall fracture is unusual. MR imaging in direct coronal, sagittal, and axial orthogonal planes is helpful in the evaluation of acetabular columns and subchondral marrow.[111] The lateral aspect of the acetabulum is formed by the anterior and posterior columns with the intervening superior dome of the acetabulum. Anterior column fractures are associated with external rotation of the femoral head, and posterior column fractures are associated with internal rotation of the femoral head.[112] Retained fragments within the hip joint are usually seen on axial T1- and T2-weighted images. Disarticulation of the femoral head on 3D CT renderings can be used to identify size, morphology, and number of osseous fragments. The association of AVN in posterior fractures (18%) can also be evaluated with MR imaging. In detecting injuries to the sciatic nerve and occult capital fractures, MR imaging is preferable to CT.[111] Intraarticular fragments may be better displayed on thin section CT, however.[111]

Capital fractures are often radiographically occult, especially when the spherical morphology of the femoral head is maintained or when an area of impacted trabecular (subchondral) bone is involved (Fig. 6-80). Axial and sagittal images may provide better delineation of fracture morphology than coronal plane images (Fig. 6-81).

With fractures of the proximal femur, including femoral neck stress fractures, radiographic signs of cortical disruption may be subtle, especially if there is either an incomplete fracture or a complete fracture without displacement of the medial trabeculae (Fig. 6-82).[113,114] MR examination is particularly useful in identifying nondisplaced femoral neck fractures that require surgical treatment but are not detected on routine radiography (Fig. 6-83). Although bone scintigraphy is also sensitive to fractures, it is nonspecific. With MR imaging, it is possible to demonstrate the morphology of the fracture segment not detectable on bone scans. Early

text continues on page 173

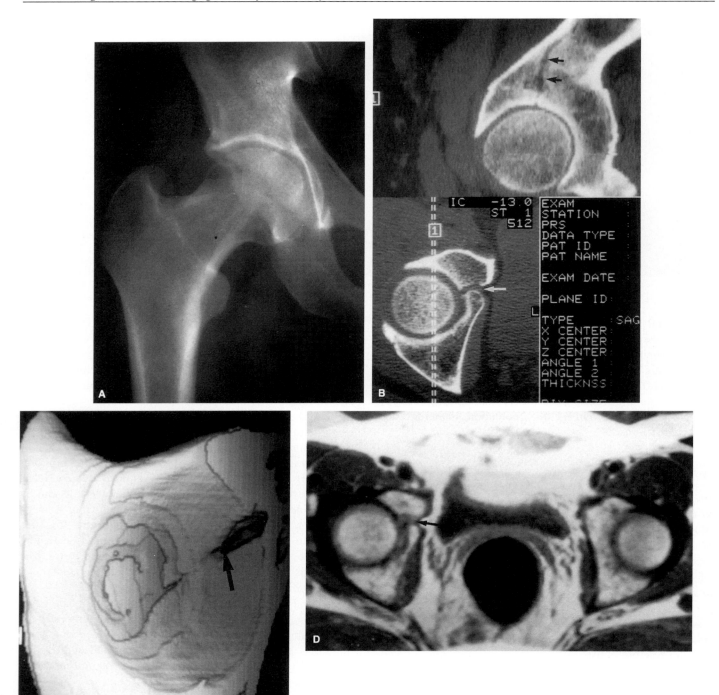

FIGURE 6-79. (A) AP radiograph does not reveal the acetabular anterior ilio-pubic column fracture. (B) Fracture morphology and extent are optimally displayed on 2D axial (*white arrow*) and reformatted (*black arrows*) CT scans. (C) Three-dimensional CT rendering allows identification of the anterior column fracture (*arrow*) with disarticulated femur. (D) The corresponding axial T1-weighted image also displays the low signal intensity anterior column fracture (*arrow*) (TR, 600 msec; TE, 20 msec).

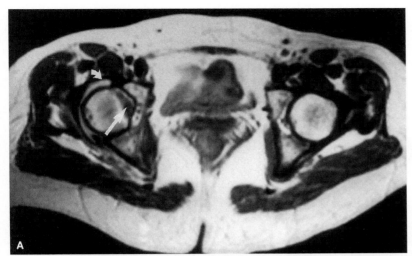

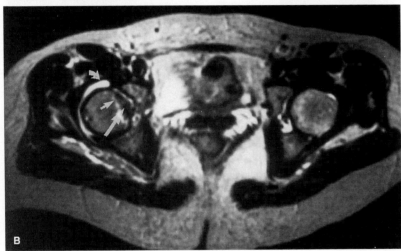

FIGURE 6-80. On axial (**A**) intermediate weighted and (**B**) T2-weighted images, a capital (ie, femoral head) impaction fracture is displayed with a wide band of low signal intensity (*large arrows*), peripheral hemorrhage (*small arrow*), and associated effusion (*curved arrows*). A wide band instead of a thin linear segment is consistent with a larger area of trabecular microfracture (TR, 2000 msec; TE, 20, 80 msec).

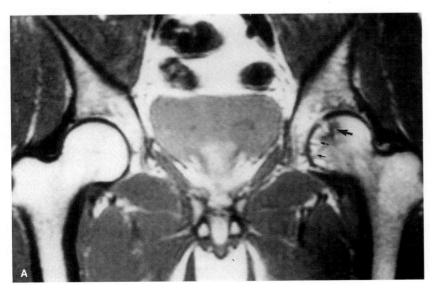

FIGURE 6-81. (**A**) A radiographically occult capital fracture (*large arrow*) is shown with associated bright signal intensity marrow hemorrhage (*small arrows*) on a T1-weighted coronal image.   *continued*

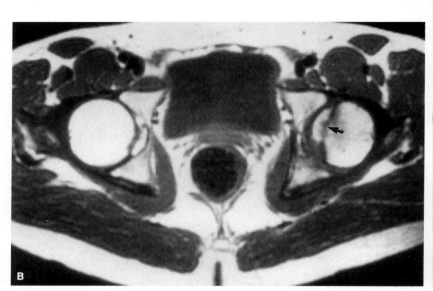

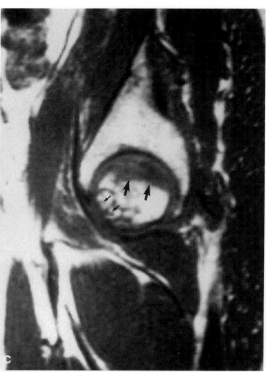

FIGURE 6-81. *Continued.* (**B**) T1-weighted axial image also reveals the fracture (*arrow*). (**C**) T1-weighted sagittal image accurately depicts the linear area of decreased signal intensity at the fracture site (*large arrows*) and marrow signal inhomogeneity anteriorly and inferiorly (*small arrows*), (TR, 500 msec; TE, 20 msec).

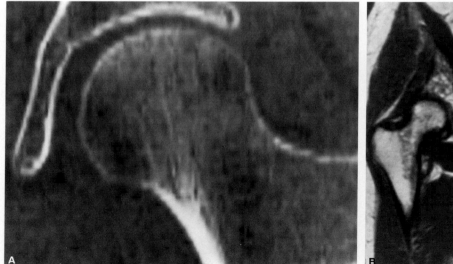

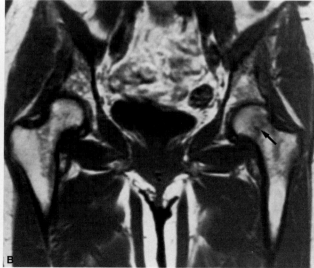

FIGURE 6-82. Early stage of left femoral neck stress fracture involving trabecular bone without cortical interruption. Coronal reformatted CT scan (**A**) is negative whereas T1-weighted (**B**) and fast STIR image (**C**) display the linear fracture morphology (*straight arrow*) and hyperintense marrow edema (*curved arrow*).

continued

intensity in the proximal femoral diaphysis, femoral neck, and head.[117] MR imaging can differentiate an osteoporotic-related subcapital fracture of the femoral neck from a pathologic fracture. The radiographic appearance of a subcapital fracture may mimic a pathologic fracture secondary to rotation displacement of the fracture fragments.[118] 3D CT or MR rendering can display varus or valgus deformities and postoperative screw placement. In displaced fractures, complicating osteonecrosis can be excluded on an MR image, and viability of the femoral head can be assessed (Figs. 6-84 through 6-86). T1-weighted images provide the best contrast for the low signal intensity fracture segment in contrast to adjacent bright signal intensity marrow fat. STIR images have shown greater sensitivity than gradient-echo techniques in displaying associated hemorrhage and edema at the fracture site.

Stress fractures about the acetabulum, ilium, pubis, and femur may be associated with extension edema, which demonstrates low signal intensity on T1-weighted images and high signal intensity on T2-weighted, T2*-weighted, fat-suppressed T2-weighted fast spin-echo or STIR images when there is no identifiable fracture segment (Fig. 6-87).[119] Thin section, high resolution CT may be necessary to achieve the precise cortical detail needed to display subtle cortical discontinuities (Figs. 6-88 and 6-89).

MR imaging affords direct visualization of cartilage prior to the appearance of ossification centers, which facilitates the identification of physeal fractures. In complex hemipelvis fracture-dislocations, MR imaging or CT can be used to assess interruptions of both the anterior and posterior pelvic ring segments and sacroiliac joint separation (Fig. 6-90).

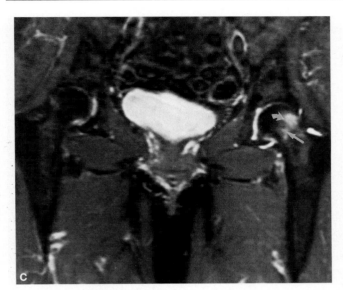

FIGURE 6-82. *Continued.*

microtrabecular stress fracture, with intact medial and lateral cortices and a negative CT finding, can also be identified on MR images. T1-weighted coronal fat-suppressed fast spin-echo and STIR sequences are sensitive in detecting occult femoral and pelvic fractures.[115,116] Associated soft tissue abnormalities, including adjacent edema and hemorrhage, are common. Contrast-enhanced MR imaging is useful for assessment of femoral head perfusion after femoral neck fracture. Intact perfusion is shown as a uniform increased signal

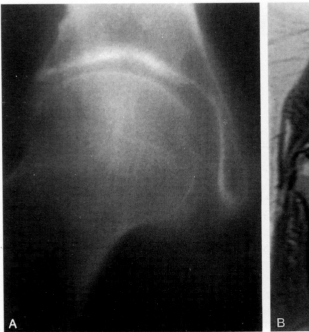
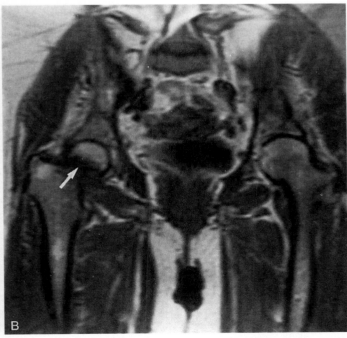

FIGURE 6-83. **(A)** This nondisplaced femoral neck fracture was missed on plain film tomography. **(B)** The fracture was detected as a low signal intensity segment (*arrow*) on a T1-weighted coronal image. The patient's fracture was subsequently pinned at surgery (TR, 800 msec; TE, 20 msec).

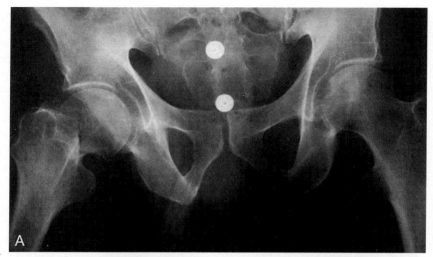

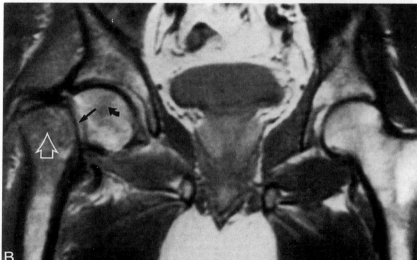

FIGURE 6-84. (**A**) AP radiograph demonstrating a right femoral neck fracture in varus deformation. (**B**) T1-weighted coronal image displaying a linear cervical neck fracture (*straight solid arrow*) and low signal intensity proximal femoral marrow edema (*open arrow*). Mild asymmetry in the femoral head marrow signal intensity is observed at this stage (*curved solid arrow*) (TR, 600 msec; TE, 20 msec).

Dislocations

Dislocation of the femoral head is usually associated with a fracture of the acetabulum, the femoral head, or both. Anterior dislocations are less frequent than posterior dislocations, and are most commonly identified anteroinferiorly.[119,120] Traumatic anterior dislocations are classified into superior and inferior types. Associated impaction fractures may lead to development of traumatic arthritis.[121] Anterior cortical fractures of the femoral head and fractures of the acetabular rim are associated with posterior dislocations.[122,123]

Chronic arthritis and AVN may complicate dislocations and fractures of the hip, and MR imaging is helpful in their early identification. In one case of posterior fracture-dislocation of the hip, MR imaging revealed an impacted femoral head fracture (low signal intensity on T1-weighted images), an acetabular rim fracture (high signal intensity hemorrhage), and multiple intraarticular fragments that were subsequently removed through an arthroscope (Fig. 6-91). At a 6-month follow-up, MR imaging showed the development of osteonecrosis at the initial site of fracture. Thus, it may be difficult to predict the subsequent development of osteonecrosis in a patient sustaining a low signal intensity compression fracture of the femoral head.

Axial MR images may be used to follow the course of the sciatic nerve, which is injured in 8% to 19% of posterior hip dislocations. Treatment of fracture-dislocations involves reduction of the hip and treatment of the associated fracture. Open surgery is required to debride osteochondral fragments. Immediate reduction of dislocation may decrease the incidence of AVN.

text continues on page 181

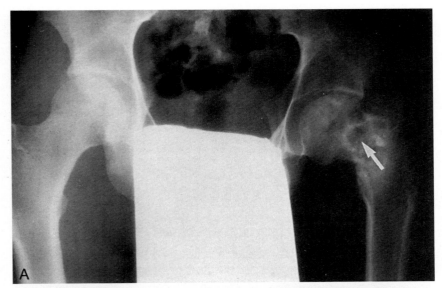

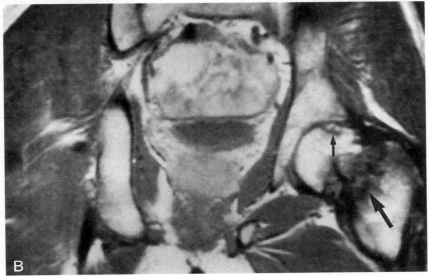

FIGURE 6-85. (A) AP radiograph shows an untreated left femoral neck fracture (*arrow*). (B) Corresponding T1-weighted coronal image demonstrates the low signal intensity sclerotic fracture site (*large arrow*) and associated focus of femoral head avascular necrosis (*small arrow*) (TR, 800 msec; TE, 20 msec).

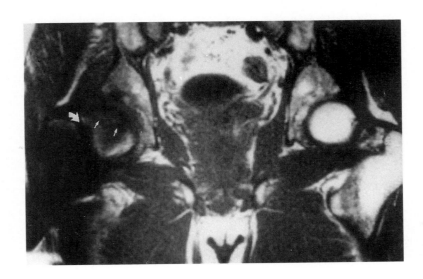

FIGURE 6-86. AVN as a complication of a midcervical femoral neck fracture after operative fixation. The metallic artifact does not preclude identification of the fracture site (*curved arrow*) or the osteonecrosis (*straight arrows*) on a T1-weighted coronal image (TR, 500 msec; TE, 20 msec).

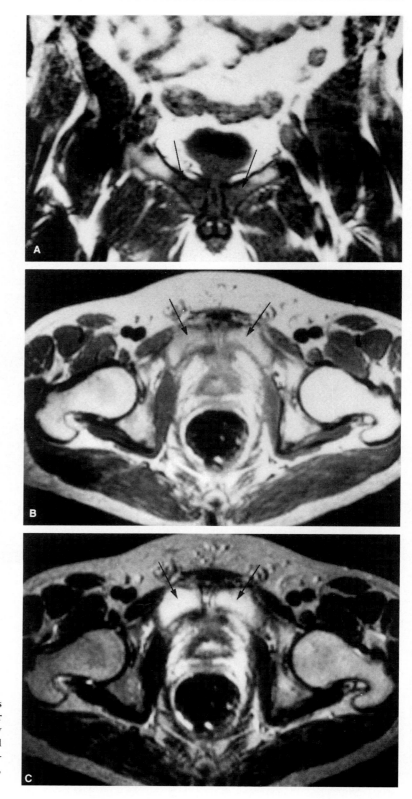

FIGURE 6-87. Bilateral superior pubic rami stress fractures (*arrows*) in an ultramarathon runner. Diffuse trabecular marrow edema and hemorrhage show low signal intensity on (**A**) a T1-weighted coronal image and increased signal intensity on (**B**) axial intermediate weighted and (**C**) T2-weighted images (**A:** TR, 600 msec TE, 20 msec; **B, C:** TR, 2000 msec; TE, 20, 80 msec).

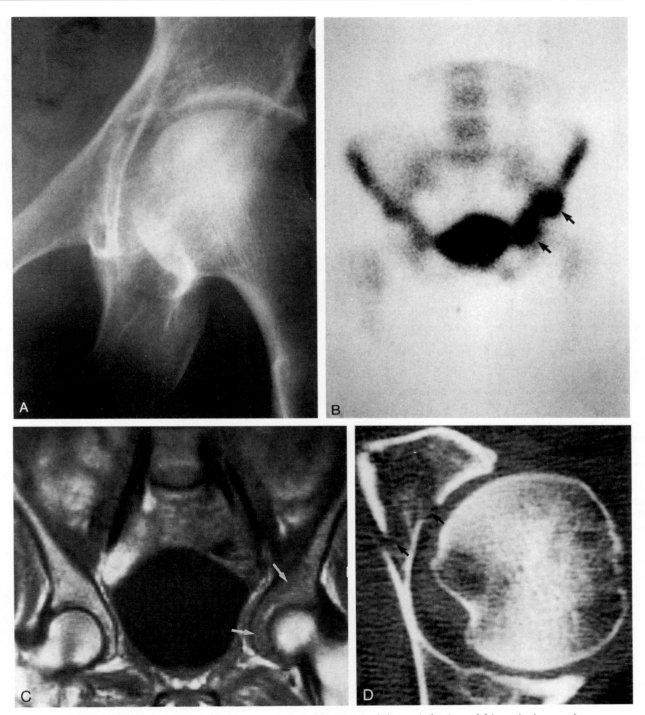

FIGURE 6-88. (**A**) AP radiograph in a patient with primary biliary cirrhosis and hip pain is negative for acetabular stress fracture. (**B**) ^{99m}TC-MDP bone scan shows uptake indicative of fracture in the left supraacetabular area (*arrows*). (**C**) T1-weighted coronal image displays diffuse low signal intensity marrow edema in the left acetabular roof (*arrows*) (TR, 1000 msec; TE, 40 msec). (**D**) Thin section CT shows multiple sites of cortical disruption, revealing the anterior column stress fracture (*arrows*).

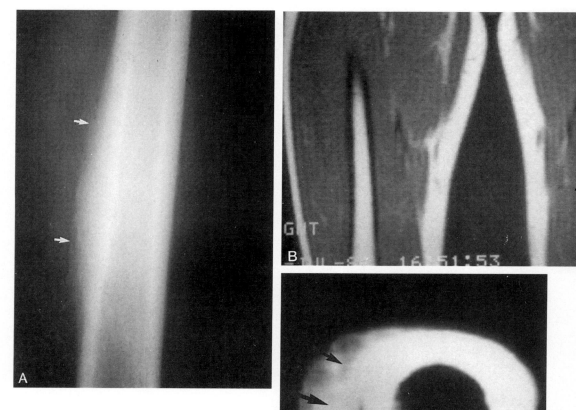

FIGURE 6-89. (**A**) AP radiograph shows thickened periosteal reaction in the medial femoral shaft in response to a stress fracture (*arrows*). (**B**) Corresponding T1-weighted coronal image demonstrates thickened medial cortex (*black arrows*) and marrow edema (*white arrow*) as low signal intensity (TR, 1000 msec; TE, 20 msec). (**C**) Axial CT allows identification of the stress fracture (*small arrows*) and the adjacent periosteal reaction (*large arrows*).

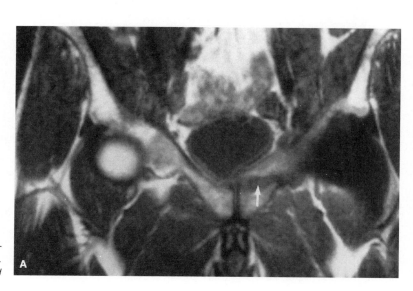

FIGURE 6-90. Malgaigne fracture. Coronal T1-weighted image shows (**A**) a superior left pubic ramus fracture (*arrow*).

continued

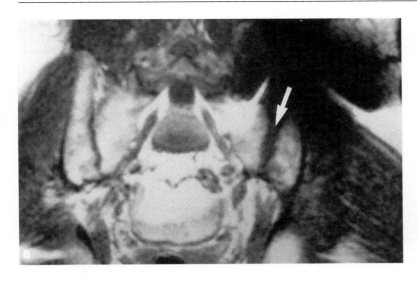

FIGURE 6-90. *Continued.* **(B)** Coronal T1-weighted image shows a separation of the ipsilateral sacroiliac joint (*arrow*). The extent of sacroiliac involvement was not initially recognized on conventional radiographs. A low signal intensity metallic artifact can be seen overlying the left hip and sacroiliac joint (TR, 600 msec; TE, 20 msec).

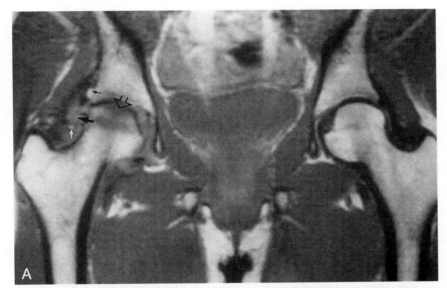

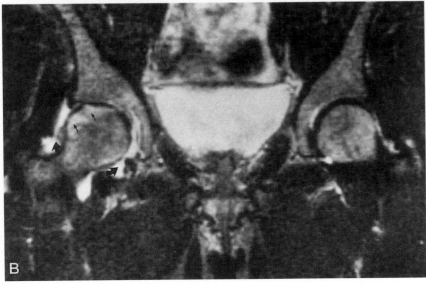

FIGURE 6-91. Posterior hip dislocation after reduction. **(A)** T1-weighted coronal image demonstrates femoral head compression fracture (*open arrow*), acetabular rim fracture (*small black arrow*), joint effusion (*large black arrow*), and intraarticular loose bodies (*white arrow*) (TR, 100 msec; TE, 20 msec). **(B)** The corresponding T2-weighted coronal image displays high signal intensity capsular effusion (*curved arrows*) and edema in the area of the compression fracture (*straight arrows*) (TR, 2000 msec; TE, 60 msec). *continued*

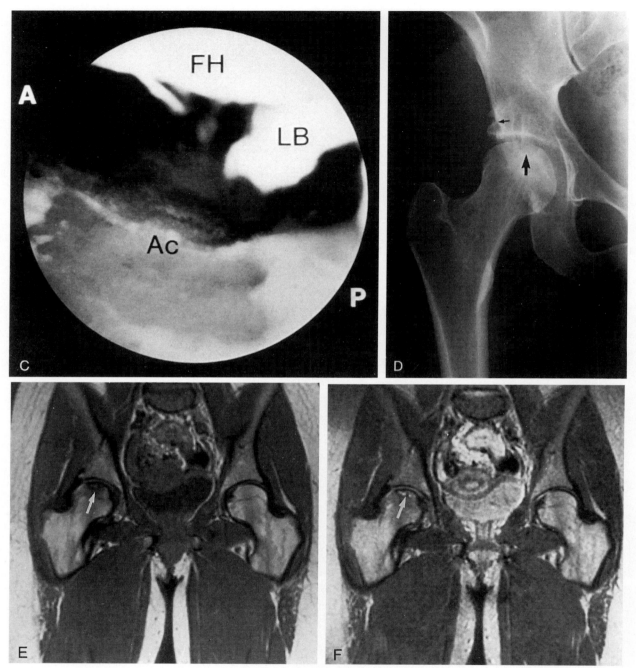

FIGURE 6-91. *Continued.* (**C**) Hip arthroscopy allows identification of the acetabular fracture (Ac), loose body (LB), and femoral head (FH) (A, anterior, P, posterior). (**D**) A follow-up radiograph taken at 6 months postinjury shows the sclerotic focus within the femoral head (*large arrow*). The site of the old acetabular rim fracture is marked (*small arrow*). The corresponding coronal (**E**) T1-weighted and (**F**) T2-weighted images demonstrate the interval progression of AVN at 6 months postinjury (*arrows*) (**E:** TR, 600 msec; TE, 20 msec; **F:** TR, 2000 msec; TE, 60 msec).

Labral Tears

By performing MR examination with a surface coil placed over the hip joint, it is possible to define the anatomic detail of the acetabular labrum (Fig. 6-92).[2] The normal labrum, variably triangular in cross section, is seen on coronal planar images as a low signal intensity triangle located between the lateral acetabulum and the femoral head (Fig. 6-93). The labrum covers the hyaline cartilage at the lateral peripheral margin of the acetabulum.[8] At arthroscopy, a groove can be seen separating the acetabular labrum from the hyaline cartilage at the margin of the acetabular fossa. The synovium lined perilabral sulcus extends around the periphery of the labrum (Fig. 6-94). The labrum demonstrates a more triangular morphology and is most substantial in its posterior superior extent; it is thinner anteroinferiorly. The labrum is usually inverted, but may be everted, and may also be mobile, as determined arthroscopically. Except for the synovium in the perilabral sulcus, the labrum is nonvascularized and without associated synovial tissue. It may not be continuous with the transverse ligament at the margins of the acetabular fossa. A demarcation or groove of acetabular articular cartilage separates the labrum and transverse ligament.

Labral tears present with symptoms of pain, decreased range of motion, and clicking. Neither conventional radiographs nor arthrography are satisfactory for accurate identi-fication of labral defects, but MR evaluation of labral tears shows potential. In patients with persistent pain and clicking with hip flexion and rotation, increased signal intensity or disruption of the labrum may be identified on T2*-weighted images using 16 to 20 cm FOVs (Figs. 6-95 and 6-96). These labral tears can be confirmed at hip arthroscopy. Abutment of acetabular labral cartilage along the medial aspect of the fibrous labrum should not be mistaken for a partial labral tear or detachment. Subchondral degeneration within the lateral acetabular roof may be associated with chronic labral disruptions (Fig. 6-97).

With MR arthrography of the hip, visualization of the labral complex is improved, and surface irregularities and abnormalities near the labral base are visualized.[124] Histology at the labral base has shown an irregular interface between the labral fibrocartilage and subchondral bone. Acetabular roof hyaline cartilage does not extend beneath the labral base. Connective tissue and degeneration, however, can be seen in the transitional zone between acetabular roof hyaline cartilage and labral fibrocartilage. Increased signal intensity can be seen through the labral base on gradient-echo sequences (Fig. 6-98), including spoiled gradient recalled acquisition in steady state (SPGR), and is attributed to cartilage degeneration, transitional zone fissures (between the labrum and subchondral bone), and partial labral detach-

text continues on page 184

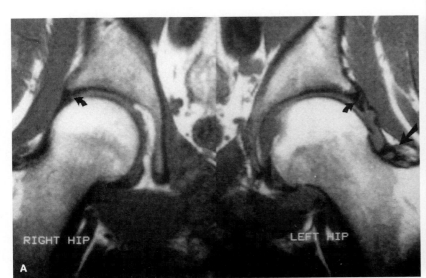
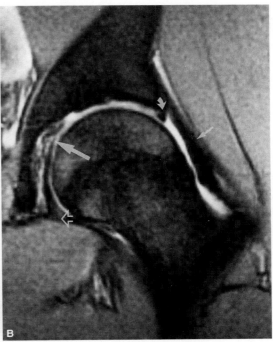

FIGURE 6-92. Normal labral anatomy. **(A)** T1-weighted coronal image shows the low signal intensity triangular-shaped acetabular labrum (*curved arrow*) and the iliofemoral ligament (*straight arrow*) (TR, 600 msec; TE, 20 msec). **(B)** A T2*-weighted image shows the low signal intensity labrum extending from the lateral acetabulum (*curved arrow*), the iliofemoral ligament (*small straight arrow*), the ligamentum teres (*large straight arrow*), and the transverse ligament (*open arrow*) (TR, 400 msec; TE, 20 msec; flip angle, 25°).

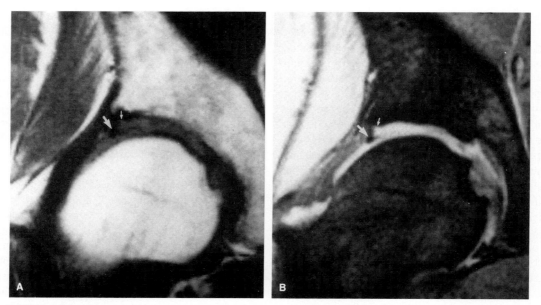

FIGURE 6-93. The normal acetabular labrum appears as a low signal intensity focus (*large arrows*) on (**A**) T1-weighted and (**B**) T2*-weighted images. The adjacent articular cartilage (*small arrows*) appears bright on a T2*-weighted image and should not be mistaken for a tear (**A:** TR, 600 msec: TE, 20 msec; **B:** TR, 400 msec; TE, 20 msec; flip angle, 25°).

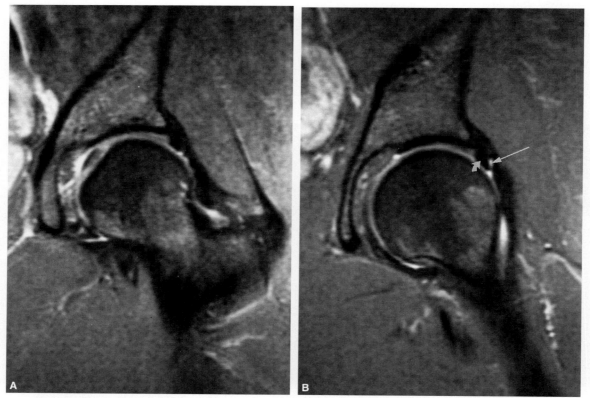

FIGURE 6-94. (**A**) Intact morphology of the acetabular labrum. (**B**) Fluid is shown in the normal recess (*straight arrow*) identified between the labrum (*curved arrow*) and joint capsule with the hip positioned in partial abduction and external rotation. Fat-suppressed T2-weighted fast spin-echo coronal images.

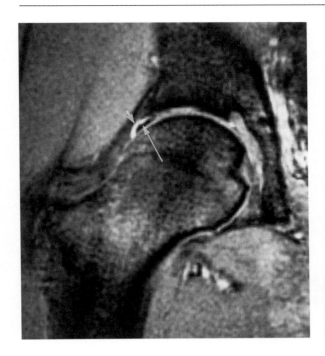

FIGURE 6-95. High signal intensity linear fluid collection (*short arrow*) in communication with a partial labral detachment (*long arrow*). This localized fluid collection represents a paralabral cyst. Note that the fluid undermines the labrum and should not be mistaken for labral recess. T2*-weighted coronal image.

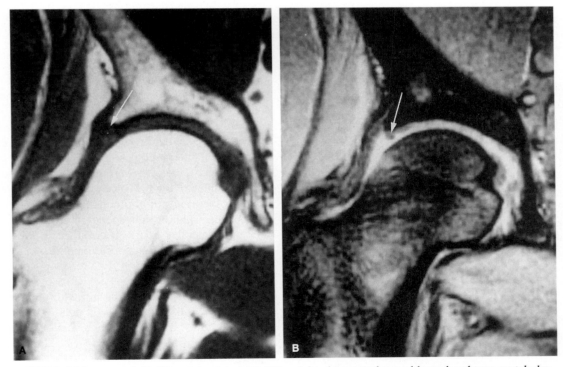

FIGURE 6-96. Coronal (**A**) T1-weighted and (**B**) T2*-weighted images show a blunted and torn acetabular labrum with absence of normal low signal intensity triangular morphology (*arrows*) (**A:** TR, 600 msec; TE, 20 msec; **B:** TR, 400 msec; TE, 20 msec; flip angle, 25°).   *continued*

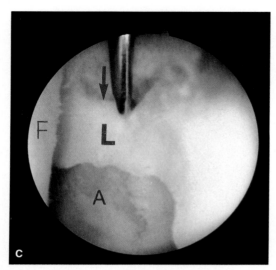

FIGURE 6-96. *Continued.* **(C)** An arthroscopic view of the lateral tear (*arrow*) shows degenerative acetabular articular cartilage in transition from white hyaline cartilage to yellow exposed bone surfaces (F, femoral head; A, acetabulum; L, labrum).

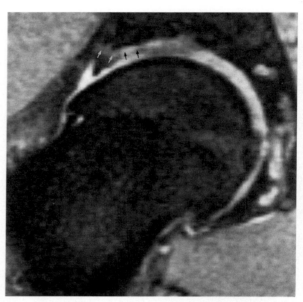

FIGURE 6-98. Increased signal intensity (*white arrows*) is seen at the base of the labrum at the labral-subchondral bone interface. This interface of hyperintensity is thought to represent basal fibro-cartilage degeneration or small transitional zone tissues (there is also mild irregularity of the morphology of the interface between the labral base and the subchondral bone). Acetabular hyaline artic-ular cartilage (*black arrows*) does not extend beneath the base labral fibrocartilage. T2*-weighted coronal image.

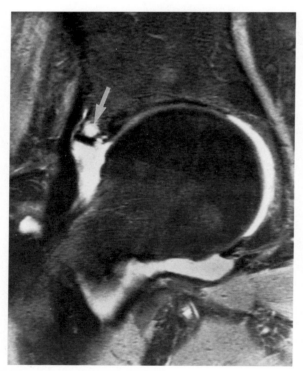

FIGURE 6-97. Complete labral disruption (absent labrum) with asso-ciated hyperintense subchondral cystic degeneration of the lateral acetabulum (*arrow*). Fat-suppressed T2-weighted fast spin-echo MR arthrogram.

ment. Labral surface irregularities (hyperintensity) may be associated with labral base degeneration. Histology shows that degenerative changes in the substance of the labrum are common and include eosinophilic, mucinous, and mucoid types. MR correlation with histology of intrasubstance labral degeneration is poor, however, compared with the ability to define labral morphology on MR scans. This limitation of MR imaging in the diagnosis of intrasubstance degeneration may be related to the presence of fibrovascular bundles or an irregular labral insertion producing signal intensity changes without corresponding degeneration. MR arthrography, how-ever, demonstrates excellent accuracy in the detection and staging of acetabular labral lesions compared to conventional MR imaging.[125]

A modified Bankart-type repair is useful for treatment of recurrent dislocation of the hip with an associated labral lesion.[126] Stability of the hip is thought to be associated with reconstruction of the labrum and reduction in capsular laxity.

Arthritis

Joint Effusions

The volume of joint fluid in the normal hip is small, and it does not generate sufficient signal for detection. Joint effusions, however, demonstrate low signal intensity on T1-weighted images and increased signal intensity on T2-weighted images. On coronal images, small collections of

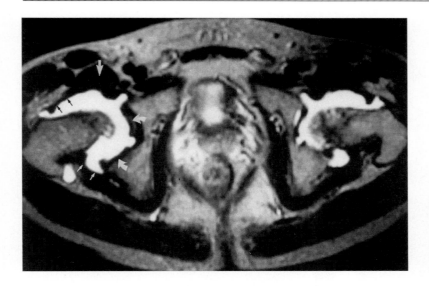

FIGURE 6-99. Distribution of joint effusion at the level of the femoral neck is shown on a T2-weighted axial image. The iliopsoas muscle (*large white arrow*), iliofemoral ligament (*small black arrows*), ischiofemoral ligament (*small white arrows*), and acetabular cortical ridge (*curved arrows*) are identified (TR, 2000 msec; TE, 80 msec).

joint fluid first accumulate superiorly in the recess border by the labrum of the acetabulum and inferomedially by the transverse ligament. With larger effusions, the medial and lateral joint capsule is distended and has convex margins. Joint effusions are also easily identified on axial and sagittal images (Fig. 6-99).

Osteoarthritis

Osteoarthritis is by far the most common form of articular cartilage degeneration. In general, incidence increases with age, and, although the etiology remains unclear, two mechanical theories predominate: (1) excessive stress on normal tissue, and (2) abnormal response to normal forces.

In addition, the biologic response resulting in inflammation undoubtedly contributes to cartilage degeneration. Many cases of osteoarthritis in the hip are thought to be secondary to an underlying condition such as an old SCFE, dysplasia, Legg-Calvé-Perthes disease in childhood, DDH, or anatomic variants such as an intraacetabular labrum.

DIAGNOSIS AND TREATMENT. The diagnosis of osteoarthritis is made by radiographic evaluation. Classically, there is loss of the joint space and sclerosis of the subchondral bone. Other changes include osteophyte and cyst formation.

The first line of treatment involves activity modification and support (eg, a cane) and nonsteroidal antiinflammatory medications. When these modalities are no longer effective, surgery may be considered. The most common surgical procedure performed is total joint replacement, but osteotomies and arthrodesis remain viable options in appropriately selected patients.

MAGNETIC RESONANCE IMAGING. T1, T2*, fat-suppressed T2-weighted fast spin-echo, and STIR sequences of the hip are used to detect the early changes of osteoarthritis (Figs. 6-100 and 6-101). Articular cartilage attenuation is best demonstrated on either sagittal or coronal fat-suppressed T2-weighted fast spin-echo images, but separation of acetabular and femoral head articular cartilage is better displayed in the

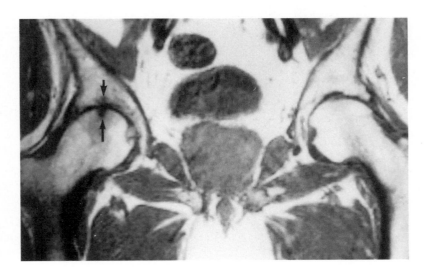

FIGURE 6-100. T1-weighted coronal image of osteoarthritis reveals superior joint-space narrowing, loss of articular cartilage, and subchondral sclerosis in the opposing surfaces of the femoral head (*large arrow*) and acetabulum (*small arrow*) (TR, 600 msec; TE, 20 msec).

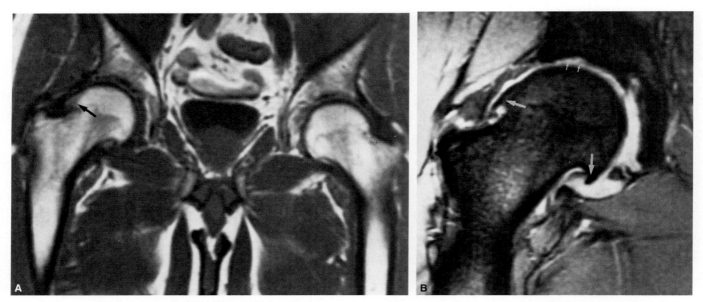

FIGURE 6-101. In osteoarthritis of the right hip, coronal **(A)** T1-weighted and **(B)** T2*-weighted surface coil images demonstrate superior joint space narrowing with attenuated articular cartilage (*small arrows*) and subcapital osteophytes (*large arrows*).

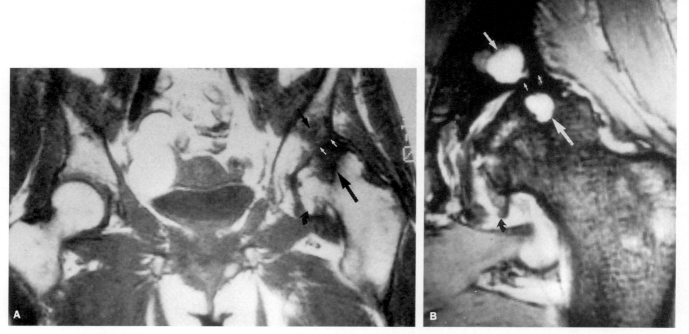

FIGURE 6-102. In osteoarthritis, coronal **(A)** T1-weighted and **(B)** T2*-weighted surface coil images display the advanced changes of osteoarthritis with acetabular and femoral head subchondral cysts (*black arrows*), sclerosis, medial subcapital osteophyte (*curved arrow*), and denuded articular cartilage (*white arrows*). Characteristic superior joint-space narrowing is present (**A:** TR, 600 msec; TE, 20 msec; **B:** TR, 400 msec; TE, 20 msec; flip angle, 25°).

sagittal plane. Stress-thickened trabeculae show low signal intensity on T1- and T2-weighted images, before there is evidence of subchondral sclerosis on conventional radiographs. Small subchondral cystic lesions can be identified on MR scans before superior joint-space narrowing, lateral acetabular and femoral head osteophytes, and medial femoral buttressing occur. Herniation pits of the femoral neck are not part of the spectrum of osteoarthritis of the hip and are considered incidental findings on conventional radiographs. These pits are related to mechanical or pressure effects of the anterior hip capsule on the proximal femoral neck.[127] These small cortical defects or cavities (<1 cm in diameter), are located in the anterior superior aspect of the lateral femoral neck. They are defined by a low signal intensity sclerotic border and display either the low signal intensity of fibrous tissue or the high signal intensity of fluid on T2-weighted images. Synovium-filled degenerative cysts about the hip are identified with low signal intensity on T1-weighted images and with uniform high signal intensity on T2-weighted or T2*-weighted images (Fig. 6-102). These cysts may be present within the subchondral bone of the acetabulum and are referred to as Egger's cysts.[128]

Osteoarthritis may also be associated with or superimposed on osteonecrosis of the femoral head. In osteonecrosis, there is greater involvement of the femoral head prior to joint-space narrowing and reciprocal changes within the acetabulum.

In selected cases, MR arthrography may be required to identify small posttraumatic or degenerative chondral lesions (Fig. 6-103). Fat-suppressed T2-weighted fast spin-echo sequences will additionally demonstrate signal abnormalities within the articular cartilage surface.

Synovial Chondromatosis and Loose Bodies

The hip is commonly involved in synovial chondromatosis (osteochondromatosis), a monarticular synovium-based cartilage metaplasia.[129] Development of intraarticular loose bodies may result in destruction of the hyaline cartilage and progress to osteoarthritis. On T2-weighted MR images, the multiple ossified loose bodies in synovial chondromatosis are seen as foci of intermediate signal intensity, bathed in the surrounding joint effusion that is bright in signal intensity. These nodules may demonstrate the high signal intensity characteristics of fatty marrow on T1- and T2-weighted images (Fig. 6-104).

Surface coil imaging of the hips has improved the identification of intraarticular loose bodies, which may be missed on images acquired with body coils and larger FOVs. On axial images, interruption of the low signal intensity space between the femoral head and the acetabulum is interposed with cartilaginous or osteocartilaginous tissue (Fig. 6-105). A cartilaginous loose body demonstrates low-to-intermediate signal intensity and is not detectable on corresponding radiographs (Fig. 6-106). The haversian fat pad or pulvinar in the

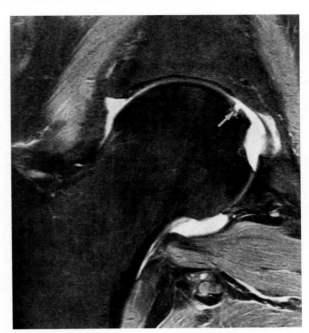

FIGURE 6-103. A focal chondral lesion (*arrow*) can be seen superior to the fovea on a coronal fat-suppressed T2-weighted fast spin-echo MR arthrogram.

acetabular fossa should not be confused with a loose body when viewing a T2*-weighted contrast image.

Rheumatoid Arthritis

Rheumatoid arthritis is a systemic disease that most frequently affects the small joints of the hands and feet. The etiology remains unknown, but the disorder is associated with HLA-DR4 and has been classified as an autoimmune disease. Although articular cartilage contains immune complexes in this disease, these complexes have not been shown to stimulate inflammatory reactions in peripheral blood lymphocyte or monocytes in vitro.[130] An infectious etiology has also been postulated.

DIAGNOSIS. The criteria for the diagnosis of rheumatoid arthritis were established in 1958 and modified in 1987.[131] These criteria include the following:

- Morning stiffness
- Arthritis of three or more joints
- Arthritis of the hand joints
- Symmetric arthritis
- Rheumatoid nodules
- Serum rheumatoid factor
- Radiographic changes.

Although rheumatoid factor is estimated to be positive in approximately 75% of rheumatoid arthritis cases, a positive rheumatoid factor alone is not sufficient for a diagnosis of rheumatoid arthritis. Conversely, the diagnosis can be made in a patient who tests negative for rheumatoid factor.

text continues on page 190

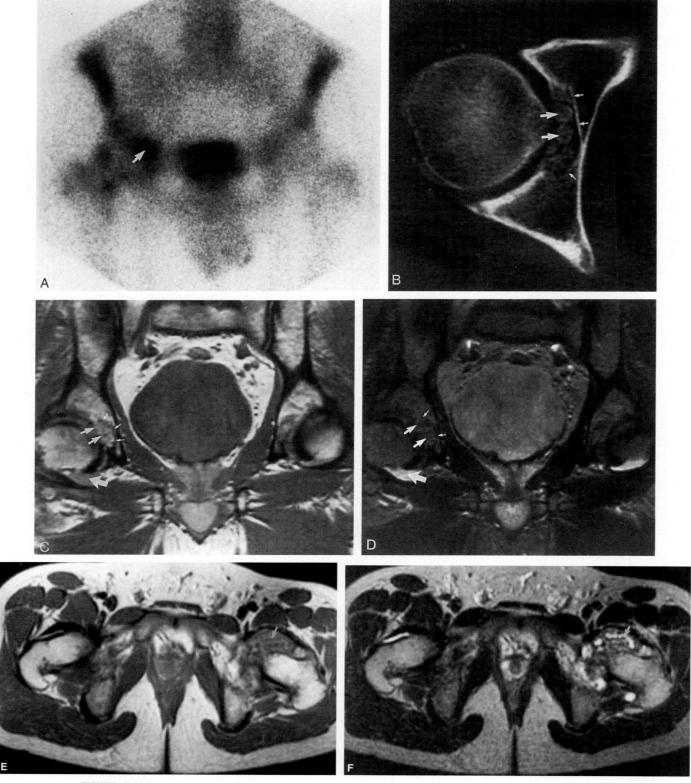

FIGURE 6-104. Synovial chondromatosis (osteochondromatosis). (A) ^{99m}TC-MDP bone scan shows uptake of bone tracer in the right hip (*arrow*). (B) Axial CT scan reveals multiple intraarticular loose bodies (*large arrows*) contained within the acetabular convexity (*small arrows*). The corresponding coronal (C) T1-weighted and (D) T2-weighted images demonstrate marrow signal intensity in the synovium-based fragments (*medium arrows*). The inner wall of the acetabulum is demarcated (*small arrows*). A joint effusion (*large arrows*) generates increased signal intensity with T2 weighting. In a separate case of synovial chondromatosis, multiple small hypointense noncalcified cartilaginous bodies (*arrows*) are visualized within the joint capsule on (E) intermediate and (F) fat-suppressed T2-weighted fast spin-echo images.

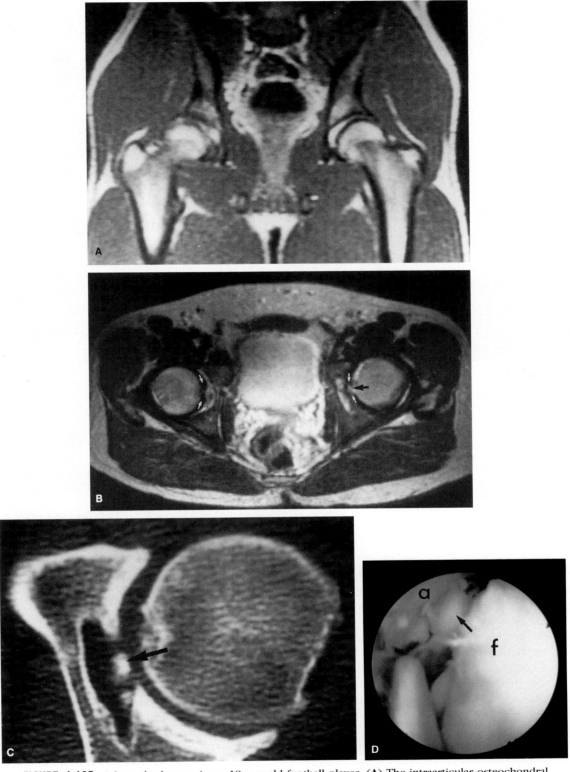

FIGURE 6-105. A loose body seen in an 18-year-old football player. (**A**) The intraarticular osteochondral fragment was not seen on the T1-weighted image (TR, 600 msec; TE, 20 msec). (**B**) On the T2-weighted axial image, an intraarticular loose body (*black arrow*) blocks the normal low signal intensity left hip joint space (*white arrows*) (TR, 2000 msec; TE, 80 msec). (**C**) Cortical detail of the osteochondral fragment (*arrow*) is shown on a 1.5-mm axial CT scan. (**D**) The corresponding arthroscopic view allows identification of the position of the loose body (*arrow*) between the acetabulum (a) and femoral head (f).

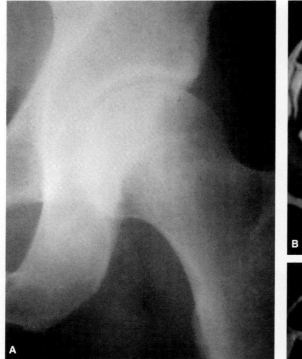

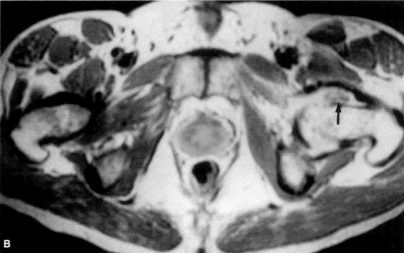

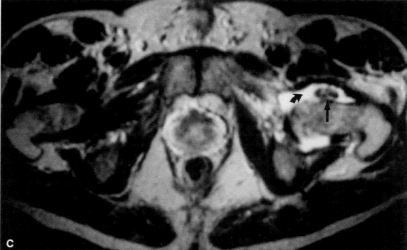

FIGURE 6-106. (**A**) AP radiograph of the left hip is negative for a cartilaginous loose body. The intermediate signal intensity cartilaginous intraarticular fragment (*straight arrow*) is revealed within the anterior joint capsule anterior to the femoral neck on (**B**) intermediate weighted and (**C**) T2-weighted axial images. The corticated low signal intensity peripheral rim cannot be seen. Associated joint effusion demonstrates high signal intensity on the T2-weighted axial image (*curved arrow*) (TR, 2000 msec; TE, 20, 80 msec).

Approximately 50% of patients with rheumatoid arthritis have radiographic evidence of hip disease, although plain film radiographs may be negative early in the course of the disease.[132,133] Radiographic changes in the hip are usually bilateral, although unilateral lesions have been described and may confuse the initial diagnosis.[134] The earliest radiographic findings are symmetric loss of joint space reflecting cartilage loss and periarticular osteopenia. With complete loss of joint space, bony erosion can occur and result in protrusio acetabuli. Protrusio acetabuli may also be associated with steroid therapy.

TREATMENT. Drug therapy is useful in decreasing symptoms of rheumatoid arthritis, but has not been proven to alter the natural history of the disease. When drug therapy fails to control the synovitis, synovectomy is an option. When radiographic evidence of significant joint destruction is found, synovectomy is less likely to be beneficial, and the precise role of synovectomy in the hip has not been established. When medical management fails to control symptoms in the hip, total hip replacement provides good pain relief.

MAGNETIC RESONANCE IMAGING. MR examination of the hip joint in patients with juvenile chronic (juvenile rheumatoid) arthritis demonstrates irregularities of the femoral capital epiphysis and growth plate, as well as osseous erosions that may be underestimated on conventional radiographs (Fig. 6-107).[135,136] Thinning of the hyaline articular cartilage can be identified on coronal and sagittal images before there is radiographic evidence of joint-space narrowing (Fig. 6-108). Synovial hypertrophy, seen as low to intermediate signal intensity, is not a common finding. Rheumatoid arthritis patients on corticosteroid therapy who are at risk for osteonecrosis can be evaluated with MR imaging during acute episodes of pain (Fig. 6-109). Hip protrusio secondary to rheumatoid arthritis is more common than idiopathic protrusio acetabuli (Fig. 6-110).

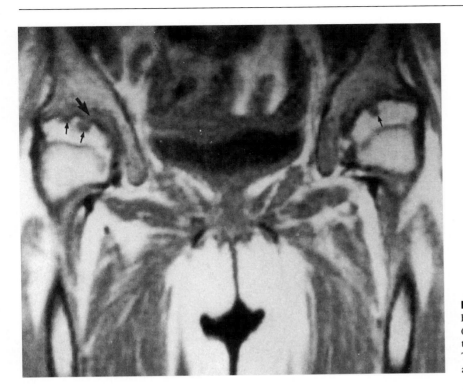

FIGURE 6-107. T1-weighted coronal image of the hips showing low signal intensity subchondral cysts (*small arrows*) and denuded intermediate signal intensity hyaline articular cartilage (*large arrow*). These findings are characteristic of juvenile chronic arthritis (TR, 800 msec; TE, 20 msec).

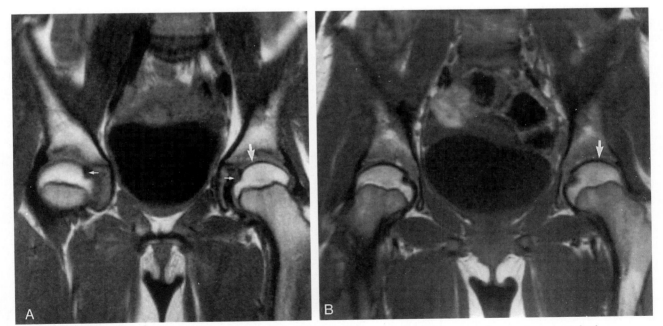

FIGURE 6-108. Early juvenile chronic arthritis. **(A)** T1-weighted coronal images of normal, age-matched control hips in a 9-year-old child with intact, intermediate signal intensity articular cartilage (*large arrow*). Normal low signal intensity fovea are present (*small arrows*). **(B)** T1-weighted coronal image shows attenuated articular cartilage in the early stages of juvenile rheumatoid arthritis (*arrow*) (TR, 600 msec; TE, 20 msec).

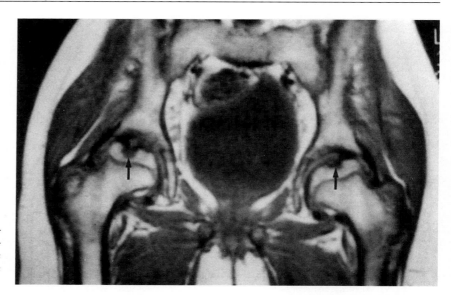

FIGURE 6-109. T1-weighted image showing bilateral osteonecrosis in a juvenile chronic arthritis patient on steroid therapy. Necrotic foci demonstrate low signal intensity on the weight-bearing surface (*arrows*) (TR, 600 msec; TE, 20 msec).

Ankylosing Spondylitis

Ankylosing spondylitis is an autoimmune disorder associated with HLA-B27. Although not diagnostic, approximately 90% of Caucasian patients with ankylosing spondylitis are HLA-B27 positive. Unlike rheumatoid arthritis, which predominantly affects small joints, ankylosing spondylitis involves the spine and larger joints. The hip is frequently affected and may be the site of initial involvement. Overall, 17% to 35% of patients with ankylosing spondylitis have hip disease.[137] Hip disease is most commonly found in patients with adolescent onset of disease. The role of MR imaging in ankylosing spondylitis has not been defined, and initial evaluation with conventional radiography is the standard for diagnostic evaluation.

Pigmented Villonodular Synovitis

Pigmented villonodular synovitis (PVNS) results from an abnormal proliferation of synovial cells. The etiology is unknown and, although similar lesions can be induced experimentally in animals by repeated intraarticular injections of blood, patients usually deny significant trauma in the clinical situation. Histologically, there is a hyperplastic layer of synovial cells with large numbers of histiocytes and giant cells containing hemosiderin, which causes the pigmentation.

The disease usually presents in the third to fifth decade of life, with clinical complaints of joint pain aggravated by activity. Although the knee is the joint most commonly affected, the hip joint may also be involved. The diagnosis

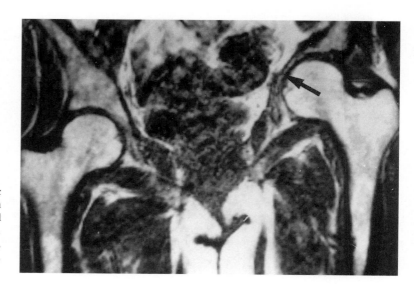

FIGURE 6-110. T1-weighted coronal image of idiopathic protrusio acetabuli shows gross medial convex protrusion of the acetabular wall into the pelvis (*arrow*) with a medial position of the acetabular line relative to the ilioischial line. No history of rheumatoid arthritis, ankylosing spondylitis, osteoarthritis, or infection was noted (TR, 500 msec; TE, 20 msec).

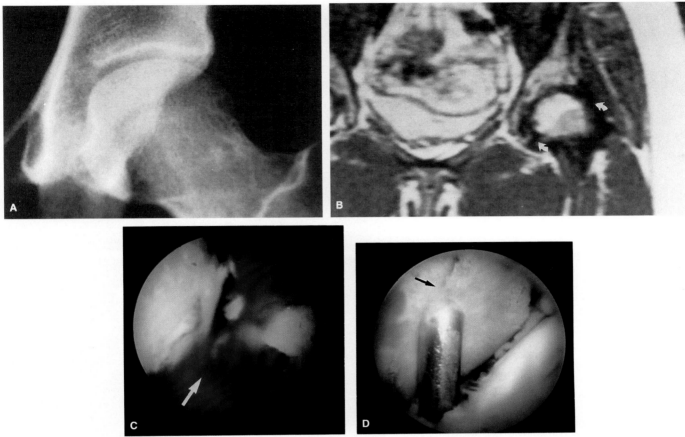

FIGURE 6-111. (**A**) AP radiograph of the left hip negative for hemorrhagic synovium. (**B**) On the T1-weighted image, low signal intensity hemosiderin and thickened synovium (*curved arrows*) are seen (TR, 600 msec; TE, 20 msec). Arthroscopy shows (**C**) hemorrhagic synovium (*arrow*) and (**D**) a detached sheet of acetabular cartilage (*arrow*).

can be difficult, and delay in diagnosis is common. In a study by Chung and Janes, the delay in diagnosis ranged from 2.5 to 11 years after the onset of symptoms.[138]

Early in the disease, radiographic findings are often negative. Later, multiple cystic areas can be seen in the acetabulum and femoral head and neck. Unlike the cysts in osteoarthritis, cysts in ankylosing spondylitis are often located away from the areas of maximum weight-bearing. Arthrography can be very helpful diagnostically. The arthrogram usually demonstrates a large joint space with many irregularities. On aspiration, blood-stained yellow joint fluid is noted.

MR images using T1- and T2*-weighted sequences are very sensitive to the presence of hemosiderin in a hemorrhagic effusion or in PVNS of the hip (Fig. 6-111).[2,139] It may be difficult, however, to differentiate hemorrhagic effusion or hemorrhagic synovium from the repeated bouts of hemosiderin deposition that occur in PVNS. The MR characteristics of PVNS reflect the proportions of hemorrhage, hemosiderin, fibrous tissue, inflamed synovium, and effusion. Thus, low-to-intermediate signal intensity areas may be de-fined on T2-weighted, T2*-weighted, or STIR images (Fig. 6-112).

Synovectomy is the treatment of choice for PVNS. Radiation is now used sparingly and reserved for recurrent lesions or incomplete resections.[140] Eventually, articular cartilage damage may necessitate a salvage procedure. Arthrodesis or total joint replacement are viable alternatives, depending on the patient's clinical status.

Amyloid Hip

Patients receiving long-term hemodialysis are at risk for an osteoarthropathy that affects the hand, wrist, and less commonly, the spine.[2,141] Large cystic erosions have also been observed in the hip. These lesions are thought to represent a spectrum of amyloid (ie, β-microglobulin) deposition occurring in synovium, tendons, and cysts. In a chronic hemodialysis patient with amyloid of the hips, MR examination reveals intermediate signal intensity masses in the femoral head and neck on T1-weighted images (Fig. 6-113). Only

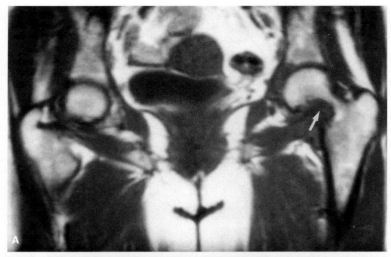

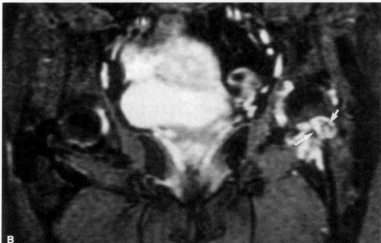

FIGURE 6-112. Pigmented villonodular synovitis presents as a cystic erosion (*large arrow*) of the medial femoral neck on (**A**) T1-weighted and (**B**) short TI inversion recover (STIR) coronal images. Central low signal intensity hemosiderin deposits (*small arrow*) are demonstrated on the STIR image. Synovial inflammation, hemorrhage, and capsular effusion also contribute to signal heterogeneity.

minimal increase in signal intensity occurs on T2-weighted images. MR examination also reveals an associated soft tissue component not evident on plain radiographs.

Miscellaneous Disorders of the Hip

Gaucher's Disease

Gaucher's disease is a rare hereditary disorder of lipid metabolism resulting in an accumulation of glucocerebroside in the reticuloendothelial system. The adult chronic nonneuropathic form can present at any age. In this form, hypersplenism with bone and skin involvement is present. The femur is the most common bone involved, and the hip joint is the most common symptomatic joint. Histologic sections demonstrate foamy histiocytes in marrow biopsies. Clinically, patients present with bone pain, and the picture can be confused with osteomyelitis. It is not uncommon for patients with Gaucher's disease to present with a low-grade fever as well as an elevated sedimentation rate and white blood cell count. In addition, on physical examination, erythema in the hip or thigh region may be found. Actual infection is rare and is usually iatrogenic. AVN of the femoral head is a common complication in these patients and often necessitates joint replacement, the results of which are not reliable. A thick, fibrous membrane often forms at the bone-cement interface and leading to early aseptic loosening in these patients.

In addition to the usefulness of MR imaging in identifying complicating AVN of the femoral head, marrow changes seen in Gaucher's disease of the pelvis and femur can be characterized by coarse hypointense signal inhomogeneity of marrow on T1-weighted images and low to intermediate signal intensity on STIR or fat-suppression images.

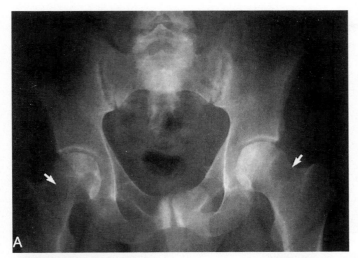

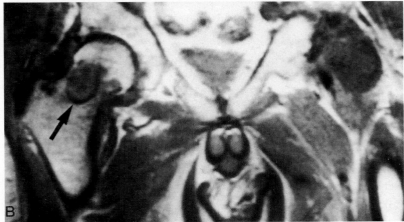

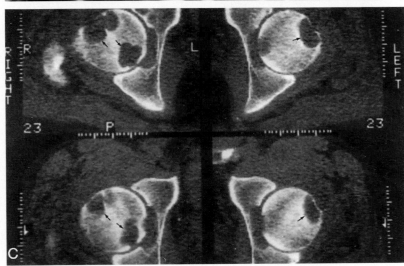

FIGURE 6-113. (A) Large cystic erosions of the femoral neck as seen on an AP radiograph in a patient on chronic renal dialysis (*arrows*). (B) T1-weighted coronal image shows intermediate signal intensity amyloid deposits in the femoral head and neck (*arrow*) (TR, 600 msec; TE, 20 msec). (C) Axial CT shows multiple cystic erosions of the femoral head (*arrows*).

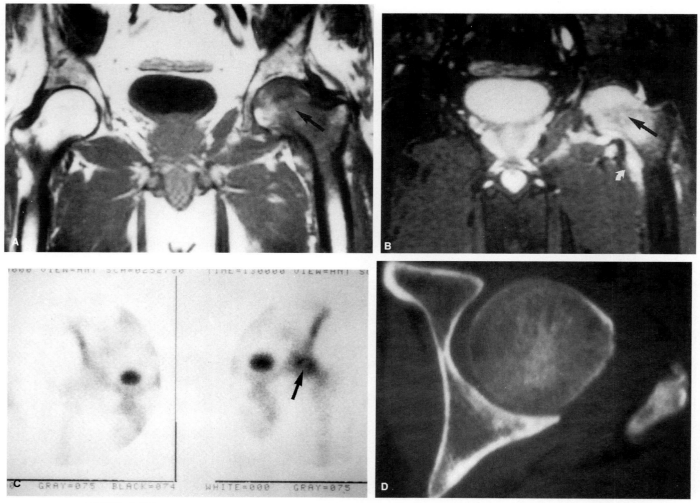

FIGURE 6-114. Various types of imaging reveal different characteristics of transient osteoporosis of the hip. (**A**) T1-weighted coronal image shows bone marrow edema with diffuse low signal intensity within the left femoral head and neck (*arrow*) (TR, 600 msec; TE, 20 msec). (**B**) A coronal short TI inversion recovery image displays the increased signal intensity of marrow (*straight arrow*) and associated effusion (*curved arrow*) (TR, 2000 msec; TI, 160 msec; TE, 43 msec). (**C**) ^{99m}TC-MDP bone scan shows uptake in the left femoral head (*arrow*). (**D**) Axial CT scan demonstrates demineralization of trabecular bone.

Bone Marrow Edema Pattern, Including Transient Osteoporosis of the Hip, Transient Bone Marrow Edema Syndrome, and Osteonecrosis

The term *bone marrow edema pattern* refers to nonspecific MR signal intensity changes, including hypointensity on T1-weighted images and hyperintensity on conventional T2-weighted images, fat-suppressed T2-weighted fast spin-echo, or STIR sequences.[142] BME encompasses the entities of transient osteoporosis of the hip, transient BME syndrome, and osteonecrosis. A nonspecific BME pattern can also be observed in cases of occult osseous trauma, infection, and neoplasms; although these entities can usually be distinguished.

Transient osteoporosis of the hip is a rare disorder that was originally described in women in the third trimester of pregnancy.[143] Since then, it also has been described in both men and nonpregnant women.[144,145] The cause is unknown, but its similarity to reflex sympathetic dystrophy suggests a neurogenic origin.[143] The disease may be bilateral in men, but in women the left hip is almost exclusively involved. The disease is self-limited but may take months to resolve. The patient presents with hip pain and limp in the absence of infection or trauma. On physical examination, hip motion is limited, and passive range of motion is painful. Treatment, which can include steroids, nonsteroidal antiinflammatory drugs, and non–weight-bearing or partial weight-bearing, is provided on the basis of symptoms, and recovery can be expected.

Transient osteoporosis of the hip must be differentiated from AVN, tuberculosis, stress fracture, malignancy, synovial chondromatosis, and PVNS. The laboratory evaluation is unremarkable except for intermittent elevation in the sedimentation rate. Although radiographs reveal osteopenia around the hip joint, these changes may lag 3 to 6 weeks behind the development of groin pain. Radiographic changes frequently develop after positive findings are made on bone scintigraphy, which shows intense homogeneous uptake within the femoral head and the neck. Although demineralization is present in the active phase of the disease, the radiographic picture eventually returns to normal. The pain resolves and motion is restored.

Transient BME syndrome refers to a reversible BME pattern without the associated radiographic changes of osteopenia. Transient BME syndrome, like transient osteoporosis of the hip, is self-limited and may in fact represent a form of transient osteoporosis of the hip. Osteonecrosis may also present with a diffuse BME pattern that either partially obscures a poorly defined subchondral focal lesion (pseudohomogeneous edema pattern) or precedes the development of a discrete well-demarcated focus of osteonecrosis. Patients with transient osteoporosis of the hip or transient BME syndrome do not have the associated common risk factors usually seen in osteonecrosis. Histologically, transient osteoporosis of the hip and AVN may show similar findings of edema, necrosis, and a fibrovascular reaction. Transient osteoporosis of the hip may thus represent an early reversible form of osteonecrosis.[146] Initial reports show that treatment of BME syndrome with drilling shortens the duration of pain and illness compared with conservative management.

In transient osteoporosis of the hip, MR imaging is useful for characterization of the low signal intensity seen on T1-weighted images and the uniform increased signal intensity seen on conventional T2-weighted, fat-suppressed T2-weighted fast spin-echo, or STIR (including fast spin-echo STIR) images (Fig. 6-114). Signal intensity changes may be seen extending from the femoral head to the intertrochanteric line.[147] Associated joint effusions are commonly seen on T2-weighted and STIR images.[145,148] There is usually resolution of clinical and MR abnormalities within 6 to 10 months. Since biopsy reveals histopathologic evidence of increased bone turnover and a mild inflammatory reaction, the signal intensity changes in transient osteoporosis of the hip are thought to be related to an increased amount of free water. Extension of marrow involvement to the epiphysis and lack of soft tissue involvement are characteristic on MR imaging.

Although the MR findings in preosteonecrosis marrow edema, reflex sympathetic dystrophy, and regional migratory osteoporosis may be similar to those described for transient osteoporosis of the hip (Fig. 6-115),[149] corresponding conventional radiography and CT do not usually demonstrate demineralization in AVN. Even with an associated BME pattern in early AVN, there is often a discrete focus of necrosis in the superior weight-bearing portion of the femoral head. Identification of such a focus may require careful examination of T1- and T2-weighted images, since it may be masked by an extensive hyperemia on fat-suppressed T2-weighted fast spin-echo or STIR images. Follow-up or sequential MR studies may be required to demonstrate the development of a discrete focus of necrosis with interval resolution of adjacent marrow hyperemia.[47] Contrast-enhanced MR imaging with intravenous gadolinium may help in demonstrating hypovascular marrow and AVN, sepa-

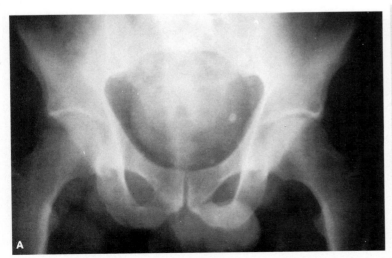
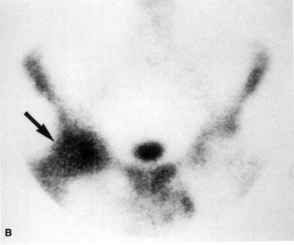

FIGURE 6-115. The appearance of transient osteoporosis of the hips is similar to that of avascular necrosis in imaging. **(A)** On an AP radiograph of the pelvis, subtle demineralization of right femoral head can be seen. **(B)** A ^{99m}TC-MDP bone scan shows increased uptake (*arrow*) in the right femoral head and neck.

continued

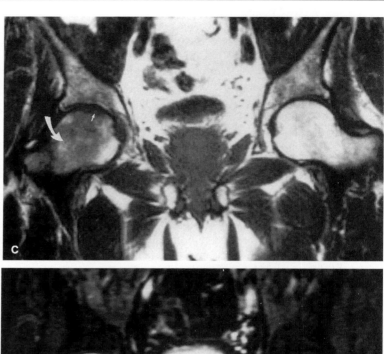

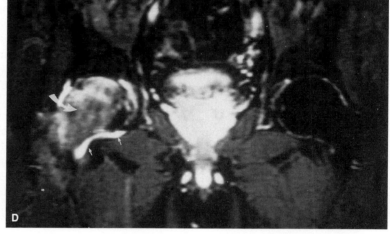

FIGURE 6-115. *Continued.* (**C**) On a T1-weighted coronal image, low signal intensity alteration of fat marrow (*curved arrow*) is seen diffusely throughout right femoral head and neck. A small area of decreased signal in the left femoral head may represent the initial focus of osteonecrosis (*straight arrow*). However, the patient's symptoms resolved within 4 months (TR, 600 msec; TE, 20 msec). (**D**) A coronal short TI inversion recovery image demonstrates high signal intensity marrow hyperemia (*curved arrow*). An associated joint effusion is present (*straight arrows*), and no osteonecrosis developed on follow-up examination (TR, 2000 msec; TI, 160 msec; TE, 43 msec).

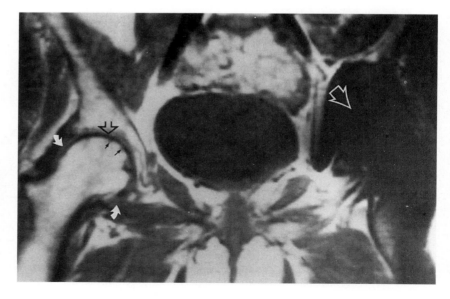

FIGURE 6-116. T1-weighted image in degenerative osteoarthritis of the right hip shows superior joint-space narrowing, attenuated intermediate signal intensity articular cartilage (*open black arrow*), and small low signal intensity subchondral cysts (*straight arrows*). There is signal void from the total hip prosthesis (*open white arrow*), and minimal joint effusion, which demonstrates intermediate signal intensity (*curved arrows*) (TR, 600 msec; TE, 20 msec).

rate from homogeneous hypervascularization in BME. In contrast to transient osteoporosis, AVN usually demonstrates a focal lesion in the anterosuperior femoral head, which initially may be poorly defined but will become well demarcated over time.[57]

Joint Prostheses

Metallic total joint prostheses or arthroplasties generate sufficient low signal intensity artifact to prevent an accurate determination of component loosening or infection (Fig. 6-116).[150,151] Proximal and medial migration of the prosthesis into the pelvis, however, which complicates prosthetic revision and replacement, can be assessed by MR imaging. In such instances, proximity to neurovascular structures can be assessed without invasive angiography. Osteolysis around total hip replacement components represents a major problem in total joint arthroplasty. Osteolysis refers to particle-induced bone resorption. Because of the geometry of the pelvis and acetabular components, it is often difficult to determine the extent of these lesions. Due to prohibitive magnetic susceptibility artifact associated with the total hip replacement components, CT may provide more information regarding the extent of lysis.

References

1. Conway WF, Totty WG, McEnery KW. CT and MR imaging of the hip. Radiology 1996;198:297.
2. Stoller DW, Genant HK. Magnetic resonance imaging of the knee and hip. Arthritis Rheum 1990;33:441.
3. Pitt MJ, Lung PJ, Speer DP. Imaging of the pelvis and hip. Orthop Clin North Am 1990;21(3):545.
4. Porter BA, et al. Low field STIR imaging of avascular necrosis, marrow edema, and infarction. Radiology 1987;165:83.
5. Gillepsy T III, et al. Magnetic resonance imaging of osteonecrosis. Radiol Clin North Am 1986;24:193.
6. Berquist TH, ed. Imaging of orthopedic trauma and surgery. Philadelphia: WB Saunders, 1986:181.
7. Wrazidlo W, Schneider S, et al. Imaging of the hip joint hyaline cartilage with MR tomography using a gradient echo sequence with fat-water phase coherence. ROFO 1990;152:56.
8. Keane GS, Villa RN. Arthroscopic anatomy of the hip: an in vivo study. Arthroscopy 1994;10:392.
9. Johnson ND, Wood BP, et al. MR imaging anatomy of the infant hip. AJR 1989;153:127.
10. Bos CF, et al. A correlative study of MR images and cryo-sections of the neonatal hip. Surg Radiol Anat 1990;12:43.
11. Steinberg MA. Management of avascular necrosis of the femoral head: an overview. In: Bassett FH, ed. Instructional course lectures, vol 37, 1988:41.
12. Jones JP. Fat embolism and osteonecrosis. Orthop Clin North Am 1985;16:595.
13. Cruess RL. Osteonecrosis of bone: current concepts as to etiology and pathogenesis. Clin Orthop 1986;208:30.
14. Gotschalk F. Indications and results of intertrochanteric osteotomy in osteonecrosis of the femoral head. Clin Orthop 1989;249:219.
15. Jacobs B. Epidemiology of traumatic and nontraumatic osteonecrosis. Clin Orthop 1978;130:51.
16. Mitchell DG, et al. Femoral head avascular necrosis: correlation of MR imaging, radiographic staging, radionuclide imaging and clinical findings. Radiology 1987;162:709.
17. Mont MA, Hungerford DS. Non-traumatic avascular necrosis of the femoral head. J Bone Joint Surg 1995;77:459.
18. Beltran J, et al. Femoral head avascular necrosis: MR imaging with clinical-pathologic and radionuclide correlation. Radiology 1988;166:215.
19. Mitchell MD, et al. Avascular necrosis of the hip: comparison on MR, CT and scintigraphy. AJR 1986;147:67.
20. Glickstein MR, et al. Avascular necrosis versus other diseases of the hip: sensitivity of MR imaging. Radiology 1988;169:213.
21. Shuman WP, et al. MR imaging of avascular necrosis of the femoral head: value of small-field-of-view sagittal surface-coil images. AJR 1988;150:1073.
22. Ficat R. Treatment of avascular necrosis of the femoral head in the hip. Proceedings of the 11th Open Scientific Meeting of the Hip Society. St Louis: CV Mosby, 1983:279.
23. Ficat RP, Arlet J. Necrosis of the femoral head. In: Hungerford DS, ed. Ischemia and necrosis of the bone. Baltimore: Williams & Williams, 1980.
24. Jones JP. Osteonecrosis. In: McCarthy DJ, ed. Arthritis and allied conditions, 10th ed. Philadelphia: Lea & Febiger, 1985:1356.
25. Springfield DS, Enneking WF. Idiopathic aseptic necrosis. In: Bones and joints. Baltimore: Williams & Williams, 1976:61.
26. Fishman EK, et al. Multiplanar (MPR) imaging of the hip. Radio-Graphics 1986;6:7.
27. Dee R, et al. Ischemic necrosis of the femoral head. In: Dee R, ed. Principles of orthopaedic practice, vol 2. New York: McGraw-Hill, 1989:1357.
28. Markisz JA, et al. Segmental patterns of avascular necrosis of the femoral heads: early detection with MR imaging. Radiology 1987;162:717.
29. Steinberg MD, Hayken GD, Steinberg DR. The conservative management of avascular necrosis of the femoral head. In: Arlet J, Ficat RP, Hungerford DS, eds. Bone circulation. Baltimore: Williams & Wilkins, 1984:334.
30. Bonfiglio M, Voke E. Aseptic necrosis of the femoral head and non-union of the femoral neck. J Bone Joint Surg [Am] 1968;50:48.
31. Camp JF, Colwell CW. Core decompression of the femoral head for osteonecrosis. J Bone Joint Surg [Am] 1986;68:1213.
32. Hungerford DS. Bone marrow pressure, venography, and core decompression in ischemic necrosis of the femoral head. Proceedings of the Seventh Open Scientific Meeting of the Hip Society. St Louis: CV Mosby, 1979:218.
33. Marcus ND, Enneking WF, Massam RA. The silent hip in idiopathic aseptic necrosis: treatment by bone grafting. J Bone Joint Surg [Am] 1973;55:1351.
34. Steinberg MD, Brighton CT, et al. Osteonecrosis of the femoral head: results of core decompression and grafting with and without electrical stimulation. Clin Orthop 1989;249:199.
35. Stulberg BN, Bauer TW, Belhobek GH. Making core decompression work. Clin Orthop 1990;261:186.
36. Sugioka YU, Kaysuki T, Hotokebuchi T. Transtrochanteric rotational osteotomy of the femoral head for treatment of osteonecrosis. Clin Orthop 1982;169:115.
37. Aaron RK, Lennox D, Bunce GE, Ebert T. The conservative treatment of osteonecrosis of the femoral head. Clin Orthop 1989;249:209.
38. Steinberg MD. Early results in the treatment of avascular necrosis of the femoral head with electrical stimulation. Orthop Clin North Am 1984;15:163.
39. Smith SW, Fehring TK, Griffin WL, Beaver WB. Core decompression of the osteonecrotic femoral head. J Bone Joint Surg [Am] 1995;77a:674.
40. Phemister DB. Treatment of the necrotic head of the femur in adults. J Bone Joint Surg 1949;31A:55.
41. Urbaniak J, Nunley JA, Goldner RD, et al. Treatment of avascular

necrosis of the femoral head by vascularized graft. Presented at 8th Combined Meeting of Orthopedic Associations of the English Speaking World, Washington, DC, May 3–8, 1987.

42. Urbaniak JR, Coogan PG, Gunneson EB, Nunley JA. Treatment of osteonecrosis of the femoral head with free vascularized fibular grafting. J Bone Joint Surg 1995;77a:681.

43. Brown TD, Pedersen DR, Baker KJ, Bland RA. Mechanical consequences of core drilling and bone-grafting on osteonecrosis of the femoral head. J Bone Joint Surg 1993;75a:1358.

44. Cabanela MD. Bipolar versus total hip arthroplasty for avascular necrosis of the femoral head: a comparison. Clin Orthop 1990;261:59.

45. Lang P, et al. 2.0 T MR imaging of the femoral head in avascular necrosis: histologic correlation [abstract]. Sixth Annual Meeting and Exhibition of the Society of Magnetic Resonance in Medicine, New York, August 17, 1987.

46. Vande Berg BE, Malghem J, Labaisse MA, Noel H. Avascular necrosis of the hip: comparison of contrast-enhanced and nonenhanced MR imaging with histologic correlation. Radiology 1992;182:445.

47. Vande Berg BE, Malghem JJ, Labaisse MA, Noel HM. MR imaging of avascular necrosis and transient marrow edema of the femoral head. Radiograpics 1993;13:501.

48. Bluemke DA, Petri M, Zerhouni EA. Femoral head perfusion and composition: MR imaging and spectroscopic evaluation of patients with systemic lupus erythematosus and at risk for avascular necrosis. Radiology 1995;197:433.

49. Beltran J, et al. Core decompression for avascular necrosis of the femoral head: correlation between long-term results and preoperative MR staging. Radiology 1990;175:533.

50. Shimizu K, Moriya H, Akita T, Sakamoto M. Prediction of collapse with magnetic resonance imaging of avascular necrosis of the femoral head. J Bone Joint Surg 1994;76a:215.

51. Mankey M, et al. Comparison of magnetic resonance imaging and bone scan in the early detection of osteonecrosis of the femoral head. Presented to the Academy of Orthopedic Surgeons, January 1987.

52. Turner DA, et al. Femoral capital osteonecrosis: MR finding of diffuse marrow abnormalities without focal lesions. Radiology 1989;171:135.

53. Stulberg BN, et al. Multimodality approach to osteonecrosis of the femoral head. Clin Orthop 1989;240:181.

54. Genez BM, et al. Early osteonecrosis of the femoral head: detection in high-risk patients with MR imaging. Radiology 1988;168:521.

55. Tervonen O, Mueller DM, Matteson EL, Velosa JA. Clinically occult avascular necrosis of the hip: prevalence in an asymptomatic population at risk. Radiology 1992;182:845.

56. Mulliken BD, Renfrew DL, Brand RA, Whitten CG. Prevalence of previously undetected osteonecrosis of the femoral head in renal transplant recipients. Radiology 1994;192:831.

57. Jiang CC, Shih TT. Epiphyseal scar of the femoral head: risk factor of osteonecrosis. Radiology 1994;191:409.

58. Coleman BG, et al. Radiographically negative avascular necrosis: detection with MR imaging. Radiology 1988;168:525.

59. Lafforgue P, Dahan E, Chagnaud C, Schiano A. Early stage avascular necrosis of the femoral head: MR imaging for prognosis in 31 cases with at least 2 years of follow-up. Radiology 1993;187:199.

60. Wynee-Davies R, Gormley J. The etiology of Perthes disease. J Bone Joint Surg [Br] 1978;60:6.

61. Catterall A, Lloyd-Roberts GC, Wynne-Davies R. Association of Perthes disease with congenital anomalies of the genitourinary tract and inguinal region. Lancet 1971;i:996.

62. Catterall A. The natural history of Perthes disease. J Bone Joint Surg [Br] 1971;53:37.

63. Salter RB, Thompson GH. Legg-Calvé-Perthes disease: the prognostic significance of the subchondral fracture and a two-group classification of the femoral head involvement. J Bone Joint Surg [Br] 1978;60:6

64. Green NE, Beauchamp RD, Griffin PD. Epiphyseal extrusion as a prognostic index in Legg-Calvé-Perthes disease. J Bone Joint Surg [Am] 1981;63:900.

65. Catterall A, Pringle H, Byers PD, et al. A review of the morphology of Perthes disease. J Bone Joint Surg [Br] 1982;64:269.

66. Dolman CL, Bell HM. The pathology of Legg-Calvé-Perthes syndrome. J Bone Joint Surg [Am] 1973;55:184.

67. Herring JA. The treatment of Legg-Calvé-Perthes disease. J Bone Joint Surg 1994;76a:448.

68. Weinstein SL. Legg-Calvé-Perthes disease: results of long-term follow-up. In: The Proceedings of the 13th Open Scientific Meeting of the Hip Society. St Louis: CV Mosby, 1985:28.

69. Easton EJ Jr, et al. Magnetic resonance imaging and scintigraphy in Legg-Perthes' disease: diagnosis, treatment and prognosis. Radiology 1987;165:35.

70. Heuck A, et al. Magnetic resonance imaging in the evaluation of Legg-Perthes' disease. Radiology 1987;165:83.

71. Jamamillo D, Kasser JR, Villegas-Medina OL, Garry E. Cartilaginous abnormalities and growth disturbance in Legg-Calvé-Perthes disease: evaluation with MR imaging. Radiology 1995;187:767.

72. Rush BH, Bramson RT, Ogden JA. Legg-Calvé-Perthes disease: detection of cartilaginous and synovial changes with MR imaging. Radiology 1988;167:473.

73. Ranner G. Magnetic resonance imaging in children with acute hip pain. Pediatr Radiol 1989;20:67.

74. Wilcox PG, Weiner DS, Leighley D. Maturation factors in slipped capital femoral epiphysis. J Pediatr Orthop 1988;8:196.

75. Gelberman RH, Cohen MS, Shaw BA, et al. The association of femoral retroversion with slipped femoral epiphysis. J Bone Joint Surg [Am] 1986;68:1000.

76. Agamanolis DP, Weiner DS, Lloyd JK. Slipped capital femoral epiphysis: a pathological study. II. An ultrasound study of 23 cases. J Pediatr Orthop 1985;5:47.

77. Crawford AH. The role of osteotomy in the treatment of slipped capital femoral epiphysis. In: Barr JS, ed. Instruction course lectures, vol 38. Las Vegas: American Academy of Orthopaedic Surgeons, 1989:273.

78. Swiontkowski MF. Slipped capital femoral epiphysis: complications relative to internal fixation. Orthopaedics 1983;6:705.

79. Wiener DS. Bone graft epiphysiodesis in the treatment of slipped capital femoral epiphysis. In: Barr JS, ed. Instruction course lectures, vol 38. Las Vegas: American Academy of Orthopaedic Surgeons, 1989:63.

80. Stuhlberg SD, Cordell LD, et al. Unrecognized childhood hip disease: a major cause of idiopathic osteoarthritis of the hip. In: The hip: proceedings of the Hip Society. St Louis: CV Mosby, 1975:212.

81. Johnson ND, et al. Complex infantile and congenital hip dislocation: assessment with MR imaging. Radiology 1988;168:151.

82. Dunn PM. The anatomy and pathology of congenital dislocation of the hip. Clin Orthop 1976;119:23.

83. Soboleski DA, Babyn P. Sonographic diagnosis of developmental dysplasia of the hip: importance of increased thickness of acetabular cartilage. AJR 1993;161:839.

84. Eggli KO, King SH, Boal DKB, Quioque T. Low-Dose CT of developmental dysplasia of the hip after reduction: diagnostic accuracy and dosimetry. AJR 1994;163:1441.

85. Atar D, Lehman WB, Grant AD. 2-D and 3-D computed tomography and magnetic resonance imaging in developmental dysplasia of the hip. Orthopedic Review 1992:1189.

86. Hubbard AM, Dormans JP. Evaluation of developmental dysplasia, Perthes disease, and neuromuscular dysplasia of the hip in children before and after surgery: an imaging update. AJR 1995;164:1067.

87. Lang P, et al. Three-dimensional digital displays in congenital dislocation of the hip: preliminary experience. J Pediatr Orthop 1989;9:532.

88. Lang P, et al. Three-dimensional CT and MR imaging in congenital dislocation of the hip: technical considerations. Radiology 1987;165:279.

89. Hillman JS, et al. Proximal femoral focal deficiency: radiologic analysis of 49 cases. Radiology 1987;165:769.

90. Ehman RI, Berquist TH. Magnetic resonance imaging of musculoskeletal trauma. Radiol Clin North Am 1986;24:291.

91. Fisher MK, et al. MRI of the normal and pathological musculoskeletal system. Magn Reson Imaging 1986;4:491.

92. Doons GC, et al. MR imaging of intramuscular hemorrhage. J Comput Assist Tomogr 1985;9:908.

93. Hasselman CT, Best TM, Hughes C, Martinez S. An explanation for various rectus femoris strain injuries using previously undescribed muscle architecture. Am J Sports Med 1995;23:493.

94. Hughes C, Hasselman CT, Best TM, Martinez S. Incomplete intrasustance strain injuries of the rectus femoris muscle. Am J Sports Med 1995;23:500.

95. Brandser EA, El-Khoury GY, Kathol MH, Callaghan JJ. Hamstring injuries: radiographic, conventional tomographic CT and MR imaging characteristics. Radiology 1995;197:257.

96. Vaccaro JP, Sauser DD, Beals RK. Iliopsoas bursa imaging: efficacy in depicting abnormal iliopsoas tendon motion in patients with internal snapping hip syndrome. Radiology 1995;197:853.

97. Paletta GA, Andrish JT. Injuries about the hip and pelvis in the young athlete. Clinics in Sports Medicine 1995;14:591.

98. Micheli LJ. The young athlete. Clin Sports Med 1995;14(3).

99. Cleaves EN. Fracture avulsion of the anterior superior iliac spine of the ilium. J Bone Joint Surg [Am] 1938;20:490.

100. Milch H. Avulsion fracture of the tuberosity of the ischium. J Bone Joint Surg [Am] 1926;8:832.

101. Rogge EA, Romano RL. Avulsion of the ischial apophysis. J Bone Joint Surg [Am] 1956;38:442.

102. Tile M, Kellam J, Joyce M. Fractures of the acetabulum, classification, management protocol and results of treatment. J Bone Joint Surg [Br] 1985;67:173.

103. Fairclough J, et al. Bone scanning for suspected hip fractures. Radiology 1987;164:886.

104. Griffiths HJ, et al. Computed tomography in the management of acetabular fractures. Radiology 1985;154:567.

105. Devas M. Stress fractures. New York: Churchill-Livingstone, 1975.

106. Gilbert RS, Johnson HA. Stress fractures in military recruits: a review of 12 years' experience. Milit Med 1966;131:716.

107. Blickenstaff LD, Morris JM. Fatigue fracture of the femoral neck. J Bone Joint Surg [Am] 1966;48:1031.

108. Morris JM, Blickenstaff LD. Fatigue fractures. Springfield, IL: Charles C Thomas, 1967.

109. DeLee JC. Dislocations and fracture-dislocations of the hip. In: Rockwood CA Jr, Green DP, eds. Fractures and dislocations, 2nd ed. Philadelphia: JB Lippincott, 1984:1287.

110. Potok PS, Hopper KD, Umlauf MJ. Fractures of the acetabulum: imaging, classification, and understanding. Radiographics 1995;15:7.

111. Potter HG, Montgomery KD, Heise CW, Helfet DL. MR imaging of acetabular fractures: value in detecting femoral head injury, intraarticular fragments, and sciatic nerve injury. AJR 1993;163:881.

112. Tile M. Fractures of the acetabulum. In: Steinberg ME, ed. The hip and its disorders. Philadelphia: WB Saunders, 1991:201.

113. Deutsch AL, et al. Occult fractures of the proximal femur: MR imaging. Radiology 1989;170(1 pt 1):113.

114. Berger PE, et al. MRI demonstration of radiographically occult fractures: what have we been missing? Radiographics 1989;9:407.

115. Bogost GA, Lizerbram EK, Crues JV III. MR imaging in evaluation of suspected hip fracture: frequency of unsuspected bone and soft tissue injury. Radiology 1995;197:263.

116. Quinn SF, McCarthy JL. Prospective evaluation of patients with suspected hip fracture and indeterminate radiographs: use of T1-weighted MR images. Radiology 1993;187:469.

117. Lang P, Mauz M, Schorner W, Schwellick G. Acute fracture of the femoral neck: assessment of femoral head. Perfusion with gadopentetate dimeglumine-enhanced MR imaging. AJR 1993;160:335.

118. Schwappach JR, Murphey MD, Kokmeyer SF, Rosenthal HG. Subcapital fractures of the femoral neck: prevalence and cause of radiographic appearance simulating pathologic fracture. AJR 1994;162:651.

119. May DA, Purins JL, Smith DK. MR imaging of occult traumatic fractures and muscular injuries of the hip and pelvis in elderly patients. AJR 1996;166:1075.

120. Berquist TH, Coventry MB. The pelvis and hips. In: Berquist TH, ed. Imaging of orthopaedic trauma and surgery. Philadelphia: WB Saunders, 1986:181.

121. Erb RE, Steele JR, Nance EP, Edwards JR. Traumatic anterior dislocation of the hip: spectrum of plain film and CT findings. AJR 1995;165:1215.

122. Richardson P, et al. CT detection of cortical fracture of the femoral head associated with posterior hip dislocation. AJR 1990;155:93.

123. Tehranzadah J, et al. Osteochondral impaction of the femoral head associated with hip dislocation: CT study in 35 patients. AJR 1990;155:1049.

124. Hodler J, Yu JS, Goodwin D, Haghigh P. MR arthrography of the hip: improved imaging of the acetabular labrum with histologic correlation in cadavers. AJR 1995;165:887.

125. Czerry C, Hoffmann S, Neuhold A, et al. Lesions of the acetabular labrum: accuracy of MR imaging and MR arthrography in detection and staging. Radiology 1996;200:225.

126. Lieherman JR, Altchek DW, Salvati EA. Recurrent dislocation of a hip with a labral lesion: treatment with a modified Bankart-type repair. J Bone Joint Surg 1993;75a:1524.

127. Mokes SR, Volger JB, Spritzer CE, et al. Herniation pits of the femoral neck: appearance at MR imaging. Radiology 1989;172:231.

128. Haller J, et al. Juxtaacetabular ganglionic (or synovial) cysts: CT and MR features. J Comput Assist Tomogr 1989;13:976.

129. Szpryt P, et al. Synovial chondromatosis of the hip joint presenting as a pathological fracture. Br J Radiol 1986;59:399.

130. Schurman DJ, Palathumpat MC, et al. Biochemistry and antigenicity of osteoarthritic and rheumatoid cartilage. J Orthop Res 1986;4:255.

131. Arnett FC, Edworthy SM, et al. The American Rheumatism Association 1987 revised criteria for the clarification of rheumatoid arthritis. Arthritis Rheum 1988;31:315.

132. Duthie R, Harris C. A radiographic and clinical survey of hip joints in seropositive rheumatoid arthritis. Acta orthop Scand 1969;40:346.

133. Glick EN, Mason RM, Wely WG. Rheumatoid arthritis affecting the hip joint. Ann Rheum Dis 1963;22:416.

134. Resnick D, Williams D, Weisman MH, Slaughter L. Rheumatoid arthritis and pseudo-rheumatoid arthritis in calcium pyrophosphate crystal deposition disease. Radiology 1981;140:615.

135. Stoller DW. MRI in juvenile (chronic) arthritis. Presented to the Association of University Radiologists, Charleston, SC, March 22, 1987.

136. Senac MO Jr, et al. MR imaging in juvenile rheumatoid arthritis. AJR 1988;150:873.

137. Wilkinson M, Bywaters EGL. Clinical features and course of ankylosing spondylitis as seen in a follow up of 222 hospital referred cases. Ann Rheum Dis 1958;17:209.

138. Chung SMK, Janes JM. Diffuse pigmented villonodular synovitis of the hip joint. J Bone Joint Surg [Am] 1965;47:293.

139. Jelinek JS, et al. Imaging of pigmented villonodular synovitis with emphasis on MR imaging. AJR 1989;152:337.

140. McMaster PE. Pigmented villonodular synovitis with invasion of bone. J Bone Joint Surg [Am] 1960;42:1170.

141. Brancaccio D, et al. Amyloid arthropathy in patients on regular dialysis: a newly discovered disease. Radiology 1987;65(P):335.

142. Bloem JL. Transient osteoporosis of the hip: MR imaging. Radiology 1988;167:753.

143. Curtiss PH, Kincaid WE. Transitory demineralization of the hip in pregnancy. J Bone Joint Surg [Am] 1959;41:1327.

144. Lequesne M. Transient osteoporosis of the hip: a nontraumatic variety of Sudeck's atrophy. Ann Rheum Dis 1968;27:463.

145. Pantazopoulos T, Exarchou E, Hartofilikidis-Garofalidis G. Idiopathic transient osteoporosis of the hip. J Bone Joint Surg [Am] 1973;55:315.

146. Imhof H, Kramer J, Hofmann S, Plenk H, et al. MRI of osteonecrosis:

transient bone marrow edema. Abstract presentation at the 1st International Symposium, Musculoskeletal Magnetic Resonance Imaging, San Francisco, 1996.

147. Guerra JJ, Steinberg ME. Current concepts review: distinguishing transient osteoporosis from avascular necrosis of the hip. J Bone Joint Surg 1995;77a:616.

148. Kerr R. Transient osteoporosis of the hip. Orthopaedics 1990;13:485.

149. Hayes CW, Conway WF, Daniel WW. MR imaging of bone marrow edema pattern: transient osteoporosis, transient bone marrow edema syndrome, or osteonecrosis. Radiographics 1993;13:1001.

150. Feldman F, et al. MR imaging of soft-tissue reaction to prostheses. Radiology 1987;165(P):84.

151. Laakman RW, et al. MR imaging in patients with metallic implants. Radiology 1985;157:711.

Magnetic Resonance Imaging in Orthopaedics & Sports Medicine, Second Edition,
edited by David W. Stoller. Lippincott-Raven Publishers, Philadelphia, © 1997.

Chapter 7

The Knee

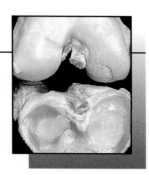

David W. Stoller
W. Dilworth Cannon, Jr.
Lesley J. Anderson

Many advances have been made in magnetic resonance (MR) imaging of the knee since its initial application, in 1984, for evaluation of the meniscus, and MR examination is now routinely used to assess a wide spectrum of internal knee derangements and articular disorders.[1–4] A noninvasive modality, MR has replaced conventional arthrography in the evaluation of the menisci and the cruciate ligaments and has decreased both the morbidity and the cost associated with arthroscopic examinations that yield negative results.[5,6] MR imaging has also proved beneficial in the selection of patients, in preoperative planning, in diagnosis, and in improved patient–doctor communication (resulting in more meaningful informed consent). The decrease in the cost of MR knee studies also has contributed to their acceptance by the orthopaedic community as a noninvasive replacement for arthrography and nontherapeutic arthroscopy.

With MR imaging, the anatomic and pathologic definition of soft tissue, ligaments, fibrocartilage, and articular cartilage is superior to that seen with computed tomography (CT). Fast spin-echo imaging, used in conjunction with fat-suppression MR techniques, has extended the sensitivity and specificity of MR for the detection of articular cartilage injuries. In addition, three-dimensional (3D) volume techniques have demonstrated the versatility of MR imaging in the evaluation of meniscal tears. 3D acquisitions of the meniscus can be used to reformat images of meniscal tears in orthogonal and nonorthogonal planes. Additional advantages of MR imaging are multiplanar and thin-section capabilities and the ability to evaluate subchondral bone and marrow. As a result, MR imaging is recommended instead of CT for the evaluation of bone contusions and occult knee fractures, including tibial plateau fractures of the knee. MR has supplanted nuclear scintigraphy in the characterization of osteonecrosis and, furthermore, can be used to assess the integrity of the overlying articular cartilage surfaces.

Kinematic and dynamic MR techniques provide an improved perspective for assessing the biomechanics of the patellofemoral joint and the normal function of the ligamentous structures of the knee. Fast-scan techniques, including 3D Fourier transform (FT) volume imaging with submillimeter capability, can produce more than 120 images through the knee in a single acquisition. 3D gradient-echo and fast spin-echo images can be reformatted retrospectively in any orthogonal or prescribed oblique orientation.

MR imaging is unique in its ability to evaluate the internal structure as well as the surface of the meniscus.[7] With conventional arthrography, intraarticular injection of contrast media permits visualization of surface anatomy but does not allow delineation of fibrocartilage structure or subchondral bone. Intravenous gadolinium contrast (gadolinium-diethylenetriamine pentaacetic acid [DTPA]) MR imaging, which is used to enhance areas of pannus in cases of inflammatory arthritis, allows more precise evaluation of articular cartilage surfaces, and both meniscal repairs and cruciate reconstructions may be facilitated by either the intraarticular (MR arthrography) or intravenous administration of gadolinium. Joint capsule distention with an MR contrast agent or saline also improves the identification of synovial plicae.

IMAGING PROTOCOLS FOR THE KNEE

Routine MR examinations are performed in the axial, sagittal, and coronal planes. Although there is no single optimal or correct technique for MR protocols, several general principles assist in the development of sequences for a comprehensive knee examination. Some form of T2 weighting should be used in each of the three acquisition planes (axial, sagittal, and coronal). Conventional T2-weighted images are usually supplemented with a short inversion time (TI) inversion recovery (STIR) sagittal acquisition to improve visualization of osseous contusions and muscle trauma. When fast spin-echo techniques are used, fat suppression is added to improve visualization of edema fluid and contusions. To prevent blurring with fast spin-echo and to allow accurate detection of meniscal degenerations and tears, the echo train, which represents the number of echoes per repetition time (TR), must be relatively short (eg, <4). Fat-suppressed T2-weighted fast spin-echo images are sensitive to articular car-

tilage lesions in all three compartments of the knee. A T1 or T2 gradient-echo sagittal sequence (two-dimensional [2D] or 3D FT) improves the accuracy of detection of meniscal lesions by compensating for the blurring inherent in most fast spin-echo acquisitions. (The image blurring seen in fast spin-echo MR represents a decrease in spatial resolution along the phase-encoded axis and is more severe with short echo times [TEs].[8])

Manipulation of the knee joint, which is necessary to perform an arthrogram, is not required in MR studies. This advantage is particularly important in the examination of patients who have sustained trauma with associated joint effusions and who cannot tolerate physical examination without anesthesia. Radial imaging, in which multiple planes are rotated from the center of each meniscus or the center of the tibia, can section portions of both the medial and lateral meniscus, in views similar to a conventional arthrogram. Radial images best display the anatomy of the meniscocapsular junction, including the meniscofemoral and meniscotibial attachments of the deep capsular layer of the knee. 3D FT volume acquisitions through the knee can be reformatted and displayed in radial planes, eliminating the need to perform dedicated 2D radial acquisition. 3D rendering techniques permit disarticulation of specified areas of pathology, generating surface and volume detail (Fig. 7-1).

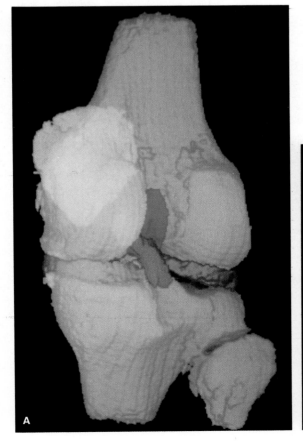

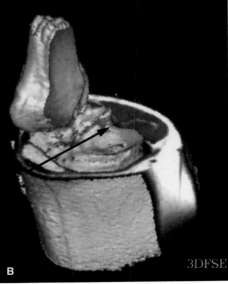

FIGURE 7-1. (A) A 3D MR rendering in a posterior oblique projection shows the ACL (*dark blue*), the PCL (*green*), and the meniscal structures (*yellow*). (B) A 3D MR rendering (from a 3D fast spin-echo acquisition) showing axial and sagittal cross sections. *Arrow*, posterior horn of the medial meniscus; *purple*, PCL.

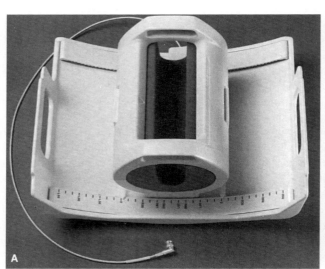

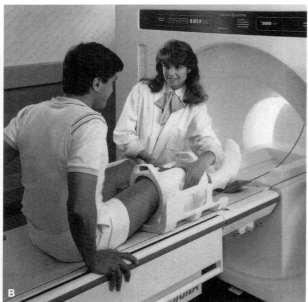

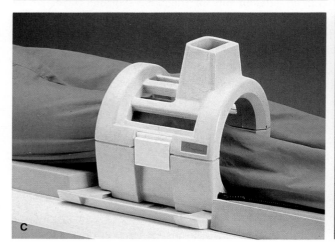

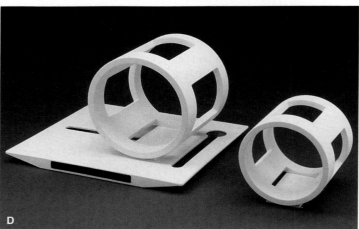

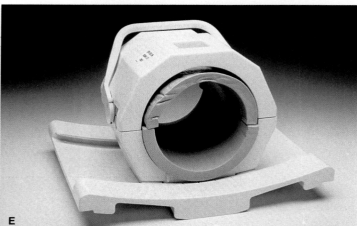

FIGURE 7-2. (**A**) A circumferential transmit-and-receive surface coil used in imaging the knee. (**B**) The coil as it is positioned on the patient. Quadrature (**C** and **D**) and phased-array (**E**) coils of different design.

Soft-tissue discrimination with MR imaging is excellent, and differentiations can be made among cortex, marrow, ligaments, tendons, muscle, synovium, and vascular and cartilage elements. This differentiation is not possible with conventional radiographic techniques.[9,10]

Routine Protocols

A circumferential extremity coil (with a send–receive, quadrature, or phased-array design) provides a uniform signal-to-noise ratio across the knee (Fig. 7-2). Field homogeneity can be improved and image artifacts minimized by the imaging enhancement options selected. For the evaluation of internal knee derangements, our routine protocols include T1-weighted images in the axial, sagittal, and coronal planes. Fat-suppressed T2-weighted fast spin-echo contrast images also are obtained in the axial, sagittal, and coronal planes. T2*-weighted 2D or 3D FT gradient-echo sagittal images replace or complement routine T1-weighted sagittal images in the evaluation of the meniscus. Compared with T2*-weighted images, conventional T2, STIR, and especially fat-suppressed T2-weighted fast spin-echo techniques are more sensitive in the detection of fluid in areas of articular cartilage injury (Fig. 7-3). An acquisition matrix of 256 (number of phase encodings), a field of view of 10 to 14 cm, and 1 to 2 number of excitations (NEX) are routinely used. In children, the field of view should be 12 cm or less to increase spatial resolution. Gradient-echo images are acquired with an acquisition matrix of 192 or 256. When T2-weighted fast spin-echo acquisitions are used in conjunction with fat suppression, the TE should be less than 40 milliseconds to maintain a high signal-to-noise ratio.

Imaging Planes

An axial acquisition through the patellofemoral joint is used as the initial localizer for subsequent sagittal and coronal plane images. Meniscal pathology is evaluated primarily on sagittal plane images. However, the morphology and signal intensity of meniscal cartilages should be assessed secondarily on coronal plane images. The cruciate ligaments are best seen on sagittal plane images, with coronal and axial views for secondary visualization and confirmation of pathology. The medial and lateral collateral ligaments (MCL and LCL) are clearly displayed on coronal and axial images and can also be routinely identified on 1-mm-thick 3D FT sagittal images. The articular cartilage surfaces of the medial and lateral compartments are assessed in both coronal and sagittal planes. The patellofemoral joint, including patellar facet and trochlear groove articular cartilage, is best seen on axial and sagittal images.

Patient Positioning

Although imaging studies are routinely performed with the knee placed in 10° to 15° of external rotation (to realign the anterior cruciate ligament [ACL] parallel with the sagittal imaging plane), this external rotation becomes less important when thinner sections (≤3 mm) are used. Excessive external rotation of the knee results in elongation of the anterior-to-posterior dimensions of the femoral condyle (especially the lateral femoral condyle) and may decrease accurate visualization of meniscal anatomy. An alternative is to use sagittal images in an oblique plane parallel to the orientation of the ACL as assessed on an axial localizer.

Slice Thickness

Four-millimeter sections are used for axial and coronal plane images, and 3- to 4-mm-thick sections are used for sagittal images. When needed, submillimeter resolution can be obtained with 3D FT volume protocols. The maximum slice thickness for evaluation of the meniscus is 5 mm. 3D FT gradient-echo axial images at 0.7-mm thickness provide six to eight sections through the meniscus and display circumferential tear patterns (eg, longitudinal versus flap versus radial tear patterns). In children's knees, 3-mm slices allow optimum medial-to-lateral joint coverage in the sagittal plane and anterior-to-posterior coverage in the coronal plane. In cases of inadequate imaging of the ACL on orthogonal sagittal views, oblique sagittal images through the ACL, which is identified on the axial localizer, may better display its femoral and tibial attachments.[11] 3D FT volume protocols using a 1- to 2-mm slice thickness, however, obviate the need for oblique cruciate imaging.

Application and Techniques for Routine Protocols

Conventional T2-weighted images are generated with a TR of 2000 milliseconds; a TE of 20, 80 milliseconds; a 256 × 192 (or 256 × 256) acquisition matrix, and 1 NEX. The use of fast spin-echo and STIR (including the fast spin-echo version of STIR, or fast inversion recovery) techniques has increased the routine application of long TR protocols while reducing overall imaging time. Effective T2 or T2* contrast can be obtained with refocused 2D FT gradient-echo images, a TR of 400 to 600 milliseconds, a TE of 15 to 25 milliseconds, a flip angle of 20° to 30°, and an acquisition matrix of 256 × 192. Imaging time can be reduced by using 3D FT gradient-echo volume imaging and a slice thickness of less than 1 mm. Axial 3D FT images are acquired with a TR of 55 milliseconds, a TE of 15 milliseconds, and a flip angle of 10°. These images can be reformatted without loss

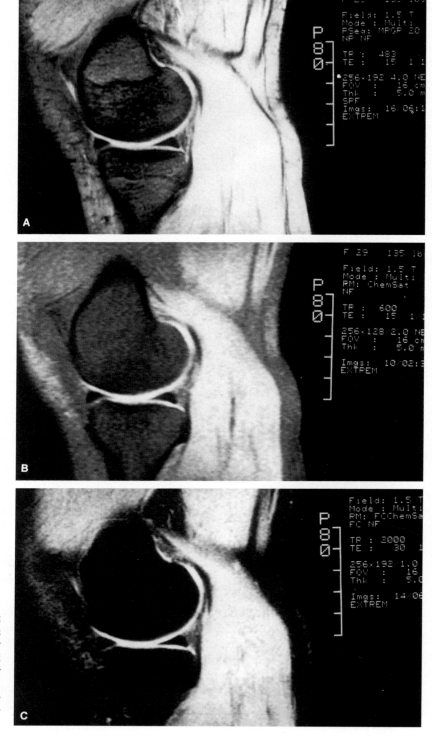

FIGURE 7-3. A comparison of T2*-weighted contrast (**A**) with fat-saturation protocols (**B** and **C**). Although marrow fat is of low signal intensity in all images, only the ChemSat images show low signal intensity from all fat-containing tissues (ie, subcutaneous fat). The longer the TR and TE, the greater the degree of fat saturation. ChemSat is used to apply a frequency-selective presaturation pulse to fat before the excitation pulse, destroying the longitudinal magnetization of fat.

of spatial resolution.[12] 3D FT T2*-weighted sagittal images can be performed with a TR of 33 milliseconds, a TE of 13 milliseconds, and a field of view of 10 cm at a 256 × 192 matrix with 2 NEX.

T2*-weighted radial images demonstrate meniscocapsular anatomy and are used to evaluate peripheral meniscal tears. T2 (including fat-suppressed T2-weighted fast spin-echo) contrast is helpful in highlighting ligamentous edema and hemorrhage in collateral ligaments in the coronal imaging plane or cruciate ligaments in the sagittal imaging plane. In patients with degenerative or inflammatory arthritis, sagittal images provide the most information in early synovial reactions (defining the free-edge contour of Hoffa's fat pad) and cartilage erosions. For identification of trabecular bone contusions and fractures, STIR and fat-suppressed T2-weighted fast spin-echo weighted images are more sensitive than conventional T2- or T2*-weighted protocols. T2* gradient-echo contrast is not helpful in the detection of subchondral bone and marrow pathology. Susceptibility artifacts, secondary to postoperative meniscal or ACL repair, are accentuated on gradient-echo images because of the absence of a 180° refocusing pulse.[13] Although high-resolution 3D spoiled-grass (SPGR) images display increased anatomic detail at small fields of view (eg, 4 cm), unless they are obtained in conjunction with fat-suppression techniques (fat-suppressed SPGR) they are not as sensitive to subchondral bone and articular cartilage abnormalities as are STIR or fat-suppressed T2-weighted fast spin-echo sequences.

Fat-suppressed T2-weighted fast spin-echo protocols use a TR of 3000 to 4000 milliseconds, with a TE of 40 to 50 milliseconds. This proton-density weighted TE ensures an adequate signal-to-noise ratio when fat suppression is used. Fast spin-echo protocols require either a prolonged TE (>120 milliseconds) or a proton-density–like TE (approximately 40 milliseconds) to maintain dynamic contrast between fat and fluid (because of the increased signal intensity from fat compared with that on conventional T2-weighted spin-echo images). Blurring or decreased resolution is increased with fast spin-echo techniques when an echo train length greater than 4 and shorter TE sequences are used. For this reason, fast spin-echo images are not adequate to identify meniscal degenerations and tears. With TR values less than 2900 milliseconds, fluid–articular cartilage interfaces may become difficult to differentiate, even with fast spin-echo and fat suppression.

Magnetization transfer methods can be used in conjunction with 3D grass acquisitions to emphasize articular cartilage–fluid interfaces. With these techniques, tissues with a high macromolecular content or slow macromolecular dynamics, such as cartilage, demonstrate decreased signal intensity in contrast to tissues with a lower macromolecular content, such as blood and synovial fluid.[14,15] Overall, fat-suppressed T2-weighted fast spin-echo contrast is the preferred technique for a survey of articular cartilage pathology.

STIR (fast inversion recovery) protocols use a TR of 4000 milliseconds, a TE of 18 milliseconds, a TI of 140 milliseconds, and an echo train length of 4. Evaluation of neoplastic lesions, both benign and malignant, requires a combination of T1-, T2- (conventional or fast spin-echo), STIR-, or T2*-weighted images in the axial plane to demonstrate compartment and neurovascular

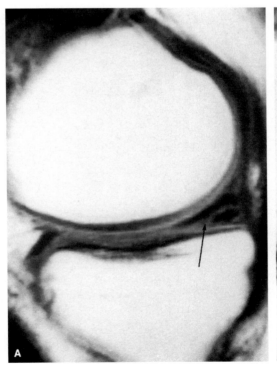
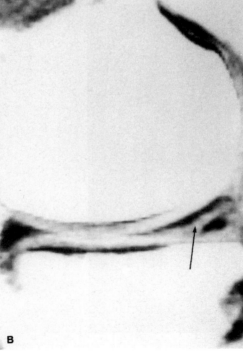

FIGURE 7-4. **(A)** An MR image, grade 3 signal intensity, shows a posterior horn medial meniscal tear (*arrow*). **(B)** The tear (*arrow*) is also shown with high-contrast photography.

anatomy. Fat-suppressed T2-weighted fast spin-echo or fast inversion-recovery sagittal or coronal images delineate the proximal-to-distal extent of a tumor on one complete image. Although fat suppression eliminates the high signal intensity of fat, it still does not provide the sensitivity of STIR images with T1 and T2 added. Fat-suppressed T1-weighted images are used when an intraarticular MR contrast agent, such as gadolinium, is used to highlight joint surfaces and distend the capsule. Fat-suppressed T2-weighted fast spin-echo contrast provides excellent visualization of fluid (which demonstrates high signal intensity) in cases in which intraarticular saline is used instead of a paramagnetic contrast agent in MR arthrography.

Artifacts and Photography

Popliteal artery pulsation artifacts can be minimized by exchanging the phase and frequency-encoded directions in the sagittal imaging plane.[16]

Although high-contrast, narrow–window-width photography is useful for emphasizing or highlighting internal signal intensities within the fibrocartilaginous meniscus, it is not routinely necessary (Fig. 7-4).[17] Gradient-echo images adequately display the spectrum of meniscal degenerations and tears without contrast adjustment.

NORMAL GROSS AND MR ANATOMY OF THE KNEE

Axial Images

Axial plane images have an important role in routine knee evaluation. The medial and lateral patellar facets and articular cartilage, because of their oblique orientation, are most accurately demonstrated on axial images through the patellofemoral joint. Patellofemoral disease (ie, chondromalacia) may be over- or underestimated on sagittal images alone. Submillimeter 3D FT axial images are used to define circumferential meniscal tear patterns and to create 3D composite images using a workstation. Axial plane images are also used as a localizer to determine sagittal and coronal coverage. Although the axial plane can be used to display meniscal structure, routine axial images at 4 or 5 mm are not sensitive

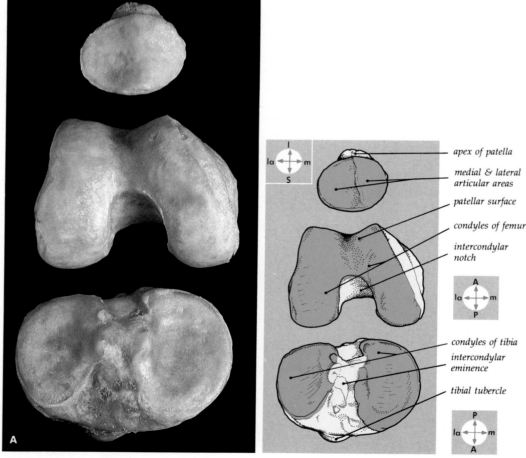

apex of patella

medial & lateral articular areas

patellar surface

condyles of femur

intercondylar notch

condyles of tibia

intercondylar eminence

tibial tubercle

FIGURE 7-5. (A) The articular surfaces of the patella, femur, and tibia.

continued

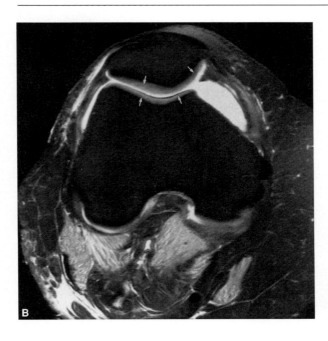

FIGURE 7-5. *Continued.* (**B**) Visualization of the patellar facet and trochlear groove articular cartilage surfaces (*arrows*) on a fat-suppressed T2-weighted fast spin-echo MR arthrogram. Articular cartilage is gray or intermediate in signal intensity relative to the hyperintense joint fluid.

to meniscal pathology because the sections are too thick. Sagittal images, which section the meniscus perpendicular to its surface, provide the best demonstration of internal meniscal anatomy and pathology.

Axial joint dissection displays the osseous relations among the patella, femur, and tibia (Fig. 7-5). The medial femoral condyle is longer than the lateral condyle and is oriented toward the lateral aspect of the knee as it extends from the posterior to anterior.[18] The medial tibial articular facet has a greater anterior-to-posterior dimension than the lateral tibial articular facet, as assessed in the sagittal plane. Both tibial plateau articular facets have a mild concavity in the coronal plane, although the lateral facet displays a convexity in the sagittal plane. The osseous contribution to the screw-home mechanism causes the tibia to undergo external rotation during the last degrees of full extension as it rolls anteriorly, more on the medial femoral condyle than on the lateral. The trochlear groove or surface is continuous inferiorly and posteriorly with the intercondylar notch. The two patellar facets are divided by a median ridge, and the lateral facet is usually larger than the medial facet. The supratrochlear tubercle represents the nonarticular area of the anterior distal femur, in which the patella rests in full extension. Outerbridge's ridge describes the sharp or distinct drop-off between the distal femur articular cartilage and the supratrochlear tubercle. These anatomic features contribute to the superolateral movement of the patella in full knee extension.

The circumferential surface anatomy of the menisci and attachments of the cruciate and collateral ligaments is shown by disarticulation of the femur from the tibia (Fig. 7-6) and is directly visualized on corresponding axial plane images (Fig 7-7). The anterior and posterior horns of the lateral meniscus are attached to the nonarticular area of the tibial plateau, contributing to its relatively circular appearance.[18] The anterior and posterior horns of the C-shaped medial

meniscus are attached forward on the anterior aspect of the proximal tibia and on the posterior tibia above the posterior cruciate attachment, respectively. The transverse ligament is a fibrous band that connects the anterior horns of the medial and lateral menisci. The ligament of Wrisberg and the ligament of Humphrey (the posterior and anterior meniscofemoral ligaments, respectively) are variably present and pass from the posterior horn of the lateral meniscus to the medial aspect of the intercondylar notch. The ligament of Wrisberg passes posterior to the posterior cruciate ligament (PCL), and the ligament of Humphrey passes anterior to it.

The tibial plateau is seen on inferior axial images through the knee joint. The posterior cruciate insertion is displayed on the posterior tibial surface and demonstrates low signal intensity on cross section. The popliteus muscle is seen posterior to the tibia at the level of the superior tibiofibular joint. At the midjoint level, the medial and lateral menisci are seen with uniform low signal intensity. The medial meniscus has an open C-shaped configuration with a narrow anterior horn and wider posterior horn. The lateral meniscus has a more circular shape and consistent width. Sections that are 3 mm or less in thickness display both menisci on axial images.

The transverse ligament of the knee is seen as a band of low signal intensity connecting the anterior horn of the lateral and medial menisci. It can be identified where it transverses Hoffa's infrapatellar fat pad, which, in contrast to the ligament, demonstrates bright signal intensity.

The semimembranosus and semitendinosus tendons are seen as circular structures of low signal intensity located lateral to the medial head of the gastrocnemius muscle and posterior to the medial tibial plateau. The semimembranosus tendon appears larger than the semitendinosus tendon. The elliptical sartorius muscle and the circular gracilis tendon

text continues on page 220

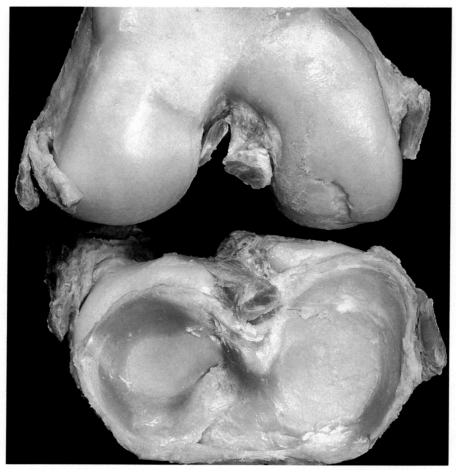

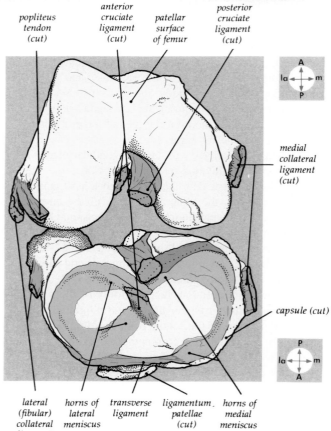

popliteus tendon (cut)

anterior cruciate ligament (cut)

patellar surface of femur

posterior cruciate ligament (cut)

medial collateral ligament (cut)

capsule (cut)

lateral (fibular) collateral ligament (cut)

horns of lateral meniscus

transverse ligament

ligamentum patellae (cut)

horns of medial meniscus

FIGURE 7-6. The attachments of the cruciate ligaments and the shape and attachments of the menisci. Cutting of the cruciate and collateral ligaments allows the femur to be separated from the tibia.

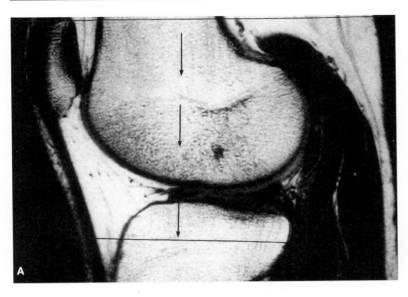

FIGURE 7-7. Normal axial MR anatomy. **(A)** This T1-weighted sagittal localizer was used to identify image locations graphically, from **(B)** superior to **(N)** inferior.

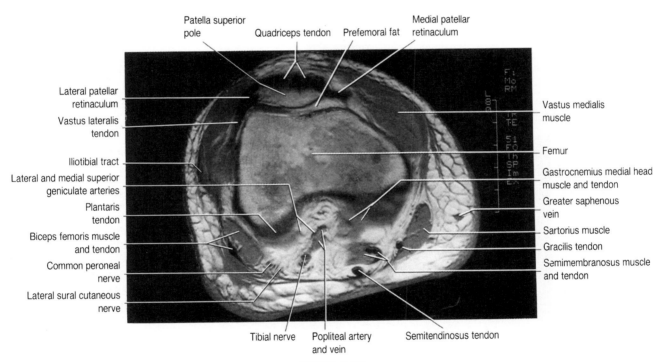

Patella superior pole

Quadriceps tendon

Prefemoral fat

Medial patellar retinaculum

Lateral patellar retinaculum

Vastus lateralis tendon

Iliotibial tract

Lateral and medial superior geniculate arteries

Plantaris tendon

Biceps femoris muscle and tendon

Common peroneal nerve

Lateral sural cutaneous nerve

Vastus medialis muscle

Femur

Gastrocnemius medial head muscle and tendon

Greater saphenous vein

Sartorius muscle

Gracilis tendon

Semimembranosus muscle and tendon

Tibial nerve

Popliteal artery and vein

Semitendinosus tendon

FIGURE 7-7B.

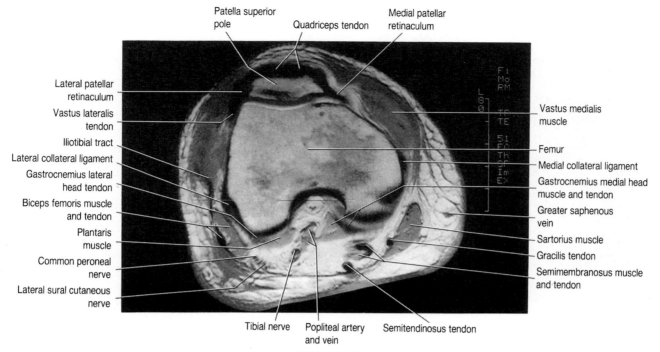

FIGURE 7-7C.

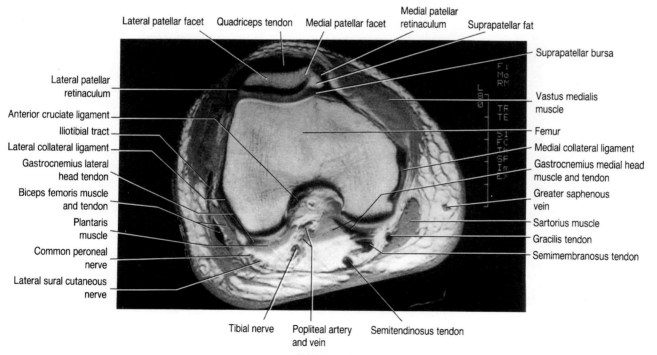

FIGURE 7-7D.

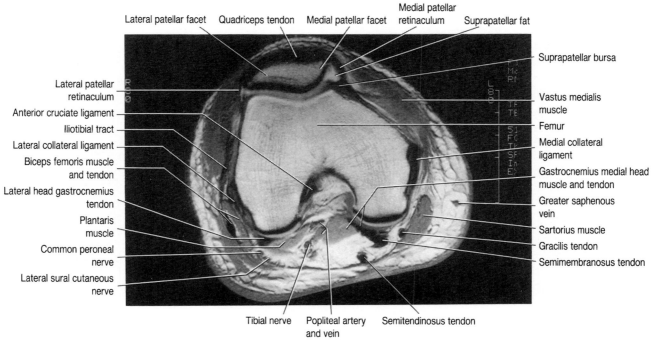

Lateral patellar facet Quadriceps tendon Medial patellar facet Medial patellar retinaculum Suprapatellar fat

Suprapatellar bursa

Lateral patellar retinaculum

Anterior cruciate ligament

Iliotibial tract

Lateral collateral ligament

Biceps femoris muscle and tendon

Lateral head gastrocnemius tendon

Plantaris muscle

Common peroneal nerve

Lateral sural cutaneous nerve

Vastus medialis muscle

Femur

Medial collateral ligament

Gastrocnemius medial head muscle and tendon

Greater saphenous vein

Sartorius muscle

Gracilis tendon

Semimembranosus tendon

Tibial nerve   Popliteal artery and vein   Semitendinosus tendon

FIGURE 7-7E.

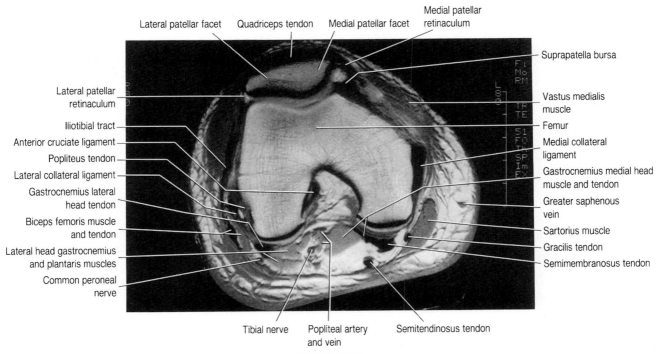

Lateral patellar facet   Quadriceps tendon   Medial patellar facet   Medial patellar retinaculum

Suprapatella bursa

Lateral patellar retinaculum

Iliotibial tract

Anterior cruciate ligament

Popliteus tendon

Lateral collateral ligament

Gastrocnemius lateral head tendon

Biceps femoris muscle and tendon

Lateral head gastrocnemius and plantaris muscles

Common peroneal nerve

Vastus medialis muscle

Femur

Medial collateral ligament

Gastrocnemius medial head muscle and tendon

Greater saphenous vein

Sartorius muscle

Gracilis tendon

Semimembranosus tendon

Tibial nerve   Popliteal artery and vein   Semitendinosus tendon

FIGURE 7-7F.

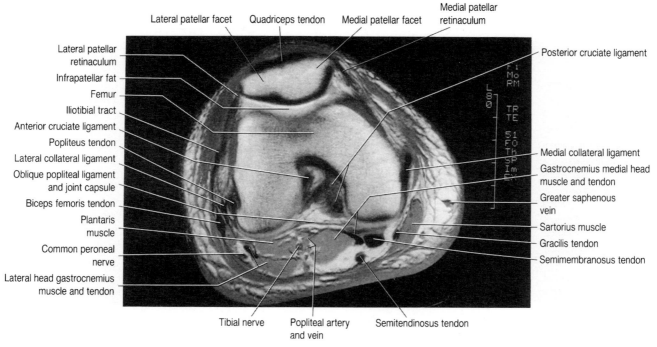

Lateral patellar facet Quadriceps tendon Medial patellar facet Medial patellar retinaculum

Lateral patellar retinaculum
Infrapatellar fat
Femur
Iliotibial tract
Anterior cruciate ligament
Popliteus tendon
Lateral collateral ligament
Oblique popliteal ligament and joint capsule
Biceps femoris tendon
Plantaris muscle
Common peroneal nerve
Lateral head gastrocnemius muscle and tendon

Posterior cruciate ligament
Medial collateral ligament
Gastrocnemius medial head muscle and tendon
Greater saphenous vein
Sartorius muscle
Gracilis tendon
Semimembranosus tendon

Tibial nerve Popliteal artery and vein Semitendinosus tendon

FIGURE 7-7G.

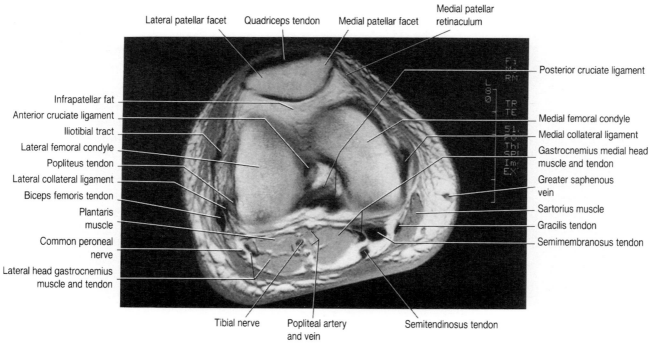

Lateral patellar facet Quadriceps tendon Medial patellar facet Medial patellar retinaculum

Infrapatellar fat
Anterior cruciate ligament
Iliotibial tract
Lateral femoral condyle
Popliteus tendon
Lateral collateral ligament
Biceps femoris tendon
Plantaris muscle
Common peroneal nerve
Lateral head gastrocnemius muscle and tendon

Posterior cruciate ligament
Medial femoral condyle
Medial collateral ligament
Gastrocnemius medial head muscle and tendon
Greater saphenous vein
Sartorius muscle
Gracilis tendon
Semimembranosus tendon

Tibial nerve Popliteal artery and vein Semitendinosus tendon

FIGURE 7-7H.

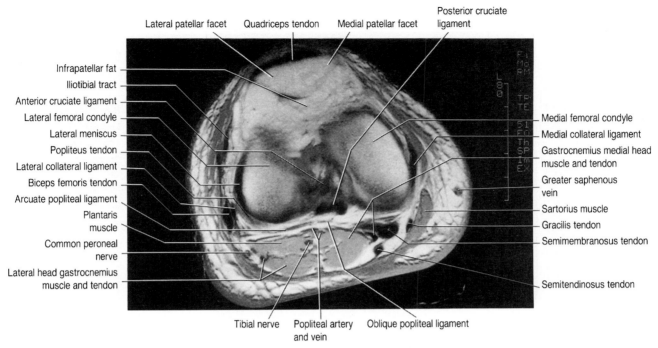

Lateral patellar facet   Quadriceps tendon   Medial patellar facet   Posterior cruciate ligament

Infrapatellar fat
Iliotibial tract
Anterior cruciate ligament
Lateral femoral condyle
Lateral meniscus
Popliteus tendon
Lateral collateral ligament
Biceps femoris tendon
Arcuate popliteal ligament
Plantaris muscle
Common peroneal nerve
Lateral head gastrocnemius muscle and tendon

Medial femoral condyle
Medial collateral ligament
Gastrocnemius medial head muscle and tendon
Greater saphenous vein
Sartorius muscle
Gracilis tendon
Semimembranosus tendon
Semitendinosus tendon

Tibial nerve   Popliteal artery and vein   Oblique popliteal ligament

FIGURE 7-7I.

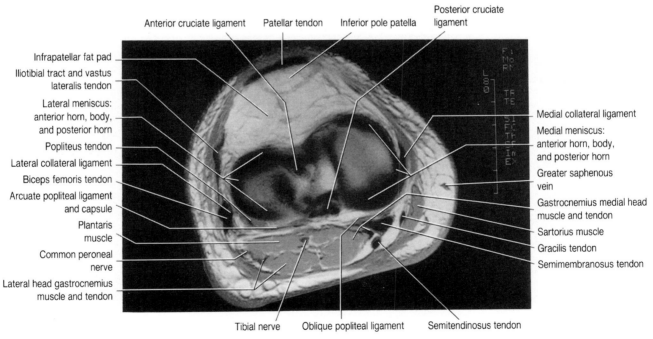

Anterior cruciate ligament   Patellar tendon   Inferior pole patella   Posterior cruciate ligament

Infrapatellar fat pad
Iliotibial tract and vastus lateralis tendon
Lateral meniscus: anterior horn, body, and posterior horn
Popliteus tendon
Lateral collateral ligament
Biceps femoris tendon
Arcuate popliteal ligament and capsule
Plantaris muscle
Common peroneal nerve
Lateral head gastrocnemius muscle and tendon

Medial collateral ligament
Medial meniscus: anterior horn, body, and posterior horn
Greater saphenous vein
Gastrocnemius medial head muscle and tendon
Sartorius muscle
Gracilis tendon
Semimembranosus tendon

Tibial nerve   Oblique popliteal ligament   Semitendinosus tendon

FIGURE 7-7J.

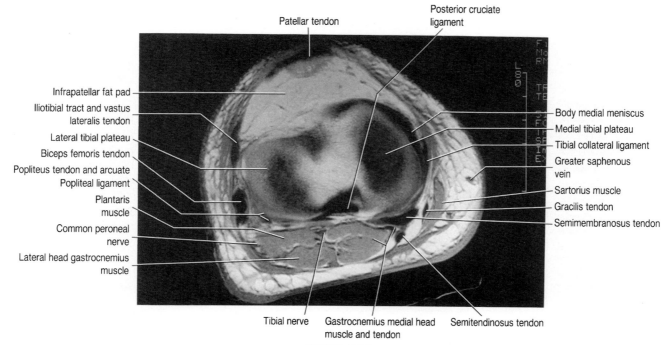

Patellar tendon

Posterior cruciate ligament

Infrapatellar fat pad

Iliotibial tract and vastus lateralis tendon

Lateral tibial plateau

Biceps femoris tendon

Popliteus tendon and arcuate popliteal ligament

Plantaris muscle

Common peroneal nerve

Lateral head gastrocnemius muscle

Body medial meniscus

Medial tibial plateau

Tibial collateral ligament

Greater saphenous vein

Sartorius muscle

Gracilis tendon

Semimembranosus tendon

Tibial nerve

Gastrocnemius medial head muscle and tendon

Semitendinosus tendon

FIGURE 7-7K.

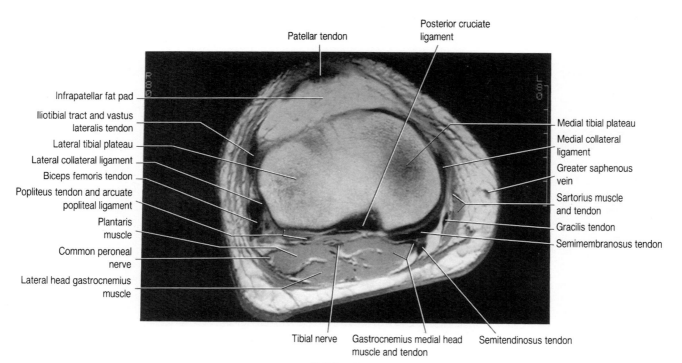

Patellar tendon

Posterior cruciate ligament

Infrapatellar fat pad

Iliotibial tract and vastus lateralis tendon

Lateral tibial plateau

Lateral collateral ligament

Biceps femoris tendon

Popliteus tendon and arcuate popliteal ligament

Plantaris muscle

Common peroneal nerve

Lateral head gastrocnemius muscle

Medial tibial plateau

Medial collateral ligament

Greater saphenous vein

Sartorius muscle and tendon

Gracilis tendon

Semimembranosus tendon

Tibial nerve

Gastrocnemius medial head muscle and tendon

Semitendinosus tendon

FIGURE 7-7L.

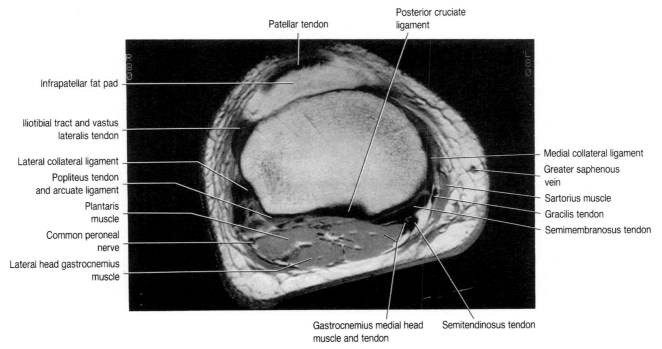

Patellar tendon

Posterior cruciate ligament

Infrapatellar fat pad

Iliotibial tract and vastus lateralis tendon

Lateral collateral ligament

Popliteus tendon and arcuate ligament

Plantaris muscle

Common peroneal nerve

Lateral head gastrocnemius muscle

Medial collateral ligament

Greater saphenous vein

Sartorius muscle

Gracilis tendon

Semimembranosus tendon

Gastrocnemius medial head muscle and tendon

Semitendinosus tendon

FIGURE 7-7M.

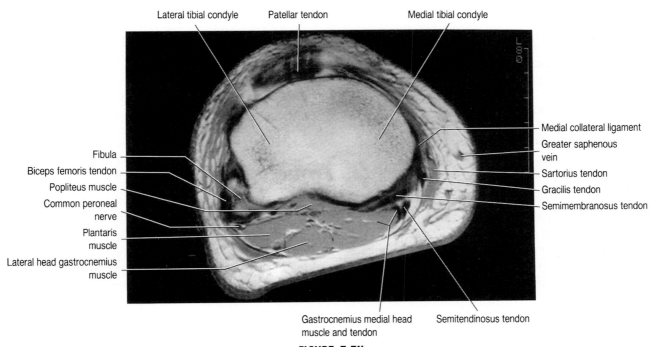

Lateral tibial condyle

Patellar tendon

Medial tibial condyle

Fibula

Biceps femoris tendon

Popliteus muscle

Common peroneal nerve

Plantaris muscle

Lateral head gastrocnemius muscle

Medial collateral ligament

Greater saphenous vein

Sartorius tendon

Gracilis tendon

Semimembranosus tendon

Gastrocnemius medial head muscle and tendon

Semitendinosus tendon

FIGURE 7-7N.

are located more medial and posterior than the semimembranosus and semitendinosus tendons and are in line with the MCL, which crosses the peripheral joint line. Proximal to its insertion on the fibular head, the biceps femoris tendon is positioned anterolateral to the lateral head of the gastrocnemius muscle. The popliteal artery is found anterior to the popliteal vein, anterior to and between the two heads of the gastrocnemius muscle. Because it is located posterior to the posterior horn of the lateral meniscus, it is potentially at risk for injury during meniscal repair.

In cross section, the low-signal-intensity LCL, or fibular collateral ligament, may be surrounded by high-signal-intensity fat. The ACL and PCL insertions can be seen within the intercondylar notch. The ACL can be identified superior to the joint line, 15° to 20° off axis, in an anteromedial orientation.[19] The PCL is circular in cross section. The origin of the ACL can be seen on the medial aspect of the lateral femoral condyle, and the PCL can be seen on the lateral aspect of the medial femoral condyle.

Hoffa's infrapatellar fat pad is bordered by the low-signal-intensity iliotibial band laterally, the medial retinaculum medially, and the thick patellar tendon anteriorly. The common peroneal nerve is located lateral to the plantaris muscle, demonstrates low-to-intermediate signal intensity, and is encased in fat. At the level of the femoral condyles, the tibial nerve is located posterior to the popliteal vein and demonstrates intermediate signal intensity.

The larger lateral patellar facet and the oblique medial patellar facet are also seen in the axial plane. The thick articular cartilage surfaces of the patella show intermediate signal intensity on T1- and T2-weighted images. Both the medial and lateral patellar retinacular attachments are seen at the level of the patellofemoral joint and are of low signal intensity. Medial and lateral reflections of the suprapatellar bursa should not be mistaken for retinacular attachments or plicae.

Sagittal Images

Sagittal plane dissection displays the components of the medial (Fig. 7-8) and lateral (Fig. 7-9) collateral ligaments and adjacent capsule. The patellofemoral compartment, quadriceps, and patellar tendon are demonstrated on midsagittal dissections (Fig. 7-10). The suprapatellar bursa (pouch) extends 5 to 7 cm proximal to the superior pole of the patella.[18] Superficial medial dissection displays the conjoined pes anserinus tendons (semitendinosus, gracilis, and sartorius) as they course along the posteromedial aspect of the knee. The pes anserinus runs superficial to the distal MCL and inserts into the anteromedial tibial crest distal to the joint line. On the lateral aspect of the knee, the LCL and the more posteriorly located fabellofibular ligament (structures of the posterolateral corner of the knee) are shown. The fabellofibular and arcuate ligaments have insertions on the posterior aspect of the fibular styloid, posterior and deep to the LCL. These

ligaments course superficially and posteriorly, blending with the origin of the lateral head of the gastrocnemius and the oblique popliteal ligament. The arcuate ligament extends toward the popliteus capsular hiatus.

The ACL and PCL are best displayed on sagittal images (Figs. 7-11 and 7-12). The LCL, or fibular collateral ligament, and the biceps femoris tendon also may be seen on peripheral sagittal sections. Images in the sagittal plane are key in evaluating meniscal anatomy for both degenerations and tears. The MCL is usually not defined in the sagittal plane unless thin-section 3D FT volume images are acquired. Complex meniscal and bucket-handle tears may require examination of coronal images to identify displaced meniscal tissue or fragments.

On medial sagittal images, the low-signal-intensity semimembranosus tendon and intermediate-signal-intensity muscle are seen posteriorly. The vastus medialis muscle makes up the bulk of the musculature anterior to the medial femoral condyle. On T1-weighted images, fatty (ie, yellow) marrow demonstrates bright signal intensity, whereas adjacent cortical bone demonstrates uniform low signal intensity. Femoral and tibial hyaline articular cartilage demonstrates intermediate signal intensity on T1- and conventional T2-weighted images, bright signal intensity on T2*-weighted images, and low to intermediate signal intensity on fat-suppressed T2-weighted fast spin-echo images. The anterolateral femoral articular cartilage, which is particularly thick, is frequently the site of early erosions or attenuation in osteoarthritis (trochlear groove chondromalacia). The tibial cortex appears thicker than the femoral cortical bone because of a chemical-shift artifact.

The medial meniscus, which is composed of fibrocartilage, demonstrates uniform low signal intensity. The body of the medial meniscus has a continuous bow-tie shape on at least one or two consecutive sagittal images taken in 5-mm sections. In medial compartment images approaching the intercondylar notch, the separate anterior and posterior horns of the medial meniscus can be seen. The meniscal horns appear as opposing triangles on a minimum of two or three consecutive sagittal images. The posterior horn of the medial meniscus is larger than the opposing anterior horn. The medial head of the gastrocnemius muscle sweeps posteriorly from its origin along the distal femur. A small band of high-signal-intensity fat, representing the bursa, is seen between the posterior horn of the medial meniscus and the low-signal-intensity posterior capsule.

When sagittal images are viewed in the medial to lateral direction, the PCL is seen before the ACL comes into view. The thick, uniform, low-signal-intensity PCL arcs from its anterolateral origin on the medial femoral condyle to its insertion on the posterior inferior tibial surface. With partial knee flexion, the convex curve of the PCL becomes taut as the anterolateral band or bundle of the PCL is lax in extension. The anterior and posterior meniscofemoral ligaments (the ligaments of Humphrey and Wrisberg, respectively) are seen individually or together on either side of the PCL.

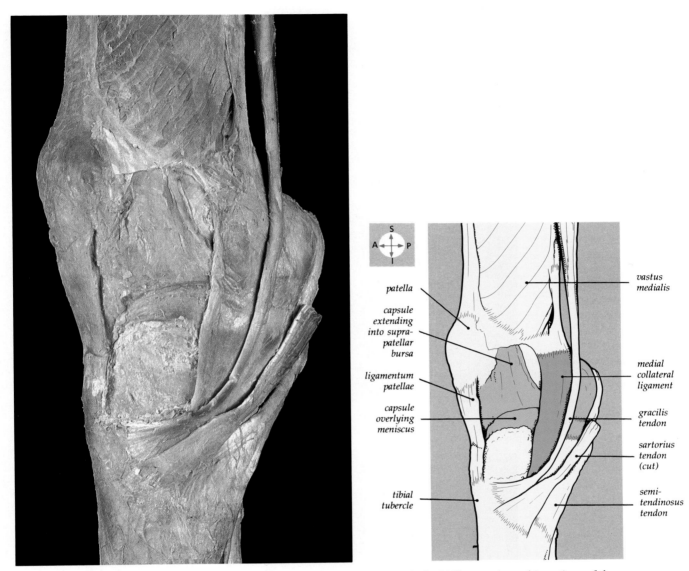

FIGURE 7-8. Superficial dissection from the medial aspect reveals the MCL, capsule, and insertions of the sartorius, gracilis, and semitendinosus tendons.

In the lateral portion of the intercondylar notch, the ACL extends obliquely from its semicircular origin on the posteromedial aspect of the lateral femoral condyle to its insertion, which starts 15 mm from the anterior border of the tibial articular surface (between the tibial spines). On average, it is 30 mm in length through the anterior intercondylar area.[20,21]

Although the ACL is composed of two functional bands of fibers (the anteromedial and posterolateral bands [AMB and PLB]), these bands cannot be differentiated on sagittal images. ACL fibers may display a minimally higher signal intensity than those of the PCL, and this difference is seen independent of a partial-volume effect with the lateral femoral condyle. Normally, the ACL is seen on at least one sagittal image when the knee is properly positioned in 10° to 15°

of external rotation and 5-mm-thick sections are used. With 1-mm-section 3D FT protocols, the ACL can be seen on several sagittal images. Fiber-bundle striations of the ACL are prominent at femoral and tibial attachments, especially when oblique sagittal images are performed to display attachment sites.

Portions of both cruciate ligaments may be observed on the same sagittal section. Excessive external rotation of the knee causes elongation of the anterior-to-posterior dimensions of the femoral condyles. Excessive internal rotation also causes elongation of the anterior-to-posterior dimensions of the condyles (lateral femoral condyle) with foreshortening of the medial femoral condyle. Excessive internal rotation also prevents adequate visualization of the ACL.

text continues on page 236

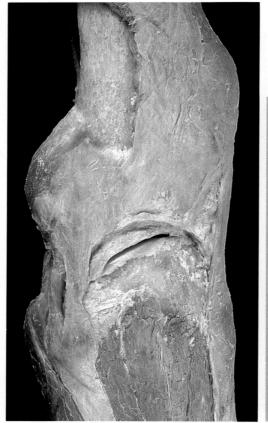
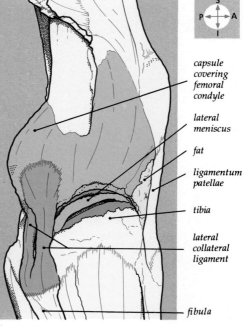

FIGURE 7-9. Dissection from the lateral aspect shows the LCL and the meniscus, which are revealed by removing part of the capsule.

capsule covering femoral condyle

lateral meniscus

fat

ligamentum patellae

tibia

lateral collateral ligament

fibula

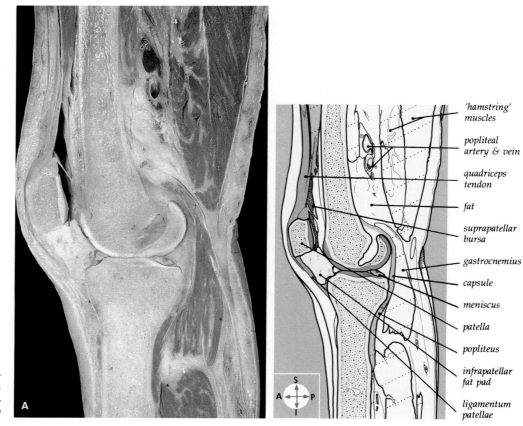

FIGURE 7-10. (**A**) A sagittal section through the knee joint shows the articular surfaces and suprapatellar pouch.   *continued*

'hamstring' muscles

popliteal artery & vein

quadriceps tendon

fat

suprapatellar bursa

gastrocnemius

capsule

meniscus

patella

popliteus

infrapatellar fat pad

ligamentum patellae

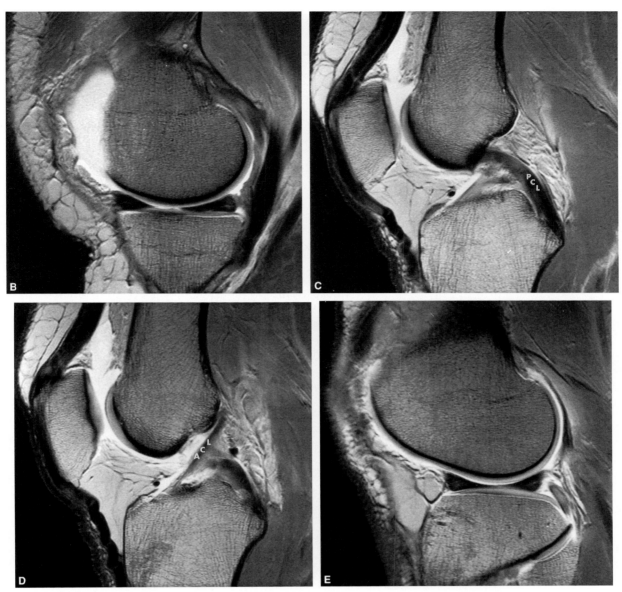

FIGURE 7-10. *Continued.* Representative sagittal MR arthrographic images through the medial compartment (**B**), PCL (**C**), ACL (**D**), and lateral compartment (**E**).

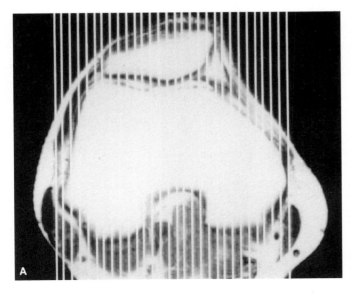

FIGURE 7-11. Normal sagittal MR anatomy of the medial compartment. (**A**) This T1-weighted localizer was used to identify image locations (**B**) medial through (**P**) the plane of the intercondylar notch.

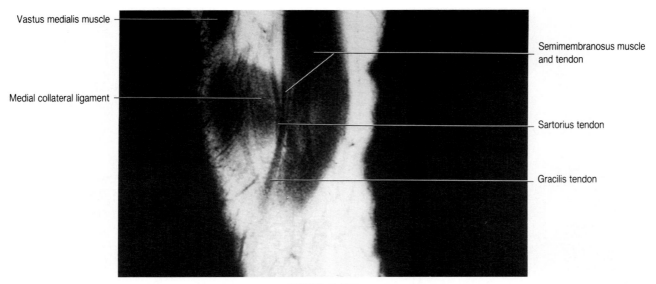

Vastus medialis muscle

Medial collateral ligament

Semimembranosus muscle and tendon

Sartorius tendon

Gracilis tendon

FIGURE 7-11B.

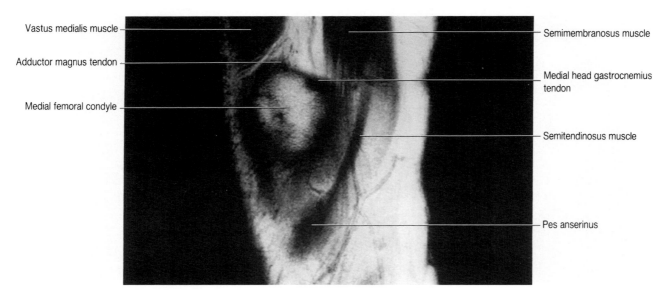

Vastus medialis muscle

Adductor magnus tendon

Medial femoral condyle

Semimembranosus muscle

Medial head gastrocnemius tendon

Semitendinosus muscle

Pes anserinus

FIGURE 7-11C.

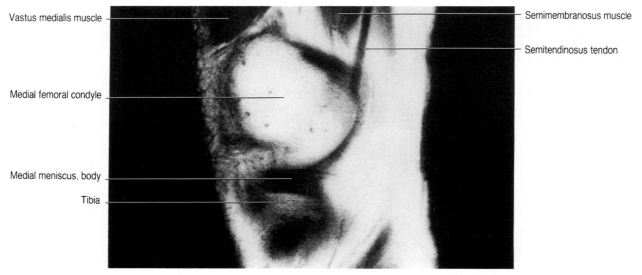

Vastus medialis muscle

Medial femoral condyle

Medial meniscus, body

Tibia

Semimembranosus muscle

Semitendinosus tendon

FIGURE 7-11D.

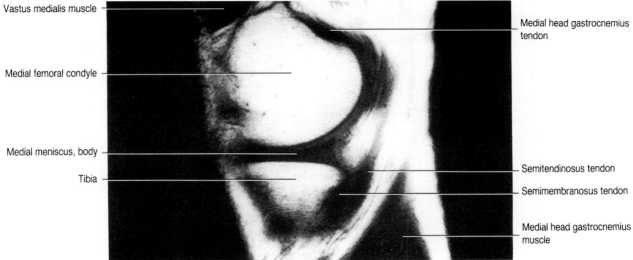

Vastus medialis muscle

Medial femoral condyle

Medial meniscus, body

Tibia

Medial head gastrocnemius tendon

Semitendinosus tendon

Semimembranosus tendon

Medial head gastrocnemius muscle

FIGURE 7-11E.

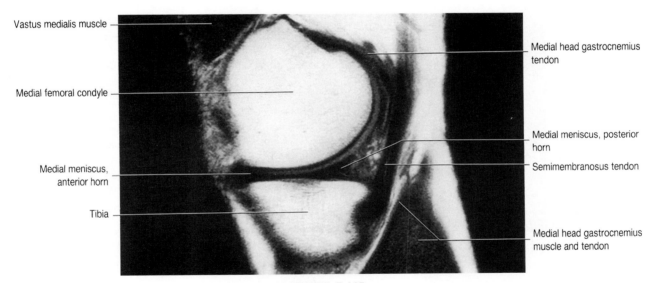

Vastus medialis muscle

Medial femoral condyle

Medial meniscus, anterior horn

Tibia

Medial head gastrocnemius tendon

Medial meniscus, posterior horn

Semimembranosus tendon

Medial head gastrocnemius muscle and tendon

FIGURE 7-11F.

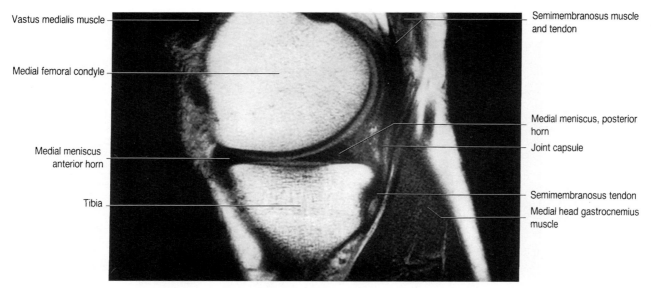

Vastus medialis muscle

Medial femoral condyle

Medial meniscus anterior horn

Tibia

Semimembranosus muscle and tendon

Medial meniscus, posterior horn

Joint capsule

Semimembranosus tendon

Medial head gastrocnemius muscle

FIGURE 7-11G.

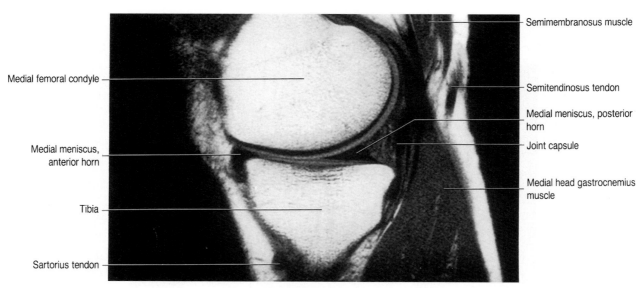

Medial femoral condyle

Medial meniscus, anterior horn

Tibia

Sartorius tendon

Semimembranosus muscle

Semitendinosus tendon

Medial meniscus, posterior horn

Joint capsule

Medial head gastrocnemius muscle

FIGURE 7-11H.

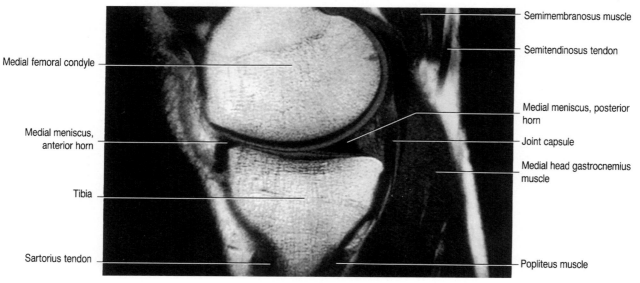

Medial femoral condyle

Medial meniscus, anterior horn

Tibia

Sartorius tendon

Semimembranosus muscle

Semitendinosus tendon

Medial meniscus, posterior horn

Joint capsule

Medial head gastrocnemius muscle

Popliteus muscle

FIGURE 7-11I.

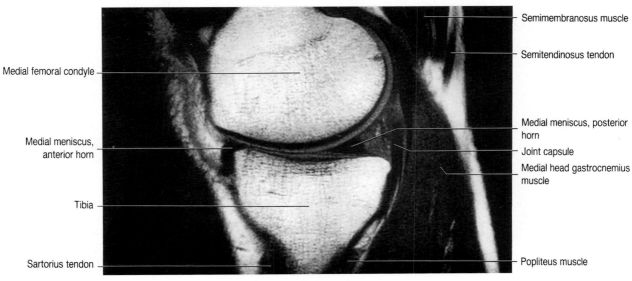

Medial femoral condyle

Medial meniscus, anterior horn

Tibia

Sartorius tendon

Semimembranosus muscle

Semitendinosus tendon

Medial meniscus, posterior horn

Joint capsule

Medial head gastrocnemius muscle

Popliteus muscle

FIGURE 7-11J.

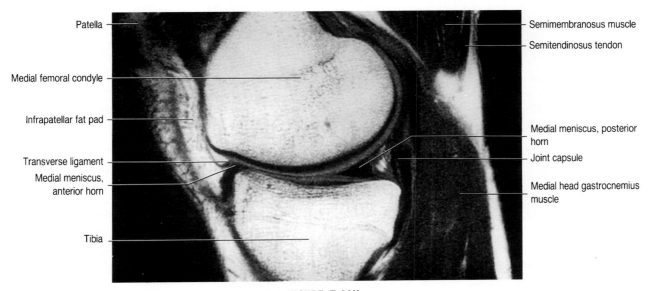

Patella

Medial femoral condyle

Infrapatellar fat pad

Transverse ligament

Medial meniscus, anterior horn

Tibia

Semimembranosus muscle

Semitendinosus tendon

Medial meniscus, posterior horn

Joint capsule

Medial head gastrocnemius muscle

FIGURE 7-11K.

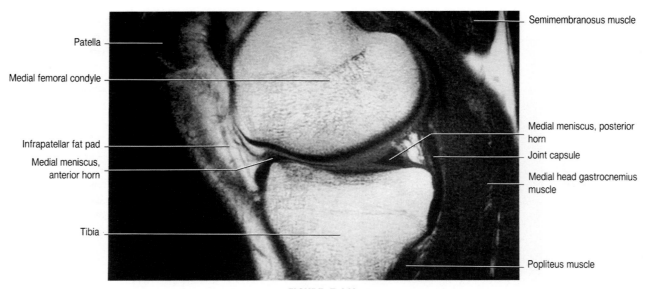

Patella

Medial femoral condyle

Infrapatellar fat pad

Medial meniscus, anterior horn

Tibia

Semimembranosus muscle

Medial meniscus, posterior horn

Joint capsule

Medial head gastrocnemius muscle

Popliteus muscle

FIGURE 7-11L.

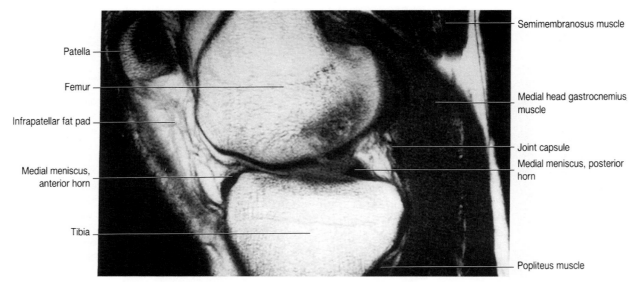

Patella

Femur

Infrapatellar fat pad

Medial meniscus, anterior horn

Tibia

Semimembranosus muscle

Medial head gastrocnemius muscle

Joint capsule

Medial meniscus, posterior horn

Popliteus muscle

FIGURE 7-11M.

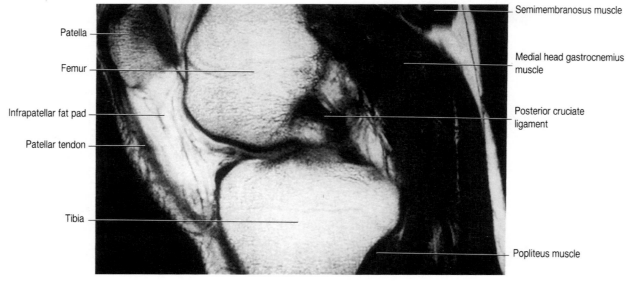

Patella

Femur

Infrapatellar fat pad

Patellar tendon

Tibia

Semimembranosus muscle

Medial head gastrocnemius muscle

Posterior cruciate ligament

Popliteus muscle

FIGURE 7-11N.

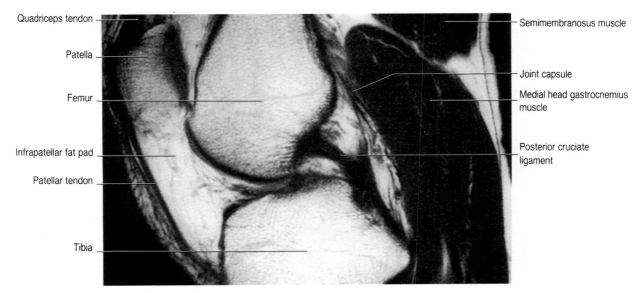

Quadriceps tendon —
Patella —
Femur —
Infrapatellar fat pad —
Patellar tendon —
Tibia —

Semimembranosus muscle
Joint capsule
Medial head gastrocnemius muscle
Posterior cruciate ligament

FIGURE 7-11O.

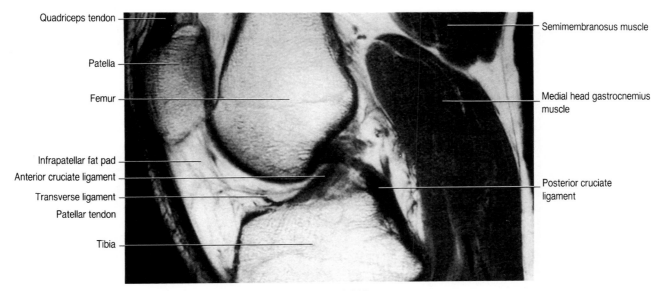

Quadriceps tendon —
Patella —
Femur —
Infrapatellar fat pad —
Anterior cruciate ligament —
Transverse ligament —
Patellar tendon —
Tibia —

Semimembranosus muscle
Medial head gastrocnemius muscle
Posterior cruciate ligament

FIGURE 7-11P.

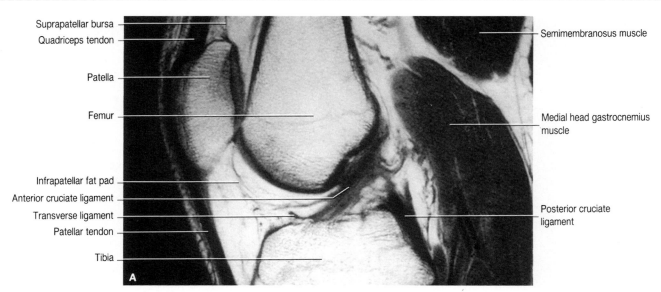

FIGURE 7-12. Normal sagittal MR anatomy of lateral compartment. See Figure 7-11*A* for the localizer that was also used to prescribe image locations from (**A**) the plane of the intercondylar notch through (**P**) the lateral aspect of the lateral compartment.

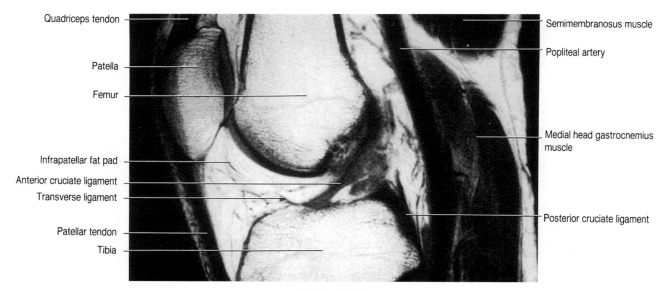

FIGURE 7-12B.

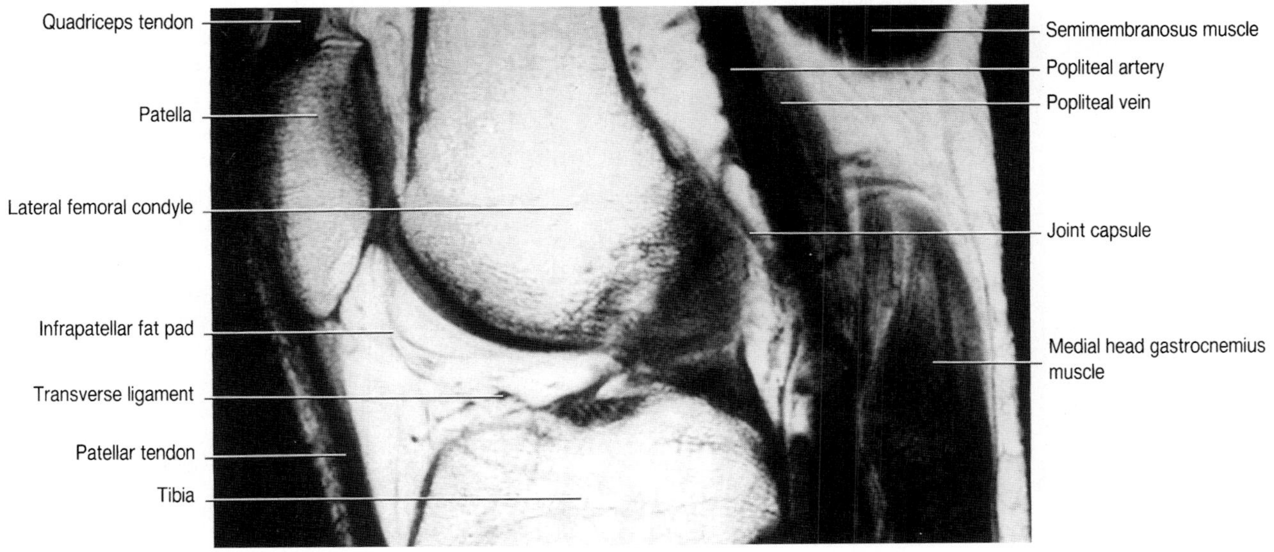

Quadriceps tendon

Patella

Lateral femoral condyle

Infrapatellar fat pad

Transverse ligament

Patellar tendon

Tibia

Semimembranosus muscle

Popliteal artery

Popliteal vein

Joint capsule

Medial head gastrocnemius muscle

FIGURE 7-12C.

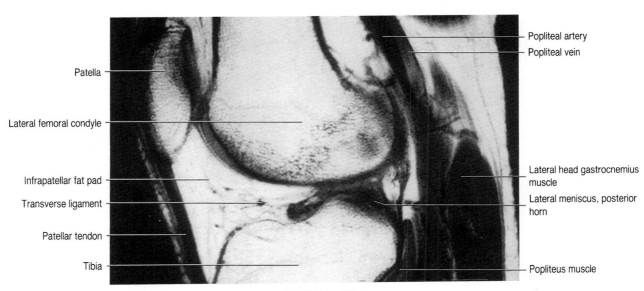

Patella

Lateral femoral condyle

Infrapatellar fat pad

Transverse ligament

Patellar tendon

Tibia

Popliteal artery

Popliteal vein

Lateral head gastrocnemius muscle

Lateral meniscus, posterior horn

Popliteus muscle

FIGURE 7-12D.

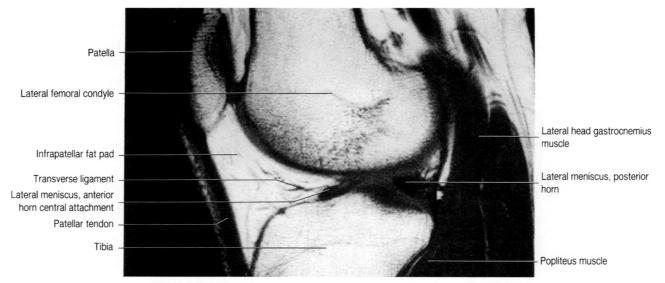

Patella

Lateral femoral condyle

Infrapatellar fat pad

Transverse ligament
Lateral meniscus, anterior horn central attachment
Patellar tendon

Tibia

Lateral head gastrocnemius muscle

Lateral meniscus, posterior horn

Popliteus muscle

FIGURE 7-12E.

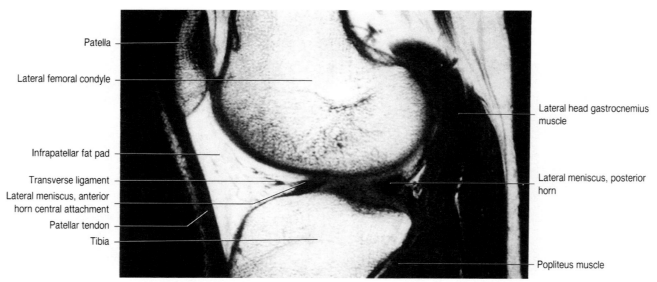

Patella

Lateral femoral condyle

Infrapatellar fat pad

Transverse ligament
Lateral meniscus, anterior horn central attachment
Patellar tendon

Tibia

Lateral head gastrocnemius muscle

Lateral meniscus, posterior horn

Popliteus muscle

FIGURE 7-12F.

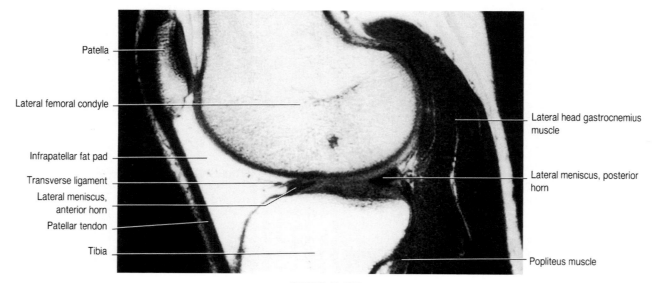

Patella

Lateral femoral condyle

Infrapatellar fat pad

Transverse ligament
Lateral meniscus, anterior horn
Patellar tendon

Tibia

Lateral head gastrocnemius muscle

Lateral meniscus, posterior horn

Popliteus muscle

FIGURE 7-12G.

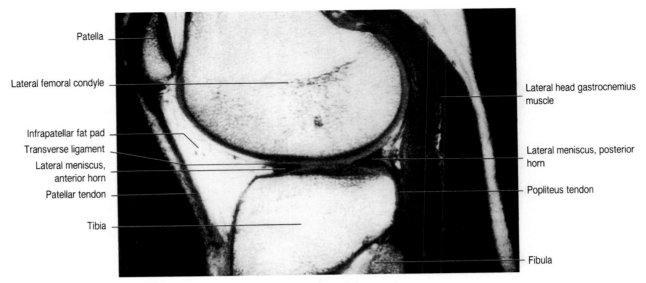

Patella

Lateral femoral condyle

Infrapatellar fat pad
Transverse ligament
Lateral meniscus,
anterior horn
Patellar tendon

Tibia

Lateral head gastrocnemius
muscle

Lateral meniscus, posterior
horn

Popliteus tendon

Fibula

FIGURE 7-12H.

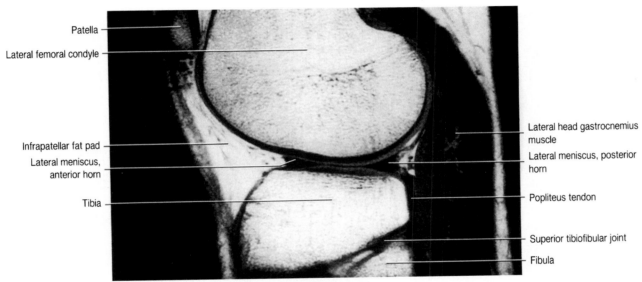

Patella

Lateral femoral condyle

Infrapatellar fat pad
Lateral meniscus,
anterior horn

Tibia

Lateral head gastrocnemius
muscle

Lateral meniscus, posterior
horn

Popliteus tendon

Superior tibiofibular joint

Fibula

FIGURE 7-12I.

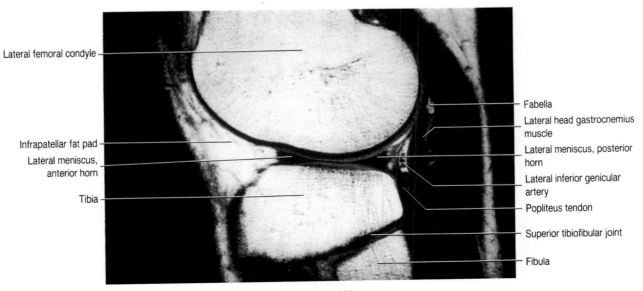

Lateral femoral condyle

Infrapatellar fat pad
Lateral meniscus,
anterior horn

Tibia

Fabella

Lateral head gastrocnemius
muscle

Lateral meniscus, posterior
horn

Lateral inferior genicular
artery

Popliteus tendon

Superior tibiofibular joint

Fibula

FIGURE 7-12J.

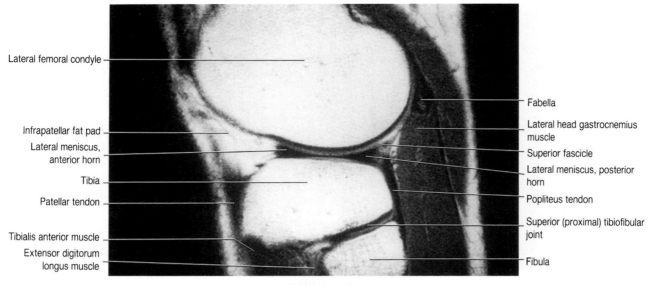

Lateral femoral condyle

Infrapatellar fat pad

Lateral meniscus, anterior horn

Tibia

Patellar tendon

Tibialis anterior muscle

Extensor digitorum longus muscle

Fabella

Lateral head gastrocnemius muscle

Superior fascicle

Lateral meniscus, posterior horn

Popliteus tendon

Superior (proximal) tibiofibular joint

Fibula

FIGURE 7-12K.

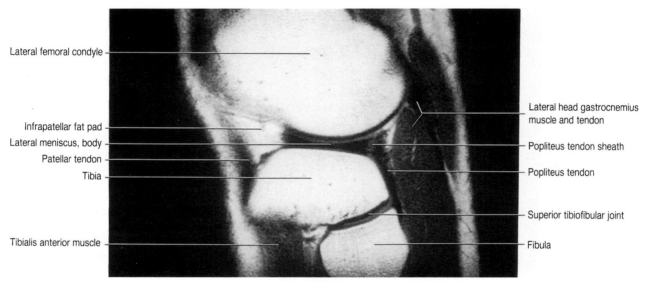

Lateral femoral condyle

Infrapatellar fat pad

Lateral meniscus, body

Patellar tendon

Tibia

Tibialis anterior muscle

Lateral head gastrocnemius muscle and tendon

Popliteus tendon sheath

Popliteus tendon

Superior tibiofibular joint

Fibula

FIGURE 7-12L.

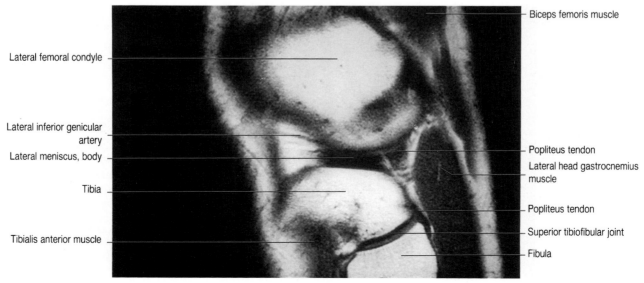

Lateral femoral condyle

Lateral inferior genicular artery

Lateral meniscus, body

Tibia

Tibialis anterior muscle

Biceps femoris muscle

Popliteus tendon

Lateral head gastrocnemius muscle

Popliteus tendon

Superior tibiofibular joint

Fibula

FIGURE 7-12M.

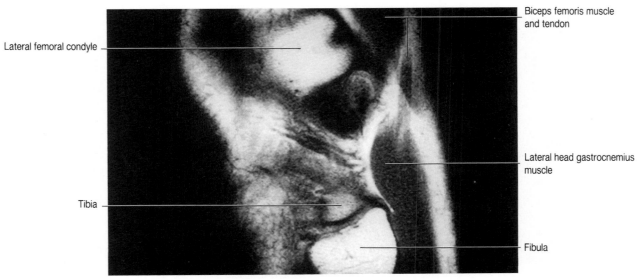

Biceps femoris muscle
and tendon

Lateral femoral condyle

Lateral head gastrocnemius
muscle

Tibia

Fibula

FIGURE 7-12N.

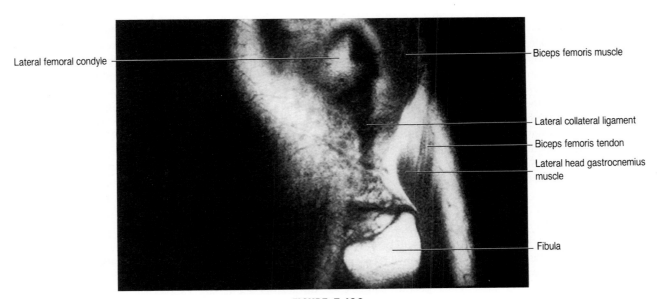

Lateral femoral condyle

Biceps femoris muscle

Lateral collateral ligament

Biceps femoris tendon

Lateral head gastrocnemius
muscle

Fibula

FIGURE 7-12O.

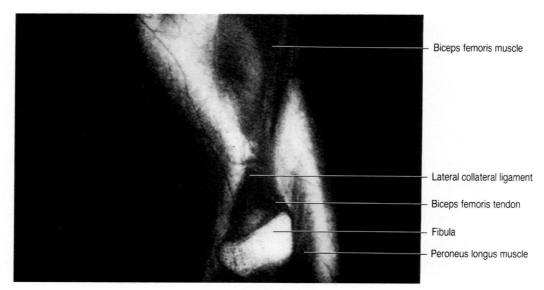

Biceps femoris muscle

Lateral collateral ligament

Biceps femoris tendon

Fibula

Peroneus longus muscle

FIGURE 7-12P.

On midsagittal sections, the quadriceps and patellar tendons, which demonstrate low signal intensity, are seen at their anterior attachments to the superior and inferior patellar poles, respectively. Hoffa's infrapatellar fat pad is directly posterior to the patellar tendon and demonstrates bright signal intensity. The posterior patellar articular cartilage displays a smooth or a convex arc on sections through the medial and lateral patellar facets. In the absence of joint fluid, the collapsed patellar bursa is not seen proximal to the superior pole of the patella.

On intercondylar sagittal images, the popliteal vessels are seen in long axis, with the artery in an anterior and the vein in a posterior position.

On extreme sagittal sections, the conjoined insertion of the LCL and the biceps femoris tendon on the fibular head can be identified. The lateral head of the gastrocnemius muscle is seen posterior to the fibula and follows an inferior course from the distal lateral femoral condyle behind the popliteus muscle. The low-signal-intensity popliteus tendon and its intermediate-signal-intensity sheath are seen in their expected anatomic location, between the capsule and the periphery of the lateral meniscus. Separate synovium-lined fascicles, or struts, of the menisci allow intraarticular passage of the popliteus tendon. In its middle third (ie, body), the C-shaped lateral meniscus also demonstrates a bow-tie shape. On more medial sections through the lateral compartment, the separate triangular shapes of the anterior and posterior horn, which are oriented toward each other and are nearly symmetric in size and shape, can be distinguished. The MCL is not routinely defined on 3- or 5-mm sagittal sections.

Coronal Images

Posterior-to-anterior coronal anatomic dissection demonstrates the posterior capsule (Fig. 7-13), the popliteus tendon (Fig. 7-14), the cruciate ligaments and menisci (Fig. 7-15),

the collateral ligaments (Figs. 7-16 and 7-17), and the extensor mechanism (see Fig. 7-17). Coronal plane images (Fig. 7-18) are most frequently used to identify collateral ligament anatomy. Images in this plane also display the posterior femoral condyles, which are common sites of articular erosions. The cruciate ligaments, although displayed to best advantage in the sagittal plane, can also be identified on coronal and axial images. The oblique popliteal ligament and arcuate popliteal ligament define the posterior capsule.

The low-signal-intensity popliteal vessels are also identified on posterior coronal images. The LCL (fibular collateral ligament) is seen as a low-signal-intensity cord stretching from its insertion on the fibular head to the lateral epicondyle of the femur. It is separated from the lateral meniscus by the thickness of the popliteus tendon.

At the level of the femoral condyles, the meniscofemoral ligaments (the ligaments of Wrisberg and Humphrey) may be observed as thin, low-signal-intensity bands extending from the posterior horn of the lateral meniscus to the lateral surface of the medial femoral condyle. The ligament of Humphrey is variable in size. Although one or the other of the branches of the meniscofemoral ligament may be identified on one third of knee studies, the coexistence of the two is seen in only 3% of examinations.[22]

The functional location of the AMB and PLB of the ACL may be discerned on anterior and posterior coronal images, respectively. The PCL is circular and of uniform low signal intensity on anterior and midcoronal sections. On posterior coronal images, the triangular attachment to the PCL can be differentiated as it fans out from the lateral aspect of the medial femoral condyle. The MCL, or tibial collateral ligament, is identified on midcoronal sections, anterior to sections in which the femoral condyles appear to fuse together with the distal metaphysis. The MCL is seen as a band of

text continues on page 251

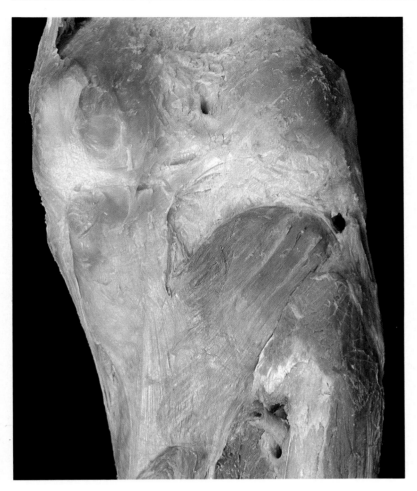

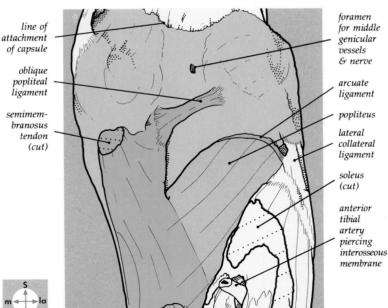

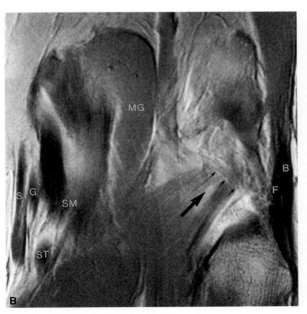

FIGURE 7-13. (**A**) Superficial dissection from the posterior aspect reveals the capsule, semimembranosus insertion, oblique popliteal ligament, popliteus tendon, and arcuate ligament. The oblique popliteal ligament is a tendinous expansion of the semimembranosus muscle. The arcuate ligament arches over the popliteus muscle. (**B**) Posterior coronal image identifying location of the arcuate ligament (*small arrow*) and popliteus muscle (*large arrow*). *B,* biceps femoris tendon; *F,* fibular collateral ligament; *MG,* medial head gastrocnemius muscle; *SM,* semimembranosus tendon; *ST,* semitendinosus tendon; *G,* gracilis tendon; and *S,* sartorius tendon.

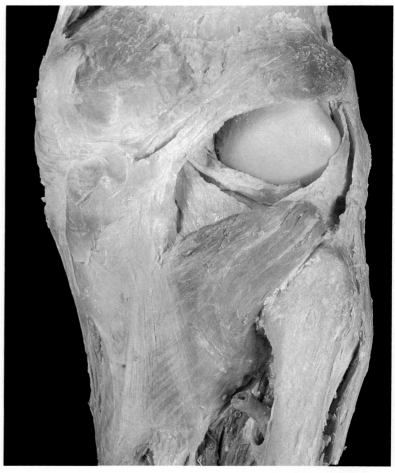

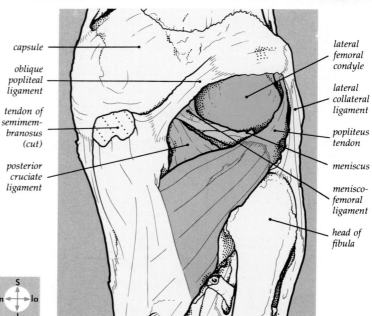

FIGURE 7-14. The posterior part of the capsule has been removed to reveal the meniscofemoral ligament, the PCL, and the popliteus tendon.

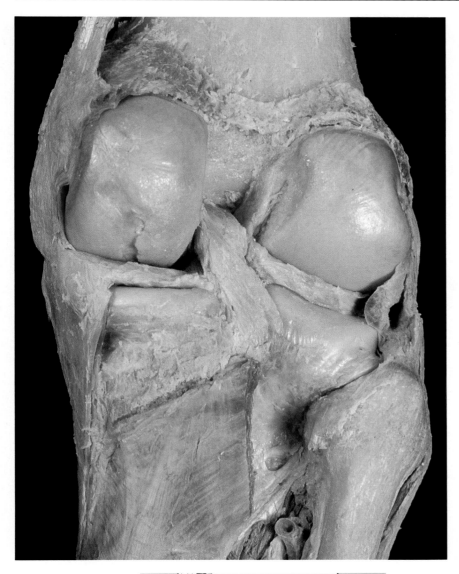

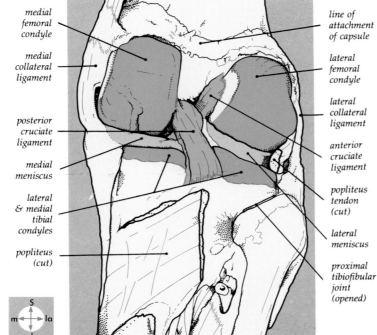

medial
femoral
condyle

medial
collateral
ligament

posterior
cruciate
ligament

medial
meniscus

lateral
& medial
tibial
condyles

popliteus
(cut)

line of
attachment
of capsule

lateral
femoral
condyle

lateral
collateral
ligament

anterior
cruciate
ligament

popliteus
tendon
(cut)

lateral
meniscus

proximal
tibiofibular
joint
(opened)

A

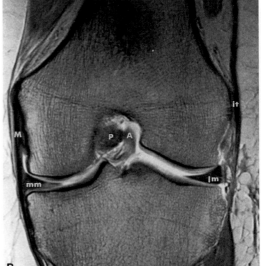

B

FIGURE 7-15. (**A**) The posterior part of the capsule has been removed to reveal the ACL and PCL and menisci. (**B**) A coronal image obtained more anteriorly in the plane of the MCL (*M*) and iliotibial tract (*it*). *P*, PCL; *A*, ACL; *mm*, medial meniscus; *lm*, lateral meniscus.

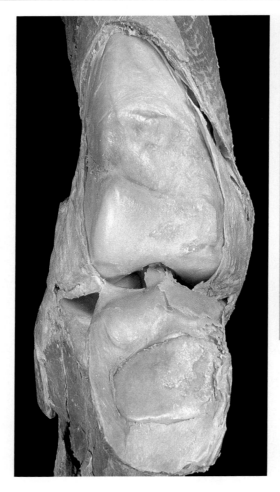

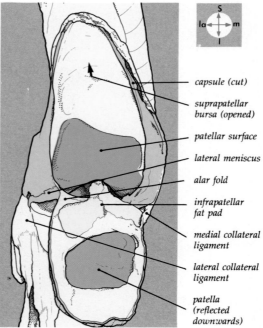

capsule (cut)

suprapatellar
bursa (opened)

patellar surface

lateral meniscus

alar fold

infrapatellar
fat pad

medial collateral
ligament

lateral collateral
ligament

patella
(reflected
downwards)

FIGURE 7-16. The interior of the joint and the suprapatellar pouch are exposed by opening the capsule anteriorly and reflecting the patella downward.

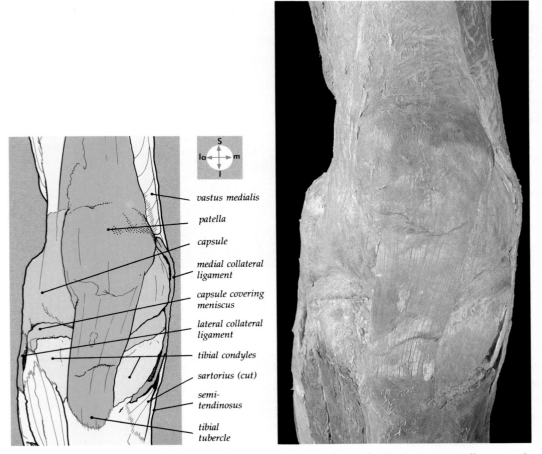

FIGURE 7-17. Superficial dissection from the anterior aspect shows the ligamentum patellae, capsule, and MCL and LCL.

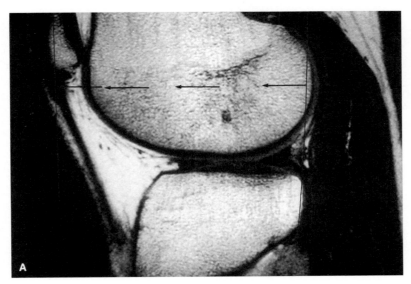

FIGURE 7-18. Normal coronal MR anatomy. (A) This T1-weighted sagittal localizer was used to identify image locations from posterior (B) to anterior (X).

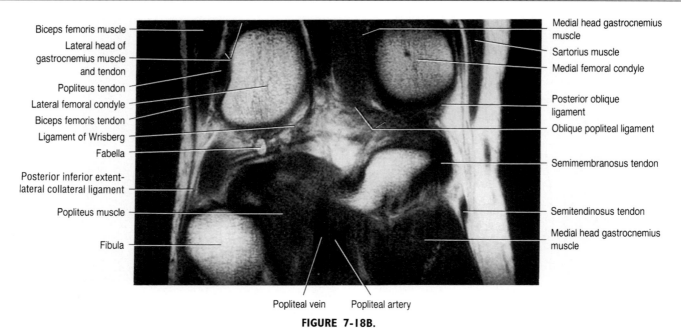

Biceps femoris muscle

Lateral head of gastrocnemius muscle and tendon

Popliteus tendon

Lateral femoral condyle

Biceps femoris tendon

Ligament of Wrisberg

Fabella

Posterior inferior extent-lateral collateral ligament

Popliteus muscle

Fibula

Medial head gastrocnemius muscle

Sartorius muscle

Medial femoral condyle

Posterior oblique ligament

Oblique popliteal ligament

Semimembranosus tendon

Semitendinosus tendon

Medial head gastrocnemius muscle

Popliteal vein   Popliteal artery

FIGURE 7-18B.

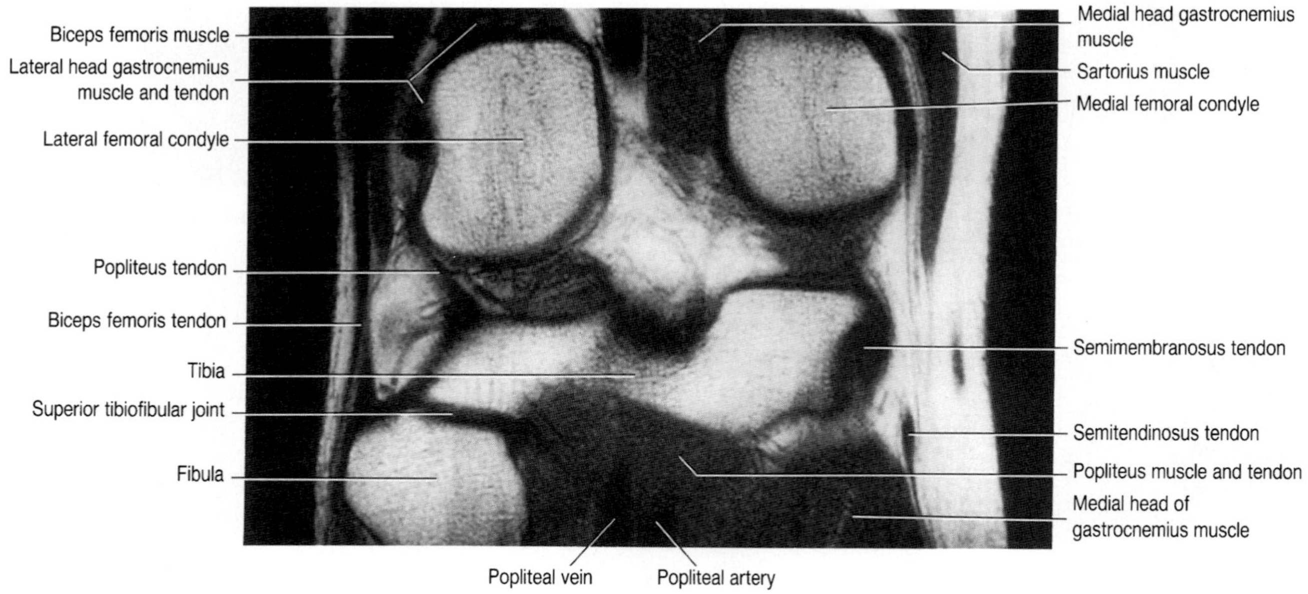

Biceps femoris muscle

Lateral head gastrocnemius muscle and tendon

Lateral femoral condyle

Popliteus tendon

Biceps femoris tendon

Tibia

Superior tibiofibular joint

Fibula

Medial head gastrocnemius muscle

Sartorius muscle

Medial femoral condyle

Semimembranosus tendon

Semitendinosus tendon

Popliteus muscle and tendon

Medial head of gastrocnemius muscle

Popliteal vein   Popliteal artery

FIGURE 7-18C.

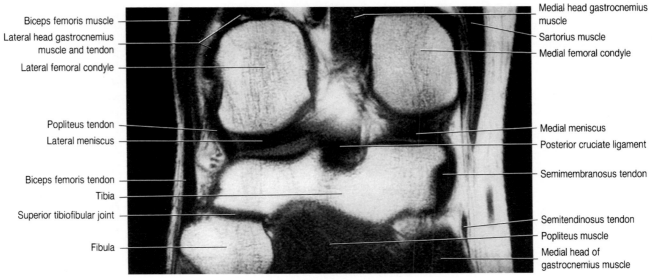

Biceps femoris muscle

Lateral head gastrocnemius muscle and tendon

Lateral femoral condyle

Popliteus tendon

Lateral meniscus

Biceps femoris tendon

Tibia

Superior tibiofibular joint

Fibula

Medial head gastrocnemius muscle

Sartorius muscle

Medial femoral condyle

Medial meniscus

Posterior cruciate ligament

Semimembranosus tendon

Semitendinosus tendon

Popliteus muscle

Medial head of gastrocnemius muscle

FIGURE 7-18D.

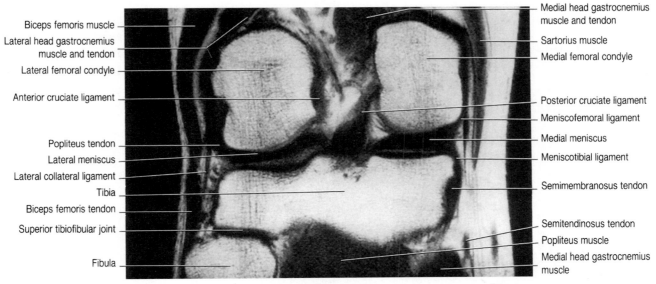

Biceps femoris muscle

Lateral head gastrocnemius muscle and tendon

Lateral femoral condyle

Anterior cruciate ligament

Popliteus tendon

Lateral meniscus

Lateral collateral ligament

Tibia

Biceps femoris tendon

Superior tibiofibular joint

Fibula

Medial head gastrocnemius muscle and tendon

Sartorius muscle

Medial femoral condyle

Posterior cruciate ligament

Meniscofemoral ligament

Medial meniscus

Meniscotibial ligament

Semimembranosus tendon

Semitendinosus tendon

Popliteus muscle

Medial head gastrocnemius muscle

FIGURE 7-18E.

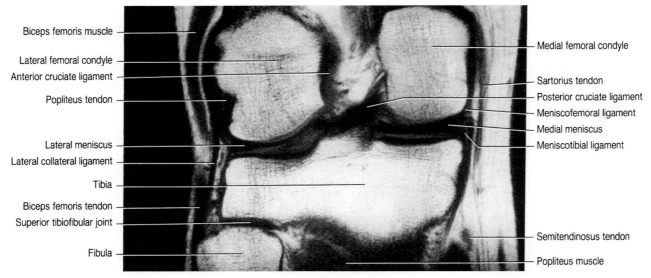

Biceps femoris muscle
Lateral femoral condyle
Anterior cruciate ligament
Popliteus tendon
Lateral meniscus
Lateral collateral ligament
Tibia
Biceps femoris tendon
Superior tibiofibular joint
Fibula

Medial femoral condyle
Sartorius tendon
Posterior cruciate ligament
Meniscofemoral ligament
Medial meniscus
Meniscotibial ligament
Semitendinosus tendon
Popliteus muscle

FIGURE 7-18F.

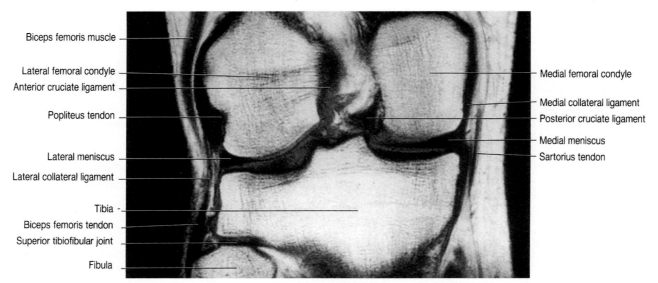

Biceps femoris muscle
Lateral femoral condyle
Anterior cruciate ligament
Popliteus tendon
Lateral meniscus
Lateral collateral ligament
Tibia
Biceps femoris tendon
Superior tibiofibular joint
Fibula

Medial femoral condyle
Medial collateral ligament
Posterior cruciate ligament
Medial meniscus
Sartorius tendon

FIGURE 7-18G.

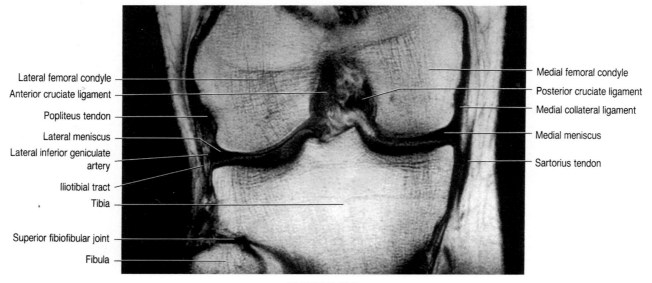

Lateral femoral condyle
Anterior cruciate ligament
Popliteus tendon
Lateral meniscus
Lateral inferior geniculate artery
Iliotibial tract
Tibia
Superior fibifibular joint
Fibula

Medial femoral condyle
Posterior cruciate ligament
Medial collateral ligament
Medial meniscus
Sartorius tendon

FIGURE 7-18H.

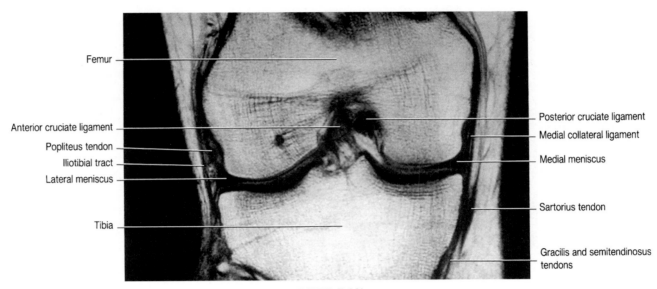

Femur

Anterior cruciate ligament
Popliteus tendon
Iliotibial tract
Lateral meniscus

Tibia

Posterior cruciate ligament
Medial collateral ligament

Medial meniscus

Sartorius tendon

Gracilis and semitendinosus
tendons

FIGURE 7-18I.

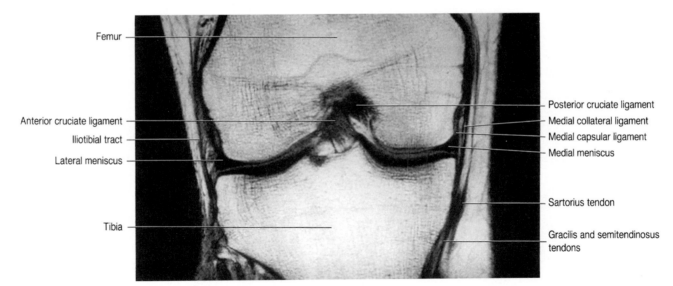

Femur

Anterior cruciate ligament
Iliotibial tract
Lateral meniscus

Tibia

Posterior cruciate ligament
Medial collateral ligament
Medial capsular ligament
Medial meniscus

Sartorius tendon

Gracilis and semitendinosus
tendons

FIGURE 7-18J.

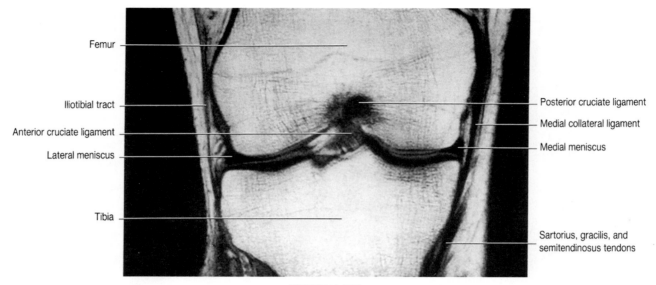

Femur

Iliotibial tract

Anterior cruciate ligament

Lateral meniscus

Tibia

Posterior cruciate ligament

Medial collateral ligament

Medial meniscus

Sartorius, gracilis, and semitendinosus tendons

FIGURE 7-18K.

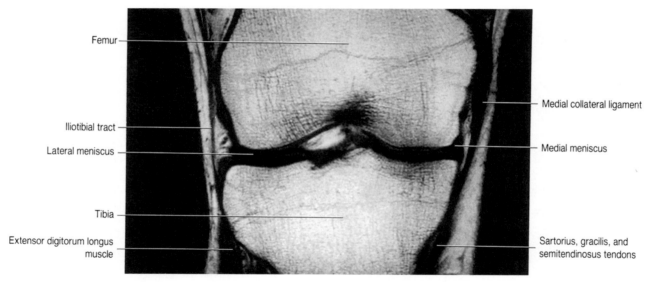

Femur

Iliotibial tract

Lateral meniscus

Tibia

Extensor digitorum longus muscle

Medial collateral ligament

Medial meniscus

Sartorius, gracilis, and semitendinosus tendons

FIGURE 7-18L.

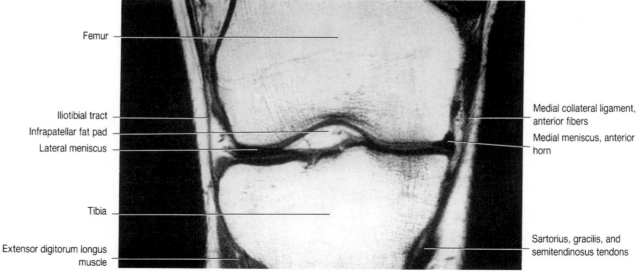

Femur

Iliotibial tract

Infrapatellar fat pad

Lateral meniscus

Tibia

Extensor digitorum longus muscle

Medial collateral ligament, anterior fibers

Medial meniscus, anterior horn

Sartorius, gracilis, and semitendinosus tendons

FIGURE 7-18M.

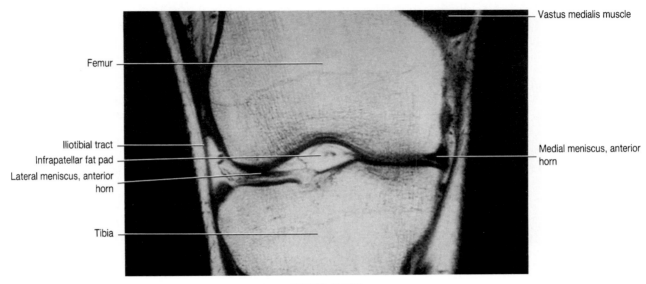

Vastus medialis muscle

Femur

Iliotibial tract

Infrapatellar fat pad

Lateral meniscus, anterior horn

Medial meniscus, anterior horn

Tibia

FIGURE 7-18N.

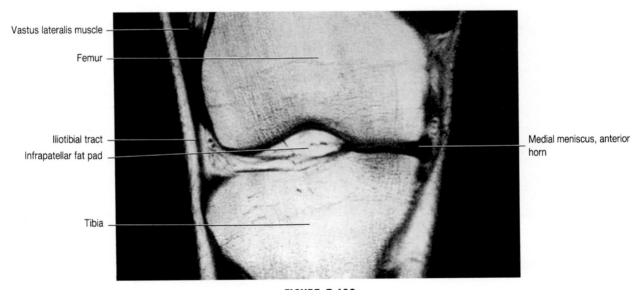

Vastus lateralis muscle

Femur

Iliotibial tract

Infrapatellar fat pad

Medial meniscus, anterior horn

Tibia

FIGURE 7-18O.

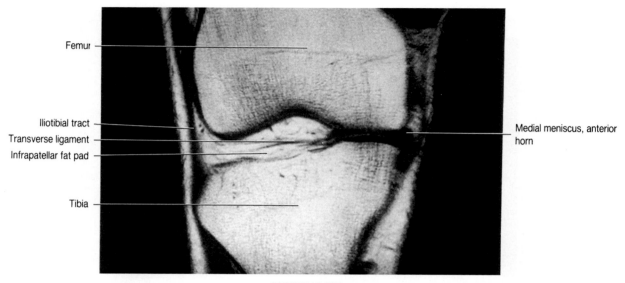

Femur

Iliotibial tract
Transverse ligament
Infrapatellar fat pad

Tibia

Medial meniscus, anterior
horn

FIGURE 7-18P.

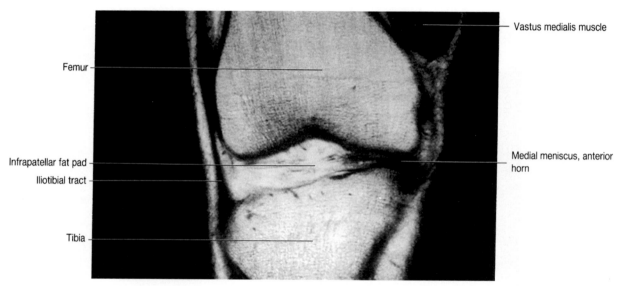

Vastus medialis muscle

Femur

Infrapatellar fat pad
Iliotibial tract

Tibia

Medial meniscus, anterior
horn

FIGURE 7-18Q.

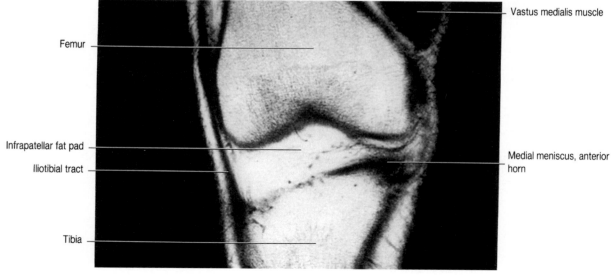

Vastus medialis muscle

Femur

Infrapatellar fat pad
Iliotibial tract

Tibia

Medial meniscus, anterior
horn

FIGURE 7-18R.

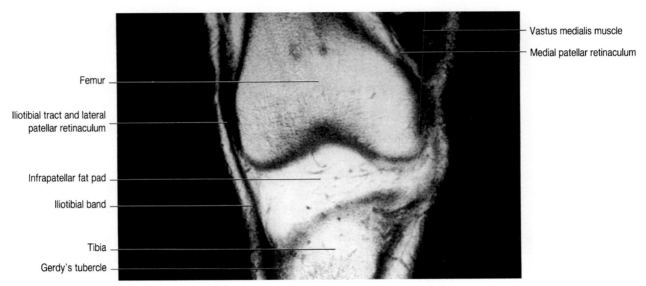

Vastus medialis muscle

Medial patellar retinaculum

Femur

Iliotibial tract and lateral patellar retinaculum

Infrapatellar fat pad

Iliotibial band

Tibia

Gerdy's tubercle

FIGURE 7-18S.

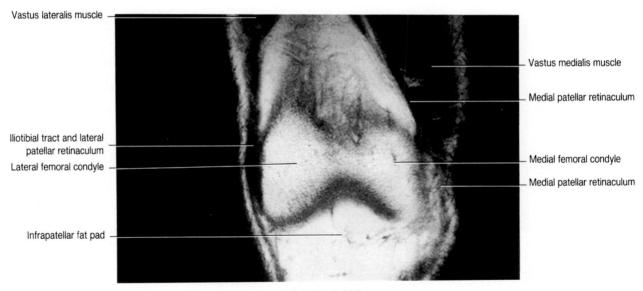

Vastus lateralis muscle

Vastus medialis muscle

Medial patellar retinaculum

Iliotibial tract and lateral patellar retinaculum

Lateral femoral condyle

Medial femoral condyle

Medial patellar retinaculum

Infrapatellar fat pad

FIGURE 7-18T.

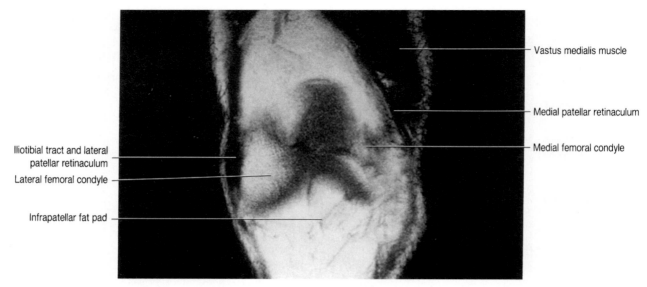

Vastus medialis muscle

Medial patellar retinaculum

Medial femoral condyle

Iliotibial tract and lateral patellar retinaculum

Lateral femoral condyle

Infrapatellar fat pad

FIGURE 7-18U.

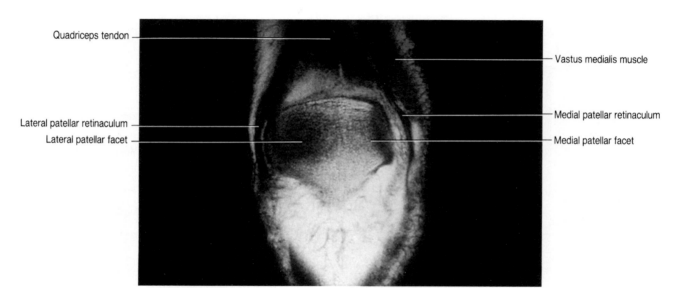

Quadriceps tendon

Vastus medialis muscle

Lateral patellar retinaculum

Lateral patellar facet

Medial patellar retinaculum

Medial patellar facet

FIGURE 7-18V.

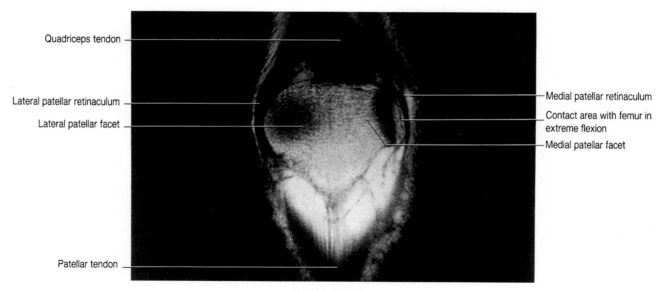

Quadriceps tendon

Lateral patellar retinaculum

Lateral patellar facet

Medial patellar retinaculum

Contact area with femur in extreme flexion

Medial patellar facet

Patellar tendon

FIGURE 7-18W.

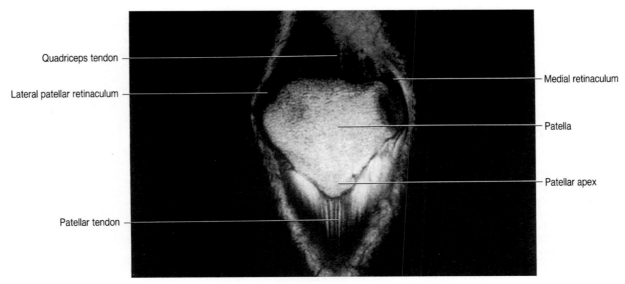

Quadriceps tendon

Lateral patellar retinaculum

Patellar tendon

Medial retinaculum

Patella

Patellar apex

FIGURE 7-18X.

low signal intensity extending from its femoral epicondylar attachment to the medial tibial condyle. It consists of superficial and deep layers attached to the periphery of the medial meniscus.

The femoral and tibial attachments of the uninjured or intact MCL are uniformly dark (low signal intensity) and are indistinguishable from underlying cortical bone. From the plane of the posterior femoral condyle, the MCL can be seen on at least two to three coronal images if they are acquired with 5-mm sections and no interslice gap. A line of intermediate signal intensity separating the medial meniscus from the deep layer of the MCL represents a small bursa. The body and the anterior and posterior horns of the medial and lateral meniscus are seen as distinct segments and not as opposing triangles as on sagittal images. On posterior coronal images, the plane of section is parallel with the posterior curve of the C-shaped menisci, and the posterior horn may be seen as a continuous band of low signal intensity.

Midcoronal sections display the anterior tibial spine, whereas anterior images are marked by the high signal intensity of Hoffa's infrapatellar fat pad anterior to the lateral knee compartment. Anteriorly, the iliotibial band blends with the lateral patellar retinaculum, and the vastus medialis is in continuity with its medial retinacular patellar attachment. The low-signal-intensity fibers of the quadriceps and patellar tendons can be identified on most anterior sections in the same plane as the patella.

THE MENISCUS

Imaging Protocols

T1- or intermediate-weighted (ie, proton-density weighted) images were at one time considered optimal for detecting meniscal lesions, which are sensitive to the T1 shortening of imbibed synovial fluid in tears and mucinous degenerations.[23,24] Short-TE images (T1-, intermediate-, or T2*-gradient weighted) are more sensitive than longer TE images (T2-weighted) in the detection of meniscal degenerations and tears.[25] Newer techniques such as gradient-echo T2*-weighted 2D FT or 3D FT images, however, are sensitive not only to grade 1 (focal) and 2 (linear) intrasubstance degenerations but also to meniscal tears.[26] However, T1, STIR or fat-suppressed T2-weighted fast spin-echo sequences are more sensitive than heavily T2*-weighted images to subchondral marrow edema in osseous contusions. The chronic subchondral sclerosis seen in degenerative arthrosis and chondromalacia also is better seen on T1- than T2*-weighted images. Bright-signal-intensity fat-marrow is also better displayed on T1-weighted images. The rate of false-positive results in the detection of meniscal pathology is lower with 3D FT gradient-echo sequences than with conventional 2D spin-echo sequences (TR of 2000 milliseconds and TE of 20, 80 milliseconds).[27] Although fast spin-echo images offer the advantage of faster data acquisition, they are less sensitive to meniscal pathology than conventional T2 spin-echo pulse sequences.[28] Even with shorter echo train lengths (≤ 4) to reduce image blurring, the sensitivity (65%) and specificity (96%) for meniscal pathology are decreased with fast spin-echo techniques. Rubin and colleagues[28] have postulated that the presence of a ghosting artifact (secondary to phase differences between even and odd echoes in the echo train) or loss of meniscal signal intensity in tears secondary to an increased magnetization transfer with the fast spin-echo sequence may be responsible for the lower sensitivity of this sequence. Long TE fast spin-echo sequences, however, may be used to partially reduce blurring and loss of meniscal signal intensity. Although useful for the evaluation of the morphology of the meniscus (especially in complex tears, postoperative partial meniscectomies, and pri-

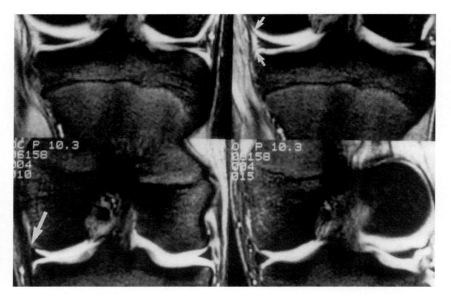

FIGURE 7-19. These T2*-weighted radial images progress from the posterior (*top left*) to the anterior (*bottom right*) horn of the medial meniscus. Normal meniscofemoral and meniscotibial attachments (*small arrows*) of the deep medial capsular layer (ie, ligament) are present. The closely applied meniscal attachment to the capsule and the MCL are shown (*large arrow*).

mary repairs), fast spin-echo images are not recommended for the primary diagnosis of meniscal degenerations or tears.

There are three approaches to sagittal protocols for evaluation of the meniscus. In one technique, the first echo of a conventional T2-weighted pulse sequence is used to produce intermediate contrast images for the identification of meniscal lesions. The second echo is used to identify soft tissue and osseous pathology. Another approach is the use of a T1-weighted protocol to identify meniscal degenerations and tears (displayed as areas of intermediate to increased signal intensity). The third approach is the use of either 2D or 3D FT T2* images to demonstrate increased signal intensities in grades 1 and 2 and grade 3 meniscal signal intensities. T2*-weighted images offer several advantages: they reduce scanning time; they provide thin, contiguous slices; and they allow 3D reformatting from 3D FT sequences.[12] Radial images acquired with gradient-echo contrast show the meniscus perpendicular to the orthogonal sagittal plane and can be used to evaluate peripheral meniscal tears and equivocal grade 2 or 3 signal intensities. This technique is also sensitive in identifying the meniscocapsular junction (Fig. 7-19). Radial MR images are as accurate as conventional T2 sagittal spin-echo images.[29]

The interpretative sensitivity and specificity for the meniscus are increased when both radial MR and sagittal spin-echo are used as complementary sequences. Simultaneous acquisition of radial and coronal or sagittal images is possible with multisection gradient-echo contrast. Reformatted 3D FT gradient-echo images can also be used to generate radial planes of section. In addition, intravenous gadolinium is useful for the identification of the postoperative meniscus interface of meniscal implants functioning as artificial menisci. Intraarticular gadolinium is also proving useful in differentiating healing from repeated injury after primary meniscal repair or partial meniscectomy.[30] Steady-state free procession images (ie, with TR shorter than T2) display heavily weighted T2 contrast. Although it may not be possible to detect

grades 1 and 2 degenerations on these scans, they are sensitive to small amounts of fluid in meniscal tears or cysts.

Normal Anatomy and MR Imaging of the Meniscus

The C-shaped fibrocartilaginous menisci or semilunar cartilages are attached to the condylar surface of the tibia and provide added mechanical stability to femorotibial gliding (Figs. 7-20 and 7-21). The meniscus protects the joint articular cartilage (by acting as a buffer between femoral and tibial surfaces with loading) and provides joint lubrication and increases joint stability (by providing congruity between femoral and tibial articular surfaces). This congruity is assisted by deepening of the articular surfaces of the tibial plateaus to accommodate the articulation between the femoral condyles.[31] The proximal or superior meniscal surface is smooth and concave, producing greater contact with the femoral condyles. The inferior meniscal surface is flat and rests on the opposing surface of the tibia.[31] The periphery of the menisci are convex and thick and attach to the inside of the joint capsule. Facing the intercondylar notch, the meniscus tapers to a thin, free edge. Tibial attachments to the meniscus are made through the meniscofemoral, meniscotibial, or coronary ligaments of the joint capsule. Except for the peripheral 10% to 25% of the meniscus, which is supplied by the perimeniscal capillary plexus, the meniscus in adults is relatively avascular.[32,33] In children's knees, the vascularity of the meniscus is already restricted to the peripheral third, whereas the inner two thirds of the meniscus are relatively avascular.[34]

Intact menisci demonstrate uniform low signal intensity on T1-, T2- (by conventional and fast spin-echo techniques),

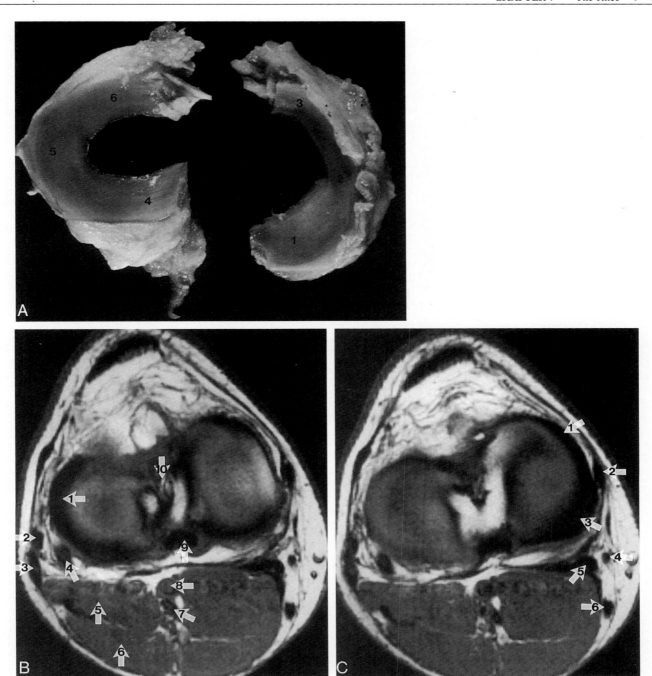

FIGURE 7-20. Axial anatomy of the menisci. (**A**) Gross anatomy of the lateral meniscus (*left*) and medial meniscus (*right*). The larger posterior horn of the medial meniscus is evident. *1*, posterior horn of medial meniscus; *2*, body of meniscus; *3*, anterior horn of medial meniscus; *4*, posterior horn of lateral meniscus; *5*, body of lateral meniscus; *6*, anterior horn of lateral meniscus. (**B**) An axial image made in the plane of the lateral meniscus. *1*, lateral meniscus; *2*, fibular collateral ligament; *3*, biceps femoris tendon; *4*, popliteus tendon; *5*, plantaris muscle; *6*, lateral head of gastrocnemius muscle; *7*, popliteal vein; *8*, popliteal artery; *9*, PCL; *10*, ACL. (**C**) An axial image made in the plane of the medial meniscus. *1*, anterior horn of medial meniscus; *2*, medial tibial collateral ligament; *3*, posterior horn of medial meniscus; *4*, gracilis tendon; *5*, semimembranosus tendon; *6*, semitendinosus tendon.

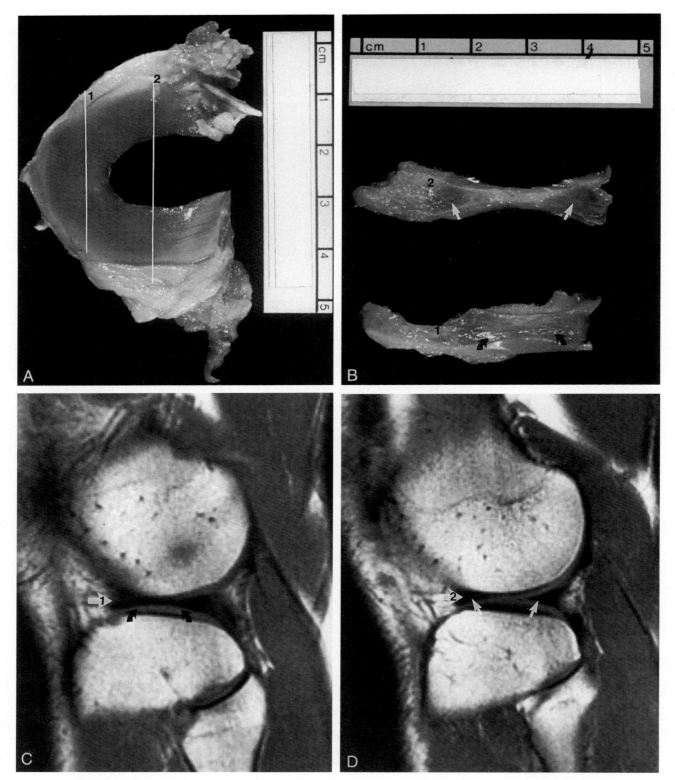

FIGURE 7-21. Normal anatomy of the meniscus. (**A**) Gross specimen of the lateral meniscus. *Line 1,* the sagittal plane of section through the body of the lateral meniscus; *line 2,* the sagittal plane of section through the anterior and body of the lateral meniscus. (**B**) The corresponding gross sagittal sections (*1* and *2*) are seen through the body (*curved black arrows*) and anterior and posterior horns (*straight white arrows*) of the lateral meniscus. The periphery or body of the meniscus has a continuous bow-tie appearance. The anterior and posterior horns are oriented as opposing triangles of fibrocartilage. (**C** and **D**) The corresponding sagittal plane images (*1* and *2*) demonstrate the low signal intensity body (*curved black arrows*) and anterior and posterior horns (*straight white arrows*) of the lateral meniscus.

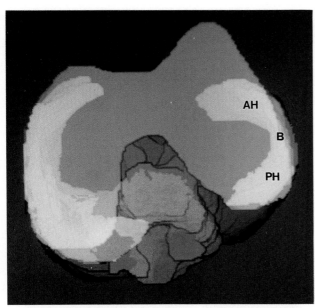

FIGURE 7-22. This 3D MR rendering demonstrates the division of the lateral meniscus into the anterior horn (*AH*), body (*B*), and posterior horn (*PH*). *Salmon-colored area*, a posterior tibial fracture, seen from a superior view.

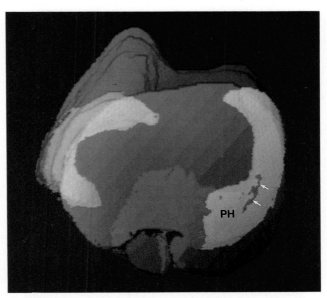

FIGURE 7-23. Normal morphology of the posterior horn (*PH*) of the medial meniscus. A longitudinal tear pattern (*arrows*) is shown. A posterior tibial fracture fragment can be seen from below when looking toward the femur from inferior to superior.

and T2*-weighted images. They are triangular in cross section, with an outer convex curve. The apex is directed toward the intercondylar notch. The meniscus is arbitrarily divided into thirds: the anterior horn, the body, and the posterior horn (Fig. 7-22). Peripherally, the meniscus has a bow-tie appearance. On sagittal sections close to the intercondylar notch, the meniscus is visualized with opposing triangular shapes representing the anterior and posterior horns.

Functions of the menisci include:[35]

- Transmission of axial and torsional forces across the joint
- Cushioning of mechanical loading
- Limitation of comprehensive displacement
- Distribution of synovial fluid
- Increasing of the surface area for femoral condylar motion
- Prevention of synovial impingement.

The stabilizing effect and vascularization of the peripheral third of the meniscus is the basis for attempts to preserve this tissue in partial meniscectomies. However, its preservation may not protect the joint from degenerative changes.[32,36]

Medial Meniscus

The semicircular medial meniscus has a wide posterior horn, narrows anteriorly, and has a more open C-shaped configuration than the more circular lateral meniscus (Fig. 7-23). Anterior to the tibial attachment of the ACL, the anterior horn of the medial meniscus is attached to the area of the intercondylar fossa of the tibia.[31] The posterior fibers of the anterior horn attachment of the medial meniscus attach to

the transverse ligament. The transverse ligament of the knee connects the anterior horns of the medial and lateral meniscus. The attachment of the posterior horn of the medial meniscus is located at the posterior intercondylar fossa of the tibia.[31,37,38] It can be identified between the attachment of the posterior horn of the lateral meniscus and the PCL. The medial meniscus is attached to the joint capsule along its entire peripheral circumference. The less mobile medial meniscus attachment to the deep layer of the MCL and capsule render the medial meniscus more susceptible to injury. A small intermediate-signal-intensity bursa separates the posterior horn of the medial meniscus from the joint capsule.

Lateral Meniscus

The lateral meniscus forms a tight C shape (more circular than the medial meniscus) and is relatively symmetric in width from anterior to posterior. It accommodates the popliteus tendon posteriorly (Fig. 7-24), is separated from the lateral collateral (ie, extracapsular) ligament, and has posterior horn attachments to the PCL and medial femoral condyle through the ligament of Wrisberg (posterior to the PCL) and ligament of Humphrey (anterior to the PCL). The ligaments of Wrisberg and Humphrey represent branches of the meniscofemoral ligament attaching the posterior horn of the lateral meniscus to the lateral aspect of the medial femoral condyle. The lateral meniscus is relatively mobile and covers two thirds of the tibial articular surface.[7] The anterior horn of the lateral meniscus is attached between the tibial intercondylar eminence and the anterior attachment of the ACL.[31,37,38] The

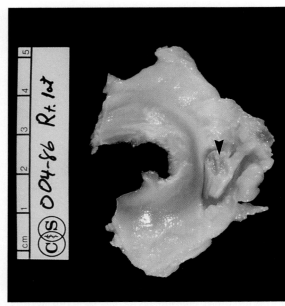

FIGURE 7-24. Gross anatomy of the lateral meniscus and associated popliteus tendon (*arrowhead*).

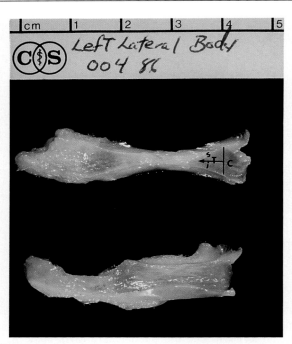

FIGURE 7-25. The circumferential (*C*) and transverse (*T*) zones of the meniscus. The middle perforating collagen bundle (*arrow*) divides the transverse zone into superior (*s*) and inferior (*i*) leaves.

posterior horn of the lateral meniscus is attached between the tibial intercondylar eminence and the posterior medial meniscus. Except for the passage of the popliteus tendon, the lateral meniscus has a loose peripheral attachment to the joint capsule. There is no direct attachment of the lateral meniscus to the fibular collateral ligament, or LCL. The popliteus recess allows passage to the popliteus tendon through a 1-cm hiatus in the posterolateral attachment of the lateral meniscus. The superior fascicle is seen medial to the inferior fascicle as the popliteus tendon penetrates the meniscocapsular junction. The function of the popliteal tendon attachments to the lateral meniscus is to pull the lateral meniscus posterior when the knee is flexed.[39] Whereas the popliteus tendon can effectively rotate the tibia with the knee in extension, this unlocking of the knee from full extension is the reverse of the screw-home mechanism of the knee. The screw-home mechanism functions to lock the knee in extension with internal rotation of the femur relative to the tibia.[40,41]

Microstructure of the Meniscus

The microstructure of the fibrocartilaginous meniscus is organized so that the collagen bundles form two distinct zones, the circumferential and the transverse (Fig. 7-25).[42] The circumferential fibers or bundles are bound in the peripheral third of the meniscus. The transverse collagen fibers bridge the circumferential zone of the meniscus peripherally to the free edge of the meniscus. Radial fibers within the meniscus contribute to structural rigidity and provide resistance to longitudinal splitting of the meniscus.[31] On cross section,

the transverse zone of the meniscus is divided into superior and inferior leaves by the middle perforating collagen bundle (Fig. 7-26). Middle perforating collagen fibers normally cannot be distinguished from adjacent meniscal tissue on MR images. Secondary vertical collagen fibers, which function as secondary stabilizers, may be present within the transverse

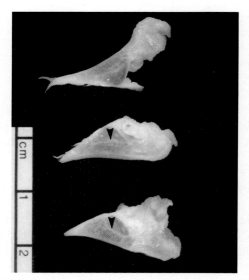

FIGURE 7-26. Gross meniscal sections identify the location of the middle perforating collagen bundle and the site of preferential horizontal mucinous degeneration (*arrowheads*).

zone. The middle perforating bundle may demarcate the sheer plane of the meniscus. In internal degenerations, the middle perforating collagen bundle corresponds to the location of the predominantly horizontal signal intensity seen in grade 2 menisci. The meniscocapsular junction is peripheral to the circumferential zone. The function of the circumferential collagen fibers is to resist longitudinal loading (ie, hoop stresses).[43]

Vascular Supply of the Meniscus

The perimeniscal capillary plexus originates from branches of the lateral and medial geniculate arteries and supplies the periphery of the meniscus throughout its attachment to the joint capsule.[31] It penetrates the peripheral border of the meniscus with a circumferential network and radial branches oriented toward the center of the joint. In the adult meniscus, vascular penetrations may extend to 30% of the width of the meniscus.

Meniscal Degenerations and Tears

Pathogenesis and Clinical Presentation

The meniscal cartilages support 50% of the load transmission in the medial compartment and more than 50% in the lateral compartment.[44] The menisci are thus clearly important in joint stabilization and in reduction of compressive forces acting on the articular cartilage. Conservation of meniscal tissue does minimize the development of degenerative joint changes.[45]

The rotation of the femur against a fixed tibia during flexion and extension places the menisci at risk for injury.[46] Tears involving the medial meniscus usually start on the inferior surface of the posterior horn. The lateral meniscus is more prone to transverse or oblique tears. Related hemorrhage and tearing of the peripheral meniscal attachments may contribute to the pain perceived in meniscal tears. Meniscal injury may be associated with a history of twisting, squatting, or cutting.[47] Abnormal shear forces may be generated during compression and rotation at the knee, leading to meniscal damage. Clinical signs of meniscal pathology include joint pain (at the joint line), giving way, clicking, and effusions.[44] Locking of the joint in fixed flexion may occur immediately after displacement of a meniscal fragment or pseudolock secondary to hamstring muscle spasms.[47] The differential diagnosis of a meniscal tear includes osseous bone contusions (occult bony injuries), plica syndromes, popliteal tendinitis, osteochondritis and chondral lesions, loose bodies, patellofemoral pain and instability, fat-pad impingement syndrome, inflammatory arthritis, physeal or tibial spine fractures, meniscotibial ligament sprain, synovial lesions or tumors, and discoid menisci.[47]

Sequelae of complete meniscectomy include degenerative joint disease as well as increased instability, especially in the ACL-deficient knee.[36,43,48,49] These changes are less likely to occur with partial meniscectomy and are minimized with primary meniscal repair.

MR of Meniscal Degenerations and Tears

The normal meniscus demonstrates homogeneous low signal intensity on T1-, T2- (conventional and fast spin-echo), gradient-echo, and STIR-weighted images. The low signal intensity of the intact meniscus is attributed to the lack of mobile protons (water molecules within the meniscus are closely related to or absorbed within larger collagen macromolecules).[25] Subsequent dephasing of hydrogen nuclei results in shortening of T2 times, contributing to the low signal intensity of meniscal tissue on all pulse sequences. Degenerations and tears of the meniscus demonstrate increased signal intensity, attributed to imbibed synovial fluid.[23] As synovial fluid diffuses through the meniscus, areas of degeneration and tears trap water molecules onto surface boundary layers, increasing the local spin density. This interaction of synovial fluid with large macromolecules in the meniscus slows the rotational rates of protons and shortens T1 and T2 values.[23] This phenomenon explains the sensitivity of T1-weighted and intermediate weighted (ie, proton-density weighted images) in revealing meniscal degenerations and tears. Degenerative changes and tears also result in local increases in the degree of freedom of trapped water molecules, resulting in increased T2 times and allowing detection of increased signal intensity on short TE sequences.[25] Therefore, the increased intrameniscal signal intensity seen in degeneration and tears is best visualized on short TE images using T1, intermediate weighted, or gradient-echo sequences. Increased signal intensity in synovial fluid gaps has been confirmed in surgically induced tears in animal models.[50] In the absence of a joint effusion, meniscal degenerations and tears may actually decrease in signal intensity on T2-weighted images. On T2*-weighted gradient-echo images, however, intrasubstance degeneration and tears generate increased signal intensities.[24] Therefore, gradient-echo sequences are extremely sensitive to the spectrum of meniscal degenerations and tears. The fast spin-echo sequence is not as useful in the diagnosis of intrasubstance meniscal signal intensity and tears, even when performed with echo train lengths (number of echoes per TR) of 4 or less.[28] Fast spin-echo images may underestimate the extent or grades of MR signal intensity and thus mask the presence of a tear (Fig. 7-27). Rubin and colleagues[28] have attributed this blurring, which limits the usefulness of fast spin-echo images, to a ghosting artifact or an increase in magnetization transfer. Blurring is more pronounced with the use of a shorter effective TE, a larger echo train length, and a smaller acquisition matrix. Short effective TE-related blurring occurs secondary

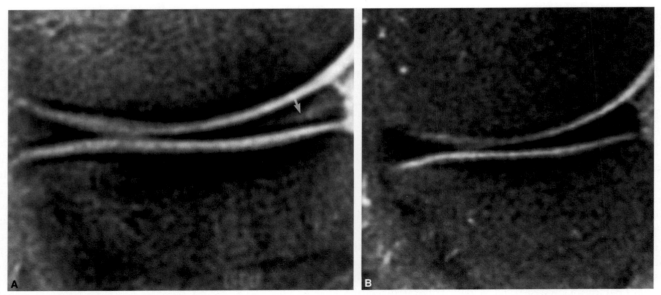

FIGURE 7-27. Grade 2 signal intensity (*arrow*) seen in the posterior horn of the medial meniscus on T2*-weighted image (**A**) is not apparent on corresponding fat-suppressed T2-weighted fast spin-echo image (**B**).

to attenuation by T2 decay of later echoes (high spatial-frequency data) at the edges of K-space.

To understand the significance of increased signal intensity in meniscal abnormalities, an MR grading system has been developed and correlated with a pathologic (ie, histologic) model (Fig. 7-28).[23] Areas of degeneration demonstrate increased signal intensity in a spectrum of patterns or grades that are based on the signal distribution (morphology) relative to an articular meniscal surface or meniscal apex, exclusive of the peripheral capsular margin of the meniscus, which is considered nonarticular. The articular meniscal surfaces refer to the superior and inferior aspects of the meniscus opposite the distal femoral and proximal tibial articular cartilage surfaces, respectively.

In MR grade 1, a nonarticular focal or globular intrasubstance increased signal intensity is seen (Fig. 7-29). Histologically, grade 1 signal intensity correlates with foci of early mucinous degeneration and chondrocyte-deficient or

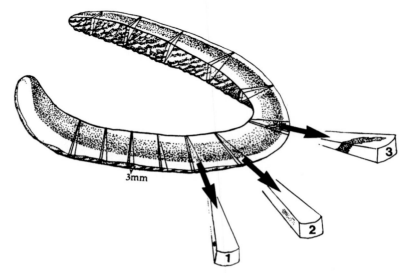

FIGURE 7-28. Representative signal intensity grades of meniscal degeneration (grades 1 and 2) and tear (grade 3) are shown in relation to the gross meniscus.

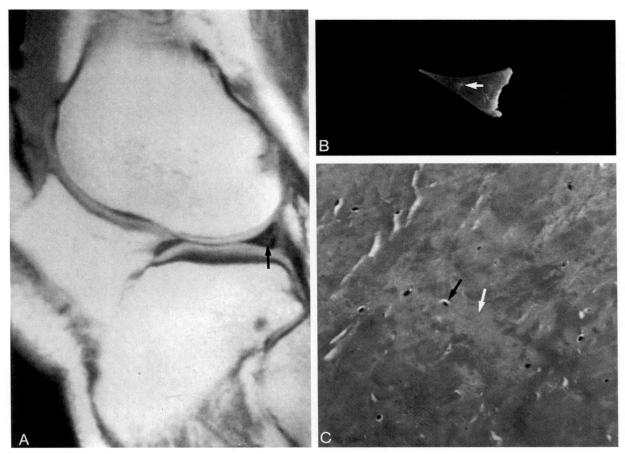

FIGURE 7-29. (A) A T1-weighted sagittal image shows grade 1 signal intensity (*arrow*) in the posterior horn of the lateral meniscus. (B) On a cut gross section, a focus of meniscal degeneration (*arrow*) can be seen. (C) The corresponding photomicrograph shows hypocellularity, with decreased numbers of chondrocytes (*black arrow*) in pale-staining areas (*white arrow*). (Hematoxylin and eosin stain.)

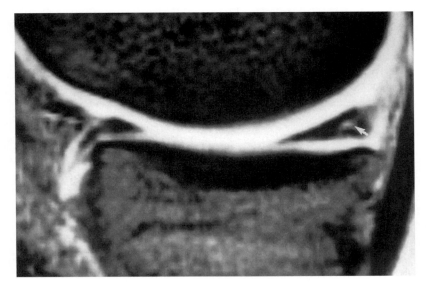

FIGURE 7-30. A T2*-weighted sagittal image shows grade 1 signal intensity (*arrow*) in the posterior horn of the medial meniscus in an athlete without medial compartment pain.

hypocellular regions that are pale staining on hematoxylin and eosin preparations. The terms "mucinous," "myxoid," and "hyaline" degeneration can be used interchangeably to describe the accumulation of increased production of mucopolysaccharide ground substance in stressed or strained areas of the meniscal fibrocartilage.[51,52] These changes usually occur in response to mechanical loading and degeneration. Grade 1 signal intensity may be observed in asymptomatic athletes and normal volunteers and is not clinically significant (Fig. 7-30).

In MR grade 2, a horizontal, linear intrasubstance increased signal intensity usually extends from the capsular periphery of the meniscus but does not involve an articular meniscal surface (Fig. 7-31). Areas and bands of mucinous degeneration are more extensive in MR grade 2 than in MR grade 1 (Fig. 7-32). Although no distinct cleavage plane or tear is observed in grade 2 menisci, microscopic clefting and collagen fragmentation may be seen in hypercellular regions of the fibrocartilaginous matrix. The middle perforating collagen bundle, a structure not ordinarily seen on MR images, sends out fibers that horizontally divide the meniscus into superior and inferior leaves.[53] The low–spin-density meniscus and middle perforating collagen fibers cannot be differentiated in the normal knee, because they both demonstrate low signal intensity. The middle perforating collagen bundle creates a neutral or buffer plane for the superior femoral and inferior tibial frictional forces and is a site for preferential accumulation of mucinous ground substance that displays grade 2 signal intensity (Fig. 7-33). It also represents the shear plane of the meniscus and is the site of horizontal degenerative tears of the meniscus. Grade 2 signal intensity in menisci is a continuation of progressive degeneration from grade 1 and is not a discrete isolated histologic occurrence.

Patients with images of grade 2 signal intensity are usually asymptomatic. Although the posterior horn of the medial meniscus is the most common location of grade 2 signal intensity, the finding of grade 2 signal intensity cannot be used as a prognostic indicator for temporal development of grade 3 signal intensity.[54] The presence of mucinous degeneration is, however, thought to represent potential structural weakening within collagen fibers, and when grade 3 signal intensity tears do develop, they are adjacent to or in continuity with areas of grade 2 meniscal degenerations. This finding is consistent with the posterior horn of the medial meniscus as the most common location for the occurrence of a meniscal tear. Although it is has been suggested that grade 2 meniscal signal intensity is a risk factor for the development of symptomatic meniscal tears, this possibility may be difficult to quantify.[25,54–59] In a 3-year follow-up study evaluating grade 2 meniscal abnormalities in the stable knee, no progression was identified.[60]

Postexercise studies have shown increased signal intensity in meniscal degenerations without alterations in morphology or grade of signal intensity.[61] In a separate prospective study of asymptomatic football players over a 1-year period, the progression of grades of meniscal degenerations were recorded.[59] Again, these preliminary findings cannot be used to predict the temporal occurrence of meniscal tears from preexisting areas of intrasubstance degenerations. The increased prevalence (24.1%) of grade 2 signal intensity in the posterior horn of the medial meniscus (as determined in a study sample of 54 asymptomatic patients with an average age of 28.5 years) is consistent with the increased frequency of grade 2 findings in this location found in cadaver menisci.[23,62] Grade 2 signal intensity and discoid menisci may represent cystic areas or cavities of mucinous degeneration, which can be symptomatic and may require treatment with partial meniscectomy. With the exception of discoid menisci, as mentioned, it is not common practice to surgically treat menisci with grade 2 intrasubstance signal intensity even in a symptomatic patient.

In the immature meniscus, vascular ingrowth that has been primarily reabsorbed cannot fully explain the finding of grade 2 signal intensity in young children without associated fibrocartilaginous degeneration.[34] In the adult, however, the finding of increased signal intensity distinctly correlates with areas of mucinous degeneration.

A meniscus is considered MR grade 3 when the area of increased signal intensity communicates or extends to at least one articular surface (Fig. 7-34). A meniscus may contain multiple areas of grade 3 signal intensity or the entire meniscal segment (horn) may be involved, with irregular morphology. Fibrocartilaginous separation or tears can be found in all menisci with grade 3 signal intensity. In less than 5%, these disruptions represent what has been referred to in the orthopaedic literature as confined intrasubstance cleavage tears (Fig. 7-35).[63] Diagnosis of these closed meniscal tears requires surgical probing during arthroscopy and might be missed altogether on a routine arthroscopic examination if surface extension is not identified. These lesions may also partially explain some of the false-positive interpretations of grade 3 signal intensity when correlated with arthroscopy. Because the meniscus is an innervated structure, intrasubstance tears may present with pain in these rheologically abnormal menisci.[25] In addition, false-negative correlations with arthroscopy may be related to spurious interpretation of areas of fraying or fibrillation as meniscal tears. Even without joint locking, the resultant edema and inflammation created by confined horizontal cleavage tears may be responsible for the clinical presentation of acute knee pain. Meniscal tears frequently occur adjacent to areas of intrasubstance degeneration (Fig. 7-36).

In addition to observing increased signal intensity within tears, the morphology (ie, size and shape) of the meniscus should be assessed when evaluating meniscal lesions (Figs. 7-37 and 7-38). The normal meniscus measures 3 to 5 mm in height. The medial meniscus varies in width from 6 mm at the anterior horn to 12 mm at the posterior horn. The lateral meniscus is approximately 10 mm in width throughout its length.[64]

Regenerative chondrocytes and synovial development represent attempts at meniscus healing along the tear–meniscus interface (Fig. 7-39). In fact, arthroscopic rasping is performed to induce a neovascular response by abrading synovium and creating a blood supply. Synovial ingrowth in degenerative tears is

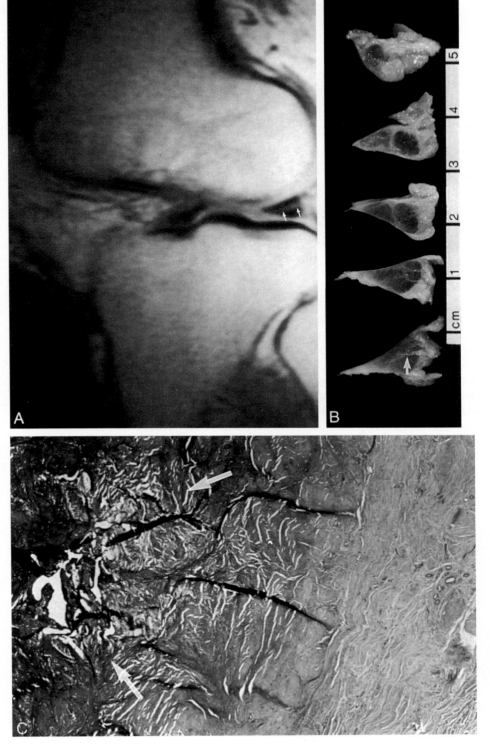

FIGURE 7-31. (A) A T1-weighted sagittal image demonstrates grade 2 signal intensity in the posterior horn of the lateral meniscus (*arrows*). (B) The corresponding gross section demonstrates linear mucinous meniscal degeneration (*arrow*). (C) The corresponding histologic study shows a focus of mucinous degeneration within the meniscal fibrocartilage (*arrows*).

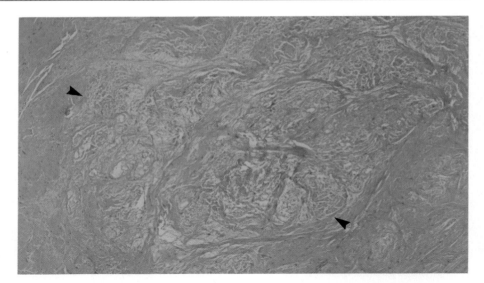

FIGURE 7-32. The region of mucinous degeneration (*arrowheads*) corresponds to grade 2 meniscal intrasubstance degeneration. (Hematoxylin and eosin stain.)

thought to contribute to the development of acute and chronic pain (Fig. 7-40). Hyperplasia of the synovium may also occur, secondary to joint debris in degenerative osteoarthritis, and is arthroscopically resected. Peripheral perimeniscal capillary ingrowth may be seen perforating areas of degeneration and fibrocartilaginous separation, supporting preferential healing in this location (Fig. 7-41). Acute traumatic tears have less predictable orientations and smaller areas of associated mucinous degeneration as sites for structural weakening than degenerative horizontal, cleavage, or flap tears (Fig. 7-42).[65] Grade 3 signal intensity is most frequent in the posterior horn of the medial meniscus, a finding supported by the observations of increased stress and

strain generated on the undersurface of the medial meniscus with femoral tibial rotations.

MR makes a significant contribution in imaging of this frequently injured site. The accuracy of arthroscopy in identifying inferior surface tears of the posterior medial meniscus is reported to be as low as 45% to 65%.[66,67] Furthermore, arthrographic and arthroscopic surface evaluation are insensitive to grade 1 and 2 intrasubstance degenerations as precursors to the formation of a defined meniscal tear.[68] MR also detects multiple meniscal tears that may be overlooked on arthrography.

Classification of Meniscal Tears

CROSS-SECTIONAL PATTERNS: VERTICAL AND HORIZONTAL TEARS. The present system of classifying meniscal tears as grade 3 signal intensity relative to a meniscal articular surface does not address the anatomy of various horizontal and vertical tear patterns as identified during arthroscopic surgery of the knee.[69] By using the cross-sectional anatomy of the meniscus as demonstrated on sagittal images, meniscal tears can be classified into two primary tear planes, vertical or horizontal (Fig. 7-43). However, because most meniscal tears are not exclusively perpendicular or parallel with the tibial plateau surface, tears classified as either vertical (Fig. 7-44) or horizontal (Fig. 7-45) may have secondary tear patterns (ie, horizontal or vertical, respectively). For example, most horizontal tears extend to the inferior surface of the meniscus and do not extend to the meniscal apex as a cleavage tear (see Fig. 7-45).

An accurate description of the morphology and location of the tear is particularly useful in choosing between primary meniscal repair and partial meniscectomy. It is possible to display meniscal anatomy and pathology with 3D composite images, spatially disarticulated from the knee joint and processed from

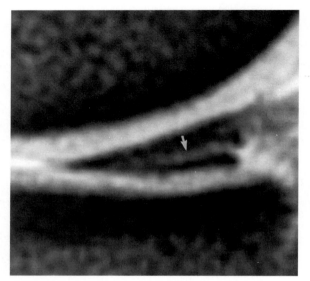

FIGURE 7-33. Grade 2 signal intensity (*arrow*) is seen in the posterior horn of the medial meniscus on this T2*-weighted sagittal image.

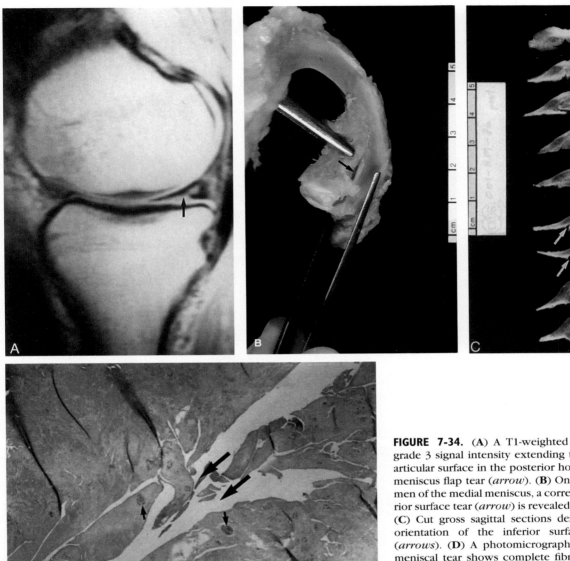

FIGURE 7-34. (A) A T1-weighted image shows grade 3 signal intensity extending to the inferior articular surface in the posterior horn of a medial meniscus flap tear (*arrow*). (B) On a gross specimen of the medial meniscus, a corresponding inferior surface tear (*arrow*) is revealed with probing. (C) Cut gross sagittal sections demonstrate the orientation of the inferior surface flap tear (*arrows*). (D) A photomicrograph of a grade 3 meniscal tear shows complete fibrocartilaginous separation (*large arrows*) with regenerative chondrocytes along the free edge of the torn meniscus (*small arrows*).

3D FT T2*-weighted images. With this technique, rotation of the meniscus and internal tear patterns are displayed.

CIRCUMFERENTIAL OR SURFACE PATTERNS: LONGITUDINAL, RADIAL, AND OBLIQUE TEARS. As viewed from the surface of the meniscus at arthroscopy, and relative to its circumference, three tear patterns can be seen: longitudinal, radial or transverse, and oblique or flap (Fig. 7-46).[42]

Vertical tears extend to the meniscal surface as either longitudinal, radial, or oblique tears. Horizontal tears display either longitudinal or oblique surface tear patterns unless the tear remains in the plane of the middle perforating collagen bundle and extends to the meniscal apex as a degenerative horizontal cleavage tear with similar sized superior and infe-

rior leaves (Fig. 7-47). Although horizontal tears are sometimes referred to as "fish-mouth" tears, the description is imprecise. Horizontal cleavage tears are most frequently associated with meniscal cysts, and treatment of the underlying meniscal tear leads to involution of the cyst (Fig. 7-48). Complex tears display combinations of vertical and horizontal tear patterns (Fig. 7-49).

Longitudinal Tears. A tear seen from the surface of the meniscus as longitudinal, may be either vertical or horizontal on sagittal images (Figs. 7-50 and 7-51). Internal probing of a longitudinal surface tear during arthroscopy confirms these findings. Longitudinal tears extend cir-

text continues on page 273

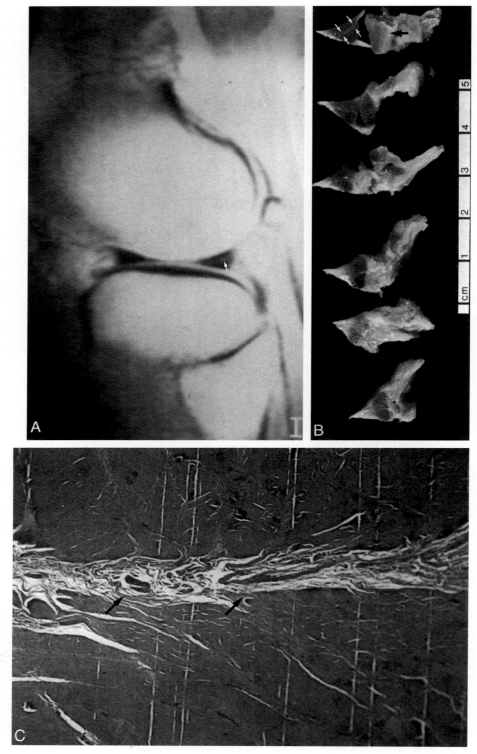

FIGURE 7-35. Closed meniscal tear. **(A)** On a T1-weighted sagittal image, a horizontal intrasubstance cleavage tear has grade 3 signal intensity (*white arrow*). **(B)** The sagittal gross section shows degeneration approaching the inferior surface of the meniscus without a visible surface tear (*white arrows*). *Black arrow*, the popliteus tendon. **(C)** The corresponding photomicrograph demonstrates confined fibrocartilaginous separation (*arrows*).

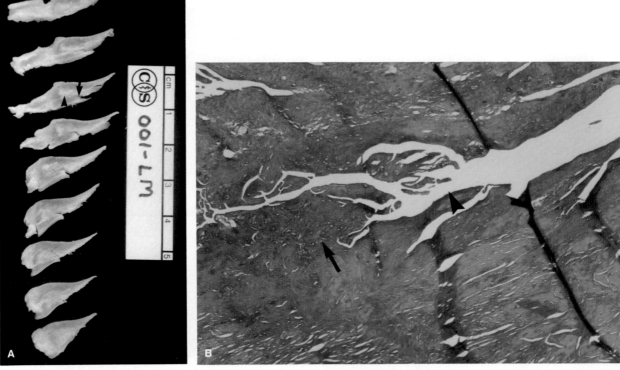

FIGURE 7-36. (A) A gross specimen of the posterior horn of the medial meniscus shows an inferior surface tear (*arrow*) adjacent to an area of intrasubstance degeneration (*arrowhead*). (B) The corresponding photomicrograph demonstrates a fibrocartilaginous tear (*arrowhead*) and surrounding (*blue*) mucinous degeneration (*arrow*). (Alcian blue stain.)

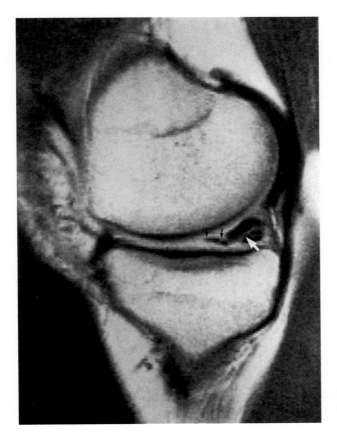

FIGURE 7-37. Intermediate weighted sagittal image is used to demonstrate a grade 3 flap tear of the posterior horn of the medial meniscus (*white arrow*) with a truncated meniscal apex (*black arrows*).

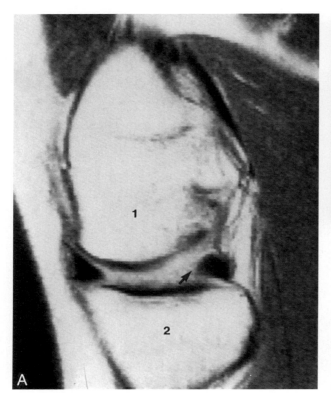

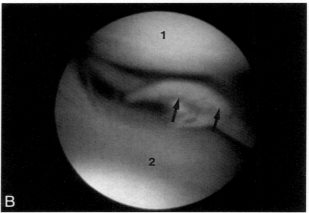

FIGURE 7-38. This torn medial meniscus shows abnormal morphology. **(A)** The T1-weighted sagittal image shows a blunted and foreshortened apex of the posterior horn of the medial meniscus (*arrow*). *1*, femur; *2*, tibia. **(B)** The arthroscopic view demonstrates a complete flap tear (*arrows*) that extends to the truncated medial meniscus. *1*, femur; *2*, tibia.

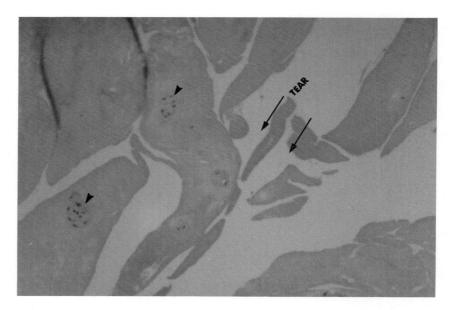

FIGURE 7-39. A high-power photomicrograph shows large regenerative chondrocytes (*arrowheads*) at the tear site (*long arrows*). (Hematoxylin and eosin stain.)

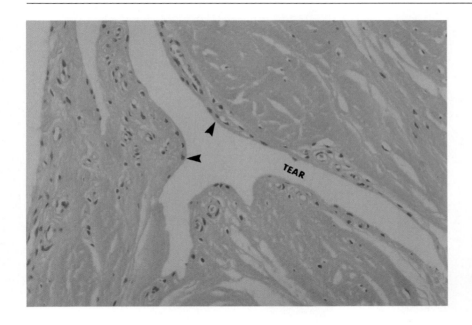

FIGURE 7-40. A photomicrograph shows peripheral synovial ingrowth into the meniscal tear cleavage plane. (Hematoxylin and eosin stain.)

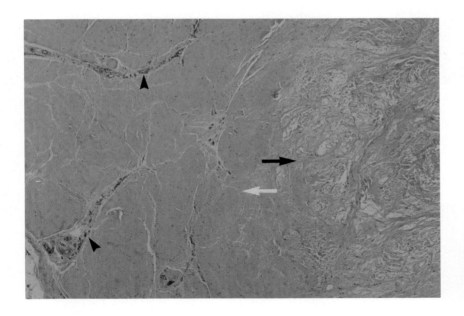

FIGURE 7-41. Perimeniscal capillary ingrowth (*arrowheads*) is directed toward an area of mucinous degeneration (*black arrow*). *White arrow*, normal adjacent meniscal tissue.

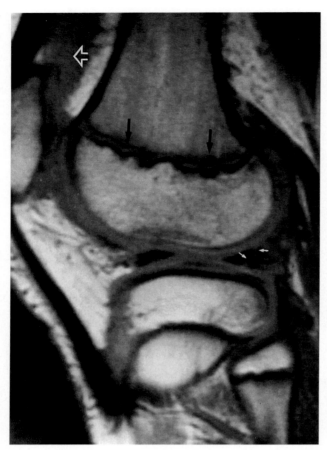

FIGURE 7-42. A traumatic meniscal tear in a 12-year-old child. This complex tear of the posterior horn of the lateral meniscus communicates with both the superior and the inferior articular surfaces (*white arrows*). A physeal scar (*black arrows*) and associated joint effusion (*open arrow*) are shown.

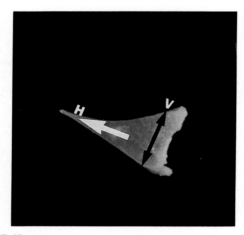

FIGURE 7-43. Idealized directions of horizontal (*H, white arrow*) and vertical (*V, black arrows*) tear patterns in a gross cross section of the meniscus.

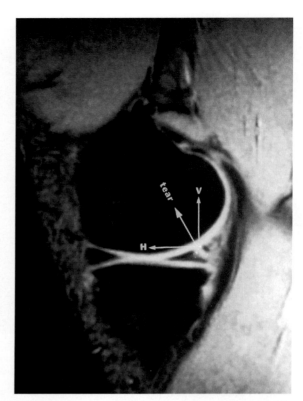

FIGURE 7-44. The vertical primary tear pattern (*tear*) is shown with both vertical (*V*) and horizontal (*H*) vector components. The tear is directed more than 45° from the horizontal component.

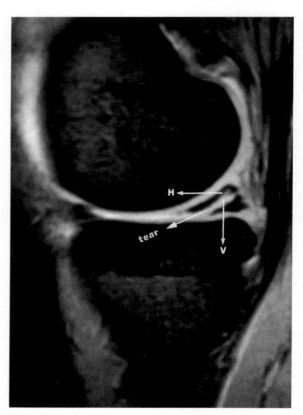

FIGURE 7-45. A horizontal primary tear pattern (*tear*) has both horizontal (*H*) and vertical (*V*) vector components. The direction of the tear is close to but less than 45° from the horizontal, indicating almost equal contributions from the horizontal and vertical vectors.

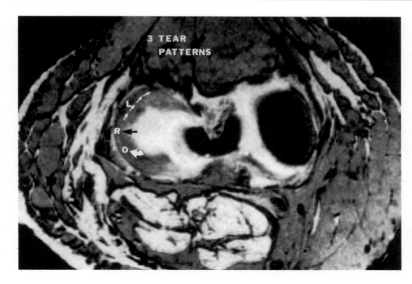

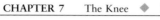

FIGURE 7-46. Longitudinal (*L, straight white arrows*), transverse or radial (*R, black arrow*), and oblique (*O, curved white arrow*) tear patterns as seen from the surface of the lateral meniscus.

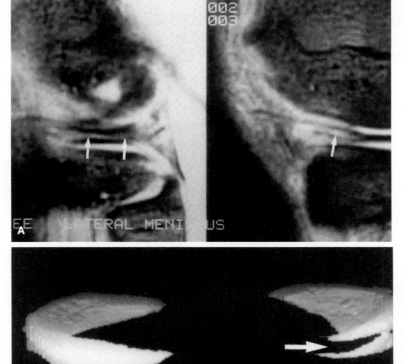

FIGURE 7-47. (**A**) A T2*-weighted sagittal image shows a horizontal tear (*arrows*) of the body (*left*) and anterior horn (*right*) of the lateral meniscus parallel with the tibial surface. (**B**) A 3D MR rendering displays a horizontal tear pattern (*arrow*) dividing the meniscus into superior and inferior leaves (ie, halves). Although most meniscal tears have horizontal components, a pure cleavage tear parallel with the tibial articular surface and extending to the apex is less common.

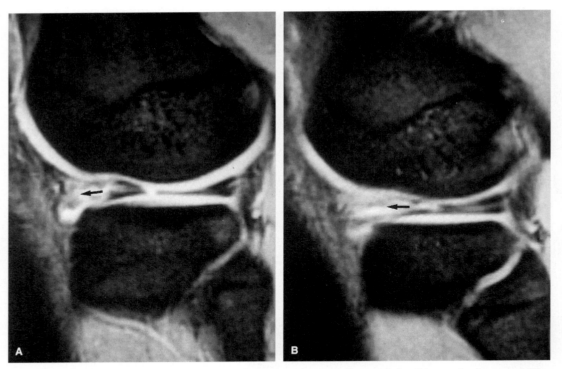

FIGURE 7-48. On these T2*-weighted sagittal images, a horizontal tear of the (**A**) anterior horn and (**B**) body of the lateral meniscus decompresses into an anterolateral meniscal cyst (*arrows*).

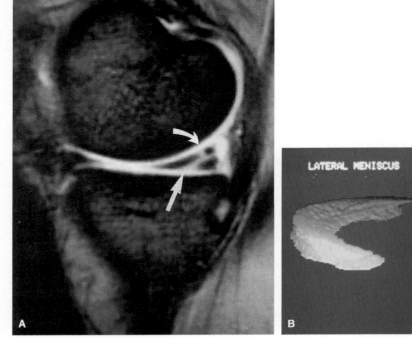

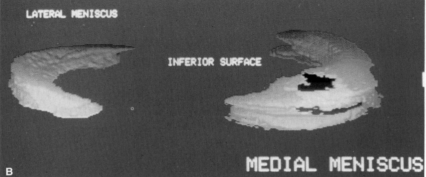

FIGURE 7-49. (**A**) A T2*-weighted image displays a complex tear pattern with superior (*curved arrow*) and inferior (*straight arrow*) meniscal tear extension. (**B**) A 3D MR rendering shows both vertical and horizontal components (*red*) in this complex oblique tear pattern.

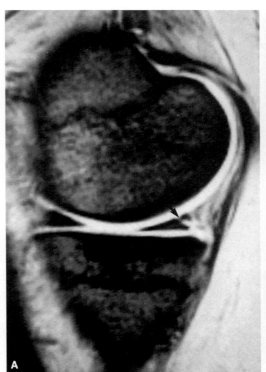

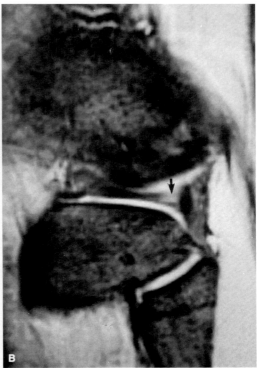

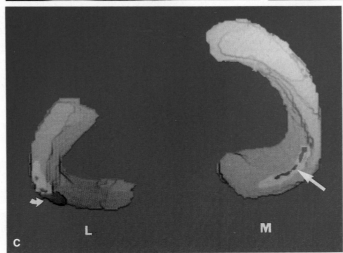

FIGURE 7-50. A longitudinal tear with the primary vertical tear pattern can be seen on the meniscal cross section in the sagittal plane. Peripheral (ie, involving the outer one third of the meniscus) vertical tears of the posterior horn of the **(A)** medial and **(B)** lateral meniscus can be seen on T2*-weighted sagittal images. **(C)** The corresponding 3D MR rendering demonstrates superior surface extension of the medial meniscus (*M*), the longitudinal tear (*straight arrow*), and the peripheral location of the tear (*curved arrow*) of the lateral meniscus (*L*).

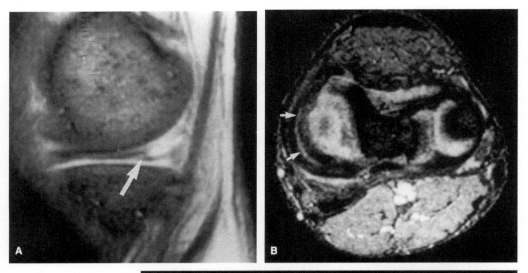

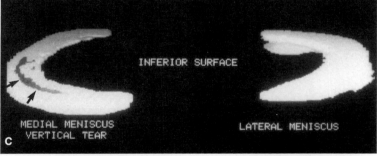

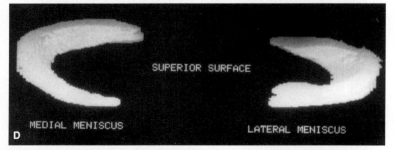

FIGURE 7-51. A longitudinal tear with a primary horizontal tear pattern as seen on the meniscal cross section in the sagittal plane. (**A**) A T2*-weighted sagittal image shows a tear (*arrow*) of the posterior horn of the medial meniscus with a primary horizontal morphology. (**B**) A 0.7-mm 3D FT axial image shows a longitudinal tear pattern (*arrows*). (**C** and **D**) A 3D MR rendering displays an inferior surface longitudinal tear (**C**) with an intact superior meniscal surface (**D**). (**E**) Two months after the MR study, arthroscopic examination revealed a displaced longitudinal tear (*all arrows*) with a bucket-handle morphology. *F*, femur. (**F**) A partial meniscectomy with remaining horizontal cleavage component (*arrows*) was performed after resection of the displaced bucket-handle fibrocartilage. Longitudinal tears can have either vertical or horizontal components. *F*, femoral condyle; *T*, tibia.

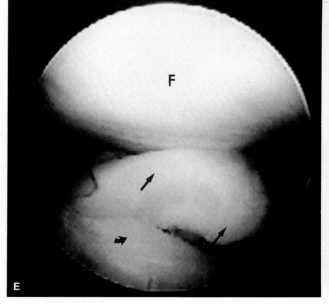

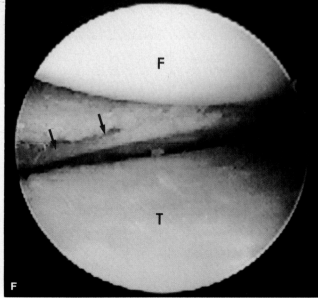

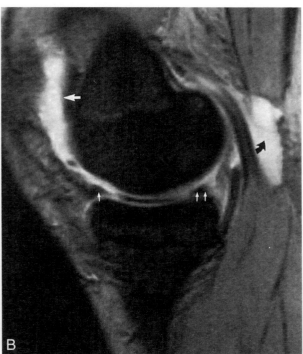

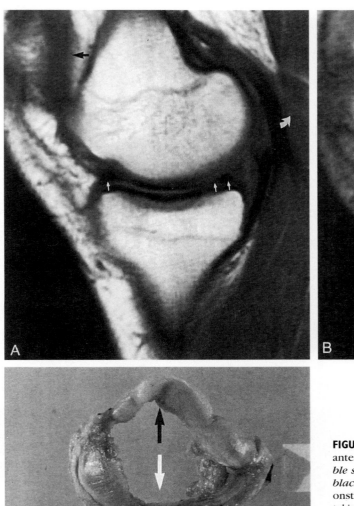

FIGURE 7-52. A bucket-handle tear with foreshortened anterior (*single small white arrows*) and posterior (*double small white arrows*) horns. Suprapatellar fluid (*large black arrows*) and a popliteal cyst (*curved arrows*) demonstrate (**A**) low signal intensity on the T1-weighted sagittal image and (**B**) high signal intensity on the T2*-weighted sagittal image. (**C**) A gross specimen demonstrates a displaced longitudinal bucket-handle tear (*black arrows*) from the medial meniscus (*white arrow*).

cumferentially along the anteroposterior extent of the meniscus (parallel to the meniscus margin).[45] Peripheral vertical tears are successfully treated with primary meniscal repair, whereas horizontal tears that extend into avascular fibrocartilage are treated with partial meniscectomy. The peripheral extension of MR grade 3 signal intensity to the stable meniscal rim may assist the arthroscopist in performing a partial meniscectomy but may not be appreciated at arthroscopy. This observation is consistent with the frequent appearance of grade 3 signal intensity in an asymptomatic partial meniscectomy meniscal remnant on MR.

Bucket-Handle Tears.   A displaced longitudinal tear of the meniscus, usually the medial meniscus, is called a bucket-handle tear because the separated central fragment resembles the handle of a bucket (Fig. 7-52).[23] The remaining larger

peripheral section of the meniscus is the bucket. Vertical longitudinal tears are further classified as single vertical longitudinal tears, displaced bucket-handle–type tears, broken bucket-handle tears, and double and triple vertical longitudinal bucket-handle tears.[70] On MR images it can be further shown that a bucket-handle tear may originate from either primary vertical or horizontal longitudinal tear patterns. Bucket-handle tears frequently occur in young patients secondary to significant trauma.[71]

Medial meniscus bucket-handle tears are three times more frequent than bucket-handle tears involving the lateral meniscus. The central fragment of a bucket-handle tear may be completely displaced into the intercondylar notch or, as may occur with a shorter tear of the posterior meniscus, may be only partially displaced. A bucket-handle tear effectively

text continues on page 276

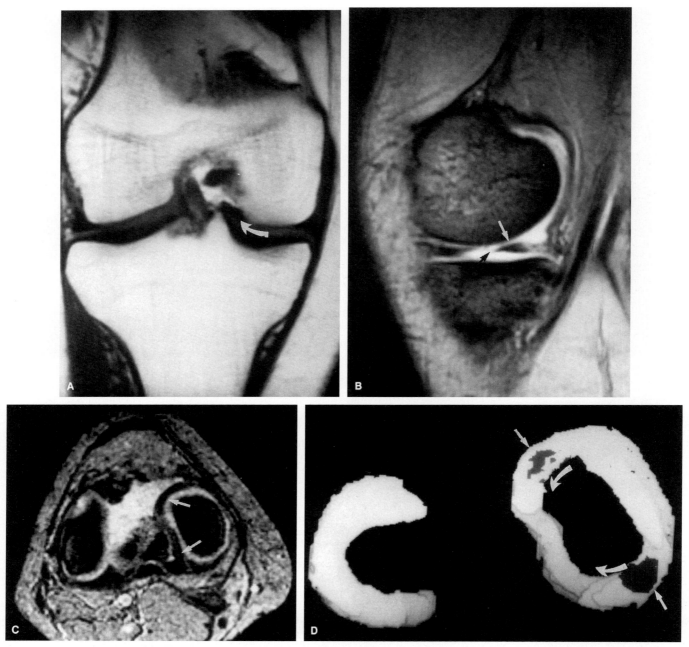

FIGURE 7-53. A bucket-handle tear. (**A**) Displaced medial meniscal tissue is seen in the intercondylar notch on a T1-weighted coronal image (*curved arrow*). (**B**) A T2*-weighted sagittal image shows a tear (*black arrow*) with foreshortening of the posterior horn of the medial meniscus (*white arrow*). (**C**) A 0.7-mm 3D FT T2*-weighted axial image reveals an intercondylar displaced meniscal tissue fragment (*arrows*). (**D**) A 3D MR rendering shows the bucket-handle tear pattern (*curved arrows*) with anterior and posterior tear points (*straight arrows*).

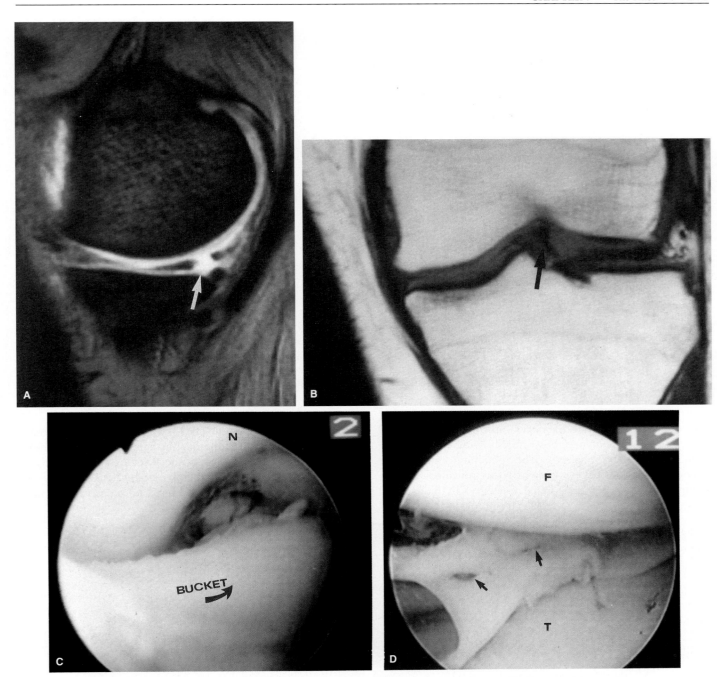

FIGURE 7-54. Displaced vertical longitudinal bucket-handle tear. (**A**) A T2*-weighted saggital image displays a peripheral one-third vertical tear of the posterior horn of the medial meniscus (*arrow*). (**B**) On a T1-weighted coronal image, the bucket fragment (BUCKET) in intercondylar notch (*arrow*) demonstrates low signal intensity. (**C**) The arthroscopic photograph allows identification of the intercondylar notch (N) and bucket-handle fragment (*curved arrow*). (**D**) Another arthroscopic photograph shows primary arthroscopic repair approximating the separated meniscal fragments. Suture points are indicated (*arrows*). (F, femoral condyle; T, tibia.)

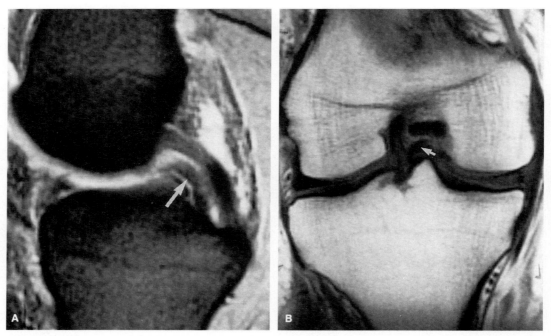

FIGURE 7-55. A bucket-handle tear. (**A**) A T2*-weighted sagittal image shows the pseudo-PCL created by the displaced bucket-handle tear of the medial meniscus (*arrow*). (**B**) The corresponding T1-weighted coronal image allows identification of the displaced bucket meniscal fragment in the intercondylar notch (*arrow*).

reduces the width of the meniscus, and peripheral sagittal images fail to demonstrate the normal bow-tie configuration of the body of the meniscus. The remaining anterior and posterior horns are often hypoplastic or truncated, with or without increased internal signal intensity. In the normal medial meniscus without tear, the posterior horn is wider and thus has greater height than the anterior horn. Foreshortening of the posterior horn of the medial meniscus without history of previous partial meniscectomy is associated with bucket-handle morphology. A displaced meniscal fragment

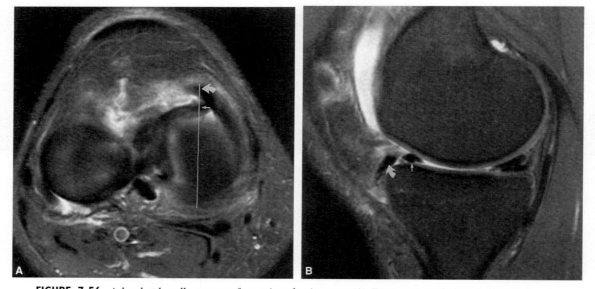

FIGURE 7-56. A bucket-handle tear on fast spin-echo images. (**A**) Fat-suppressed T2-weighted fast spin-echo axial image identifies the location of the displaced anterior fragments of a bucket-handle tear (*curved* and *straight arrows*). *Straight line*, the sagittal plane of section, intersecting the anterior horn, bucket-handle fragment, and posterior horn. (**B**) Fat-suppressed T2-weighted fast spin-echo sagittal image shows the corresponding displaced anterior horn (*curved arrow*) and bucket (*small arrow*) fragments.

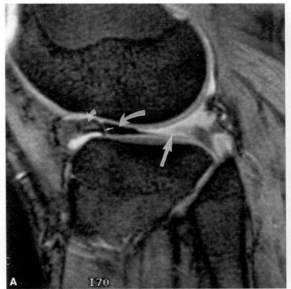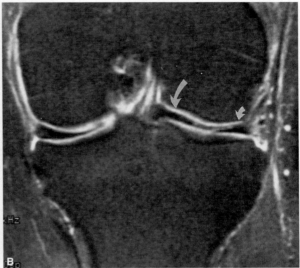

FIGURE 7-57. A bucket-handle tear of the lateral meniscus. **(A)** Sagittal T2*-weighted and **(B)** fat-suppressed T2-weighted fast spin-echo coronal images show an anteriorly displaced posterior horn of the lateral meniscus (*large curved arrow*). Note the absence of meniscal tissue in the expected location (the posterior horn of the lateral meniscus) (*large straight arrow*). This deformity, with blunting of the apex (*small straight arrow*) of the anterior horn segment (*small curved arrow*), is commonly seen as a result of compression by the displaced posterior horn.

can frequently be identified within the intercondylar notch on coronal images (Figs. 7-53 and 7-54).[72]

The displaced fragment of a bucket-handle tear is displayed on sagittal images as a low-signal-intensity band parallel and anterior to the PCL, but we have not found this to be the most common presentation (Fig. 7-55).[73] In complex bucket-handle tears, 3D FT (3D gradient-echo or fast spin-echo) axial images show the relation of the displaced tear to the remaining meniscus in a single section (Fig. 7-56). The lateral meniscus may also be the site of bucket-handle tears in which the body of the lateral meniscus is displaced into the intercondylar notch (Fig. 7-57).[74]

Patients with bucket-handle tears may present with a locked knee or may lack full extension. These tears may also be associated with ACL injuries,[71] and single or multiple flaps of meniscal tissue may be generated. As previously discussed, bucket-handle tears may start as a longitudinal tear with a primarily horizontal tear pattern. A displaced vertical component subsequently generates a bucket-handle morphology. This pathogenesis is supported by the finding that residual peripheral horizontal grade 3 signal intensity may persist after a partial meniscectomy performed to treat a bucket-handle tear. More commonly, bucket-handle tears are displaced vertical, longitudinal tears. A partial meniscectomy is performed for nonseparated symptomatic tears. A meniscal repair may be considered in certain double bucket-handle tears. Excision of a displaced fragment of a bucket-handle tear is considered when (1) there is a significant radial split tear in the displaced bucket-handle component; (2) the

meniscal rim size is 5 mm or greater, placing the tear clearly in the avascular zone of the meniscus; or (3) the tear is chronic, with deformed (twisted) morphology.[70]

Radial or Transverse Tears.   A radial or transverse tear is, by definition, a vertical tear perpendicular to the free edge of the meniscus (Fig. 7-58). On sagittal images (because the sagittal plane sections the meniscus perpendicular to the free edge orientation of the tear), the only evidence of a radial tear may be increased signal intensity (focal grade 3) on one or two peripheral sections.[75] The middle third of the lateral meniscus is a common location for radial tears, probably because of its more circular shape and decreased radius of curvature, its increased mobility (the posterior horn is pulled posteriorly in flexion), and excessive loading during valgus stress.[64,76,77] Radial tears located near the posterior horn origin of the lateral meniscus may be associated with ACL sprains and tears.[70] Radial tears of the medial meniscus usually occur in the posterior horn and present in older patients. Tears 3 mm or less may be asymptomatic, whereas tears greater than 5 mm in length may be symptomatic.[71] Symptomatic tears can be treated by trimming the anterior and posterior leaves adjacent to the tear site. Some radial tears are associated with more complex meniscal tears, including a vertical longitudinal tear or horizontal cleavage component peripherally (Fig. 7-59). We prefer not to use the term "parrot-beak" tear, which is sometimes used to describe a free edge tear with both vertical and horizontal compo-

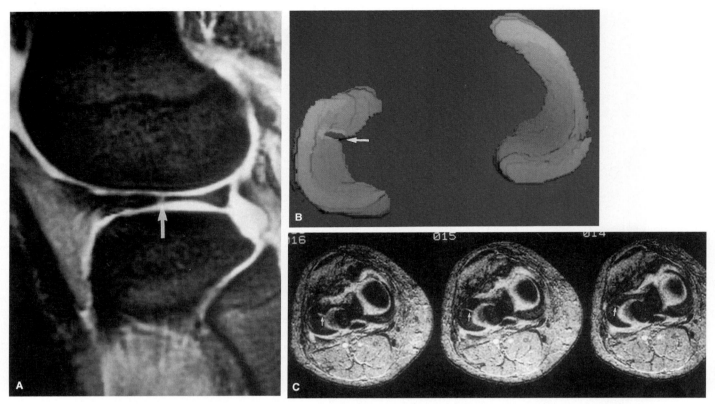

FIGURE 7-58. (A) A transverse or radial tear (*arrow*) with grade 3 signal intensity is seen in the anterior horn–body junction of the lateral meniscus on a T2*-weighted image. (B) A 3D MR rendering reveals the free-edge radial tear (*arrow*). (C) Corresponding 0.7-mm axial images show the radial tear (*arrow*) of the free edge of the lateral meniscus in three images.

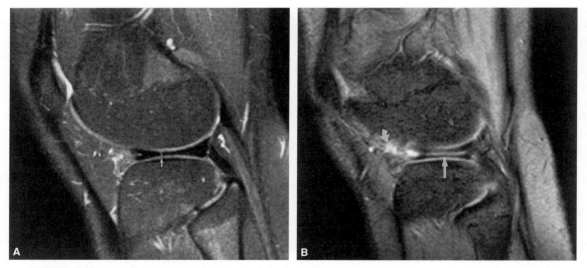

FIGURE 7-59. A radial tear (*small arrow*) of the lateral meniscus (A) seen in association with a more peripheral horizontal tear (B). The horizontal tear (*large straight arrow*) communicates with a small meniscal cyst (*curved arrow*). (A, fat-suppressed T2-weighted fast spin-echo sagittal image; B, T2*-weighted sagittal image.)

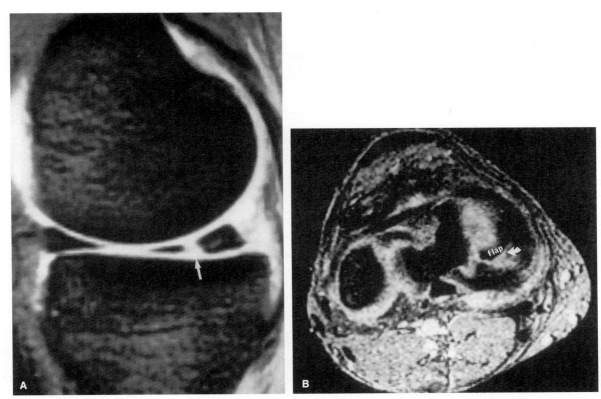

FIGURE 7-60. Vertical oblique or flap tear. (**A**) A T2*-weighted sagittal image shows a vertical tear (*arrow*) dividing the posterior horn of the medial meniscus. (**B**) The corresponding 0.7-mm 3D FT T2*-weighted axial image reveals flap-tear morphology and allows identification of the oblique tear site (*curved arrow*).

nents. This term is confusing and does not accurately describe the tear pattern of the meniscus. A parrot-beak pattern is also sometimes classified as an oblique (flap) tear with a smaller horizontal component.

Oblique or Flap Tears.   An oblique tear, which represents a composite of a longitudinal and transverse or radial tear, starts on the free edge of the meniscus and curves obliquely into the meniscal fibrocartilage. These tears are also referred to as flap tears. Oblique or flap tears represent the most common meniscal tear type and are usually associated with a horizontal tear pattern on sagittal plane meniscal cross section (eg, grade 3 signal intensity extending to the inferior surface of the posterior horn of the medial meniscus). On

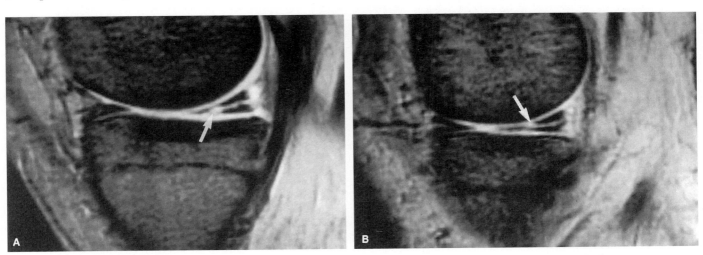

FIGURE 7-61. A change in direction of the posterior horn medial meniscus tear (*arrow*) from (**A**) the inferior surface to (**B**) the superior surface is frequently seen in oblique or flap-tear morphology on T2*-weighted sagittal images.

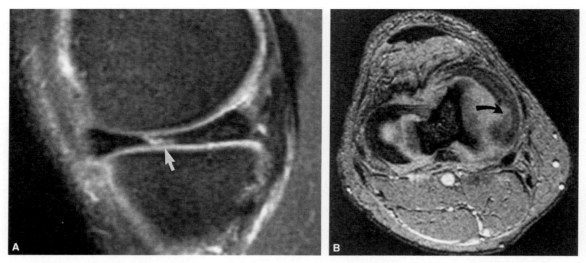

FIGURE 7-62. (**A**) Peripheral flap tear (*arrow*) with extension to both superior and inferior meniscal surfaces on a fat-suppressed T2-weighted fast spin-echo sagittal image. (**B**) Flap-tear morphology (*curved arrow*) is demonstrated on a 0.7-mm 3D FT T2* axial image.

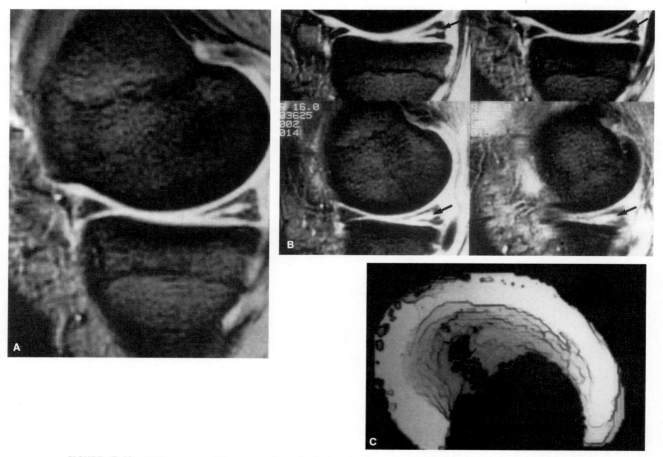

FIGURE 7-63. Oblique tear. The tear, of grade 3 signal intensity, of the posterior horn of the medial meniscus is shown (**A**) on a single T2*-weighted sagittal image and (**B**) on a series of T2*-weighted sagittal images from the meniscal body to the posterior horn (*arrows*). When a change in the direction of grade 3 signal intensity from the inferior to the superior surface of the meniscus is not apparent, it is difficult to differentiate an oblique from a longitudinal tear. (**C**) A 3D MR rendering demonstrates an oblique or flap tear pattern.

continued

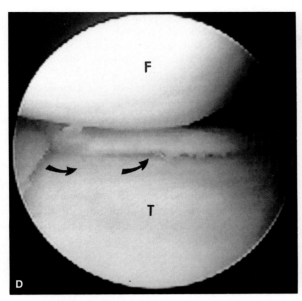 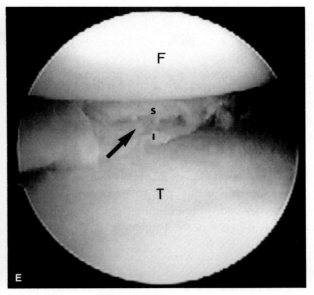

FIGURE 7-63. *Continued.* (**D**) An arthroscopic photograph shows a flap tear with displacement of the meniscal flap toward the intercondylar area (*curved arrows*). *F*, femur; *T*, tibia. (**E**) Another arthroscopic photograph shows a stable meniscal rim, postmeniscal contouring, and flat excision with residual horizontal components (*arrow*) between stable superior (*S*) and inferior (*I*) meniscal leaves. *F*, femur; *T*, tibia.

sagittal images, flap tears may display either a primary vertical or horizontal tear pattern (Fig. 7-60). However, without the use of thin-section axial images or a 3D composite image of the meniscus, it is difficult to differentiate between oblique (flap) and longitudinal tear morphology on sagittal images (Figs. 7-61 and 7-62). When grade 3 signal intensity is seen to extend to the superior and inferior surface of the meniscus on separate sagittal images, oblique morphology may be inferred (see Fig. 7-61). Oblique tears may generate an anterior- or posterior-based flap of meniscus.[42]

A flap tear often involves the avascular inner edge of the meniscus and is irreparable.[70] Treatment is partial meniscectomy with transection through the base and contouring of the remaining attachment to a stable rim.[76] Residual peripheral horizontal grade 3 signal intensity is often seen after arthroscopic resection of the flap (Fig. 7-63).

MR Accuracy

Compared with that of arthroscopy, the sensitivity of MR imaging of meniscal tears has been reported to be between 80% and 100%.[6,24,26,29,49,62,78–87] In a series by Mink and colleagues, 600 menisci were studied with an accuracy rate of 92%; there were nine false-negative and 18 false-positive findings.[88] With fast 3D MR imaging, there is a 95% concurrence between MR imaging and arthroscopy in detection of meniscal tears and a 100% correlation for meniscal degeneration.[89] Li and colleagues studied 459 menisci and reported an arthroscopic correlation of 93%.[19]

For excluding tears on normal MR examinations of the meniscus, the negative predictive value of MR imaging approaches 100%. In a large multicenter series of 1014 patients, the MR imaging accuracy of diagnosis was 89% for the medial meniscus and 88% for the lateral meniscus.[90] In a prospective study of 561 patients who also underwent arthroscopy, Justice and Quinn reported an accuracy rate of 93% for the lateral meniscus and 95% for the medial meniscus.[87] In a retrospective study by De Smet and colleagues of 400 MR examinations (800 menisci), there were 83 original diagnostic errors, yielding an accuracy rate of 90%.[83] De Smet's group also provided an analysis of causative errors. Errors were classified as unavoidable errors (40%) and errors related to equivocal MR findings (21%) and interpretation errors (21%). Unavoidable errors (discordant MR-arthroscopic correlation) were represented by 21 false-negative and 12 false-positive diagnoses. Subtle or equivocal MR findings resulted from interobserver differences in interpretations. Of the interpretation errors, 38% were attributed to normal MR variants mistaken for a meniscal tear. Even in retrospective review, 6% of the meniscal tears could not be diagnosed. Of note was a small (1.5%) false-positive diagnosis attributed to healed tears or tears overlooked at arthroscopy. This study emphasizes that observer variation as represented in the equivocal MR finding category can affect MR accuracy rates in diagnosis of meniscal tears. Other studies have minimized differences in observer performance.[84] Increased observer experience may improve accuracy with subtle or equivocal MR findings, including grade 1 versus grade 2 signal intensities, flap tears, and peripheral tears. Correlating peripheral meniscal signal intensity on sagittal MR images with coronal plane images of the corresponding menisci may reduce false-positive MR interpretations, especially in the posterior horn of the medial meniscus.

In addition, in cases in which there are multiple knee lesions, the accuracy of the clinical knee examination drops from 72% for a single lesion to 30%.[91] These results support the use of MR in the proper clinical setting. The ability to detect an associated meniscal tear in the presence of a clinically deficient ACL knee or an existing MCL tear are clinical indications for MR referral. The improved sensitivity of MR in the detection of chondral lesions using fat-suppression fast spin-echo techniques may further improve clinical diagnostic accuracy for treatment and patient care. Although it has been suggested that a pattern of intrameniscal signal intensity extending to the meniscal surface is less likely to represent a tear if it is seen only on one image,[86] the morphology of the signal intensity and techniques used must be taken into consideration. It is not unusual to identify a meniscal tear in only one imaging plane.

La Prade and colleagues found meniscal tears in 5.6% of asymptomatic patients.[62] Lateral meniscal tears were twice as common as medial meniscal tears. In addition, grade 2 signal intensity involving the posterior horn of the medial meniscus was found in 24.1% of cases. MR findings of grade 2 signal intensity in the posterior horn of the medial meniscus correlate with histologic studies showing that the posterior horn of the medial meniscus receives the greatest femoral tibial forces during biomechanical loading and is the most frequent site of grade 2 signal intensity. Nonetheless, depiction of grade 2 signal intensity in asymptomatic patients cannot be used to prospectively predict progression to fibrocartilaginous weakening, which may eventually result in a meniscal tear. Although this study reported accuracy rates of 98.6% for the medial meniscus and 90.3% for the lateral meniscus as correlated with arthroscopy, it is essential that clinical exam findings be coordinated with MR studies based on the 5.6% prevalence of meniscal tears in asymptomatic persons.

3D MR rendering techniques can be used to display meniscal pathology and to follow changes in morphology after surgery, but we have not found these techniques to be accurate in measuring meniscal volume or in replacing direct diagnosis on 2D MR images.[92,93]

In addition, although radial images of the knee have been shown to be as accurate as sagittal images, we recommend that radial images be used as an additional or adjunct sequence or acquisition because of potential pitfalls related to section thickness and observer error.[29]

Variations in the accuracy rates of MR compared with those of arthroscopy may be due to the following factors:

- Differences in the learning curves of radiologists in interpreting MR signal intensities
- Differences in the experience of several arthroscopists participating in the correlative studies
- False interpretation of areas of fibrillation or fraying as meniscal tears
- Inability of arthroscopy to detect intrasubstance degenerative cleavage tears
- Obstructed arthroscopic visualization of the posterior horn of the medial meniscus by the medial femoral condyle

- Difficulty in accurately imaging the periphery of the meniscus at the meniscocapsular junction
- Variability in examinations using different MR imaging equipment and surface coils at a variety of field strengths.

The cost effectiveness of MR has been addressed in several studies. Rowe and colleagues reported that in 51.4% of 103 patients studied during a 9-month period, MR examination was instrumental in avoiding unnecessary diagnostic arthroscopy, resulting in a savings of $103,700.[6] In another (prospective) study of 58 patients, basing interventions on MR findings produced a 29% reduction in unnecessary arthroscopic examinations. MR thus reduces not only the overall cost of patient care but also the morbidity associated with unnecessary arthroscopic examinations or those yielding negative results.[5]

Discoid Meniscus

A discoid meniscus is a dysplastic meniscus that has lost its normal or semilunar shape and has a broad disclike configuration.[94–96] Lateral discoid menisci are more common than medial discoid menisci, and the degree of enlargement varies from mild hypertrophy to a bulky slab of fibrocartilage (Fig. 7-64). The incidence of discoid menisci is reported to be between 1.4% and 15.5%.[97] The rare medial discoid meniscus is found in 0.3% of meniscectomies (Fig. 7-65).[25] Watanabe's classification groups discoid menisci into complete, incomplete, and Wrisberg-ligament type (Fig. 7-66). Complete and incomplete refer to the degree or extent to which the meniscus demonstrates discoid morphology with an intact posterolateral meniscotibial ligament.[25,98] The Wrisberg-ligament type discoid meniscus completely lacks the posterior capsular attachment, the posterior meniscotibial ligament. This deficiency or lack of posterior capsular attachment is thought to result in incomplete mediolateral motion, trauma, and secondary hypertrophy of the hypermobile meniscus.[99] There is no medial meniscus counterpart to the Wrisberg-ligament type discoid lateral meniscus.

Discoid menisci are considered congenital deformities and are frequently bilateral. They present as fibrocartilaginous masses with an oval or circular shape. The thickness of the fibrocartilage varies from 5 to 13 mm.[97] A complete discoid meniscus extends to the intercondylar notch. An anterior megahorn discoid meniscus is seen when the posterior horn is normal but the anterior horn and body form a solid mass of fibrocartilage. Discoid menisci are susceptible to tears and cysts, and young patients often present with symptoms of torn cartilage (see Fig. 7-64). Pain, clicking or snapping, and locking are common presenting clinical findings in children.[42,100] Clinical symptoms of a discoid lateral meniscus may not develop until adolescence. The Wrisberg ligament–type of discoid meniscus may, however, present earlier with lateral joint pain with or without an audible or palpable ''clunk.'' The result of McMurray's test may be

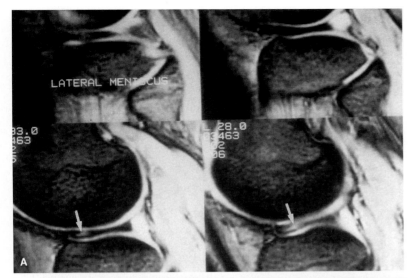

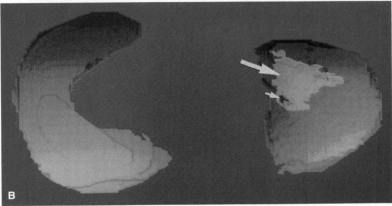

FIGURE 7-64. **(A)** A lateral discoid meniscus. The fibro-cartilage of the separate anterior and posterior horns has a slablike morphology as seen on consecutive T2*-weighted sagittal images. A superior surface tear (*arrow*) is demonstrated with associated intrasubstance degeneration. **(B)** A 3D MR rendering shows intrasubstance degeneration (*orange and large arrow*) and a superior surface tear (*red and small arrow*).

negative on examination, and in fact most discoid menisci are asymptomatic.

The differential diagnosis of a discoid meniscus includes any condition that presents as a "snapping knee" on physical examination (a snapping sound during knee flexion and extension). Patellofemoral joint subluxation or dislocation; meniscal cysts; congenital subluxation of the tibiofemoral joint; subluxation or dislocation, or both, of the proximal tibiofibular joint; and snapping of the tendons about the knee (ie, on an osteophyte or roughened surface) all need to be considered.

Treatment of the unstable inner segment of a discoid meniscus requires saucerization or resection (partial meniscectomy) to a stable rim. The Wrisberg ligament–type discoid lateral meniscus is prone to medial displacement into the intercondylar notch and is best treated with a total meniscectomy.[43,101] Some patients with symptomatic discoid menisci have undergone saucerization and partial resection in the presence of intrasubstance degeneration without a surface tear.[98] On MR examination these menisci demonstrate prominent or thick horizontal grade 2 signal intensity oriented along the middle collagen bundle or shear plane of the meniscus. Except for cases of discoid lesions, menisci with grade 2 signal intensity are not usually treated at arthroscopy.[98,102]

Plain-film radiographs of the discoid menisci (although usually of limited value) may show widening (Fig. 7-67) of the involved compartment (lateral joint space), a hypoplastic lateral femoral condyle, a high fibular head, chondromalacia, cupping of the lateral tibial plateau, and a squared-off lateral femoral condyle.[103] Arthrography demonstrates an elongated and enlarged meniscus that extends toward the intercondylar notch. On sagittal images, using a 4- to 5-mm slice thickness, a discoid meniscus exhibits a continuous or bow-tie appearance on three or more consecutive images (see Fig. 7-64).[100,104] Demonstration of the anterior and posterior horns is limited to one or two sagittal sections adjacent to the intercondylar notch. Central tapering, seen in the normal meniscus on sagittal images, is lost in discoid fibrocartilage. The increased inferior-to-superior dimensions of the meniscus can be appreciated on both coronal and sagittal MR images. A discoid meniscus may be as much as 2 mm higher than the opposite meniscus.[104] Coronal images show the extension of the discoid meniscus apex toward or into the

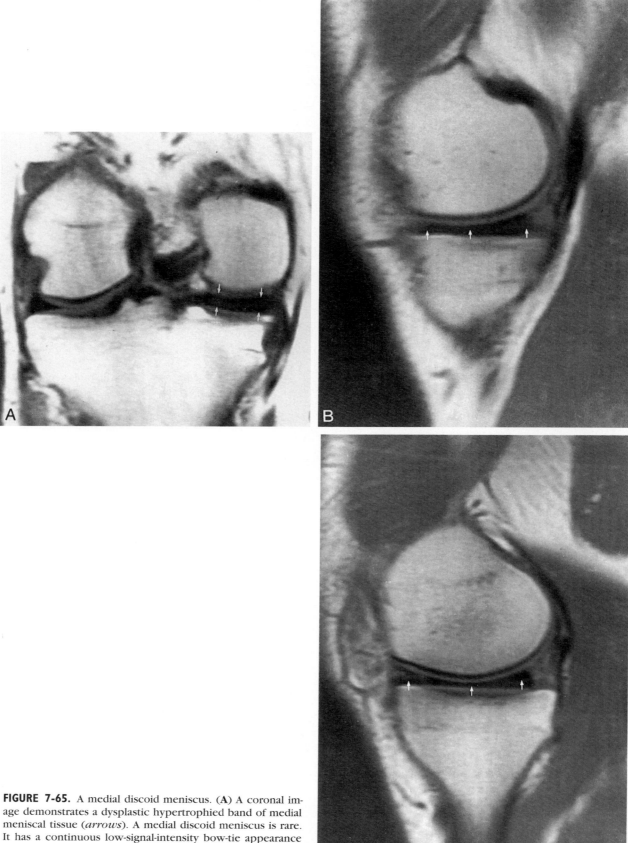

FIGURE 7-65. A medial discoid meniscus. (**A**) A coronal image demonstrates a dysplastic hypertrophied band of medial meniscal tissue (*arrows*). A medial discoid meniscus is rare. It has a continuous low-signal-intensity bow-tie appearance (*arrows*) on multiple sagittal images from (**B**) the periphery toward (**C**) the intercondylar notch.

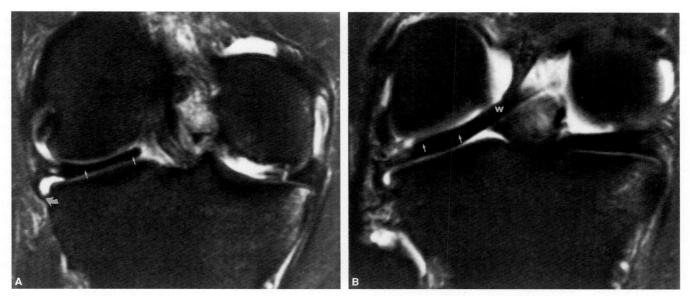

FIGURE 7-66. (**A** and **B**) A complete discoid meniscus (*small arrows*) interposed between the lateral femoral condyle and tibial plateau on fat-suppressed T2-weighted fast spin-echo coronal images. An intact meniscotibial ligament (**A**, *curved arrow*) and Wrisberg-ligament (**B**, *W*) are shown. The Wrisberg-ligament type of discoid lateral meniscus lacks the posterior meniscotibial ligamentous attachment.

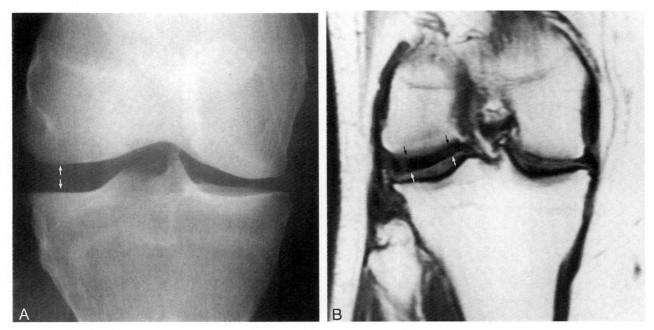

FIGURE 7-67. A lateral discoid meniscus. (**A**) An anteroposterior radiograph reveals a widened lateral joint compartment (*arrows*). The thick slab of lateral meniscal fibrocartilage is seen as a continuous low-signal-intensity band in corresponding (**B**) coronal images (*arrows*).   *continued*

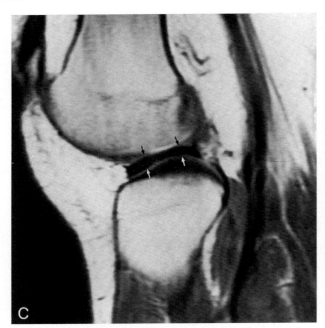

FIGURE 7-67. *Continued.* (C) The thick slab of lateral meniscal fibrocartilage is seen as a continuous low-signal-intensity band in corresponding sagittal images (*arrows*).

intercondylar notch. In a complete discoid meniscus, meniscal fibrocartilage without distinct anterior and posterior horns is usually interposed between the femoral condyle and the tibial plateau on every sagittal image through the involved compartment. In the more common incomplete discoid type meniscus, the meniscus does not extend into the intercondylar notch on coronal images. If the radial diameter, as shown on coronal images through the body or central third of the meniscus, measures 13 mm from the capsular margin to the free edge, a discoid meniscus is probable.[25] Normally, the central coronal image displays the smallest radial cross section of the meniscal body, thus making this image sensitive to the enlargement seen in discoid menisci. In the presence of an effusion, the enlarged meniscus is outlined with high-signal-intensity fluid on T2-, T2*-, or STIR-weighted images. 3D FT axial images at less than 1-mm section thickness demonstrate the circumferential morphology of both incomplete and complete discoid menisci. Grade 2 signal intensity and discoid menisci may correlate with intrameniscal cavitation or cysts, and many orthopaedic surgeons recommend meniscectomy for a symptomatic discoid meniscus, even without grade 3 signal intensity. These menisci usually demonstrate a prominent and thickened grade 2 signal intensity that may correlate with an intrasubstance cleavage tear.

Pitfalls in Interpreting Meniscal Tears

Knowledge of the more common pitfalls encountered in MR imaging of the meniscus helps to maintain high specificity and accuracy of diagnostic interpretations of meniscal tears.[85,105–109]

GRADE 2 VERSUS GRADE 3 SIGNAL INTENSITY. In some cases, less than 5% in our experience, it may be difficult to distinguish articular surface extension of signal intensity. In such cases, evaluation of the morphology of the meniscus as well as the degree and thickness of increased intensity may facilitate a more accurate interpretation. Weakening or decreased signal intensity of a grade 3 lesion as it approaches an articular surface, for example, favors a diagnosis of an intrasubstance cleavage tear that, at arthroscopy, might require surgical probing for detection. In the presence of a joint effusion, the grade 3 signal, which becomes more conspicuous on conventional T2 weighting, corresponds to a disrupted meniscal surface, which facilitates the influx of free water molecules (ie, T2 prolongation).

Radial imaging or radial reformatting of a 3D sequence may be helpful in patients with peripheral signal intensity or when grade 2 and grade 3 signal intensities cannot be differentiated. By providing a plane perpendicular to that seen on orthogonal sagittal images, extension to the superior or inferior surface of the meniscus or meniscal apex can be more easily determined.[29]

A less common pitfall involves a truncation artifact, which may mimic a meniscal tear when a 128×128 matrix with a 128-pixel phase-encoded axis is oriented in the superior-to-inferior direction.[110] These artifacts are minimized when a 192 or 256×256 matrix is used. A pseudotear may be seen when the high-signal-intensity artifact is projected over the low-signal-intensity meniscus.[111] This artifact is most conspicuous 2 pixels from the high contrast interface between the meniscus and the articular cartilage.

TRANSVERSE LIGAMENT. The transverse ligament of the knee, which connects the anterior horns of the medial and lateral meniscus, can simulate an oblique tear adjacent to the anterior horn of the lateral meniscus (Fig. 7-68). The transverse ligament originates anterolateral to the central rhomboid attachment of the lateral meniscus. The central rhomboid attachment of the anterior horn of the lateral meniscus may normally demonstrate linear increased signal intensity. On sagittal or axial images, the transverse ligament can be identified coursing between the tibial attachment of the ACL and Hoffa's infrapatellar fat pad to its insertion on the anterior superior aspect of the anterior horn of the medial meniscus (Fig. 7-69).

The transverse ligament varies in diameter and is absent in 40% of gross specimens. In up to 30% of MR examinations, the fat that surrounds the low-signal-intensity ligament mimics grade 3 signal intensity. In 15% of MR examinations, the transverse ligament can be followed in its entire medial-to-lateral extent.[111] Infrequently the medial extent of the transverse ligament may simulate a tear adjacent to the anterior horn of the medial meniscus (Fig. 7-70). 3D FT axial images, 1 mm or less, are most successful in demonstrating the entire course of the transverse ligament as a low-signal-intensity band traversing Hoffa's infrapatellar fat pad. 2D axial images obtained at thicker

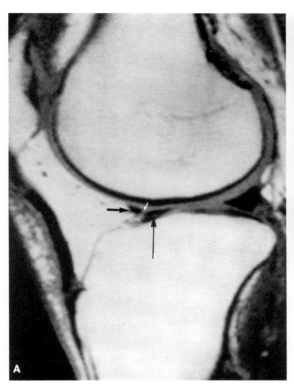

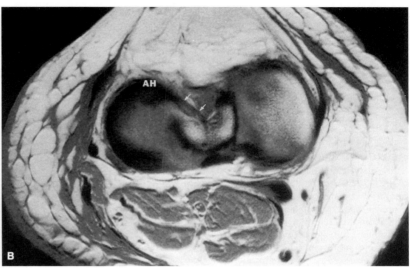

FIGURE 7-68. (A) A T1-weighted sagittal image of the transverse ligament of the knee shows an oblique pseudotear created by fat (*white arrow*) associated with the low-signal-intensity transverse ligament of the knee (*short black arrow*). Normal signal intensity is identified in the central rhomboid attachment of the anterior horn of the lateral meniscus (*long black arrow*). (B) A T1-weighted axial image shows central rhomboid attachment (*small arrows*) of the anterior horn (*AH*) of the lateral meniscus.

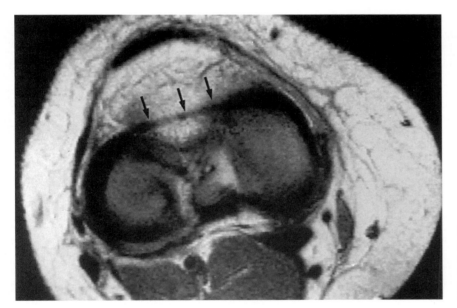

FIGURE 7-69. The low-signal-intensity transverse ligament of the knee is shown connecting the anterior horns of the medial and lateral menisci (*arrows*) on a T1-weighted axial image. The ligament is surrounded by high-signal-intensity fat in Hoffa's infrapatellar fat pad.

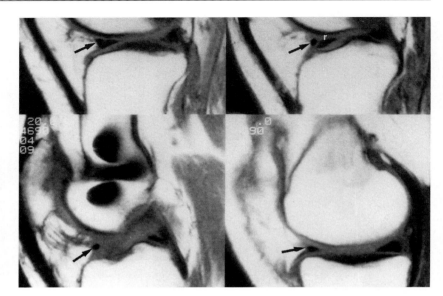

FIGURE 7-70. T1-weighted sagittal images show the transverse ligament (*arrows*) of the knee producing a pseudotear adjacent to the anterior horn of the lateral meniscus and the medial meniscus as it courses directly posterior to Hoffa's infrapatellar fat pad. Note the characteristic oblique line of intermediate signal intensity between the transverse ligament and lateral meniscus. The anterior horn of the lateral meniscus assumes a more rhomboid (*r*) shape at the site of its central ligamentous attachment to the tibia.

section show the course of the transverse ligament less reliably. On serial sagittal images, the round transverse ligament may be traced from the anterior horn of the lateral meniscus to the anterior horn of the medial meniscus.

Isolated tears of the anterior horn of the lateral meniscus can be easily differentiated from the transverse ligament pseudotear and are relatively uncommon compared to other meniscal tear locations. The central anterior ligamentous attachment of the anterior horn of the lateral meniscus may be mistaken for a meniscal tear. This attachment, which is

a rhomboid in shape, is normally directed obliquely upward on sagittal images and frequently contains increased internal signal intensity. It may be visualized on one or two sagittal images adjacent to the intercondylar notch and occurs near the origin of the transverse ligament.

Rarely, a prominent branch vessel from a lateral inferior geniculate artery will produce a pseudotear adjacent to the anterior horn of the lateral meniscus (Fig. 7-71). In the presence of a joint effusion, increased signal intensity may be present in the interface between the transverse ligament and

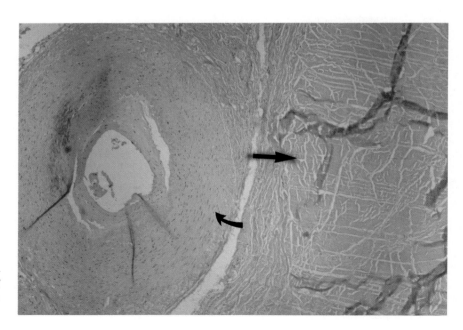

FIGURE 7-71. A photomicrograph shows proximity of the lateral inferior geniculate artery (*curved arrow*) to the lateral meniscus (*straight arrow*). (Hematoxylin and eosin stain.)

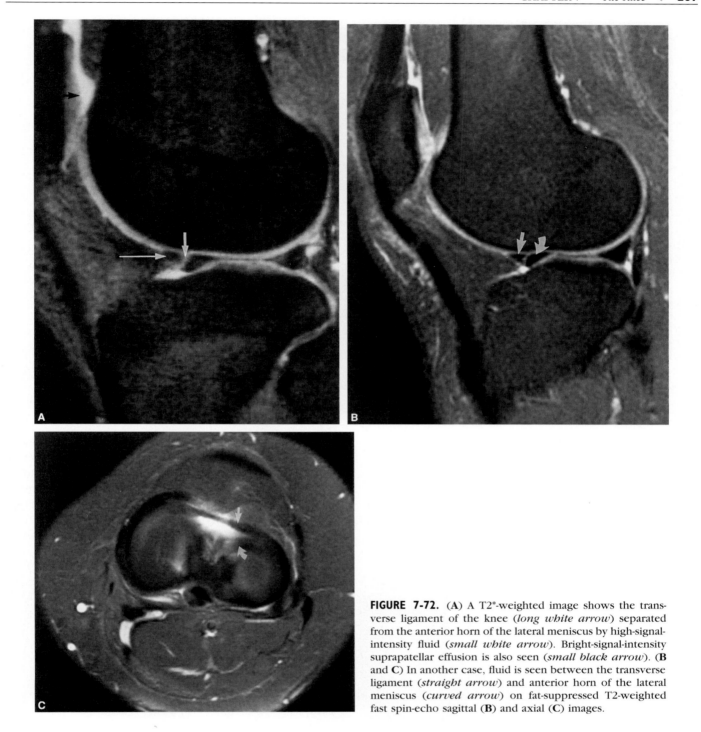

FIGURE 7-72. (A) A T2*-weighted image shows the transverse ligament of the knee (*long white arrow*) separated from the anterior horn of the lateral meniscus by high-signal-intensity fluid (*small white arrow*). Bright-signal-intensity suprapatellar effusion is also seen (*small black arrow*). (**B** and **C**) In another case, fluid is seen between the transverse ligament (*straight arrow*) and anterior horn of the lateral meniscus (*curved arrow*) on fat-suppressed T2-weighted fast spin-echo sagittal (**B**) and axial (**C**) images.

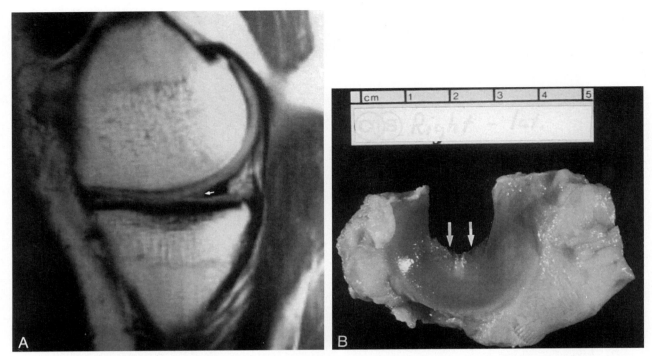

FIGURE 7-73. (**A**) Increased signal intensity restricted to the apex of the meniscus represents degenerative fibrillation or fraying (*arrows*). (**B**) The gross specimen shows a meniscus with fibrillation along the concave free edge (*arrows*).

the anterior horn of the lateral meniscus, especially on T2- or T2*-weighted images (Fig. 7-72).

FIBRILLATION. Fibrillation or fraying of the concave free edge of the meniscus facing the intercondylar notch is seen as increased signal intensity restricted to the apex of the meniscus in the presence of normal meniscal morphology

(Figs. 7-73 and 7-74). If, however, there is abnormal morphology (truncation or foreshortening of the meniscus), a meniscal tear is likely. Fat-suppressed T2-weighted fast spin-echo images are useful in defining the meniscal outline or morphology but are less sensitive to the detection of intrameniscal signal intensity. There may be cases where differentiation between MR characteristics of fraying and tearing

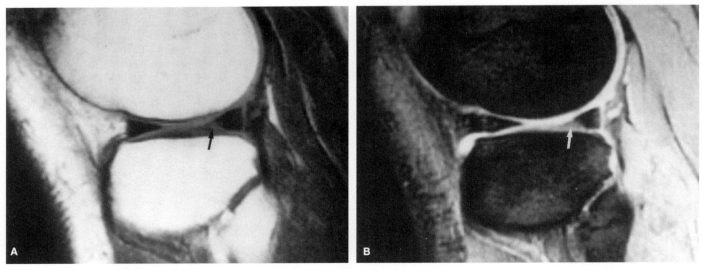

FIGURE 7-74. Free-edge fibrillation of the posterior horn of the lateral meniscus with an apex of increased signal intensity is seen on (**A**) T1-weighted and (**B**) T2*-weighted sagittal images. *continued*

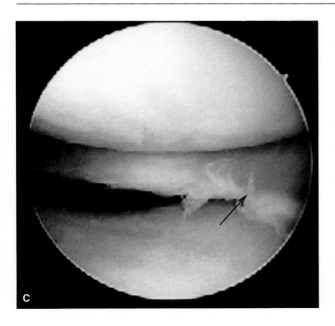

FIGURE 7-74. *Continued.* (**C**) The arthroscopic view also shows lateral meniscal fibrillation.

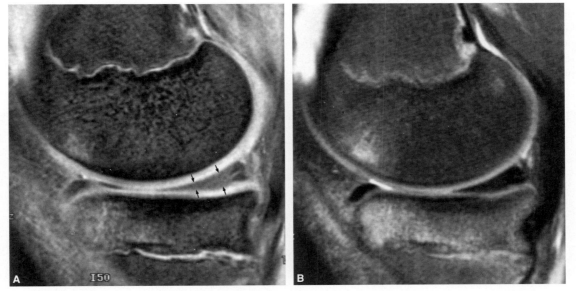

FIGURE 7-75. (**A**) Acute posttraumatic diffuse "meniscal edema" (*arrows*) is hyperintense on this T2*-weighted sagittal image. (**B**) The posterior horn of the medial meniscus, however, demonstrates normal morphology without tearing on a corresponding fat-suppressed T2-weighted fast spin-echo sagittal image. Associated anterior medial compartment bone contusions can be seen on this sequence.

of the meniscus are difficult.[87] A macerated meniscus imbibes synovial fluid throughout its substance and demonstrates a diffuse increase in signal intensity (multiple grade 3 tears). We have observed posttraumatic diffuse increased intrameniscal signal intensity without a discrete meniscal tear (Fig. 7-75).

POPLITEUS TENDON. In the posterior horn of the lateral meniscus, the popliteus tendon sheath may be mistaken for grade 3 signal intensity and can be falsely interpreted as a tear (Fig. 7-76). The popliteus tendon sheath is intermediate in signal intensity on T1- and T2-weighted images and courses in an oblique, anterosuperior-to-posteroinferior direction, anterior to the low-signal-intensity popliteus tendon (Fig. 7-77). In the presence of a joint effusion, fluid in the popliteus sheath demonstrates bright signal intensity on T2- or T2*-weighted images. In addition, the superior and inferior fascicles of the posterior horn of the lateral meniscus are best displayed on T2-weighted images (including fat-suppressed T2-weighted fast spin-echo or T2*-weighted sequences) in the presence of a joint effusion (Fig. 7-78). A fascicle tear should not be confused with the normal superior and inferior meniscocapsular defects, which allow passage of the popliteus tendon through the popliteus hiatus (Fig. 7-79). In the sagittal plane, the most lateral image through the popliteus tendon displays the anatomy of the inferior fascicle, with normal deficiency of the superior fascicle. More

medially, both the superior and inferior fascicles are visualized. The most medial image through the popliteus tendon and sheath displays the superior fascicle with normal deficiency of the inferior fascicle. The course of the popliteus muscle and tendon can be followed on serial axial, sagittal, and posterior coronal images. The thickness of the popliteus tendon sheath is variable and may be identified as a thin line or a thick band. A true peripheral lateral meniscal tear usually presents with a different obliquity than that described for the popliteus tendon sheath (Fig. 7-80). A vertical tear of the posterior horn of the lateral meniscus, however, may parallel the popliteus tendon sheath. In such cases, the popliteus tendon should be used as a landmark for the location of the peripheral edge of the meniscus. After lateral meniscectomy, the low-signal-intensity popliteus tendon may be mistaken for a retained posterior horn remnant. Continuity with the popliteus tendon helps to avoid this misdiagnosis.

PARTIAL VOLUME AVERAGING. The concave peripheral meniscal edge may produce the appearance of grade 2 signal intensity on peripheral sagittal images through the body of the meniscus.[107] This appearance is more commonly seen in the medial meniscus and is caused by partial volume averaging of fat and neurovascular structures lying in the concavity of the meniscus. This artifact has been reported in up to 29% of medial and 6% of lateral menisci.[111] Corresponding thin-section radial or coronal images, however, display an

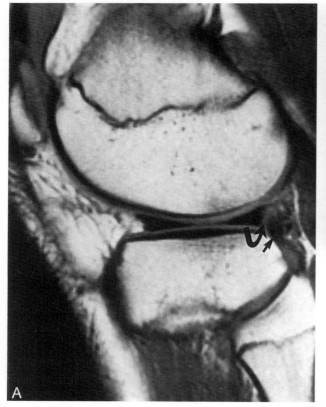

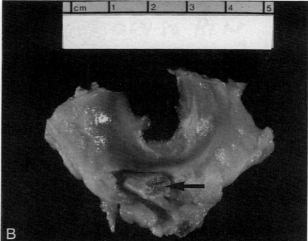

FIGURE 7-76. Popliteus tendon and sheath. **(A)** On a T1-weighted sagittal image, the popliteus tendon sheath (*curved arrow*) demonstrates intermediate signal intensity, and the popliteus tendon (*straight arrow*) demonstrates low signal intensity. **(B)** The corresponding gross specimen shows the course of the popliteus tendon (*arrow*) along the posterior horn of the lateral meniscus.

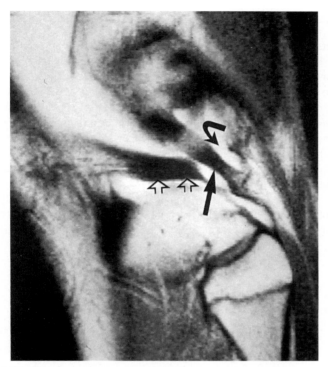

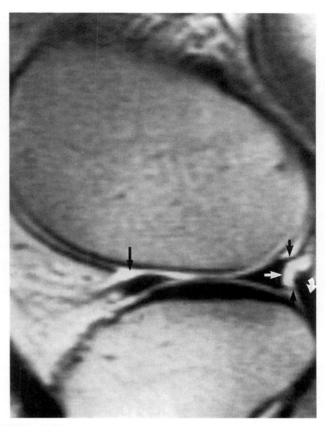

FIGURE 7-77. A T2-weighted peripheral sagittal image allows identification of the oblique course of the popliteus tendon (*straight arrow*) to its superior attachment along the lateral femoral condyle. The adjacent body of the lateral meniscus (*open arrows*) and high-signal-intensity synovial effusion (*curved arrow*) are shown.

FIGURE 7-78. A T2-weighted sagittal image demonstrates high-signal-intensity joint fluid reflected over the lateral meniscus (*large black arrow*) and contained within the popliteus sheath (*straight white arrow*). Lateral meniscal struts (*small black arrows*) and the popliteus tendon (*curved white arrow*) are also seen.

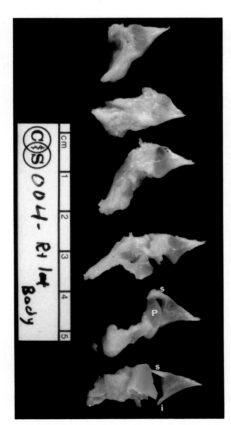

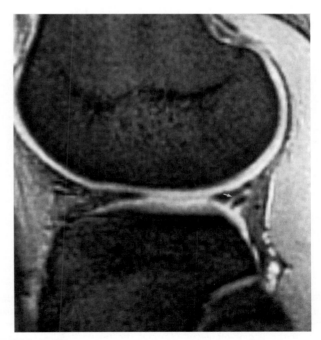

FIGURE 7-79. Examination of a gross anatomic specimen allows identification of the superior (*s*) and inferior (*i*) fascicles. The popliteus tendon (*P*) passes normally through defects in the inferior and superior fascicles.

FIGURE 7-80. A tear (*arrow*) of the posterior inferior corner of the lateral meniscus on a T2*-weighted sagittal image. The oblique direction of the tear is opposite to the expected course of the popliteus tendon.

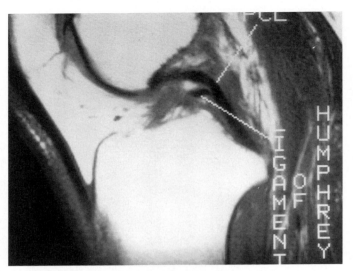

FIGURE 7-81. The low-signal-intensity ligament of Humphrey is prominent on a T1-weighted sagittal image.

intact meniscal structure and may display the concave margin of the meniscus.

MENISCOFEMORAL LIGAMENTS. Laterally, the meniscofemoral ligament (MFL) consists of the ligament of Humphrey, which extends anterior to the PCL, and a posterior branch of the ligament of Wrisberg, seen posterior to the PCL (Figs. 7-81 and 7-82). The MFL most commonly has direct attachment to the lateral meniscus and is obliquely oriented to its insertion on the medial femoral condyle. The posterior branch of the MFL, the ligament of Wrisberg, is the larger of the two branches and may appear to be half the cross-sectional diameter of the PCL.[111] The anterior me-

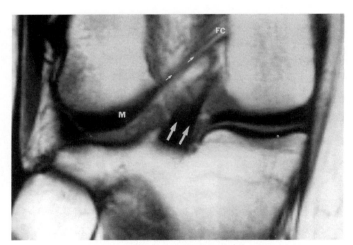

FIGURE 7-82. The ligament of Wrisberg (*small arrows*) and the PCL (*large arrows*) are seen on a T1-weighted posterior coronal image. The attachments of the ligament of Wrisberg to the posterior horn of the lateral meniscus (*M*) and the posteromedial femoral condyle (*FC*) are evident.

niscofemoral ligament has been reported to be present in 34% of anatomic dissections and the posterior meniscofemoral ligament in 60%. MR visualization has been reported in 33% of cases for either ligament, and in 3% of MR examinations both structures are identified. One branch of the meniscofemoral ligament usually predominates. The ligament of Humphrey can be best seen on sagittal images, whereas the ligament of Wrisberg is best shown on posterior coronal images. The ligament of Humphrey can, however, be identified on coronal images (Fig. 7-83).

Meniscal insertion of the meniscofemoral ligament may mimic the appearance of a vertical tear in the posterior horn of the lateral meniscus (Fig. 7-84).[108] This pseudotear, the

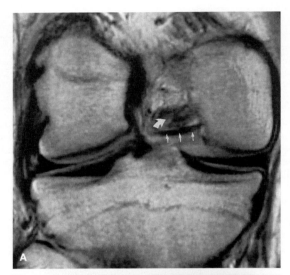

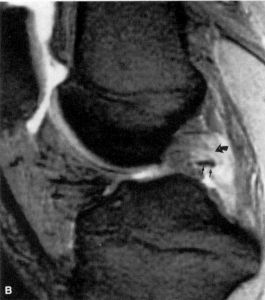

FIGURE 7-83. (**A**) Intermediate weighted coronal and (**B**) T2*-weighted sagittal images show the anatomy of the ligament of Humphrey (*straight arrows*). A complete tear of the PCL (*curved arrow*) is also present.

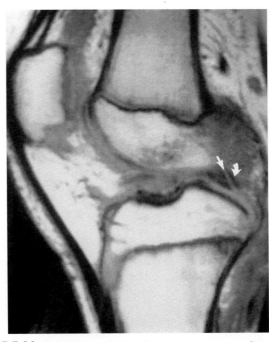

FIGURE 7-84. A pseudotear (*straight arrow*) is seen as a linear band of increased signal intensity on a T1-weighted sagittal image. This band is located between the superior articular surface of the posterior horn of the lateral meniscus and the meniscofemoral ligament (*curved arrow*).

result of fat interposed between the meniscus attachment and the meniscofemoral ligament, can be seen extending obliquely from the superior meniscal surface and is directed posteriorly and inferiorly toward the inferior meniscal surface. Less commonly, this pseudotear is seen as a vertical line parallel with the periphery of the meniscus.

PSEUDO–BUCKET-HANDLE TEAR.   Separate portions of the posterior horn may be mistaken for a lateral bucket-handle tear, because posterior coronal images traverse both the body and the posterior horn of the lateral meniscus, especially with the knee positioned in external rotation. This appearance is not usually encountered on posterior coronal images through the medial meniscus. Correlation with sagittal images will show normal meniscal morphology without tear.

PSEUDOHYPERTROPHY OF THE ANTERIOR HORN.   Complex meniscal tears may present with a unique MR appearance. In the lateral meniscus, the posterior horn may be absent or truncated, or it may be displaced or flipped anteriorly, occupying the space adjacent to the anterior horn (Fig. 7-85), creating pseudohypertrophy of the anterior horn fibrocartilage. This pattern is commonly seen in bucket-handle tears of the lateral meniscus.[74] The two meniscal horns are separated by an interface of fluid. The flipped posterior horn tissue is posterior to the anterior horn.

LAX MENISCAL SIGN.   Sometimes a lax or redundant folding or buckling of the meniscus contour is present without any associated fibrocartilage tear (Fig. 7-86). This finding is usually seen in the medial meniscus and is associated with a joint effusion and joint laxity, often secondary to fractures or ligamentous trauma. The lax or "buckled meniscus" may simulate a central or peripheral meniscal tear. However, this phenomenon may disappear with joint manipulation or subsequent imaging.

VACUUM PHENOMENON.   The magnetic susceptibility of normal amounts of intraarticular gas may produce a low-signal-intensity void or blooming artifact on gradient-echo images (Fig. 7-87). This artifact may be mistaken for a meniscal tear or articular cartilage injury.

PSEUDO–LOOSE BODY.   Normal intercondylar notch signal intensity may be mistaken for a loose body on T2*-weighted or fat-suppressed coronal or sagittal images. This pitfall is not a problem when T1-weighted images are correlated with corresponding gradient-echo or fat-suppressed images.

MCL BURSA.   The bursa of the MCL is seen between the periphery of the body of the medial meniscus and the MCL.[8]

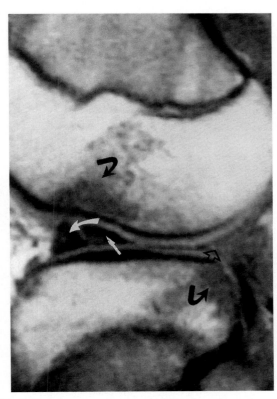

FIGURE 7-85. The posterior horn of the lateral meniscus (*open arrow*) is displaced toward (*straight arrow*) the anterior horn of lateral meniscus (*curved arrow*). Trabecular bone contusions are of low signal intensity relative to the adjacent bright fatty marrow epiphysis on a T1-weighted sagittal image.

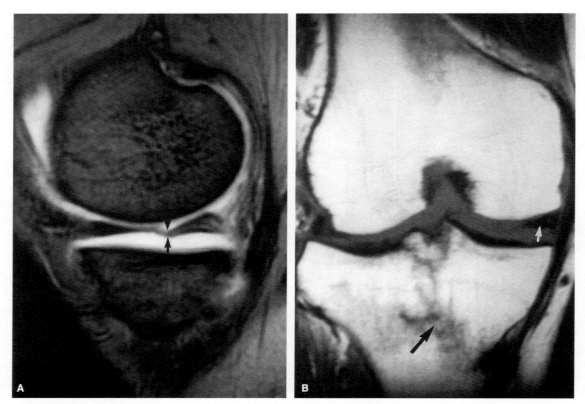

FIGURE 7-86. **(A)** A T2*-weighted sagittal image demonstrates that a wavy or folded contour may be a normal variant of the intact medial meniscus (*arrows*). **(B)** The corresponding T1-weighted coronal image reveals low-signal-intensity trabecular microfractures (*black arrow*) and a normal medial meniscus (*white arrow*).

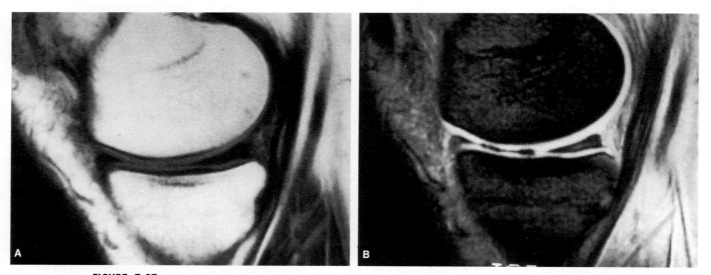

FIGURE 7-87. **(A)** A T1-weighted sagittal image shows the medial compartment vacuum phenomenon, with normal intraarticular gas identified as a thin linear area of signal void between the femoral and tibial articular cartilage. **(B)** A T2*-weighted sagittal image demonstrates blooming of the signal void, caused by magnetic-susceptibility effects of the intraarticular gas.

On T2-weighted images, fluid within the bursa may be falsely mistaken for a peripheral meniscocapsular tear.

MAGIC-ANGLE PHENOMENON. On short TE images, the magic-angle phenomenon may be responsible for increased signal intensity in the upward-sloping portion, or medial segment, of the posterior horn of the normal lateral meniscus.[109] This effect is demonstrated in meniscal sections oriented at approximately 55° relative to the static magnetic field (Bo) along the long axis of the magnet bore.

Treatment of Meniscal Tears

Meniscal repairs are frequently performed in conjunction with ACL reconstructions because of the association of meniscal tears with ACL-deficient knees. Results of meniscal repairs per-

formed in conjunction with ACL reconstructions are better than those of isolated meniscal repairs. The vascularity of the posterior horn of the lateral meniscus permits repair of complex tears. Injection of a fibrin clot can be used as an adjunct to certain repairs.[112,113] Meniscal tears that are considered definitely reparable are traumatic, are located within the peripheral third (the vascular zone), and have relative preservation of the body segment of the meniscus. These tears include vertical longitudinal and peripheral tear patterns (Fig. 7-88). Tears involving the avascular zone may not be suitable for repair. Open meniscal repair may be indicated for peripheral tears that occur within 1 to 2 mm of the meniscosynovial junction and involve the posterior third of the medial or lateral meniscus.[31] Nonoperative treatment may be indicated for partial-thickness split tears that involve less than 50% of the meniscal width and for full-thickness tears less than 5 mm in size with vertical or oblique tear patterns. Tears

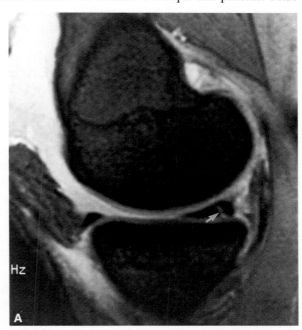

FIGURE 7-88. Meniscal repair. (**A**) A vertical tear (*arrows*) of the posterior horn of the medial meniscus located in the peripheral one third of the meniscus. (**B**) Corresponding arthroscopic views probing the peripheral meniscal tear (*arrow*). (**C**) Arthroscopic view of the primary suture repair (*arrow*).

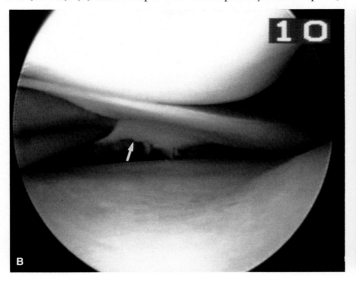

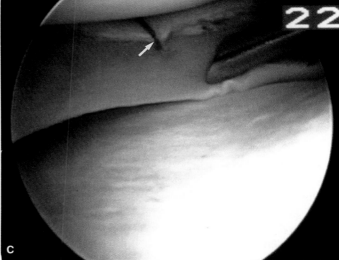

stable to arthroscopic probing (<3 mm of translation on arthroscopic palpation) and short radial tears less than 5 mm in length may not require resection.[47] There have been reports of patients in whom certain lateral meniscal tears (posterior horn avulsion tears, vertical tears posterior to the popliteus tendon, and stable vertical longitudinal and radial tears) were identified during ACL reconstruction and who had remained asymptomatic without treatment of their meniscal lesions.[114]

Partial meniscectomy is used to treat complex tears, degenerative tears, and large radial and flap tears.[47] In addition, avascular tears and tears associated with unstable ACL-deficient knees in patients older than 40 years are frequently treated by partial meniscectomy.[47] Meniscal repair may be used for vascular zone tears and for unstable peripheral longitudinal vertical tears greater than 1 cm in length, including displaced bucket-handle tears.[47] Indications for meniscal repair may be expanded to include tears in avascular portions of the meniscus in communication with peripheral synovium and perimeniscal capsular plexus. Techniques such as abrasion of the perimeniscal synovium, meniscal rasping, and implantation of exogenous fibrin clots have increased and expanded the criteria for meniscal repair. Most tear types with rim widths of up to 5 mm are considered candidates for meniscal repair, provided or contingent on their ability to be stabilized and coapted. Because of the importance of the lateral meniscus in load transmission and potential for severe degenerative disease in patients undergoing total lateral meniscectomy, meniscal repair techniques are usually attempted for most lateral meniscal tears.[44] The decision to perform a partial meniscectomy depends on the morphology of the tear and its extension to the free edge of the meniscus.[76] Horizontal tears should not be treated with primary meniscal repair. For longitudinal, vertical or bucket-handle tears, when meniscal repair is not indicated, a partial meniscectomy is performed in which the displaced portion of the meniscus is reduced with a probe before resection of the meniscus until stable tissue is exposed. A horizontal component is often present at the meniscal rim. Radial tears greater than 5 mm may be symptomatic and partially resected at arthroscopy. Although usually associated with horizontal tears, meniscal cysts may be associated with deep radial tears. Partial meniscectomy with removal of a flap is performed in oblique tears. The stability of the remaining portion of the meniscus can be tested with a probe at arthroscopy and varies as a function of the horizontal and vertical component to the tear. In horizontal cleavage tears, if one leaf is unstable, it is resected leaving the stable leaf. A 3-mm flap may be left.

MENISCAL TRANSPLANTATION. Meniscal transplantation, developed by Garrett and associates, is used to delay the development of degenerative disease after meniscectomy.[115] In this procedure, age and size matched allograft menisci are sutured to the resected meniscal rim. The anterior and posterior meniscal horn and meniscotibial attachments are preserved so that they can function as firm anchors for the

generation of hoop stresses. This technique is indicated in young patients who have undergone total meniscectomy and who are likely to develop degenerative arthrosis by middle age. Degenerative arthrosis develops more rapidly after lateral meniscectomy than after medial meniscectomy.

Meniscal transplantation also contributes to stability in ACL-deficient knees with absent medial menisci and fibrocartilage. It may also contribute to preservation of joint function as part of a three-stage reconstruction that includes the repair of the meniscus, the ACL, and any associated osteochondral lesion.

MR is presently used to evaluate the integrity of the transplant and allograft, to determine proper sizing, and to follow peripheral healing at the suture site. During the process of peripheral revascularization after meniscal transplantation, persistent grade 3 signal intensity may be seen (Fig. 7-89).

POSTOPERATIVE APPEARANCE OF THE MENISCUS. The postoperative evaluation of partial meniscectomies and primary repair offers unique challenges for MR imaging (Fig. 7-90). Correlation of MR findings with preoperative MR studies or details of the arthroscopic surgery is useful in increasing the accuracy of MR diagnosis of a retear (Fig. 7-91), persistent tear (Fig. 7-92), or a normal healing response to the meniscal fibrocartilage. It may be difficult to identify tears in the meniscal remnants after a partial meniscectomy. Even in the absence of a retear, the meniscal remnant may demonstrate a residual grade 3 signal intensity. Long TE or T2-weighted spin-echo images or T2* gradient-

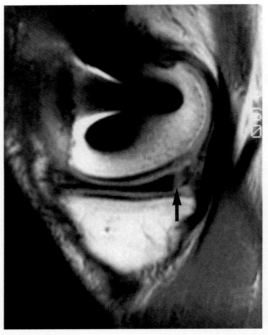

FIGURE 7-89. A T1-weighted sagittal image shows that peripheral grade 3 signal intensity (*arrow*) in a postmeniscal transplant represents suture attachment with healing, not a vertical tear.

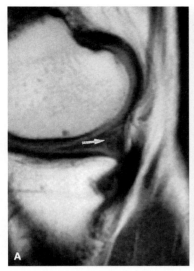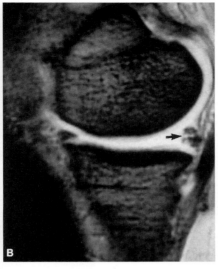

FIGURE 7-90. (**A**) Sagittal T1-weighted and (**B**) T2*-weighted images show normal residual grade 3 signal intensity (*arrow*) in a partial remnant from a posterior horn medial meniscectomy. This intensity does not represent a retear in this stable meniscal rim.

echo images can be used to identify fluid directly extending into the cleavage plane of a tear in a meniscal remnant. This finding is more specific than the presence of grade 3 signal intensity on short TE or T1-weighted images. A sharp, blunt, surgical truncation of the apex of the meniscus with foreshortening is often seen with partial meniscectomy (Fig. 7-93). The meniscal tissue, however, may be contoured so that the remnant is identified without obvious blunting (Figs. 7-94 and 7-95). There may also be residual signal intensity if one or both leaves of a cleavage component of a tear are removed. We have successfully used fat-suppressed T2-weighted fast spin-echo images to display the morphology of the postoperative meniscus with decreased magnetic sus-

ceptibility artifact in comparison with gradient-echo techniques. It is important, however, to recognize the limitation of fast spin-echo technique in accurately identifying intrameniscal signal intensity and it should be used in conjunction with either T1, T2 or gradient-echo images. Postoperative meniscal fragments adjacent to the site of a meniscectomy may also be identified with MR imaging, especially using techniques of fast spin-echo with fat suppression or conventional T2 spin-echo images. No meniscal tissue is seen after a total meniscectomy (Fig. 7-96). The joint space left after removal of fibrocartilage may be occupied with fluid. Associated MR findings after meniscectomy include joint space

text continues on page 302

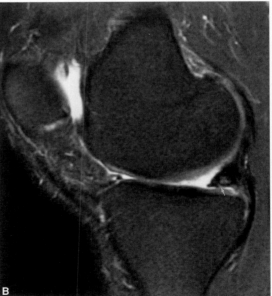

FIGURE 7-91. A retear (*arrow*) of the posterior horn remnant at the meniscal free edge. (**A**, T2*-weighted sagittal image; **B**, fat-suppressed T2-weighted fast spin-echo sagittal image.)

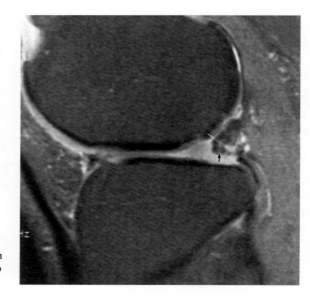

FIGURE 7-92. Persistent grade 3 signal intensities (*arrows*) in the posterior horn remnant of the lateral meniscus. (Fat-suppressed T2-weighted fast spin-echo sagittal image.)

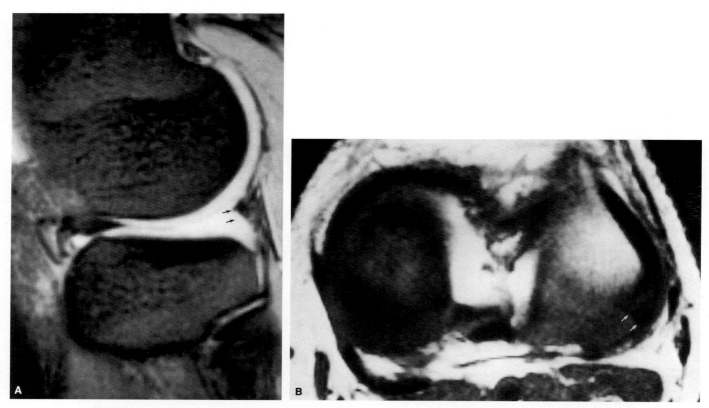

FIGURE 7-93. (**A**) A partial lateral meniscectomy with a posterior horn remnant (*arrows*) is seen on a T2*-weighted sagittal image. (**B**) An abrupt lateral meniscus surgical defect (*arrows*) is revealed on a T1-weighted axial image.

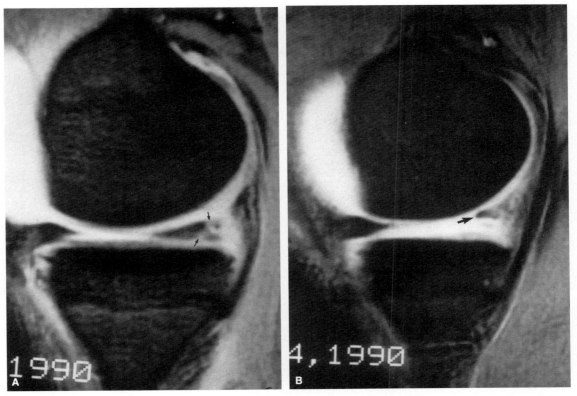

FIGURE 7-94. **(A)** A complex tear (*arrows*) that involves the posterior horn of the medial meniscus is shown on a T2*-weighted sagittal image. Superior and inferior surface extension are present. **(B)** A small, contoured posterior horn remnant (*arrow*) remains after partial meniscectomy, as demonstrated on a T2*-weighted sagittal image.

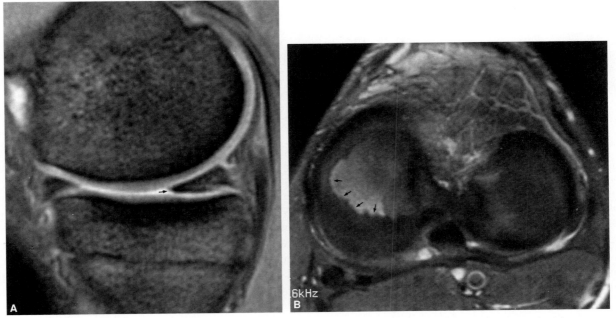

FIGURE 7-95. **(A)** Minimal blunting of the posterior horn of the medial meniscus (*arrow*) on a T2*-weighted sagittal image. **(B)** An area of meniscal contouring (*arrows*) is shown on a fat-suppressed T2-weighted fast spin-echo axial image.

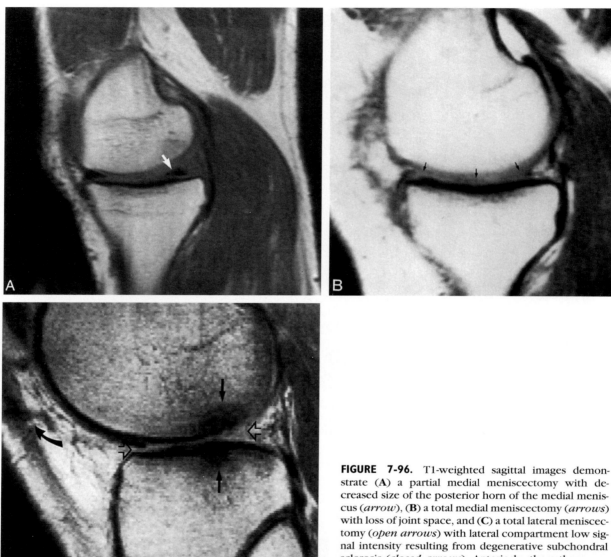

FIGURE 7-96. T1-weighted sagittal images demonstrate **(A)** a partial medial meniscectomy with decreased size of the posterior horn of the medial meniscus (*arrow*), **(B)** a total medial meniscectomy (*arrows*) with loss of joint space, and **(C)** a total lateral meniscectomy (*open arrows*) with lateral compartment low signal intensity resulting from degenerative subchondral sclerosis (*closed arrows*). Anteriorly, the arthroscopy track is seen as an area of low signal intensity (*curved arrow*).

narrowing with articular cartilage loss (Fig. 7-97) and subchondral low signal intensity in the involved compartment before the appearance of plain-film sclerosis. Subchondral changes may display increased signal intensity on corresponding STIR or fat-suppressed fast spin-echo images during stages of reactive hyperemia. Flattening or posterior ridging of the femoral condyles and tibial marginal spurring and sclerosis (indicative of previous meniscectomy) are later findings that have also been reported in plain-film evaluation.[47]

Smith and colleagues have divided the MR characteristics of partial meniscectomy into three groups.[116] Group 1 menisci demonstrate near-normal length but no osteoarthri-

tis. Group 2 menisci are significantly shortened, also without osteoarthritis (see Fig. 7-94). Group 3 menisci may be any length but they demonstrate the development of osteoarthritis (Fig. 7-98). In group 2 menisci, contour irregularities simulated meniscal fragmentation in 40% of segments studied; therefore, no rigid criteria for diagnosis of tearing in meniscal segments with partial meniscectomy contour irregularities were established in this study. Regenerated meniscal tissue (ie, rim) is composed of fibrous tissue, is smaller than normal, and demonstrates low to intermediate signal intensity on T1-, T2-, or T2*-weighted images.

Applegate and colleagues have reported an 88% accuracy for the diagnosis of recurrent tears in the postoperative me-

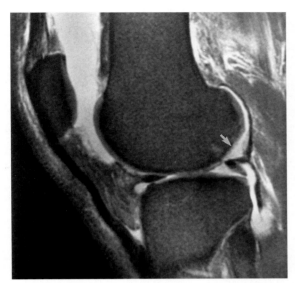

FIGURE 7-97. Loss of lateral femoral condyle articular cartilage (*arrow*) opposite the lateral meniscus posterior horn remnant as shown on a fat-suppressed T2-weighted fast spin-echo sagittal image.

niscus with MR arthrography compared with an overall accuracy of 66% when conventional MR imaging was used.[30] MR arthrography was particularly useful in characterizing small meniscal remnants.

Primary meniscal repairs may show grade 1, grade 2, or persistent grade 3 signal intensities on postoperative MR (Fig. 7-99).[117-119] Second-look arthroscopy has shown that healed meniscal repair may demonstrate grade 3 signal intensity, making postoperative characterization of primary repairs difficult (Fig. 7-100).[117] Intraarticular gadolinium may be helpful in identifying imbibed synovial fluid extending into menisci that are retorn after primary repair (Fig. 7-101), according to the same principle underlying the use of long

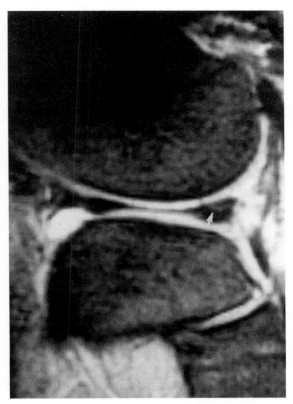

FIGURE 7-99. A T2*-weighted sagittal image made after primary repair of the lateral meniscus shows absence of signal intensity in the posterior horn.

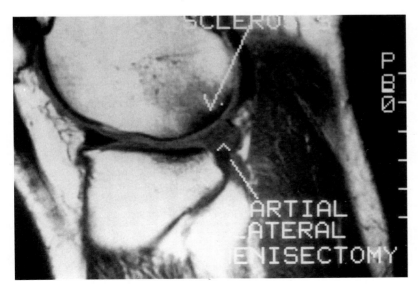

FIGURE 7-98. On a T1-weighted sagittal image, low-signal-intensity subchondral sclerosis is seen in the posterior lateral femoral condyle after a partial lateral meniscectomy.

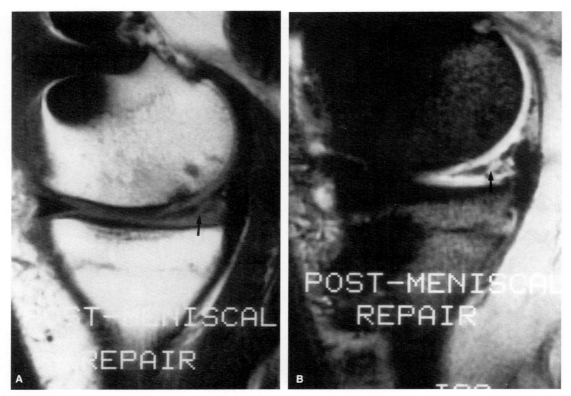

FIGURE 7-100. (**A**) Sagittal T1-weighted and (**B**) T2*-weighted images show residual grade 3 signal intensity (*arrow*) after primary repair of the meniscus. No retear was found at second-look arthroscopy.

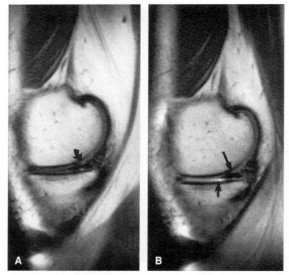

FIGURE 7-101. (**A**) Pre- and (**B**) postintraarticular gadolinium-enhanced T1-weighted sagittal images show an intact posterior horn after primary meniscal repair of a bucket-handle tear. High-signal-intensity gadolinium coats the articular cartilage (*small straight arrow*) adjacent to the intact posterior horn (*large straight arrow*). A suture artifact is shown on the unenhanced image (*curved arrow*).

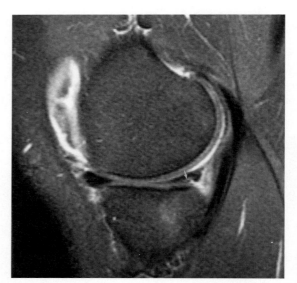

FIGURE 7-102. Intravenous gadolinium enhancement facilitates identification of grade 3 signal intensity (*arrow*) extending to the irregular inferior surface of the postoperative meniscus on a fat-suppressed T1-weighted image.

TE or T2-weighted images to identify the direct extension of fluid into the cleavage plane of a tear to help increase diagnostic accuracy. Both intravenous and intraarticular gadolinium have already been used to improve characterization of recurrent tears and meniscal surfaces (Fig. 7-102).[30,120]

Second-look arthroscopic examination of postprimary menisci has also shown that there may be conversion of grade 3 signal intensity into lower grades of signal intensity, primarily in areas of fibrovascular healing corresponding to the conversion of granulation or scar tissue to normal fibrocartilage. This process is known to occur over a period of months. Arnoczky and colleagues evaluated MR signals in healing menisci in dogs.[119] They found that in full-thickness radial tears, the normal fibrovascular scar tissue or repair tissue generated increased signal intensity on MR that persisted at 26 weeks even though this fibrovascular repair tissue had converted from scar into fibrocartilage. This study supports the observation that normal fibrovascular repair tissue as well as conversion of fibrovascular repair tissue to fibrocartilage may demonstrate persistent grade 3 signal intensity in healing menisci. The findings, by Deutsch and colleagues, of persistent signal intensity up to 27 months

postoperatively demonstrate that the repair process from fibrovascular tissue to fibrocartilage is protracted and may even be chronic.[117] It has been suggested that characterization of the time course for meniscal repair and its relation to persistent MR signal intensity needs further study.[30]

Miscellaneous Meniscal Pathology

Meniscocapsular Separations

Meniscocapsular separations or tears usually involve the less mobile medial meniscus (Fig. 7-103).[105] The thick medial third of the joint capsule or medial capsular ligament is divided into meniscofemoral and meniscotibial components.[121] These fibers are separated from the superficial fibers of the MCL by an interposed bursa and can best be seen on radial images through the medial compartment of the knee. The meniscocapsular junction is poorly seen on routine orthogonal coronal images, especially when using a T1-weighted technique. The posterior horn of the medial meniscus, fixed to the tibia by meniscotibial or coronary ligaments,

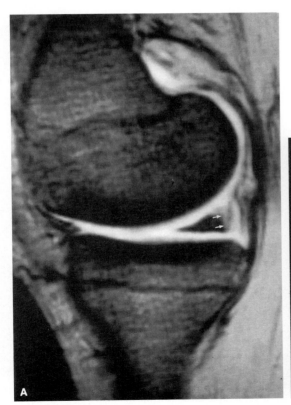

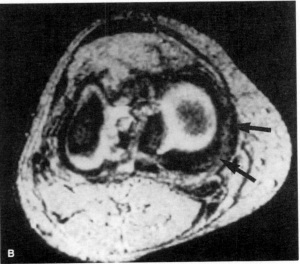

FIGURE 7-103. A meniscocapsular tear. **(A)** A T2*-weighted sagittal image shows a thin linear vertical signal in the posterior horn of the medial meniscus (*arrows*). **(B)** A 0.7-mm 3D FT T2*-weighted axial image shows peripheral meniscocapsular increased signal intensity. **(C)** The corresponding 3D MR rendering reveals a meniscocapsular tear (*arrows*). **(D)** On arthroscopy, separation of the meniscus from the capsule (*curved arrow*) is seen. *F*, femur; *T*, tibia.

continued

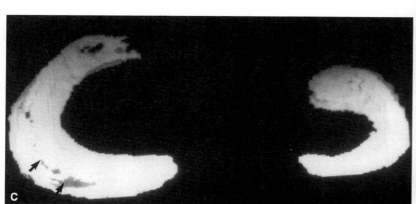

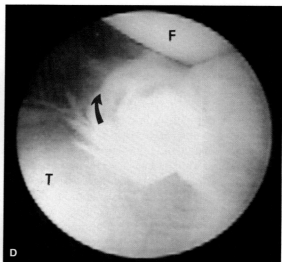

FIGURE 7-103. *Continued*

is especially susceptible to tearing at its capsular attachment. Even in the absence of grade 3 signal intensity through the meniscus, a separation at the meniscocapsular junction may have clinical significance in patient care if associated with pain.

Small or nondisplaced meniscocapsular tears may heal without surgical intervention because these tears occur through the vascularized periphery of the meniscus, adjacent to the perimeniscal capillary plexus.[64] Minor repair of these lesions also has a high success rate because of their peripheral location.

On sagittal MR images, the tibial plateau articular cartilage should be covered by the posterior horn of the medial meniscus without an exposed articular cartilage surface. Displacement of the posterior horn of the medial meniscus by 5 mm or more, uncovered tibial articular cartilage, or fluid interposed between the peripheral edge of the meniscus and capsule are suggestive of peripheral detachment.[64] Uncovering of the tibial articular cartilage, however, is not a specific sign for meniscocapsular injury, and quantitative measurements of meniscal displacement may be unreliable (Fig. 7-104). In addition, the meniscus may have fluid within the superior and inferior capsular recesses without violation of the meniscocapsular junction (Fig. 7-105). In cases of meniscocapsular separations, T2, fast spin-echo T2, or gradient-echo sagittal images may show fluid between the peripheral portion of the posterior horn of the medial meniscus and the joint capsule. Coronal images, and especially radial coronal images, best display the anatomy of the deep capsular layer and its relation to the meniscus for identification of disruptions of the meniscofemoral and meniscotibial ligaments. MCL tears may be associated with meniscocapsular tears; in these patients radial imaging is also useful to supplement

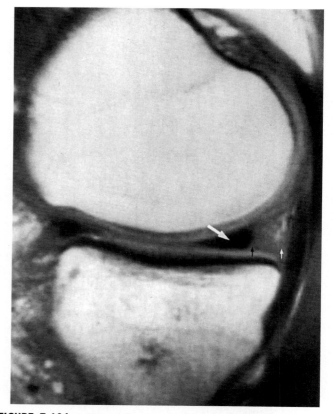

FIGURE 7-104. A T1-weighted sagittal image shows meniscocapsular separation with exposure of tibial cartilage. The periphery of the meniscus (*black arrow*) should cover the periphery of the hyaline cartilage surface (*small white arrow*). The posterior horn of the medial meniscus (*large white arrow*) is identified. This finding may be nonspecific and should be correlated with T2-weighted coronal images.

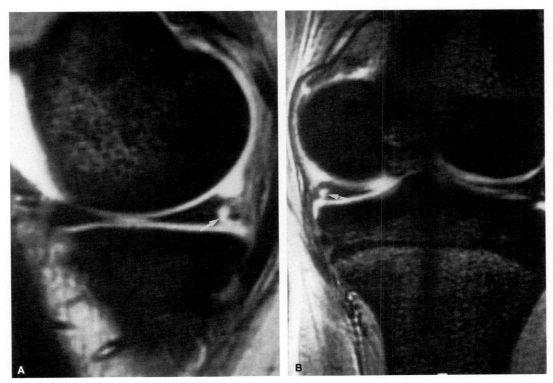

FIGURE 7-105. A peripheral vertical tear (*arrow*) involving the inferior surface of the posterior horn of the medial meniscus as seen on T2*-weighted (**A**) sagittal and (**B**) radial images. This degree of vertical signal intensity is abnormal and does not represent a meniscal recess.

coronal and sagittal images. A complete peripheral detachment of the posterior horn is seen as a free-floating meniscus, especially if it is associated with a MCL tear (Figs. 7-106 and 7-107).

Meniscal Cysts

Cysts of the meniscus have been reported in 1% of meniscectomies.[8,25] Cysts associated with the meniscus can be classified into intrameniscal cysts, parameniscal cysts, and synovial cysts. Meniscal cysts are also referred to as ganglion cysts, a nonspecific and less descriptive term. Intrameniscal cysts are uncommon and represent intrameniscal fluid collections in continuity with meniscal tears (Fig. 7-108). The more common parameniscal cysts most frequently present as loculated or simple fluid collections located at the periphery of the meniscus, commonly with a horizontal cleavage tear pattern on cross section. Synovial cysts are rare and are not associated with meniscal tears. They represent cystic outpouchings of the joint capsule.[25]

Parameniscal cysts usually present at the level of the joint line, either as a focal mass or a swelling. They may develop in response to trauma or degeneration and are associated with meniscectomy.[122,123] One theory holds that injuries or trauma generate tangential or compressive forces that initiate necrosis in the central peripheral aspect of the meniscus leading to mucoid degeneration and cyst development.

Lateral parameniscal cysts are three to seven times more common than medial cysts, and they often present at the medial third of the peripheral margin of the meniscus. The difference in the prevalence of lateral and medial meniscal cysts may be exaggerated because of underreporting of medial cysts, which are less likely to cause symptoms. Diagnostic use of MR for meniscal lesions should provide more accurate statistics about these cysts.

Medial cysts tend to be larger than lateral meniscal cysts and dissect through soft tissue (ie, joint capsule and MCL), often presenting in a different location than the meniscus tear origin. Medial meniscal cysts can been seen extending from the posterior horn and dissecting peripherally to present in a more anterior location (Fig. 7-109). A thin stalk in continuity with the meniscus can usually be identified in these cases. A horizontal meniscal tear or flap tear with a primarily horizontal component frequently communicates with a meniscal cyst with decompression of synovial fluid (see Fig. 7-108). Ninety percent of lateral meniscal cysts are associated with a horizontal flap or a horizontal cleavage tear. Lateral meniscal cysts are usually located anterior to the LCL or between the LCL and popliteus tendon. Medial meniscal cysts are usually found deep to the MCL or in the posteromedial corner deep to the posterior oblique ligament. In the medial meniscus, if

text continues on page 311

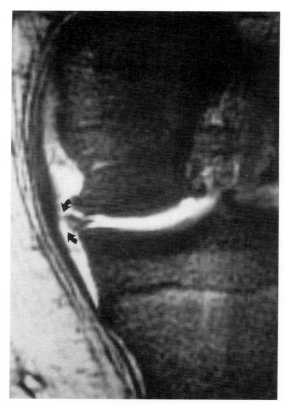

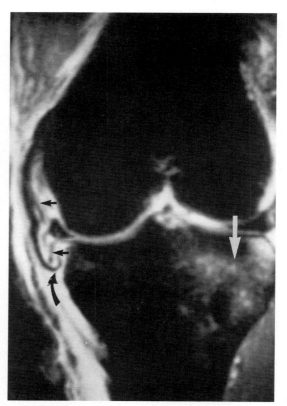

FIGURE 7-106. Meniscocapsular separation occurs with peripheral capsular detachment to the medial meniscus. Fluid signal intensity extends freely between the MCL and the meniscus (*arrows*) on all T2*-weighted radial images.

FIGURE 7-107. A complete tear (*curved arrow*) of the superficial layer of the distal MCL is shown on a STIR coronal image. The deep medial capsular layer is represented by the torn meniscofemoral and meniscotibial attachments (*small straight black arrows*). A lateral tibial plateau contusion is also shown (*white arrow*).

FIGURE 7-108. A horizontal tear of the medial meniscus communicates with a posteromedial meniscal cyst (*arrow*). The cyst is of low signal intensity on the T1-weighted coronal image (**A**) and is hyperintense on the T2*-weighted sagittal image (**B**).

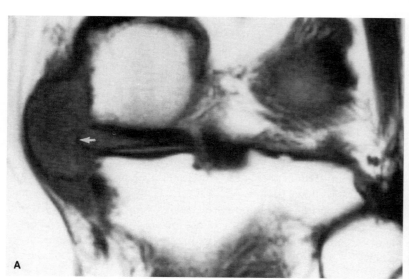

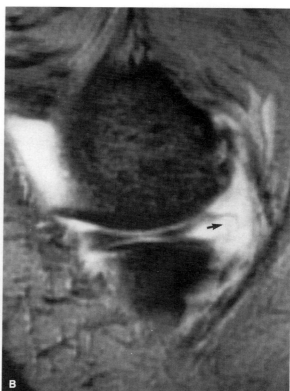

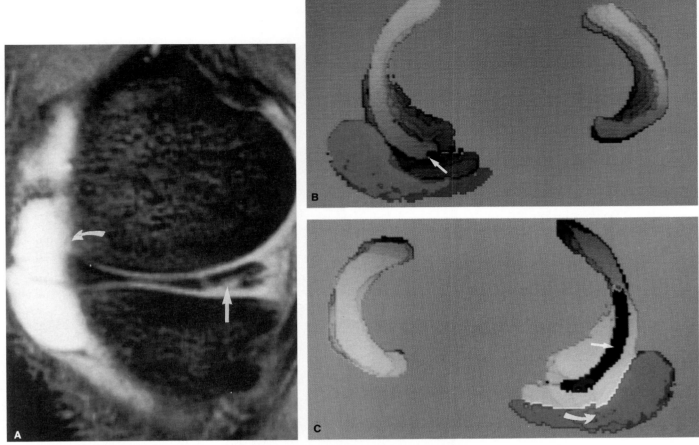

FIGURE 7-109. (**A**) A T2*-weighted sagittal image shows a complex tear (*straight arrow*) of the posterior horn of the medial meniscus. The tear has both horizontal and vertical components. An associated hyperintense meniscal cyst (*curved arrow*) projects anteriorly with a peripheral extension following the convex contour of the posterior horn and body of the meniscus. (**B** and **C**) On a 3D MR rendering, the superior (**B**) and the inferior (**C**) surface views show a corresponding meniscal cyst (*blue and curved arrow*) in communication with a posterior horn medial meniscus tear (*straight arrow*).

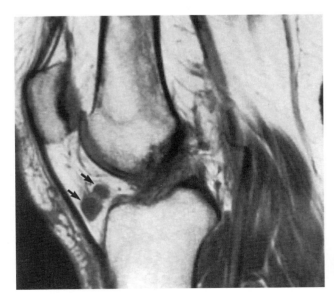

FIGURE 7-110. A bilobed meniscal cyst (*arrows*) is seen dissecting through Hoffa's infrapatellar fat pad. The synovial fluid contents are of low signal intensity on this T1-weighted sagittal image.

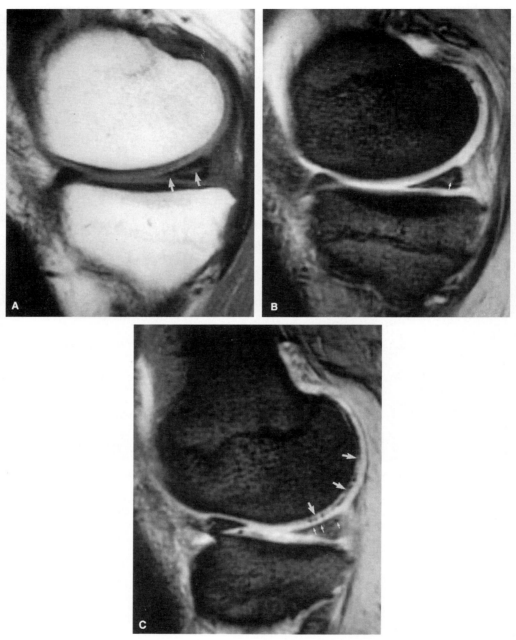

FIGURE 7-111. Chondrocalcinosis. (**A**) On a T1-weighted sagittal image the posterior horn of the medial meniscus shows grade 3 signal intensity (*arrows*). (**B**) On the corresponding T2*-weighted sagittal image, chondrocalcinosis dampens the meniscal signal intensity (*arrow*) as a result of localized magnetic susceptibilities. (**C**) On a T2*-weighted sagittal image through the lateral compartment, multiple foci of deposition resulting from calcium pyrophosphate disease are evident within the articular cartilage (*large arrows*) and the meniscus (*small arrows*).

continued

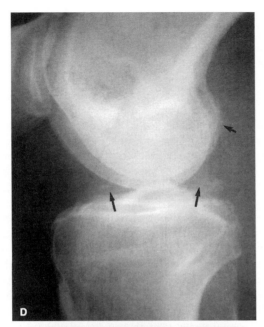

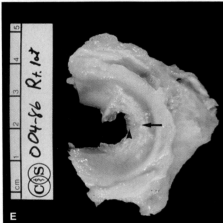

FIGURE 7-111. *Continued.* (**D**) On the corresponding lateral radiograph, chondrocalcinosis is evident in a region of meniscal fibrocartilage (*large arrows*) and articular cartilage (*small arrow*). (**E**) On a gross meniscal specimen, deposition resulting from chondrocalcinosis is seen in the lateral meniscus (*arrow*). Degenerative free edge of the meniscus is shown (*arrowhead*).

there is peripheral propagation of mucoid degeneration, the meniscus may appear intact without tear in the presence of an associated external cyst.

Meniscal cysts are uniformly low in signal intensity on T1-weighted images and increase in signal intensity on fat-suppressed T2-weighted fast spin-echo images, T2* gradient-echo images, or STIR images. Because cysts may also contain bloody or gelatinous fluid with an increased protein content, there may be some variation in their signal intensity properties on T2-type sequences relative to the appearance and imaging characteristics of free synovial fluid.[8] Loculations or septations may be seen, especially in complex

meniscal cysts, usually in those cysts removed in distance from their site of origin (meniscal tear) (Fig. 7-110).

The differential diagnosis for parameniscal cysts should include osteophytic spurring, synovial cyst formation, proximal tibiofibular cysts, traumatic bursitis, and masses (including pigmented villonodular synovitis [PVNS], hemangioma, lipoma, and synovial sarcoma).[124] Although aggressive malignant lesions such as synovial sarcomas may show hyperintensity on T2-weighted images, they tend to have a lower and more inhomogeneous signal intensity relative to that of synovial fluid. Sometimes synovial sarcomas mimic the appearance of a hemorrhagic or highly proteinaceous fluid collection.

Chondrocalcinosis

In chondrocalcinosis, meniscal calcifications are usually identified with conventional radiographic techniques. In patients with calcium pyrophosphate disease, MR studies using high contrast settings for photography revealed focal, low-signal-intensity calcification separate from adjacent low-signal-intensity meniscus. On T2*-weighted images, local susceptibility artifacts are seen around the foci of calcium pyrophosphate deposition, making them easier to identify (Fig. 7-111). Because of local magnetic susceptibility, however, crystals resulting from calcium pyrophosphate disease in either the meniscus or articular cartilage may dampen the signal intensity for meniscal degenerations and tears, falsely producing grade 2 signal intensity in a patient with grade 3 signal intensity on corresponding T1-weighted images. This possibility limits the usefulness of gradient-echo imaging in the evaluation of degenerative menisci. Dicalcium phosphate dihydrate, hydroxyapatite, and calcium oxalate are also responsible for cartilaginous calcifications.[43] A meniscal ossicle is larger and occurs as an isolated focus in asymptomatic patients without a history of antecedent trauma (Fig. 7-112).[119] On MR the marrow-containing corticated ossicle can be seen within the posterior horn of the medial meniscus.

CRUCIATE LIGAMENTS

Anterior Cruciate Ligament (ACL)

Functional Anatomy of the ACL

The cruciate ligaments are intracapsular and extrasynovial. The ACL and PCL are enveloped by a fold of synovium that takes origin from the posterior intercondylar area of the knee.[125] Proximally, the ACL is attached to a fossa on the posteromedial aspect of the lateral femoral condyle.[121,125] At its origin, the ACL is 16 to 24 mm in diameter, located posteriorly within the intercondylar notch.[125] Distally the ACL extends inferior and medial to the anterior tibial intercondylar area and attaches to a fossa anterior and lateral to

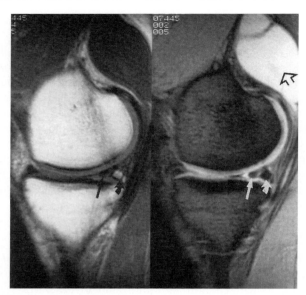

FIGURE 7-112. The meniscal ossicle (*curved arrow*) shows bright marrow-fat signal intensity on a T1-weighted sagittal image (*left*) and low signal intensity on a T2*-weighted sagittal image (*right*). The blunted apex of the posterior horn (*straight arrow*) is indicated. A popliteal cyst is seen with increased signal intensity on the T2*-weighted sagittal image (*open arrow*).

the anterior tibial spine, between the anterior attachments of the menisci. The center of origin of the ACL is 15 mm from the junction of the posterior femoral shaft and the proximal aspect of the lateral femoral condyle (defined as the "over-the-top" position). This over-the-top position is a critical landmark in the placement of the femoral tunnel when reconstructing the ACL. The ACL is 11 mm wide and 31 to 38 mm long.[20] The tibial attachment of the ACL (broader or larger than the femoral attachment) passes deep to the transverse ligament of the knee.[125] It begins as the ACL starts to fan out in its proximal third.

The individual fascicles of the ACL are divided into two functional fiber bundles that do not exist as distinct structures on gross examination.[125–127] The longer and stronger AMB tightens with knee flexion, whereas the smaller and shorter PLB tightens with knee extension.[35] With knee flexion, the femoral attachment of the ACL assumes a more horizontal orientation resulting in AMB tightening and PLB loosening.[125] In flexion, the anteromedial fibers twist or spiral over the posterolateral fibers.[77] The continuum of dynamics between the AMB and PLB, results in some portion of the ACL being taut in both flexion and extension.[125] The ACL prevents anterior translation of the tibia and resists posterior translation of the femur. Both the anterior and PCLs regulate the screw-home mechanism of the knee.[128]

Mechanism of Injury of the ACL

ACL failure can occur during external rotation and abduction with hyperextension, direct forward displacement of the tibia, or internal rotation with the knee in full extension.[45]

With varus or valgus stress, the ACL is injured after collateral ligament failure. Forced valgus in external rotation is the most common mechanism of injury and causes disruption of the MCL and medial supporting structures.[20,129–131] Most ACL injuries are caused by a direct or contact mechanism of injury versus an indirect mechanism.[131] O'Donoghue's triad of ACL, MCL, and medial meniscus injuries is associated with the mechanism of valgus in external rotation, or the clip injury. Tears of the posterior horn of the lateral meniscus are also associated with these lesions and are considered more serious. The second most common mechanism of injury (occurring in 30% of patients) is hyperextension associated with a meniscus tear. A direct blow to the flexed knee with the ankle plantar flexed, as seen in turf injuries represents the third most common pattern of injury to the ACL. The PCL and posterior capsule may be damaged in severe contact hyperextension images. Posterolateral instability may be associated with disruption of the posterolateral complex. The frequency of noncontact or indirect mechanisms of injuries, as occur in downhill skiing, has significantly increased in the past 10 years. Isolated ACL injuries are less common but can occur with pivoting during deceleration, which causes forced internal rotation of the femur. The classic knee injury in skiing is a forward fall catching the inside edge of the ski, placing the knee in external rotation in valgus stress. There may be associated posterolateral complex and lateral meniscus injuries. In skiers, a forceful quadriceps contraction with passive anterior force applied through the forward movement of the ski boot may result in an isolated ACL injury.[20] Basketball and football players who suddenly decelerate to change direction can also produce an anterior drawer force on the proximal tibia from forceful quadriceps contraction. Noncontact isolated tears of the ACL are also seen in hyperextension injuries in basketball players who rebound and in gymnasts who miss a dismount.[131]

Associated Intraarticular Pathology

Meniscal tears are associated with 41% to 68% of acute isolated ACL injuries.[20,132–133] When this association occurs, the prognosis for successful meniscal repair performed in conjunction with the ACL reconstruction is improved.[134] Meniscal pathology is associated with 85% to 91% of chronic ACL-deficient knees.[135] Patients with acute ACL injuries are found to have a higher incidence of lateral meniscal tears, whereas medial meniscal tears are more common in patients with chronic ACL injuries.[136,137] Injury to the meniscus and articular cartilage, especially in the medial compartment of the knee, is associated with episodic anterior tibial subluxation.[20] Articular cartilage lesions, including erosions and chondral fractures of both medial and lateral compartments, have been observed in 23% of acute and 54% of chronic injuries.[133] In contrast to O'Donoghue's triad of injury to the ACL, MCL, and medial meniscus, Shelbourne and Nitz have demonstrated that present mechanisms of injury are more frequently represented by the triad of injury to the ACL, MCL, and lateral meniscus.[136]

Clinical Assessment of ACL Injury

Acute ACL tears are associated with acute hemarthrosis (75%) and an audible pop (34%) at the time of injury.[20,43] Hemarthrosis is evident within the first several hours in more than 70% of patients.[131] As the primary stabilizer for anterior tibial displacement, the ACL can resist loads as great as 2000 N with maximum loading.[20,138] The AMB of the ACL must be disrupted before a positive anterior drawer sign performed in 90° of knee flexion is demonstrated. The anterior drawer sign, however, usually requires associated disruption of the medial capsule.[139] In almost all patients with an ACL disruption, Lachman's sign is positive (ie, the result of an anterior drawer test performed between 15° to 30° of flexion is positive) and the result of the pivot-shift test performed with valgus stress and flexion is positive. Tests for anterolateral rotatory instability are designed to elicit the pivot-shift phenomenon (a momentary anterior subluxation of the tibia relative to the femur at 25° of knee flexion). However, the pivot-shift test is difficult to perform in an acutely injured knee with pain and muscle spasm producing guarding.[131] In isolated tears of the ACL, the classic anterior drawer sign may give a false-negative result because the medial tibial plateau and meniscus abut the convex surface of the medial femoral condyle in flexion, which limits anterior tibial translation. These isolated tears are best identified with Lachman's test.[46]

In subacute tears, adhesions or attachments to the PCL may result in decreased laxity on clinical testing. Partial tears of the ACL are present in 24% to 39% of ACL injuries and frequently involve the AMB. These tears commonly progress to complete tears within 1 year of the initial injury.[140] The KT-1000 arthrometer (Medmetric, San Diego, CA) and knee laxity tester (Ortho System, Hayward, CA) are instrument measurement systems that document anterior or posterior tibial displacement by tracking the tibial tubercle in relation to the patella.[131] When the knee is subjected to a 28 to 40 pound anterior load test, ACL ligament disruption is associated with anterior tibial translation or subluxation 3 mm greater in the involved knee than in the uninvolved knee. A grade I ACL tear represents intraligamentous injury without a change in ligament length. In a grade II ACL tear, there is intraligamentous injury and an increase in ligament length. A grade III ACL tear represents complete ligamentous disruption.

The ACL has limited intrinsic healing capacity possibly because of the heterogeneity of its collagen fibers or fibroblast function within a synovial environment.[128] This poor capacity for healing of the torn ACL may lead to chronic disability including stretching of secondary knee restraints, articular cartilage destruction and meniscal tearing.[140]

The majority of ACL injuries can be diagnosed from the history and physical examination by an experienced clinician. MR arthrometer measurements are usually used for confirmation. MR, in fact, is used primarily to evaluate associated lesions including the meniscal and chondral lesions in the ACL-deficient knee.[137] Arthroscopy may be indicated when examination results are equivocal. At arthroscopy, the ACL may appear to be intact if the proximal stump has remained within the intercondylar notch, adherent to the PCL.[131] Proper placement of the knee to identify the empty lateral wall and vertical strut signs (vertical orientation of retracted ligament fibers) can improve visualization of the torn ligament. In an animal model study to evaluate partially torn ACLs, positive findings on MR for ACL pathology combined with a normal arthroscopy did not necessarily represent a false-positive MR result. Instead, MR may be identifying intrasubstance tears not detected on gross inspection and examination of the ACL during arthroscopy.[141]

Radiography and Arthrography of the ACL

In routine radiography of acute ACL injuries, soft-tissue swelling and a joint effusion may be present. The lateral knee radiograph frequently shows irregularity in the contour of Hoffa's fat pad, similar to the irregular fat-pad sign on MR sagittal images in the presence of synovitis. This feature is evaluated by observing the irregular free edge of the fat-pad density in contrast to the adjacent fluid. The synovitis is a result of hemarthrosis, which acts as a synovial irritant. Other causes of acute hemarthrosis must be considered and include patellar dislocation and osteochondral fractures. An avulsion off the anterior tibial eminence, a lateral tibial rim fracture (Segond fracture), a posterior fracture of the lateral tibial plateau, and an osteochondral fracture of the lateral femoral condyle all may be associated with ACL injuries and can be identified on plain radiographs.[8]

On arthrography, the ACL can only be indirectly assessed by observing air and contrast along the reflected synovial surface. Direct visualization of ligamentous fibers is not possible. An absent or wavy anterior synovial surface on lateral radiographs represents an abnormal ACL on arthrography. The normal ligamentum mucosum may be mistaken for an intact ACL. Arthrographic findings can be subtle, and proper examination requires a high level of technical experience to produce acceptable accuracy rates.[8]

MR Appearance of the ACL

MR IMAGING TECHNIQUES. For routine MR examinations, positioning the knee in 10° to 15° of external rotation (to orient the ACL with the sagittal imaging plane) is less critical as section thickness decreases (≤4 mm) (Fig. 7-113). However, 5-mm contiguous thick sections may need to be supplemented with oblique images parallel to the ACL or, alternatively, the entire sagittal sequence can be performed

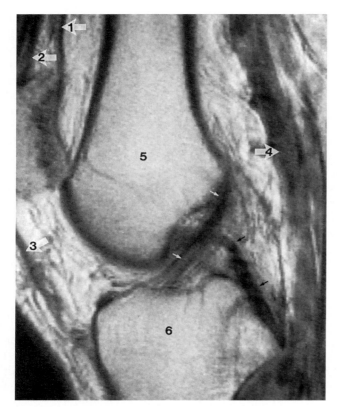

FIGURE 7-113. The sagittal plane through the intercondylar notch. *White arrows*, ACL; *black arrows*, PCL; *1*, suprapatellar bursa with fluid; *2*, quadriceps tendon; *3*, patellar tendon; *4*, popliteal artery; *5*, femur; *6*, tibia.

in an oblique sagittal plane parallel to the orientation of the ACL.

Excessive external rotation of the knee results in elongation of the anterior-to-posterior dimensions of the femoral condyles and limits accurate imaging of the meniscal carti-

lages. Excessive internal rotation of the knee may increase the partial volume effect of the proximal ACL attachment with the medial aspect of the lateral femoral condyle. This partial volume effect may produce a pseudomass at the proximal portion of the ACL. This pseudomass does not appear on corresponding coronal or axial images and does not demonstrate increased signal intensity on T2-weighted images.[140]

We routinely use all three planes (axial, sagittal, and coronal) to evaluate the ACL (Figs. 7-114 through 7-116). Sagittal scans best demonstrate the femoral and tibial attachments on one or two images and represent the primary plane for ACL analysis. Axial and coronal scans are particularly useful in demonstrating the relation of the proximal ACL attachment to the medial aspect of the lateral femoral condyle. The partial volume effect may be minimized with thin sections. We routinely use sagittal images that are 3 to 4 mm in thickness. If ligament visualization is suboptimal with this protocol, direct sagittal oblique imaging of the ACL is recommended (Fig. 7-117), with an axial localizer to display the tibial and femoral attachments of the ACL. More accurate identification of the ACL fibers is achieved by using a 3D FT volume technique, which yields a large series of thin section sagittal images (Fig. 7-118). Oblique sagittal images are also important in postoperative evaluation of ACL reconstruction. The coronal plane is used as a localizer for the course of the neoligament.

Kinematic imaging of the ACL in the sagittal plane has been attempted in partial ligamentous tears and reconstructions.[139] T1- and T2-weighted spin-echo or proton-density and T2-weighted spin-echo images are frequently used to evaluate the signal intensity changes in acute and subacute ACL injuries. We routinely use both T2*-weighted gradient-echo MR images and fat-suppressed T2-weighted fast spin-echo images to demonstrate morphology and signal intensity changes within the ACL. The fat-suppressed T2-weighted fast spin-echo images are excellent

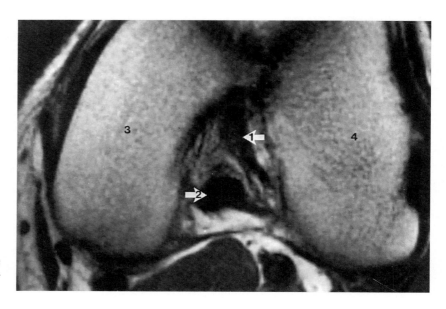

FIGURE 7-114. Axial intercondylar anatomy of the ACL and PCL. *1*, ACL; *2*, PCL; *3*, medial femoral condyle; *4*, lateral femoral condyle.

for demonstrating ACL contours, especially in ligament disruption. However, these images may not demonstrate the same degree of high signal intensity within the ligament as shown on corresponding gradient-echo images. In imaging postoperative ACL reconstructions, T2-weighted fast spin-echo images have less magnetic susceptibility artifact than is seen with corresponding T2*-weighted scans. All routine protocols for the knee include some form of T2-weighting (conventional or fast spin-echo) in all three planes to maximize the sensitivity and specificity for detecting ACL pathology. T1-weighted images alone are inadequate to appreciate areas of edema and hemorrhage in a disrupted ligament.

NORMAL ACL IMAGING CHARACTERISTICS. On coronal, sagittal, and axial images, the normal ACL is seen as a band of low signal intensity with separate fiber striations visible near attachment points. In full knee extension, the ACL is usually appears as a 3- to 4-mm-thick single low-signal-intensity band with a straight or taut anterior margin.[140] Changing the position of the knee from extension to flexion is associated with a decrease in the signal intensity of the cruciate ligaments.[142] A decrease in ACL signal intensity with applied tension and a reciprocal increase in signal intensity with the release of tension has also been shown. These findings may in part explain the higher signal intensity often observed in the ACL compared with

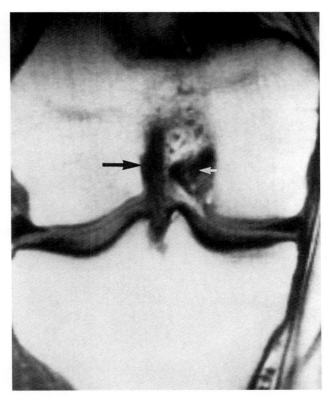

FIGURE 7-116. The anatomy of the ACL (*black arrow*) and PCL (*white arrow*) as seen on a T1-weighted coronal image. The ACL is seen as a band, whereas the PCL is circular in cross section.

the PCL, because evaluations are performed in knee extension. The ACL may show a more lax configuration on MR with knee flexion, although biomechanically the AMB tightens and the PLB loosens as the knee is flexed. The ACL parallels the orientation of the low-signal-intensity line representing the intercondylar roof on sagittal images. Depending on the obliquity of the ACL fibers, the ACL may not be displayed in its entire course on a single sagittal image. The individual low-signal-intensity fiber bundles may be separated by linear stripes of intermediate to bright signal intensity on T1-weighted images.[140] These stripes are believed to represent fat and synovium and are usually identified at the tibial attachment of the ACL.

The AMB forms the anterior border of the ACL. The PLB, representing the bulk of the ACL, may display more intermediate signal intensity on T1-weighted images. The normal ACL fibers demonstrate low signal intensity on conventional T2, fat-suppressed T2-weighted fast spin-echo, and T2*-weighted images. Areas of eosinophilic degeneration of the ACL in older persons may be visualized as regions of intermediate signal intensity.[143] The axial plane is helpful in spatially identifying sites of tears corresponding to the locations of the AMB and the PLB.

Anterior to the ACL, the ligamentum mucosum, or infrapatellar plica, arises from the superior condylar notch. It may sometimes be seen as a distinct structure on MR images. Independent of partial volume effect, the ACL may demonstrate a greater signal intensity than observed in the homoge-

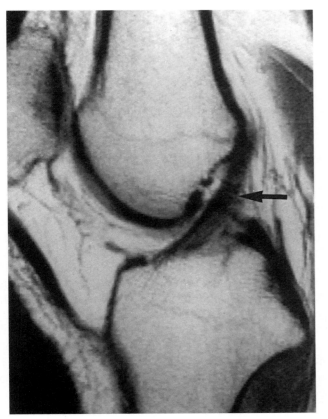

FIGURE 7-115. An intact low-signal-intensity ACL (*arrow*) is shown on a T1-weighted sagittal image.

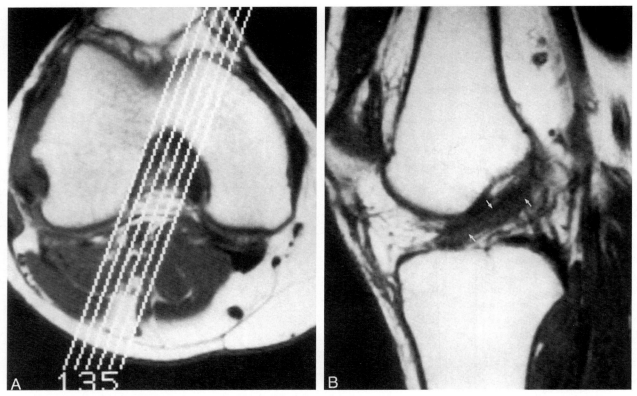

FIGURE 7-117. Oblique imaging of the ACL. The axial plane (**A**) through the intercondylar notch is used as a localizer for prescribing direct oblique sagittal 3-mm images (**B**) through the ACL (*arrows*).

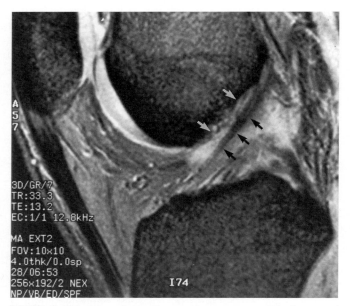

FIGURE 7-118. Normal anterior cruciate anatomy (*black arrows*) is displayed on this 3D FT volume T2* sagittal image obtained at a 10-cm field of view. The ACL fibers are straight and parallel to the intercondylar roof (*white arrows*).

neously low-signal-intensity PCL on T1-, conventional T2-, fast spin-echo T2-, and T2*-weighted images.

ACL TEARS. MR evaluation can characterize the spectrum of morphologic and signal intensity changes in ACL tears. The discontinuity of the ACL, especially as assessed in the sagittal and axial planes, and failure of ACL fascicles to parallel Blumensaat's line are considered primary and accurate signs of a ligament tear (Fig. 7-119).[144,145] Other predictors of an ACL tear include (1) discontinuity of the ACL in one plane; (2) disruption of fascicles; (3) bone contusions on the weight-bearing surface of the lateral femoral condyle and posterolateral tibial plateau; (4) buckling of the PCL, a positive PCL sign (failure of a line drawn along the posterior PCL on sagittal images to intersect the medullary cavity within 5 cm of the distal femur); and (5) a positive posterior femoral line sign (failure of a line drawn at a 45° angle from the posterosuperior corner of Blumensaat's line to intersect the flat portion of the proximal tibial surface or to intersect a point within 5 cm of its posterior margin).[144,146] The absence of secondary or indirect signs does not exclude the diagnosis of an ACL tear.[147]

The most accurate assessment for ACL tears requires

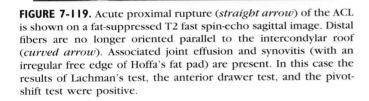

FIGURE 7-119. Acute proximal rupture (*straight arrow*) of the ACL is shown on a fat-suppressed T2 fast spin-echo sagittal image. Distal fibers are no longer oriented parallel to the intercondylar roof (*curved arrow*). Associated joint effusion and synovitis (with an irregular free edge of Hoffa's fat pad) are present. In this case the results of Lachman's test, the anterior drawer test, and the pivot-shift test were positive.

the combined use of axial, coronal and sagittal images (Fig. 7-120).[148] In an acute ACL tear, there is loss of ligament continuity associated with a wavy or lax contour (including posterior bowing or concavity of the anterior margin of the ACL). The ruptured ligament has a more horizontal orientation, as demonstrated on sagittal images. The ACL itself usually demonstrates increased signal intensity on T2- or T2*-weighted images. Changes in signal intensity may be less pronounced with fast spin-echo or fat-suppressed fast spin-echo techniques (Fig. 7-121) An edematous soft-tissue mass may be seen in the region of the torn fibers.[144] Widening of the entire ligament is associated with an interstitial tear pattern. An interstitial disruption shows variable increases in signal intensity on T2-weighted images.[140] Increased signal intensity on T2 or fat-suppressed T2-weighted fast spin-echo weighted images is usually identified within the ACL at its femoral attachment on coronal images. Axial images are excellent for showing fluid within the proximal ligament fibers or between the torn ACL and the lateral femoral condyle sidewall (medial aspect). This capability is especially helpful in evaluating injuries in skiers where the frequency of proximal ACL tears shows an increase compared with midsubstance distributions in nonskiers.[140] An acute or focal angular deformity of the middle third of the ACL usually is

identified as a discontinuous segment and is a common pattern also seen in acute ACL tears (Fig. 7-122).

Avulsions of the tibial intercondylar eminence occur in 5% of patients (Fig. 7-123). Because of minimal or no displacement of the avulsed fragment, careful evaluation of marrow signal on T1- or gradient-echo images is important. Bone marrow edema in the avulsed fragment is often minimal. Thus, avulsion injuries could be missed on T2 or fat-suppressed T2-weighted fast spin-echo images. Anterior subluxation or anterior displacement of the tibia on lateral sagittal images is a secondary sign of anterolateral instability (Fig. 7-124).[149] This anterior drawer, or more properly Lachman's sign (because the knee is in extension), is dependent on the degree of knee flexion, positioning, and the design of the extremity coil, and its usefulness is limited by lack of comparison with the contralateral knee. On sagittal images, if the ACL is intact, a vertical line drawn at a tangent to the posterolateral femoral condyle should intersect the posterolateral tibial plateau. Although anterior tibial subluxation of greater than 7 mm has been reported in ACL tears,[149] we recommend that this finding be used as a secondary sign only.

The hemarthrosis associated with acute ACL tears is characterized by synovitis with an irregular free concave edge of Hoffa's infrapatellar fat pad (Fig. 7-125). This finding occurs most often in complete acute ACL disruptions, however, it may also be present in partial ligamentous tears. Ligament edema or hemorrhage may be associated with blurring of the cruciate fascicles. Fluid within the substance of the anterior cruciate ligament or occupying the extrasynovial triangular space between the cruciate ligaments is an abnormal finding associated with injury.[150]

Accurate assessment of partial ligamentous tears is more difficult than the detection of complete disruptions. A partial tear corresponds to a grade 2 ligament injury as defined by the American Medical Association Ligament Injury Classification System (incomplete tears with a small increase in laxity).[151,152] Arthroscopy may not be as sensitive as MR to partial intrasubstance tears.[141] Specific designation of AMB versus PLB tears is frequently not possible. The detection of a discrete area or focus of increased signal intensity within the substance of the ACL is consistent with a diagnosis of a partial tear (Fig. 7-126). Although the bulk of the ligament appears to be intact, with a relatively normal axis, there may be localized angulation of the ligament at the site of fiber disruption.[140] It is difficult to grade progressive degrees of partial tears to accurately correlate with clinical grading of ACL pathology. ACL tears involving less than 25% of the substance are associated with a more favorable clinical outcome than tears involving 50% or more, which predispose to ACL deficiency and reinjury.[153,154]

The difficulty in detecting partial ACL tears is related to the nonspecificity of intrasubstance abnormal signal intensity with concomitant morphology alteration such as

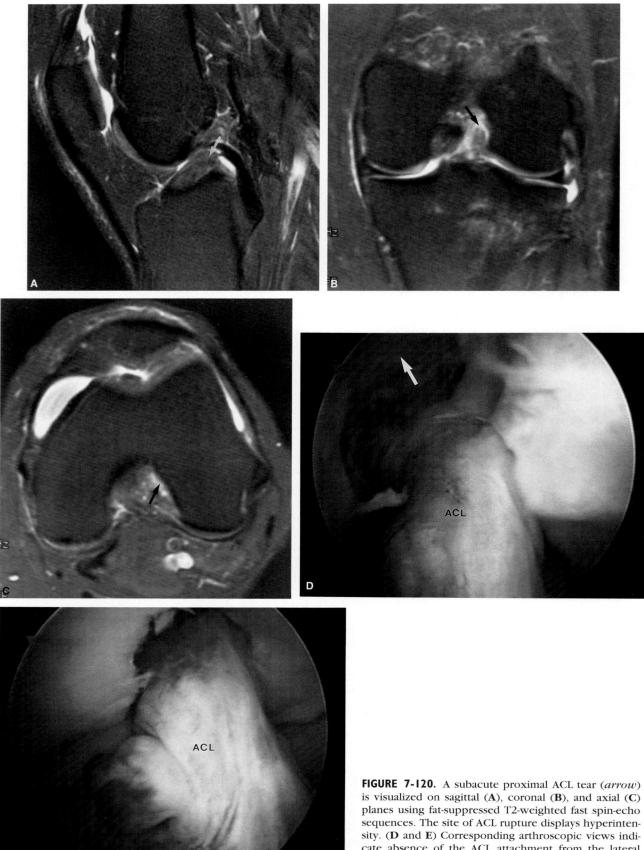

FIGURE 7-120. A subacute proximal ACL tear (*arrow*) is visualized on sagittal (**A**), coronal (**B**), and axial (**C**) planes using fat-suppressed T2-weighted fast spin-echo sequences. The site of ACL rupture displays hyperintensity. (**D** and **E**) Corresponding arthroscopic views indicate absence of the ACL attachment from the lateral femoral condyle (**D**, *arrow*) and an ACL stump in the anterior aspect of the intercondylar notch (**E**).

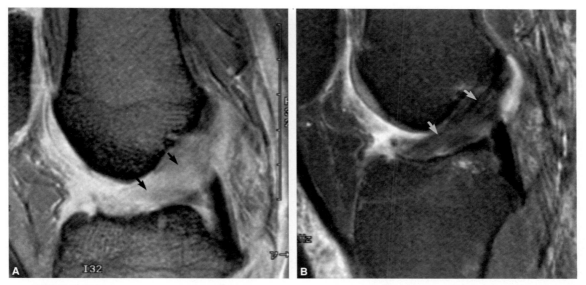

FIGURE 7-121. An interstitial tear. **(A)** An ACL interstitial tear pattern with diffuse hyperintensity (*arrows*) along the entire course of the ligament on a T2*-weighted sagittal image. **(B)** A thickened and posteriorly bowed ACL (*arrows*) is visualized with decreased signal intensity on a corresponding fat-suppressed T2-weighted fast spin-echo sagittal image.

bowing or attenuation of ACL fibers.[153] Abnormal signal intensity alone may be associated with either a ligamentous contusion or disruption of collagen fibers,[143] which may remain arthroscopically occult. We have found the

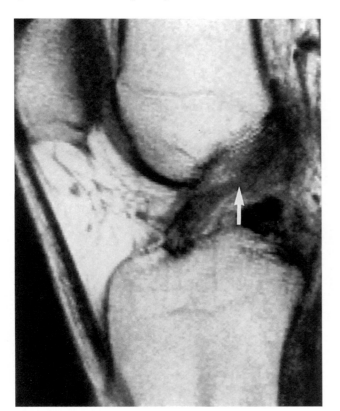

FIGURE 7-122. A midsubstance tear of the ACL (*arrow*) shows loss of continuity of its normally parallel margins.

use of fat-suppressed T2-weighted fast spin-echo or conventional T2 weighting to be more accurate in correlating areas of increased signal intensity with partial tears than is exclusive reliance on the abnormal signal intensity seen on gradient-echo images. This finding may in part explain why some MR studies using gradient-echo sequences show poor arthroscopic correlation for the detection of partial ACL tears.[153]

The AMB is most commonly involved in incomplete or partial ACL tears (see Fig. 7-126).[152] Because the AMB provides the primary (96%) restraining force to anterior drawer at 30° of knee flexion, rupture of the AMB is thought to be functionally equivalent to a complete ACL tear. Lintner and colleagues, however, were unable to clinically detect isolated tears of the AMB in cadaver knees by either physical examination or arthrometric testing after sectioning this band.[152] Thus, clinically diagnosed partial tears are more likely to represent a complete rupture of the ACL. The progression from partial tears to symptomatic instability may, in fact, involve patients who have had a functionally incompetent ACL from the time of injury.[152] MR may have an important role in defining partial ACL tears because these injuries are difficult to differentiate from complete ACL tears clinically.

In subacute ACL tears, morphology of the torn ligament fibers may be less obscured by the initial hemorrhage as the hematoma resolves (Fig. 7-127). The distal segment of the ACL often assumes a more horizontal location or orientation within the joint. Fluid interposed in the ligamentous gap of the tear site is usually more sharply defined. Associated

text continues on page 322

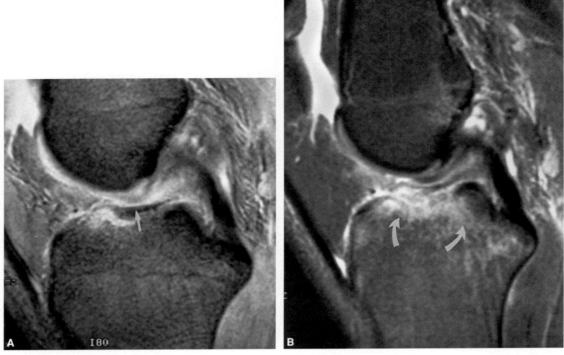

FIGURE 7-123. An avulsion fracture of the intercondylar eminence (*straight arrow*) at the insertion of the ACL is best identified on T2*-weighted sagittal images (**A**). The associated hyperintense bone marrow edema (*curved arrows*) and ACL morphology are more apparent on fat-suppressed T2-weighted fast spin-echo sagittal images (**B**).

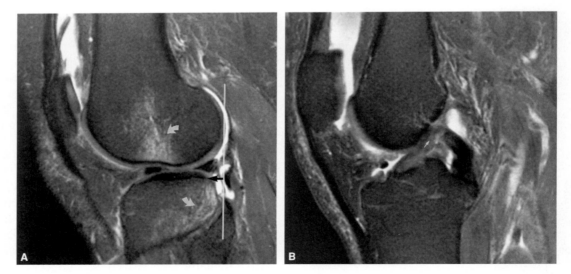

FIGURE 7-124. An acute ACL tear. (**A**) An MR anterior drawer sign (specifically, an MR Lachman's sign) on a fat-suppressed T2-weighted fast spin-echo sagittal image shows anterior displacement of the lateral tibial plateau (*straight arrow*) relative to a plum line (*long white line*) extrapolated from the posterior lateral femoral condyle. Hyperintense bone contusions (*curved arrows*) are shown in the lateral femoral condyle and posterior lateral tibial plateau. (**B** and **C**) An associated ACL tear (*arrow*) is shown on a fat-suppressed T2-weighted fast spin-echo sagittal image (**B**) and a gadolinium-DTPA–enhanced fat-suppressed T1-weighted image (**C**). The ACL is torn proximally and has irregular morphology. *continued*

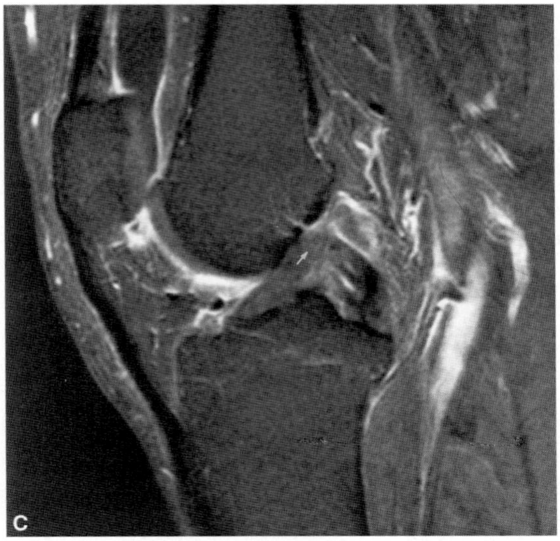

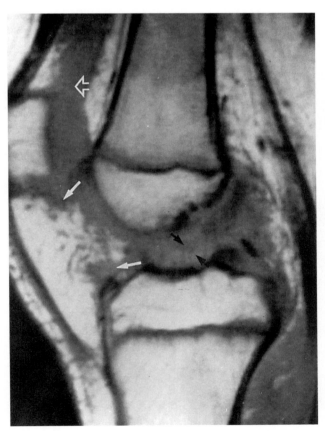

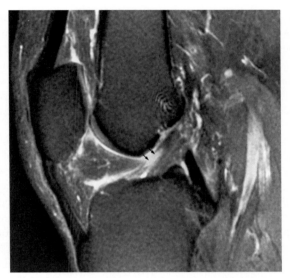

FIGURE 7-124. *Continued*

FIGURE 7-126. A focal partial tear of the anterior midportion of the ACL corresponding to the AMB fibers. The partial tear is hyperintense (*small arrows*), whereas the ACL maintains normal morphology and is parallel to the intercondylar roof on this fat-suppressed T2-weighted fast spin-echo sagittal image.

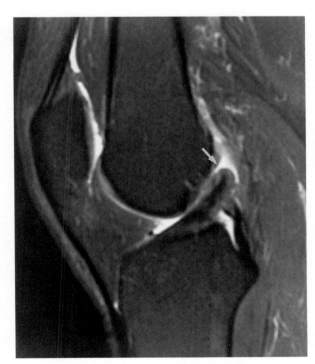

FIGURE 7-125. The presence of a disrupted ACL (*solid black arrows*) associated with hemorrhagic effusion (*open white arrow*) and synovitis is implied by the irregular edge of Hoffa's infrapatellar fat pad (*solid white arrows*).

FIGURE 7-127. A subacute ACL tear with fluid present at the site of proximal rupture (*arrow*). The ACL morphology is visible and demonstrates hypointensity on this fat-suppressed T2-weighted fast spin-echo sagittal image. There has been an interval decrease in joint effusion and synovitis since the initial injury.

bone contusions are usually persistent but may demonstrate decreased signal intensity or extent of involvement in the lateral femoral condyle and posterolateral tibial plateau. The synovitis inferred by the irregular contour of Hoffa's fat pad is frequently detected, but is decreased (see Fig. 7-127), in subacute tears. It is usually seen in association with a joint effusion that has also decreased since the initial injury.

In chronic tears of the ACL, edema and synovitis are usually not present. There is usually no irregularity of the free concave edge of Hoffa's fat pad, although there may be a small chronic joint effusion. The ACL may not be visualized on sagittal or coronal images. The absence of ACL tissue in the lateral intercondylar notch is responsible for the empty notch sign on coronal MR images ("empty lateral wall") (Fig. 7-128).[144] The chronically torn ACL is often seen with a horizontal axis, although it may display a more vertical orientation and discontinuity or retraction of its normal proximal lateral femoral condylar attachment site. It is not uncommon for the torn ACL to be adhered to the PCL,[155] producing a clinical end point on knee testing for an anterior drawer. The ACL may also appear attenuated or small in chronic tears. Anterior translation of the tibia on the femur is also associated with chronic ACL dysfunction (Fig. 7-129). This finding of the MR anterior drawer sign represents a static assessment of anterolateral instability.

Posterolateral capsular injuries seen with acute ACL injuries show no signs of fluid extravasation or edema at this stage of chronic injury. There is uncovering of the undersurface of the posterior horn of the lateral meniscus (uncovered lateral meniscus sign) and buckling of the foreshortened PCL (see Fig. 7-129) as the tibia translates anteriorly.[144] Buckling or redundancy of the patellar tendon is another indirect sign associated with ACL injury and forward tibial displacement. However, this may also be seen with hyperextension of the knee and with cases of quadriceps dysfunction.[8] These indirect findings may be specific but are not sensitive signs for the spectrum of ACL ligament pathology. Imaging with the patient in the supine position causes the tibia to fall in neutral alignment relative to the femur (because of gravity) in an ACL-deficient knee. In a PCL tear, however, the tibia tends to undergo subluxation posteriorly.

Intercondylar notch or ganglion cysts of the ACL have been described arising both on the surface (Fig. 7-130) of the ACL and within the substance of the ACL (Fig. 7-131).[156–158] These cysts are located in the mid and proximal portions of both the ACL and PCL. They are thought to represent either mucinous degeneration of connective tissue or a herniation of synovial tissue through a capsular defect.[157] The cyst may be septated and demonstrates uniform increased signal intensity on T2-weighted images. Intravenous administration of

text continues on page 325

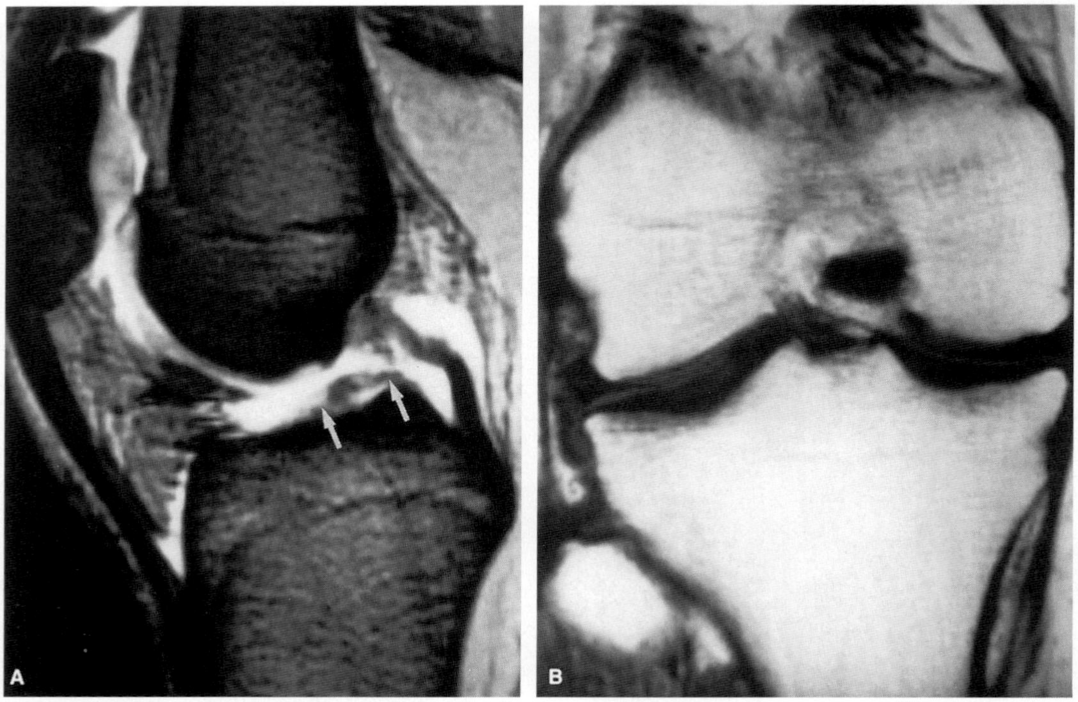

FIGURE 7-128. An empty-notch sign. (**A**) A chronic ACL tear with a horizontally oriented ligament (*arrows*) is seen on a T2*-weighted sagittal image. There is no blurring of the ligament fibers in this chronic injury. (**B**) The ACL is absent on this T1-weighted coronal image.

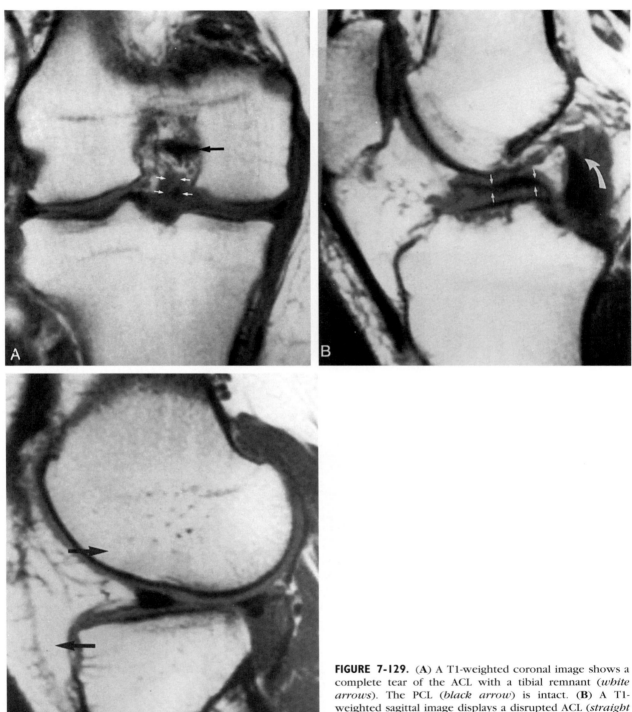

FIGURE 7-129. (A) A T1-weighted coronal image shows a complete tear of the ACL with a tibial remnant (*white arrows*). The PCL (*black arrow*) is intact. (B) A T1-weighted sagittal image displays a disrupted ACL (*straight white arrows*) associated with buckling of the PCL (*curved white arrow*). (C) A T1-weighted sagittal image demonstrates the anterior drawer sign with forward displacement of the tibia on the femur (*arrows*).

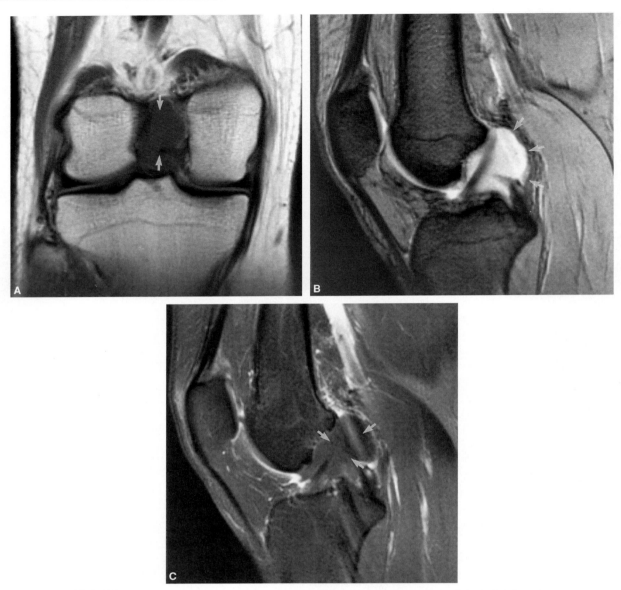

FIGURE 7-130. An intercondylar notch cyst (*arrows*) associated with the surface of the ACL is hypointense on a T1-weighted coronal image (**A**), is hyperintense on a T2*-weighted sagittal image (**B**), and is not enhanced after intravenous administration of gadolinium-DTPA on a fat-suppressed T1-weighted sagittal image (**C**).

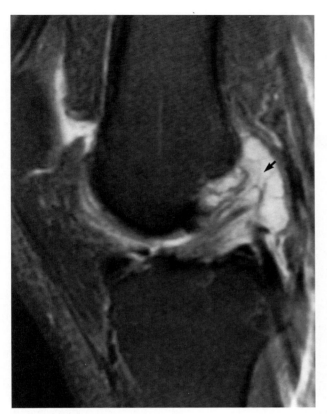

FIGURE 7-131. An intercondylar notch proximal anterior cruciate ligament cyst (*arrow*) is hyperintense on this fat-suppressed T2-weighted fast spin-echo sagittal image.

MR contrast media does not cause enhancement of the cyst contents (see Fig. 7-130). These cysts may be symptomatic, causing either pain or intermittent swelling,[156] and correspond to an ACL injury, or other associated intraarticular joint pathology; or they may present as an incidental finding. Patients often present with pain and clicking during terminal knee extension. Intercondylar notch cysts can be successfully treated with arthroscopic debridement.[157]

ACL-ASSOCIATED POSTEROLATERAL CORNER INJURIES AND OSSEOUS INJURIES. Posterolateral corner injuries are frequently associated with acute ACL (also PCL) tears (Fig. 7-132). It is uncommon for the posterolateral corner to be involved as an isolated injury.[159] Functional failure of a reconstructed ACL can occur if the reconstruction was completed without performing an associated repair of the posterolateral corner at the time of surgery. The anatomic structures of the posterolateral corner include the LCL, the arcuate ligament, the popliteus tendon, the popliteofibular ligament, the short lateral ligament, the fabellofibular ligament, and the posterolateral part of the capsule.[160,161] The arcuate ligament is a Y-shaped structure with a medial and lateral limb. Because terminology used to describe the anatomy of the posterolateral structures and arcuate complex are inconsistent, it is best to refer to the organization of the posterolateral corner anatomy as three layers as described by Seebacher and colleagues (see the section ''Functional Anatomy of the LCL,'' later in this chapter).[162] Combined sectioning of the ACL and posterolateral ligaments have shown maximal increases in primary anterior and posterior translations at 30° of knee flexion.[159] Increases have also been shown for primary varus, primary internal, and coupled external rotation. Isolated posterolateral sectioning results in primary posterior translation, varus and external rotation, and coupled external rotation maximal at 30° to 45° of knee flexion. Hyperextension is the most common mechanism in patients with a combined ACL and posterolateral injury.[160] Common MR findings in posterolateral corner injuries include fluid posterior to the popliteus tendon, edema, tearing of the popliteus muscle and muscle–tendon junction (Fig. 7-133), and direct visualization of arcuate ligament disruption as assessed on T2-weighted axial images. The extravasation of fluid along the course of the popliteus muscle and tendon is a sign of trauma to the attachment of the arcuate complex. Injuries to the arcuate ligament are indicated by the presence of fluid directly posterior to the popliteus tendon in the expected location of the medial limb of the arcuate ligament. Because the superficial fibers of the popliteus attach to the medial limb of the arcuate ligament, it is viewed as a separate but contiguous structure to the popliteus.[39] Acute repair or reconstruction of the posterolateral corner is performed at the time of ACL reconstruction. Extensive posterolateral injury may require primary repair, augmentation, or reconstruction of the popliteus-muscle/tendon unit and the LCL.[160,163]

Several different osseous injuries are also associated with tears of the ACL. Lateral compartment bone contusions, involving the weight-bearing portion of the lateral femoral condyle and the posterolateral tibial plateau, are the most common associated bone injuries in acute ACL injuries (Fig. 7-134). Murphy and colleagues have found posterolateral tibial plateau (94%) and lateral femoral condyle (91%) subchondral bone impactions to be relatively specific signs of an acute ACL tear.[164] This association with trabecular bone contusions is attributed to the impact of the lateral femoral condyle into the posterior tibia during either the initial rotatory subluxation or the recoil of the lateral femoral condyle. The combination of valgus forces with anterior subluxation of the lateral tibial plateau produces the impaction force on the weight-bearing surface or midportion of the lateral femoral condyle, opposite or over the anterior horn of the lateral meniscus.[144–147,165,166] Fat-suppressed T2-weighted fast spin-echo and STIR images are the most sensitive techniques for demonstrating the increased subchondral signal intensity in these lesions. These associated bone contusions resolve over time and are not as commonly seen 9 or more weeks after

text continues on page 329

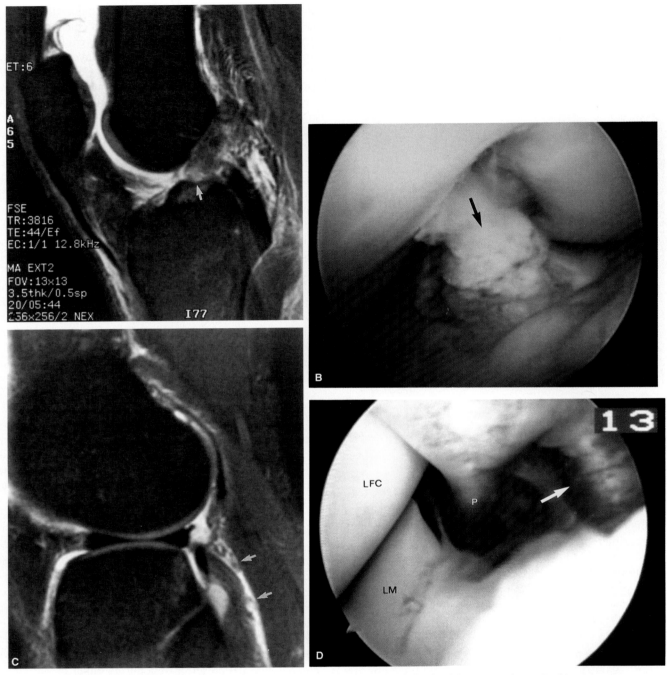

FIGURE 7-132. Posterolateral corner injury. **(A)** A fat-suppressed T2-weighted fast spin-echo sagittal image displays a complete ACL tear (*arrow*) with ligament fibers horizontally oriented in the floor of the intercondylar notch. **(B)** An arthroscopic view of the ACL tear (*arrow*) with no femoral attachment. **(C)** An associated posterolateral corner capsular tear with extravasation of fluid (*arrow*) both anterior and posterior to the popliteus muscle and tendon. **(D)** Hemorrhagic posterolateral corner (*arrow*) is viewed at arthroscopy. *LFC,* lateral femoral condyle; *LM,* lateral meniscus; *P,* popliteus tendon.

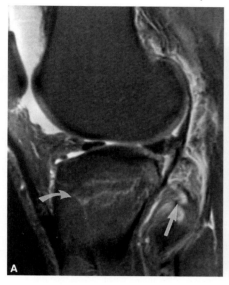
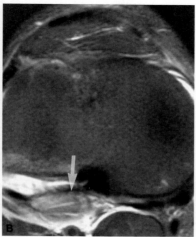

FIGURE 7-133. Posterolateral capsular trauma in association with an acute ACL tear. **(A)** A popliteus muscle tear (*straight arrow*) with hyperintense hemorrhage on a fat-suppressed T2-weighted fast spin-echo sagittal image. Note the anterior translation of the tibia relative to the femur. Osseous contusion (*curved arrow*) is indicated. **(B)** Hyperintensity of the popliteus muscle (*arrow*) on an axial fat-suppressed T2-weighted fast spin-echo image.

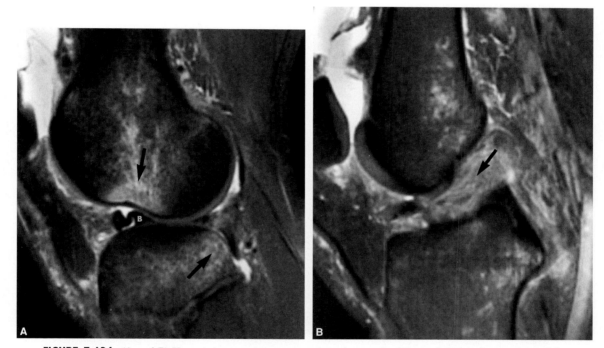

FIGURE 7-134. **(A and B)** Hyperintense osseous contusions (*arrows*) of the weight-bearing surface of the lateral femoral condyle and posterior lateral tibial plateau **(A)** associated with an acute grade 3 (*arrow*) ACL tear **(B)**. **(C)** A posterior medial tibial plateau contusion (*arrow*) is also shown. This patient also sustained a bucket-handle tear of the lateral meniscus (*B* in **A**), and a peripheral vertical tear of the posterior horn of the medial meniscus **(C)**. *continued*

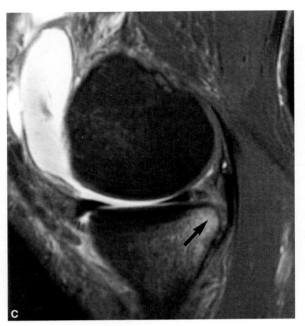

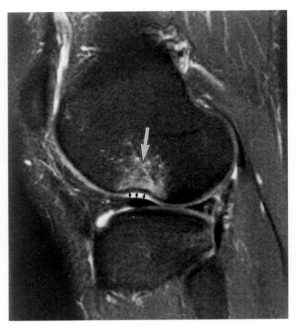

FIGURE 7-134. *Continued*

FIGURE 7-135. Lateral condylopatellar sulcus impaction (*small arrows*) with hyperintense subchondral marrow edema (*large arrow*). Smaller posterior lateral tibial plateau bone contusion and vertical tear of the posterior horn of the lateral meniscus are also present on a fat-suppressed T2-weighted fast spin-echo sagittal image.

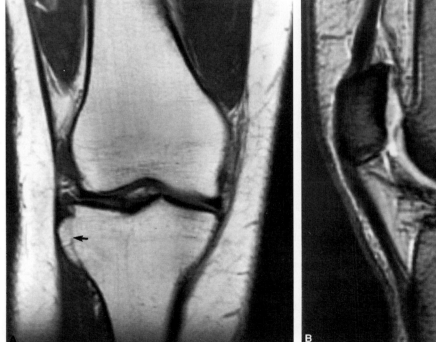

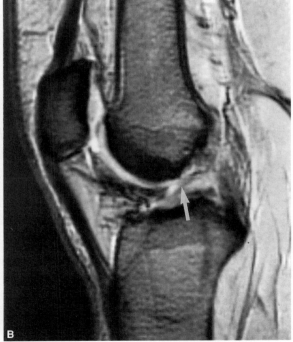

FIGURE 7-136. A Segond fracture. (**A**) A healed lateral tibial rim fracture or Segond fracture (*arrow*). On this T1-weighted coronal image, the fracture is seen to be oriented along the long axis of the tibia, lateral and immediately inferior to the joint line (posterior and proximal to Gerdy's tubercle). (**B**) A chronic ACL tear (*arrow*) is shown on T2*-weighted sagittal image.

injury.[8] However, a pattern of bone contusions may be seen in patients with chronic ACL tears secondary to persistent or continued osseous impaction or trauma from the initial injury or secondary to reinjury from recurrent subluxation of the tibia in association with ACL insufficiency.[146] Decreased signal intensity as well as a decrease in the area of subchondral bone involvement may be seen during the resolution phase of these trabecular impactions.

A lateral femoral condylar notch or cortical depression separate from the normal sulcus terminale may be visualized with ACL injuries (Fig. 7-135). This ''lateral notch sign'' is visualized as a depression or condylar indentation greater than 1.5 mm in depth at the condylopatellar sulcus. Subcortical bone is of low signal intensity on T1-weighted images and high signal intensity on fat-suppressed T2-weighted fast spin-echo or STIR images in the area of subchondral marrow edema. (Bone contusions in general may show variable increases in signal intensity on conventional T2-weighted images compared with fat-suppressed fast spin-echo or STIR techniques.) An associated ''kissing impaction'' fracture of the posterolateral tibial plateau is usually present and should be identified, especially in hyperextension mechanisms of injuries.[166] Bone contusions or impactions of the lateral tibial plateau may occur as an isolated finding, relatively specific for ACL injury, or in association with involvement of the lateral femoral condyle in acute ACL ruptures.

The Segond fracture represents a bony ligamentous avulsion of the meniscotibial portion of the middle third of the lateral capsular ligament (Fig. 7-136). It is associated with rupture of the ACL in 75% to 100% of cases.[20,167,168] On MR scans a small vertical avulsion of the LCL insertion in the lateral aspect of the proximal tibia can be identified. The elliptical fracture fragment may be seen at the fracture site on coronal images. In acute or subacute injuries, the fracture fragment demonstrates low signal intensity on T1-weighted images and hyperintensity on fat-suppressed T2-weighted fast spin-echo or STIR images. In chronic injuries, normal fatty marrow signal intensity can be visualized in the fracture fragment with cortical offset as healing ensues. The Segond fracture is seen with excessive internal rotation and varus stress, as commonly occurs in skiing, basketball, and baseball injuries.[168] The small Segond fragment may be better demonstrated on plain radiographs than on MR images.

A tibial spine avulsion is an uncommon but specific finding for ACL injury (Fig. 7-137).[168] Distal ACL injuries are frequently associated with avulsion injuries because the dis-

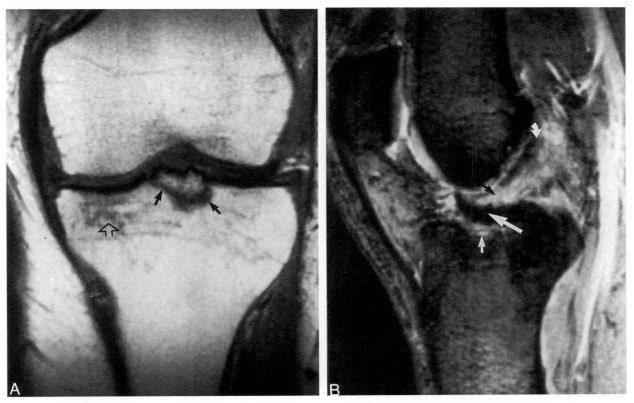

FIGURE 7-137. ACL avulsion. (**A**) A T1-weighted coronal image shows avulsion of the anterior tibial spine (*solid arrows*) caused by tension from the ACL. Associated low-signal-intensity edema is seen in a medial tibial plateau compression fracture (*open arrow*). (**B**) The corresponding T2*-weighted sagittal image reveals a high signal intensity hemorrhage in the tibial portion of the ACL (*black arrow*). Normal ACL fibers demonstrate low signal intensity (*curved arrow*). Low-signal-intensity fracture avulsion (*large white arrow*) and undermining high signal intensity fluid (*small white arrow*) are also shown.

tal ACL fibers are relatively stronger than adjacent bone.[168] Avulsion tears represent only 5% of ACL injuries in adults, however, and ACL injuries that are thought to be primarily avulsion injuries more likely are either intraligamentous or complete tears of the ACL.

A fracture of the posteromedial tibial plateau may result during external rotation and abduction force on the flexed knee, with avulsion of the posterior tibial attachment of the central tendon of the semimembranosus (see Fig. 7-134C).[140] Avulsion of the arcuate complex may produce injury of the posterior tibial rim and fibular head.

ACCURACY OF MR IMAGING. In a review of 242 arthroscopic procedures indicated by 3000 MR examinations, the accuracy of MR imaging in diagnosis of ACL pathology was 95%. Accuracy, sensitivity, and specificity increased when T2-weighted sequences were added.[169] Lee and associates reported a MR sensitivity of 94%, compared with 78% for the anterior drawer test and 89% for Lachman's test.[170] In addition, MR imaging was shown to have a specificity of 100% for tests of ACL instability. The use of nonorthogonal (oblique sagittal) compared with orthogonal imaging increased the accuracy from 61% to 66% and sensitivity from 70% to 100%; specificity remained at 100% for detection of ACL injuries.[171] MR sensitivity and specificity have shown to be 98% and 73% respectively when supplementing

sagittal images with coronal and axial images to determine the status of the ACL.[148]

MR studies have not been shown to be accurate in the differentiation of complete from partial ACL tears. Even the presence of lateral compartment bone contusions or other ancillary findings did not improve the identification of partial ACL tears, because these indirect findings occur in both partial and complete ACL injuries. Although many partial tears eventually result in instability and ACL insufficiency, they may not warrant surgery at the time of initial injury.[146] ACL deficiency also leads to intrasubstance meniscal degenerations and tears (Fig. 7-138), possibly because the menisci help to stabilize anterior tibial translation on the femur in an ACL-deficient knee.[43]

Arthroscopy should be viewed as an imperfect or relative gold standard for the diagnosis of these disorders, because stretching or intrasubstance injuries to the ACL may go undetected despite positive MR findings.[141] Our initial experience has shown more promising results in comparing arthrometric knee testing, MR, and second-look arthroscopic procedures for the assessment of partial tears of the ACL. However, this is an area that needs further study.

Treatment of ACL Injuries

The specific treatment selected for ACL injury often depends on whether an associated meniscal injury or second ligament injury is present. Associated meniscal tears, collat-

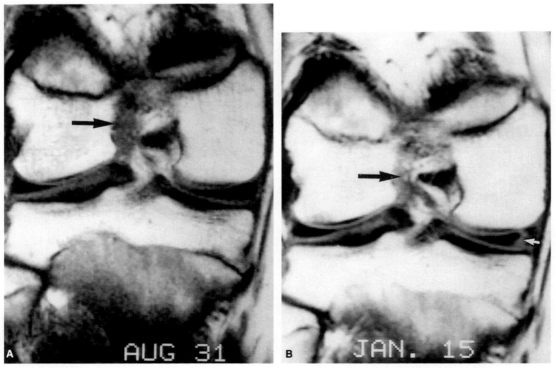

FIGURE 7-138. **(A)** An ACL tear (*arrow*) is seen on a T1-weighted coronal image. **(B)** A repeat scan 4.5 months later shows an associated vertical medial meniscus tear of grade 3 signal intensity (*white arrow*). The ACL is absent (*black arrow*).

eral ligament injuries, or patellofemoral instabilities are indications for ACL reconstructions.[172] Primary repair is most successful when avulsion occurs at either the femoral or tibial ACL attachment. Avulsion from low signal intensity cortical bone, without an associated subchondral marrow containing component, may be more difficult to visualize on T1-weighted contrast. Visualization of cortical and trabecular bone may require the use of gradient-echo sequences. Patients with midsubstance interstitial tears are not good candidates for ACL repair.

The ACL-deficient knee is reported to be at risk for osteoarthritis, articular cartilage degeneration, and secondary meniscal tears. These secondary meniscal tears can occur in as many as 20% of patients subsequent to degenerative wear.[140] Because of the potential for long term disability and progressive deterioration, treatment of ACL tears is directed to reestablishing function of the ACL through either repair or reconstruction. Nonoperative or conservative treatments of ACL injuries have yielded satisfactory results in people who are older and less active.[173] These patients may have to accept some instability and risk for meniscal tear. Factors influencing decisions related to conservative and surgical management of acute ACL injuries include the presence or absence of a torn meniscus; the patient's age, occupation, and athletic participation; and the degree of ligamentous laxity. Recreational athletes treated with aggressive rehabilitation and functional bracing for ACL injuries have shown fewer degenerative changes on roentgenography than previously reported.[174] Satisfactory outcomes (83%) have also been reported for nonoperative treatment of ruptures of the ACL in middle-aged patients.[175] Patients with combined instabilities and a desire to resume sports activity, however, were felt to be candidates for operative reconstruction.

ACL REPAIR. Bony avulsion of the distal ACL is treated successfully with direct bone-to-bone fixation. Primary repair for midsubstance tears of the ACL, however, are frequently unsuccessful and not recommended. Separate studies by Feagin and Sherman[127] have described 5-year follow-up examinations of primary repairs with signs of pain, stiffness, and instability reported in the majority of patients.[176] Primary ACL repair and intraarticular augmentation produce better results than ACL repair alone, as assessed by the pivot-shift test, arthrometric testing, and activity levels. Results of ACL repair and synthetic augmentation (an intraarticular polyester ligament augmentation or LAD device) were poor, as assessed by both the pivot-shift test and the ability to return to preinjury levels of activity.[176]

ACL RECONSTRUCTION. The goal of ACL reconstruction is to establish sufficient isometric tension to keep the distance between the tibial and femoral attachment point from

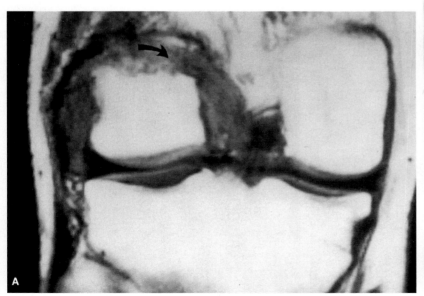
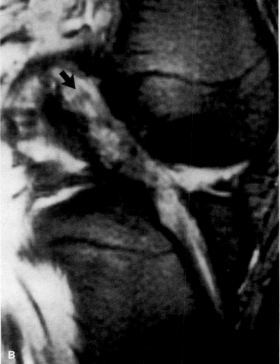

FIGURE 7-139. Lateral over-the-top repair of the ACL was made by using the iliotibial band. On **(A)** T1-weighted posterior coronal and **(B)** T2*-weighted radial oblique images, the reconstructed ligament (*arrow*) is seen over the lateral femoral condyle.

changing more than 2 to 3 mm through 0° to 90° of flexion. Surgical reconstructions are classified as extraarticular, intraarticular, or combined intra- and extraarticular.[20,177] Extraarticular procedures (eg, the MacIntosh, Ellison, and Andrews procedures) include a transfer for the pes anserinus and various lateral techniques that use the iliotibial tract to provide restraint to anterior subluxation of the lateral tibial plateau. These procedures have been used with variable success and may be associated with persistent anterior tibial translation (ie, pes transfer). The results with intraarticular reconstructions, which involve the use of a bone–patellar tendon–bone construct, are better than those achieved with extraarticular techniques. In some procedures, the iliotibial band may be transferred intraarticularly in a lateral over-

the-top reconstruction (Fig. 7-139). Other techniques use the semitendinosus and gracilis tendons doubled or the semitendinosus tendon quadrupled (Fig. 7-140).

Autogenous, allograft, xenograft, and synthetic tissues are used for ligament reconstruction for both acute and chronic ACL injuries.[20,178–180] Allograft tissues include the patellar and Achilles tendons (Fig. 7-141); synthetic allograft materials include carbon fiber, knitted Dacron, and braided polypropylene. The use of expanded polytetrafluoroethylene (Gore-Tex) has been complicated by attenuation, rupture, and stretching of the grafts (Fig. 7-142).

The bone–patellar tendon–bone graft using the central (middle) third of the patellar tendon remains the most common procedure for ACL reconstruction. Medial hamstring

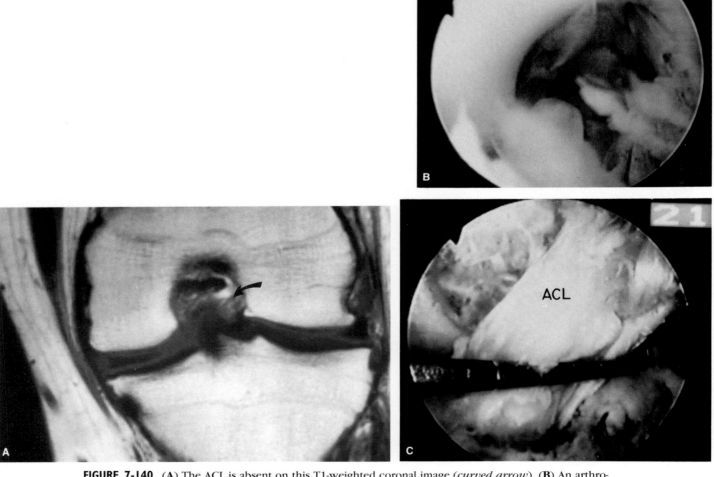

FIGURE 7-140. (A) The ACL is absent on this T1-weighted coronal image (*curved arrow*). (B) An arthroscopic view shows a shredded ACL in the intercondylar notch (*N*). (C) The ACL (*ACL*) was reconstructed using the semitendinosus tendon.

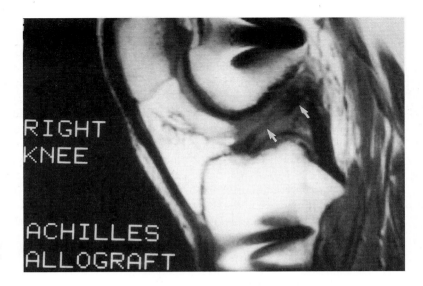

FIGURE 7-141. An Achilles tendon allograft (*arrows*) can be used for reconstruction of the ACL, as seen on this T1-weighted sagittal image.

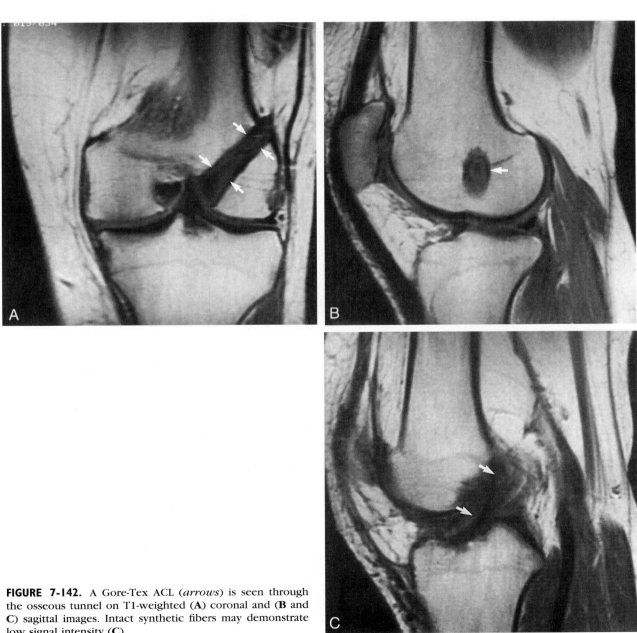

FIGURE 7-142. A Gore-Tex ACL (*arrows*) is seen through the osseous tunnel on T1-weighted (**A**) coronal and (**B** and **C**) sagittal images. Intact synthetic fibers may demonstrate low signal intensity (**C**).

tendons using the semitendinosus and gracilis are individually less strong than the patellar tendon. Therefore, when used for grafting are transferred as free double-looped (folded) grafts. Ninety percent of good results (a negative pivot-shift test result and clinical stability) with ACL reconstruction in acute injuries use the middle third of the patellar tendon (bone–patellar tendon–bone) in reconstruction.[140]

In the bone–patellar tendon–bone autograft, bone plugs are taken from the tibial tubercle and patella with a central third of the patellar tendon used as a free graft.[140] The graft can be placed arthroscopically as an endoscopic reconstruction of the ACL. The patellar tendon graft is one and a half times as strong as the normal ACL. The bone plugs and interference screws allow for stable fixation within the bone tunnels. This procedure offers the advantage of bone-to-bone healing of the graft and easy arthroscopic accessibility to the central third of the patellar tendon. Complications associated with the use of the patellar tendon include patellar fracture, tendon rupture or tendinitis, quadriceps weakness, and patellofemoral pain.

The graft is placed in a 10-mm bone tunnel after proper sizing and contouring of the bone plugs and graft. The tibial tunnel is usually located just posterior to the midpoint of the tibial ACL footprint to reduce impingement in extension and decrease the necessity for an aggressive notchplasty. An isometric point is located on the femur 5 mm anterior to the over-the-top position. The isometric point on the femur

corresponds to the 11-o'clock position for a right knee (Fig. 7-143) and a 1-o'clock position for the left knee. To limit impingement of the graft on the anterolateral aspect of the condylar notch, especially in knee extension, a notchplasty is usually performed.[172] Parallel osseous tunnels through the lateral femur and the anterior tibia are created after isometric points are selected. Incorrect placement and positioning of the graft can result in either slackening or overtension and stretching, resulting in increased laxity.[181] Isometry is relative because all of the graft fibers cannot maintain an isometric relation during knee flexion. Because selection of the femoral graft attachment is more dependent on fiber length, isometry is less affected by the selection of the tibial attachment. If the femoral tunnel is too far anterior, excessive strain may occur during knee flexion. Posterior or distal femoral attachment of the graft may produce similar strain or elongation of the graft in knee extension.[8]

Bone impingement on the graft can occur in either the roof and walls of the intercondylar fossa, or at the intraarticular exits of the bone tunnels.[181] Impingement can result in stretching, abrasion, fibrocartilaginous remodeling, or tearing of the graft, which is subjected to larger compressive stresses. Similarly, a congenitally narrow intercondylar notch may result in impingement of the native ACL.[182–184] In full knee extension, the normal ACL lies along the roof of the intercondylar fossa. The anterior distal fibers of the normal ACL curve around the junction of the intercondylar

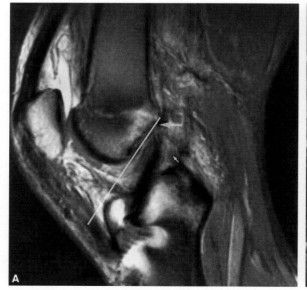
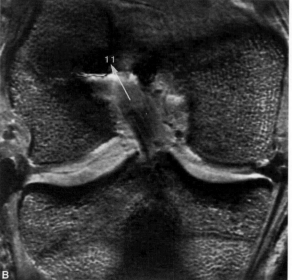

FIGURE 7-143. A stable ACL autograft. **(A)** Normal unimpinged low-signal-intensity ACL graft with the tibial tunnel posterior to the slope (*long line*) of the intercondylar roof. The PCL is straight (*small arrow*) with the knee positioned in partial flexion. The isometric placement of the graft is indicated by the posterosuperior origin of the graft on the femur (*large arrow*) at the intersection of the posterior femoral cortex and the physeal scar. (Fat-suppressed T2-weighted fast spin-echo sagittal image.) **(B)** The normal 11-o'clock position (*11*) of the femoral tunnel on a SPGR coronal image.

fossa and the trochlear groove before insertion into the tibia. Because this distal fiber curvature proximal to the tibial insertion is not present in grafts, a graft placed at the anterior edge of the ACL tibial attachment can result in impingement with the intercondylar roof at full knee extension unless adequate superior notchplasty is performed. Side wall impingement with the intercondylar fossa is related to the shape of the fossa, the graft size, and the presence of osteophytes. Impingement at intraarticular tunnel exits is caused by knee flexion and bending of the graft, which may rub or abrade at the bone tunnel exit. Chamfering at the bone tunnel exit and the drilling and alignment of the femoral tunnel through the tibial tunnel minimize this potential source of impingement.

Revascularization of the ACL Graft. Healing of the native ACL is poor and is significantly different from the improved healing response seen in extraarticular ligaments such as the MCL.[185] In animal models, autogenous patellar tendon grafts have been shown to be necrotic and without vascular or synovial attachment 2 weeks after intraarticular implantation.[185] Graft swelling, to two to three times the original size, occurred 4 weeks after implantation. Decreased graft swelling and the presence of a synovial envelope occurred at 6 weeks. No further gross changes were shown at 30 weeks. The term ''ligamentization'' is used to describe the histologic stages of incorporation of the patellar tendon graft after reconstruction of the ACL. The patellar tendon graft progresses through four stages of transformation: avascular necrosis (stage I), revascularization (stage II), cellular prolif-

eration (stage III), and remodeling (stage IV). After remodeling (stage IV), the morphology and histology of the ACL graft closely resembles that of the native ACL. There is evidence that further graft maturation occurs after the first year.

Fibroblast healing is thought to occur through the synovial membrane. This healing is not intrinsic to the patellar tendon graft. Revascularization of the patellar tendon graft occurs from the synovial fold and the endosteal vessels in the bone tunnels of the ACL graft. Graft revascularization is complete at 20 weeks, having progressed from a vascular synovial covering at 6 weeks, and intrinsic vessel formation at 6 to 10 weeks postoperatively. Comparison with patellar tendon autografts and allografts have shown delayed vascularity of the allograft. Abe and colleagues have confirmed that when assessed by arthroscopy and light microscopy, autogenous patellar tendon grafts from ACL reconstructions appeared to be revascularized in the early postoperative period, similar to the original ACL 1 year postoperatively.[186] However, electron microscopic ultrastructural study suggests that the grafts were still immature 1 year postoperatively, based on the presence of active fibroblasts with a higher cytoplasm-to-nucleus ratio than that of the normal ACL. This finding indicates that it may be necessary to reexamine aggressive rehabilitation programs that emphasize early return to full activity.

The mechanical properties of the patellar tendon autograft also change with time after implantation. In a canine model of ACL reconstruction, the ACL graft showed de-

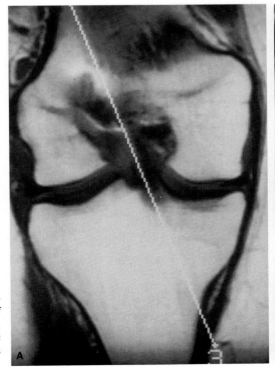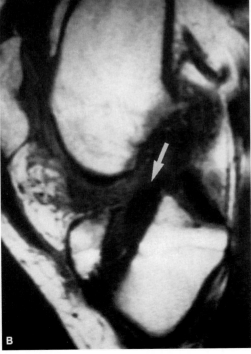

FIGURE 7-144. **(A)** A coronal localizer indicates the location of **(B)** a sagittal oblique image, which shows the position of the ACL reconstruction (*arrow*) on these T1-weighted images.

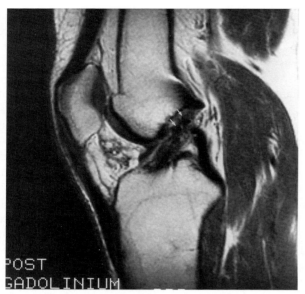

FIGURE 7-145. Proximal ACL nodularity (*arrow*) from suture material artifact in a primary repair with femoral fixation. (Gadolinium-DTPA–enhanced T1-weighted sagittal image.)

creased ability to restrict anterior tibial translation 4 weeks after surgery.[185] Improvement to the postoperative level of ability, however, had occurred at 6 months, although the graft did show a loss in strength compared with controls. Patients who are encouraged to move immediately postoperatively demonstrate a greater range of motion than patients

treated with prolonged immobilization.[185] However, the mechanical properties of the graft in these two patient populations are unaffected by mobilization.

MR Evaluation of ACL Reconstructions. Thin section (≤3 mm) sagittal or sagittal oblique MR scans (Fig. 7-144), parallel to the orientation of the ACL graft as assessed on coronal images, are recommended for accurate visualization of the course of the neoligament. Conventional T2 or fat-suppressed T2-weighted fast spin-echo images show less susceptibility artifact than do gradient-echo images and demonstrate fluid and edema as areas of increased signal intensity. Depending on the magnitude of obliquity used in the sagittal oblique images, a separate sagittal orthogonal plane may be required to prevent distortion and to aid in interpreting meniscal pathology.

Nonaugmented primary repair of the ACL has not been highly successful, primarily because of poor healing of the ACL.[185] A successful sutured ACL ligament maintains low signal intensity except for focal areas of susceptibility artifact (Fig. 7-145). Recent repairs may display edema and fluid within the ACL. The orientation of the primary repair should restore the parallel relation with the intercondylar roof that existed with the native ligament.

Extraarticular reconstructions of the ACL, which use a segment of the iliotibial band to stabilize the tibia, show thickening or micrometallic or ferromagnetic artifact of the distal iliotibial-band donor site on anterior coronal images.[187]

MR assessment of intraarticular reconstructions permits evaluation of tunnel placement (Fig. 7-146), graft impinge-

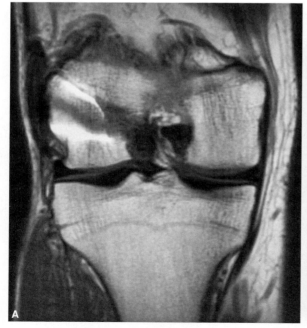

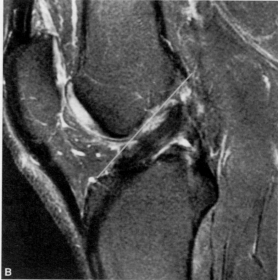

FIGURE 7-146. T1-weighted coronal (**A**) and fat-suppressed T2-weighted fast spin-echo sagittal (**B**) images demonstrate a stable, low-signal-intensity ACL autograft without impingement. The tibial tunnel is placed posterior to the slope (*long white line*) of the intercondylar roof.

ment, and rupture. The criteria for MR evaluation of ACL graft tunnel positions have been extrapolated from standards developed with conventional radiographic studies. Isometry is primarily controlled by the tunnel placement in the femoral condyle whereas graft roof impingement is reflected in the location of the tibial tunnel.[188-190] The femoral tunnel cannot be more than a few millimeters anterior or inferior to the anatomic origin of the ACL on the lateral wall of the intercondylar notch without compromising isometry. In the sagittal plane, the intersection of the low-signal-intensity posterior femoral cortical line with the posterior intercondylar roof represents the intraarticular point of reference of the femoral tunnel (see Fig. 7-143).[8] The posterior superior edge of the intercondylar roof closely corresponds to the posterior edge of the physeal scar on sagittal MR images.[187] The opening of the femoral tunnel is identified by either the 11-o'clock (right knee) or 1-o'clock (left knee) positions on coronal MR images. A femoral tunnel placed too far anteriorly contributes to tautness of the graft in knee flexion and increased laxity in extension. Placement of the graft in the over-the-top position, causes increased tension in extension. Compared with the small isometric zone for the femoral tunnel, isometry on the tibia is greater in the sagittal plane and is less sensitive to the site of the graft's tibial attachment.[191]

Graft Impingement.   Using serial MR scans, Howell and Taylor found that both centering the tibial tunnel 5 mm anterior and medial to the center of the ACL insertion and placing it within the ACL insertion put the graft at risk for impingement.[190] Centering the tibial tunnel 2 to 3 mm posterior to the center of the ACL insertion, however, helped to avoid potential roof impingement. Excessive lateral positioning of the tunnel is also likely to result in impingement. The tibial tunnel least likely to result in impingement is located with its distal opening inferior to the tibial tubercle and extends posterosuperiorly immediately anterior to the anterior tibial spine on flat tibia.[187] The center of the correctly placed tibial tunnel is 42% of the sagittal distance from the anterior aspect of the tibial plateau. Roof impingement occurs in grafts that are only 30% of the anterior-to-posterior distance of the tibial plateau.[187,190] Howell and Taylor have shown that if the entire articular opening of the tibial tunnel is anterior to the slope of the intercondylar roof (as seen on a lateral roentgenogram or sagittal MR), there is severe roof impingement on the graft (Fig. 7-147).[190] When a portion of the articular opening of the tibial tunnel is located anterior to the slope of the intercondylar roof, there is moderate graft impingement (Fig. 7-148). There is no impingement when the entire articular opening of the tibial tunnel is posterior to the slope of the intercondylar roof (see Figs. 7-143 and 7-146). Because the slope of the intercondylar roof may change with knee flexion (see Fig. 7-143), it is recommended that the tibial tunnel be placed parallel to the slope of the intercondylar roof with the knee in full extension.[192] The opening of the properly placed tibial tunnel into the joint

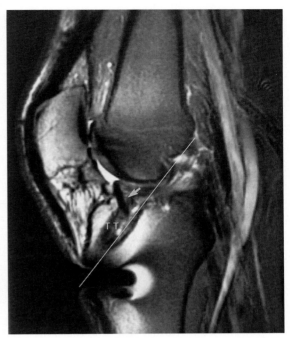

FIGURE 7-147. Graft failure and roof impingement is demonstrated on a fat-suppressed T2-weighted fast spin-echo sagittal image. The anteriorly displaced graft (*arrow*) is directed toward Hoffa's fat pad. The tibial tunnel (*TT*) is anterior to the projected slope of the intercondylar roof (*long straight line*).

is centered on the intercondylar eminence on coronal MR images,[187] and the exit sites do not correspond to the location or position of the interference screws, staples, or bone plugs used for the ACL reconstruction.

Studies have shown that the unimpinged ACL graft has no discernible blood supply for as long as 2 years after implantation.[193] The periligamentous soft tissues, however, are vascularized (enhanced on MR contrast studies) and cover the graft by 1 month (Fig. 7-149). Synovial diffusion and not revascularization may thus be more important in the viability of the unimpinged ACL graft. Unimpinged grafts demonstrate low signal intensity on T1, proton-density, and T2 (including fast spin-echo T2) images. Except for MR changes in the donor site, ACL reconstructions with bone–patellar tendon–bone grafts, hamstring tendons, and Achilles tendons are thought to have similar imaging characteristics in the unimpinged and impinged conditions.[187] The normal hypovascular appearance of the postoperative ACL graft is characterized by low signal intensity, similar to the adjacent PCL.[32,187] The portions of the graft within the osseous tunnels also demonstrate low signal intensity. Ten percent of clinically assessed normal or stable grafts may demonstrate intermediate signal intensity (Fig. 7-150).[187] This intermediate signal intensity does not indicate retear of the graft, especially in the absence of associated signs of impingement (eg, an anteriorly positioned tibial tunnel).

Rak and colleagues have studied the accuracy of MR in evaluating ACL allograft reconstructions. They used 3-mm

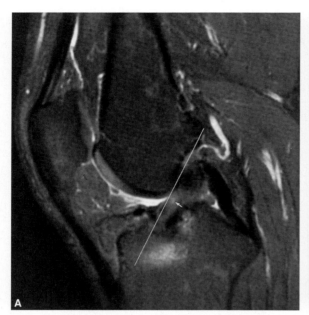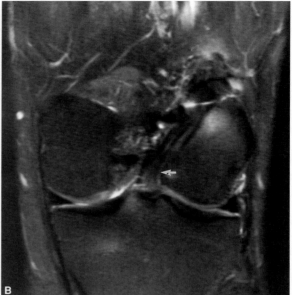

FIGURE 7-148. Graft impingement. (**A**) Distal graft hyperintensity on fat-suppressed T2-weighted fast spin-echo sagittal image in an impinged ACL graft. The tibial tunnel intraarticular opening is partially anterior to the slope of the intercondylar roof (*long straight line*). (**B**) The distal graft curves around the medial aspect of the lateral femoral condyle (*arrow*). This finding may predispose the ACL graft to sidewall impingement.

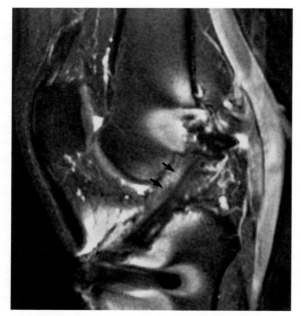

FIGURE 7-149. A fat-suppressed T2-weighted fast spin-echo sagittal image with intermediate signal intensity periligamentous soft tissue (*arrows*) between the intercondylar roof and the anterior aspect of the unimpinged ACL graft.

sections to evaluate patellar tendon autografts,[194] and found excellent correlations between MR findings and clinical examination (92%). They also found a 100% correlation between MR findings and second-look arthroscopy in ACL reconstructions using patellar bone–tendon–tibial bone autografts. Buckling of the PCL was associated with ACL laxity in these cases. Less satisfactory MR results were reported by Moeser and colleagues in observing ACL reconstructions performed with fascia latae from the iliotibial band and a MacIntosh lateral substitution over-the-top repair.[195,196] In 84% of studies by Fezoulidis and associates, carbon fiber ligament augmentation of the ACL was accurately imaged on MR scans of intraarticular and extraarticular grafts.[197]

Maywood and colleagues confirmed the usefulness of MR in identifying intact, partially torn, and complete tears of ACL autografts as correlated with the results of clinical examination and arthroscopy.[198] Imaging the ACL autograft in its anatomic plane and use of T2 weighting was necessary to determine graft integrity and to differentiate partial from complete tears. The process of ligamentization, including the development of a synovial envelope, may be responsible for temporal changes of increased signal intensity seen in unimpinged ACL grafts in some studies. However, these changes may also represent the earliest signs of clinically occult roof impingement. These changes are best appreciated on T1- or proton density weighted images.

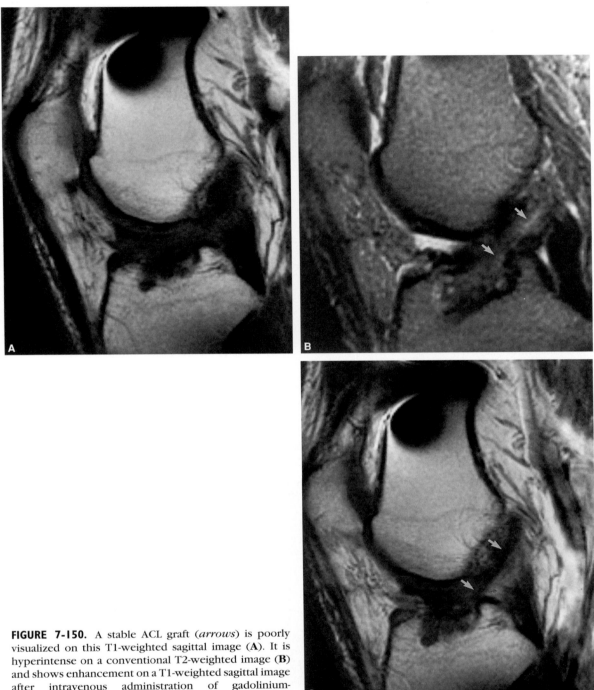

FIGURE 7-150. A stable ACL graft (*arrows*) is poorly visualized on this T1-weighted sagittal image (**A**). It is hyperintense on a conventional T2-weighted image (**B**) and shows enhancement on a T1-weighted sagittal image after intravenous administration of gadolinium-DTPA (**C**).

MR evaluation of ACL reconstructions using hamstring tendons in children with open physes has shown grafts with areas of increased signal intensity despite clinical stability.[199,200]

Clinical findings suggestive of roof impingement are knee joint effusion, extension deficit, recurrent instability, anterior knee pain, or a combination of these findings.[201] MR findings in roof impingement include a regionally increased signal intensity in the distal two thirds of the graft and posterior bowing of the graft caused by direct contact of the graft against the intercondylar roof. MR findings of placement of a portion of the tibial tunnel anterior to the slope of the intercondylar roof in a fully extended knee confirm roentgenographic diagnosis.[201]

Arthroscopic patterns of graft injury associated with roof impingement include the development of a fibrocartilaginous nodule or Cyclops lesion anterior to the distal third of the ACL graft, fractured bundles of the graft, guillotined fibers at the entrance into the notch, parallel fragmentation of graft fibers (lax bundles), and extrusion or molding of the graft by the distal end of the notch.[201] The localized fibrocartilaginous or Cyclops lesion may limit knee extension after ACL reconstruction. Cyclops lesions are graded 1, 2, or 3 depending on their anterior extent along the femoral condyle.[202] Fibrocartilaginous tissue shows low to intermediate signal intensity on T1, T2, and fast spin-echo images; and is best visualized in the sagittal plane, between Hoffa's fat pad and the leading edge of the distal ACL graft (Fig. 7-151). Fractured bundles involving the anterior portion of the graft are reported to be the most common injury present in

graft impingement (Fig. 7-152). This finding is consistent with intercondylar roof impingement affecting the anterior surface of the graft before extension of damage to the posterior fibers, as is seen in cases of modest or severe impingement in unstable knees. On MR scans it is possible to identify a ruptured anterior bundle separate from intact but impinged posterior bundle fibers. Because the process of graft rupturing removes the site of impingement on that portion of the graft, the ruptured portion may demonstrate lower signal intensity than the remaining intermediate-signal-intensity impinged fibers. Dislodged bone plugs may require the use of gradient-echo contrast to improve the visualization of the low-signal-intensity osseous components or osseous ends of the ruptured ACL graft within or displaced anterior to the intercondylar notch (see Fig. 7-152). In addition to the characteristic increased signal intensity visualized in graft impingement, there may be associated graft angulation and elongation caused by impingement from the intercondylar roof. The increased signal intensity observed in the distal two thirds of the ACL graft may persist for 1 to 3 years after implantation.[203] Enlargement of the roof can alleviate the signs of graft impingement, including a return (within 12 weeks) to a normal low signal intensity appearance. Although increased signal intensity may occur in an ACL graft with roof impingement but without initial evidence of clinical instability, patients with an impinged graft who subsequently regain a complete range of extension do become clinically unstable.[190] Gradual graft elongation secondary to roof impingement precedes this development of instability.

On coronal MR images, side wall impingement can be seen with the graft indented as it curves over the medial

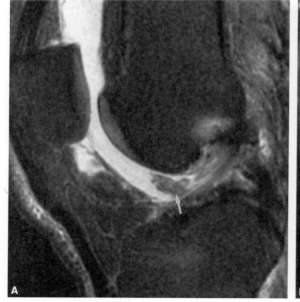
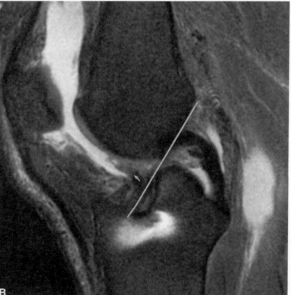

FIGURE 7-151. A cyclops lesion as shown on fat-suppressed T2-weighted fast spin-echo sagittal images. **(A)** A low signal intensity cyclops lesion (*arrow*) located between Hoffa's fat pad and the anterior surface of the ruptured ACL graft. **(B)** ACL graft rupture (*arrow*) associated with roof impingement. The tibial tunnel is anterior to the slope (*long white line*) of the intercondylar roof. A cyclops lesion may be associated with either an intact or a ruptured ACL graft and may produce a loss of knee extension.

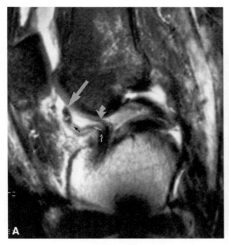
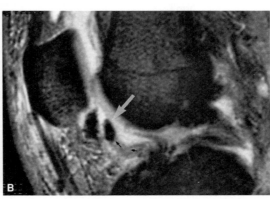
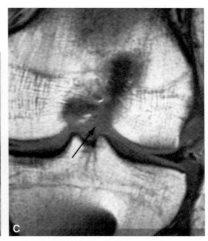

FIGURE 7-152. Graft rupture (*small arrow*) on fat-suppressed T2-weighted fast spin-echo (**A**) and T2*-weighted (**B**) sagittal sequences. The proximal bone plug (*large straight arrow*) remains attached to the anterior bundle (*large arrow*). The bone plug is best visualized on the T2*-weighted image because of a susceptibility effect. The ruptured posterior bundle (*curved arrow*) is also identified. The torn graft is displaced anteriorly and is hypointense: no impingement is present, as the graft is free of the intercondylar roof). (**C**) The corresponding T1-weighted coronal image shows absence of the ACL within the intercondylar notch.

aspect of the lateral femoral condyle. Sidewall impingement may be associated with the opening of the femoral tunnel positioned low in the intercondylar notch. The finding of sidewall impingement is usually apparent at arthroscopy.

Gadolinium contrast studies may not only confirm synovial envelope vascularity but may also improve the conspicuity of the ACL graft by enhancing the anterior and posterior borders of the graft relative to its synovial envelope. Intraligamentous enhancement of the ACL graft is thought to represent occult or unrecognized roof impingement and is not present in normal unimpinged grafts.[187] Enhancement in the impinged graft may be related to intrinsic revascularization (a phenomenon that does not occur in the unimpinged graft)

or replacement of injured graft tissue by vascularized periligamentous tissue.[193] The most common cause of a failed ACL reconstruction is an anteriorly placed femoral tunnel, which creates a nonisometric graft that will elongate with knee flexion.

MR changes in the patellar tendon are seen immediately after ACL reconstruction.[204] Initially, the patellar tendon demonstrates increased signal intensity on T1- and T2-weighted images with an associated thickening in the anteroposterior plane (Fig. 7-153). At the end of 12 months, uncomplicated donor sites show normal low signal intensity or, sometimes, a residual line of higher signal intensity parallel to the patellar tendon at its harvest site. There may also

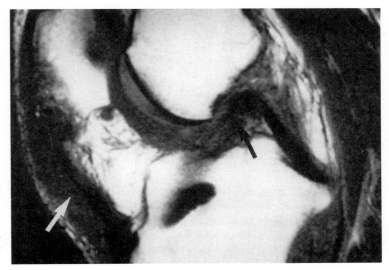

FIGURE 7-153. A T1-weighted image of patellar tendon ACL reconstruction shows the donor site (*white arrow*) and the reconstructed ligament (*black arrow*).

be residual thickening of the tendon. Symptomatic patellar tendons measure greater than 10 mm in the anteroposterior dimension at 12 months.[187] Patella baja, secondary to associated adhesion and fibrosis, may be seen during the first 6 months postoperatively. Patellar tendon donor site complications include patellar fracture, tendinitis, tendon rupture, patellar entrapment, and reflex sympathetic dystrophy. These changes can all be evaluated by MR.

Posterior Cruciate Ligament (PCL)

The PCL originates in the lateral aspect of the medial femoral condyle, crosses the ACL and attaches to the posterior intercondyloid fossa of the tibia.[205,206] It averages 38 mm in length and 13 mm in width at the midportion.[207] The cross-sectional area of the PCL decreases from its proximal-to-distal attachments. The smaller tibial insertion of the PCL attaches onto an inclined recessed shelf, posterior and inferior to the articular plateau of the tibia. The large femoral origin is on the lateral wall of the medial femoral condyle (Fig. 7-154) where the PCL attaches to a flat upper border and a convex lower border that parallels the articular surface of the medial femoral condyle. The PCL, similar to the ACL, is intraarticular but is extrasynovial and enveloped by a fold of synovium reflected from the posterior capsule. The PCL is composed of an anterolateral and posteromedial band that tightens on flexion and extension respectively. With progressive

knee flexion, the posteromedial bundle or band of the PCL passes anterior to and under the anterolateral bundle. The larger cross-sectional anterior band (anterolateral) tightens with knee flexion and relaxes with knee extension. The smaller cross-sectional posterior (posteromedial) band is lax in flexion and tightens in extension. A smaller posterior oblique band or bundle has also been described in the PCL. Functional and morphologic descriptions of the PCL divide the ligament first into an anterior and central portion, which constitutes the bulk of the ligament. Posterior longitudinal and posterior oblique components represent 10% to 15% of the substance of the ligament. The PCL is viewed as a central stabilizer of the knee, restraining posterior tibial displacement on the femur. It stabilizes the joint against excessive varus or valgus angulation and resists internal rotation of the tibia on the femur. Isolated rupture of the PCL (which is rare), has little effect on tibial rotational laxity or varus and valgus angulation without associated injury of the extraarticular restraints. A combined injury of the PCL and posterolateral (arcuate) complex results in a significant increase in both varus angulation and tibial external rotation, maximal at 90 degrees of knee flexion. Most PCL fibers are not isometric, except in the posterior oblique fiber region located at the posterosuperior margin of the anterior femoral PCL attachment.

Posterior to the PCL, the ligament of Wrisberg connects the posterior horn of the lateral meniscus to the lateral aspect of the medial femoral condyle near the origin of the PCL. The ligament of Humphrey passes anterior to the PCL. Either the anterior or posterior meniscofemoral ligament is found

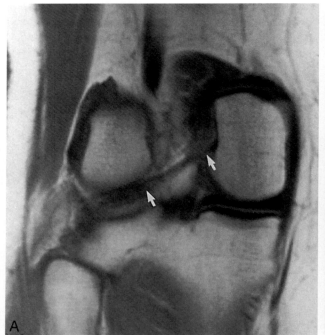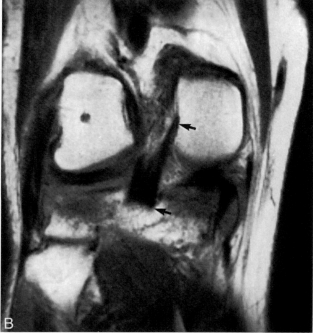

FIGURE 7-154. (A) A coronal T1-weighted image shows the low signal intensity ligament of Wrisberg (*arrows*, meniscofemoral ligament) extending from the posterior horn of the lateral meniscus to the medial femoral condyle. (B) The coronal anatomy of the PCL (*arrows*) is seen immediately anterior to the insertion of the ligament of Wrisberg on the medial femoral condyle.

in 80% of knee joint specimens,[208] and both meniscofemoral ligaments are present in 6% to 88% of knees.[209] The ligaments of Humphrey and Wrisberg are taut in flexion and extension respectively. With internal rotation of the tibia, both meniscofemoral ligaments tighten; therefore, the posterior drawer test should be performed in neutral or external tibial rotation.[43,210] These ligaments are considered stabilizers of the posterior horn of the lateral meniscus. The meniscofemoral ligament increases in congruity between the meniscotibial socket and the lateral femoral condyle during knee flexion and may function as a secondary restraint to posterior tibial translation after complete rupture of the PCL.[207]

Location and Mechanism of Injury of the PCL

The PCL is twice as strong as the ACL, with a larger cross-sectional area and higher tensile strength. These features account for a lower incidence of rupture of the PCL.[43,211,212] Injuries to the PCL represent only 5% to 20% of all knee ligament injuries.[213] Tears of the PCL are most common in the midportion (76%), followed by avulsions from the femur (36% to 55%), and the tibia (22% to 42%).[205,214,215] Rupture can be caused by excessive rotation, hyperextension, dislocation, or by direct trauma while the knee is flexed.[216,217] Motor vehicle accidents (dashboard injuries) and injuries sustained in contact sports (eg, football) are the most common causes of damage to the PCL.[218,219] Injuries to the PCL are usually associated with tears of either the ACL, the meniscus, or collateral ligaments.[210,220] When there is a lateral shift of the normal center of the axis of rotation of the joint, PCL insufficiency may lead to articular cartilage degeneration in the medial compartment of the knee. A positive posterior drawer sign indicating posterior tibial displacement can be seen in up to 60% of cases.[43]

The posterolateral capsule and popliteus complex are secondary restraints to posterior tibial displacement with a less important contribution made by the MCL.[43] Posterolateral instability may thus be associated with PCL injuries; posteromedial instability is less common. In direct trauma, PCL injuries are associated with acute hemarthrosis, although not as severe as that seen with ACL injuries.[221] The frequent lack of soft-tissue swelling may lead to a delay in clinical diagnosis. Unlike ACL injuries, associated meniscal abnormalities in the PCL-deficient knee are relatively uncommon.[219] Isolated injuries (30%) of the PCL may be associated with lateral compartment pathology or patellar articular cartilage injury.[222] The incidence of meniscal tears and articular cartilage injuries in the medial compartment increases in chronic PCL injuries.[222] In cases of knee dislocation with the PCL injury as one component of a combined injury, it is important to conduct a neurovascular evaluation.[218] The posterior sag sign is seen in complete tears of the PCL. The tibia sags into posterior subluxation relative to the femur with the patient supine and the knee flexed to 90°.[218] Other clinical tests used to indicate PCL injury include the quadriceps active test, which results in translation of the tibia anteriorly during quadriceps contraction, and various versions of the reverse pivot-shift test.

Arthroscopic Evaluation of PCL Injury

Direct arthroscopic findings include damage to the PCL involving both midsubstance and interstitial tears with ligament stretching and avulsion of bony insertions. Indirect arthroscopic findings include degenerative changes of the patellofemoral joint and medial compartment. The "sloppy-ACL sign" at arthroscopy describes the increased relative laxity of the ACL secondary to posterior tibial drop-back. Posterior tibial drop-back is the phenomenon of gravity-assisted posterior tibial subluxation produced by the absence of the restraining function of the PCL.[223] Limitations of arthroscopy are related to poor visualization of the PCL in the presence of an intact ACL, the misinterpretation of a normal ligament of Humphrey (meniscofemoral ligament) as an injury, and the location of the arthroscopic portals selected to visualize the PCL. The inferolateral patellar portal and occasionally the posteromedial arthroscopic portal should allow complete visualization of the entire PCL.[224]

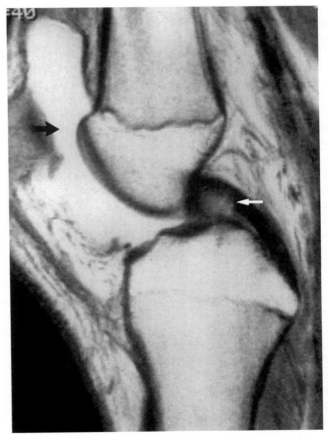

FIGURE 7-155. An intact low-signal-intensity PCL (*white arrow*) shows adjacent high-signal-intensity joint effusion (*black arrow*) on a T2-weighted sagittal image.

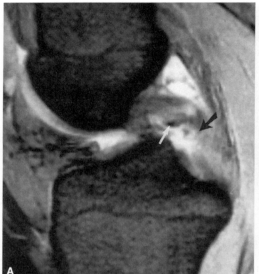 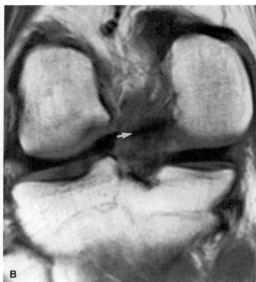

FIGURE 7-156. (A) A T2*-weighted sagittal image shows a hyperintense complete PCL tear (*black arrow*). The ligament of Humphrey (*white arrow*) is seen anterior to the PCL. (B) The corresponding T1-weighted coronal image shows the ligament of Humphrey (*arrow*) located anterior to the expected location of the absent PCL.

MR Imaging of the PCL

The normal PCL is seen as a uniform low-signal-intensity band. The morphology and signal intensity of the PCL are routinely evaluated on axial, coronal, and sagittal images. In the sagittal plane, the PCL has an arcuate shape with the knee positioned in neutral or minimal flexion (Fig. 7-155).[8] The PCL is visualized on one or two consecutive sagittal images in its entire length. The PCL becomes taut with knee flexion and more lax with hyperextension. In the posterior coronal plane, the PCL demonstrates a more vertical orientation as it is sectioned in the downward slope of its curved arc. Mid- and anterior-coronal images display the more circular cross-section of the ligament. Axial images can be used to follow the sectioning of the ligament from the posterior tibia to its broad anterior medial femoral condyle attachment. The low signal intensity anterior and posterior meniscofemoral ligaments are identified in up to 60% of MR examinations. Although the meniscofemoral ligaments are more commonly seen on sagittal images (midportion of the PCL), they are often identified on coronal and axial images. Their visualization may improve in the presence of the edema and hemorrhage associated with a torn PCL (Fig. 7-156). An abnormally high arc or buckling of the PCL may indicate a tear of the ACL with secondary forward tibial displacement.

We use the same protocols for evaluation of PCL and ACL injuries. A combination of T1 and fat-suppressed T2-weighted fast spin-echo images in all three planes (axial, coronal, and sagittal) provides sufficient information to differentiate an intact ligament from a partial or complete tear. Depiction of both normal PCL morphology and tears is excellent on MR images as confirmed by arthroscopy and arthrotomy.[225] Findings of increased signal intensity with normal PCL morphology on T1-weighted images requires the addition of conventional T2, T2*, or fat-suppressed T2-weighted fast spin-echo images to identify the sites of ligamentous pathology. Hemorrhage and edema, seen in acute injuries, are bright on T2- (including fast spin-echo) and T2*-weighted images and cause less distortion or mass effect than do tears of the ACL.

Any increase in PCL signal intensity on T1, T2, T2*, or fat-suppressed T2-weighted fast spin-echo images is abnormal (Fig. 7-157). In an interstitial tear, the entire ligament or long segment may be difficult to identify because of diffuse widening and increased signal intensity (Fig. 7-158). In complete tears, there is an amorphous high signal intensity with-

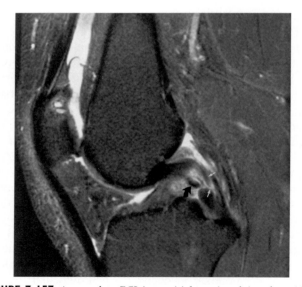

FIGURE 7-157. A complete PCL interstitial tear involving the middle one third of the ligament (*straight arrow*) on a fat-suppressed T2-weighted fast spin-echo sagittal image. A hyperintense fluid signal is insinuated between the planes of the torn fibers. The intact hypointense ligament of Humphrey is present (*curved arrow*).

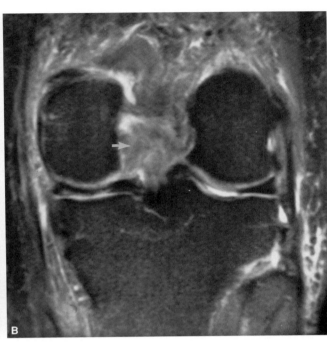

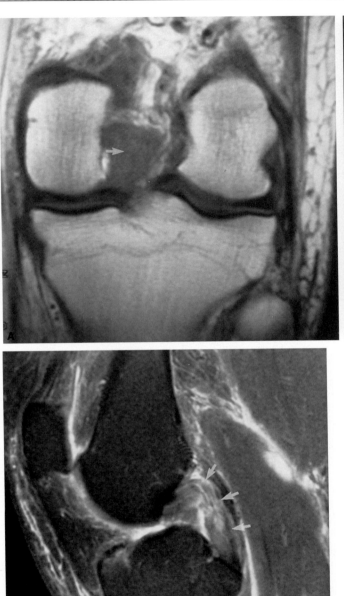

FIGURE 7-158. Acute rupture of the PCL with a diffuse interstitial tear pattern (*arrows*) associated with widening of the ligament. The PCL is intermediate in signal on a T1-weighted coronal image (**A**) and inhomogeneously hyperintense on fat-suppressed T2-weighted fast spin-echo coronal (**B**) and sagittal (**C**) images.

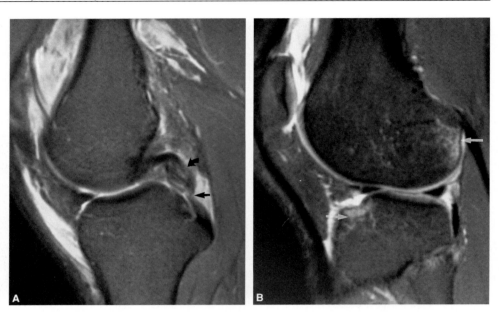

FIGURE 7-159. (**A**) Fat-suppressed T2-weighted fast spin-echo sagittal image of a PCL tear with focal discontinuity (*straight arrow*). Note the enlarged end of the torn proximal segment (*curved arrow*), which has associated interstitial tearing. The identification of a discrete gap or ligament discontinuity is a less common presentation of a ruptured PCL. (**B**) Associated bone contusions (*arrows*) involve the anterior lateral tibia and posterior lateral femoral condyle.

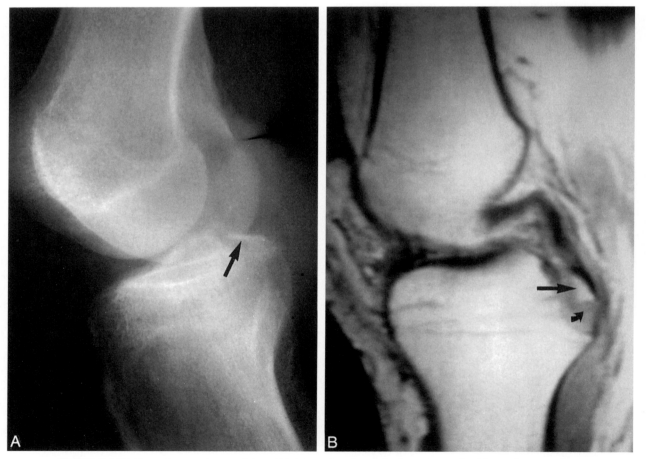

FIGURE 7-160. Posterior cruciate avulsion. (**A**) A lateral radiograph shows an avulsed bony fragment from the posterior tibial plateau (*arrow*). (**B**) The corresponding T1-weighted sagittal image shows avulsed bone containing high signal intensity yellow marrow from the attachment site of the PCL (*straight arrow*). Intermediate signal intensity is generated by associated edema and hemorrhage (*curved arrow*).

out definable ligamentous fibers.[226] Less commonly, a focal discontinuity or gap may be seen (Fig. 7-159). Partial tears display increased signal intensity with discernible fibers identified along the course of the ligament. A chronic partial tear may be difficult to identify on MR, even in the presence of a clinically positive posterior sag sign.[218]

It is easier to assess ligament morphology on fat-suppressed T2-weighted fast spin-echo images than on gradient-echo images, which tend to display a greater degree of hyper-

intensity in regions of edema and hemorrhage. An avulsion tear off the tibial plateau may be associated with high-signal-intensity ligamentous hemorrhage and a bone fragment containing marrow (Figs. 7-160 and 7-161). Subchondral marrow edema and hemorrhage between the avulsed fragment and tibia are frequently seen on fat-suppressed T2-weighted fast spin-echo and STIR images.

Bone contusions in the anterolateral tibia and posterior lateral femoral condyle are consistent with a forced posterior

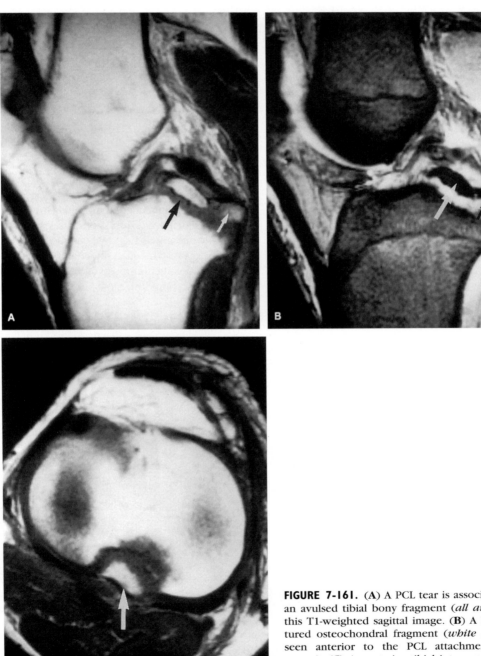

FIGURE 7-161. (A) A PCL tear is associated with an avulsed tibial bony fragment (*all arrows*) on this T1-weighted sagittal image. (B) A large fractured osteochondral fragment (*white arrow*) is seen anterior to the PCL attachment (*black arrow*). (C) A posterior tibial intercondylar fracture is revealed on a T1-weighted axial image (*arrow*).

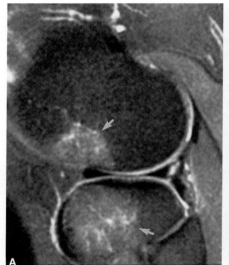
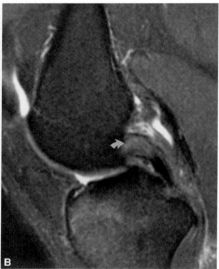

FIGURE 7-162. (**A**) Anterior bone contusions (*straight arrows*) of the lateral compartment associated with a partial interstitial tear (*curved arrow*) of the proximal PCL. (Fat-suppressed T2-weighted fast spin-echo sagittal image.) (**B**) Anterior tibial bone contusions are commonly associated with PCL injuries. The mechanism of injury in this patient was hyperextension. (Fat-suppressed T2-weighted fast spin-echo sagittal image.)

displacement of the tibia in a flexed knee (see Fig. 7-159).[227] Hyperextension injuries may demonstrate contusions of the anterotibial articular surface and the anterior aspect of the femoral condyle (Fig. 7-162). There may be an associated ACL rupture. Sonin and colleagues retrospectively reviewed MR findings in PCL injuries[226] and found that 38% of patients with PCL injuries had complete tears; 55% had partial tears; and 63% had midsubstance injuries. Of these injuries, 20% were proximal and 3% were distal. Isolated PCL injury were found in 24% of patients, and tibial insertion avulsion injuries were found in 7% of patients. Associated findings included involvement of the MCL injury more often than LCL and the medial meniscus more commonly than the lateral meniscus. In the majority of patients, joint effusions are relatively small.

Coronal plane images can be used to confirm regions of signal abnormality identified on sagittal images (see Fig. 7-158). Linear intrasubstance splits and regions of hyperintensity are displayed in cross-section through the vertical and horizontal portions of the ligament. Chronic tears result in abnormal ligamentous morphology, with intermediate signal intensity on T1- and T2-weighted images, and sometimes an apparent continuity across an area of ligamentous scarring (Fig. 7-163). Chronic disruption may also be indicated by abnormal laxity of the fibers or failure of the PCL to become taut during flexion. A magic angle effect could produce inhomogeneity of signal intensity in an arthroscopically normal PCL, based on the orientation of the PCL to the magnetic field.

Sensitivity and specificity of MR in identifying complete tears of the PCL has been reported to be 100%.[219] In severe posterolateral disruptions, there may be avulsion off the fibular head or Gerdy's tubercle. Osteoarthritis of the medial, lateral, and patellofemoral compartments can be seen in chronic injuries.

Treatment of PCL Injury

PCL tears with tibial plateau avulsions require surgical treatment and direct repair. Midsubstance and femoral avulsions require augmentation and reconstruction with the use of free or vascularized grafts from the patellar tendon or semitendinosus and gracilis tendons, or allografts.[43,210] Nonoperative treatment is recommended for acute isolated PCL injuries, with surgical reconstruction reserved for symptomatic chronic PCL injuries, acute bony avulsions, and acute combined injuries.[219]

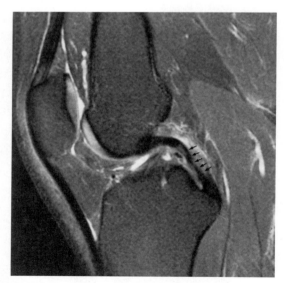

FIGURE 7-163. A chronic PCL tear with irregular ligament morphology and contour (*small arrows*) on a fat-suppressed T2-weighted fast spin-echo sagittal image. PCL continuity, however, is partially maintained. Both fibrous scar tissue and the normal PCL may display hypointensity on T1- and T2-weighted sequences. Contour irregularities, including ligamentous redundancy or tapering, are associated with chronic PCL disruptions. The intact PCL is taut in partial knee flexion.

The isolated PCL tear requires surgical reconstruction, however, when the posterior tibial drop-back is greater than 10 to 15 mm. PCL tears associated with ACL tears or extensive capsular disruptions are also surgically treated. One of the more serious complications associated with PCL reconstruction is neurovascular injury during tibial tunnel preparation. In addition, delayed complications related to PCL reconstruction include loss of motion, avascular necrosis involving the medial femoral condyle, and recurrent laxity.[219]

COLLATERAL LIGAMENTS

Medial Collateral Ligament (MCL)

Warren and Marshall have divided the medial aspect of the knee into three layers, from superficial to deep.[228] Layer 1 consists of the deep fascia surrounding the sartorius muscle and overlying the gastrocnemius. Layer 2 is the superficial MCL, and layer 3 is the medial capsular ligament (ie, the true capsule of the knee joint that forms the deep layer of the MCL in its midportion). Posteriorly, layers 2 and 3 merge to form the posterior oblique ligament (oblique portion of the tibial collateral ligament).

Functional Anatomy of the MCL

The MCL, or tibial collateral ligament, is 8 to 10 cm long and extends from its medial epicondylar origin to attach 4 to 5 cm inferior to the tibial plateau and posterior to the pes anserinus insertion. The insertion of the MCL on the tibia is covered by the muscle group of the pes anserinus. The MCL is considered to be composed of two layers: (1) deep fibers, corresponding to layer 3, that attach to the capsule and medial meniscus peripherally and (2) more superficial fibers, corresponding to layer 2.

In general, the term "MCL" refers to layer 2 (the superficial MCL). The superficial MCL can be further divided into anterior and posterior portions. The anterior fibers of the superficial MCL tighten with knee flexion of 70° to 105°.[128] When the knee is extended, the fibers of the MCL are taut and limit hyperextension. When the knee is flexed, the MCL provides primary valgus stability. The MCL remains taut through flexion. It is separated from the underlying capsular ligament and medial meniscus by a bursa that reduces friction during knee flexion. MCL function is tested with applied valgus stress in partial knee flexion, with the tibia in external rotation (allowing relaxation of the cruciate ligaments). The importance of MCL function increases with increasing flexion, as the posterior capsular structures become lax, and its contribution decreases with increasing valgus movement and rotation, as the posteromedial aspect of the capsule becomes more involved.[128]

The medial capsular ligament (layer 3) is composed of meniscofemoral and meniscotibial attachments to the menis-

cus. The superficial MCL provides the primary valgus restraint relative to the deep capsular ligament.[43] If the MCL fails at 10 to 15 mm of joint opening, the cruciate ligaments become the primary restraints to valgus stress. In the ACL-deficient knee, the superficial MCL and medial capsule function as secondary restraints to anterior tibial translation.

Location and Mechanism of Injury of the MCL, Including the Posteromedial Corner

Usually, the MCL is injured with a valgus force applied to the flexed knee. Partial ruptures or sprains frequently involve fibrous attachments to the medial femoral condyle. Complete MCL rupture may be associated with tears of the medial and posterior capsule, the ACL, and the medial meniscus.[46] Peripheral medial meniscal tears are more common in isolated MCL injuries, whereas substance tears are more frequently seen with combined MCL and ACL injuries.[229] A contusion or fracture caused by the impact of the lateral femoral condyle on the lateral tibial plateau during valgus injury is common.

A grading system for MCL ligament injuries classifies grade I lesions as minimal tears without instability, grade II injuries as partial tears with increased instability, and grade III injuries as complete ruptures with gross instabilities.[43] Quantification of joint space opening has led to an additional classification system that can be applied to partial tears or sprains. Grade I joint-space opening is 0 to 5 mm; grade II is 6 to 10 mm; grade III is 11 to 15 mm; and grade IV is 16 to 20 mm. Stress testing in an extremity coil should be performed with the knee in partial flexion to produce maximum medial joint-space opening.

The posteromedial corner of the knee is an important and anatomically complex region frequently injured in association with other medial supporting structures and the medial meniscus.[8] The posteromedial corner receives an important contribution from the semimembranosus tendon. The posterior oblique ligament, formed by the merging of the previously described layers 2 and 3 of the knee, represents the connection between the capsular attachment of the semimembranosus tendon and oblique fibers of the superficial MCL. The five arms of insertion of the semimembranosus tendon are (1) the attachment to the posteromedial aspect of the tibia just distal to the joint line, (2) the more anterior attachment to the tibia deep to the superficial MCL, (3) an attachment of its tendon sheath to the posteromedial capsule, (4) an oblique popliteal ligament attachment, and (5) a distal attachment to the fascia of the popliteus muscle. Functionally, the posteromedial corner resists valgus laxity in knee extension. Injuries of the posteromedial corner frequently involve the posterior horn of the medial meniscus (peripheral aspect), the popliteal oblique ligament, and the MCL. Although the semitendinosus tendon does not directly contribute to the posteromedial corner, however, injuries of this structure may present with posteromedial knee pain (Fig. 7-164).

MR Appearance of MCL Injury

TEARS AND SPRAINS. Arthrography is limited in the ability to detect MCL injuries, especially after 48 hours when extravasation of contrast media can no longer be seen. MR

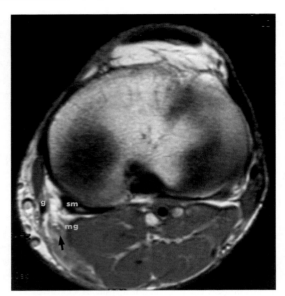

FIGURE 7-164. A T1-weighted axial image of a torn and retracted semitendinosus tendon in a soccer player. The semitendinosus tendon is not present in its usual location (*arrow*) medial to the medial head of the gastrocnemius muscle (*mg*), posterior to the semimembranosus tendon (*sm*), and lateral to the gracilis tendon (*g*) at the level of the tibial plateau.

evaluation of these injuries is best accomplished with coronal images that demonstrate the low-signal MCL and its attachment points, where it merges with low signal intensity cortical bone. Occasionally, separation of the deep and superficial layers can be distinguished on T2-weighted images. A thin band of intermediate signal intensity, originally thought to be fat, is actually an intraligamentous bursa between layers 2 and 3 and is often seen between the anterior portion of

the MCL and the deep medial capsular ligament complex.[230] This bursa may be seen to extend proximal and distal to the level of the joint line medially. Although this line does not represent meniscocapsular separation, increased signal intensity above or below the level of the meniscus may represent pathologic change, especially if it is seen posteriorly where layers 2 and 3 fuse.

Edema and hemorrhage, which extend into subcutaneous fat, are identified parallel to the superficial MCL and may occur in acute grade I sprains (Fig. 7-165). The MCL is of normal thickness and is closely applied to the underlying cortical bone. Partial tears or grade II sprains of the MCL demonstrate displacement of ligament fibers from adjacent cortical bone with varying degrees of edema and hemorrhage (Fig. 7-166). T2, T2*, fat-suppressed fast spin-echo, and STIR images demonstrate high signal intensity edema, hemorrhage, or both around low signal intensity ligamentous fibers, which are superficial and deep to the MCL. Usually there is some degree of ligamentous attenuation or areas of fluid separating partially torn fibers in grade II injuries. In grade III lesions or tears, there is complete loss of continuity of the ligamentous fibers with or without extension into the capsular layer (Fig. 7-167). It may be difficult to distinguish between high grade partial tears and complete tears of the MCL, however. Complete biomechanical failure of the MCL is associated with disruption of the medial capsular layer or ligament.[231,232]

Schweitzer and colleagues have reported that fascial edema and loss of demarcation from adjacent fat are the most sensitive signs of grade II MCL injury.[233] Although findings in this study also indicated that MR grading may not be highly accurate for classification of MCL injuries, it

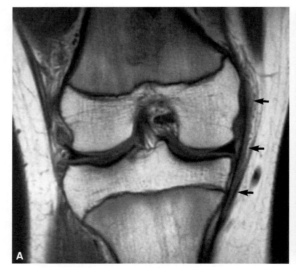
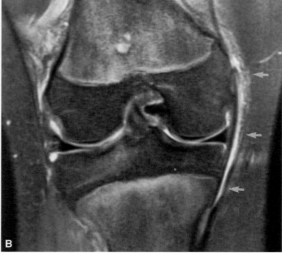

FIGURE 7-165. Grade I MCL sprain with fluid (*arrow*) superficial to the MCL is hypointense on a T1-weighted coronal image (**A**) and hyperintense on a fat-suppressed T2-weighted fast spin-echo coronal image (**B**). There is no displacement or thickening of the low signal intensity ligament. A grade I tear is primarily a periligamentous injury with associated microscopic tearing of ligament fibers.

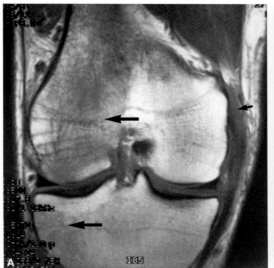

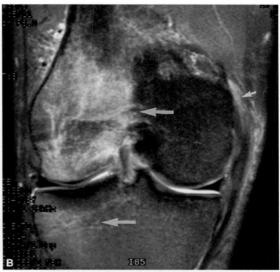

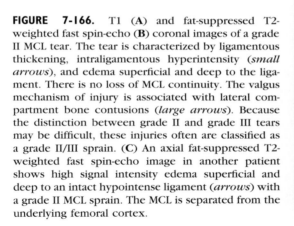

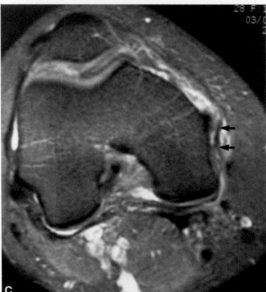

FIGURE 7-166. T1 (**A**) and fat-suppressed T2-weighted fast spin-echo (**B**) coronal images of a grade II MCL tear. The tear is characterized by ligamentous thickening, intraligamentous hyperintensity (*small arrows*), and edema superficial and deep to the ligament. There is no loss of MCL continuity. The valgus mechanism of injury is associated with lateral compartment bone contusions (*large arrows*). Because the distinction between grade II and grade III tears may be difficult, these injuries often are classified as a grade II/III sprain. (**C**) An axial fat-suppressed T2-weighted fast spin-echo image in another patient shows high signal intensity edema superficial and deep to an intact hypointense ligament (*arrows*) with a grade II MCL sprain. The MCL is separated from the underlying femoral cortex.

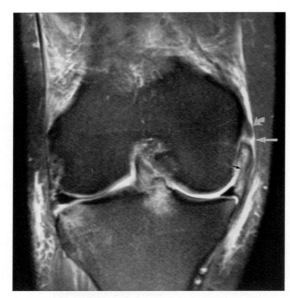

FIGURE 7-167. A grade III MCL tear with discontinuity of the proximal ligament fibers (*large straight arrow*). High signal intensity fluid fills the tear site. A small stump of proximal epicondylar fibers remains (*curved arrow*). The meniscofemoral ligament is torn (*small straight arrow*), whereas the meniscotibial ligament is intact. Hyperintense lateral tibial plateau contusion and tibial spine avulsion also are seen on this fat-suppressed T2-weighted fast spin-echo coronal image.

was limited by lack of correlation with T2-weighted coronal images and lack of comparison with clinical grading of MCL injuries.

MCL tears may be associated with extensive joint effusion (from hemarthrosis) and extravasation of joint fluid, which tracks along the ligament fibers. An associated capsular disruption may be related to diminished or absent joint swelling. Focal hemorrhage can be visualized at the femoral epicondylar attachment in complete ligamentous avulsions (Fig. 7-168). In these cases, there may be subchondral marrow hyperemia or hemorrhage in the adjacent bone. Subacute hemorrhage demonstrates increased signal intensity on T1- and T2-weighted images. A tear of the distal or tibial attachment of the MCL may be associated with a wavy or serpiginous ligamentous contour (Figs. 7-169 and 7-170). T2-weighted images, including fat-suppressed T2-weighted fast spin-echo and gradient-echo images are useful in documenting interval healing with reattachment of the torn MCL. The process of religamentization or healing of the MCL may be associated with intermediate signal intensity in a region of increased thickness of the ligament.

Tearing of the MCL with capsular disruption may be associated with a peripheral meniscal tear and widening of the medial joint space. In response to chronic tears, the MCL is thickened but does not demonstrate increased signal intensity. Axial images are particularly useful in documenting the separation of the distal MCL fibers from the underlying tibia. They are also helpful, in conjunction with coronal images,

in documenting the extent of injury and involvement of either the anterior or posterior portions of the superficial MCL. This information may be useful in distinguishing between partial and complete tears of the MCL.

Calcification of the femoral epicondylar or proximal attachment of the MCL is thought to be the result of trauma and is referred to as Pellegrini-Stieda disease. The calcified deposit in Pellegrini-Stieda disease is low in signal intensity on T1- and T2-weighted images. Thickened ligamentous healing may be demonstrated at the same time calcification or periarticular ossification is detected (Fig. 7-171). Acute avulsions of the MCL may also be associated with a low-signal-intensity fractured cortical fragment (see Fig. 7-171).

In the acute setting, nondisplaced compression fractures of the lateral tibial plateau may be seen in conjunction with MCL injuries secondary to valgus injury (see Figs. 7-166 and 7-169). These fractures or bone contusions demonstrate low signal intensity on T1-weighted images and increased signal intensity on T2-weighted, fat-suppressed fast spin-echo, and STIR images. MR is sensitive to the identification of these injuries, and they may be detected even when radiographic findings are normal.[234] Contusions may also be identified in the lateral femoral condyle.

Separation of the meniscofemoral and meniscotibial components of the medial capsular ligament are poorly displayed on routine orthogonal coronal images. Radial images of the knee are preferable for displaying attachments of the MCL and meniscofemoral and meniscotibial ligaments. Radial images, however, should not replace routine coronal images, because MCL disruptions may be misdiagnosed unless the full posterior-to-anterior extent of the ligament is identified. Axial images can also be used to identify the course of the oblique popliteal ligament at the level of the distal femoral condyle and at the level of the joint line. The oblique popliteal ligament is visualized as a linear area of low signal intensity often appearing at the same level as the arcuate ligament complex.

MCL OR TIBIAL COLLATERAL LIGAMENT BURSITIS. Medial or tibial collateral ligament bursitis can be demonstrated on MR images in patients presenting with medial joint pain (Fig. 7-172). Bright signal intensity on T2-, T2*-, or fast spin-echo T2-weighted scans is demonstrated between layer 2 (superficial MCL) and layer 3 (medial capsular ligament). A well-defined, elongated collection of fluid extending predominantly inferior to the joint line may be observed without associated pathology in the medial meniscus, capsular ligament, or MCL. In addition, there may be fluid in a bursa deep to the pes anserinus bursa (see Fig. 7-172). Fluid in this region (anterior to the conjoined tendons of the sartorius, semitendinosus, and gracilis tendons) demonstrates low signal intensity on T1-weighted images and hyperintensity on T2-weighted images. There may be a septation or hemorrhage within this bursa.[235]

text continues on page 355

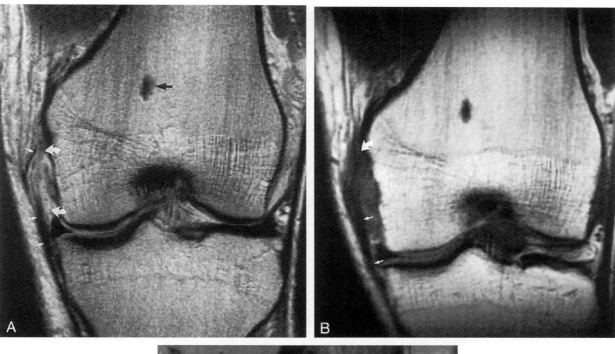

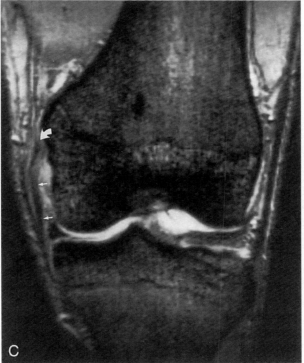

FIGURE 7-168. MCL avulsion. (**A**) An intermediate weighted coronal image shows subacute avulsion of the MCL from its femoral epicondylar cortical attachment (*straight white arrows*). Focal hemorrhage (*curved white arrows*) exhibits high signal intensity. An incidental bone island is seen as a focus of low signal intensity (*black arrow*). (**B** and **C**) After 6 months of brace treatment, the MCL (*straight arrows*) is in continuity with its thickened proximal portion (*curved arrows*). Delineation of the femoral cortical attachment improves as weighting progresses from a T1-weighted sequence (**B**) to a T2*-weighted sequence (**C**).

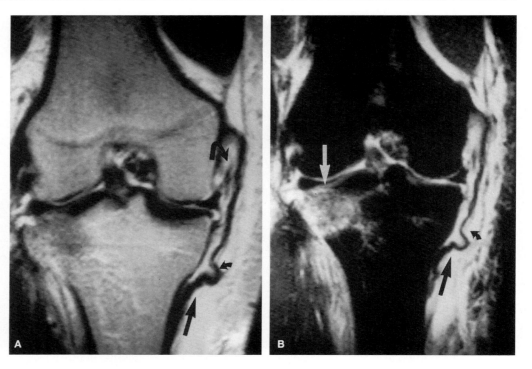

FIGURE 7-169. (A) Coronal T2-weighted and (B) coronal STIR images show avulsion of the distal tibial attachment of the MCL with proximal ligament retraction (*straight black arrow*) and increased ligamentous laxity (*small curved arrow*). Lateral tibial plateau impaction is best demonstrated by STIR contrast, which reveals hyperintense marrow hemorrhage (*straight white arrow*). Associated disruption of the meniscofemoral attachment of the deep capsular ligament (*large curved arrow*) is present. The extracapsular soft-tissue edema and hemorrhage is evident on the STIR image.

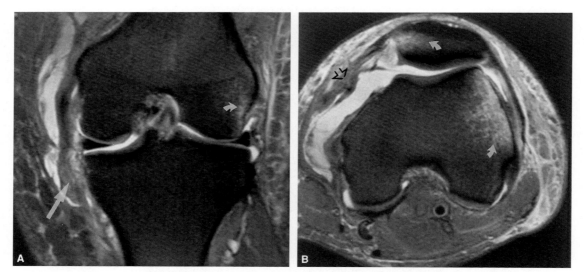

FIGURE 7-170. Fat-suppressed T2-weighted fast spin-echo coronal (**A**) and axial (**B**) images of a distal MCL (*straight arrow*) and medial retinacular disruption (*open arrow*) after lateral patellar dislocation. The MCL is grossly thickened, demonstrates increased laxity, and is displaced medial to the femur and tibia (**A**). Associated medial patellar and lateral femoral condylar contusions (*curved arrows*) characteristic of patellar dislocation are shown. The coronal view (**A**) demonstrates valgus instability with opening of the medial joint space.

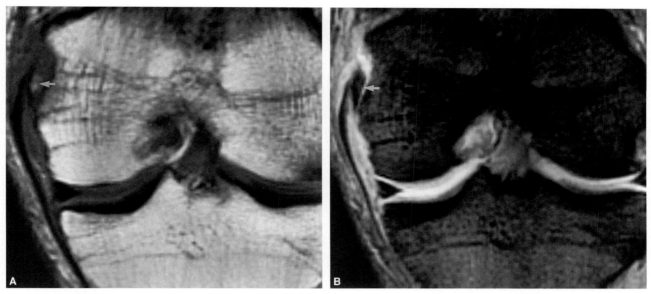

FIGURE 7-171. A grade III MCL tear with an avulsed bone fragment (*arrow*) from the femoral epicondyle is seen on T1- (**A**) and T2*- (**B**) weighted coronal images. The associated extracapsular hemorrhage is hyperintense on the T2*-weighted image.

Healing and Treatment of MCL Injury

Healing of the MCL occurs best when the disrupted ends of the ligaments are in direct contact or proximity. The size of the gap between the torn ends affects the potential of the ligament to heal. Tension has been shown to have a positive effect on ligament healing. The ligament recovers only 50% of its original modulus and tensile strength after 12 months. The load and stiffness of the MCL bone complex, however, may be normal as the healed tissue is thickened with a larger cross-sectional area.[128]

Grades I, II, and III isolated MCL sprains are treated with early functional rehabilitation. In isolated grade III MCL tears, operative and nonoperative treatment is equally effective. The posterior oblique ligament assists the MCL in resisting valgus and external rotation forces in extension and flexion. Combined MCL and ACL injuries are usually treated with surgical repair of only the ACL, thus converting the ACL to an isolated MCL injury.

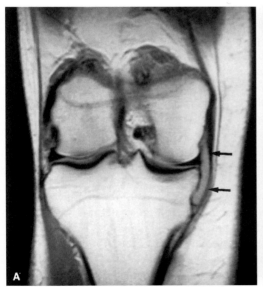
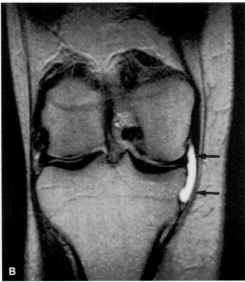

FIGURE 7-172. Coronal (**A**) intermediate weighted and (**B**) T2-weighted images of tibial collateral ligament bursitis (*arrows*) show no associated pathologic findings in the medial meniscus or collateral ligament. Fluid is hyperintense on the T2-weighted image.   *continued*

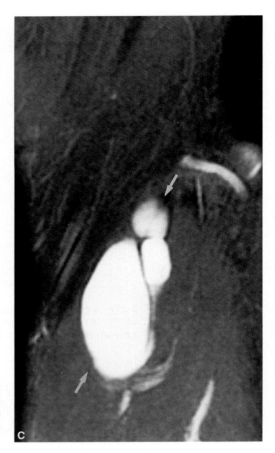

FIGURE 7-172. *Continued.* **(C)** In another patient, a multiseptal ganglion cyst (*arrows*) appears as pes anserinus bursitis. The fluid-filled mass originates deep to the pes anserinus tendons (the semitendinosus, gracilis, and sartorius tendons) and is hyperintense on this fatsuppressed T2-weighted fast spin-echo medial sagittal image.

Lateral Collateral Ligament (LCL) and Posterolateral Corner

The lateral aspect of the knee is divided into three structural layers.[43,162] Layer 1 is the most superficial layer and consists of the iliotibial tract with its anterior expansion and the superficial portion of the biceps femoris with its posterior expansion. Layer 2 consists of the quadriceps retinaculum anteriorly and two patellofemoral ligaments or retinacula posteriorly. Layers 1 and 2 merge at the lateral aspect of the patella. Layer 3 is the deepest layer and consists of the lateral joint capsule, including attachments to the lateral meniscus, and the lateral capsular ligament with its meniscofemoral and meniscotibial components. The LCL is located posteriorly between the superficial and deep divisions of layer 3. The ligament itself is considered a layer 2 structure.

The posterolateral (arcuate) complex includes the LCL, the popliteus tendon, the lateral head of the gastrocnemius muscle, and the arcuate ligament.[236]

The posterolateral complex also includes the popliteofibular (Fig. 7-173) and fabellofibular ligaments (Fig. 7-174).

The arcuate ligament (in layer 3) spans the posterolateral joint and extends distally, parallel with the LCL (see Fig. 7-174*A*). The Y-shaped arcuate ligament has a medial limb that extends from the posterior capsule at the level of the distal femur and extends medially on the popliteus muscle to the oblique popliteal ligament. The oblique popliteal ligament formed by the reflected portion of the semimembranosus tendon makes up the primary portion of the posterior capsule (Fig. 7-175). The lateral limb of the arcuate ligament extends from the posterior capsule and courses laterally over the popliteus muscle and tendon to insert on the posterior aspect of the fibula.[160] The popliteofibular ligament (see Fig. 7-173), also a layer 3 structure, is deep to the lateral limb of the arcuate ligament. This ligament takes origin from the posterior aspect of the fibula (posterior to the biceps insertion) and extends toward the junction of the popliteus muscle and tendon.[40] Proximal to the musculotendinous junction of the popliteus, the popliteofibular ligament joins the popliteus tendon. The popliteofibular ligament thus connects the fibula to the femur through the popliteus tendon. The fabellofibular (see Fig. 7-174) or short lateral ligament courses parallel to

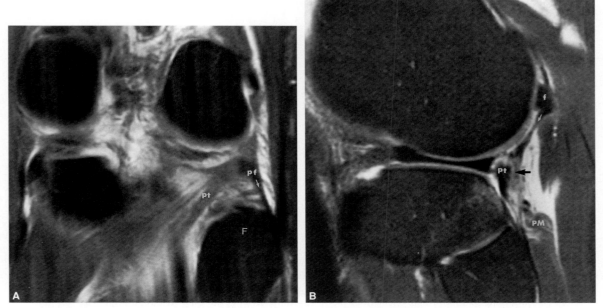

FIGURE 7-173. Posterolateral capsular structures on fat-suppressed T2-weighted fast spin-echo (**A**) coronal and (**B**) sagittal images. As a normal variant, the arcuate ligament may not be visualized in the presence of a fabellofibular ligament. (**A**) *pt*, popliteus tendon; *pf* and *arrow*, popliteofibular ligament; *F*, fibula. (**B**) *pt*, popliteus tendon; *f*, fabella; *small arrow*, fabellopopliteal ligament; *large arrow*, torn arcuate ligament; *PM*, partial torn popliteus muscle.

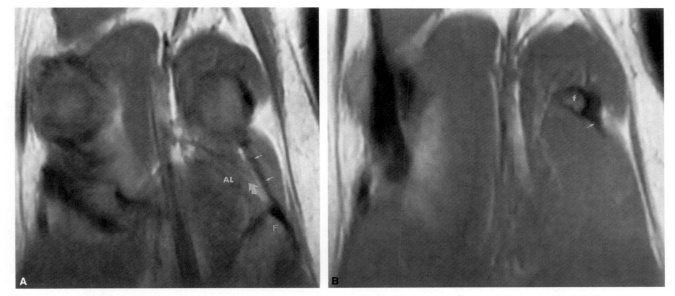

FIGURE 7-174. (**A** and **B**) The normal course of the fabellofibular ligament (*arrows*) between the fabella (*f*) and fibular head (*F*) on T1-weighted coronal images. The fabella is identified on the more posterior coronal view (**B**). The fabellofibular ligament is visualized posterior to the plane of the LCL. The arcuate ligament (*AL*) and its course (*curved arrow*) are shown. In this case, the prominent fabellofibular ligament acts as the lateral limb of the arcuate ligament.

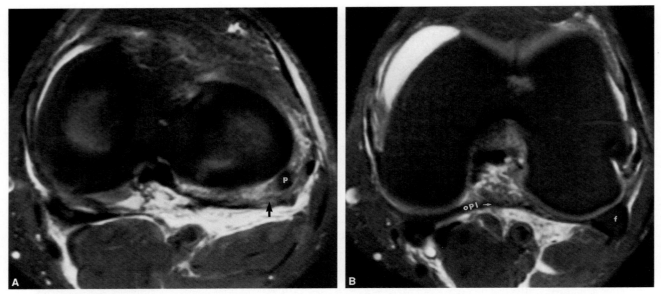

FIGURE 7-175. (A and B) Fat-suppressed T2-weighted fast spin-echo axial images showing the relation of the popliteus tendon (*P*) and arcuate ligament sprain (*arrow*) at the level of the joint line (**A**) and the normal visualization of the oblique popliteal ligament (*op* and *arrow*) on a more superior axial image at the level of the femoral condyles (**B**). *f*, fabella.

the LCL from the fabella to the fibula and inserts posterior to the biceps femoris tendon. If the fabella is absent, the short lateral ligament may be either attenuated or absent. When present, it is found adjacent to the lateral limb of the arcuate ligament, coursing from the femoral condyle over the lateral head of the gastrocnemius to the fibula. There may be an inverse relation between the size of the fabellofibular and arcuate ligaments. In the presence of a large fabella, the fabellofibular ligament is prominent and the arcuate ligament may be attenuated or absent. The fabellofibular ligament, when present, thus functions as the lateral limb of the arcuate ligament.[39] In the absence of the fabella, the lateral limb of the arcuate ligament is known as the short lateral ligament. Sagittal MR images have also documented the existence of a fabellopopliteal ligament (see Fig. 7-173).

Functional Anatomy of the LCL

The LCL, or fibular collateral ligament, is 5 to 7 cm long. It is extracapsular and free from meniscal attachment in its course from the lateral femoral epicondyle to its conjoined insertion with the biceps femoris tendon on the fibular head.[90] The intracapsular popliteus tendon passes medial to the LCL, and the posterior fibers of the LCL blend with the deep capsule, which contributes to the arcuate ligament.

Location and Mechanism of Injury of the LCL and Posterolateral Structures

The arcuate ligament and complex stabilize the posterolateral aspect of the knee against varus and external rotation.[160] With the leg in internal rotation, an applied varus

force can cause injury to the LCL and capsule. Injury or disruption of the LCL is significantly less common than injury to the MCL. Injury to the posterolateral corner can result from direct or noncontact forces that cause knee hyperextension or hyperextension and external rotation. A direct blow to the tibia with the knee flexed or extended or a twisting injury could produce posterolateral instability. These injuries may be seen in conjunction with either an ACL or PCL injury. Combined posterior cruciate and pos-

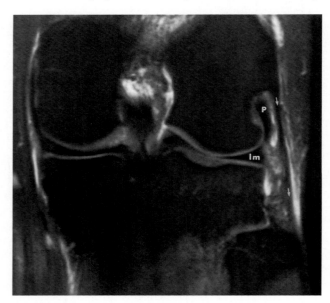

FIGURE 7-176. An intact LCL (*arrows*) displays low signal intensity on a fat-suppressed T2-weighted fast spin-echo coronal image. The popliteus tendon (*P*) and lateral meniscus (*lm*) are shown.

terolateral capsular injuries are often missed at initial clinical presentation. Posterolateral pain, buckling into hyperextension with weight-bearing, and instability are seen on clinical presentation. Cruciate and lateral meniscal tears may be associated with lateral compartment ligament tears. Conventional radiographs may reveal widening of the joint space, a fracture of the fibular head, and a Segond fracture (ie, avulsion of the tibial insertion of the lateral capsule ligament). A Segond fracture or a lateral capsular sign is also associated with ACL injuries.[43]

MR Appearance of the LCL

The LCL is best seen on posterior coronal images and appears as a band of low signal intensity (Fig. 7-176). Peripheral sagittal images demonstrate LCL anatomy at the level of the fibular head (Figs. 7-177 and 7-178). One-millimeter 3D volume protocols routinely image the LCL on at least two sagittal images. Edema and hemorrhage, although less frequent in this location, are seen as ligamentous thickening with increased signal intensity on T2- or fast spin-echo T2-weighted images (with fat suppression). Edema and hemorrhage may also be confirmed on peripheral sagittal images. Signal intensity is not as high in LCL injuries as in MCL disruptions, perhaps because the normal capsular separation of the LCL excludes accumulation of extravasated

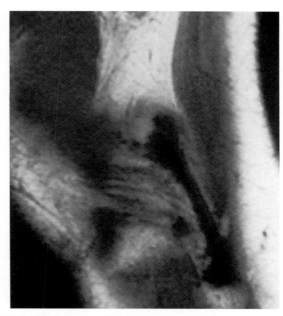

FIGURE 7-178. Low signal intensity identifies the LCL on a peripheral sagittal T1-weighted image.

joint fluid. In complete disruptions, the LCL demonstrates a wavy or serpiginous contour and loss of ligamentous continuity (Figs. 7-179 through 7-181). There may be proximal migration of the avulsed ligament from its fibular attachment. Radial images improve characterization of the LCL

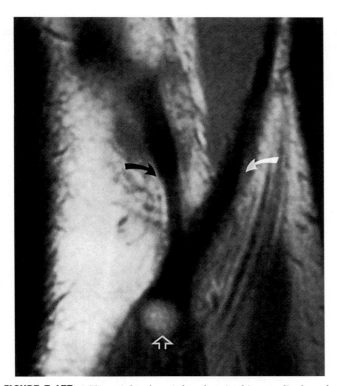

FIGURE 7-177. A T1-weighted peripheral sagittal image displays the conjoined insertion on the fibular head (*open arrow*) of the separate LCL (*curved black arrow*) and biceps femoris tendon (*curved white arrow*).

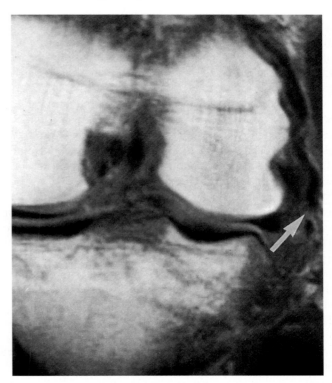

FIGURE 7-179. A complete tear of the LCL near its distal fibular attachment (*arrow*) can be seen on a T1-weighted coronal image. The disrupted ligament has a wavy contour.

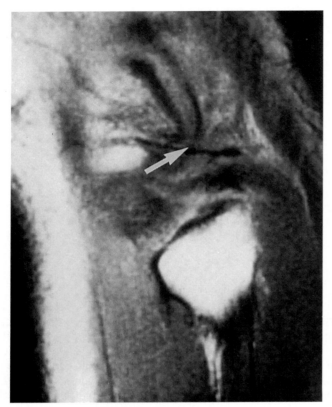

FIGURE 7-180. Complete disruption of the fibular LCL at the level of the joint line (*arrow*) is revealed on a T1-weighted sagittal image.

when 3D FT protocols are not used. T2 axial images are also important in diagnosing ligament tears when the course of the entire LCL cannot be visualized on coronal images. LCL injuries are graded by a system similar to that described for MCL injuries.

Associated medial plateau compression fractures can also be detected on MR scans and are often seen with significant varus or axial injuries.[234] Tears of the iliotibial band may also be associated with LCL disruptions. Inclusion of the iliotibial band on anterior coronal images is important if this structure is to be used to reconstruct the LCL. The iliotibial band, which provides lateral compartment support, is seen as a thin band of low signal intensity, parallel to the femur, with an anterolateral tibial insertion on Gerdy's tubercle. The iliotibial band friction syndrome (see the section "Retinacular Attachments," later in this chapter) is caused by abnormal contact of the iliotibial band and the lateral femoral condyle. Patients may present with pain in the lateral aspect of the thigh and knee, especially in 30° of knee flexion.[8,237] The biceps femoris muscle also plays an important role as a lateral stabilizer.

Popliteus muscle and tendon injuries are best displayed on fat-suppressed T2-weighted fast spin-echo or STIR sagittal and axial images. Areas of muscle edema and hemorrhage can be evaluated in these planes. Focal enlargement of the popliteus muscle may be secondary to by hemorrhage or

tearing of muscle fibers. Areas of increased signal intensity can be visualized at the muscle–tendon junction on sagittal images in conjunction with ACL and posterolateral corner injuries. The popliteus muscle and tendon are associated with concomitant injuries to the posterolateral complex. Although rare, there are reports of isolated cases of popliteus tendon rupture.[238] Normally, the popliteus tendon resists external rotation of the tibia acting as both a static and active restraint.

Treatment of LCL Injury

Acute injuries of the LCL are represented by avulsions from the femur or fibula or interstitial ligament injuries. Avulsion injuries can be treated with suture repair. An interstitial injury to the LCL can be treated by augmentation with the biceps tendon. Associated injuries of the posterolateral corner, with either acute or chronic posterolateral instability, are often associated with cruciate ligament injuries. These injuries are best treated with surgical reconstructions that initially address the cruciate ligaments and then concentrate on operative repair of the posterolateral structures. The LCL, the popliteal attachment to the tibia, and the popliteofibular ligament are important posterolateral static stabilizers and are thus anatomically repaired or reconstructed in both acute and chronic posterolateral instability.[239]

Surgical repair of the LCL may be necessary when there are associated acute ACL injuries.[43] Surgery is also used to treat grade III tears without an associated ACL tear when both the primary (ie, LCL) and secondary (ie, posterolateral or arcuate complex) restraints are injured. The results of surgical reconstructions performed in cases of acute posterolateral instability are superior to those performed in cases of chronic posterolateral instability.[239]

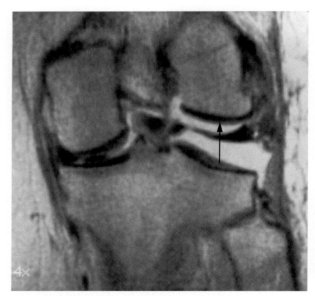

FIGURE 7-181. Disruption of the LCL, popliteus tendon, and ACL, with lateral instability, is shown by opening the lateral compartment (*arrow*). (Conventional T2-weighted coronal image.)

PATELLOFEMORAL JOINT AND THE EXTENSOR MECHANISM

Axial images are required to characterize patellofemoral articulation. The lateral and medial facets are obliquely oriented and cannot be accurately characterized on sagittal or coronal images. Patellar cartilage, the femoral or trochlear groove, and retinacular attachments are defined on axial sections through the patellofemoral joint. The quadriceps muscles and tendons can be seen on sagittal or axial images. The patellar tendon is seen en face in the coronal plane, in profile in the sagittal plane, and in cross section in the axial plane.

Chondromalacia

Chondromalacia patellae is characterized by patellofemoral (ie, retropatellar) joint pain, accentuated during knee flexion, and associated crepitus. Softening of the articular cartilage with associated degenerative changes is responsible for the spectrum of changes seen. Chondromalacia most often affects adolescents and young adults and may be primary and idiopathic or occur subsequent to patellar trauma.[240]

Patella alta, an increased valgus angle, and femoral condyle hypoplasia may predispose the patient to cartilage changes involving both the medial and lateral facets. Sclerosis or hyperemia of the subchondral bone may be associated with articular cartilage changes including softening, edema, and fissuring. Symptoms of chondromalacia may in some cases mimic meniscal pathology. Degenerative chondromalacia secondary to osteoarthritis may affect either the medial or the lateral patellar facets, depending on the underlying cause.

The causes of acute chondromalacia include instability, direct trauma, and fracture. The causes of chronic chondromalacia include subluxation, an increased quadriceps angle (Q-angle), quadriceps imbalance, posttraumatic malalignment, excessive lateral pressure syndrome, late effects of direct trauma or pressure, and PCL injuries. Chronic chondromalacia may also result from inflammatory arthritis, synovitis, and infection.[43] Four arthroscopic grades of chondromalacia are classified by Outerbridge.[241,242] In grade 0 chondromalacia, the articular cartilage is normal. In grade 1, discoloration of the articular cartilage occurs and may include blistering, usually without fragmentation or fissuring. Blistering represents separation of the superficial layer of articular cartilage. Localized softening, swelling, and fibrillation is limited to an area of 0.5 cm or less in diameter. In grade 2 disease, fissuring and fibrillation within soft areas of the articular cartilage may extend to a depth of 1 to 2 mm and to an area of 1.3 cm or less in diameter. In grade 3 chondromalacia, fissuring and fibrillation may involve more than half of the depth of the articular cartilage thickness and an area greater than 1.3 cm in diameter. The articular carti-

lage surface resembles crab meat, with fasciculation of multiple cartilaginous fragments attached to the underlying subchondral bone. There is no involvement of subchondral bone, however. In grade 4 (ie, end-stage) chondromalacia, complete loss or erosion of the articular cartilage surface results in exposed subchondral bone. Advanced patellofemoral arthrosis and end-stage chondromalacia have the same appearance.

Chondromalacia may also present with either a basilar or superficial degenerative pattern.[243] Basal degeneration affects young people and is associated with posttraumatic disruption of basal collagen. This condition leads to cartilage softening and subsequent blisters, ulcers, and fragmentation. The pattern of superficial degeneration of patellar articular cartilage occurs in older people, beginning with a loss of ground substance or cartilage matrix and leading to fissuring, fragmentation, and eventual exposure of subchondral bone.[244] Although thought to be more common in the age groups mentioned above, either pattern of degeneration may be seen in both young and older people. The primary abnormality in chondromalacia is a decrease in sulfated mucopolysaccharides within the ground substance. This decrease leads to an unstable collagen framework.[245]

Another arthroscopic grading system, developed by Shahriaree and colleagues, incorporates both traumatic and nontraumatic types of chondromalacia and has been useful in correlating arthroscopic findings with MR findings.[243,245] In this four part classification, grade 1 chondromalacia caused by trauma shows softening whereas nontraumatic chondromalacia demonstrates fibrillation. In grade 2 there is separation of the superficial from the deep layer of articular cartilage in a blister lesion. There may be associated fissures as vertical collagen fibers become exposed. In grade 3, there is ulceration, fragmentation, and cartilage fibrillation in larger areas of cartilage. In grade 4, there is frank cartilage ulceration with craters of exposed bone and progression to involvement of the subchondral bone.

MR Appearance of Chondromalacia

We use fat-suppressed T2-weighted fast spin-echo images (routinely) or MR arthrography (optional) to evaluate and define the fluid–cartilage interface in chondromalacia of the patellofemoral joint. Conventional T2-weighted images may be associated with false-positive diagnoses, and, in our experience, this sequence does not provide enough contrast differentiation between articular cartilage and cortical bone.[245] The SPGR technique with fat suppression has not been routinely used, although it is sensitive to fluid in areas of damaged articular cartilage. SPGR without fat suppression is not sensitive to cartilage degeneration and is thus insensitive in the detection of fluid in areas of fibrillation or fragmentation. STIR sequences can be used to improve sensitivity in the differentiation of high-signal-intensity synovial fluid from intermediate-signal-intensity articular carti-

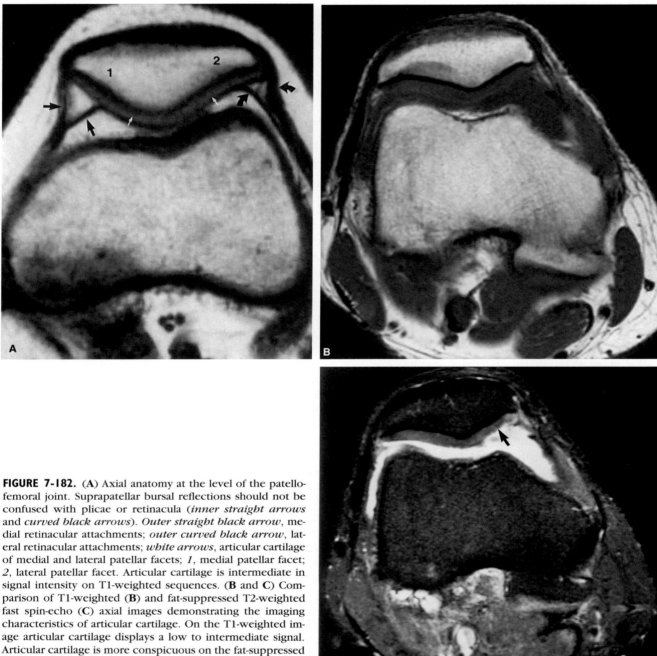

FIGURE 7-182. (A) Axial anatomy at the level of the patello-femoral joint. Suprapatellar bursal reflections should not be confused with plicae or retinacula (*inner straight arrows* and *curved black arrows*). *Outer straight black arrow*, medial retinacular attachments; *outer curved black arrow*, lateral retinacular attachments; *white arrows*, articular cartilage of medial and lateral patellar facets; *1*, medial patellar facet; *2*, lateral patellar facet. Articular cartilage is intermediate in signal intensity on T1-weighted sequences. (**B** and **C**) Comparison of T1-weighted (**B**) and fat-suppressed T2-weighted fast spin-echo (**C**) axial images demonstrating the imaging characteristics of articular cartilage. On the T1-weighted image articular cartilage displays a low to intermediate signal. Articular cartilage is more conspicuous on the fat-suppressed T2-weighted fast spin-echo image, in contrast to hypointense patellar subchondral bone.

lage. T2* gradient-echo images are no longer used to evaluate articular cartilage lesions, because the high signal intensity of the articular cartilage does not allow enough contrast resolution to successfully detect areas of articular cartilage softening and inhomogeneity. Small fissures with imbibed synovial fluid may be missed on images obtained using gradient-echo techniques.

Fat signal intensity anterior to the trochlear groove may produce false-positive interpretations of articular cartilage irregularities when using fat-suppressed axial images or STIR images. Corresponding T1-weighted axial images or sagittal images can be used to confirm the morphology of the articular cartilage. Sagittal images, which are less sensitive to cartilage erosions, may show a straightening or loss of the convex curve normally seen in cartilage when viewed in profile. Subchondral low signal intensity, which represents sclerosis, may be associated with irregular surface erosions. Patellar cysts may be seen in the early stages of patellar softening, before cartilage erosions occur.

On T1-weighted axial images the patellar facet articular cartilage surface displays a homogeneous intermediate signal intensity (Fig. 7-182). A thin layer of overlying fluid, however, is often difficult to separate from the underlying articular cartilage surface. T1-weighted images alone are not accurate in characterizing the spectrum and progression of articular cartilage changes described in the arthroscopic gross classifications. The normal patellar articular cartilage is homogeneous and smooth in contour. The superficial layer of articular cartilage has a bilaminar or laminated appearance, with a light gray or intermediate signal intensity on

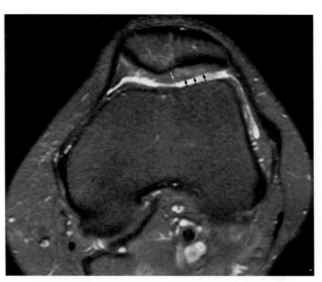

FIGURE 7-184. Early softening and swelling of the lateral patellar facet articular cartilage (*black arrows*), corresponding to findings in arthroscopic grade 1 chondromalacia. Hyperintensity within normal thickness lateral facet articular cartilage is shown on this fat-suppressed T2-weighted fast spin-echo axial image. More advanced changes of surface irregularity and fibrillation are present in the medial facet. Less than 1-mm superficial surface irregularity is identified (*white arrow*).

T1 MR arthrograms (Fig. 7-183).[245] This bilaminar appearance may be due either to the higher water content in superficial cartilage compared with deeper layers of articular cartilage or to an anisotropic arrangement of collagen fibers, which is thought to produce different zones on MR.[245] Articular cartilage demonstrates lower signal intensity on proton-density and conventional T2-weighted images. On SPGR images with fat suppression or fat saturation articular cartilage is of uniform bright signal intensity in contrast to dark bone and marrow fat. On fat-suppressed T2-weighted fast spin-echo images, it displays low to intermediate signal intensity or gray signal intensity similar to that seen with STIR sequences. Fat-suppressed T2-weighted fast spin-echo may be more sensitive to basal articular cartilage changes than MR arthrography, which is better for the detection of articular cartilage surface irregularity. Joint effusions are commonly associated with patellofemoral chondromalacia and demonstrate low signal intensity on T1-weighted images and bright signal intensity on T2, fast spin-echo T2, and STIR images. Cartilage erosions may be the source and donor site of loose bodies. Associated thinning of articular cartilage or articular cartilage chondromalacia of the trochlear groove, including both the anterolateral femoral condyle and anteromedial femoral condyle, as well as subchondral sclerosis of the trochlear groove should be evaluated as associated pathology.

The arthroscopic grades of chondromalacia have been correlated with findings on MR imaging.[246,247] These early descriptions, however, relied primarily on the use of

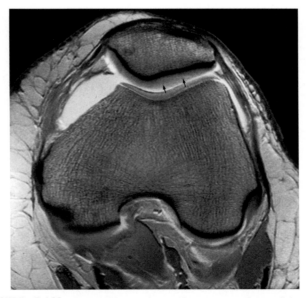

FIGURE 7-183. MR arthrography with intraarticular gadolinium-DTPA outlines the articular cartilage surfaces of the patella and trochlear groove on a T1-weighted axial image. The MR arthrogram demonstrates the subtle bilaminar appearance of the lateral patellar facet articular cartilage, which shows higher signal intensity in the more superficial layer of cartilage (*arrows*).

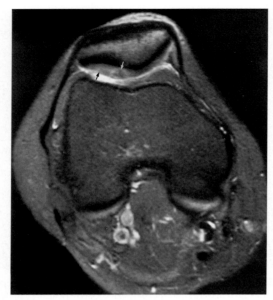

FIGURE 7-185. Fat-suppressed T2-weighted fast spin-echo axial image displays lateral facet articular cartilage softening as shown by a diffuse area of cartilage hyperintensity (*black arrow*). A more focal, circular hypointense (*white arrow*) area is seen in the medial aspect of the lateral facet. With the use of fat-suppressed T2-weighted fast spin-echo sequences, changes of focal areas of hypointensity are a less common finding in grade 1 chondromalacia than are areas of diffuse hyperintensity.

T1-weighted images without the use of fat-suppressed T2-weighted fast spin-echo or STIR techniques or MR arthrography.

In arthroscopic grade 1 chondromalacia, T1-weighted images show focal areas of decreased signal intensity without cartilage surface or subchondral bone extension. Fat-suppressed T2-weighted fast spin-echo images display focal areas of hyperintensity in the absence of any change in the smooth superficial cartilage contour (Figs. 7-184 and 7-185). Fat-suppressed T2-weighted fast spin-echo images also detect small, less than 1-mm (see Fig. 7-184), irregularities of the articular cartilage surface. These findings represent the earliest changes of softening and swelling of articular cartilage. The histologic changes of articular cartilage softening (closed chondromalacia) occur in the transitional zone deep to the superficial zone of articular cartilage. Changes in the collagen matrix include reorientation of collagen fibers into collapsed segments associated with a decrease in matrix proteoglycans[243] These early changes of softening—not routinely appreciated on T1-, conventional T2-, or gradient-echo T2-weighted images—can usually seen on images obtained with fat-suppressed T2-weighted fast spin-echo contrast. Focal basal or deep layer hyperintensity is also seen in this early stage. In grade 2 chondromalacia, indicated by blisterlike swelling, T1-weighted images show areas of decreased signal intensity extending to the articular cartilage surface. A sharp margin is preserved between the patellar and trochlear articular cartilage surfaces. Fat-suppressed T2-weighted fast spin-echo images demonstrate the blister lesion (Fig. 7-186), which may or may not be associated with underlying articular cartilage signal inhomogeneity (usually increased signal intensity). This finding represents a focal separation of superficial and deep layers of articular cartilage. On T1-weighted images, the surface irregularity and attenuation seen in arthroscopic grade 3 lesions directly correlate with focal areas of decreased signal intensity associated with loss of the sharp articular margin between the patellar and trochlear sur-

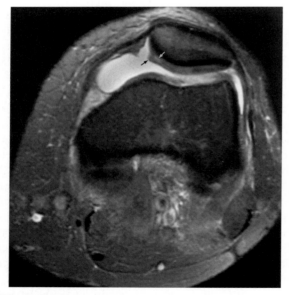

FIGURE 7-186. Focal blister formation with surface convexity (*black arrow*) and intracartilaginous hyperintensity (*white arrow*) on a fat-suppressed T2-weighted fast spin-echo axial image.

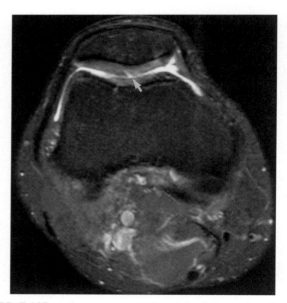

FIGURE 7-187. A fat-suppressed T2-weighted fast spin-echo axial image showing a discrete fissure (*arrow*) with linear hyperintensity in the medial aspect of the lateral patellar facet. This fissure extends through 50% of the depth of the articular cartilage. Note the focus of medial facet articular cartilage softening.

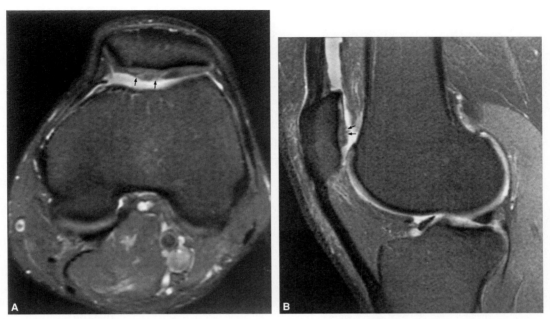

FIGURE 7-188. Cartilage fibrillation with a hyperintense crab-meat lesion (*black arrows*) on fat-suppressed T2-weighted fast spin-echo axial (**A**) and sagittal (**B**) images. The individual fronds of cartilage fibrillation are identified on the sagittal image.

faces. Fat-suppressed T2-weighted fast spin-echo images show the imbibed fluid in surface articular cartilage defects as high-signal-intensity sites (Fig. 7-187). Identification of focal ulcerations and resolution of "crab meat" lesions benefits from the use of fat-suppressed T2-weighted fast spin-echo contrast (Fig. 7-188). Ulceration and exposure of subchondral bone seen in arthroscopic grade 4 are represented on MR images by frank

articular cartilage defects, exposed subchondral bone, and underlying fluid in subchondral bone (Fig. 7-189). On T1-weighted images there are low-signal-intensity changes in the subchondral bone of the medial and lateral patellar facets. These areas may be hyperintense on fat-suppressed T2-weighted fast spin-echo or STIR images. Gradient-echo contrast is less sensitive to changes in underlying subchondral signal intensity. The

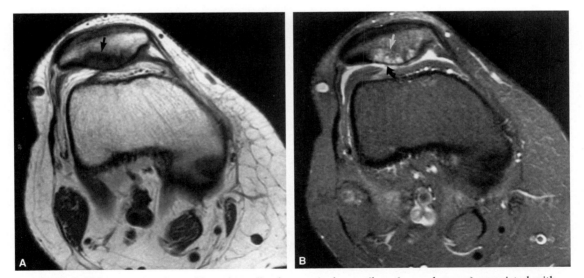

FIGURE 7-189. Complete loss of lateral patellar facet articular cartilage (*curved arrow*) associated with subchondral bone erosions (*straight arrow*) on T1-weighted axial (**A**) and fat-suppressed T2-weighted fast spin-echo axial (**B**) images in grade 4 chondromalacia. The subchondral bone changes are hypointense on the T1-weighted sequence (**A**) and hyperintense on the fat-suppressed T2-weighted fast spin-echo sequence (**B**).

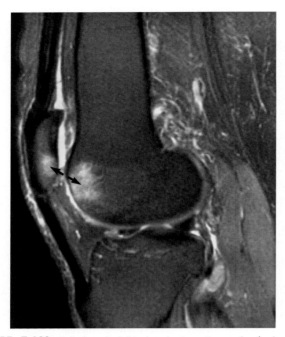

FIGURE 7-190. Subchondral kissing lesions in grade 4 chondromalacia demonstrate subchondral and cancellous hyperintensity (*arrows*) in the anterolateral femoral condyle and inferior pole of the lateral patellar facet on a fat-suppressed T2-weighted fast spin-echo sagittal image. The articular cartilage surfaces are denuded in these lesions.

precise depth of articular cartilage fissures or ulceration is best determined on fat-suppressed T2-weighted fast spin-echo images. MR sagittal images often demonstrate reciprocal subchondral bone changes in the femoral trochlear groove and patellar facet (Fig. 7-190).

Correlation with pathologic specimens has also demonstrated the ability of MR to characterize cartilage morphology, particularly ulcerations of the cartilage surfaces (ie, fibrillation).[248]

Treatment of Chondromalacia

Treatment of chondromalacia requires an initial conservative period of rehabilitation.[43] Instabilities or malalignments may require surgical intervention if conservative treatment fails. Arthroscopic shaving or removal of fibrillated and traumatized areas of articular cartilage, especially in posttraumatic chondromalacia, may improve the patient's symptoms, although results may deteriorate with time. Treatment by shaving of the patellar cartilage surface can be identified on MR studies as an artificially straight articular surface with macroscopic metallic artifacts. Other surgical procedures include chondroplasty with subchondral drilling (Fig. 7-191), spongialization realignment procedures, tibial tubercle elevation (Fig. 7-192), patellectomy (Fig. 7-193) and patellar resurfacing.

Dorsal Defect of the Patella

Dorsal defect of the patella involves the superolateral aspect of the articular surface of the patella. This well-defined benign lesion has sclerotic margins with an intact overlying

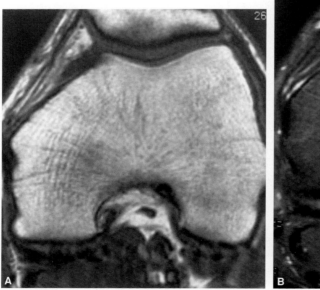

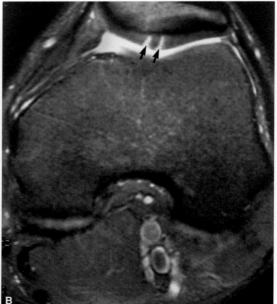

FIGURE 7-191. Postoperative drilling in the medial aspect of the lateral facet is not apparent on a T1-weighted axial image (**A**). However, it can be visualized as linear hyperintensity (*arrow*) on a fat-suppressed T2-weighted fast spin-echo axial image (**B**).

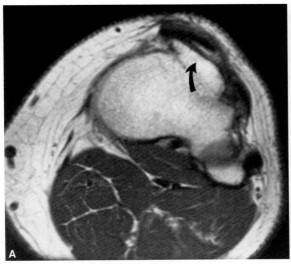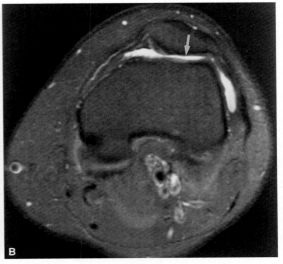

FIGURE 7-192. Fulkerson osteotomy (*curved arrow*) of the tibial tubercle on a T1-weighted axial image (**A**). This patient had denuded articular cartilage (*straight arrow*) of the lateral patellar facet, which can be seen on a fat-suppressed T2-weighted fast spin-echo axial image (**B**).

articular cartilage surface.[243] It is usually circular, about 1 cm in diameter, and appears radiolucent on conventional radiographs. The etiology is unclear but may be related to a vastus lateralis traction injury in the ossification process of the patella, similar to the pathophysiology of a bipartite

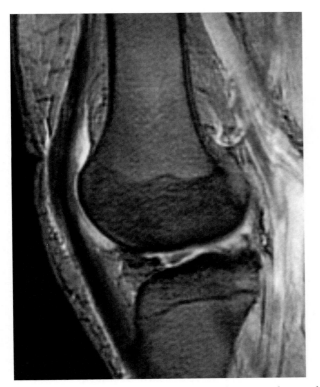

FIGURE 7-193. Patellectomy with continuity between the quadriceps and patellar tendon on a T2*-weighted sagittal image.

patella.[249] Fifty percent of cases of dorsal defect of the patella are asymptomatic. Histologic findings include necrotic bone and fibrous tissue. The lesion is low to intermediate in signal intensity on T1-weighted images, and there may be central areas of increased signal intensity within the lesion. Cases with arthroscopically visible cartilage surface perforations have been documented. The differential diagnosis of dorsal defect of the patella includes Brodie's abscess, osteochondritis dissecans, and neoplastic bony lesions.

Osteochondritis Dissecans Patellae

Osteochondritis dissecans (Fig. 7-194) patellae may be associated with patellar subluxation.[250] The subchondral fragment usually remains in situ, causing retropatellar crepitus and pain. A loose body, however, may be present. A loose or partially detached articular fragment is treated by excision and drilling of the subchondral bone. In contrast to dorsal defect of the patella, osteochondritis dissecans has a predilection for the medial facet of the patella. It is characterized by an articular cartilage lesion (separation) with or without localized involvement of subchondral bone. Osteochondritis affecting the femoral condyle is discussed in the section "Osteochondritis Dissecans," later in this chapter.

Patellar Subluxation and Dislocation

Subluxation refers to the partial lateral displacement of the patella early in the process of knee flexion.[251] It may be associated with patellar tilt. Lateral patellar subluxations in-

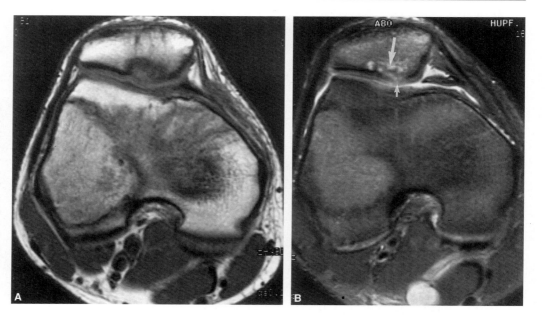

FIGURE 7-194. Osteochondritis dissecans involving the medial aspect of the lateral patellar facet on T1-weighted (**A**) and fat-suppressed T2-weighted fast spin-echo (**B**) axial images. The localized involvement of the articular cartilage and subchondral bone are characteristic. The mid- and inferior poles are commonly involved with sparing of the upper pole. The full-thickness articular cartilage lesion (*small arrow*) and the hyperintense interface of the subchondral fragment (*large arrow*) are shown.

clude recurrent subluxation (associated with patellofemoral incongruence, dislocation, or patella alta), habitual subluxation (occurring with all knee movements), permanent lateral subluxation, and subluxation in extension (uncommon). Medial patellar subluxations may occur secondary to overcorrection in operations for the realignment of the extensor mechanism, including lateral release.

Dislocations of the patella can be recurrent (Fig. 7-195), permanent (no contact between the patella and articular carti-

lage of the distal femur), congenital, medial (a rare condition, possibly resulting from surgical overcorrection of a lateral dislocation), or traumatic (lateral).[251]

The patellar groove or sulcus has a median depth of 5.2 mm. The quadriceps angle, or Q-angle, is determined by the intersection of a line connecting the center of the patella with the anterior superior iliac spine (approximating the line of pull of the quadriceps tendon) with a second line (in the direction of the patellar tendon) that connects the center of

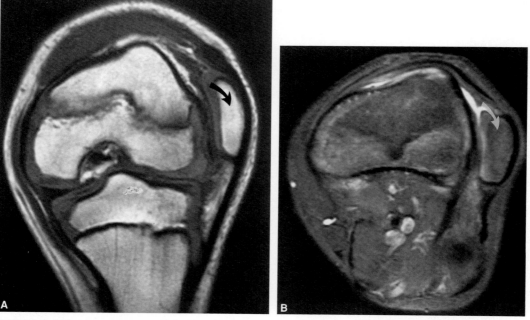

FIGURE 7-195. Complete lateral dislocation (*curved arrow*) of the patella on T1-weighted coronal (**A**) and fat-suppressed T2-weighted fast spin-echo axial (**B**) images in a child with a history of recurrent dislocations. There is still relative preservation of patellar articular cartilage.

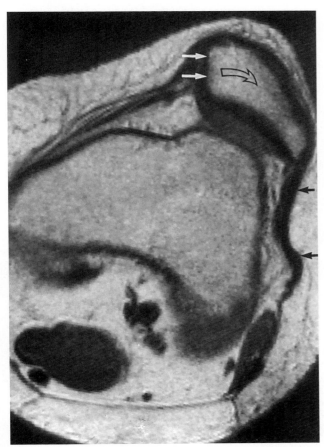

FIGURE 7-196. A T1-weighted axial image shows lateral subluxation (*curved open arrow*) of a dysplastic patella with a missing medial facet (*white straight arrows*). This defect is referred to as a "Jagerhut patella." A lax lateral retinaculum is also seen (*black straight arrows*).

the lateral femoral condyle, is a known cause of patellar dislocation or subluxation.

Radiographic measurements of patellofemoral congruence include the sulcus angle, the congruence angle, the lateral patellofemoral angle, and the patellofemoral index.[253] Those measurements can also be adapted to MR to assess the alignment between the patella and trochlear groove. The sulcus angle (depth of the trochlea) is formed by the condyles and sulcus and has a mean value of 138° with a standard deviation of 6°. The sulcus angle correlates with dysplasia and recurrent dislocation as an indication of instability. A larger angle indicates dysplasia and a greater likelihood of malalignment. The congruence angle, which measures the degree of patellar subluxation, is determined by the anterior distance between the articular ridge of the patella and a reference line that bisects the sulcus angle. The mean congruence angle is −6°, with a standard deviation of 6°. The lateral patellofemoral angle is formed by the angle between the intercondylar line and the lateral facet. This angle should open laterally and measures tilt with subluxation if the lines become parallel or open medially. The patellofemoral index measures tilt and subluxation by comparing the closest distance of the lateral facet with the medial facet expressed as a ratio. The normal ratio is 1:6 or less.

Malalignment patterns of the patella include patellar tilt, with or without associated subluxation.[254] Chronic patellar tilt may lead to excessive lateral pressure syndrome. Subluxation or dislocation can be caused by trauma without a preex-

the patella to the tibial tubercle. The normal Q-angle measures between 14° and 15°; measurements greater than 14° to 15° are abnormal. The Q-angle defines the proximal-to-distal forces that act on and through the patella.[251,252]

Recurrent and habitual subluxation or dislocation may be seen with ligamentous laxity. An abnormal iliotibial band and vastus lateralis attachment may produce a lateral patellar pull. Intrinsic muscle abnormalities and soft-tissue damage, including medial patellar retinaculum injuries, may also lead to recurrent dislocation, as may a hypoplastic femoral sulcus and lateral femoral condyle. Variation of patellar shapes (Weiberg types), especially a small and convex medial patellar facet (Weiberg type 3), may have a tendency to produce recurrent dislocations. We have used MR to identify dysplastic patellae without a medial facet or central ridges as a cause for lateral subluxation associated with a shallow or hypoplastic femoral groove. This condition is classified as a Weiberg type 5 (ie, Jagerhut) patella (Fig. 7-196). Other patellar types are demonstrated using axial plane images (Fig 7-197). Patella alta, with loss of the buttressing effect of

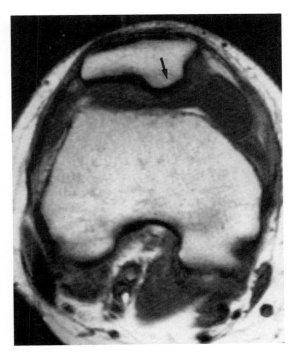

FIGURE 7-197. A Weiberg type 2 patella is indicated by concave surfaces, a smaller medial facet, and a prominent central ridge (*arrow*), as seen on a T1-weighted axial image.

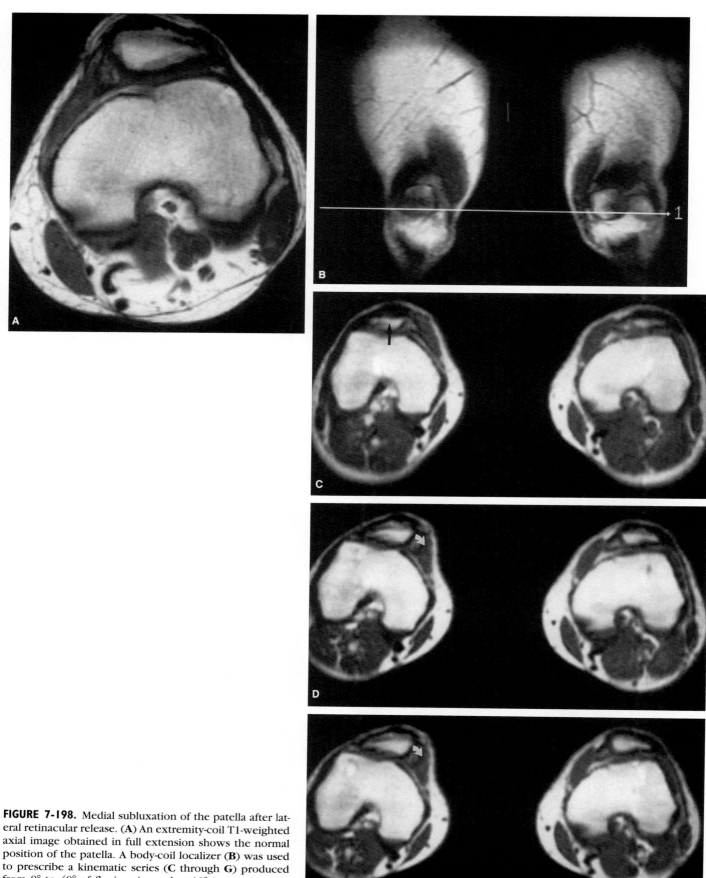

FIGURE 7-198. Medial subluxation of the patella after lateral retinacular release. **(A)** An extremity-coil T1-weighted axial image obtained in full extension shows the normal position of the patella. A body-coil localizer **(B)** was used to prescribe a kinematic series **(C** through **G)** produced from 0° to 40° of flexion, imaged at 10° increments. *All arrows*, position of the patella.

continued

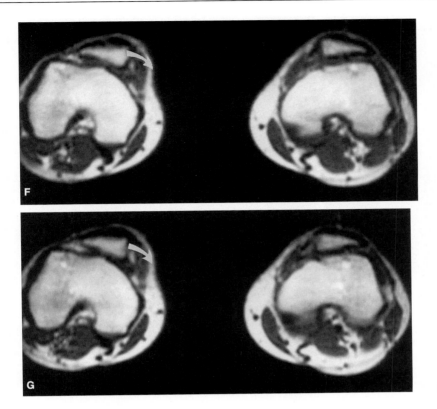

FIGURE 7-198. *Continued*

isting malalignment. Permanent dislocation is often associated with congenital or traumatic dysplasia of the extensor mechanism and trochlea.

MR is sometimes used to complement CT studies in the assessment of patellar tracking, with the application of both kinematic and dynamic techniques (Fig. 7-198). MR is especially useful for evaluation of the patellofemoral mechanism during the first 30° of knee flexion in recurrent dislocation of the patella.[251] Another method for detecting patellar subluxation, described by Laurin and colleagues, uses axial radiography of the patellofemoral joint at 25°.[255] With this technique a perpendicular line is erected to the apex of the medial femoral condyle from a transcondylar line. The medial facet should be between 0 and 2 mm of this line to be normal. Cine-MR imaging (motion-triggered cine-MR) is useful for the evaluation of patellar tracking for patellar malalignment,[256] and kinematic MR may be used to evaluate the efficacy of a patellar realignment brace in counteracting patellar subluxation.[257]

Treatment of recurrent patellar dislocation and patellar instability attempts to realign and stabilize the extensor mechanism, including the patella. Bony operations include transfer of the lateral tuberosity, elevation of the tibial tuberosity (Maquet's procedure) (Fig. 7-199), femoral osteotomy, and patellectomy. Soft-tissue operations include lateral retinacular release, fascioplasty, patellar ligament procedures, tendon (gracilis, semitendinosus, and sartorius) and muscle transfers, and capsulorrhaphy.[251]

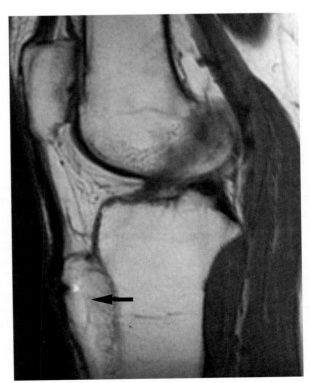

FIGURE 7-199. Maquet's procedure with advancement of the tibial tuberosity by elevation of the tibial crest, as seen on a T1-weighted sagittal image (*arrow*).

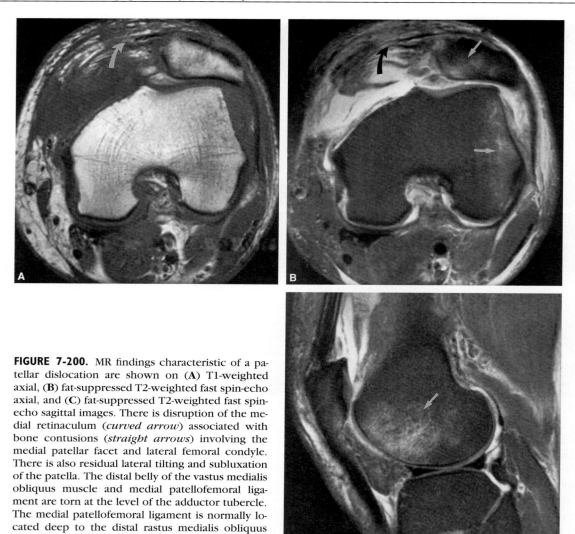

FIGURE 7-200. MR findings characteristic of a patellar dislocation are shown on (**A**) T1-weighted axial, (**B**) fat-suppressed T2-weighted fast spin-echo axial, and (**C**) fat-suppressed T2-weighted fast spin-echo sagittal images. There is disruption of the medial retinaculum (*curved arrow*) associated with bone contusions (*straight arrows*) involving the medial patellar facet and lateral femoral condyle. There is also residual lateral tilting and subluxation of the patella. The distal belly of the vastus medialis obliquus muscle and medial patellofemoral ligament are torn at the level of the adductor tubercle. The medial patellofemoral ligament is normally located deep to the distal rastus medialis obliquus muscle and represents the superior extent of the second layer of the medial side of the knee.

Traumatic Dislocations

The mechanisms of injury for traumatic patellar dislocations are twisting, valgus stress, or a direct blow to the knee.[251] A direct contact injury to the patella is less common and may produce the rare intraarticular (trapped within the joint) and superior patellar dislocations. Operative findings in acute patellar dislocations include hemarthrosis, medial retinacular rupture, stretch of the medial retinaculum, medial marginal fracture of the patella, intraarticular fracture of the patella, fracture of the chondral or osseous portions of the lateral femoral condyle, or partial patellar tendon detachment. Associated articular cartilage injuries may result in late posttraumatic arthritis.

MR imaging is an excellent modality for demonstrating the constellation of findings that characterizes a patellar dislocation (Fig. 7-200)[258,259] Patellar dislocation is frequently not clinically considered before MR imaging.[259] In a series of patients studied by Kirsch and colleagues,[259] MR findings included disruption or sprain of the medial retinaculum (96%), lateral patellar tilt or subluxation (92%), lateral femoral condyle contusion (81%), osteochondral injury (58%), and joint effusion (100%). Associated major ligament or meniscal injury was also reported (31%). The combination of T1 and fat-suppressed T2-weighted fast spin-echo or T1 and STIR images in the axial, coronal, and sagittal planes displays the osseous- and soft-tissue findings characteristic of acute patellar dislocations. Occasionally, a single axial image may demonstrate the entire spectrum of findings including contusions in the lateral aspect of the lateral femoral condyle, medial facet contusion (with or without articular cartilage injury), medial retinacular tears, joint effusion, and lateral patellar subluxation. Sallay and colleagues have shown the importance of additional MR findings in acute dislocations of the patella to include tearing of the medial patellofemoral ligament, at the level of the adductor tubercle and edema with tearing of the distal muscle belly of the rastus medialis obliquus (VMO).[260]

The medial retinaculum injury ranges from a sprain to complete disruption or avulsion from its patellar attachment.

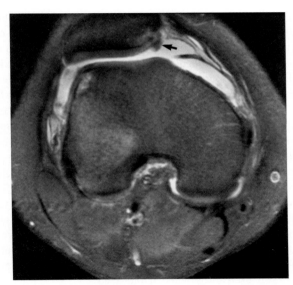

FIGURE 7-201. Medial patellar facet chondral injury with disrupted and dislocated articular fragment (*arrow*) after patellar dislocation. This fat-suppressed T2-weighted fast spin-echo axial image also demonstrates the pattern of medial facet and lateral femoral condyle bone contusions and medial retinacular injury.

Avulsion injuries may be associated with a small displaced osseous fragment (retracted). Fat-suppressed T2-weighted fast spin-echo images show areas of disruption or defect in patellar articular cartilage (Fig. 7-201). The pattern of contusions displayed on MR images results from the impact of the medial facet of the patella on the lateral aspect of the lateral femoral condyle. In extension, the patella spontaneously reduces back into the trochlear groove. Careful evalua-

tion for osteochondral fragments and loose bodies, including cartilage and osseous fragments, should be performed in assessing T2 axial, coronal, and sagittal images (fat-suppressed T2-weighted fast spin-echo or STIR). A partially torn medial retinaculum is often poorly visualized and may be difficult to distinguish from a complete retinacular disruption (Fig. 7-202). Presentation may include poor visualization of the medial retinaculum, with the appearance of wavy fibers; the medial retinaculum as a whole is generally thickened, because of interdigitated fluid within disrupted fibers. Those fibers that are seen in continuity may be thin or wispy. The articular injury to the patella usually occurs during the actual dislocation but may also occur during the subsequent phase of recoil of the patella.

Nonoperative treatment is important in treating patients with acute patellar dislocations.[251] Cast immobilization and rehabilitation represent time-honored conservative treatment, although recently the importance of early return of the range of motion and strength has been recognized. Arthroscopy is used in the diagnosis and treatment of osteochondral fragments and associated intraarticular pathology and in performing selective lateral retinacular releases. If there is no underlying malalignment or significant patellar tilt, however, lateral retinacular release is not performed. Redislocation (eg, defects in the vastus obliquus insertion) is treated more aggressively.

Retinacular Attachments

The medial and lateral retinacula (Fig. 7-203) are fascicle extensions of the vastus medialis and lateralis muscle groups, respectively.[16] The retinacula reinforce and guard normal

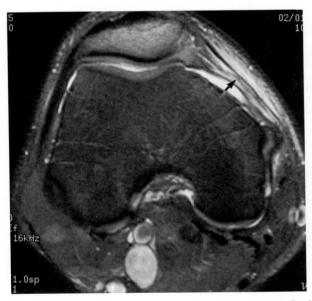

FIGURE 7-202. A partially torn medial retinaculum (*arrow*) displays thickening and hyperintensity on a fat-suppressed T2-weighted fast spin-echo axial image. Continuity of the retinacular fibers, however, is maintained.

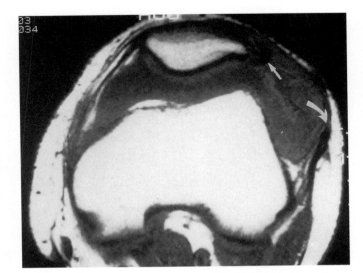

FIGURE 7-203. Traumatic disruption of the lateral patellar retinaculum is seen on a T1-weighted axial image. Torn, low-signal-intensity fibers are revealed at the lateral aspect of the patella (*straight arrow*). A retracted vastus lateralis tendon (*curved arrow*) is shown.

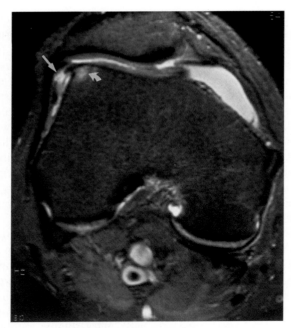

FIGURE 7-204. Iliotibial band friction syndrome with fluid and soft-tissue thickening (*straight arrow*) deep to the iliotibial band on a fat-suppressed T2-weighted fast spin-echo axial image. Subchondral hyperemia (*curved arrow*) also is demonstrated, at the site of an anterolateral osteophyte adjacent to the area of inflammation.

patellar tracking. On anterior coronal images, the retinacular attachments are seen as low-signal-intensity structures converging on the medial and lateral patellar fascicles. The medial and lateral retinacula, however, are best evaluated on axial images through the patellofemoral joint. The medial retinaculum is commonly torn after patellar dislocation (see Fig. 7-200). Axial MR images demonstrate either a free-floating retinaculum without patellar attachment or a mass-like effect caused by compressed torn retinacular fibers or chondral fragments. Associated edema and hemorrhage produce high signal intensity on T2, fat-suppressed T2-weighted fast spin-echo, or STIR images. In addition to patellar dislocations, retinacular tears may be associated with severe tears of the proximal portion of the patellar tendon or distal quadriceps tendon. These retinacular disruptions may involve either the medial or lateral retinacular fibers. Valgus hyperextension stress injuries can also result in retinacular disruptions as well as tears of the MCL.

A tight lateral retinaculum (ie, excessive lateral pressure syndrome) tilts the patella in a lateral direction and may be accompanied by patellar subluxation. A retinacular release may be performed to minimize the development of lateral facet degenerative disease. The site of retinacular division after release can be evaluated with MR.

Separate from the lateral retinaculum is the iliotibial band, representing the distal tendon of the tensor fascia lata, which may become inflamed proximal to its insertion onto the anterolateral tibia (Gerdy's tubercle). This condition oc-

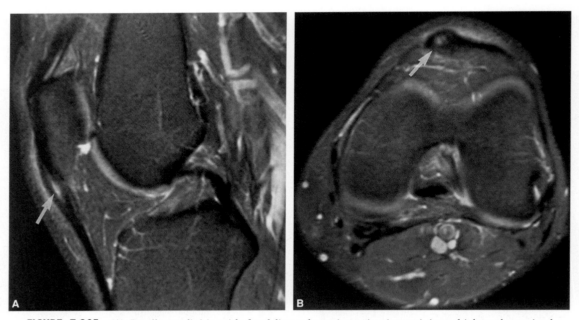

FIGURE 7-205. (A) Patella tendinitis with focal linear hyperintensity (*arrow*) in a thickened proximal patellar tendon on a fat-suppressed T2-weighted fast spin-echo sagittal image. (B) Preferential medial involvement (*arrow*) of the patellar tendon is shown on the corresponding fat-suppressed T2-weighted fast spin-echo axial image. Tendon widening is associated with the development of intrasubstance longitudinal splits and mucinous degeneration. Superimposed chronic tears with inflammation and necrosis result in increased signal intensity on T2, T2*, STIR, and T2-weighted fast spin-echo sequences.

curs in the iliotibial-band friction syndrome, which is usually seen in long-distance runners, cyclists, football players, and weight lifters, and is thought to be caused by friction and inflammation between the iliotibial tract and the anterolateral femoral condyle.[261] T2-weighted images show high signal intensity deep to the iliotibial band, lateral to the lateral femoral condyle (Fig. 7-204). Tenderness and pain present proximal to the lateral joint line.

The Extensor Mechanism and Patellar Tendon Abnormalities

Patellar Tendinitis

Chronic patellar tendinitis, also referred to as jumper's knee, usually affects the patellar tendon at its proximal insertion. Malalignment of the extensor mechanism, instability associated with forces generated in jumping sports, and overuse all may lead to the inflammatory changes.[43] The tendinitis usually occurs in adults. Findings include microtears of the tendon tissue, devitalization, and areas of focal degeneration adjacent to the point of the bone–tendon insertion.[262] A proposed clinical classification relates patients' symptomatic pain in four phases relative to activity levels. Phase 4 represents complete tendon rupture. Other causes of anterior knee pain are included in the differential diagnosis.

On axial and sagittal MR images, patellar tendinitis usually demonstrates focal thickening in the proximal third of the patellar tendon (Fig. 7-205). The medial to central portion of the tendon is most frequently involved (Fig. 7-206),[263] as is best appreciated on axial images, which demonstrate the convexity associated with localized tendon thickening. The lesion in chronic patellar tendinitis may also be associated with a more diffuse tendon thickening or enlargement (Fig. 7-207). T1- and proton-density weighted images of the affected area are low to intermediate in

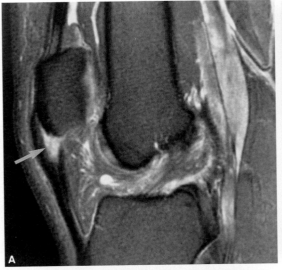

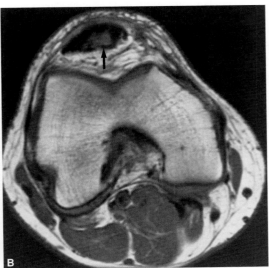

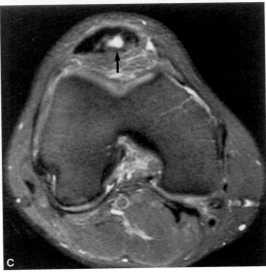

FIGURE 7-206. (**A**) Chronic patellar tendinitis involving the proximal tendon with hyperintensity on a fat-suppressed T2-weighted fast spin-echo sagittal image. There is marked thickening of the proximal tendon, associated with greater involvement of the posterior fibers and margin of the tendon. (**B** and **C**) Tendon thickening and the focus of increased signal intensity are central, showing intermediate signal on T1-weighted axial images (**B**) and hyperintensity on fat-suppressed T2-weighted fast spin-echo axial images (**C**).

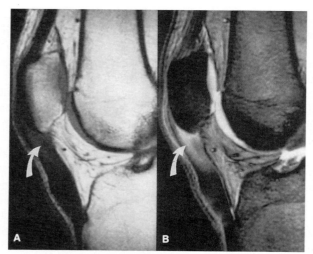

FIGURE 7-207. Patellar tendinitis (jumper's knee) results in proximal patellar tendon edema (*curved arrows*). This edema exhibits (**A**) intermediate signal intensity on a T1-weighted sagittal image and (**B**) increased signal intensity on a T2*-weighted sagittal image. There is diffuse thickening of the entire patellar tendon.

signal intensity with increased signal intensity shown on T2, fat-suppressed T2-weighted fast spin-echo, T2*, and STIR images. T2*-weighted and STIR sequences, however, tend to show a greater extent of tendon hyperintensity than do comparable fast spin-echo images before the development of chronic tears associated with inflammation and necrosis. The tendon may maintain hypointensity or isointensity on T1- and T2-weighted images. The posterior tendon margin is poorly defined at the level of thickening. The low signal intensity anterior border of the tendon may be preserved. The areas of increased signal intensity correspond to tenocyte hyperplasia, angiogenesis with endothelial hypoplasia, loss of longitudinal collagen architecture, and microtears with collagen fiber separation.[263] The degree of hyaline degeneration appears to correlate with the duration of the patient's symptoms. McLoughlin and colleagues have used gadolinium-enhanced MR images to grade patellar tendinitis based on fibrovascular repair in the enthetic region of the proximal patellar tendon.[264]

Acute patellar tendinitis (symptoms for <2 weeks) may demonstrate greater signal abnormalities in the peritenon region, without significant intrasubstance tendon changes in either signal intensity or morphology. As discussed, in chronic patellar tendinitis (symptoms for >6 weeks), an area of low signal intensity with enlargement may be seen within the tendon before the development of associated chronic tears within the tendon.[243] The high-signal-intensity MR appearance of chronic patellar tendinitis complicated by the development of chronic tears with inflammation and necrosis may be similar to the presentation of acute partial intrasubstance patellar tendon tears on T2-weighted sequences. Subcutaneous edema, however, is commonly present in the setting of acute partial tears.

Patellar Tendon Tears

Patellar tendon tears, which result in a loss of extension and a high-riding patella, can occur with avulsion injuries from the tibial tubercle (Fig. 7-208) or inferior pole of the patella (Fig. 7-209).[265] Most tendon ruptures occur in the proximal patellar tendon at the inferior patellar pole junction. Midsubstance ruptures are unusual and are related to severe trauma with forced knee flexion against a contracted quadriceps muscle (Fig. 7-210).[258] Distal tears near the lower pole are seen in young people. MR images demonstrate disruption and loss of continuity of the normal low-signal-intensity tendon. Superior retraction or patella alta is associated with complete tears. The area of disruption frequently demonstrates high signal intensity on T2, fat-suppressed T2-weighted fast spin-echo, and STIR images secondary to the influx of fluid from edema and hemorrhage. Frequently the patellar tendon has a lax or wavy contour as a function of the degree of tendon retraction (Fig. 7-211). The entire tendon may appear thickened, especially if there is an underlying or predisposing tendinitis. Bony fragments, with or without the signal intensity of marrow, may be identified on sagittal MR images. T2*-weighted sagittal images are sensitive to small avulsed bony fragments that may be overlooked on T1- or conventional T2-weighted images (Fig. 7-212).

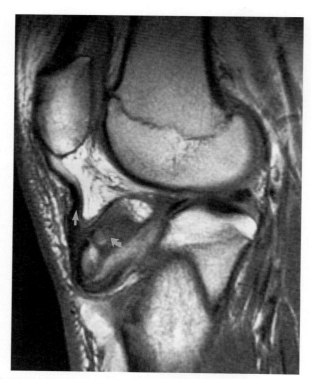

FIGURE 7-208. A T1-weighted sagittal image of a displaced anterior tibial fracture with an attached patellar tendon. Proximal retraction of the tendon (*straight arrow*) and osseous fragment (*curved arrow*) are shown.

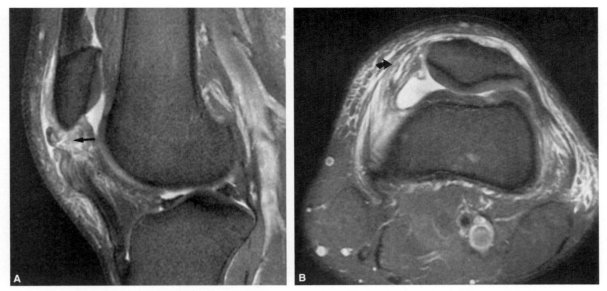

FIGURE 7-209. Acute proximal patellar tendon rupture (*straight arrow*) associated with a medial retinacular tear (*curved arrow*) on fat-suppressed T2-weighted fast spin-echo sagittal (**A**) and axial (**B**) images.

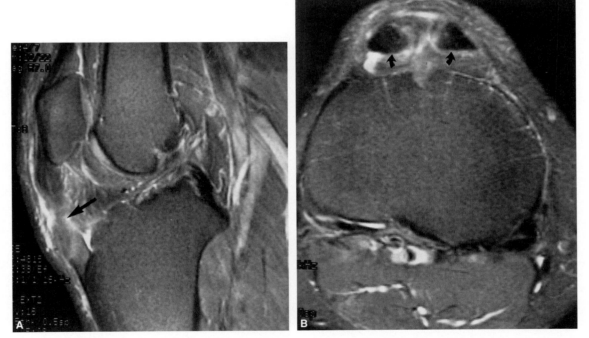

FIGURE 7-210. (**A**) A fat-suppressed T2-weighted fast spin-echo mid-sagittal image shows focal narrowing in the midsubstance of the patellar tendon caused by a high-grade partial tear (*straight arrow*) of the middle one third of the tendon. (**B**) A fat-suppressed T2-weighted fast spin-echo axial image shows the peripheral portions of the intact tendon (*curved arrows*) as two separate structures.

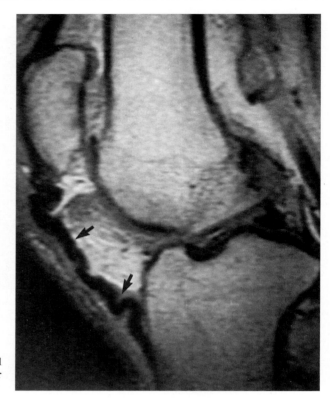

FIGURE 7-211. A T1-weighted sagittal image shows a tear of the proximal patellar tendon that results in increased laxity and redundant contour (*arrows*).

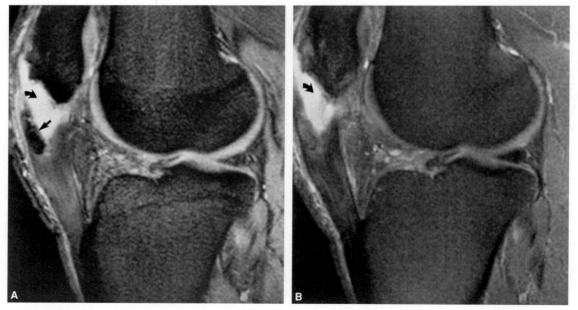

FIGURE 7-212. T2* (**A**) and fat-suppressed T2-weighted fast spin-echo (**B**) sagittal images of a proximal patellar tendon rupture (*curved arrow*) associated with diffuse tendon thickening. The avulsed inferior pole osseous fragment (*straight arrow*) is best visualized on the T2*-weighted sequence (**A**) because of the bone susceptibility effect. The greater degree of diffuse tendon hyperintensity is also shown on the T2*-weighted sequence.

Partial tears of the patellar tendon typically involve proximal fibers and are associated with tendon thickening. In acute partial tears, the thickness of the tendon may be normal, and there may be edema in the subcutaneous tissues anterior to the patellar tendon or edema involving the adjacent portion of Hoffa's fat pad deep to the proximal patellar tendon. Typically, these partial tears involve the posterior fibers of the patellar tendon in its proximal extent. The patellar tendon may also appear thickened after arthroscopy.

Treatment of patellar tendon ruptures includes direct tendon repair, reconstruction with semitendinosus tendon, or bony reattachment.[43]

Patella Alta and Baja

The patellar tendon–to–patella ratio is considered abnormal when the lengths of the patella and patellar tendon are unequal (when the ratio of the length of the patella to the patellar tendon exceeds 1:2).[265] Patella alta (high position of the patella) and patella baja (low position of the patella) can

be determined on direct sagittal images that show the entire length of the patellar tendon and the superior-to-inferior dimensions of the patella. Patella alta has been associated with subluxation, chondromalacia, Sinding-Larsen-Johansson syndrome, cerebral palsy, and quadriceps atrophy (Figs. 7-213 and 7-214).[266] Patella baja is most commonly seen as a postoperative complication of ACL surgery or lateral retinacular release. It may also be associated with polio, achondroplasia, and juvenile chronic arthritis (previously known as juvenile rheumatoid arthritis [JRA]) (Figs. 7-215 and 216).

Osgood-Schlatter Disease

In Osgood-Schlatter disease, osteochondrosis of the developing tibial tuberosity (ie, apophysis) is thought to be secondary to repetitive microtears during adolescent growth. There is activity-related pain about the tibial tubercle.[267] There may be clinical swelling and tenderness of the tibial tubercle, patellar tendon, and peripatellar soft tissues. Radiographic changes include soft-tissue edema anterior to the

text continues on page 382

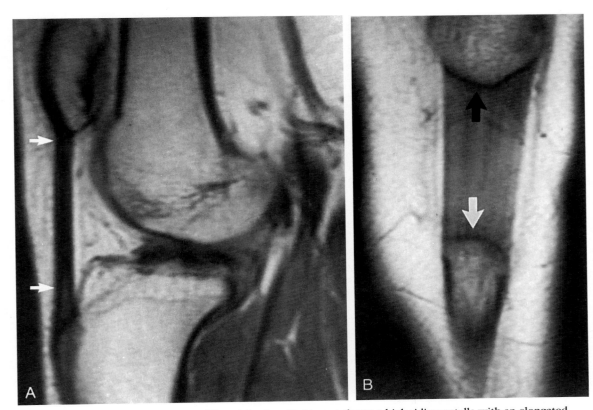

FIGURE 7-213. Patella alta. **(A)** A T1-weighted sagittal image shows a high-riding patella with an elongated patellar tendon (*arrows*) in a patient with atrophy of the quadriceps muscle. **(B)** The corresponding T1-weighted coronal image demonstrates a stretched patellar tendon en face. Patellar attachments (*black arrow*) and tibial tubercle attachments (*white arrow*) are identified.

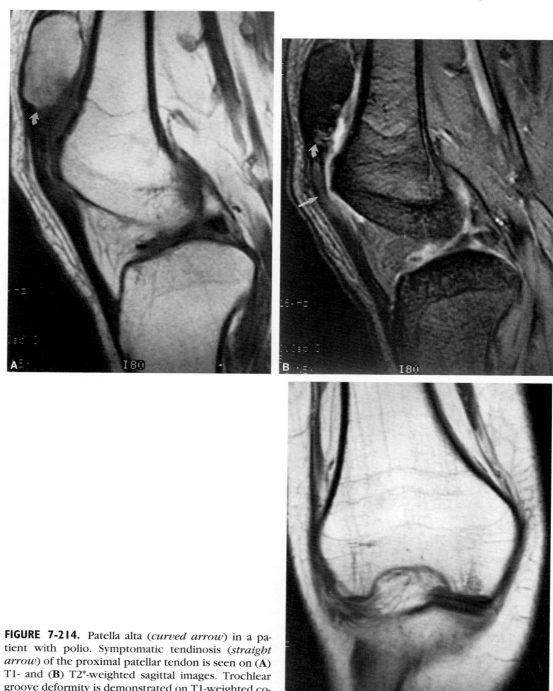

FIGURE 7-214. Patella alta (*curved arrow*) in a patient with polio. Symptomatic tendinosis (*straight arrow*) of the proximal patellar tendon is seen on (**A**) T1- and (**B**) T2*-weighted sagittal images. Trochlear groove deformity is demonstrated on T1-weighted coronal image (**C**).

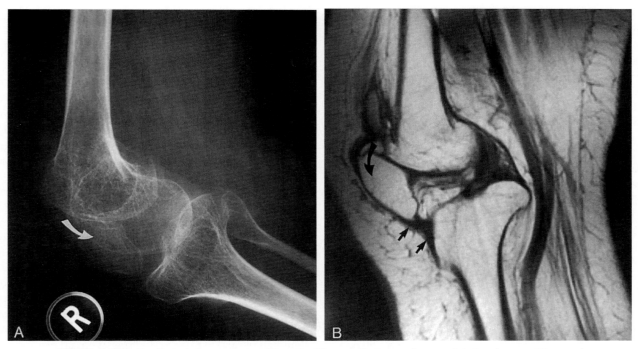

FIGURE 7-215. Patella baja in a patient with polio. The patella (*curved arrows*) is in a low position, and a shortened patellar tendon (*straight arrows*) is seen on (**A**) a lateral radiograph and (**B**) a T1-weighted sagittal image.

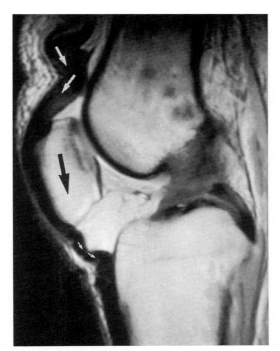

FIGURE 7-216. A proximal quadriceps tendon rupture results in patella baja (*black arrow*), lax quadriceps tendon (*white arrows*), and foreshortened patellar tendon.

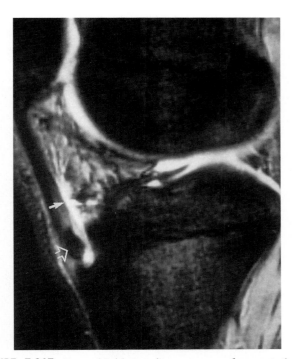

FIGURE 7-217. Osgood-Schlatter disease causes fragmentation of the tibial tubercle (*open arrow*) and development of a hyperintense fluid collection directly posterior to the patellar tendon (*solid arrow*) on a T2-weighted sagittal image. Signal intensity is mildly increased in the adjacent fibers of the patellar tendon.

tibial tuberosity and avulsion and fragmentation of the tibial tubercle ossification center. MR findings include irregularity of the distal patellar tendon with localized hyperintensity on T2, fat-suppressed T2-weighted fast spin-echo, STIR, and gradient-echo images. There may be adjacent edema within Hoffa's fat pad or fluid interposed between the patellar tendon tibial tubercle and inferior aspect of Hoffa's fat pad. MR findings in Osgood-Schlatter disease include multiple small ossicles or a single fragment anterior to the tibial tuberosity that display the high signal intensity of marrow fat on T1-weighted images and low signal intensity on T2* or fat-suppressed T2-weighted fast spin-echo images (Figs. 7-217 and 7-218). Patellar tendon thickening and low-signal-intensity sclerosis in underlying subchondral bone may also be seen.

Sinding-Larsen-Johansson Syndrome

In Sinding-Larsen-Johansson syndrome, osteochondrosis involves the distal patellar pole at the insertion of the patellar tendon. Persistent traction at the cartilaginous junction of the inferior pole of the patella (a traumatic origin) is thought to be the cause. Similar to Osgood-Schlatter disease, Sinding-Larsen-Johansson syndrome usually occurs in the preteen or teen-age years and with a greater incidence in boys. Differential diagnosis includes a stress fracture of the patella, patellar sleeve fracture (through the cartilaginous bone junction), and a type 1 bipartite patella. In Sinding-Larsen-Johansson syndrome sagittal images display an area of low signal intensity on T1-weighted sequences and hyperintensity on gradient-echo or fat-suppressed T2-weighted fast

spin-echo images (Figs. 7-219 and 7-220). Fragmentation of the inferior pole of the patella may be associated with areas of signal alteration in the adjacent proximal fat pad or proximal patellar tendon.

Patellar Bursa

Prepatellar bursitis ("housemaid's knee") may involve one of the anterior subcutaneous bursa over the patella and anterior to the patellar tendon. The superficial or subcutaneous infrapatellar bursa is located between the skin and the tibial tuberosity (Fig. 7-221). The deep infrapatellar bursa is bordered by the distal patellar tendon, the tibial tuberosity, and the inferior extent of Hoffa's fat pad (Fig. 7-222).[16] Although increased amounts of fluid of homogeneous signal intensity can be identified in the deep infrapatellar bursa, the subcutaneous infrapatellar bursa demonstrates either edema or a more localized fluid collection. When inflamed, the appearance of the prepatellar bursa ranges from edema, to a simple fluid collection, to a more complex septated fluid-filled collection that may contain areas of hemorrhage and proteinaceous condensations. Prolonged stress or inflammation related to an underlying synovial process including rheumatoid arthritis may predispose to patellar bursal inflammation. Inflammation (ie, bursitis) with fluid demonstrates low signal intensity on T1-weighted images and high signal intensity on T2, fat-suppressed T2-weighted fast spin-echo, and STIR images. Areas of more complex fluid collections including hemorrhage may demonstrate areas of susceptibility or intermediate-signal-intensity changes on T2-weighted images intermixed with areas of hyperintensity.

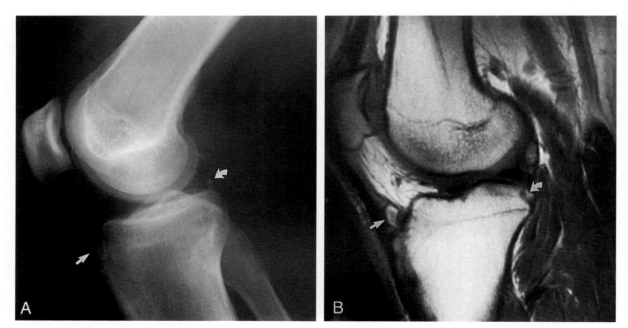

FIGURE 7-218. Unresolved or chronic Osgood-Schlatter disease is associated with avulsion and irregularity of the tibial tuberosity ossicle (*straight arrows*) as seen on (**A**) a lateral radiograph and (**B**) a T1-weighted sagittal image. An unrelated posterior osteochondral fragment (*curved arrows*) is also identified.

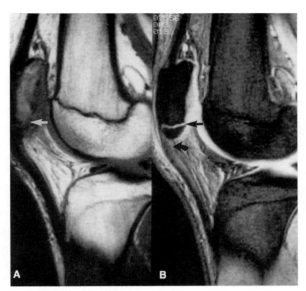

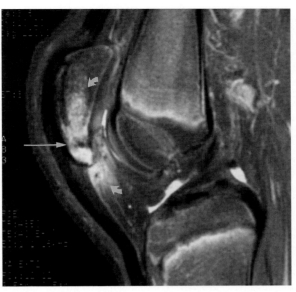

FIGURE 7-219. Sagittal (**A**) T1-weighted and (**B**) T2*-weighted images of the patella in a patient with Sinding-Larsen-Johansson syndrome. Note the separation of the lower pole of the patella (*straight arrows*) and mild thickening and hyperintensity of the proximal patellar tendon (*curved arrow*).

FIGURE 7-220. A fat-suppressed T2-weighted fast spin-echo sagittal image in a case of Sinding-Larsen-Johansson syndrome. The cause is identified as trauma with reactive marrow edema (*curved arrows*) of the inferior pole of the patella and Hoffa's fat pad adjacent to the patellar fracture (*straight arrow*).

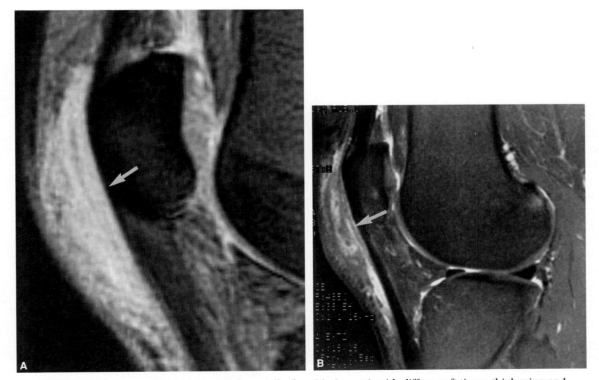

FIGURE 7-221. Prepatellar bursitis. (**A**) Prepatellar bursitis (*arrow*) with diffuse soft-tissue thickening and hyperintensity on a T2*-weighted sagittal image. (**B**) Chronic prepatellar bursitis (*arrow*) in another patient is shown with signal inhomogeneity on a fat-suppressed T2-weighted fast spin-echo sagittal image. Inhomogeneity may also be seen in infectious fluid collections.

continued

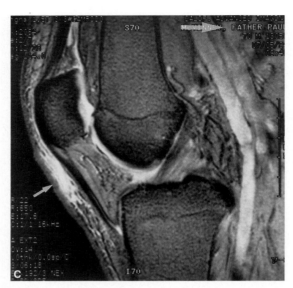

FIGURE 7-221. *Continued.* (**C**) Subcutaneous edema and a poorly demarcated fluid collection (*small arrow*) is seen in a case of "clergyman's knee" (*large arrow*). Because involvement is primarily proximal, within the prepatellar bursa, this MR appearance represents housemaid's knee in contrast to the more distal involvement usually seen in clergyman's knee.

or direct trauma. Myositis ossificans can be a sequela to injury, especially when the vastus medialis is involved. Acute quadriceps tendon rupture is treated with direct surgical repair, with or without reinforcement of the tendon, and may include transverse drill holes across the patella for suture fixation.

For MR evaluation of extensor muscle injuries and tears of the quadriceps tendon, an initial set of coronal or sagittal images is used to display the longitudinal extent of muscle involvement (Fig. 7-223). Axial images are used to identify both the precise muscle group involved and its adjacent anatomic relations. Axial images are also useful in differentiating complete muscle tears with diastasis from partial tears with associated atrophy. Atrophy is best displayed on T1-weighted images. Areas of edema and hemorrhage are best shown on either fat-suppressed T2-weighted fast spin-echo or STIR images. Gradient-echo images can be useful in showing susceptibility in hemosiderin deposits in chronic hematomas. MR imaging is sensitive to both acute and chronic hemorrhage in extensor muscle tears. Subacute hematomas may demonstrate areas of increased signal intensity on T1-weighted images secondary to the paramagnetic effect of methemoglobin. Areas of chronic hemorrhage demonstrate low signal intensity, especially on gradient-echo images.

Selected Patellofemoral Surgical Procedures

Patellectomy may be required to treat unmanageable chondromalacia with severe pain and comminuted fracture of the patella.[43] This procedure usually is reserved for patients who are not candidates for a patellofemoral replacement or Maquet's procedure (described below).[268] After patellectomy, sagittal MR images display the absence of the patella and the continuity of the quadriceps and patellar tendons. Residual bone chips or calcification may still be present in the quadriceps expansion.

Maquet's procedure, or anterior tibial tubercle elevation, is performed to decrease loading forces across the patellofemoral joint by raising the insertion of the patellar tendon. It is not used as a primary treatment for patellar malalignment. The Elmslie-Trillat procedure, or medialization of the tibial tubercle, is a commonly performed procedure for lateral subluxations or recurrent patellar dislocations.[268] The Fulkerson osteotomy not only medializes the tibial tubercle but also provides elevation with one osteotomy.

Quadriceps Tendon and Muscle Tears

The quadriceps muscle group is composed of the rectus femoris and vastus intermedius muscles, which insert on the base of the patella, and the vastus lateralis and medialis muscles, which insert on the lateral and medial aspects of the patella, respectively. Quadriceps tears or ruptures occur in the young athlete with either forced muscle contraction

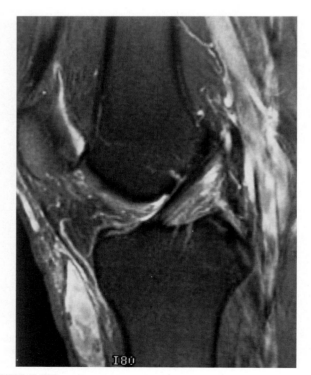

FIGURE 7-222. A fat-suppressed T2-weighted fast spin-echo sagittal image showing bursitis of the subcutaneous infrapatellar bursa between the skin and tibial tuberosity.

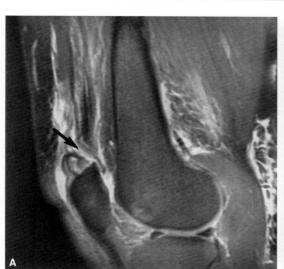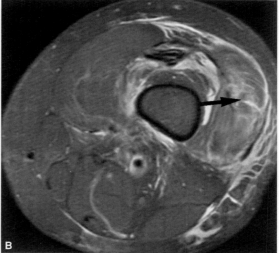

FIGURE 7-223. (A) A fat-suppressed T2-weighted fast spin-echo sagittal image shows acute rupture of the quadriceps tendon with high signal intensity fluid filling the tendon gap (*arrow*). There is associated patellar baja secondary to the distal pull from the patellar tendon. (B) A fat-suppressed T2-weighted fast spin-echo axial image shows diffuse vastus lateralis muscle edema (*arrow*).

These differences in signal characteristics may be important in distinguishing between areas of suspected hemorrhage and other soft-tissue masses, such as synovial sarcoma. Intravenous gadolinium can also be used to help clarify a differential diagnosis if an area of hemorrhage cannot be clearly characterized. After contrast administration, hemorrhage demonstrates peripheral enhancement without central hyperintensity, whereas a malignant neoplasm, such as a synovial sarcoma, demonstrates increased intake of gadolinium centrally within the lesion. Edema and areas of fraying in the affected muscle demonstrate intermediate signal intensity on T1-weighted images and increased signal intensity on T2, STIR, and fat-suppressed T2-weighted fast spin-echo images. Muscle atrophy and fatty infiltration are seen as regions of increased signal intensity on T1-weighted images. A retracted proximal or distal muscle bundle can be identified as a soft-tissue mass with higher signal intensity than the native muscle.

Any increase in signal intensity within the quadriceps tendon is abnormal. Increases range from intrasubstance signal in degeneration or tendinitis to high signal intensity hemorrhage or edema in complete avulsions or ruptures of the tendon. MR imaging is also used to document an intact quadriceps tendon in superficial injuries associated with subcutaneous edema or hemorrhage.

Secondary signs of quadriceps insufficiency include patellar tilting and redundancy or laxity of the patellar tendon. However, laxity of the patellar tendon may be secondary to positioning of the knee.

GENERAL PATHOLOGIC CONDITIONS AFFECTING THE KNEE

Arthritis

Assessment of the extent, progression, and therapeutic response in arthritic disorders in adults and in JRA is enhanced by MR imaging of articular cartilage.[269] Joint effusions, synovial reactions, popliteal cysts, and osteonecrosis can be demonstrated and evaluated with MR studies, even in patients with negative findings on conventional radiographs.

Cartilage Evaluation

The function of articular cartilage is to assist in the distribution of loads and to decrease stress in subchondral bone. It is composed of chondrocytes and an extracellular matrix. There are no nerve cells or blood vessels within articular cartilage.[270] Chondrocytes are nourished through the diffusion of nutrients and metabolites through the matrix, which consists of macromolecules containing water. The structural macromolecules include collagen and proteoglycans and noncollagenous proteins. Collagens in a fibrillar meshwork provide tensile strength and form to articular cartilage. Type II collagen represents 90% to 95% of articular cartilage collagen. Type IX (surface binding) and type XI (internal core formation) collagen help to organize and stabilize type II collagen fibers.

The lamellar organization of articular cartilage consists of four zones, based on the proximity of chondrocytes in the composition of matrix in each of four successfully deeper zones. The most superficial, or gliding, zone forms the articular surface of the joint. Flattened or ellipsoid chondrocytes and collagen fibers are parallel to the articular surface deep to a thin cell-free layer of overlying matrix. The next zone, deep to the superficial zone, is the larger transitional zone, which has a more random distribution of collagen fibers. The largest layer of articular cartilage is the radial, or deep, zone, with its cells arranged or aligned into short columns. The radial zone contains the largest collagen fibers, the highest proteoglycan content, and the lowest water content. The thin calcified zone (the deepest zone) divides the articular cartilage from the underlying subchondral bone (including subchondral plate and deeper cancellous bone). The tidemark, or calcification line, demarcates the transition from the radial zone to the calcified zone of cartilage.

Pathology

The early changes of osteoarthritis include localized fibrillation, which represents disruption of superficial articular cartilage layers.[270,271] When extensive, fibrillation may have deep projections that reach subchondral bone. Disruption of the molecular framework of the matrix leads to an increase in water content and a decrease in proteoglycan content.[270] Consequently, there is an increase in permeability and a decrease in stiffness of the matrix. These changes may make the articular cartilage more susceptible to further damage. As articular cartilage fissures develop, the tips of fibrillated cartilage tear. The release of cartilage fragments and the enzymatic degradation of the matrix contribute to a decrease in overall cartilage thickness and volume. Simultaneously, anabolic cytokines stimulate the production of matrix macromolecules and proliferation of chondrocytes in an attempt to repair cartilage degeneration. An unsuccessful repair response leads eventually to end-stage changes in degenerative articular cartilage, which include exposed subchondral bone, sclerosis, subchondral cysts, joint space narrowing, and osteophytes.

Imaging of Articular Cartilage

Cartilage of the patellar, femoral, and tibial articular surfaces is routinely observed on MR images.[269,272] Because of its hydropic composition, normal hyaline cartilage demonstrates intermediate signal intensity on T1-weighted images, compared with the low signal intensity of cortex and fibrocartilaginous menisci (Fig. 7-224). It is believed that changes in the signal intensity of cartilage are caused by a loss of water-binding proteoglycan molecules. On conventional T2-weighted images, hyaline cartilage displays an intermediate signal intensity. In the presence of a joint effusion, T2-weighted images create an arthrogram-like effect, with hyperintense synovial fluid improving the delineation of thinner cartilage surfaces (eg, medial and lateral compartments) (Fig. 7-225). There is poor contrast, however, between articular cartilage and subchondral bone on conventional T2-weighted images, and in the absence of a joint effusion, surface or contour irregularities may not be resolved.[8] With gradient-

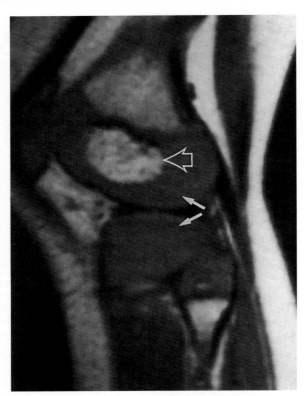

FIGURE 7-224. Normal thick hyaline articular cartilage demonstrates intermediate signal intensity (*solid arrows*) on a T1-weighted sagittal image. The femoral ossific nucleus is seen with high signal intensity fatty marrow (*open arrow*). The tibial ossific nucleus has not yet developed.

echo, chemical-shift, and fast low-angle–shot techniques, hyaline cartilage demonstrates high signal intensity. Although articular cartilage defects smaller than 3 mm have been identified with T2*-weighted images, in general these techniques may underestimate articular cartilage degeneration because it may be difficult to distinguish high-signal-intensity fluid from high-signal-intensity articular cartilage with accuracy. Surface articular cartilage fissures and early articular cartilage softening may be missed on T2*-weighted images, and we do not recommend this sequence as a routine cartilage imaging protocol, although a dual-echo gradient-echo sequence may optimize visualization of fluid–cartilage interfaces. A T2*-weighted echo technique shows the delineation of the fluid–cartilage interface because effusions generate higher signal intensity than do adjacent cartilage surfaces.

3D sequences provide thin-section capability with multiplanar reformatting. The fat-suppressed 3D SPGR technique has been shown to have a 95% accuracy rate (with 96% sensitivity and 95% specificity) in evaluating patellofemoral articular cartilage defects in cadavers with the use of intraarticular saline.[8,273] Fat-suppressed 3D SPGR sequences can also be used to demonstrate positive contrast between articular cartilage and adjacent structures.[274] SPGR without fat suppression, however, may be insensitive to pathologic articular cartilage signal alterations (Fig. 7-226).[275,276]

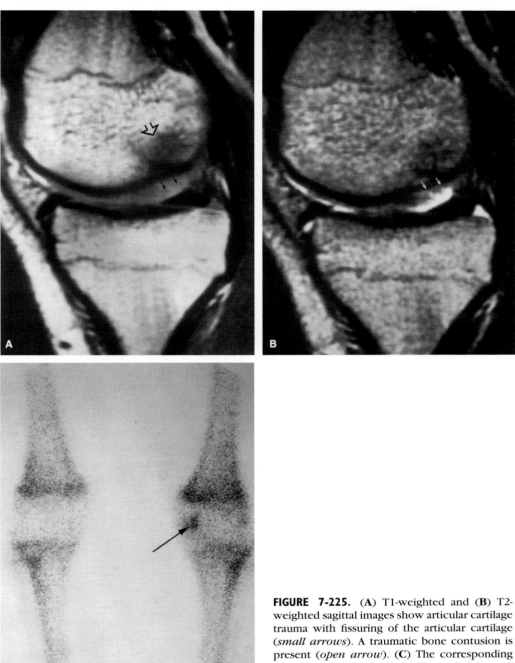

FIGURE 7-225. (A) T1-weighted and (B) T2-weighted sagittal images show articular cartilage trauma with fissuring of the articular cartilage (*small arrows*). A traumatic bone contusion is present (*open arrow*). (C) The corresponding bone scan shows uptake in the medial femoral condyle (*arrow*).

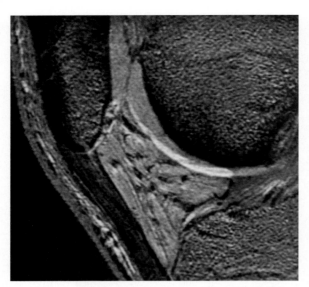

FIGURE 7-226. A sagittal 3D SPGR image obtained without fat suppression shows the patellofemoral articular cartilage in excellent anatomic detail. However, the sensitivity of this technique for surface and intrasubstance degeneration is limited.

On spin-echo and gradient-echo sequences, articular cartilage is sometimes seen to have a bilaminar or trilaminar appearance.[272] Cartilage has a trilaminar appearance on fat-suppressed SPGR images.[273] This trilaminar appearance consists of a superficial region of high signal intensity, an intermediate area of low signal intensity, and a deep area of high signal intensity.[273,274] The outer area of high signal intensity is thought to represent the superficial gliding zone of the articular cartilage. The isotropic arrangement of collagen and its position relative to the magnetic field is thought to influence the MR imaging characteristics of the three layers of articular cartilage. The middle layer visualized on MR scans may represent the transitional zone, whereas the deep layer seen on MR corresponds to a combination of the radial (deep) zone, the calcified zone, and subchondral bone.[8] Fat-suppressed T2-weighted fast spin-echo techniques are more successful in separating the cartilage–fluid interface and identifying early changes of articular cartilage degeneration (Fig. 7-227).[277,278] Fast spin-echo images, however, may suffer from a loss of spatial resolution along the phase-encoded axis (increased blurring occurs with short TEs). This blurring effect can be minimized and resolution increased by using a 256 or 512 matrix and sequences with lower echo train lengths (<4) and higher TEs. Without fat-suppression techniques, fast spin-echo images are limited by a higher signal intensity from fat-containing tissues relative to conventional T2 spin-echo sequences. This limitation requires the use of longer TR (>4000 millisecond) and TE

(>100 millisecond) sequences to produce a T2 effect. With STIR image contrast it is possible to differentiate the brighter signal intensity of fluid from the intermediate to high signal intensity of articular cartilage.[272] This sequence is also effective for demonstrating early changes in subchondral bone in areas of overlying articular cartilage damage. Areas of fluid within articular cartilage fissures and fragmentation can also be visualized on STIR images. The cartilage–fluid interface and changes of early articular cartilage softening may not be as well delineated compared with fat-suppressed T2-weighted fast spin-echo sequences.

Conventional T1 spin-echo sequences, combined with fat suppression and the use of gadolinium as a contrast agent, are used in intraarticular MR arthrography. With the use of intraarticular studies with an MR contrast agent, it may be possible to identify smaller chondral lesions than with intraarticular MR studies performed with saline.[279] However, gadolinium studies (compared with fat-suppressed T2-weighted fast spin-echo sequences) may not be as useful for the detection of internal articular cartilage alterations or deep or basal layer changes in the articular cartilage. Intraarticular gadolinium studies appear to be more sensitive to superficial articular cartilage changes and do not accurately reflect the internal changes of water composition within degenerating articular cartilage.

Magnetization transfer contrast is sensitive to the interaction between water molecules improving contrast on gradient-echo sequences (eg, SPGR).[280] Magnetization transfer contrast techniques have not yet been shown to be supe-

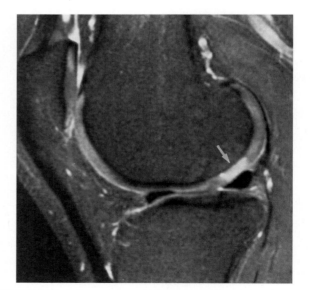

FIGURE 7-227. A fat-suppressed T2-weighted fast spin-echo sagittal image displays a high signal intensity area of degeneration (*arrow*) of the lateral femoral condyle articular cartilage opposite the superior surface of the posterior horn of the lateral meniscus. Normal articular cartilage is low to intermediate in signal intensity.

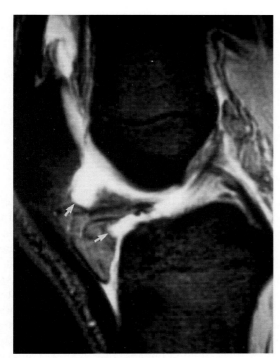

FIGURE 7-228. Confirmed hemorrhagic joint effusion results in synovial irritation with irregularity of the concave free edge of Hoffa's infrapatellar fat pad (*arrows*), as seen on a T2*-weighted sagittal image. In the absence of arthritis or infection, a nonhemorrhagic effusion is not usually associated with a positive Hoffa's infrapatellar fat-pad sign.

rior to fat-suppressed T2-weighted fast spin-echo contrast in routine articular cartilage visualization.[14,272,280]

With 3D faster techniques, there is a high signal intensity fluid interface with intermediate signal intensity on T1-weighted contrast. T1 hybrid fat-suppressed images have been recommended by Chandnani and colleagues to more accurately characterize hyaline articular cartilage structures.[281]

In children, the articular cartilage is thicker, allowing increased sensitivity in detection of focal erosions and cartilage thinning. In infants, the articular cartilage is seen before the appearance of the distal femoral and proximal tibial ossific nuclei, and it demonstrates higher signal intensity than the adjacent marrow. Before any radiographic evidence of joint-space narrowing is found, focal erosions and uniform attenuation of articular cartilage can be observed in MR studies in patients with JRA, hemophilia, or degenerative joint disease. Loss of subchondral signal intensity has also been observed in association with initial cartilage loss in patients with sclerosis. These areas of suspected subchondral sclerosis may show regions of high signal intensity on fat-suppressed T2-weighted fast spin-echo or STIR images. Interosseous cysts and hemorrhage, which demonstrate increased signal intensity on T2-weighted images, may develop at sites of denuded hyaline cartilage.

Synovium Evaluation and the Irregular Hoffa's Infrapatellar Fat-Pad Sign

Synovial reaction and proliferation are characterized on MR images by changes in the contour of synovial reflections. Irregularity with loss of the smooth posterior concave free

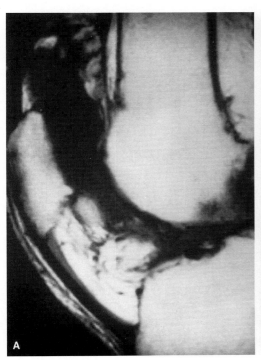

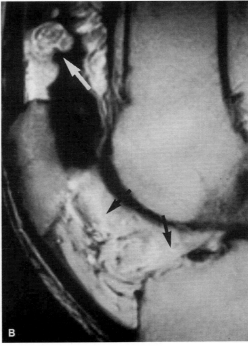

FIGURE 7-229. Lateral compartment pannus is shown (**A**) before and (**B**) after intravenous gadolinium administration. A comparison of these T1-weighted sagittal images demonstrates selective high signal intensity enhancement of pannus tissue. Thickened suprapatellar synovium (*white arrow*) and hypertrophied synovium posterior to Hoffa's infrapatellar fat pad (*black arrows*) are shown.

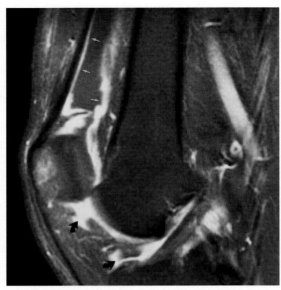

FIGURE 7-230. Fat-suppression techniques improve visualization of high signal intensity inflamed synovial tissue (*straight arrows*) on a T1-weighted sagittal image enhanced by intravenous administration of gadolinium-DTPA contrast. Note the irregular contour of Hoffa's fat pad (*curved arrows*).

ondary to trauma, there are areas of signal alterations with hyperintensity on T2, fat-suppressed T2-weighted fast spin-echo, STIR, and gradient-echo images. Areas of scarring and fibrosis demonstrate low signal intensity on T1- and T2-weighted images. Hypertrophy of the fat pad in Hoffa's disease occurs after trauma when the fat pad enlarges beyond the margins of the patellar tendon. Impingement can then occur and produce pain and inflammation.

Juvenile Chronic Arthritis (JRA)

JRA is subgrouped into Still's disease (systemic onset), polyarticular onset, and pauciarticular onset.[283] In the initial stages of clinical presentation, MR studies demonstrate synovitis with irregularity of Hoffa's infrapatellar fat pad (Fig. 7-231).[284] Articular cartilage erosions and synovial hypertrophy can be identified before joint-space narrowing is evident on plain-film radiography. Posterior popliteal cysts of the gastrocnemius and semimembranosus bursae, associated with JRA, demonstrate low signal intensity on T1-weighted images and uniform high signal intensity on T2-weighted images (Fig. 7-232). Thickening

border of Hoffa's infrapatellar fat pad can be observed in a variety of synovial reactions and is referred to as the irregular infrapatellar fat-pad sign (Fig. 7-228).[269] Although the synovium cannot be imaged directly in early synovitis, a corrugated surface along Hoffa's infrapatellar fat pad is evident in the early stages of synovial irritation. This irregular infrapatellar fat-pad sign has been seen in patients with hemophilia, rheumatoid arthritis, PVNS, Lyme arthritis, inflammatory osteoarthritis, and hemorrhagic effusions (caused by arthritis or trauma) with reactive synovium. In addition to these synovial reactions, swelling of the retropatellar fat pad has been seen in chronic patellofemoral chondromalacia and instability.[43]

Gadolinium-DTPA contrast–enhanced T1-weighted images are useful in the accurate identification of pannus tissue, which can be seen as areas of increased signal intensity adjacent to low signal intensity joint fluid (Fig. 7-229).[282] Fat-suppressed gadolinium-enhanced studies improve the contrast differentiation between bright-signal-intensity pannus and low-signal-intensity joint fluid (Fig. 7-230). On T1, T2, fat-suppressed T2-weighted fast spin-echo, and T2*-weighted protocols, synovial hypertrophy and pannus demonstrate low to intermediate signal intensity and are more difficult to identify. Fluid associated with synovial masses generates increased signal intensity on T2-weighted images. The irregular infrapatellar fat-pad sign should be distinguished from Hoffa's disease, which represents an impingement of the fat pad characterized by both inflammation and subsequent fibrosis. In Hoffa's disease, which may be sec-

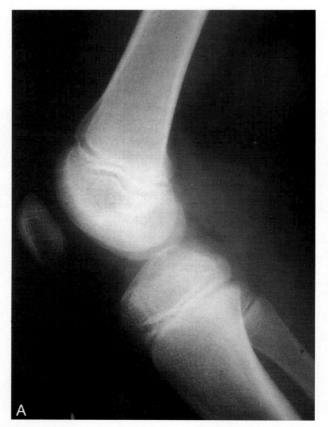

FIGURE 7-231. Early JRA. **(A)** A lateral radiograph taken at the initial clinical evaluation showed no abnormalities. *continued*

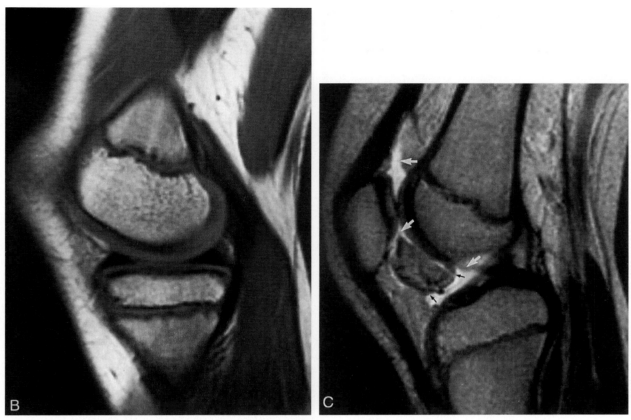

FIGURE 7-231. *Continued.* (**B**) A T1-weighted sagittal image shows that the hyaline articular cartilage is intact. (**C**) A T2-weighted sagittal image reveals the initial stages of synovitis with an irregular Hoffa's infrapatellar fat pad (*black arrows*) and high-signal-intensity effusion (*white arrows*).

of the synovium of the suprapatellar bursa can be seen with low signal intensity on T1- and T2-weighted images (Fig. 7-233). In more advanced disease, MR studies show subarticular cysts, subchondral cysts, and osteonecrosis on both femoral and tibial surfaces (Figs. 7-234 and 7-235). These changes are frequently not evident on conventional radiographs. Hypoplastic menisci, with small anterior and posterior horns and body, have also been observed on MR studies in patients with JRA. This finding may be related to an alteration in the fluid composition of synovial fluid that impairs normal fibrocartilage development. An enlarged epiphysis, widening of the intercondylar notch, and squaring of the inferior margin of the patella are conventional radiographic findings also detected on MR. With the increasing use of more aggressive treatment protocols, including drugs such as methotrexate, MR evaluation of signs of disease progression, such as pannus-tissue changes, may be a cost-effective way of monitoring the effectiveness of therapy. MR studies may also replace or complement serial radiographic surveys for assessment of the functional status of patients with JRA.

Rheumatoid Arthritis

In adult patients with rheumatoid arthritis, bicompartmental and tricompartmental disease is displayed on MR images through the medial and lateral femorotibial compartments and patellofemoral joint (Fig. 7-236).[269] Marginal and subchondral erosions with diffuse loss of hyaline articular cartilage are evident on both medial and lateral femoral articular surfaces. Large joint effusions with popliteal cysts are commonly seen and demonstrate uniform high signal intensity on T2, fat-suppressed T2-weighted fast spin-echo, and T2*-weighted images. Less frequently, signs of degenerative arthritis with osteophytosis and subchondral sclerosis demonstrate low signal intensity on MR scans. An irregular fat pad may be seen in the more active stages of the disease. Hypertrophied synovial masses remain relatively low in signal intensity on T1- and T2-weighted contrast images.

Gadolinium-DPTA contrast–enhanced images are useful in identifying the pannus or granulation tissue that grows over the surfaces of articular cartilage in rheumatoid arthritis.[285–287] Contrast-enhanced images are more effective than

text continues on page 394

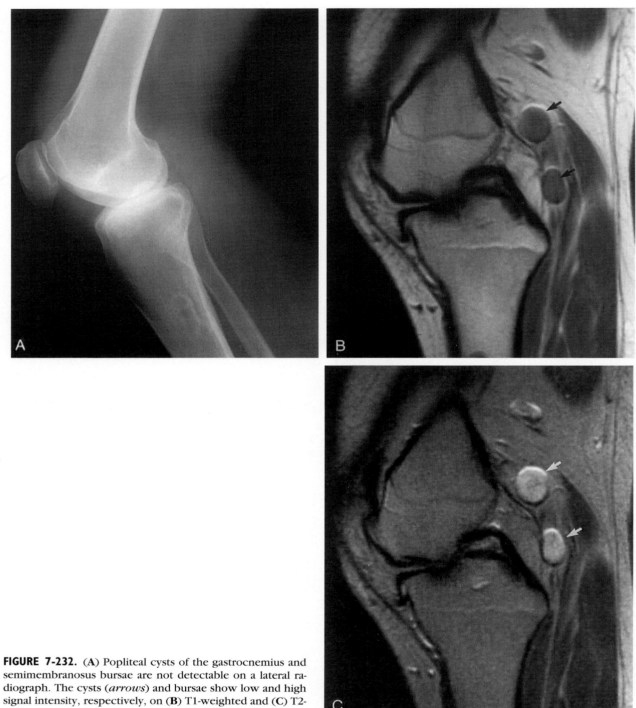

FIGURE 7-232. (A) Popliteal cysts of the gastrocnemius and semimembranosus bursae are not detectable on a lateral radiograph. The cysts (*arrows*) and bursae show low and high signal intensity, respectively, on (**B**) T1-weighted and (**C**) T2-weighted sagittal images.

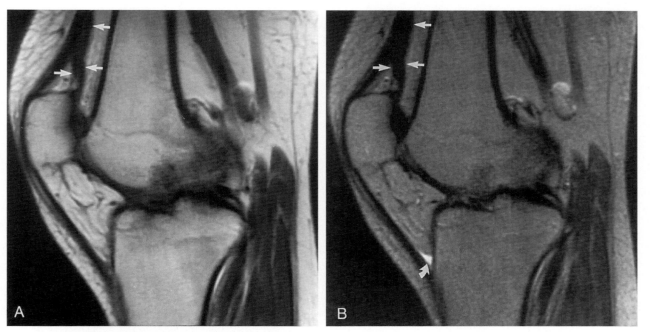

FIGURE 7-233. JRA causes suprapatellar synovial hypertrophy (*white arrows*), seen as low signal intensity on both (**A**) T1-weighted and (**B**) T2-weighted sagittal images. In contrast, a focus of fluid demonstrates bright signal intensity (*curved arrow*) on the T2-weighted image.

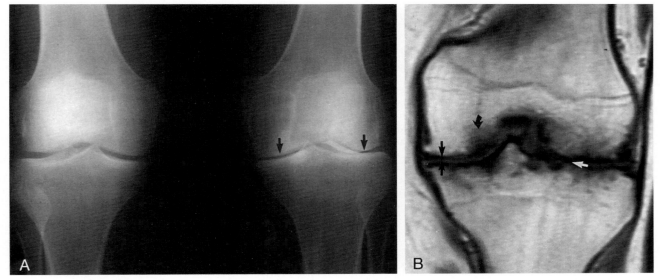

FIGURE 7-234. Advanced JRA with marked joint-space narrowing (*black arrows*) is seen on (**A**) an anteroposterior radiograph and (**B**) a T1-weighted coronal image. Articular cartilage erosion (*white arrow*) and subchondral sclerosis (*curved arrow*) are best seen on MR images.

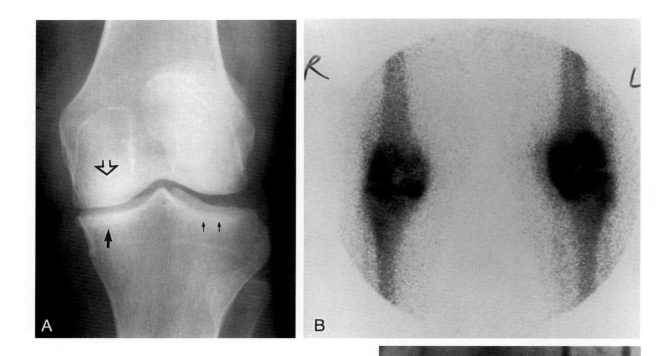

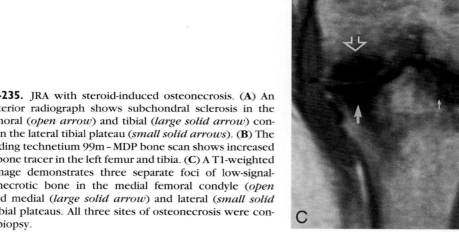

FIGURE 7-235. JRA with steroid-induced osteonecrosis. **(A)** An anteroposterior radiograph shows subchondral sclerosis in the medial femoral (*open arrow*) and tibial (*large solid arrow*) condyles and in the lateral tibial plateau (*small solid arrows*). **(B)** The corresponding technetium 99m–MDP bone scan shows increased uptake of bone tracer in the left femur and tibia. **(C)** A T1-weighted coronal image demonstrates three separate foci of low-signal-intensity necrotic bone in the medial femoral condyle (*open arrow*) and medial (*large solid arrow*) and lateral (*small solid arrows*) tibial plateaus. All three sites of osteonecrosis were confirmed at biopsy.

non–contrast-enhanced T1, T2, fat-suppressed T2-weighted fast spin-echo, T2* or STIR images for separating fluid from adjacent pannus. Pannus tissue may be underestimated without the use of intravenous gadolinium enhancement. The ability to map out pannus is useful in examining patients with severe inflammatory arthritis when synovectomy is considered before total joint arthroplasty.

Osteonecrosis and infarcts in rheumatoid patients can be identified on MR scans before corresponding radiographic changes are evident.

Pigmented Villonodular Synovitis (PVNS)

PVNS is a monarticular synovial proliferative disorder. It usually presents as a nonpainful soft-tissue mass, and the knee is a common site of involvement, especially in the diffuse form of the disease. Hemosiderin-laden macrophages are frequently deposited in hyperplastic synovial masses, and sclerotic bone lesions may be associated.

Several reports have correlated MR findings in PVNS with surgically confirmed pathologic changes.[288–291] The hemosiderin-infiltrated synovial masses demonstrate low signal intensity on T1, T2, fat-suppressed T2-weighted fast spin-echo, and T2*-weighted images because of the paramagnetic effect of iron (Figs. 7-237 through 7-239). Adjacent synovial fluid, however, may be seen with increased signal intensity on T2-weighted images. Hemosiderin deposits may be observed in thickened synovial reflections supe-

text continues on page 398

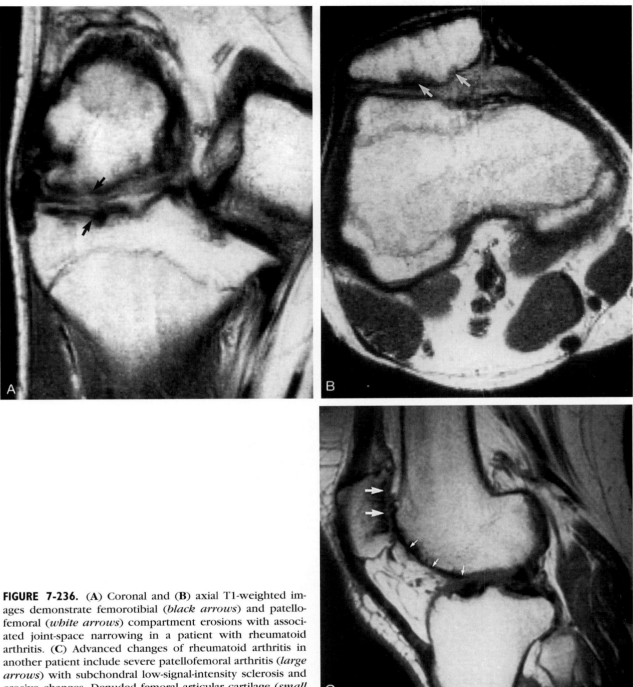

FIGURE 7-236. (**A**) Coronal and (**B**) axial T1-weighted images demonstrate femorotibial (*black arrows*) and patellofemoral (*white arrows*) compartment erosions with associated joint-space narrowing in a patient with rheumatoid arthritis. (**C**) Advanced changes of rheumatoid arthritis in another patient include severe patellofemoral arthritis (*large arrows*) with subchondral low-signal-intensity sclerosis and erosive changes. Denuded femoral articular cartilage (*small arrows*) is also present on this T1-weighted sagittal image.

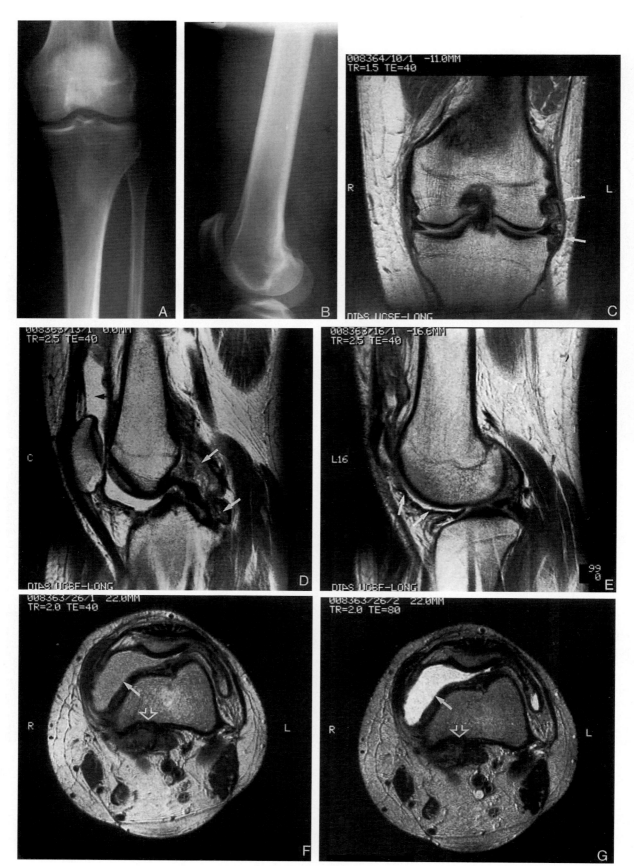

FIGURE 7-237.

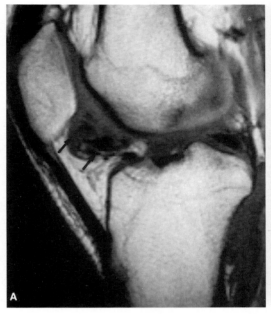

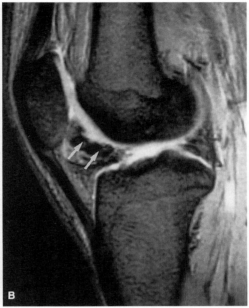

FIGURE 7-238. On sagittal (**A**) T1-weighted and (**B**) T2*-weighted images, PVNS is characterized by low signal intensity hemosiderin deposits in thickened synovium along the free edge of Hoffa's infrapatellar fat pad (*arrows*). The paramagnetic effect of hemosiderin results in a decreased T2 relaxation time.

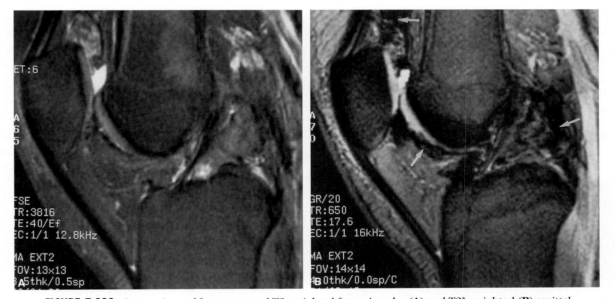

FIGURE 7-239. Comparison of fat-suppressed T2-weighted fast spin-echo (**A**) and T2*-weighted (**B**) sagittal images used in the assessment of the diffuse form of PVNS. The fat-suppressed T2-weighted fast spin-echo sequence (**A**) is less sensitive to hemosiderin (*arrow*) in pannus tissue and synovium than is the T2*-weighted sequence (**B**).

FIGURE 7-237. (**A**) Anteroposterior and (**B**) lateral radiographs of the distal femur and proximal tibia are unremarkable in a patient with PVNS. (**C**) On an intermediate weighted coronal image, a low signal intensity hyperplastic synovium is revealed on the lateral aspect of the knee (*arrows*). (**D**) On a T2-weighted sagittal image, a synovial mass of fibrous tissue and hemosiderin (*white arrows*) remains low in signal intensity, whereas an adjacent effusion demonstrates bright signal intensity (*black arrow*). (**E**) On another T2-weighted sagittal image, low-signal-intensity hemosiderin has been deposited in a thickened synovial reflection along the concave surface of Hoffa's infrapatellar fat pad (*arrows*). (**F**) Intermediate weighted and (**G**) T2-weighted axial images of the posterior hemosiderin-laden synovial mass demonstrate no change in signal intensity (*open arrows*). A suprapatellar effusion (*solid arrows*) increases in signal intensity on a T2-weighted image.

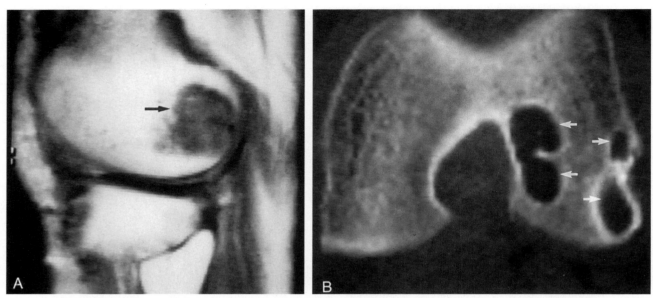

FIGURE 7-240. (**A**) On a T1-weighted sagittal image, a PVNS mass (*black arrow*) is seen in the posterolateral femoral condyle. (**B**) On an axial CT scan, femoral erosion (*white arrows*) is apparent.

rior to Hoffa's infrapatellar fat pad. Condylar erosions may be associated with a synovial mass and fibrous tissue (Fig. 7-240). A more localized nodular form of PVNS, seen as a well-described mass, may be seen within or posterior to Hoffa's infrapatellar fat pad or within the posterior capsule of the knee joint. Intravenous gadolinium-DTPA enhancement is effective in differentiating areas of pannus tissue from hemosiderin deposits and joint fluid in patients with

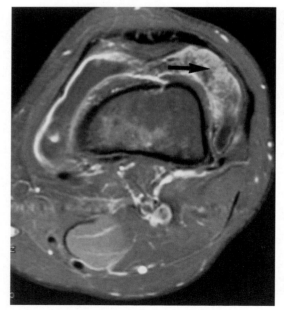

FIGURE 7-241. Enhancement of pannus tissue (*arrow*) associated with PVNS on a fat-suppressed T1-weighted axial image after intravenous administration of gadolinium-DTPA.

PVNS (Fig. 7-241). This differentiation is especially useful in identifying active sites of involvement including the suprapatellar bursa, medial and lateral compartments, and popliteal cysts.

Hemophilia

In MR studies in patients with hemophilic arthropathy, hemosiderin and fibrous tissue, formed from repeated episodes of joint hemorrhage, demonstrate low signal intensity on T1- and T2-weighted images (Fig. 7-242).[292,293] Irregular contours of Hoffa's fat pad and markedly thickened, hemosiderin-laden synovial reflections of low signal intensity are common findings (Fig. 7-243). Although conventional radiographs are normal, articular cartilage irregularities and erosions can be detected on MR scans in the early stages of disease.

Subchondral and intraosseous cysts or hemorrhage can be identified on coronal and sagittal MR images (Fig. 7-244). Fluid-filled cysts generate high signal intensity on T2-weighted images. Areas of fibrous tissue remain low in signal intensity on T1-, T2-, and T2*-weighted images, and low-signal-intensity synovial effusions can be differentiated from adjacent hemosiderin and fibrous depositions on T2-weighted sequences. Articular and subchondral abnormalities of the femoral condylar and tibial surfaces are relatively common findings, seen in 75% to 85% of cases (Fig. 7-245).

Lyme Arthritis

Lyme disease and resultant arthritis are transmitted by *Ixodes dammini* ticks and are characterized by the delayed appearance of an oligo- or polyarticular inflammatory arthri-

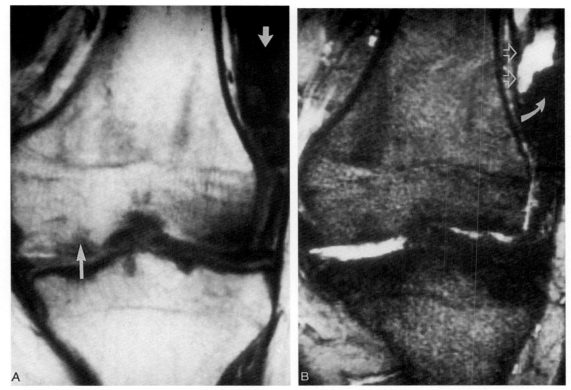

FIGURE 7-242. (**A**) A T1-weighted coronal image demonstrates erosive changes (*long arrow*) and surrounding low-signal-intensity areas along the lateral femur (*short arrow*) in a patient with hemophilia. (**B**) A T2*-weighted image distinguics01sshes high-signal-intensity fluid or hemorrhage (*open arrows*) from chronic hemosiderin deposition (*curved arrow*).

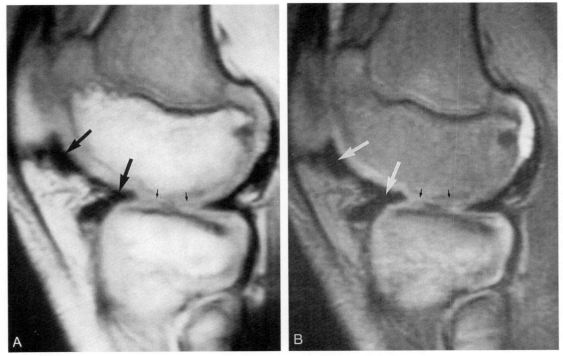

FIGURE 7-243. The knee of a patient with hemophilia shows early cartilage erosions (*small arrows*) and a thickened hemosiderin-laden synovium that demonstrates low signal intensity (*large arrows*) on (**A**) T1-weighted and (**B**) T2-weighted images. The irregularity of Hoffa's infrapatellar fat pad indicates synovial irritation.

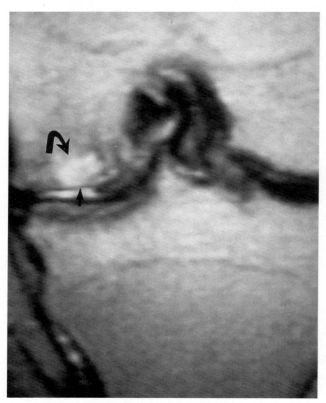

FIGURE 7-244. An intraosseous cyst (*curved arrow*) has formed through a defect in the femoral articular cartilage (*straight arrow*) in this patient with hemophilia. The cyst demonstrates high signal intensity on a T2-weighted coronal image.

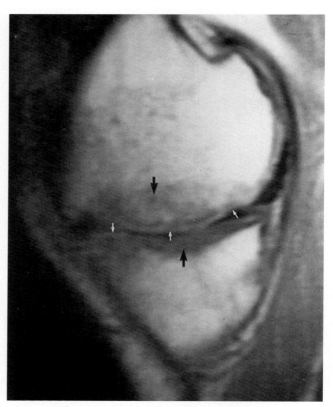

FIGURE 7-245. The knee of an adult with hemophilia shows low signal intensity subchondral sclerosis (*black arrows*) and denuded articular cartilage (*white arrows*) on a T1-weighted sagittal image.

tis.[294] The knee is most commonly affected, with development of inflammatory synovial effusions, synovial hypertrophy, infrapatellar fat-pad edema, and, in severe chronic cases, cartilage erosions. In one patient, examined 3 months after a documented tick bite, MR scans revealed an extensive joint effusion and an irregular, corrugated Hoffa's infrapatellar fat pad (Fig. 7-246).[269] After the MR studies, contrast material was injected into the joint to confirm scalloping of the synovium, characteristic of synovitis, which was first identified on MR imaging. No cartilage erosions were identified. In another patient with Lyme arthritis, an irregular fat pad was seen in association with popliteal cysts present for several years. There was no associated intraarticular pathology. Enthesopathic changes may occur in tendons (quadriceps and patellar), and new bone may form at capsular insertion sites. Loss of articular cartilage appears in 25% of patients with chronic Lyme arthritis.[295,296]

Osteoarthritis

The MR findings in degenerative arthrosis vary from osteophytic spurring, which demonstrates the bright signal intensity of marrow, to compartment collapse, denuded articular cartilage, torn and degenerative meniscal fibrocartilage, and

diminished marrow signal intensity in areas of subchondral sclerosis (Fig. 7-247).[297] Fat-suppressed T2-weighted fast spin-echo and STIR images frequently display areas of hyperintensity in subchondral bone corresponding to areas of diminished marrow signal intensity on T1-weighted images (see Fig. 7-247). These regions of bone remodeling are associated with degenerative articular cartilage and represent subchondral sclerosis, subchondral cystic cavities (with myxoid, fibrous, or cartilaginous tissue), regenerative cartilage, and new layers of bone formation.[270] The ability to accurately assess hyaline cartilage surfaces may give MR imaging an advantage over plain-film radiography in preoperative planning for joint replacement procedures, especially in unicondylar arthroplasties for osteoarthritis. A posterior-to-anterior bent-knee standing radiograph of both knees, however, allows accurate assessment of the remaining articular cartilage in the tibiofemoral compartments of the knee.[298] Chondral fragments (intermediate signal intensity) and loose bodies (high signal intensity of marrow fat) may be associated with more advanced degenerative disease (Fig. 7-248). It is important to have T1-weighted images in at least one plane to improve the identification of loose bodies that do contain marrow fat. The exclusive use of fat-suppressed–type sequences may result in confusion between areas of fat and marrow-containing loose bodies. The

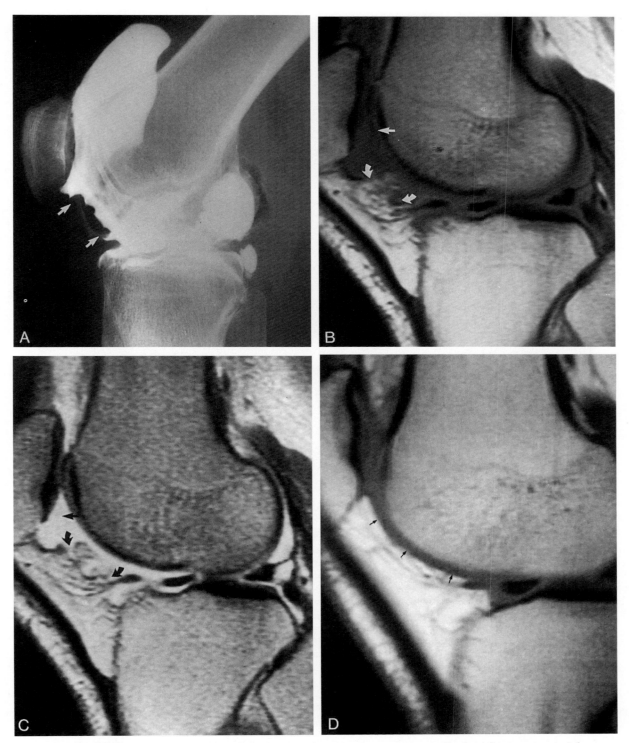

FIGURE 7-246. Lyme arthritis. (**A**) A lateral-view arthrogram demonstrates scalloping of contrast material (*arrows*), indicating synovitis. (**B**) T1-weighted and (**C**) T2-weighted sagittal images show an irregular Hoffa's infrapatellar fat pad (*curved arrows*) with interdigitation of synovial effusion (*straight arrow*). Joint effusion is bright on the T2-weighted image. (**D**) On an intermediate weighted sagittal image, the asymptomatic knee in the same patient displays the normal concave contour of the free edge of Hoffa's infrapatellar fat pad (*arrows*).

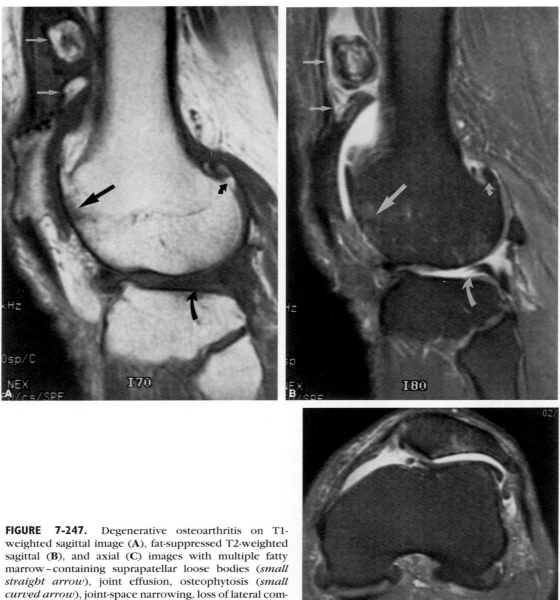

FIGURE 7-247. Degenerative osteoarthritis on T1-weighted sagittal image (**A**), fat-suppressed T2-weighted sagittal (**B**), and axial (**C**) images with multiple fatty marrow–containing suprapatellar loose bodies (*small straight arrow*), joint effusion, osteophytosis (*small curved arrow*), joint-space narrowing, loss of lateral compartment articular cartilage, a torn lateral meniscus (*large curved arrow*), subchondral sclerosis and edema (*large straight arrow*), and patellofemoral involvement (**C**). Inflammatory osteoarthritis is seen with synovitis and an irregular fat-pad sign.

fatty marrow contrast of osteochondral fragments is decreased on T2*-weighted, fat-suppressed T2-weighted fast spin-echo and STIR images. In addition to the patellofemoral, medial, and lateral compartment of the knee, the tibiofibular joint may be affected by degenerative arthrosis, ganglia, or trauma (Fig. 7-249).

Broderick and colleagues have compared arthroscopy with fat-suppressed T2-weighted fast spin-echo MR imaging for the evaluation of the severity of articular cartilage abnormalities in osteoarthritis. Their results suggest that this technique can be used to evaluate articular cartilage abnormalities.[278]

In synovial chondromatosis, multiple synovium-based chondral fragments demonstrate low to intermediate signal intensity (Fig. 7-250). In primary chondromatosis, the metaplastic fragments are usually similar to one another in size. In secondary chondromatosis, however, they occur in a variety of sizes. Synovitis in inflammatory osteoarthritis may simulate multiple loose bodies in visualizing the irregular, corrugated fat-pad surfaces.

text continues on page 406

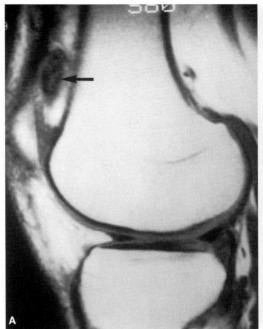
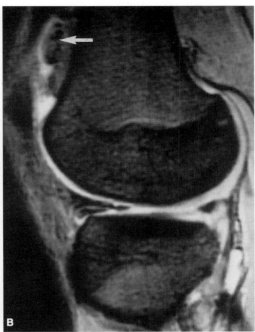

FIGURE 7-248. A low-signal-intensity cartilaginous loose body in the suprapatellar bursa (*arrows*) is revealed on (**A**) T1-weighted and (**B**) T2*-weighted sagittal images. No fatty marrow signal intensity occurs in pure cartilaginous lesions.

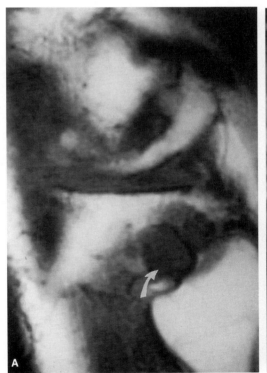
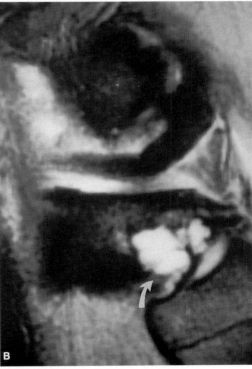

FIGURE 7-249. A degenerative synovial fluid-filled cyst (*curved arrows*) of the superior tibiofibular joint demonstrates (**A**) low signal intensity on a T1-weighted image and (**B**) high signal intensity on a T2*-weighted image. The lateral meniscus is completely absent, and there is associated joint-space narrowing.

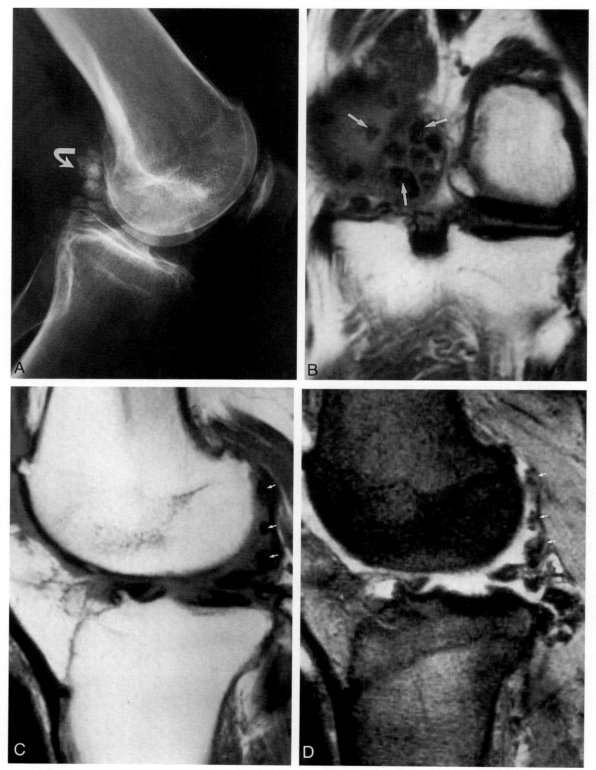

FIGURE 7-250. Synovial chondromatosis. **(A)** A lateral radiograph shows multiple calcified loose bodies (*curved arrow*). **(B)** On a T1-weighted coronal image, osteochondral loose bodies (*arrows*) are seen collecting in the posteromedial joint capsule. **(C and D)** On T1-weighted **(C)** and T2*-weighted **(D)** sagittal images, synovium-based osteochondral fragments (*arrows*) are revealed. The surrounding joint effusion demonstrates bright signal intensity with T2*-weighted contrast.

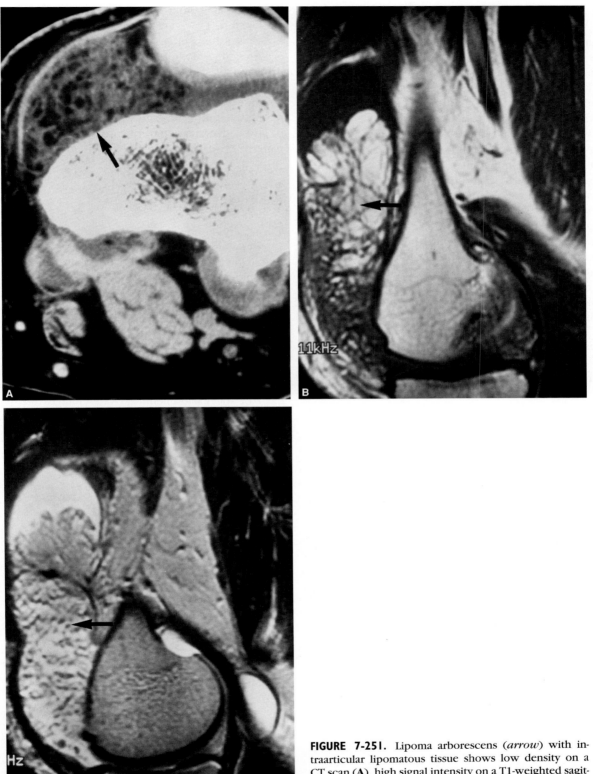

FIGURE 7-251. Lipoma arborescens (*arrow*) with intraarticular lipomatous tissue shows low density on a CT scan (**A**), high signal intensity on a T1-weighted sagittal MR image (**B**), and intermediate signal intensity on a T2-weighted fast spin-echo sagittal MR image (**C**).

Lipoma Arborescens

Lipoma arborescens is a rare intraarticular lesion consisting of villous lipomatous proliferation of the synovium that usually occurs in the knee. Arthroscopically, the lesion has numerous fatty-appearing globules and villous projections.[299] MR demonstrates large frondlike masses originating from the synovium. These intraarticular masses have signal characteristics similar to fat in all pulse sequences (Fig. 7-251).[300] Although joint effusions are common, there is no magnetic susceptibility effect from hemosiderin. MR is useful in differentiating lipoma arborescens from other causes of a chronic swollen and painful joint, including rheumatoid arthritis, PVNS, and synovial chondromatosis.[299] MR of an intraarticular hemangioma may show a susceptibility artifact and be associated with recurrent hemarthrosis. An intraarticular hemangioma may present with either a local or diffuse presentation. The diffuse variety may display a series of vascular channels that are predominantly venous in origin. These channels may result in low signal intensity penetrations within the infrapatellar fat pad.[301]

Joint Effusions

Joint effusions are characterized by low signal intensity on T1-weighted images and bright signal intensity on corresponding conventional T2, fat-suppressed T2-weighted fast spin-echo, gradient-echo T2*, and STIR images. With the knee in 10° of external rotation, the effusion may be more prominent in the lateral compartment of the knee, simulating an artificial ballottement. Fluid preferentially accumulates in the suprapatellar recess and central portions of the joint in the traumatized knee.[302] Layers of postaspiration fat–fluid, fluid–fluid, and air–fluid levels can be demonstrated in suprapatellar fluid collections. When MR imaging is performed after arthrography, contrast material can be seen coating the articular cartilage and extending into the suprapatellar recess. On T2-weighted images, fluid, initially trapped between meniscal surfaces, is seen with a bright-signal-intensity interface that does not interfere with evaluation of the meniscal fibrocartilage. As little as 1 mL of fluid can be detected within the joint on MR scans. A normal knee contains 4 mL or less of synovial fluid.

The MR appearance of an inflammatory effusion is indistinguishable from that of a noninflammatory effusion. On coronal images the distribution of fluid in the medial and lateral gutters extends into the suprapatellar bursa, taking on a saddle-bag appearance. A bland or simple joint effusion (not associated with hemorrhage or synovitis) does not result in an irregular free edge contour of Hoffa's fat pad. Hemorrhagic synovial fluid is associated with an irregular fat pad and may demonstrate a serum–sediment level in subacute hemorrhagic effusions. A fat–serum–sediment level in lipo-

hemarthrosis is often associated with severe bone contusion and fracture. Low-signal-intensity artifacts may be seen after knee aspirations or secondary to MR arthrography.

An arthrographic effect can be produced by intraarticular diffusion of gadolinium after intravenous injection.[120] Increased signal intensity can be seen within 10 minutes of contrast administration and immobilization of the knee, and it peaks within 30 minutes. This technique can be used to improve identification of meniscal surfaces and various tear patterns.

Popliteal Cysts

Classically, popliteal (Baker's) cysts of the gastrocnemius–semimembranosus bursae arise between the medial head of the gastrocnemius muscle and the more medial semimembranosus tendon (Fig. 7-252).[303,304] These cysts demonstrate low signal intensity on T1-weighted images and uniformly increased signal intensity on T2-weighted images, including fat-suppressed T2-weighted fast spin-echo. Septations that divide the cysts into compartments may also be seen, usually in atypical locations. A narrow neck connecting the cyst to the joint is usually identified on axial images, and is usually found just below the proximal attachment site of the medial head of the gastrocnemius. Axial images are particularly useful in identifying the relation of the medial head of the gastrocnemius muscle, semitendinosus, and semimembrano-

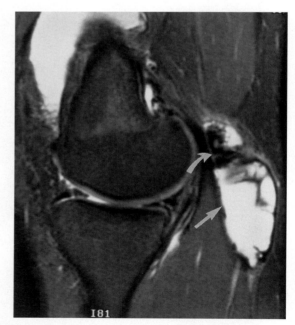

FIGURE 7-252. A fat-suppressed T2-weighted fast spin-echo sagittal image of a popliteal cyst adjacent to the medial head of the gastrocnemius muscle. This cyst is hyperintense (*straight arrow*) except for the low signal intensity foci of hemosiderin (*curved arrow*) resulting from PVNS.

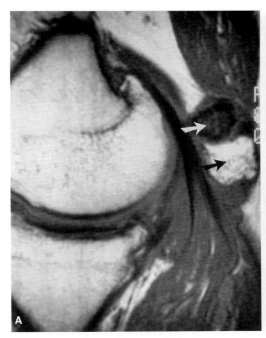
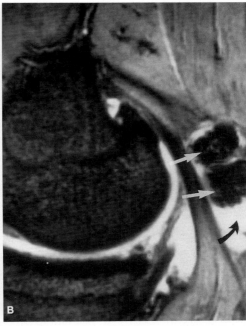

FIGURE 7-253. A popliteal cyst. (**A**) A T1-weighted sagittal image reveals a low signal intensity sclerotic loose body (*white arrow*) and a high signal intensity loose body (*black arrow*) that contains fatty marrow. (**B**) Fat contrast is lost on a T2*-weighted sagittal image. *Straight white arrows*, loose bodies; *curved black arrow*, popliteal cyst.

sus tendons. Popliteal cysts may arise from any condition that causes an increase in synovial fluid within the joint and are frequently seen in association with tears of the posterior horn of the medial meniscus. Intraarticular communication and associated pathology may be seen on contiguous sagittal images. Hemorrhagic joint effusions may also be observed, with a fluid–fluid level in the cyst, and loose bodies may collect in a posterior popliteal cyst (Fig. 7-253). A dissecting or ruptured popliteal cyst with subacute hemorrhage demonstrates increased signal intensity on T1- and T2-weighted images because of the presence of blood. This blood, however, creates areas of inhomogeneity that may generate intermediate signal intensity. Susceptibility artifact is shown as areas of low signal intensity in subacute and chronic hemorrhage on gradient-echo images.

Atypical locations for other cysts include the tibiofibular joint and the bursa between the lateral head of the gastrocnemius muscle and biceps femoris. These cysts may also present as soft-tissue masses proximal and distal to the popliteal fossa. In very young children, popliteal cysts may occur as a primary disorder in the absence of concurrent intraarticular pathology.[305] Cysts are frequently seen in patients with JRA or adult rheumatoid arthritis. With MR evaluation, a cyst can be differentiated from a popliteal artery aneurysm (Fig. 7-254) or venous malformation (Fig. 7-255), which may have a similar clinical appearance. MR imaging also offers the advantage of evaluating both popliteal and intraarticular pathology, areas of limited diagnostic accuracy with ultra-

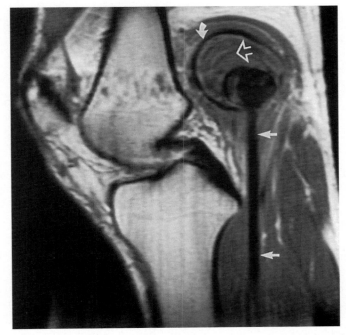

FIGURE 7-254. A T1-weighted sagittal image displays an enlarged aneurysm of the popliteal artery. The normal low-signal-intensity popliteal artery (*solid arrows*), an intermediate signal intensity thrombus (*open arrow*), and a low signal intensity peripheral rim of calcification (*curved arrow*) are identified.

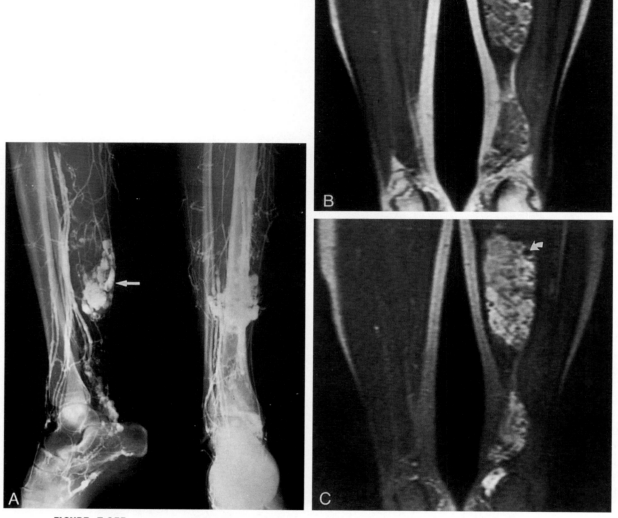

FIGURE 7-255. Venous malformation. **(A)** A venous angiogram shows a serpiginous tangle of vessels (*arrow*). T1-weighted **(B)** and T2-weighted **(C)** coronal images demonstrate inhomogeneity, with generalized increased signal intensity seen on the T2-weighted sequence **(C)**. Low-signal-intensity foci represent vessels with faster-flowing blood (*curved arrows*).

sound or conventional radiography. We have used intravenous gadolinium-DTPA to show lack of enhancement in popliteal cysts with poorly defined margins (Fig. 7-256). Frequently, a popliteal cyst may show peripheral or wall enhancement, which is a normal finding. Rarely, intraarticular gadolinium-DTPA or conventional arthrography is required to document communication with a joint. Treating the underlying joint pathology usually results in disappearance of the cyst. If a suspected soft-tissue mass shows central

or irregular gadolinium enhancement, the differential diagnosis must include soft-tissue neoplasms (eg, synovial sarcoma).

In contrast to popliteal cysts, ganglion cysts are viscous synovium-filled masses with hyaluronic acid– and mucopolysaccharide-rich contents.[306] These cysts may be intraarticular or extraarticular in location (joint capsule, pes anserinus tendons, and Hoffa's fat pad). There is usually a connection or stalk traceable to the joint. Septations are common

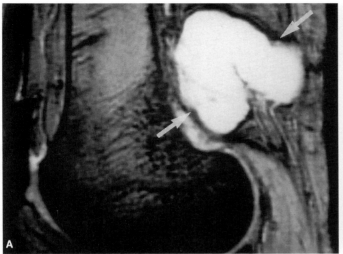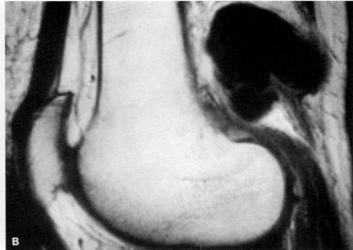

FIGURE 7-256. (A) An atypical lateral popliteal cyst (*arrow*) is hyperintense on a T2*-weighted sagittal image. (B) Lack of enhancement with intravenous administration of gadolinium on a T1-weighted sagittal image is characteristic of cystic fluid collections, not primary soft-tissue masses.

within ganglia. Unless associated with hemorrhage, ganglion cysts are low signal intensity on T1-weighted images, and hyperintense on T2-weighted images.

Plicae

Synovial plicae are one of several conditions in the differential diagnosis of anterior knee pain.[307] Plica syndrome may include anterior knee pain, clicking, catching, or locking of the knee. Synovial plicae are embryologic remnants of the septal division of the knee into three compartments.[307–309] Common plicae are suprapatellar (Fig. 7-257), medial patellar (Fig. 7-258), or infrapatellar (see Fig. 7-257), and they may be present as a large shelf in slightly fewer than 20% of knees. A medial patellar plica may be found as a normal variant in up to 60% of adult knees. Medial patellar and infrapatellar plicae are best seen on axial images, whereas the suprapatellar plica is seen on sagittal images, traversing the suprapatellar bursa. The infrapatellar plica (see Fig. 7-257) is best visualized on sagittal images anterior and parallel to the ACL. The incomplete infrapatellar plica, or ligamentum mucosum, is the most frequently occurring of the plicae, and can be confused with the ACL on arthrography. Compared with suprapatellar and medial plicae, it is probably the least well visualized. Plica tissue is seen with low signal intensity on all pulse sequences. In patients with a suprapatellar soft-tissue mass, MR studies may reveal the presence of a persistent plica dividing the suprapatellar bursa into two separate compartments containing hemorrhagic synovial fluid and debris (Fig. 7-259). There are several types of suprapatellar plicae, including a superomedial and superolateral type. A suprapatellar plica can also exist as a cord or membrane (with or without a perforation).

An inflamed medial patellar plica thickens and may interfere with normal quadriceps function and patellofemoral articulation. Erosion or abrasion of femoral condylar or patellar articular cartilage can occur as the plica loses its flexibility and gliding motion (see Fig. 7-258). On axial MR images, an abnormal medial patellar plica may be seen as a thickened band of low signal intensity with underlying

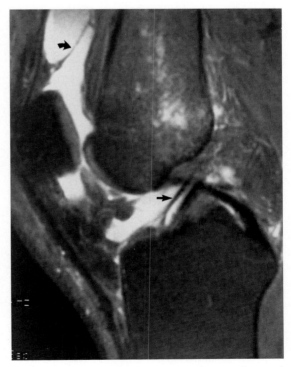

FIGURE 7-257. An infrapatellar plica (*straight arrow*), anterior and parallel to the ACL, and a suprapatellar plica (*curved arrow*) are seen on a fat-suppressed T2-weighted fast spin-echo sagittal image.

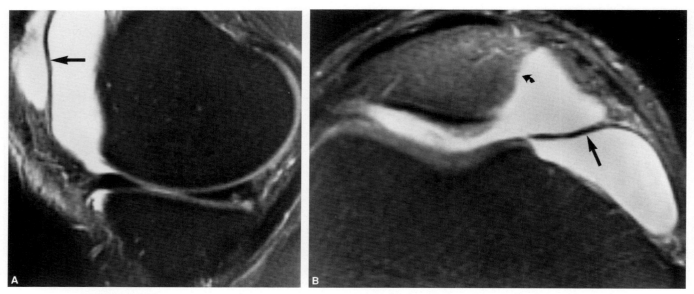

FIGURE 7-258. A thickened medial patellar plica (*straight arrow*) on fat-suppressed T2-weighted fast spin-echo (**A**) sagittal and (**B**) axial images. There is associated degeneration with loss of medial facet articular cartilage (*curved arrows*).

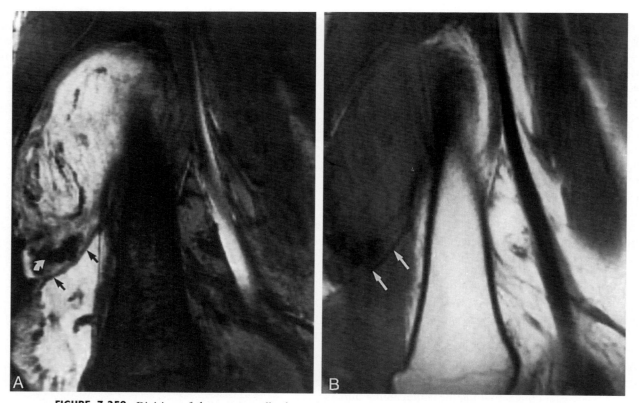

FIGURE 7-259. Division of the suprapatellar bursa into two compartments with an intact suprapatellar plica is seen as a low signal intensity band (*solid arrows*) on (**A**) T2*-weighted and (**B**) T1-weighted sagittal images. On the T2*-weighted sequence (**A**), low signal intensity hemosiderin deposits (*curved arrow*) contrast with the surrounding bright signal intensity hemorrhagic fluid.

irregularity of the medial patellar facet cartilage surface. Sagittal images through the medial compartment of the knee show the longitudinal orientation of the medial plica extending toward Hoffa's infrapatellar fat pad, anterior to the anterior horn of the medial meniscus. Although plical thickness is not measured quantitatively, fibrotic hypertrophy secondary to chronic irritation can be identified, and is considered symptomatic when impingement on the medial femoral condyle in knee flexion is present.

Osteonecrosis and Related Disorders

Spontaneous Osteonecrosis

Osteonecrosis can occur spontaneously or in association with medical conditions including steroid use, renal transplantation, alcoholism, hemoglobinopathies, Gaucher's disease, Caisson's decompression sickness, and systemic lupus erythematosus.[310] Steroid-induced osteonecrotic lesions tend to be larger than those seen in spontaneous osteonecrosis, possibly because of the frequent development of a bone infarct pattern in steroid-related osteonecrosis. Spontaneous (idiopathic) osteonecrosis of the knee typically affects older, predominantly female, patients who present with acute medial joint pain.[50,311,312] Spontaneous osteonecrosis often involves the weight-bearing surface of the medial femoral condyle (Fig. 7-260), however, the medial and lateral tibial

plateaus and the lateral femoral condyle may also be affected.[313] In tibial involvement, the weight-bearing surface may or may not be affected (Fig. 7-261). The entity of osteonecrosis of the tibial plateau is similar to that described for osteonecrosis of the femoral condyle. Meniscal tears are often associated with spontaneous osteonecrosis. The differential diagnosis of osteonecrosis includes osteochondritis dissecans, osteoarthritis, meniscal tears, stress fractures and pes anserinus bursitis.

Conventional radiographs are not sensitive in evaluating an osteonecrotic focus before the development of sclerosis and osseous collapse. Radiographic classification of the necrotic lesion consists of five stages.[13,314] Stage 1 radiographs are normal. Stage 2 shows mild flattening of the weight-bearing aspect of the femoral condyle. Stage 3 demonstrates an area of radiolucency with sclerosis distal to the lesion. In stage 4, there is a radiolucent area surrounded by a sclerotic halo. Collapsed subchondral bone is visible as a calcified plate. Stage 5 has secondary degenerative changes and erosions with subchondral sclerosis of both the femur and tibia. The two theories of pathogenesis of osteonecrosis include vascular and traumatic etiologies.[314] In the vascular model, there is interruption of the microcirculation of the femoral condyle resulting in edema. Increased interosseous pressure further impairs the vascular supply to subchondral bone leading to ischemic necrosis. Revascularization with new vessel ingrowth may weaken remaining bone architec-

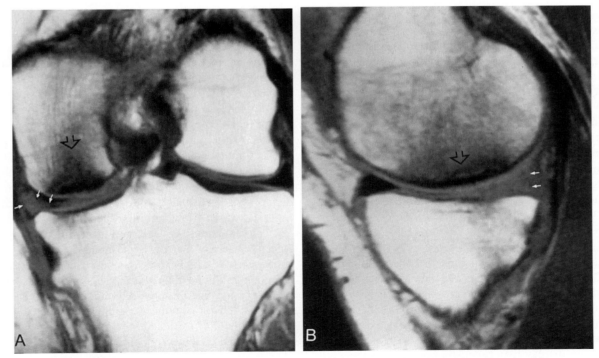

FIGURE 7-260. Spontaneous osteonecrosis of the medial femoral condyle demonstrates low signal intensity (*open arrows*) on T1-weighted (**A**) coronal and (**B**) sagittal images. The posterior horn of the medial meniscus is macerated and torn (*white arrows*).

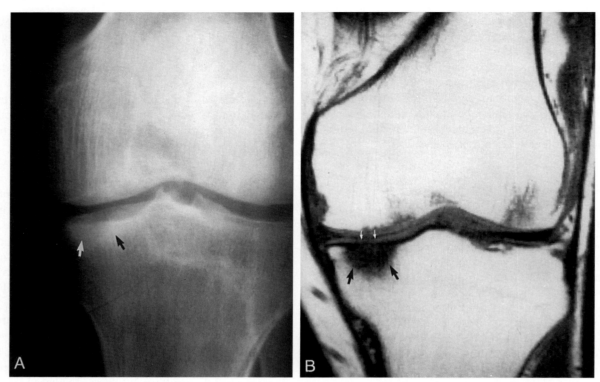

FIGURE 7-261. (A) On an anteroposterior radiograph, a sclerotic focus in the medial tibial plateau (*arrows*) indicates osteonecrosis. (B) On a T1-weighted coronal image, a well-defined region of subchondral low signal intensity is seen in the medial tibial plateau (*black arrows*). Thinning of overlying hyaline articular cartilage (*white arrows*) also is observed.

ture causing subchondral collapse and articular destruction. If revascularization is successful, however, it does not lead to collapse of the healing necrotic segment. In the trauma model, there is microfracture through osteoporotic subchondral bone. The secondary reflux of synovial fluid through damaged articular cartilage contributes to increased interosseous pressure and resultant compromise of the vascular supply to the subchondral bone. The clinical history of osteonecrosis frequently includes intense pain for 2 to 3 months with pain dissipating by 12 to 15 months. Subsequent problems are related to the development of osteoarthritis. Lesions comprising an area of greater than 50% of the condyle and measuring 5 cm or greater in diameter are classified as large and frequently progress to radiographic collapse. Small lesions (<3.5 cm in diameter or <50% of the involved condyle) may show resolution with time and have minimal radiographic sequelae.

Several patterns of spontaneous osteonecrosis can be seen on MR images. Sometimes the osteonecrotic focus is associated with adjacent bone marrow edema (Fig. 7-262), similar to that seen in transient osteoporosis of the hip. In this pattern, the necrotic focus is low signal intensity on T1- and T2-weighted images. The adjacent subchondral bone, however, may display hyperintensity on T2, fat-suppressed T2-weighted fast spin-echo, or STIR images. T2*-weighted images are less sensitive to this associated marrow edema

or hyperemia. In addition, subchondral sclerosis may be masked on T2*-weighted images. When seen, the area of adjacent marrow edema should not be used as a measure of the size of the necrotic lesion.

The marrow changes described may reflect increased interosseous pressure and early attempts at revascularization, because follow-up examinations show resolution of the marrow hyperemic pattern and a residual sharply defined necrotic focus. The necrotic focus involves the weight-bearing surface of the femoral condyle, and may involve both condyles simultaneously. The discrete morphology of the low signal intensity necrotic focus and localization to the medial femoral condyle help distinguish this pattern of osteonecrosis from that caused by traumatic trabecular bone injuries, which show a similar medullary hyperintensity on T2, fat-suppressed T2-weighted fast spin-echo, or STIR images. The area of marrow hyperintensity seen in spontaneous osteonecrosis can be much greater and deeper within the subchondral bone than would be typically expected in a region of localized trauma affecting the femoral condyle.

The focus of osteonecrosis may be detected on MR images without any associated marrow changes. In early stages of the disease, a necrotic focus itself may display some degree of hyperintensity on heavily weighted T2, fat-suppressed T2-weighted fast spin-echo, or STIR images. Even in patients with negative findings on radiographs, low signal

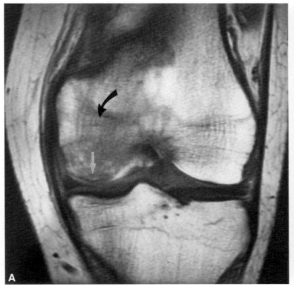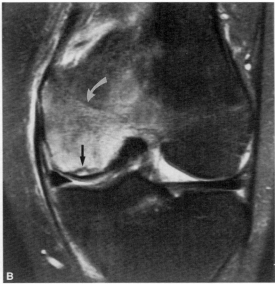

FIGURE 7-262. T1-weighted (**A**) and fat-suppressed T2-weighted fast spin-echo (**B**) coronal images exhibit a hypointense focus of osteonecrosis (*straight arrow*) associated with a larger area of reactive marrow edema (*curved arrow*) of the medial femoral condyle. In the early stages of osteonecrosis, this pattern of bone marrow edema correlates with increased pain and is hyperintense on fat-suppressed T2-weighted fast spin-echo or STIR images. Subchondral drilling may be performed in patients with symptoms at this stage. The bone marrow edema resolves in less than 1 year, leaving behind the residual necrotic focus.

intensity changes can be detected within the area of osteonecrosis on T1- and T2-weighted MR images. The overlying articular cartilage and status of the meniscal cartilage can also be evaluated on T1- and T2-weighted images. We have documented osteonecrosis in both the medial and lateral tibial plateaus with MR imaging. In one patient with JRA, osteonecrosis on the tibial plateau was observed on MR images and confirmed by biopsy. There have been several case reports of osteonecrosis occurring after arthroscopic reconstruction of the cruciate ligament and after laser-assisted arthroscopic surgery.[299,301] Changes of osteonecrosis have also been reported after arthroscopic medial meniscectomy.

Initial treatment of spontaneous osteonecrosis is conservative and includes protected weight-bearing.[313,314] Advanced stages of osteonecrosis may require surgical intervention, including arthroscopic debridement, core decompression, high tibial osteotomy, drilling with or without bone grafting, osteochondral allografts, unicompartmental arthroplasty, and total knee replacement.

Bone infarcts, in contrast to spontaneous osteonecrosis, are usually metaphyseal in location, but are also found in epiphyseal and diaphyseal locations (Fig. 7-263). The MR appearance of a bone infarct is characteristic, with a serpiginous low-signal-intensity border of reactive bone and a central component of high-signal-intensity yellow or fat marrow. On T2-weighted images, a chemical-shift artifact may be seen as a high-signal-intensity line paralleling the outline of the infarct. Fibroblastic reactive tissue, however, at the healing interface of the infarct will demonstrate hyperinten-

sity on heavily T2-weighted, fat-suppressed T2-weighted fast spin-echo and STIR images (Fig. 7-264). Epiphyseal infarcts or infarcts abutting the subchondral surface may weaken the subchondral plate resulting in microfractures and articular surface collapse. Bone infarcts can be differentiated from enchondromas on MR images. The latter lack a serpiginous border and on T1-weighted images have a central region of low signal intensity that increases with progressive T2 weighting. Calcified bone infarcts, however, demonstrate low signal intensity on T1- and T2-weighted images. Bone infarcts may be seen in association with steroid therapy when part of a chemotherapy protocol (Fig. 7-265). Bone infarcts may also demonstrate areas of mild contrast enhancement with intravenous gadolinium administration.

Osteochondritis Dissecans

Osteochondritis dissecans differs from spontaneous osteonecrosis of the knee in that it primarily affects male patients (10 to 20 years of age) and typically involves the lateral surface of the medial femoral condyle.[315–317] Osteochondritis dissecans represents an osteochondrosis characterized by necrosis of bone followed by reossification and healing.[272] A history of knee trauma is found in as many as 50% of patients. In older patients, the morphology and location of osteochondritis dissecans may overlap with the spectrum of MR findings seen in spontaneous osteonecrosis. An ischemic event has also been proposed as the cause. Granulation tissue advances into the region between the necrotic fragment and the healing bone, and the articular cartilage (the only re-

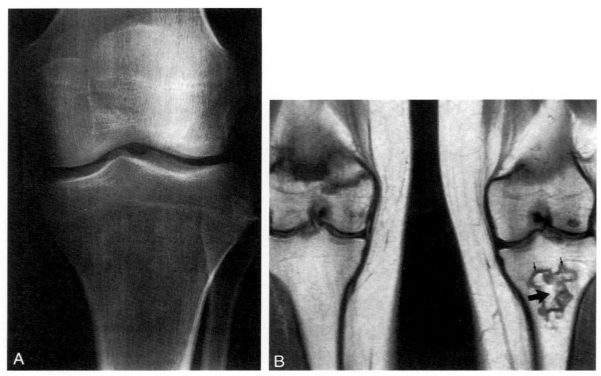

FIGURE 7-263. A bone infarct that is not seen on an anteroposterior radiograph (**A**) is revealed on a T1-weighted coronal image (**B**) with characteristic serpiginous low signal intensity peripheral sclerosis (*small arrows*) and a high signal intensity central portion (*large arrows*).

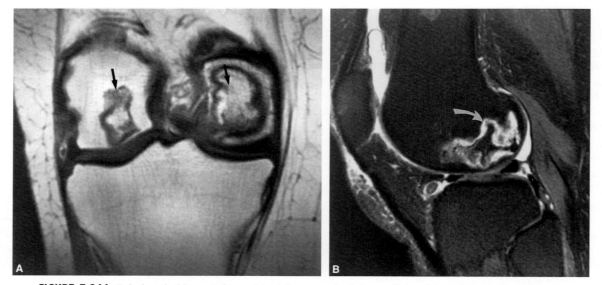

FIGURE 7-264. Subchondral bone infarcts (*straight arrows*) of the medial and lateral femoral condyle on (**A**) T1-weighted coronal image and (**B**) fat-suppressed T2-weighted fast spin-echo sagittal images. The infarcts display central fatty marrow signal characteristics and are associated with a peripheral rim (*curved arrow*) of reactive tissue (hypointense on T1-weighted images and hyperintense on T2-weighted images) that is involved in the process of gradual substitution. New bone is found at the circumference of the infarct.

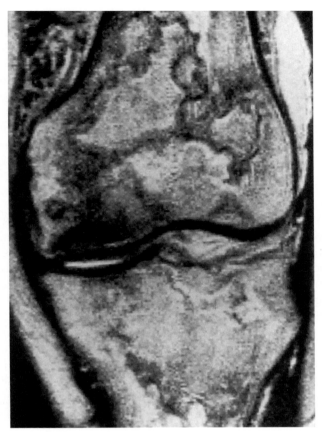

FIGURE 7-265. Multiple bone infarcts seen during steroid therapy in a patient with leukemia.

maining support for the necrotic bone) may fail and there may be detachment or fragmentation of articular cartilage into the joint. Classically, lesions are located in the lateral aspect of the medial femoral condyle (55%). Less commonly, lesions involve a central portion of the medial femoral condyle (25%). Osteochondritis dissecans may also affect the lateral femoral condyle (18%), or it may occur bilaterally (24%). An association between osteochondritis dissecans of the lateral femoral condyle and discoid lateral meniscus has been noted.

A staging system for osteochondritis was developed based on arthroscopic findings. In stage 1, the lesion is 1 to 3 cm and the articular cartilage is intact. Stage 2 is characterized by an articular cartilage defect without a loose body. In stage 3, a partially detached osteochondral fragment, with or without fibrous-tissue interposition, is found. Stage 4 demonstrates a loose body with a crater filled with fibrous tissue.[43,316]

On MR imaging, the focus of osteochondritis demonstrates low signal intensity on T1- and T2-weighted images before it can be detected on conventional radiographs. Overlying defects in the articular cartilage are best appreciated on fat-suppressed T2-weighted fast spin-echo or STIR images, where fluid is brighter than adjacent articular cartilage (Fig. 7-266). These techniques are also sensitive to subchondral bone changes, which may demonstrate areas of signal inhomogeneity, and to the direct extension of subchondral fluid. MR imaging is particularly

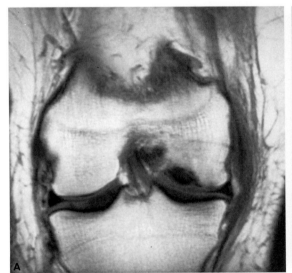
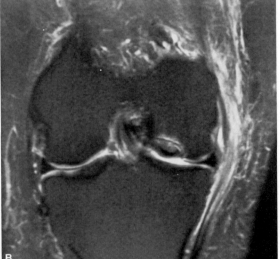

FIGURE 7-266. An osteochondral fragment in osteochondritis dissecans of the medial femoral condyle is seen on (**A**) T1-weighted coronal images and (**B**) fat-suppressed T2-weighted fast spin-echo coronal images.

continued

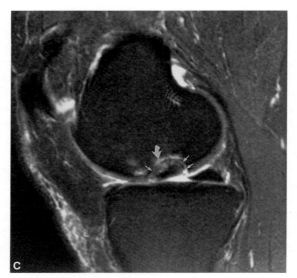

FIGURE 7-266. *Continued.* (**C**) Fat-suppressed T2 fast spin-echo sagittal images. Note the high signal intensity fluid interface (*straight arrow*) that undermines involved subchondral bone on the fat-suppressed T2-weighted fast spin-echo image. There is also increased signal intensity in both the adjacent medullary bone and fragment marrow at the fragment–donor interface (*curved arrow*).

valuable in demonstrating associated free and loose osteochondral and chondral fragments. Imbibed high-signal-intensity subchondral fluid implies fissuring of the overlying articular cartilage and has a high correlation with lesion instability, especially when this fluid circles the entire fragment in its circumference.[318] Focal cystic regions deep to the lesion are also associated with instability of the fragment. Fluid in the base of the necrotic lesion without a direct communication with the joint usually implies an abnormal overlying articular cartilage surface, which may or may not allow the extension of intraarticular injected contrast or saline across the articular cartilage surface. Hyperintensity between the lesion and adjacent bone may be visualized on T2 (including fast spin-echo and STIR) images and represents either fluid or granulation tissue. Lesion stability is related to the absence of increased signal intensity at the fragment interface on T2-weighted images. Intravenous gadolinium enhancement of granulation tissue between the necrotic fragment and parent bone also correlates with fragment loosening and instability.[287] MR arthrography with intraarticular gadolinium contrast may improve visualization of fluid across the articular cartilage surface, especially when compared with T1-weighted or T2*-weighted images.[274] Healed lesions do

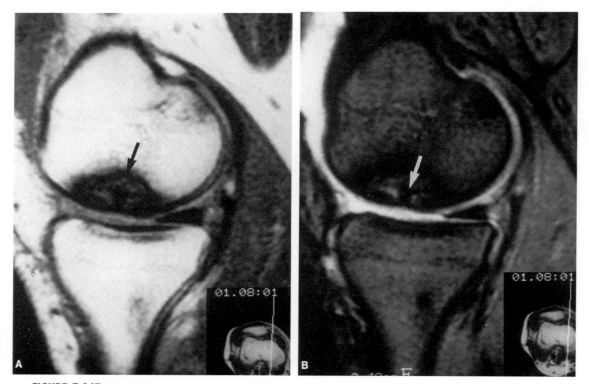

FIGURE 7-267. Medial femoral condylar osteochondritis dissecans (*arrows*) demonstrates (**A**) a low-signal-intensity focus on a T1-weighted sagittal image and (**B**) increased signal intensity in areas of subchondral bone on a T2*-weighted sagittal image.

continued

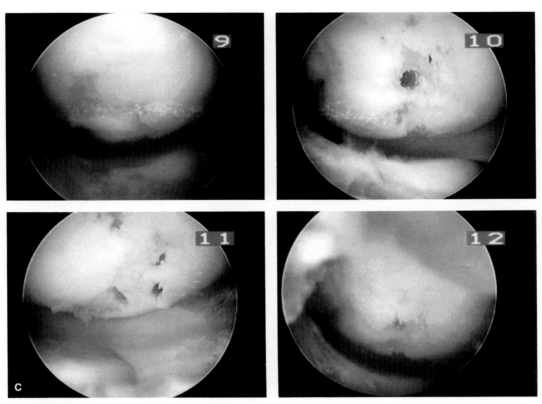

FIGURE 7-267. *Continued.* (C) This finding, in association with attenuated overlying articular cartilage, is confirmed on the corresponding arthroscopic photograph before (*frame 9*) and after (*frames 10* through *12*) arthroscopic drilling.

not demonstrate a bright-signal-intensity interface between the fragment and adjacent bone of the femoral condyle and do show the return of marrow fat signal intensity in the previously necrotic fragment. The overlying articular cartilage surface is intact without any residual contour irregularities. The location of the necrotic lesion, in either the medial or lateral femoral condylar locations or in the tibia, can be detected on MR images.

MR is also particularly useful for identifying posterocondylar lesions in children. Although it is unusual to see an extensive marrow reaction, as seen in adult spontaneous osteonecrosis, T2 or STIR imaging techniques may reveal adjacent hyperintensity of medullary bone in unstable lesions. Treatment choices in young patients range from nonoperative treatment to arthroscopic drilling of the osteochondral fragment when there is a stable intact lesion. Drilling may also be used along with internal fixation with screws or autogenous bone pegs in skeletally mature patients (Fig. 7-267). Cancellous grooves are used for internal fixation of fragments in more skeletally mature patients when fragment healing is more difficult to achieve. Loose osteochondral fragments are removed, and partially detached fragments are treated with debridement before reduction and stabilization.[272]

Fractures

Osteochondral Fractures

Osteochondral fractures (Fig. 7-268) involve trauma to the articular cartilage and underlying bone, whereas chondral fractures (Fig. 7-269) are restricted to injury of the articular cartilage alone. Osteochondral fractures are associated with trauma, including direct injury, ligament ruptures, and patellar dislocations. Indirect trauma can provide enough shearing force to fracture or avulse both articular cartilage and subchondral bone (eg, pivoting in knee extension). Osteochondral fractures of the weight-bearing condylar surfaces are associated with rotatory forces in knee flexion (eg, football and skiing injuries). A fall on the flexed knee can produce a direct shearing force on the anteromedial femoral condyle, and a kick or blow to the outside of the knee produces a direct lateral condylar shearing force. In adults, the articular cartilage is thought to tear at the junction between the calcified and uncalcified zones. In immature skeletons, where there is no calcified zone, shearing forces are transmitted directly to subchondral bone producing an osteochondral fracture. Osteochondral fractures are most commonly seen in adolescents and are thought to represent a form of osteochondritis dissecans.[319]

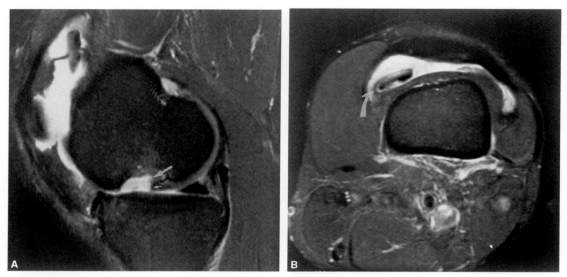

FIGURE 7-268. (A) A fat-suppressed T2-weighted fast spin-echo sagittal image shows an osteochondral fracture with involvement of both articular cartilage (*small arrow*) and subchondral bone (*large arrow*). (B) A corresponding fat-suppressed T2-weighted fast spin-echo axial image identifies the free osteochondral fragment within the suprapatellar bursa (*curved arrow*).

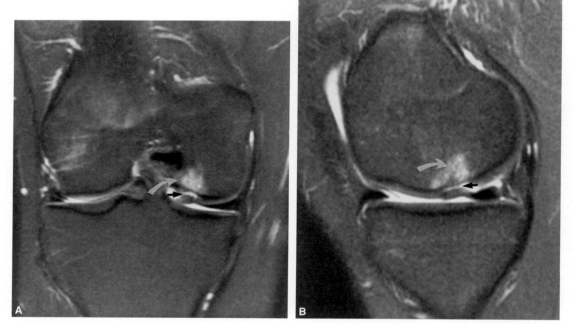

FIGURE 7-269. A chondral fracture shown on fat-suppressed T2-weighted fast spin-echo (A) coronal and (B) sagittal images. Hyperintense joint fluid (*straight arrow*) undermines the intermediate signal intensity flap of medial femoral condyle articular cartilage. Subchondral marrow edema (*curved arrow*) is present without an associated osseous fracture.

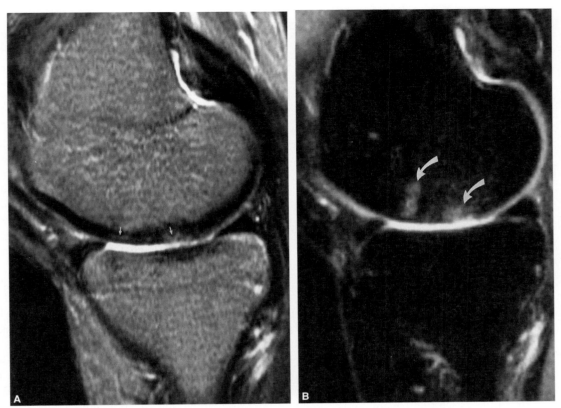

FIGURE 7-270. Application of the microfracture technique, in which a pick instrument is used to promote vascularity across the subchondral plate, is documented on (**A**) a sagittal STIR image and (**B**) a fast spin-echo version of an echo-planar imaging (EPI) image. The microfracture technique is used to create a neofibrocartilaginous surface to replace the damaged hyaline articular cartilage. The EPI image exaggerates the thickness of the subchondral plate as a result of a chemical shift artifact and allows identification of vascular areas (*straight arrows*) as distinguished from the reactive subchondral marrow edema (*curved arrow*) seen on the STIR image.

As seen in the evaluation of osteochondritis dissecans, MR is used to evaluate the integrity of articular cartilage surfaces and subchondral bone in patients with osteochondral fractures. The osteochondral fracture may parallel the joint surface and subsequently violate the integrity of the overlying articular cartilage or it may present as a periarticular osseous fracture that extends and crosses perpendicular to the articular cartilage. High signal intensity fluid is frequently identified underlying the fracture segment. Cartilage or fibrous tissue of intermediate signal intensity may be seen securing more chronic fragments. Reparative granulation tissue may be visualized in empty craters.[8] Fat-suppressed T2-weighted fast spin-echo and STIR images are most sensitive to the fracture extension across the articular cartilage surface and associated marrow edema within the fracture fragments. The size and morphology of the lesion can accurately be assessed. Absence of hyperintensity of the fragment in the junctional zone is associated with fragment stability. High signal intensity fluid surrounding the fragment indicates instability and loosening. In chondral injuries, debridement and drilled (eg, microfracture technique) have been used to

generate a congruous fibrocartilaginous healing surface (Fig. 7-270). Osteoarticular allografts are used to treat joint surface defects secondary to trauma. MR assesses the articular cartilage surface, graft interface, and complications including failure of graft incorporation and osteonecrosis (Fig. 7-271).

Osseous Fractures and Bone Contusions

Fractures about the knee can involve the femoral condyle, the tibial plateau, or the patella.[234] Tibial plateau fractures are the most common, and predominantly occur with lateral plateau involvement (Fig. 7-272).[320] The most common mechanism of injury is impaction of the anterior portion of the lateral femoral condyle in a valgus mechanism of injury. Axial loading, or pure compressive force, produces an impaction or compression fracture of the plateau, whereas a pure valgus force results in a split condylar fracture. A valgus compressive force is responsible for the frequent occurrence of lateral tibial condylar plateau fractures with tears of the medial meniscus, ACL, and MCL. Fractures of the

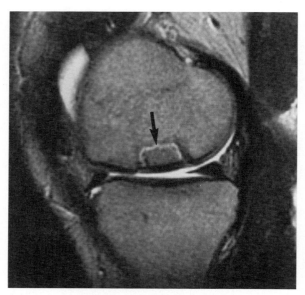

FIGURE 7-271. Medial femoral condyle osteochondral allograft. Although hyperintensity is identified at the graft interface (*arrow*), fluid did not violate the articular surface. However, this allograft eventually failed and was complicated by the development of medial femoral condyle osteonecrosis.

knee can be identified on MR scans in patients with acute or chronic knee pain and negative findings on conventional radiographs. MR imaging is also equivalent or superior to 2D CT reconstruction for displaying fracture morphology.[321] Subsequent plain-film radiography often shows areas of sclerosis or periosteal reaction at the fracture site that was initially identified on MR images. The most common MR pattern seen in fractures is sharp, well-defined, linear segments of decreased signal intensity in the distal femur or proximal tibia.

In an acute fracture, associated fluid or hemorrhage demonstrates increased signal intensity on conventional T2, fat-suppressed T2-weighted fast spin-echo, and STIR images. Gradient-echo T2 contrast images may also demonstrate hyperintensity in acute fractures. Fractures with diffuse areas of associated low signal intensity on T2-weighted images demonstrate increased signal intensity with long TR and TE settings. This reflects the prolonged T2 values in edematous or hemorrhagic marrow. STIR images are more sensitive than gradient-echo T2*-weighted images and conventional T2-weighted images in identifying subacute fractures with associated marrow edema. T2*-weighted contrast, however, may be useful in displaying acute fracture morphology when extensive marrow hemorrhage obscures detail on T1-weighted or STIR images (Fig. 7-273). Chronic fractures remain low in signal intensity, with variable TR and TE parameters.

In animal models, posttraumatic growth-plate abnormalities, including changes in cartilage, transphyseal vascularity, and bone bridge formation, can be detected with MR imaging.[322,323] The metaphyseal–diaphyseal junction in the physis should not be mistaken for a transverse linear fracture.[324] Discontinuity of the physis may occur with trauma or epiphysiodesis (Fig. 7-274).[325] In the adult, the physeal line or scar does not demonstrate increased signal intensity on T2-weighted images. In a child, a chemical-shift artifact may display bright signal intensity parallel with the physis.

MR imaging is also used to differentiate stress fractures, common in the proximal tibia, from neoplastic processes (Fig. 7-275). The linear segment of the stress fracture in the knee is usually accompanied by marrow edema. The lack of a soft-tissue mass, cortical destruction, and characteristic marrow extension effectively excludes a tumor from the differential diagnosis. Rarely, a stress fracture is obscured on

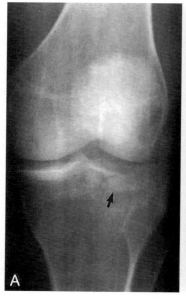
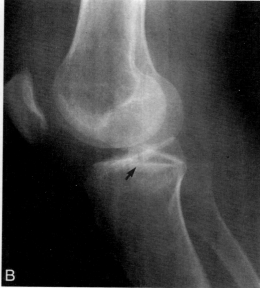

FIGURE 7-272. **(A)** Anteroposterior and **(B)** lateral radiographs demonstrating disruption (*arrows*) of the lateral tibial plateau. *continued*

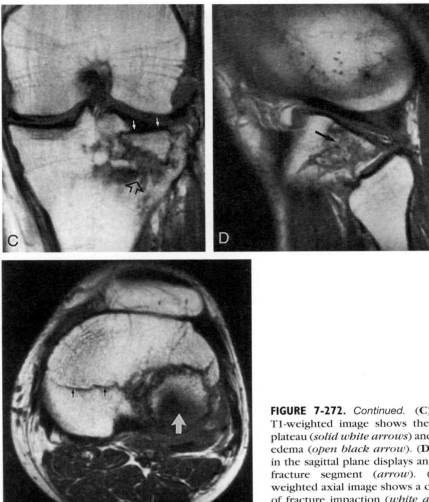

FIGURE 7-272. *Continued.* **(C)** A coronal T1-weighted image shows the depressed plateau (*solid white arrows*) and associated edema (*open black arrow*). **(D)** An image in the sagittal plane displays an edematous fracture segment (*arrow*). **(E)** A T1-weighted axial image shows a circular area of fracture impaction (*white arrow*) with radiating linear fracture extension (*black arrows*).

MR images by reactive edema, and high-resolution and thin-section CT is required to identify it.

A diffuse or localized pattern of low signal intensity on T1-weighted images without a defined fracture is seen with bone bruises or contusions at sites of microtrauma or impaction of trabecular bone.[326] Recognition of occult subcortical fractures is important because osteochondral sequelae with significant cartilage damage may develop.[327] In an acute or subacute setting, increased signal intensity is seen on T2, fat-suppressed T2-weighted fast spin-echo, or STIR images, before the appearance of sclerosis on plain-film radiographs (Fig. 7-276).[328] Normal metaphyseal–diaphyseal low-signal-intensity red marrow inhomogeneity should not be mistaken for a contusion. This marrow pattern is frequently seen in female patients and should not cross the physeal scar into subchondral bone. STIR images or heavily T2-weighted images (>3000 millisecond for conventional T2 and >5000 millisecond for fat-suppressed T2-

weighted fast spin-echo images) may demonstrate varying degrees of increased signal intensity. The morphology of bone contusions has been characterized into three types based on T1- or intermediate-weighted images.[329] In type I lesions, findings included a diffuse decrease in signal intensity in metaphyseal and epiphyseal areas (Fig. 7-277). In type II lesions, injury interruption of the low-signal-intensity cortical line is found (Fig. 7-278). In type III, a localized decrease in signal intensity in subchondral bone is seen (Fig. 7-279). Type I and II lesions are difficult to detect on radiography and arthroscopy, and are frequently associated with tears of the ACL and contralateral collateral ligament. A pathologic fracture may be complicated by internal hemorrhage that obscures the underlying lesion.

Hohl has classified tibial plateau fractures as minimally displaced (ie, <4 mm of depression or displacement) or

text continues on page 429

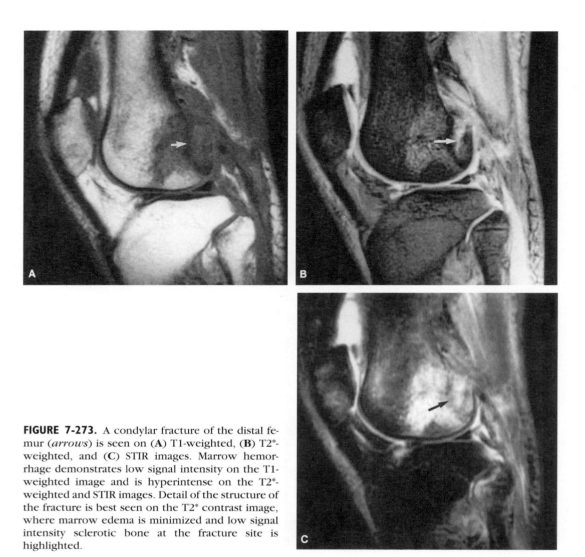

FIGURE 7-273. A condylar fracture of the distal femur (*arrows*) is seen on (**A**) T1-weighted, (**B**) T2*-weighted, and (**C**) STIR images. Marrow hemorrhage demonstrates low signal intensity on the T1-weighted image and is hyperintense on the T2*-weighted and STIR images. Detail of the structure of the fracture is best seen on the T2* contrast image, where marrow edema is minimized and low signal intensity sclerotic bone at the fracture site is highlighted.

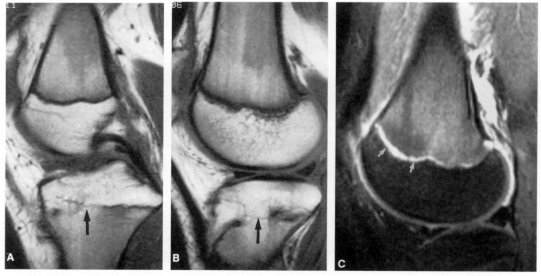

FIGURE 7-274. Epiphysiodesis is used to treat leg-length inequality. Interruption (*arrows*) of the normal low signal intensity physeal plates in the (**A**) medial and (**B**) lateral aspects of the proximal tibia is seen on T1-weighted sagittal images. (**C**) In another patient, physeal trauma is shown as a hyperintense line following the contour of the anterior lateral femoral condyle and physis (*arrows*). There is no epiphyseal involvement on this fat-suppressed T2-weighted fast spin-echo sagittal image.

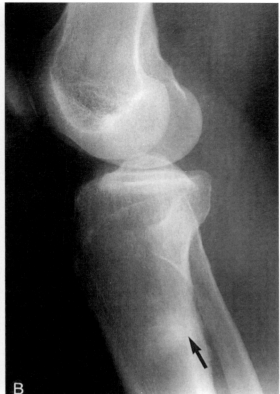

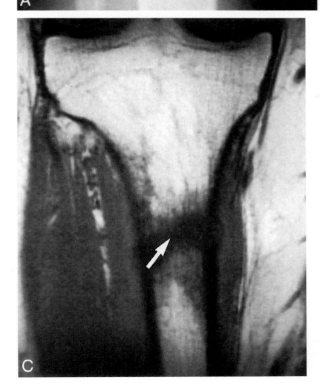

FIGURE 7-275. A stress fracture. Localized tibial sclerosis (*arrows*) is apparent on (**A**) anteroposterior and (**B**) lateral radiographs. (**C**) On a T1-weighted coronal image, the low-signal-intensity transverse fracture (*arrow*) is located in the proximal tibia.

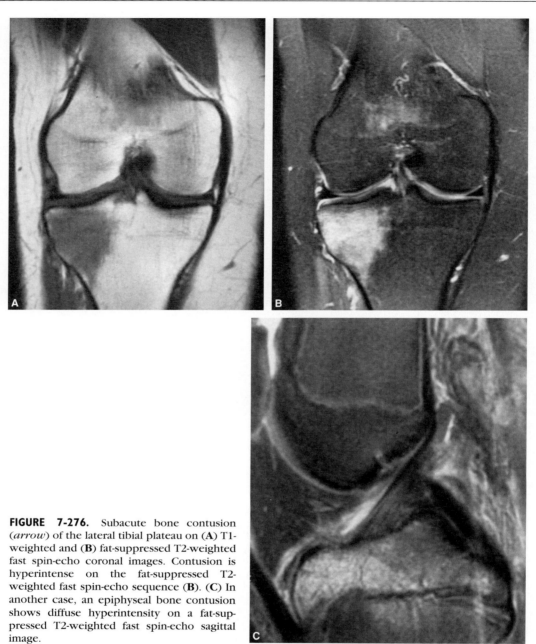

FIGURE 7-276. Subacute bone contusion (*arrow*) of the lateral tibial plateau on (**A**) T1-weighted and (**B**) fat-suppressed T2-weighted fast spin-echo coronal images. Contusion is hyperintense on the fat-suppressed T2-weighted fast spin-echo sequence (**B**). (**C**) In another case, an epiphyseal bone contusion shows diffuse hyperintensity on a fat-suppressed T2-weighted fast spin-echo sagittal image.

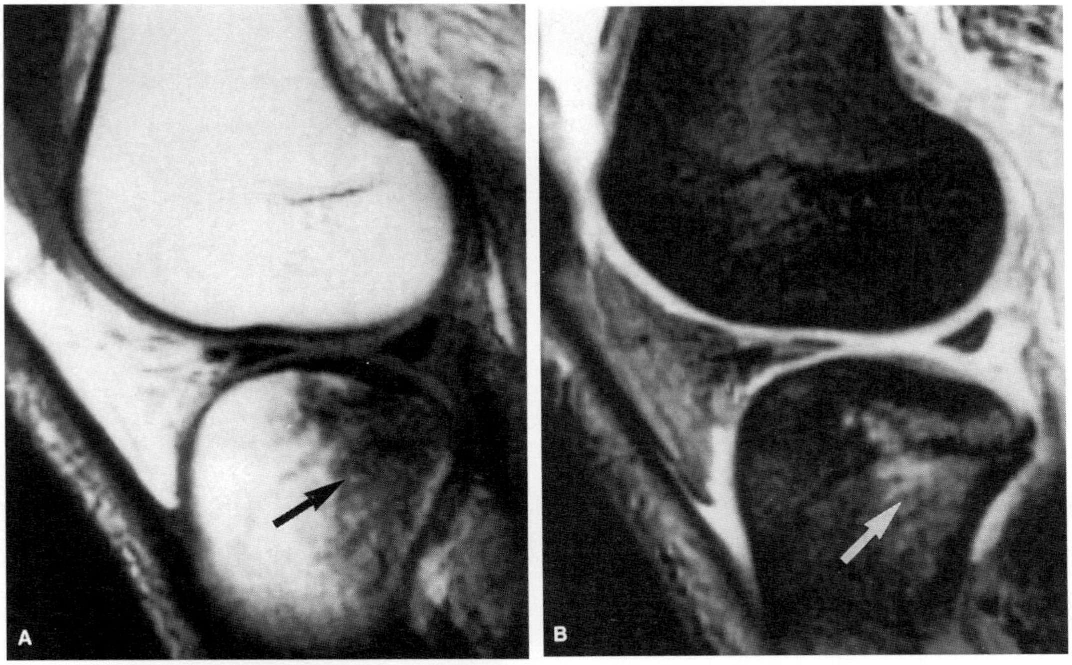

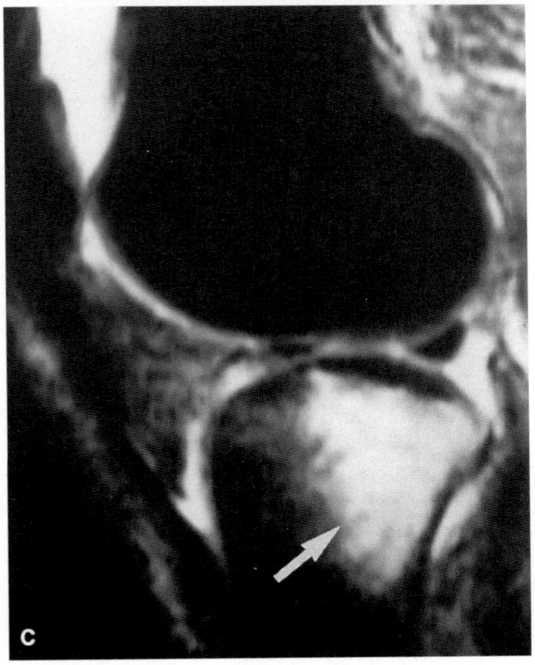

FIGURE 7-277. Marrow hemorrhage resulting from lateral plateau contusion (type I lesion) (*arrows*) is seen as a diffuse region of hyperemia demonstrating low signal intensity on (**A**) a T1-weighted sagittal image and hyperintensity on (**B**) T2*-weighted and (**C**) STIR sagittal images. Type I bone injuries appear as diffuse or reticulated low-signal-intensity areas in metaphyseal and epiphyseal regions of trabecular bone without a cortical fracture.

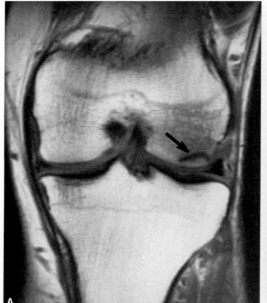
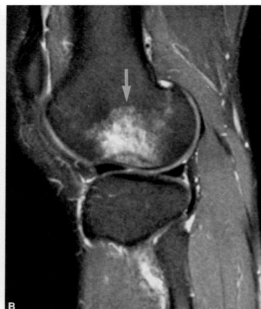

FIGURE 7-278. (**A**) A nondisplaced linear fracture of the lateral femoral condyle (*arrow*) with extension to the subchondral plate on a T1-weighted coronal image. (**B**) Corresponding fat-suppressed T2-weighted fast spin-echo sagittal image with hyperintense bone marrow edema (*arrow*) associated with the fracture site.

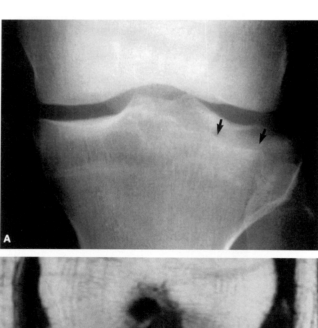
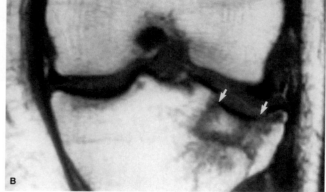

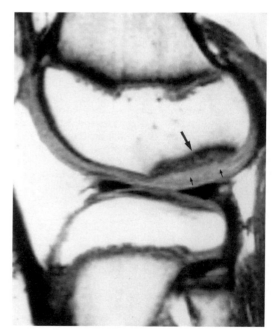

FIGURE 7-279. A T1-weighted sagittal image shows a type III bone lesion with flattening of the intermediate signal intensity articular cartilage (*small arrows*) overlying a low signal intensity focus of osteochondritis dissecans (*large arrow*). Osteonecrosis, osteochondritis dissecans, and degenerative sclerosis all are considered type III lesions not related to acute trauma.

FIGURE 7-280. A local, central-depression-type lateral tibial plateau fracture (*arrows*) is seen on (**A**) an anteroposterior radiograph and (**B**) a T1-weighted coronal image. Morphologic features of the fracture and subchondral marrow hemorrhage are best demonstrated on an MR image.

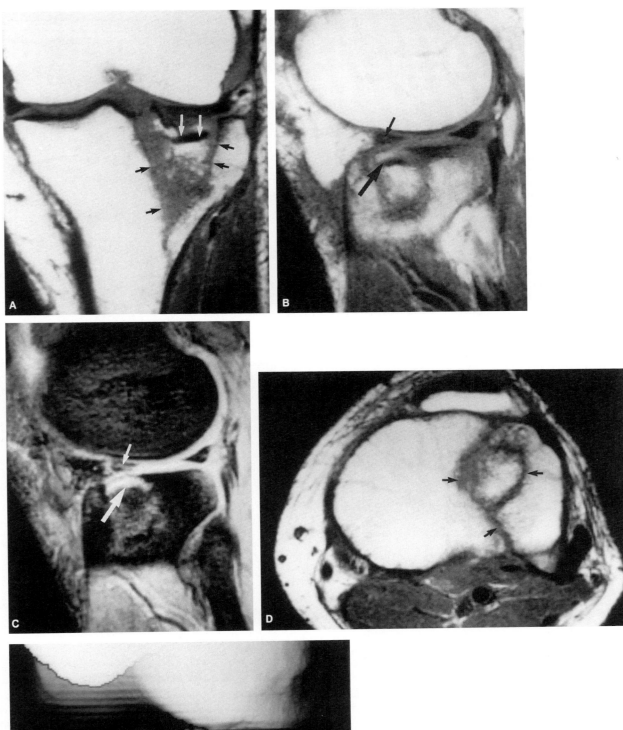

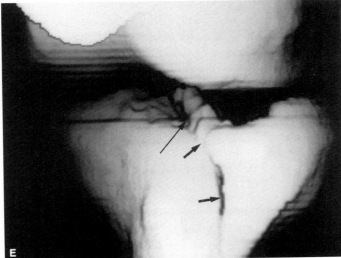

FIGURE 7-281. (**A**) A T1-weighted coronal image shows a vertical-wedge (*black arrows*) tibial plateau fracture with a central-depression component (*white arrows*) involving the lateral tibial condyle. (**B**) T1-weighted and (**C**) T2*-weighted sagittal images demonstrate cortical depression (*large arrow*) and associated meniscal tearing of the anterior horn of the lateral meniscus (*small arrow*). (**D**) A T1-weighted axial image shows the anterior-to-posterior extent of the plateau fracture and the central depression (*arrows*). (**E**) A 3D CT image displays a vertical fracture segment (*small thick arrows*) with intraarticular involvement (*long thin arrow*).

FIGURE 7-282. Depressed anterior lateral tibial plateau fracture (*curved arrow*), poorly seen on a conventional lateral radiograph (**A**), is identified with associated articular cartilage involvement (*straight black arrow*) on a fat-suppressed T2-weighted fast spin-echo sagittal image (**B**). Note the intact articular surface in the posterior lateral tibial plateau (*straight white arrow*). MR also documents the condition of the meniscus cartilages. The direct sagittal-plane evaluation of the fracture site permits accurate measurement of plateau depression.

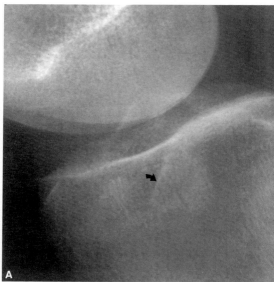
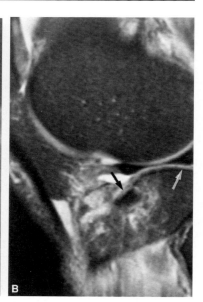

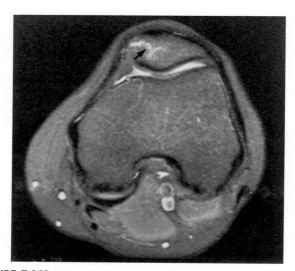

FIGURE 7-283. A nondisplaced patellar fracture (*arrow*) with linear hyperintensity in the medial facet on a fat-suppressed T2-weighted fast spin-echo axial image.

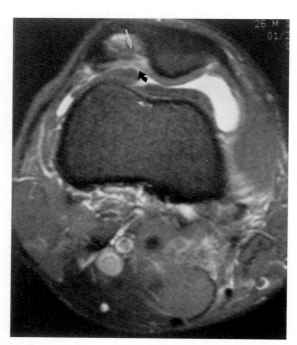

FIGURE 7-284. A fat-suppressed T2-weighted fast spin-echo axial image of a bipartite patella involving the superolateral margin of the patella. The anterior-to-posterior division represents a developmental anomaly of the accessory ossification center (*straight arrow*). Note the relative continuity of the patellar facet articular cartilage surface (*curved arrow*).

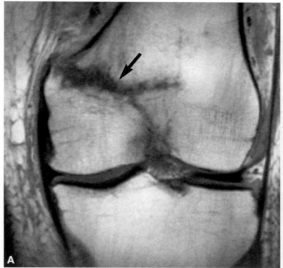

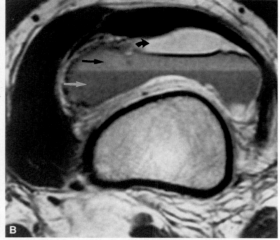

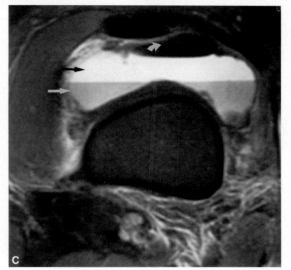

FIGURE 7-285. (**A**) T1-weighted coronal image of a medial femoral condylar fracture (*arrow*). (**B** and **C**) Lipohemarthrosis with fat–serum–cellular layering is identified in a hemorrhagic effusion. *Straight white arrow*, cellular layer; *straight black arrow*, serum layer; *curved arrow*, fat layer. (**B**, T1-weighted axial image; **C**, fat-suppressed T2-weighted fast spin-echo axial image.) Hemarthrosis is commonly seen in ACL tears and osteochondral fractures. The supernatant layer of hemorrhage is bright on long TR/TE sequences, whereas the cellular layer is dark on short and long TR/TE protocols. The fat layer is hypointense on the fat-suppressed T2-weighted fast spin-echo sequence (**C**).

displaced.[330] Displaced fractures are further subdivided into local compression (Fig. 7-280), split compression (Fig. 7-281), total condylar depression, split, rim, and bicondylar fractures. MR allows multiplanar fracture and articular cartilage characterization, which is not possible with CT (Fig. 7-282).

Patellar fractures should be differentiated from bipartite patellar morphology (Fig. 7-283). Patellar fractures are vertical, transverse, or comminuted. The bipartite patella is a developmental variant that involves accessory ossification of the superolateral margin, and not a fracture (Fig. 7-284). MR also demonstrates inferior pole avulsion fractures, which may be missed on initial radiographs and clinical evaluation.[331]

Lipohemarthrosis may be identified in fractures involv-

ing the patella, femur, or tibia (Fig. 7-285). T1 and T2 (including fat-suppressed T2-weighted fast spin-echo) images are useful in identifying fluid–fluid layers.

Compartment syndrome, a known complication of trauma, including fracture, can be identified on MR images by the presence of edema that is limited to a specified muscle group(s) (Fig. 7-286).[332] Edema may be replaced with fatty atrophy after chronic denervation (Fig. 7-287). Sudeck's atrophy, or reflex sympathetic dystrophy, can also occur as a complication of fracture (Fig. 7-288). Diffuse juxtaarticular low signal intensity on T2-weighted images is seen as aggressive osteoporosis develops with or without the presence of an associated fracture.[333] On STIR images, reflex sympathetic dystrophy demonstrates increased signal intensity sec-

text continues on page 432

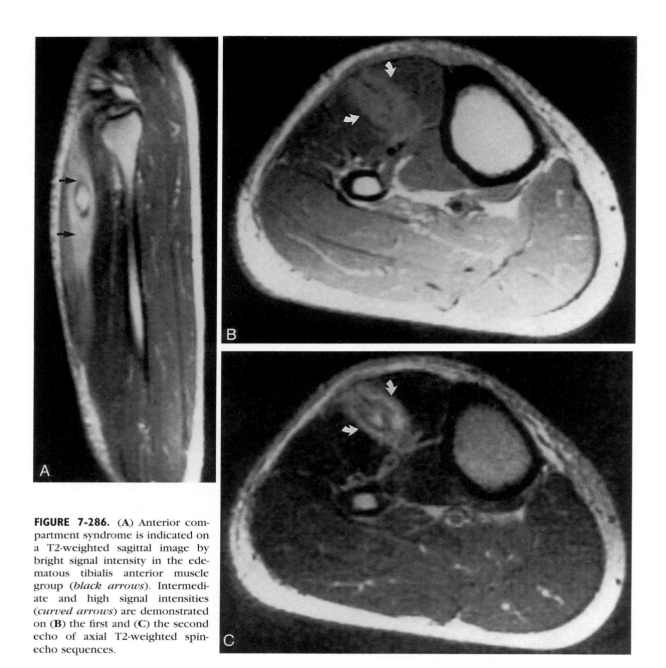

FIGURE 7-286. (**A**) Anterior compartment syndrome is indicated on a T2-weighted sagittal image by bright signal intensity in the edematous tibialis anterior muscle group (*black arrows*). Intermediate and high signal intensities (*curved arrows*) are demonstrated on (**B**) the first and (**C**) the second echo of axial T2-weighted spin-echo sequences.

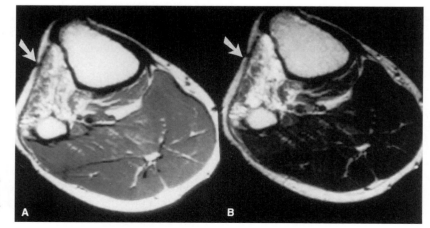

FIGURE 7-287. Fatty atrophy (*arrows*) of the muscles of the anterior fascial compartment of the leg as a result of peroneal nerve injury is seen on (**A**) intermediate weighted and (**B**) T2-weighted axial images.

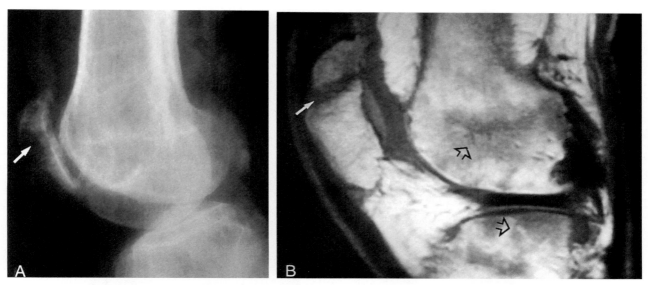

FIGURE 7-288. **(A)** A lateral radiograph shows a patellar fracture (*arrow*) and diffuse osteoporosis. **(B)** A T1-weighted sagittal image shows the transverse patellar fracture (*solid white arrow*) and patchy juxtaarticular low signal intensity (*open black arrows*) that correspond with aggressive osteoporosis in reflex sympathetic dystrophy.

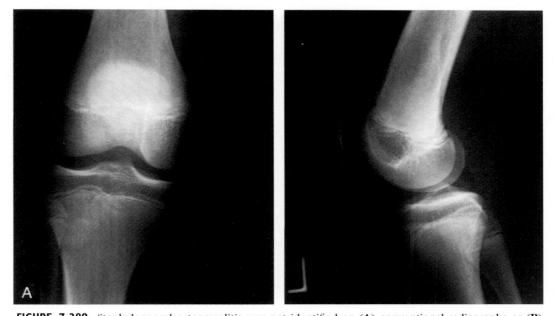

FIGURE 7-289. Staphylococcal osteomyelitis was not identified on **(A)** conventional radiographs or **(B)** bone scintigrams.   *continued*

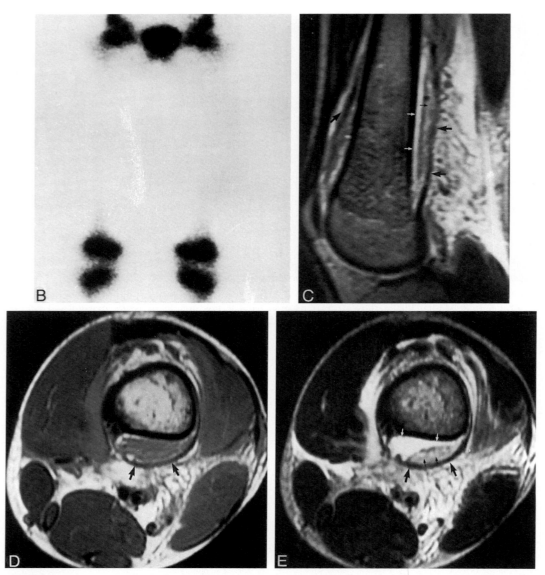

FIGURE 7-289. *Continued.* (**C**) T2-weighted sagittal, (**D**) intermediate weighted axial, and (**E**) T2-weighted axial images reveal purulent fluid (*white arrows*), necrotic tissue (*small black arrows*), and elevated low-signal-intensity periosteum (*large black arrows*). Purulent debris (ie, fluid) demonstrates increased signal intensity on T2-weighted images (*small white arrows*).

ondary to hyperemic bone marrow edema.[334] STIR imaging sequences are more sensitive and may define increased signal intensity in hyperemic bone in patients with negative findings on T2- or T2*-weighted images.

Infection

Capsular distention and joint effusions can be seen on MR scans of infected joints, but are nonspecific findings.[335] A septic joint may be further characterized by intraarticular debris and synovitis from hematogenous seeding. In osteomyelitis in the immature skeleton, a mottled pattern of yel-

low marrow stores can be seen in the epiphyseal center of the femur or tibia. This appearance should not be confused with the coarsened trabecular pattern seen in Paget's disease.[336] In cases of osteomyelitis, the metaphysis, an active site of bone formation in children, may show signal abnormalities (low signal on T1, bright signal on T2 or STIR images) restricted to this region.[337] In one case of osteomyelitis involving the distal femur, MR studies revealed collections of the infected fluid confined by elevated periosteum (Fig. 7-289). Findings on plain-film radiographs and nuclear bone scans were negative in this case, which was surgically debrided on the basis of the MR findings.

An infectious tract with fluid may simulate pathologic

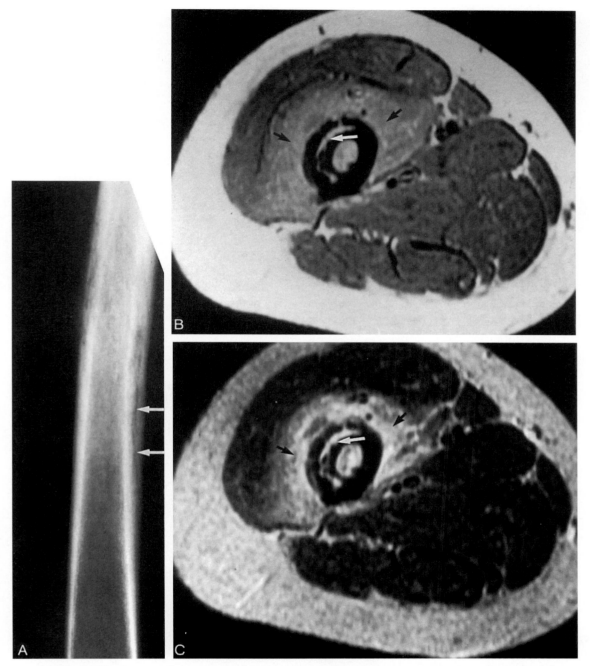

FIGURE 7-290. Osteomyelitis can resemble Ewing's sarcoma. (**A**) An anteroposterior radiograph of the midfemur demonstrates periosteal reaction and longitudinal cortical lucency (*arrows*). (**B**) Intermediate weighted and (**C**) T2-weighted axial images reveal a corresponding high-signal-intensity infectious track (*white arrows*) with perilesional edema (*black arrows*). Edema demonstrates increased signal intensity on T2-weighted sequences.

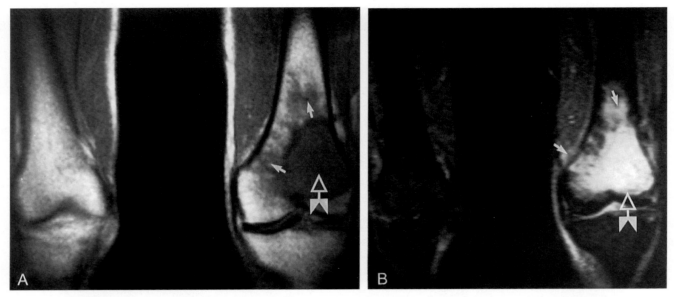

FIGURE 7-291. (**A**) T1-weighted and (**B**) STIR coronal images display a focus of staphylococcal osteomyelitis in the femoral metaphysis (*flagged arrows*). Marrow infiltration and extension (*solid arrows*) demonstrate low signal intensity on the T1-weighted image and high signal intensity on the STIR image.

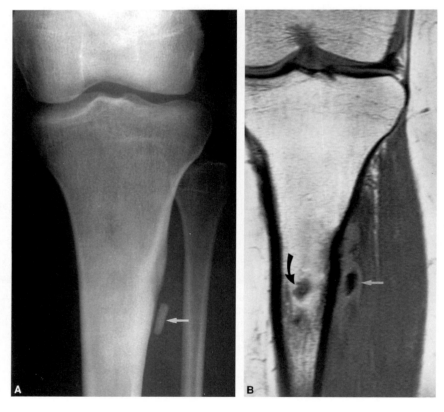

FIGURE 7-292. Chronic active osteomyelitis with a sequestrum (*straight arrow*) adjacent to the lateral tibial cortex. An anteroposterior radiograph (**A**) demonstrates irregularity of the lateral tibial cortex, the presence of the sequestrum, and medullary bone sclerosis. The active infection within the medullary cavity (*curved arrow*) is seen as hypointense foci on a T1-weighted coronal image (**B**) and as a hyperintense area on the fat-suppressed T2-weighted fast spin-echo axial image (**C**).

continued

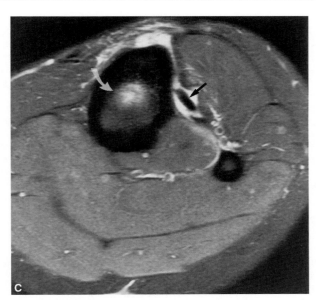

FIGURE 7-292. *Continued.* Note the chronically infected fluid associated with the sequestrum, which tracks anterolateral to the tibia. The sequestrum *(straight arrow)* is hypointense on both the T1(**B**) and the fat-suppressed T2-weighted fast spin-echo (**C**) images.

fracture or stress fracture, and when associated with extensive surrounding edema, can be confused with tumor (Fig. 7-290). This infectious tract may be associated with adjacent muscle edema, and the patient may in fact present with a condition resembling compartment syndrome. In a patient with multifocal osteomyelitis, seeding of the distal femur and proximal humerus was identified on MR scans as a central nidus of high-intensity marrow and calcified sequestra of low signal intensity. Marrow infiltration and soft-tissue extension of osteomyelitis can be demonstrated using STIR and fat-suppressed T2-weighted fast spin-echo images (Fig. 7-291). T2*-weighted images are not sensitive enough to display the reactive marrow changes in areas of osteomyelitis. Cellulitis is best identified on either STIR or fat-suppressed T2-weighted fast spin-echo images. The STIR sequence, however, may be sensitive to reactive marrow changes in the absence of active infection and in the presence of normal marrow signal intensity on T2-weighted images.[338] A low signal intensity ''rim sign'' has been described in chronic infection resulting from trauma.[338] This rim of fibrous tissue or reactive bone displays low signal intensity on T1-, T2-, and STIR-weighted images and surrounds the area of active bone disease.

MR is also used to evaluate subacute osteomyelitis including Brodie's abscess. In Brodie's abscess the focus of involvement of osteomyelitis is hyperintense on STIR and fat-suppressed T2-weighted fast spin-echo images. The sclerotic margin displays low signal intensity on all pulse sequences, and there may be fluid in communication with the central infected focus. The differential diagnosis for Brodie's abscess usually includes osteoid osteoma and stress fracture. The sequestrum or necrotic bone adjacent to or associated

with the osteomyelitis can be visualized as a low-signal-intensity fragment on MR images (Fig. 7-292). There may be areas of edema or fluid associated with the sequestrum.

References

1. Stoller DW, Genant HK. Magnetic resonance imaging of the knee and hip. Arthritis Rheum 1990;33:441.
2. Kursunoglu-Brahme S, Resnick D. Magnetic resonance imaging of the knee. Orthop Clin North Am 1990;21:561.
3. Mink JH, Deutsch AL. Magnetic resonance imaging of the knee. Clin Orthop 1989;244:29.
4. Burk DL Jr, Mitchell DG, Rifkin MD, Vinitski S. Recent advances in magnetic resonance imaging of the knee. Radiol Clin North Am 1990;28:379.
5. Spiers ASD, Meagher T. Ostlere SJ. Can MRI of the knee affect arthroscopic practice? A prospective of 58 patients. J Bone Joint Surg [Br] 1993;75:49.
6. Rowe PA, Wright J, Randall RL, Lynch JK, et al. Can MR imaging effectively replace diagnostic arthroscopy? Radiology 1992;183:335.
7. Reicher MA, et al. High resolution magnetic resonance imaging of the knee joint: normal anatomy. AJR Am J Roentgenol 1985;145:895.
8. Resnick D, Niwayama G. Internal derangements of joints. Diagnosis of bone and joint disorders, 2nd ed, vol 5. Philadelphia: WB Saunders, 1988:2899.
9. Reicher MA, et al. MR imaging of the knee: I. traumatic disorders. Radiology 1987;162:547.
10. Hartzman MD, et al. MR imaging of the knee: II. chronic disorders. Radiology 1987;162:553.
11. Buckwalter KA, Pennas DR. Anterior cruciate ligament: oblique sagittal MR imaging. Radiology 1990;175:276.
12. Adam G, Bohndorf K, Drobnitzky M, Guenther RW. MR imaging of the knee—three dimensional volume imaging combined with fast processing. J Comput Assist Tomogr 1989;13:984.
13. Mirowitz SA. Fast scanning and fat-suppression MR imaging of musculoskeletal disorders. AJR Am J Roentgenol 1993;161:1147.
14. Santyr GE, Mulkern RV. Magnetization transfer in MR imaging. J Magn Reson Imaging 1995;5:121.
15. Wolff SD, Balaban RS. Magnetization transfer imaging: practical aspects and clinical applications. Radiology 1994;192:593.
16. Crues JV, Shellock FG. Technical consideration. In: Mink JH, Reicher MA, Crues JY, eds. Magnetic resonance imaging of the knee. New York: Raven Press, 1987:3.
17. Buckwalter KA, Braunstein EM, Janizek DB, Vahey TN. MR imaging of meniscal tears: narrow versus conventional window width photography. Radiology 1993;187:827.
18. Johnson RL. Anatomy and biomechanics of the knee. In: Chapman MW, ed. Operative orthopaedics, 2nd ed. Philadelphia: JB Lippincott, 1993:2039.
19. Li DKB, et al. Magnetic resonance imaging of the ligaments and menisci of the knee. Radiol Clin North Am 1986;24:209.
20. Bessette GC, Hunter RE. The anterior cruciate ligament. Orthopaedics 1990;13:551.
21. Grigis FG, et al. The cruciate ligaments of the knee joint. Clin Orthop 1975;106:216.
22. Watanabe AT, et al. Normal variations in MR imaging of the knee: appearance and frequency. AJR Am J Roentgenol 1987;153:341.
23. Stoller DW, et al. Meniscal tears: pathological correlation with MR imaging. Radiology 1987;163:452.
24. Stoller DW, et al. Gradient echo MR imaging of the knee. Radiology 1987;165.
25. Crues JV, Stoller DW. The menisci. In: Mink JH, Reicher MA, Crues

JV, Deutsch AL, eds. MRI of the knee. New York: Raven Press, 1993:91.

26. Mandelbaum BR, et al. Magnetic resonance imaging as a tool for evaluation of traumatic knee injuries: anatomical and pathoanatomical correlations. Am J Sports Med 1986;14:361.

27. Spritzer CE, et al. MR imaging of the knee: preliminary results with a 3DFT grass pulse sequence. AJR Am J Roentgenol 1988;150:597.

28. Rubin DA, Kneeland JB, Listerud J, Underberg-Davis SJ. MR diagnosis of meniscal tears of the knee: value of fast spin-echo vs. conventional spin-echo pulse sequences. AJR Am J Roentgenol 1994; 162:1131.

29. Quinn SF, Brown TR, Szumowski J. Menisci of the knee: radial MR imaging correlated with arthroscopy in 259 patients. Radiology 1992;185:577.

30. Applegate GR, Flannigan BD, Tolin BS, Fox JM. MR diagnosis of recurrent tears in the knee: value of intraarticular contrast material. AJR Am J Roentgenol 1993;161:821.

31. Dehaven KE, Arnoczky SP. Meniscal repair: I. basic science, indications for repair, and open repair. J Bone Joint Surg 1994;76(A):140.

32. Arnoczky SP, et al. Microvasculature of the human meniscus. Am J Sports Med 1982;10:90.

33. Arnoczky SP, et al. The microvasculature of the meniscus and its response to injury. Am J Sports Med;1983;11:31.

34. Kaplan EB. The embryology of the menisci of the knee joint. Bull Hosp Joint Dis 1955;16:111.

35. Wilson R, et al. Arthroscopic anatomy. In: Scott W, et al, eds. Arthroscopy of the knee. Philadelphia: WB Saunders, 1990;49.

36. Yocum LA, et al. Isolated lateral meniscectomy: a study of 26 patients with isolated tears. J Bone Joint Surg [Am] 1979;61:338.

37. Johnson DL, Swelson TM, Livesay GA, Aizawa H. Insertion-site anatomy of the human menisci: gross, arthroscopic and topographical anatomy as a basis for meniscal transplantation. Arthroscopy 1995;11:386.

38. Kohn D, Moreno B. Meniscus insertion anatomy as a basis for meniscus replacement: a morphological cadaveric study. Arthroscopy 1995;11:96.

39. Jones CDS, Keene GCR, Christie AD. The popliteus as a retractor of the lateral meniscus of the knee. Arthroscopy 1995;11:270.

40. Hallen L, et al. The 'screw-home' movement in the knee joint. Acta Orthop Scand 1966;37:97.

41. Shaw JA, et al. The longitudinal axis of the knee and the role of the cruciate ligaments in controlling transverse rotation. J Bone Joint Surg [Am] 1974;56:603.

42. Voto S. A nomenclature system for meniscal lesions of the knee. Surgical Rounds for Orthopaedics 1989;October:34.

43. Chernye S. Disorders of the knee. In: Deer, et al, eds. Priciples of orthopaedic practice, vol 2. New York: McGraw-Hill, 1989:1283.

44. O'Meara PM. The basic science of meniscus repair. Orthop Rev 1993;June:681.

45. Newman AP, Daniels AV, Burks RT. Principles and decision making in meniscal surgery. Arthroscopy 1993;9:33.

46. Turek SL. Orthopedics: principles and their applications, 4th ed. Philadelphia: JB Lippincott, 1984:1269.

47. Cannon WD, Morgan CD. Meniscal repair: II. arthroscopic repair techniques. J Bone Joint Surg 1994;76(A):294.

48. Krause WR, et al. Mechanical changes in the knee after meniscectomy. J Bone Joint Surg [Am] 1976;58:599.

49. Warren RF, et al. Meniscal lesions associated with anterior cruciate ligament injury. Clin Orthop 1983;172:32.

50. Beltran J, et al. Meniscal tears: MR demonstration of experimentally produced injuries. Radiology 1986;158:691.

51. Tobler TH. Makroskopische und histologische befund am kniegeluk meniscus in verschiedenen lebensaiten. Schweiz Med Wochenschr 1926;56:1359.

52. Roca FA, Vilalta A. Lesions of the meniscus. I: macroscopic and histologic findings. Clin Orthop 1980;146:289.

53. Roca FA, Vilalta A. Lesions of the meniscus. II: horizontal cleavages and lateral cysts. Clin Orthop 1980;146:301.

54. Kornick JK, et al. Meniscal abnormalities in the asymptomatic population at MR imaging. Radiology 1990;177:463.

55. Dillon EH, Pope CF, Jokl P, Lynch K. The clinical significance of stage 2 meniscal abnormalities on magnetic resonance knee images. Magn Reson Imaging 1990;8:411.

56. Frija G, Schouman-Claeys E, d'Anthouard F, Feron JM, Paraire F. Grossly normal knee menisci: correlations with pathology and magnetic resonance imaging. Diagn Interv Radiol 1989;1:29.

57. Kaplan PA, Nelson NL, Garvin KL, Brown DE. MR of the knee: the significance of high signal intensity in the meniscus that does not clearly extend to the surface. AJR Am J Roentgenol 1991;156:333.

58. Negendank WG, Fernandez-Madrid FR, Heibrun LK. Magnetic resonance imaging of meniscal degeneration in asymptomatic knees. J Orthop Res 1990;8:311.

59. Reinig JW, McDevitt ER, Ove PN. Progress of meniscal degenerative changes in college football players: evaluation with MR imaging. Radiology 1991;181:255.

60. Dillon EH, Pope CF, Jokl P, Lynch JK. Follow-up of grade 2 meniscal abnormalities in the stable knee. Radiology 1991;181:849.

61. Kursundglu-Brahme S, et al. Jogging causes acute changes in the knee joint: an MR study in normal volunteers. AJR Am J Roentgenol 1990;154:1233.

62. La Prade RF, Burnett QM, Veenstra MA, Hodgman CG. The prevalence of abnormal magnetic resonance imaging findings in asymptomatic knees. Am J Sports Med 1994;22:739.

63. Smillie LS. Diseases of the knee joint, 2nd ed. London: Churchill-Livingstone, 1980;340.

64. Mink JH. The Knee. In: Mink JH, Deutsch A, eds. MRI of the musculoskeletal system: a teaching file. 1990:251.

65. Ricklin P, et al. Meniscus lesions: diagnosis, differential diagnosis and therapy. 2nd ed. New York: Stratton, 1983.

66. Levinsohn ME, Baker BE. Prearthrotomy diagnostic evaluation of the knee: review of 100 cases diagnosed by arthrography and arthroscopy. AJR Am J Roentgenol 1980;134:107.

67. Watts I, et al. Pitfalls in double contrast knee arthrography. Br J Radiol 1980;134:107.

68. Raunest J, Hotzinger H, Burrig KF. MRI and arthroscopy in the detection of meniscal degenerations. Arthroscopy 1994;10:624.

69. Stoller DW, et al. Three-dimensional rendering and classification of meniscal tears disarticulated from 3-D FT images. In: Abstracts of the 9th Annual Meeting of the Society of Magnetic Resonance in Medicine 1990;1:346.

70. Cannon WD, Vitton JM. Basic arthroscopy. In: Aichroth PM, Cannon WD, Disnitz M, eds. Knee surgery: current practice. London: Martin Dunitz, 1992:54.

71. Rosenberg TO, Pavlos LE, et al. Arthroscopic surgery of the knee. In: Chapman MW, ed. Operative orthopaedics, 2nd ed. Philadelphia: JB Lippincott, 1993:2403.

72. Singson RD, et al. MR imaging of displaced bucket-handle tear of the medial meniscus. AJR Am J Roentgenol 1991;156:121.

73. Weiss KL. Sagittal MR images of the knee: a low signal. AJR Am J Roentgenol 1991;156:117.

74. Wright DH, DeSnet AA, Norris M. Bucket-handle tears of the medial and lateral menisci of the knee: value of MR imaging in detected displaced fragments. AJR Am J Roentgenol 1995;165:621.

75. Tuckman GA, Miller WJ, Remo JW, Fritts HM. Radial tears of the menisci: MR findings. AJR Am J Roentgenol 1994;163:395.

76. Rosenberg TD. Arthroscopic diagnosis and treatment of meniscal disorders. In: Scott W, et al, eds. Arthroscopy of the knee. Philadelphia: WB Saunders, 1990:67.

77. Rosenberg TD, et al. Arthroscopic surgery of the knee. In: Chapman MW, et al, eds. Operative orthopaedics. Philadelphia: JB Lippincott, 1988:1585.

78. Crues JV III, etal. Meniscal tears of the knee: accuracy of MR imaging. Radiology 1987:164:445.

79. Jackson DW, Jennings LD, Maywood RM, Berger PE. Magnetic resonance imaging of the knee. Am J Sports Med 1988;16:29.

80. Polly DW Jr, Callaghan JJ, Sikes RA, et al. The accuracy of selective magnetic resonance imaging compared with the findings of arthroscopy of the knee. J Bone Joint Surg [Am] 1988;70:192.

81. Glashow JL, Katz R, Schneider M, Scott W. Double-blind assessment of the value of magnetic resonance imaging in the diagnosis of anterior cruciate and meniscal lesions. J Bone Joint Surg [Am] 1989;71:113.

82. Crues JV, Ryu R, Morgan FW. Meniscal pathology. The expanding role of magnetic resonance imaging. Clin Orthop 1990;252:90.

83. De Smet AA, Tuite MJ, Norris MA, Swan JS. MR diagnosis of meniscal tears: analysis of causes of errors. AJR Am J Roentgenol 1994;163:1419.

84. De Smet AA, Norris MA, Yandow DR, Graf BK. Diagnosis of meniscal tears of the knee with MR imaging: effect of observer variation and sample size on sensitivity and specificity. AJR Am J Roentgenol 1993;160:555.

85. Mesgarzadeh M, Moyer R, Leder D, Revesz G. MR imaging of the knee: expanded classification and pitfalls to interpretation of meniscal tears. Radiographics 1993;13:489.

86. DeSmet AA, Norris MA, Yandow DR, Quintana FA. MR diagnosis of meniscal tears of the knee: importance of high signal in the meniscus that extends to the surface. AJR Am J Roentgenol 1993;161:101.

87. Justice WW, Quinn SF. Error patterns in the MR imaging evaluation of menisci of the knee. RSNA 1995;196:617.

88. Mink JH, et al. MR imaging of the knee: technical factors, diagnostic accuracy, and further pitfalls. Radiology 1987;165(P):175.

89. Tyrrell R, et al. Fast three-dimensional MR imaging of the knee: A comparison with arthroscopy. Radiology 1987;166:865.

90. Fischer SP, et al. Accuracy of diagnosis from magnetic resonance imaging of the knee. J Bone Joint Surg [Am] 1991;73:2.

91. Oberlander MA, Shalvoy RM, Hughston JC. The accuracy of the clinical knee examination documented by arthroscopy. Am J Sports Med 1993;21:773.

92. Stone KR, Stoller DW, Irving SG, Elmquist C. 3D MRI volume sizing of knee meniscus cartilage. Arthroscopy 1994;10:641.

93. Disler DG, Kattapuram SC, Chew FS, Rosenthal DI. Meniscal tears of the knee: preliminary comparison of three-dimensional MR reconstruction with two-dimensional MR imaging and arthroscopy. AJR Am J Roentgenol 1993;160:343.

94. Kaplan EB. Discoid lateral meniscus of the knee joint. J Bone Joint Surg [Am] 1957;39:77.

95. Dickason JM, et al. A series of ten discoid medial menisci. Clin Orthop 1982;168:75.

96. Weiner B, Rosenberg N. Discoid medial meniscus associations with bone changes in the tibia. J Bone Joint Surg [Am] 1974;56:171.

97. Aichroth PM, Patel D. Congenital discoid lateral meniscus in children: an overview and current clinical perspectives. In: Aichroth PM, Cannon WD, Disnitz M, eds. Knee surgery: current practice. London: Martin Dunitz, 1992:521.

98. Auge WK, Kaeding CC. Bilateral discoid medial menisci with extensive intrasubstance cleavage tears: MRI and arthroscopic correlation. Arthroscopy 1994;10:313.

99. Fujikawa K. Discoid meniscus in children. In: Aichroth PM, Cannon WD, Disnitz M, eds. Knee surgery: current practice. London: Martin Dunitz, 1992:530.

100. Barnes CL, McCarthy RE, VanderSchilden JL, McConnell JR. Discoid lateral meniscus in a young child: case report and review of the literature. J Pediatr Orthop 1988;8:707.

101. Howe MA, Buckwalter KA, Braunstein EM, Wojtys EM. Case Report 483: discoid lateral meniscus (DLM), medially displaced with complex tear. Skel Radiol 1988;17:293.

102. Hamada M, Shino K, Kawano K, Araki Y. Usefulness of magnetic resonance imaging for detecting intrasubstance tear and/or degenration or lateral discoid meniscus. Arthroscopy 1994;10:645.

103. Schonholtz GJ, Koenig TM, Prince A. Bilateral discoid medial menisci: A case report and literature review. Arthroscopy 1993;9:315.

104. Silverman JM, Mink JH, Deutsch AL. Discoid menisci of the knee: MR imaging appearance. Radiology 1989;173:351.

105. Mink JH, et al. MR imaging of the knee: pitfalls in interpretation. Radiology 1987;165(P):239.

106. Kaplan PA, et al. MR of the knee: the significance of high signal in the meniscus that does not clearly extend to the surface. AJR Am J Roentgenol 1991;156:333.

107. Herman LJ, et al. Pitfalls in MR imaging of the knee. Radiology 1988;167:775.

108. Vahey TN, et al. MR imaging of the knee: pseudotear of the lateral meniscus caused by the meniscofemoral ligament. AJR Am J Roentgenol 1990;154:1237.

109. Peterfy CG, Janzen DL, Tirman PF, VanDijke CF. 'Magic angle' phenomenon: A cause of increased signal in the normal lateral meniscus on short-TE MR images of the knee. AJR Am J Roentgenol 1994;163:149.

110. Turner DA, Rapoport MI, Erwin WD, et al. Truncation artifact: a potential pitfall in MR imaging of the menisci of the knee. Radiology 1991;179:629.

111. Mink JH. Pitfalls in interpretation in MRI of the knee, 2nd ed. Mink JH, Reicher MA, Crues JV, Deutsch AL, eds. New York: Raven Press, 1993:433.

112. Cannon DW, Vittori JM. Meniscal repair. In: Aichroth PM, Cannon DW, Disnitz M, eds. Knee surgery: current practice. London: Martin Dunitz, 1992:71.

113. Henning CF, Yearout KM, Vequist, et al. Use of the fascia sheath coverage and exogenous fibrin clot in the treatment of complex meniscal tears. Am J Sports Med 1991;19:626.

114. Fitzgibbons RE, Shelbourne KD. 'Aggressive' nontreatment of lateral meniscal tears seen during anterior cruciate ligament reconstruction. Am J Sports Med 1995;23:156.

115. Garrett JC, et al. Meniscal transplantation in the human knee: a preliminary report. Arthroscopy 1991;7:57.

116. Smith DK, et al. The knee after partial meniscectomy: MR imaging features. Radiology 1990;176:141.

117. Deutsch AL, et al. Peripheral meniscal tears: MR findings after conservative treatment of arthroscopic repair. Radiology 1990;176:485.

118. Kent RH, Pope CF, Lynch JK, et al. Magnetic resonance imaging of the surgically repaired meniscus: six month follow-up. Magn Reson Imag 1991;9:335.

119. Arnoczky SP, Cooper TG, Stadelmaier DP, Hannafin JA. Magnetic resonance signal in healing menisci: an experimental study in dogs. Arthroscopy 1994;10:552.

120. Drape J-L, Thelen P, Gay-Depassier P, Silbermann O. Intraarticular diffusion of Gd-DTPA after intravenous injections in the knee: MR imaging evaluation. Radiology 1993;188:227.

121. Strobel M. Anatomy, proprioception and biomechanics in diagnostic evaluation of the knee. Berlin: Springer-Verlag, 1990:2.

122. Gallimore GW, Harmes SE. Knee injuries: high resolution MR imaging. Radiology 1986;160:457.

123. Burk DL, et al. Meniscal and ganglion cysts of the knee: MR evaluation. AJR Am J Roentgenol 1988;150:331.

124. Ryu RK, Ting AJ. Arthoscopic treatment of meniscal cysts. Arthroscopy 1993;9:591.

125. Dodds JA, Arnoczky SP. Anatomy of the anterior cruciate ligament: A blueprint for repair and reconstruction. Arthroscopy 1994;10:132.

126. Kennedy JC, et al. The anatomy and function of the anterior cruciate ligament. J Bone Joint Surg [Am] 1974;56:223.

127. Feagin JA, Curl WW: Isolated tear of the anterior cruciate ligament: 5-year follow-up study. Am J Sports Med 1976;4:95.

128. Fu FH, Harner CD, Johnson DL, Miller MD. Biomechanics of the knee ligaments. Am Acad Orthop Surg 1993;75(A):1716.

129. Fetto JF, et al. The natural history and diagnosis of anterior cruciate ligament insufficiency. Clin Orthop 1980;147:29.

130. Kennedy JC, et al. The anatomy and function of the anterior cruciate ligament as determined by clinical and morphological studies. J Bone Joint Surg [Am] 1974;56:223.

131. Johnson DL, Warner JJ. Diagnosis for ACL surgery. Clinics Sports Med 1993;October:671.

132. Cerabona F, et al. Patterns of meniscal injury with acute anterior cruciate ligament tears. Am J Sports Med 1988;16:603.

133. Indelicato PA, et al. A perspective of lesions associated with ACL insufficiency of the knee. A review of 100 cases. Clin Orthop 1985;198:77.

134. Cannon WD, Vittori JM: The incidence of healing in arthroscopic meniscal repairs in anterior cruciate ligament-reconstructed knees vs. stable knees. Am J Sports Med 1992;20:176.

135. McDaniel WJ. Untreated ruptures of the anterior cruciate ligament. J Bone Joint Surg [Am] 1980;62:696.

136. Duncan JB, Hunter R, Purnell M, Freeman J. Meniscal injuries associated with acute anterior cruciate ligament tears in alpine skiers. Am J Sports Med 1995;23:170.

137. Barber FA. Snow skiing combined anterior cruciate ligament/medial collateral ligament disruptions. Arthroscopy 1994;10:85.

138. Woo SLY, Hollis JM, ADAMS QJ, et al. Tensile properties of the human femur-anterior cruciate ligament-tibia complex: the effects of specimen age and orientation. Am J Sports Med 1991;19:217.

139. Nitsu M, et al. Tears of the cruciate ligaments and menisci: evaluation with cine MR imaging. Radiology 1991;176:276.

140. Karzel RP, Friedman MJ. Anterior cruciate ligament reconstruction using central one-third of the patellar tendon. In: Aichroth PM, Cannon DW, Disnitz M, eds. Knee surgery: current practice. London: Martin Dunitz, 1992:138.

141. Bowdy PA, Vellet KD, Fowler PJ, Marks PH. Magnetic resonance imaging of the partially torn anterior cruciate ligament: An in vitro animal model with correlative histopathology. Clin J Sports Med 1994;4:187.

142. Smith KL, Daniels JL, Arnoczky SP, Dodds JA. Effect of joint position and ligament tension on the MR signal intensity of the cruciate ligaments of the knee. J Magn Reson Imaging 1994;4:819.

143. Hodler J, Highy P, Trudell D, et al. The cruciate ligament of the knee: correlation between MR appearance and gross and histologic findings in cadaveric specimens. AJR Am J Roentgenol 1992;159:357.

144. Robertson PL, Schweitzer ME, Bartolozzi AR, Ligoni A. Anterior cruciate ligament tears: evaluation of multiple signs with MR imaging. Radiology 1994;193:829.

145. Tung GA, Davis LM, Wiggins ME, Fadale PD. Tears of the anterior cruciate ligament: primary and secondary signs at MR imaging. Radiology 1993;188:661.

146. McCauley TR, Moses M, Kier R, Lynch JK, et al. MR diagnosis of tears of anterior cruciate ligament of the knee: importance of ancillary findings. AJR Am J Roentgenol 1994;162:115.

147. Brandser EA, Riley MA, Berbaum KS, et al. MR imaging of anterior cruciate ligament injury: independent value of primary and secondary signs. AJR 1996;167:121.

148. Fitzgerald SW, Remer EM, Friedman H, Rogers LF, et al. MR evaluation of the anterior cruciate ligament: value of supplementing sagittal images with coronal and axial images. AJR Am J Roentgenol 1993;160:1233.

149. Vahey TN, Junt JE, Shelbourne KD. Anterior translocation of the tibia at MR imaging: a secondary sign of anterior cruciate ligament tear. Radiology 1993;187:817.

150. Lee SH, Petersilge CA, Trudell DJ, et al. Extrasynovial spaces of the cruciate ligaments: anatomy, MR imaging, and diagnostic implications. AJR 1996;166:1433.

151. American Medical Association Commitee on the Medical Aspects of Sport: Standard nomenclature of athletic injuries. Chicago: American Medical Association, 1968.

152. Lintner DM, Kamaric E, Moseley JB, Noble PC. Partial tears of the anterior cruciate ligament. Are they clinically detectable? Am J Sports Med 1995;23:111.

153. Umans H, Wimpfheimer O, Haramati N, Applbaum YH. Diagnosis of partial tears of the anterior cruciate ligament of the knee: value of MR imaging. AJR Am J Roentgenol 1995:165;893.

154. Noyes FR, Moor LA, Moorman CT, McGinniss GH. Partial tears of the anterior cruciate ligament. J Bone Joint Surg 1989;71(B):825.

155. Vahey TN, Broome DR, et al. Acute and chronic tears of the anterior cruciate ligament: differential features at MR imaging. Radiology 1991;181:251.

156. Kang CN, Lee SB, Kim SW. Case Report. Symptomatic ganglion cyst within the substance of the anterior cruciate ligament. Arthroscopy 1995;11:612.

157. Liu SH, Osti L, Mirzayan R. Case Report. Ganglion cysts of the anterior cruciate ligament: a case report and review of the literature. Arthroscopy 1994;10:110.

158. Deutsch A, Veltri DM, Altchek DW, Potter HG. Case Report. Symptomatic intraarticular ganglia of the cruciate ligaments of the knee. Arthroscopy 1994;10:219.

159. Veltri DM, Deng XH, Torzilli PA, Warren RF. The role of the cruciate and posterolateral ligaments in stability of the knee. Am J Sports Med 1995;23:436.

160. Veltri DM, Warren RF. Posterolateral instability of the knee. J Bone Joint Surg 1994;76(A):460.

161. Watanabe Y, Moriya H, Takahashi K, Yamagata M. Functional anatomy of the posterolateral structures of the knee. Arthroscopy 1993;9:57.

162. Seebacher J, Inglis A, Marshall J, et al. The structure of the posterolateral aspect of the knee. J Bone Joint Surg [Am] 1982;64:536.

163. Noyes FR, Barber-Westin SD. Surgical reconstruction of severe chronic posterolateral complex injuries of the knee using allograft tissues. Am J Sports Med 1995;23:2.

164. Murphy BJ, Smith RL, et al. Bone signal abnormalities in the posterolateral tibia and lateral femoral condyle in complete tears of the anterior cruciate ligament: a specific sign? Radiology 1992;182:221.

165. Speer KP, Warren RF, Wickiewicz TL, Horowitz L. Observations on the injury mechanism of anterior cruciate ligament tears in skiers. Am J Sports Med 1995;23:77.

166. Fowler PJ. Bone injuries associated with anterior cruciate ligament disruption. Arthroscopy 1994;10:453.

167. Weber WN, Nuemann CH, Barakos JA, et al. Lateral tibial rim (Segond) fractures: MR imaging characteristics. Radiology 1991; 180:731.

168. Kezdi-Rogus PC, Lomasney LM. Plain film manifestations of ACL injury. Orthopaedics 1994;17:969.

169. Mink JH, et al. Tears of the anterior cruciate ligament and menisci of the knee: MR imaging evaluation. Radiology 1988;167:769.

170. Lee JK, et al. Anterior cruciate ligament tears: MR imaging compared with arthroscopy and clinical tests. Radiology 1988;166:861.

171. Vallet AD, et al. Accuracy of nonorthogonal magnetic resonance imaging in acute disruption of the anterior cruciate ligament. Arthroscopy 1989;5:287.

172. Karzel RP, et al. Arthroscopic diagnosis and treatment of cruciate and collateral ligament injuries. In: Scott W, et al, eds. Arthroscopy of the knee. Philadelphia: WB Saunders, 1990:131.

173. Buss DD, Min R, Skyhar M, Galinat B. Nonoperative treatment of acute anterior cruciate ligament injuries in a selected group of patients. Am J Sports Med 1995;23:160.

174. Loosli A, Oshimo T. Conservatively treated anterior cruciate ligament injuries: activities, symptoms, and roentgenographic changes. Clin J Sports Med 1994;4:228.

175. Ciccotti MG, Lombardo SJ, Nonweiler B, Pink M. Non-operative treatment of ruptures of the anterior cruciate ligament in middle-aged patients. J Bone Joint Surg 1994;76(A):1315.

176. Nogalski MP, Bach BR Jr. A review of early anterior cruciate ligament surgical repair or reconstruction. Orthop Rev 1993;November:1213.

177. Boden BP, et al. Arthroscopically-assisted anterior cruciate ligament reconstruction: a follow-up study. Contemp Orthop 1990;20:187.

178. Arnoczky SP, et al. Replacement of the anterior cruciate ligament using patellar tendon allograft. J Bone Joint Surg [Am] 1986;68:376.

179. Fox JM, et al. Techniques and preliminary results in arthroscopic anterior cruciate prosthesis. Presented at the 53rd Annual Meeting of the American Academy of Orthopaedic Surgeons; February 20, 1986; New Orleans, LA.

180. Zarins B, et al. Combined anterior cruciate ligament reconstruction using semitendinosus tendon and iliotibial tract. J Bone Joint Surg [Am] 1986;68:160.

181. Grood ES. Placement of knee ligament grafts. In: Aichroth PM, Cannon WD, Disnitz M, eds. Knee surgery: current practice. London: Martin Dunitz, 1992:116.

182. Souryal TO, Freeman TR. Intercondylar notch size and anterior cruciate ligament injuries in athletes: a prospective study. Am J Sports Med 1993;21:535.

183. LaPrade RF, Burnett QM II. Femoral intercondylar notch stenosis and correlation to anterior cruciate ligament injuries: a prospective study. Am J Sports Med 1994;22:198.

184. Herzog RJ, Silliman JF, Hutton K, Rodkey WG. Measurements of the intercondylar notch by plain film radiography and magnetic resonance imaging. Am J Sports Med 1994;22:204.

185. Boynton MD, Fadale PD. The basic science of anterior cruciate ligament surgery. Orthop Rev 1993;June:673.

186. Abe S, Kurosaka M, Iguchi T, Yoshiya S, et al. Light and electron microscopic study of remodeling and maturation process in autogenous graft for anterior cruciate ligament reconstruction. Arthroscopy 1993;9:394.

187. Deutsch AL, Mink JH. The postoperative knee. In: Mink JH, Reicher MA, Crues JV, Deutsch AL, eds. MRI of the knee. New York: Raven Press, 1993:237.

188. Morgan CD, Kalman CR, Grawl DM. Definitive landmarks for reproducible tibial tunnel placement in anterior cruciate ligament reconstruction. Arthroscopy 1995;11:275.

189. Jackson DW, Gasser SI. Tibial tunnel placement in ACL reconstruction. Arthroscopy 1994;10:124131.

190. Howell SM, Taylor MA. Failure of reconstruction of the anterior cruciate ligament due to impingement by the intercondylar roof. J Bone Joint Surg 1993;75(A):1042.

191. Vergis A, Gillquist J. Graft failure in intra-articular anterior cruciate ligament reconstructions: a review of the literature. Arthroscopy 1995;11:312.

192. Howell SM, Barad SJ. Knee extension and its relationship to the slope of the intercondylar roof. Implications for positioning the tibial tunnel in anterior cruciate ligament reconstructions. Am J Sports Med 1995;23:288.

193. Howell SM, Knox KE, Farley TE, Taylor MA. Revascularization of a human anterior cruciate ligament graft during the first two years of implantation. Am J Sports Med 1995;23:42.

194. Rak KM, et al. Anterior cruciate ligament reconstruction: evaluation with MR imaging. Radiology 1991;178:553.

195. Moeser P, et al. MR imaging of anterior cruciate ligament repair. J Comput Assist Tomogr 1989;13:105.

196. MacIntosh DL, Darby JA. Lateral substitution reconstruction. In: Proceedings of the Canadien Orthopaedic Association. J Bone Joint Surg 1976;58(B):142.

197. Fezoulidis I, et al. MRI of the status following augmentation plasty of the anterior crucite ligament using carbon fibers. Radiology 1989;29;550.

198. Maywood RM, Murphy BJ, Uribe JW, Hechtman KS. Evaluation of arthroscopic anterior cruciate ligament reconstruction using magnetic resonance imaging. Am J Sports Med 1993;21:523.

199. Parker AW, Drez D, Cooper JL. Anterior cruciate ligament injuries in patients with open physes. Am J Sports Med 1994;22:44.

200. Nottage WM, Matsuura PA. Management of complete traumatic anterior cruciate ligament tears in the skeletally immature patient: current conceptrs and review of the literature. Arthroscopy 1994;10:569.

201. Watanabe BM, Howell SM. Arthroscopic findings associated with roof impingement of an anterior cruciate ligament graft. Am J Sports Med 1995;23:616.

202. Recht MP, Piraino DW, Cohen MAH, Parker RD. Localized anterior arthrofibrosis (cyclops lesion) after reconstruction of the anterior cruciate ligament: MR imaging findings. AJR Am J Roentgenol 1995;165:383.

203. Howell SM, Berns GS, Farley TE. Unimpinged and impinged anterior cruciate ligament grafts: MR signal intensity measurements. Radiology 1991;179:639.

204. Coupens SD, Yates CK, Sheldon C, et al. Magnetic resonance imaging evaluation of the patellar tendon after use of its center one-third for anterior cruciate ligament reconstruction. Am J Sports Med 1992;20:332.

205. Hughston JC, et al. Classiciation of knee ligament instabilities: I. the medial compartment and cruciate ligaments. J Bone Joint Surg [Am] 1976;58:159.

206. Kennedy JC. The posterior cruciate ligament. J Trauma 1967;7:367.

207. Covery DC, Sapega AA. Anatomy and function of the posterior cruciate ligament. Clinics Sports Med 1994;13:509.

208. Williams PL, et al. Gray's Anatomy. 37th ed, Edinburgh: Churchill-Livingstone, 1989:527.

209. Harner CD, Xerogeanes JW, Livesay GA, Carlin GJ, et al. The human posterior cruciate ligament complex: an interdisciplinary study. Ligament morphology and biomechanical evaluation. Am J Sports Med 1991;19:626.

210. Clancy WG, et al. Treatment of knee joint instability secondary to rupture of the posterior cruciate ligament: report of a new procedure. J Bone Joint Surg [Am] 1983;65:310.

211. Kennedy JC, Grainger RW. The posterior cruciate ligament. J Trauma 1966;7:367.

212. Kennedy JC, et al. Tension studies of human knee ligament. J Bone Joint Surg [Am] 1976;7:367.

213. Javadpour SM, Finegan PJ, Glacken P, O'Brien M. Anatomy of the posterior cruciate ligament ligament and its length patterns during knee flexion. Clinical Jounral Sports Medicine. New York: Raven Press, 1994;4:125.

214. Turner, et al. Acute injury of the ligaments of the knee: magnetic resonance evaluation. Radiology 1985;154:717.

215. Loos WC, et al. Acute posterior cruciat ligament injuries. Am J Sports Med 1981:9:86.

216. Seebacher JR, et al. The structures of the postero-lateral aspect of the knee. J Bone Joint Surg [Am] 1982;64:536.

217. Miller MD, Harner CD. Posterior cruciate ligament injuries. Current concepts in diagnosis and treatment. Physician Sports Med 1993;21:38.

218. Covey DC, Sapega AA. Current concepts review. Injuries of the posterior cruciate ligament. J Bone Joint Surg 1993;75(A):1376.

219. Miller MD, Johnson DL, Harner CD, Fu FH. Posterior cruciate ligament injuries. Orthop Rev 1993;November:1201.

220. Hughston JC, et al. Acute tears of the posterior cruciate ligament: results of operative treatment. J Bone Joint Surg [Am] 1980;62:438.

221. Fanelli GC. Posterior criciate ligament injuries in trauma patients. Arthroscopy 1993;9:291.

222. Giessler WB, Whipple TL. Intraarticular abnormalities in association with posterior cruciate ligament injuries. Am J Sports Med 1993;21:846.

223. Andrews JR, Edwards JC. Isolated posterior cruciate ligament injuries. Clinics Sports Med 1994:519.

224. Fanelli GC, Giannotti BF, Edson CJ. The posterior cruciate ligament. Arthroscopic evaluation and treatment. Arthroscopy 1994;10:673.

225. Grover JS, et al. Posterior cruciate ligament: MR imaging. Radiology 1990;174:527.

226. Sonin AH, Fitzgerald SW, Hoff FL, Friedman H, et al. MR imaging of the posterior cruciate ligament: Normal, abnormal, and associated injury patterns. Radiographics 1995;15:552.

227. Sonin AH, Fitzgerald SW, Friedman H, Hoff FL, et al.. Posterior cruciate ligament injury: MR imaging diagnosis and patterns of injury. Radiology 1994;190:455.

228. Cherney S. The knee. In: Dee R, et al, eds. Principles of orthopaedic practice. New York: McGraw-Hill, 1989:1054.

229. Fetto JR, et al. Medical collateral ligament injuries of the knee: a rationale for tratment. Clin Orthop 1978;132:206.

230. Anderson JE, eds. Grant's atlas of anatomy. Baltimore: Williams & Wilkins, 1983.

231. Indelicato PA, et al. Nonoperative management of complete tears of the medial collateral ligament. Orthop Rev 1989;18:947.

232. Kennedy JC, et al. Medial and anterior instability of the knee. An anatomical and clinical study using stress machines. J Bone Joint Surg [Am] 1971;53:1257.

233. Schweitzer MS, Tran D, Deely DM, Hume EL. Medial collateral ligament injuries: evaluation of multiple signs, prevalence and location of associated bone bruises and assesment with MR imaging. Radiology 1995;194:825.

234. Stoller DW, Mink J. MRI detection of knee fractures. American Roentgen Ray Society; April 15–May 1, 1987; Miami, FL. Abstract.

235. Forbes JR, Helms CA, Janzen DL. Acute pes anserine bursitis: MR Imaging. Radiology 1995;194:525.

236. Yu JS, Salonen DC, Hodler J, Haghighi O, Trudell D, et al. Posterolateral aspect of the knee: improved MR imaging with a coronal oblique technique. Radiology 1996;198:199.

237. Ekman EF, Pope T, Martin DF, Cuel WW. Magnetic resonance imaging of iliotibial band syndrome. Am J Sports Med 1994;22:851.

238. Westrich GH, Hannafin JA, Potter HG. Isolated rupture and repair of the popliteus tendon. Arthrscopy 1995;22:628.

239. Veltri DM, Warren RF. Operative treatment of posterolateral instability of the knee. Clinics Sports Med 1994;13:615.

240. Resnick D, Niwayama G. Diagnosis of bone and joint disorders, 2nd ed, vol 3. Philadelphia: WB Saunders, 1988:1455.

241. Outerbridge RE. The etiology of chondromalacia patellae. J Bone Joint Surg 1961;43(B):752.

242. Lombardo SJ, Bradley JP. Arthroscopic diagnosis and treatment of patellofemoral disorders. In: Scott W, et al, eds. Arthroscopy of the knee. Philadelphia: WB Saunders, 1990:155.

243. Deutsch AL, Shellock FG. The exterior mechanism and patellohemoral joint in MRI of the knee, 2nd ed. Mink J.H., Reichan M.A., Crues J.V. III; Deutsch A.L. New York: Raven Press, 1993:189.

244. Rose PM, Demlow TA, Szumowski J, Quinn SF. Chondromalacia patellae: Fat-suppressed MR Imaging. Radiology 1994;193:437.

245. Gagliardi JA, Chung EM, Chandnani VP, Kesling KL, Christensen KP, Null RN, Radvany MG, Hansen MF. Detection and Staging of Chondromalacia patellae: Relative efficacies of conventional MR Imaging, MR arthrography, and CT arthrography. AJR Am J Roentgenol 1994;163:629.

246. Yulish BS, et al. Chondromalacia patellae: assessment with MR imaging. Radiology 1987;164:763.

247. Conway WF, Hayes CW, Loughran T, et al. Cross-sectional imaging of the patellofemoral joint and surrounding structures. Radiographics 1991;11:195.

248. Hayes CW, et al. Patellar cartilage lesions: in vitro detection and staging with MR imaging and pathologic correlation. Radiology 1990;176:479.

249. Sueyoshi Y, Shimozaki E, Matsumoto T, Tomita K. Two cases of dorsal defect of the patella with arthroscopically visible cartilage surface perforations. Arthroscopy 1993;9:164.

250. Dandy DJ. Chondral and osteochondral legions of the hemoral condyles. In: Aichroth PM, Cannon WD, Disnitz M, eds. Knee surgery: current practice. London: Martin Dunitz, 1992:443.

251. Aichroth PM, Al-Duri, Z. Dislocation and subluxation of the patella: an overview. In: Aichroth PM, Cannon WD, Disnitz M, eds. Knee surgery: current practice. London: Martin Dunitz, 1992:354.

252. Merchant, AC. Patellohemoral disorders. In: Chapman MW, ed. Operative orthopaedics, 2nd ed. Philadelphia: JB Lippincott, 1993:2063.

253. Merchant, AC. Radiologic evaluation of the patellohemoral joint. In: Aichroth PM, Cannon WD, Disnitz M, eds. Knee surgery: current practice. London: Martin Dunitz, 1992:380.

254. Fullerson, JP. Patellar malalignment. In: Aichroth PM, Cannon DW, Disnitz M, eds. Knee surgery: current practice. London: Martin Dunitz, 1992:389.

255. Laurin CA, Dussault R, Levesque AP. The tangential X-ray investigation of the patellofemoral joint. Clin Orthop 1979;144:16.

256. Brossman J, Muhle C, Schroder C, Melchert UH, Bull CC, Spielmann RP, Heller M. Patellar tracking patterns during active and passive knee extension: Evaluation with motion-triggered cine MR Imaging. Radiology 1993;187:205.

257. Shellock FG, Mink JH, Deutsch AL, Fox J, Molnar T, Kvitne R, Ferkel R. Effect of a patellar realignment brace on patellofemoral relationships: Evaluation with kinematic MR Imaging. J Magn Reson Imaging 1994;4:590.

258. Sonin AH, Fitzgerald SW, Bresler ME, Kirsch MD, Hoff FL, Friedman H. MR Imaging Appearance of the Extensor Mechanism of the knee: Functional anatomy and Injury patterns. Radiographics 1995;15:367.

259. Lance E, Deutsch AL, Mink H. Prior lateral patellar dislocaton: MR imaging findings. Radiology 1993;189:905.

260. Kirsch MD, Fitzgerald SW, Friedman H, Rogers LF. Transient lateral patellar dislocation: Diagnosis with MR imaging. AJR Am J Roentgenol 1993;161:109.

261. Murphy BJ, Hechtman KS, Uribe JW, Selesnick H, et al. Iliotibial band friction syndrome: MR imaging findings. Radiology 1992;185:569.

262. Tortensen ET, Bray RC, Wiley JP. Patellar tendinitis: a review of current concepts and treatment. Clin J Sports Med 1994;4:77.

263. Yu JS, Popp JE, Kaeding CC, Lucas J. Correlation of MR Imaging and Pathologic findings in athletes undergoing surgery for chronic patellar tendinitis. AJR Am J Roentgenol 1995;165:115.

264. McLoughlin RF, Raber EL, Vellet AD, Wiley JP, et al. Patellar tendinitis: MR imaging fractures, with suggested pathogenesis and proposed classification. Radiology 1995;197:843.

265. Rockwood CA Jr, Green DP, Heckman JD, Bucholz RW. Fractures in Adults, 4th ed. Philadelphia: Lippincott-Raven, 1996.

266. Weissman BNW, Sledge CB. Orthopaedic radiology. Philadelphia: WB Saunders, 1986:497.

267. Stanitski CL. Anterior knee pain syndromes in the adolescent. Am Acad Orthop Surg 1993;75(A):1407.

268. Grelsamer RP, Cartier P. Comprehensive approach to patellar pathology. Orthopaedics 1990;20:493.

269. Stoller DW, Genant HK. MR Imaging of knee arthritides. Radiology 1987;165(P):233.

270. Buckwalter JA, Martin, J. Degenerative Joint Disease. Ciba Clinical Symposia 1995;47(2):

271. Mori Y, Kubo M, Okumo H, Kuroki Y. a scanning electron microscopic study of the degenerative cartilage in patellar chondropathy. Arthroscopy 1993;9:237.

272. Recht MP, Resnick D. MR Imaging of articular cartilage: Current status and future directions. AJR Am J Roentgenol 1994;163:283.

273. Recht MP, Kramer J, Marcelis S, Pathria MN, Trudell D, Haghighi P, Sartoris DJ, Resnick D. Abnormalities of articular cartilage in the knee: analysis of available MR techniques. Radiology 1993;187:473.

274. Disler DG, Peters TL, Muscoreil SJ, Ratner LM, Wagle WA, Cousins JP, Rifkin MD. Fat-suppressed spoiled GRASS imaging of knee hya-

line cartilage: technique optimization and comparison with conventional MR imaging. AJR Am J Roentgenol 1994;163:887.

275. Disler DG, McCauley TR, Wirth CR, Fuchs MD. Detection of knee hyaline cartilage defects using fat-suppressed three-dimensional spoiled gradient-echo MR imaging: comparison with standard MR imaging and correlation with arthroscopy. AJR Am J Roentgenol 1995;165:377.

276. Peterfy CG, Majumdar S, Lang P, van Dijke CF, Sack K, Genant, HK MR Imaging of the arthritic knee: improved discrimination of cartilage, synovium, and effusion with pulsed saturation transfer and fat-suppressed T1-weighted sequences. Radiology 1994;191:413.

277. Tervonen O, Dietz MJ, Carmichael SW, Ehman RL. MR Imaging of knee hyaline cartilage: evaluation of two- and three-dimensional sequences. J Magn Reson Imaging 1993;3:663.

278. Broderick LS, Turner DA, Renfrew DL, Schnitzer TJ, Huff JP, Harris, C. Severity of articular cartilage abnormality in patients with osteoarthritis: evaluation with fast spin-echo MR vs. arthroscopy. AJR Am J Roentgenol 1994;162:99.

279. Gylys-Morin VM, Hajek PC, Sortoris DJ et al; Articular cartilage defects: detectability in cadaver knees with MR. AJR Am J Roentgenol 148:1153, 1987.

280. Wolff SD, Chesnick S, Frank JA, Lim KO, Balaan RS. Magnetization Transfer Contrast: MR imaging of the knee. Radiology 1991;179:623.

281. Chandnani VP, Ho C, Chu P, et al. Knee hyaline cartilage evaluated with MR imaging: A cadaveric study involving multiple imaging sequences and intraarticular injection of gadolinium and saline solution. Radiology 1991;178:557.

282. Björkengren AG, Geborek P, Rydholm U, et al. MR imaging of the knee in acute rheumatoid arthritis: synovial uptake of gadolinium-DTPA. AJR Am J Roentgenol 1990;155:329.

283. Rodrigo JL, Gershwin ME. Management of the arthritic joint. In: Chapman MW, ed. Operative orthopaedics, 2nd ed. Philadelphia: JB Lippincott, 1993.

284. Stoller DW. MRI in juvenile rheumatoid (chronic) arthritis. Presented at the meeting of the Association of University Radiologists; March 22–27, 1987; Charleston, SC.

285. Konig H, et al. Rheumatoid arthritis: evaluation of hypervascular and fibrous pannus with dynamic MR imaging enhanced with Gd-DTPA. Radiology 1990;176:473.

286. Adam G, et al. Rheumatoid arthritis of the knee: value of gadopentetate dimeglumine-enhanced MR imaging. AJR Am J Roentgenol 1991;156(Jan):125.

287. Ostergaard M, Gideon P, Wieslander S, Henriksen O, Lorenzen I. Pannus-induced destruction of joint cartilage and subchondral bone: visualization and staging by MRI. Magma 1994;2:91.

288. Stoller DW, Genant HK. MRI of pigmented villonodular synovitis. American Roentgen Ray Society; May 8–13, 1988; San Francisco. Abstract.

289. Kottal RA, et al. Pigmented villonodular synovitis: report of MR imaging in two cases. Radiology 1987;163:551.

290. Poletti SC, et al. The use of magnetic resonance imaging in the diagnosis of pigmented villonodular synovitis. Orthopaedics 1990;13:185.

291. Muscolo DL, Makino A, Costa-Paz, M, Ayerza MA. Localized pigmented villonodular synovitis of the posterior compartment of the knee: diagnosis with magnetic resonance imaging. Arthroscopy 1995;11:482.

292. Kulkarni MV, et al. MR imaging of hemophiliac arthropathy. JCAT 1986;10:445.

293. Yulish BS, et al. Hemophilic arthropathy: assessment with MR imaging. Radiology 1987;164:759.

294. Johnston YE, et al. Lyme arthritis: spirochetes found in synovial microangiopathic lesions. Am J Pathol 1985;118:26.

295. Lawson JP, Rahn DW. Lyme disease and radiologic findings in lyme arthritis. AJR Am J Roentgenol 1992;158:1065.

296. Jouben LM, Steele RJ, Bono JV. Orthopaedic manifestations of Lyme disease. Orthop Rev 1994;May:395.

297. Kindynis P, et al. Osteophytosis of the knee: anatomic, radiologic and pathologic investigation. Radiology 1990;174:841.

298. Rosenberg, TD, Paulos, LE, Parker, RD et al. The forty-five degree, posteroanterior flexion weight-bearing radiograph of the knee. J Bone Joint Surg [Am] 1988;70:1479.

299. Blais RE, LaPrade RF, Chaljub G, Adesokan A. The arthroscopic appearance of lipoma arborescens of the knee. Arthroscopy 1995;11:623.

300. Feller JF, Rishi M, Hughes EC. Lipoma arborescens of the knee: MR demonstration. AJR Am J Roentgenol 1994;163:162.

301. Shapiro GS, Fanton GS. Intraarticular hemangioma of the knee. Arthroscopy 1993;9:464.

302. Kaneko K, De Money EH, Robinson AE. Distribution of joint effusion in patients with traumatic knee joint disorders: MRI assessment. Clin Imaging 17:176, 1993.

303. Guerra J, et al. Gastrocnemius-semimembranosus bursal region of the knee. AJR Am J Roentgenol 1981;136:593.

304. Lindgree PG, Willen R. Gastrocnemius-semimembranosus bursa and its relation to the knee joint. Anatomy and histology. Acta Radiol (Diagn) 1977;18:497.

305. Edmonson AS, Crenshaw AH, eds. Campbell's operative orthopaedics, vol 2. St. Louis: CV Mosby, 1980:1408.

306. Reich MA. The spectrum of knee joint disorders. In: Mink JH, Reich MA, Crues JV, Deutsch AL. MRI of the knee, 2nd ed. 333.

307. Johnson DP, Eastwood DM, Witherow PJ. Symptomatic synovial plicae of the knee. J Bone Joint Surg 1993;75(A):

308. Apple JS, et al. Synovial plicae of the knee. Skel Radiol 1982;7:251.

309. Calvo RD, et al. Managing plica syndrome of the knee. Physician Sports Med 1990;18:64.

310. Peterfy CG, van Dijke CF, Janzen DL, Gluer CC, Namba R, Majumdar S, Lang P, Genant HK. Quantification of articular cartilage in the knee with pulsed saturation tansfer subtration and fat-suppressed MR imaging: optimization and validation. Radiology 1994;192:485.

311. Burk DL, et al. 1.5T surface-coil MRI of the knee. AJR Am J Roentgenol 1986;147:293.

312. Williams JL, et al. Spontaneous osteonecrosis of the knee. Radiology 1973;107:15.

313. Lotke PA, Ecker MI. Osteonecrosis-like syndrome of the medial tibial plateau. Clin Orthop 1983;176:148.

314. Rahmouni A, Chosidow O, Mathieu D, Gueorguieva E, Jazaerli N, Radier C, Faivre J-M, Roujeau J-C, Vasile N. MR Imaging in acute infectious cellulitis. Radiology 1994;192:493.

315. Linden B. The incidence of osteochondritis dissecans in the condyles of the femur. Acta Orthop Scand 1976;47:664.

316. Mesgarzadah M, et al. Osteochondritis dissecans: analysis of mechanical stability with radiography, scintigraphy and MR imaging. Radiology 1987;165:775.

317. Resnick D, Niwayama G. Diagnosis of bone and joint disorders, 2nd ed, vol 5. Philadelphia: WB Saunders, 1988:3313.

318. De Smet AA, et al. Osteochondritis dissecans of the knee: value of MR imaging in determining lesion stability and pressence of articular cartilage defects. AJR Am J Roentgenol 1990;155:549.

319. Drape J-L, Thelen P, Gay-Depassier P, Silbermann O, Benacerraf R. Intraarticular Diffusion of Gd-DOTA after intravenous injection in the knee: MR imaging ealuation. Radiology 1993;188:227.

320. Berquist TH. Imaging of orthopaedic trauma and surgery. Philadelphia: WB Saunders, 1986:293.

321. Broderick LS, Turner DA, Renfrew DL, Schnitzer TJ, Huff JP, Harris C. Severity of articular cartilage abnormality in patients with osteoarthritis: evaluation with fast spin-echo MR vs. arthroscopy. AJR Am J Roentgenol 1994;162:99.

322. Peterfy CG, Majumdar S, Lang P, van Dijke CF, Sack K, Genant, HK MR Imaging of the arthritic knee: improved discrimination of cartilage, synovium, and effusion with pulsed saturation transfer and fat-suppressed T1-weighted sequences. Radiology 1994;191:413.

323. Jaramillo D, et al. Posttraumatic growth-plate abnormalities: MR imaging of bony-bridge formation in rabbits. Radiology 1990;175:767.

324. Jelinek JS, Kransdorf MJ, Shmookler BM, Aboulafia AA, Malawer MM. Giant Cell Tumor of the Tendon Sheath: MR findings in nine cases. AJR Am J Roentgenol 1994;162:919.

325. Ogilvie-Harris, DJ, Giddens J. Hoffa's disease: arthroscopic resection of the infrapatellar fat pad. Arthroscopy 1994;10:184.

326. Mink JH, et al. Occult cartilage and bone injuries of the knee: detection, classification and assessment with MR imaging. Radiology 1989;170:823.

327. Vellet AD, et al. Occult posttraumatic osteochondral lesions of the knee: prevalence, classification and short-term sequelae evaluated with MR imaging. Radiology 1991;178:271.

328. Tervonen O, Dietz MJ, Carmichael SW, Ehman RL. MR Imaging of knee hyaline cartilage: evaluation of two- and three-dimensional sequences. J Magn Reson Imaging 1993;3:663.

329. Lynch TCP, et al. Bone abnormalities of the knee: prevalence and significance of MR imaging. Radiology 1989;171:761.

330. Hohl M. Managing the challenge of tibial plateau fractures. J Muscle Med 1991;October:70.

331. Savage L, Garth WP. Intra-articular synovial cyst of the knee originating from a chondral fracture of the medial femoral condyle. J Bone Joint Surg 1994;76(A):1394.

332. Berquist TH, et al. Magnetic resonance imaging of the musculoskeletal system. New York: Raven Press, 1987:127.

333. Kressel HY, ed. Magnetic resonance imaging annual. New York: Raven Press, 1986:1.

334. Resnick D, Niwayama G. Diagnosis of bone and joint disorders, 2nd ed, vol 1. Philadelphia: WB Saunders, 1988:228.

335. Resnick D, Niwayama G. Diagnosis of bone and joint disorders, 2nd ed, vol 1. Philadelphia: WB Saunders, 1988.

336. Roberts MC, et al. Paget disease: MR imaging findings. Radiology 1989;173:341.

337. Rubenstein JD, Kim JK, Morava-Protzner I, Stanchev PL, Henkelman RM. Effects of collagen orientation on MR imaging characteristics of bovine articular cartilage. Rdiology 1993;188:219.

338. Erdman WA, Tamburro F, Jayson HT, et al. Osteomyelitis: characteristics and pitfalls of diagnosis with MR imaging. Radiology 1991;180:533.

Magnetic Resonance Imaging in Orthopaedics & Sports Medicine, Second Edition,
edited by David W. Stoller. Lippincott-Raven Publishers, Philadelphia, © 1997.

Chapter 8

The Ankle and Foot

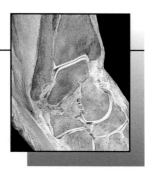

David W. Stoller
Richard D. Ferkel

Infection
> *Osteomyelitis*

Reflex Sympathetic Dystrophy
Plantar Fibromatosis
Plantar Fasciitis
Arthritis
Ganglions

Standard radiographic evaluation of the ankle joint requires anteroposterior (AP), lateral, and mortise radiographs. In patients with foot trauma, an additional oblique view may be obtained. Less frequently, arthrography and tomography may be used, primarily in the evaluation of ligamentous tears and articular cartilage defects. In tarsal coalitions and sustentacular trauma, computed tomography (CT) scans have been used to delineate talocalcaneal, transverse tarsal, and tibiotalar joint anatomy.[1] CT is limited, however, to the specific plane of section (ie, axial or angled coronal) and is dependent on reformatted images for visualization in the other orthogonal planes. Magnetic resonance (MR) imaging of the ankle and foot provides high tissue contrast and excellent spatial resolution, affording superior depiction of complex soft-tissue anatomy (eg, muscles, ligaments, tendons, and fibrous coalitions).[2–10] In addition, marrow and cortical bone definition permit increased sensitivity in the detection of fractures, cysts, inflammatory and infectious conditions, and trauma.[11] The unique ability of MR imaging to directly display hyaline articular cartilage has made it valuable in assessing arthritis and osteochondral lesions, and in identifying intraarticular loose bodies.

IMAGING PROTOCOLS FOR THE ANKLE AND FOOT

High resolution anatomic images of the ankle and foot are obtained with a dedicated extremity surface coil (quadrature or phased-array design), using a 12 to 14 cm field of view (FOV) and a 512 × 256 or 256 × 256 acquisition matrix (Fig. 8-1). Routine T1-weighted axial, sagittal, and coronal images are obtained with a repetition time (TR) of 500 to 600 msec and an echo time (TE) of 15 to 20 msec. Thin (ie, 3 mm) sections, either contiguous interleaved or with a 0.5 mm interslice gap, are preferred. T2-weighted axial images are obtained with conventional T2 or fat-suppressed T2-weighted fast spin-echo sequences. With the use of an extremity or head coil to optimize the signal-to-noise ratio, T1- and T2-weighted sequences can be performed at 1 excitation.

Effective T2*-weighted contrast can be generated with gradient-echo techniques using a partial flip angle of less than 90° (20° to 30°). Two-dimensional Fourier transform multiplanar gradient-echo protocols use a TR of 400 to 600 msec, a TE of 15 to 20 msec, and a flip angle of 20° to 30°. T1-weighted images may be supplemented with coronal and sagittal images obtained using either fast STIR or fat-suppressed T2-weighted fast spin-echo sequences. Axial three-dimensional Fourier transform (3DFT) T2* volume images with a 1 to 2 mm slice thickness may also be used to evaluate medial or lateral ligamentous structures.[12] Three-dimensional fast spin-echo using thin sections also has potential in the evaluation of medial and lateral ligamentous structures. Short TI inversion recovery (STIR and fast spin-echo STIR) images provide superior contrast in evaluating osteochondral lesions, bone contusions, and tendinitis.

To image the forefoot, the patient is placed in a prone position to orient the long axis of the foot with the orthogonal axial imaging plane or with the oblique image prescriptions parallel with the long axis of the metatarsals and cuneiform bones.

Surface coils, which allow proper placement of the foot with the patient in the supine position, can also be used to evaluate the long axis of the forefoot without drop-off of signal intensity. STIR and fast STIR sequences are useful

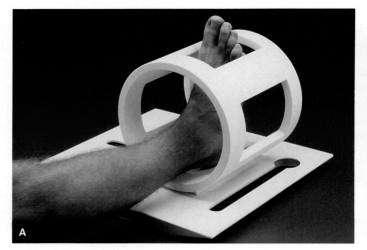
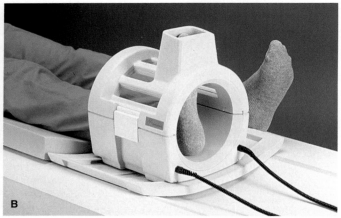

FIGURE 8-1. Quadrature design extremity coils used for ankle and foot imaging. **(A)** Open window configuration (MRI Devices, Waukesha, WI). **(B)** Forefoot extension configuration (Medical Advances, Milwaukee, WI).

in identifying forefoot lesions in the coronal plane and stress fractures in the sagittal plane.

By placing both legs within the circular extremity coil, comparison with the contralateral ankle and foot can be achieved. Alternatively, when smaller FOVs are needed, the extremities can be imaged one at a time by repositioning the surface coil. The foot is usually placed in a neutral position, although partial plantar flexion may be useful when comparing MR images to a CT ankle examination that was performed in 45° of tibiotalar angulation. A combination foot and ankle/knee coil provides adequate anatomic coverage for imaging the toes and distal metatarsals. Thin (3 mm or less) coronal T1 and STIR images are most useful. Kinematic techniques with the ankle in inversion and eversion in the coronal plane, in plantar flexion and dorsiflexion in the sagittal plane, and in internal or external rotation in the coronal or axial plane may also be used. However, these techniques are not routinely employed, and kinematic motion is not physiologic. Restricted range of motion, ligamentous instabilities, and tendon subluxations may necessitate the use of kinematic protocols.

Intravenous administration of a paramagnetic contrast agent, used in association with fat-suppression sequences, has demonstrated usefulness in the evaluation of Morton's neuroma, inflammatory synovial processes, and certain tendon pathologies (partial tear, healing, and infiltrative disorders). Intravenous and intraarticular contrast (MR arthrography) has been used on a limited basis in the study of osteochondral lesions and other intraarticular pathology. Articular cartilage is evaluated using a variety of techniques, including fat-suppressed T2-weighted fast spin-echo, fast spin-echo STIR, and MR arthrography. Fat-suppressed T2-weighted fast spin-echo and STIR contrast are the more frequently used sequences in characterizing muscle injuries.

ANATOMY OF THE ANKLE AND FOOT

Gross Anatomy

Compartments of the Leg

Anterior and posterior intermuscular septa and the interosseous membrane define the three major compartments of the lower leg (Fig. 8-2). The anterior compartment of the leg consists of the tibialis anterior, the extensor hallucis longus, the extensor digitorum longus, and the peroneus tertius muscles. The neurovascular bundle contains the deep peroneal nerve and the anterior tibial artery. The posterior compartment is divided into superficial and deep sections by deep transverse fascia. The superficial posterior compartment consists of the gastrocnemius, plantaris, and soleus muscles. The deep posterior compartment contains the popliteus, flexor digitorum longus, flexor hallucis longus, and tibialis posterior muscles. The neurovascular supply is provided by the tibial nerve and posterior tibial artery. The anterolateral compartment contains the peroneus longus and peroneus brevis muscles. The neurovascular supply is from the superficial peroneal nerve and branches of the peroneal artery.

Distal Tibiofibular Joint

The distal or inferior tibiofibular syndesmosis is a fibrous joint strongly connected by the interosseous ligament, which is continuous with the crural interosseous membrane. The tibiofibular syndesmosis is defined by the bony anatomy of the convex medial aspect of the distal fibula and corresponding concavity on the lateral aspect of the distal tibia[13,14] (Fig. 8-3). The stronger anterior and posterior inferior tibiofibular ligaments reinforce the joint anterior and posterior to the interosseous ligament. The transverse tibiofibular ligament represents the distal deep fibers of the posterior inferior tibiofibular ligament. In a recent review of 100 ankle arthroscopies (unpublished data), Ferkel and Rahhal identified four common variations of the arrangement of the posterior inferior tibiofibular ligament relative to the transverse tibiofibular ligament. The anterior inferior tibiofibular ligament extends obliquely from the anterior border of the lateral malleolus upward and medially to the anterolateral tibial tubercle more superiorly (see Fig. 8-3B).[13,14] The flat band of fibers may be divided into two or three bands, or may present as a multifasicular structure. The posterior inferior tibiofibular ligament is smaller than the anterior inferior tibiofibular ligament and is quadrilateral in shape.[13,14] Fibers originate from the posterior border of the lateral malleolus and extend superomedially onto the posterolateral tibial tubercle. The transverse tibiofibular ligament (the deep component of the posterior inferior tibiofibular ligament) is a strong thick band that extends from the posterior fibular tubercle and upper digital fossa and inserts on the posterior aspect of the tibial articular surface, reaching to the medial malleolus. The transverse tibiofibular ligament forms a posterior labrum by projecting inferiorly to the posterior tibial margin, thus deepening the tibial articular surface of the tibiotalar joint. The transverse ligament is in contact with the posterolateral talar articular cartilage surface. Posterior impingement may be caused by hypertrophy of the transverse ligament and its synovial covering.

Ankle Joint

The ankle or tibiotalar joint is a synovial articulation formed by the distal tibia and fibula. It is often described as a hinge joint between the talus and the mortise (Fig. 8-4). However, the apex of rotation of the ankle joint is not fixed, as it would be in a simple hinge joint. In fact, the apex of rotation changes during extremes of plantar flexion and dorsiflexion. The articular surfaces of the tibiotalar joint are covered with hyaline cartilage (Fig. 8-5). The fibrous capsule

text continues on page 448

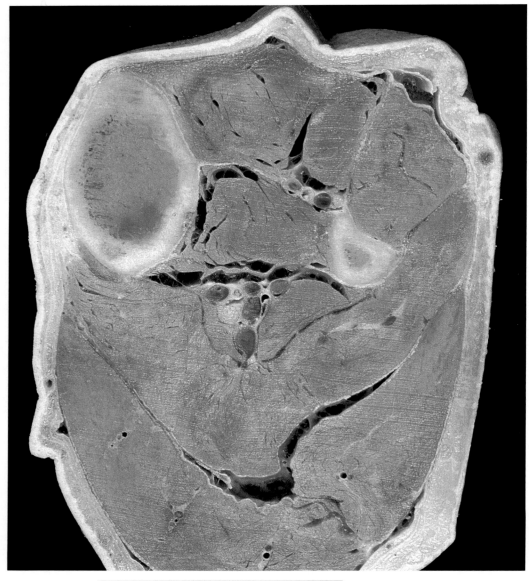

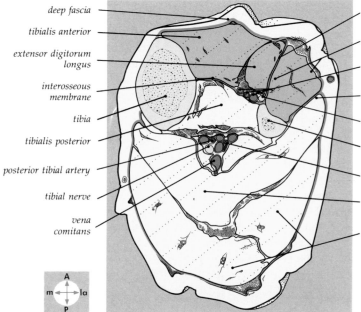

deep fascia

tibialis anterior

extensor digitorum
longus

interosseous
membrane

tibia

tibialis posterior

posterior tibial artery

tibial nerve

vena
comitans

anterior peroneal intermuscular septum

peroneus brevis & longus

anterior tibial artery & venae comitantes

posterior peroneal intermuscular septum

deep peroneal nerve

fibula

peroneal artery

soleus

medial & lateral heads of gastrocnemius

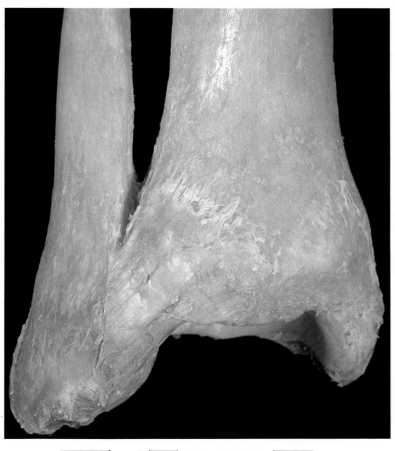

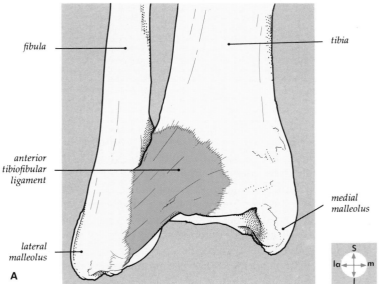

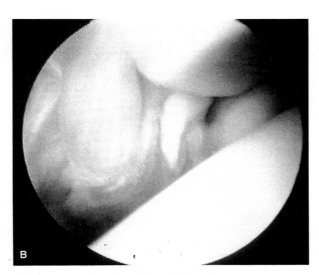

FIGURE 8-3. (**A**) The inferior tibiotalar joint is a fibrous joint. (**B**) Arthroscopic view of the right ankle demonstrating the syndesmotic ligament and the trifurcation. The trifurcation includes the fibula in the background with the tibia superior and the talus inferior. Approximately 20% of the ligament is intraarticular and it runs at a 45° angle from the tibia to the fibula.

FIGURE 8-2. A transverse section through the midcalf shows the anterior and lateral compartments and their contents.

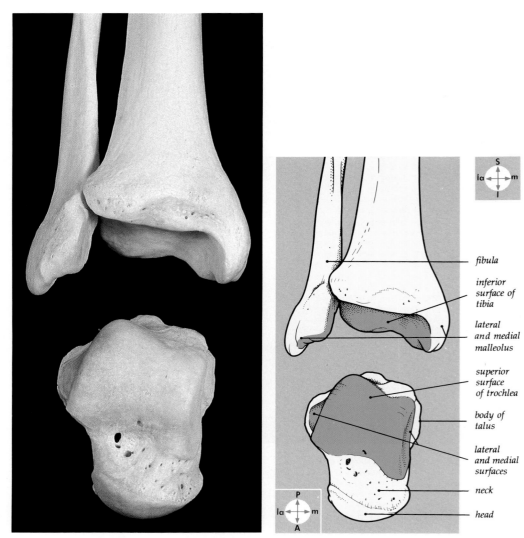

FIGURE 8-4. The bones of the ankle joint and their articular surfaces.

attaches to the articular margins of the tibia, fibula, and talus, with an anterior extension onto the talar neck. The capsule, which is thin anteriorly and posteriorly, is reinforced by strong collateral ligaments. The socket, framed by the distal tibia and medial and lateral malleoli, is wider anteriorly than posteriorly and is completed posteriorly by the transverse tibiofibular ligament (Fig. 8-6). The synovial membrane is attached to all articular margins and covers the intracapsular part of the talar neck.

Ankle Joint Ligaments

DELTOID LIGAMENT. The medial or deltoid ligament is a strong band attached by its apex to the border of the medial malleolus and consists of superficial and deep fibers (Fig. 8-7). The triangular, superficial part of the deltoid is formed by the tibionavicular fibers anteriorly, the tibiocalcaneal fibers medially (the strongest component of the superficial

deltoid), and the superficial posterior tibiotalar fibers posteriorly. Behind the navicular tuberosity, tibionavicular fibers blend with the medial margin of the plantar calcaneonavicular or spring ligament. A tibioligamentous fascicle inserts onto the superior border of the calcaneonavicular ligament. The deep part of the deltoid, which is rectangular, consists of a small anterior component (the anterior tibiotalar ligament) and a strong posterior component (the posterior tibiotalar ligament) (Fig. 8-8). The posterior tibiotalar ligament represents the strongest part of the entire medial ligament complex. The deep portion of the deltoid ligament, covered by synovium, is intraarticular.

LATERAL LIGAMENT. Three distinct bands make up the weaker lateral ligament of the ankle (Fig. 8-9). These ligamentous bands are the anterior talofibular ligament (see Fig.

text continues on page 452

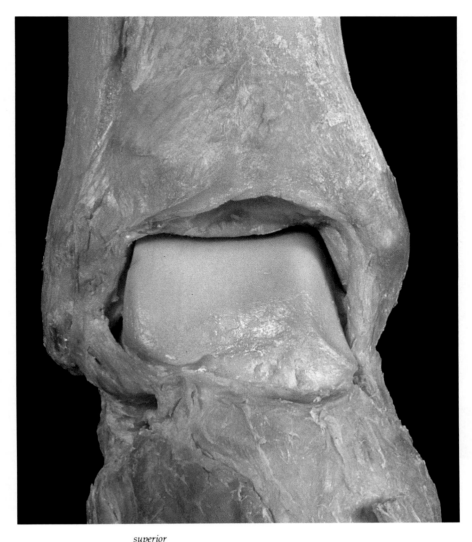

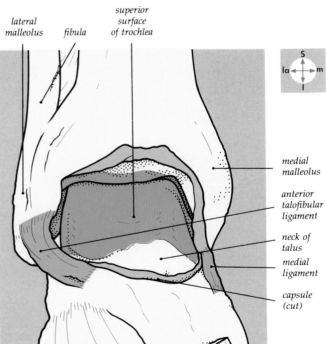

lateral malleolus

fibula

superior surface of trochlea

S

la ◆ m

l

medial malleolus

anterior talofibular ligament

neck of talus

medial ligament

capsule (cut)

FIGURE 8-5. An anterior view of the ankle joint and its articular surfaces is revealed by removal of the capsule.

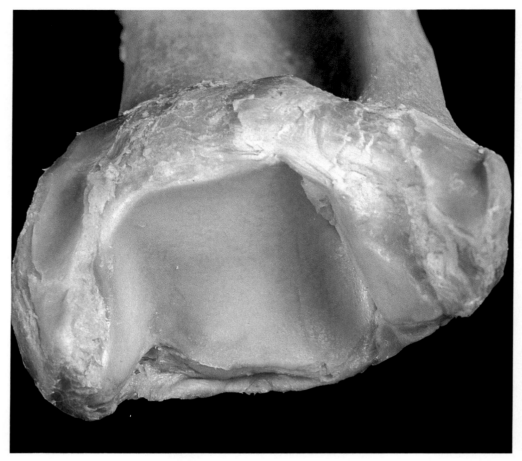

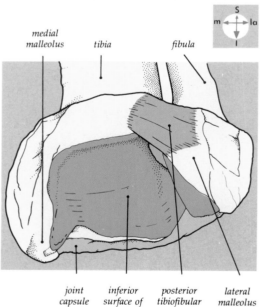

FIGURE 8-6. An oblique view of the wedge-shaped articular socket of the ankle joint.

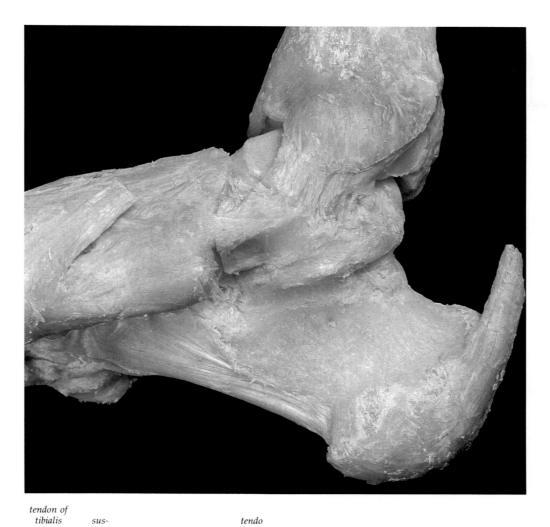

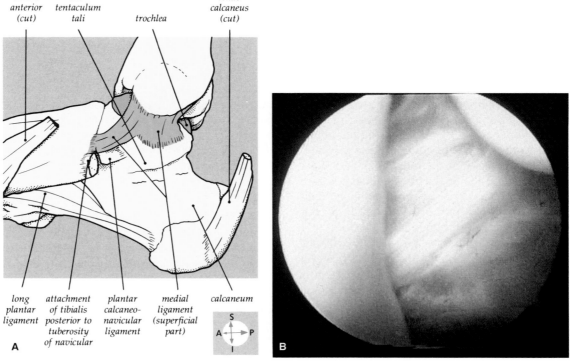

tendon of
tibialis
anterior
(cut)

sus-
tentaculum
tali

trochlea

tendo
calcaneus
(cut)

long
plantar
ligament

attachment
of tibialis
posterior to
tuberosity
of navicular

plantar
calcaneo-
navicular
ligament

medial
ligament
(superficial
part)

calcaneum

A

B

FIGURE 8-7. (**A**) The medial collateral ligament of the ankle joint can be seen after removal of the capsule. (**B**) In the right ankle, the deep portion of the deltoid ligament runs from the medial malleolus on the right to the talus on the left.

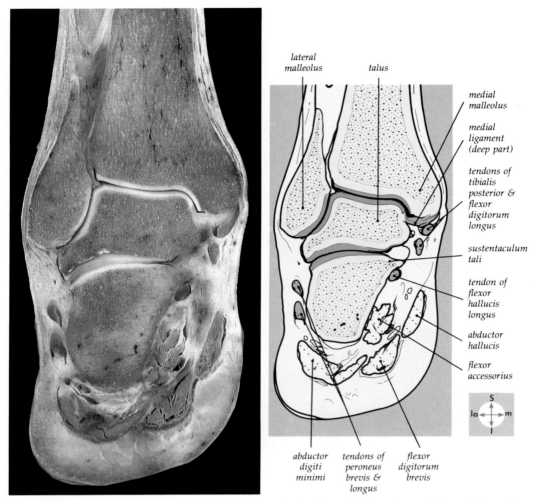

*lateral
malleolus*

talus

*medial
malleolus*

*medial
ligament
(deep part)*

*tendons of
tibialis
posterior &
flexor
digitorum
longus*

*sustentaculum
tali*

*tendon of
flexor
hallucis
longus*

*abductor
hallucis*

*flexor
accessorius*

*abductor
digiti
minimi*

*tendons of
peroneus
brevis &
longus*

*flexor
digitorum
brevis*

FIGURE 8-8. A coronal section through the ankle and talocalcaneal joints shows their articular surfaces.

8-9*B*), the calcaneofibular ligament, and the posterior talofibular ligament. The posterior inferior tibiofibular ligament lies superior to the horizontally oriented posterior talofibular ligament. The inferior part of the posterior inferior tibiofibular ligament is also referred to as the transverse tibiofibular ligament (Figs. 8-10 and 8-11). In dorsiflexion, the posterior talofibular (Fig. 8-12) and posterior inferior tibiofibular ligaments diverge like the blades of a scissors, and in plantar flexion, they lie edge to edge (see Fig. 8-10*B*).

The anterior talofibular ligament is a flat, relatively strong ligament, which may be divided into two bands. This ligament is taut in plantar flexion.[13,14] The calcaneofibular ligament is the largest of the lateral collateral ligaments, and is a strong, cord-like structure. It is deep to the peroneal tendons and their sheaths, and extends from the distal anterior border of the lateral malleolus inferiorly and posteriorly to insert on the upper part of the lateral surface of the calcaneus. The posterior talofibular ligament is the strongest and deepest portion of the

lateral ligament. It is intracapsular but extrasynovial. The posterior intermalleolar ligament or tibial slip originates on the posterior talofibular ligament, which inserts on the posterior tibia and posterior surface of the medial malleolus and blends with the transverse tibiofibular ligament.

Tarsal Joints

SUBTALAR JOINT. The subtalar or talocalcaneal joint is the posterior articulation between the talus and the calcaneus. Functionally, the subtalar joint includes the talocalcaneal part of the talocalcaneonavicular joint (Fig. 8-13). The strong talocalcaneal or interosseous ligament attaches to the sulcus tali and sulcus calcanei (see Fig. 8-13*B*). The capsule is strengthened by the medial and lateral talocalcaneal ligaments.

TALOCALCANEONAVICULAR JOINT. The talocalcaneonavicular joint is a multiaxial articulation at the triple-faceted

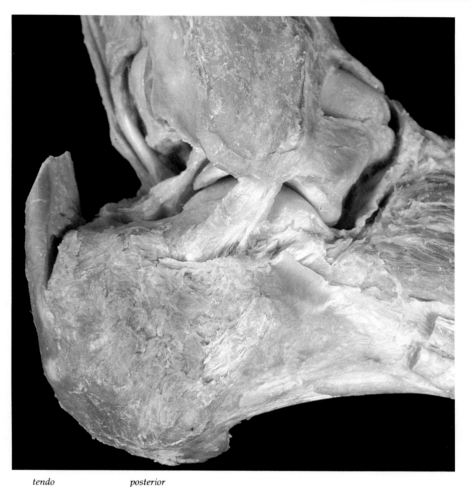

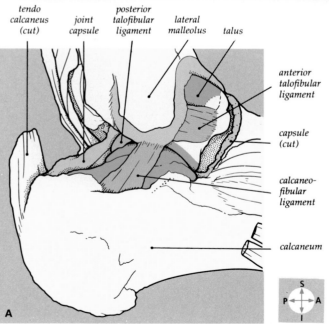

tendo
calcaneus
(cut)

joint
capsule

posterior
talofibular
ligament

lateral
malleolus

talus

anterior
talofibular
ligament

capsule
(cut)

calcaneo-
fibular
ligament

calcaneum

A

S
P ◆ A
I

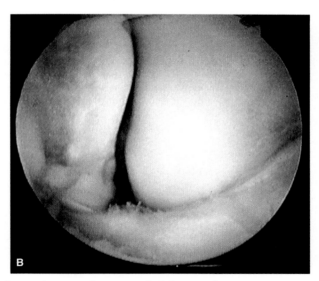

B

FIGURE 8-9. (**A**) The lateral collateral ligament of the ankle joint can he seen after removal of the capsule. (**B**) The anterior talofibular ligament is clearly demonstrated in this right ankle. The fibula is to the left, the talus is to the right. It forms the floor of the lateral gutter of the ankle.

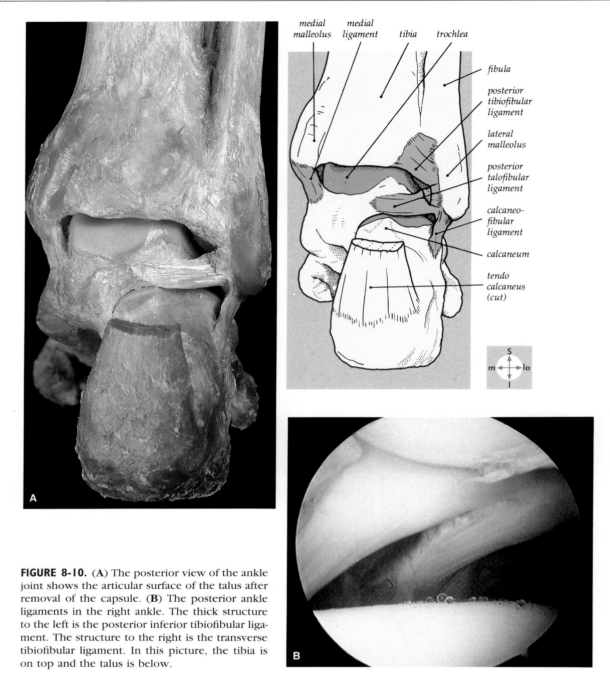

FIGURE 8-10. (**A**) The posterior view of the ankle joint shows the articular surface of the talus after removal of the capsule. (**B**) The posterior ankle ligaments in the right ankle. The thick structure to the left is the posterior inferior tibiofibular ligament. The structure to the right is the transverse tibiofibular ligament. In this picture, the tibia is on top and the talus is below.

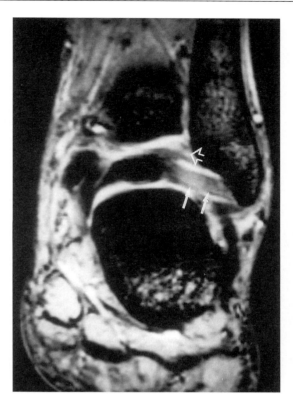

FIGURE 8-11. Transverse tibiofibular (*open arrow*) and posterior talofibular (*solid arrows*) ligaments are seen on a T2*-weighted coronal image.

anterior-inferior talar surface with the talar head, the posterior concavity of the navicular bone, the middle and anterior talar facets of the calcaneus, and the fibrocartilaginous superior surface of the plantar calcaneonavicular (ie, spring) ligament (see Fig. 8-13). The talonavicular, plantar calcaneonavicular, and calcaneonavicular parts of the bifurcated ligament support the osseous components of this joint.

CALCANEOCUBOID JOINT.   The calcaneocuboid joint is a separate joint with its own capsule between the anterior calcaneus and the posterior surface of the cuboid. The calcaneocuboid and talonavicular part of the talocalcaneonavicular joint form the midtarsal joint (Fig. 8-14). Support is provided by the fibrous capsule, the calcaneocuboid part of the bifurcated ligament, and the long plantar and plantar calcaneocuboid (ie, short plantar) ligaments. The bifurcated ligament is a strong, Y-shaped ligament on the dorsal surface of the joint, with attachments to the anterior dorsal calcaneal surface proximally, and to the dorsomedial aspect of the cuboid and dorsolateral aspect of the navicular bone distally. The long plantar ligament, also a strong ligament, is located along the plantar surface. It is attached to the undersurface of the calcaneus, the cuboid, and the bases of the third, fourth, and fifth metatarsal bones. A tunnel for the peroneus longus is created as it bridges the tendon's groove on the cuboid's plantar surface. The plantar calcaneocuboid, or short plantar

ligament, is a wide, short band attached to the anterior tubercle on the plantar aspect of the calcaneus and the adjacent surface of the cuboid.

OTHER TARSAL JOINTS.   The cuneonavicular synovial joint is formed by the navicular bone and the three cuneiform bones (see Fig. 8-14). The cuboideonavicular joint is a fibrous joint. The intercuneiform and cuneocuboid joints are synovial joints continuous with the cuneonavicular joint cavity.

Regional Anatomy of the Ankle

RETINACULA.   The extensor (Fig. 8-15) and flexor (Fig. 8-16) retinacula are formed by thickened deep fascia and maintain the position of long tendons crossing the ankle. The superior extensor retinaculum attaches to the distal anterior fibula and tibia and invests the tibialis anterior tendon medially. The Y-shaped inferior extensor retinaculum attaches to the anterolateral part of the calcaneus (the stem)

text continues on page 460

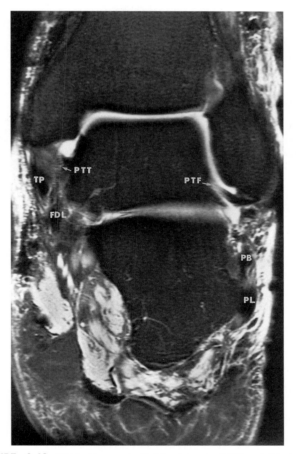

FIGURE 8-12. Posterior coronal fat-suppressed T2-weighted fast spin-echo image at the level of the posterior talofibular ligament (PTF) and posterior tibiotalar ligament (PTT). TP, tibialis posterior; FDL, flexor digitorum longus; PB, peroneus brevis tendon; PL, peroneus longus tendon.

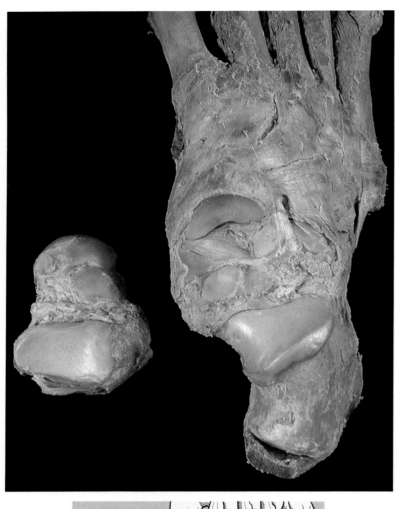

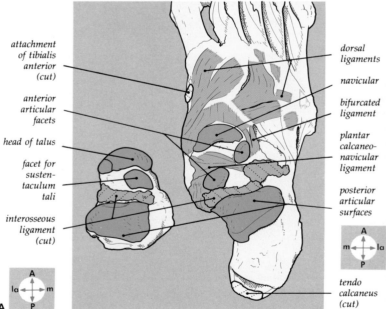

attachment of tibialis anterior (cut)

anterior articular facets

head of talus

facet for sustentaculum tali

interosseous ligament (cut)

dorsal ligaments

navicular

bifurcated ligament

plantar calcaneonavicular ligament

posterior articular surfaces

tendo calcaneus (cut)

A

B

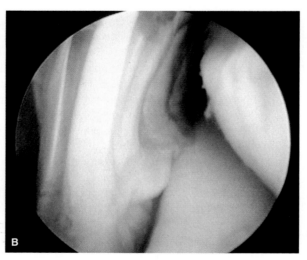

FIGURE 8-13. (A) In this gross photograph of the talocalcaneal and talonavicular joints, the talus has been disarticulated and turned over. (B) Arthroscopic picture of the interosseous ligament in the left ankle. The interosseous ligament is very thick and runs in an oblique vertical direction from the talus to the calcaneus. The talocalcaneal articulation is seen to the right of the ligament.

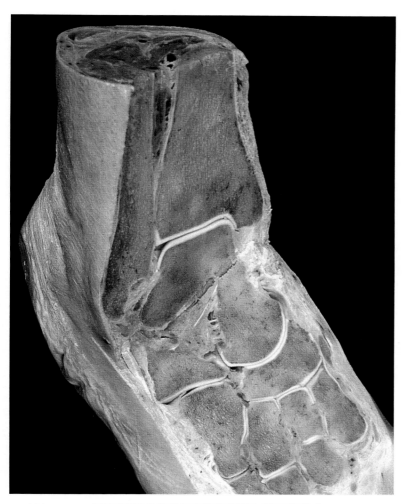

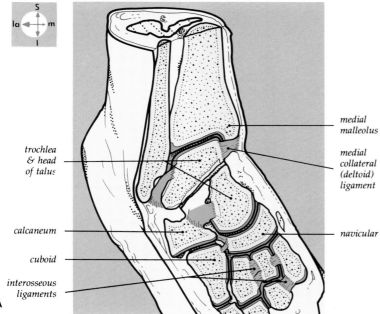

trochlea
& head
of talus

medial
malleolus

medial
collateral
(deltoid)
ligament

calcaneum

navicular

cuboid

interosseous
ligaments

A

FIGURE 8-14. (A) Vertical and horizontal sectioning of the foot and ankle reveals the interrelationships of the tarsal joints.   *continued*

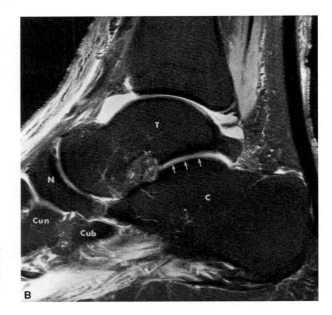

FIGURE 8-14. *Continued.* (**B**) Tibiotalar, subtalar, talonavicular, and navicular cuneiform joints are shown on a fat-suppressed T2-weighted sagittal image. The posterior facet of the subtalar joint is identified (*arrows*). T, talus; C, calcaneus; N, navicular bone; Cun, cuneiform bone; Cub, cuboid.

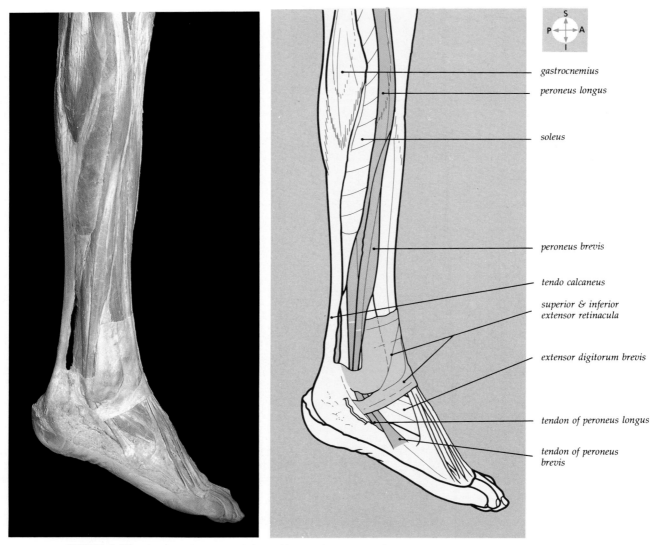

FIGURE 8-15. The lateral aspect of the ankle and foot shows the peroneal tendons and the retinacula.

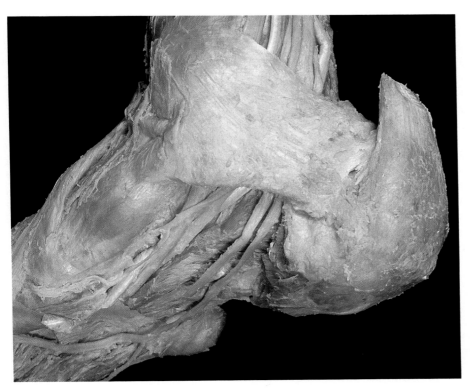

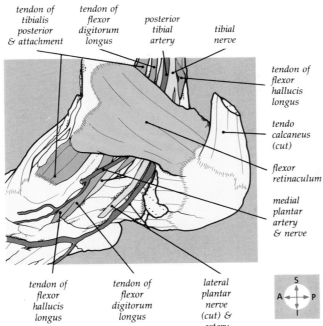

tendon of tibialis posterior & attachment   *tendon of flexor digitorum longus*   *posterior tibial artery*   *tibial nerve*

tendon of flexor hallucis longus

tendo calcaneus (cut)

flexor retinaculum

medial plantar artery & nerve

tendon of flexor hallucis longus   *tendon of flexor digitorum longus*   *lateral plantar nerve (cut) & artery*

FIGURE 8-16. The long tendons and the principal vessels and nerves from the posterior compartment of the leg pass deep to the flexor retinaculum to enter the sole of the foot.

and extends to the medial malleolus (the upper limb) and the medial plantar fascia (the lower limb) (see Fig. 8-15). The tibialis anterior, the extensor hallucis longus, the extensor digitorum longus, and the peroneus tertius tendons dividethe upper limb of the retinaculum into superficial and deep layers. The flexor retinaculum extends inferiorly and posteriorly from the medial malleolus to the medial calcaneal surface (see Fig. 8-16). The tendons of the deep calf muscles (the flexor digitorum longus, the flexor hallucis longus, and the tibialis posterior) and the neurovascular structures in the posterior compartment pass underneath the flexor retinaculum before entering the foot.

The superior peroneal retinaculum extends inferiorly and posteriorly from the lateral malleolus to the lateral calcaneal surface, binding the peroneus longus and brevis tendons (see Fig. 8-15). The inferior peroneal retinaculum is attached to the peroneal trochlea and calcaneus above and below the peroneal tendons.

ANTERIOR STRUCTURES. The saphenous nerve, the great saphenous vein, and the medial and lateral branches of the superficial peroneal nerve pass anterior to the extensor retinaculum in a medial-to-lateral direction. The tibialis anterior tendon, the extensor hallucis longus tendon, the anterior tib-

ial artery with venae comitantes, the deep peroneal nerve, the extensor digitorum longus tendon, and the peroneus tertius pass deep to or through the extensor retinaculum in a medial-to-lateral direction (Figs. 8-17 and 8-18).

POSTERIOR STRUCTURES. The tibialis posterior tendon (PTT), the flexor digitorum longus, the posterior tibial artery with venae comitantes, the tibial nerve, and the flexor hallucis longus flow in a medial-to-lateral direction and are located posterior to the medial malleolus and deep to the flexor retinaculum (see Fig. 8-18). The sural nerve and the small saphenous vein pass posterior to the lateral malleolus, superficial to the superior peroneal retinaculum. The peroneus longus and brevis tendons course posterior to the lateral malleolus deep to the superior peroneal retinaculum (see Fig. 8-18). The pre-Achilles fat pad and the Achilles tendon are located posterior to the ankle. The plantaris tendon (see Fig. 8-18*B*) is identified medial to the Achilles tendon and joins the anteromedial aspect of the Achilles tendon at the level of the subtalar joint.

Foot

MUSCLES OF THE SOLE OF THE FOOT. Deep to the plantar aponeurosis (Fig. 8-19), the muscles of the sole of the foot are divided into four layers from superficial to deep.

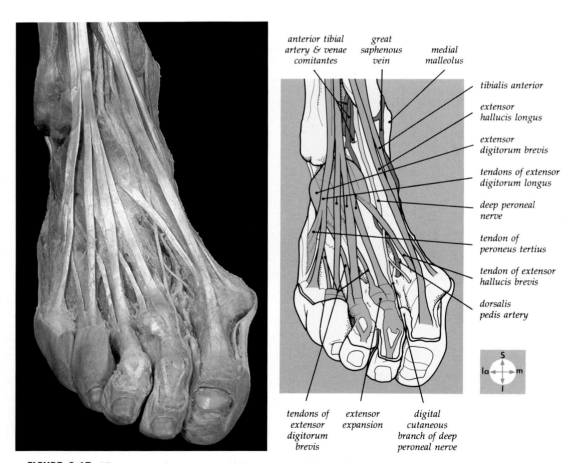

FIGURE 8-17. The principal structures of the dorsum of the ankle and foot can be seen after removal of the extensor retinaculum.

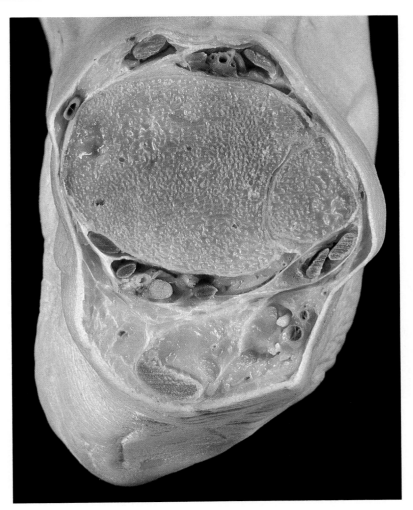

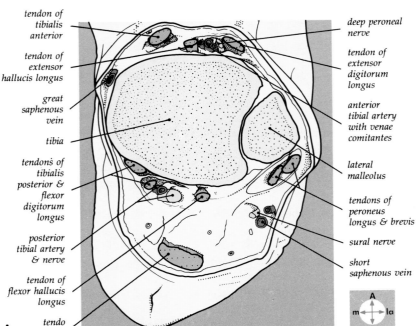

tendon of
tibialis
anterior

tendon of
extensor
hallucis longus

great
saphenous
vein

tibia

tendons of
tibialis
posterior &
flexor
digitorum
longus

posterior
tibial artery
& nerve

tendon of
flexor hallucis
longus

A   tendo
calcaneus

deep peroneal
nerve

tendon of
extensor
digitorum
longus

anterior
tibial artery
with venae
comitantes

lateral
malleolus

tendons of
peroneus
longus & brevis

sural nerve

short
saphenous vein

FIGURE 8-18. (A) A transverse section through the ankle immediately above the joint cavity shows its anterior and posterior relations.   *continued*

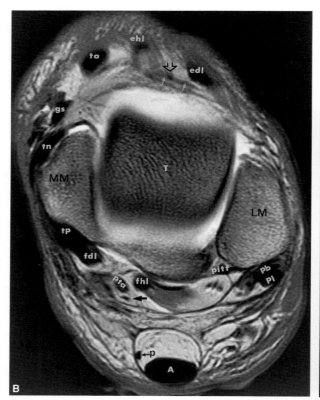
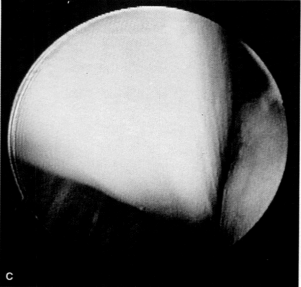

FIGURE 8-18. *Continued.* **(B)** T1 axial MR arthrographic image at the level of the talar dome. Note the position of the distal plantaris tendon (p) medial to the Achilles tendon. MM, medial malleolus; tp, tibialis posterior; fdl, flexor digitorum longus tendon; pta, posterior tibial artery; arrow, tibial nerve; fhl, flexor hallucis longus tendon; pitf, posterior inferior tibiofibular ligament; p, plantaris tendon; A, Achilles tendon; pb, peroneus brevis tendon; pl, peroneus longus tendon; LM, lateral malleolus; T, talus; edl, extensor digitorum longus tendon; open arrow, deep peroneal nerve; white arrows, anterior tibial artery; ehl, extensor hallucis longus tendon; ta, tibialis anterior; gs, greater saphenous vein; tn, tibionavicular ligament. **(C)** The flexor hallucis longus tendon is an extraarticular structure that cannot usually be seen within the ankle. It normally runs in a sheath just posterior to the ankle capsule and medial to the transverse ligament.

The first layer consists of the abductor hallucis, the flexor digitorum brevis, and the abductor digiti minimi (Fig. 8-20). The second layer consists of the quadratus plantae, the lumbricals, the flexor digitorum longus tendons, and the flexor hallucis longus tendons (Fig. 8-21). The third layer includes the flexor hallucis brevis, the adductor hallucis, and the flexor digiti minimi brevis (Fig. 8-22). The fourth layer is made up of the interossei plantares (Fig. 8-23), the peroneus longus tendon, and the tibialis posterior tendon (Fig. 8-24).

ARCHES OF THE FOOT. The arches of the foot provide support for bipedal motion and forward propulsion. The medial and lateral longitudinal arches are formed by the tarsal and metatarsal bones (Fig. 8-25). The higher medial arch, which forms the instep of the foot, consists of the

calcaneus, the talus, the navicular, the three cuneiform bones, and the medial three metatarsals (see Figs. 8-25 and 8-26). The plantar calcaneonavicular (ie, spring) ligament helps support the head of the talus, which articulates with the navicular anteriorly and the sustentaculum tali posteriorly (Fig. 8-27). The lateral arch consists of the calcaneus, the cuboid, and the lateral two metatarsals. Body weight is transmitted through the anterior and posterior pillars of the arches. The posterior pillar of the medial and lateral arches are the tubercles on the inferior calcaneal surface. The anterior pillars of the medial and lateral arches are formed by their respective metatarsal heads. The transverse arch of the foot consists of the five metatarsal bones and the adjacent cuboid and cuneiform bones.

text continues on page 469

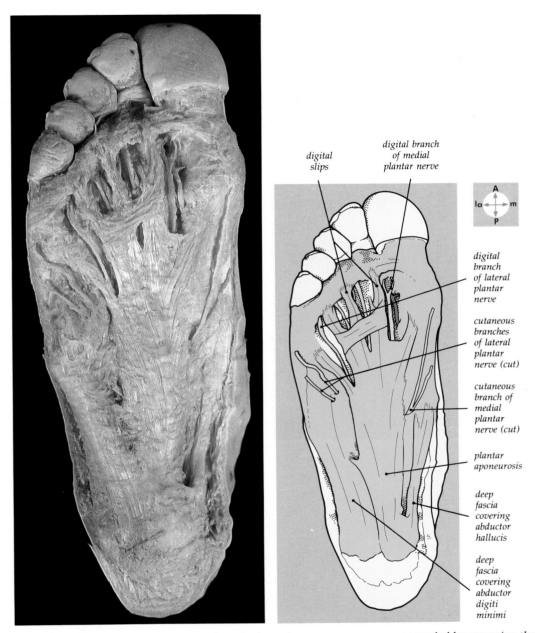

FIGURE 8-19. The plantar aponeurosis, deep fascia, and a cutaneous nerve are revealed by removing the skin of the sole of the foot.

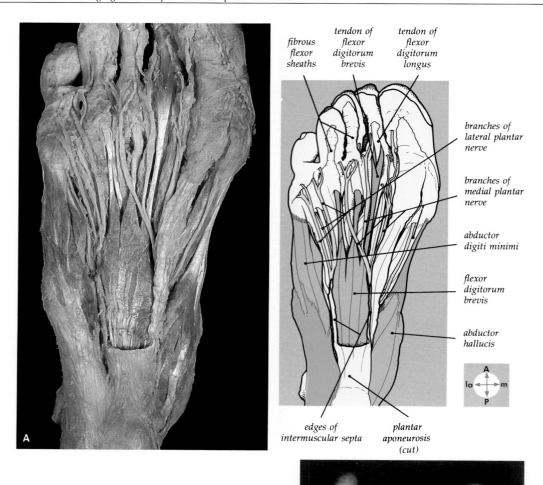

fibrous flexor sheaths

tendon of flexor digitorum brevis

tendon of flexor digitorum longus

branches of lateral plantar nerve

branches of medial plantar nerve

abductor digiti minimi

flexor digitorum brevis

abductor hallucis

edges of intermuscular septa

plantar aponeurosis (cut)

FDB

FIGURE 8-20. **(A)** The superficial intrinsic muscles and plantar nerves are shown after removal of the deep fascia, part of the plantar aponeurosis, and the second fibrous tendon sheath. In this specimen, the flexor digitorum brevis has only three tendons. **(B)** The flexor digitorum brevis (FDB) muscle and the tendons of the first layer of plantar muscles are shown on a T1-weighted axial image.

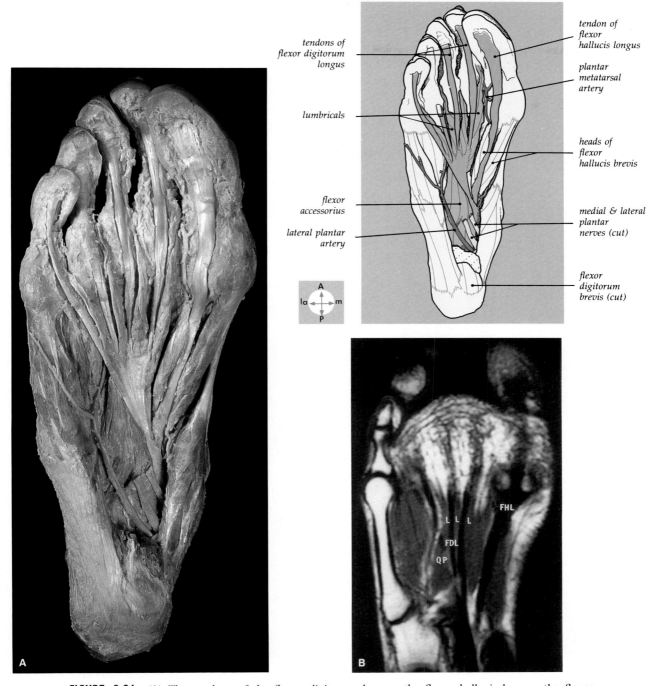

FIGURE 8-21. (A) The tendons of the flexor digitorum longus, the flexor hallucis longus, the flexor accessorius, and the lumbricals can be seen after removal of the medial and lateral plantar nerves and the tendons of the flexor digitorum brevis. (B) The quadratus plantae muscle (QP), lumbrical muscles (L), tendons of the flexor digitorum longus (FDL), and tendon of the flexor hallucis longus (FHL), all of the second layer of plantar muscles, are shown on a T1-weighted axial image.

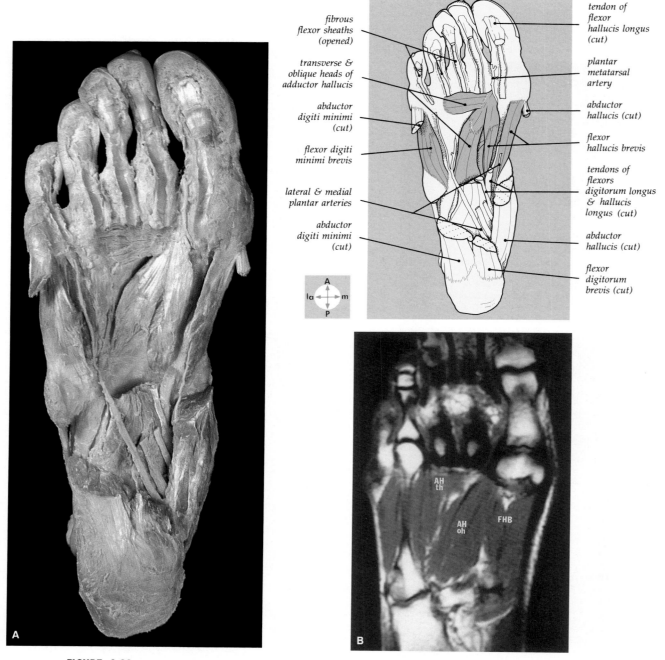

FIGURE 8-22. (A) The deep intrinsic muscles are revealed by removal of the long flexor tendon and abductors of the great and little toes. (B) The transverse head (th) and oblique head (oh) of the adductor hallucis muscle (AH) and the flexor hallucis brevis muscle (FHB) of the third layer of plantar muscles are shown on a T1-weighted axial image.

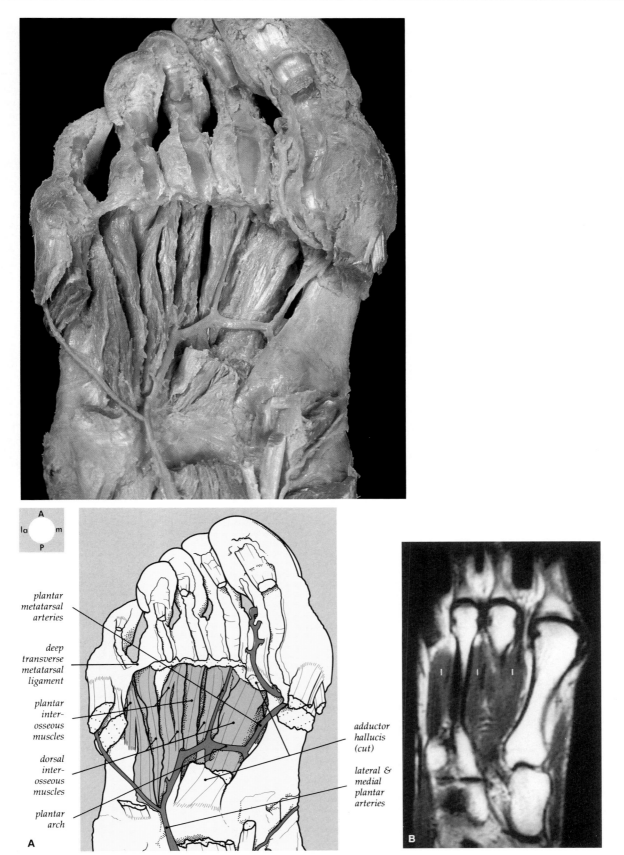

FIGURE 8-23. **(A)** The interosseous muscles and the plantar arterial arch are exposed by removal of the adductor hallucis. **(B)** The dorsal interosseous muscles (I) of the fourth layer of plantar muscles are shown on a T1-weighted axial image.

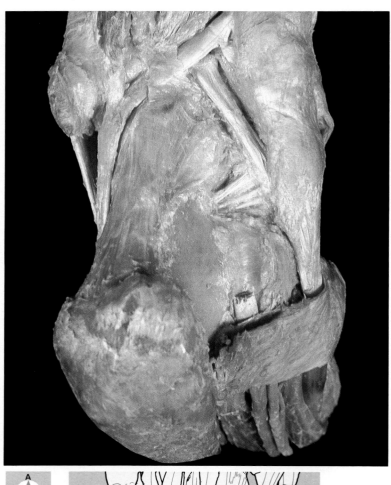

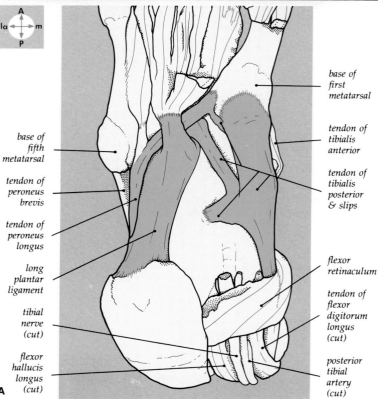

base of
first
metatarsal

tendon of
tibialis
anterior

tendon of
tibialis
posterior
& slips

flexor
retinaculum

tendon of
flexor
digitorum
longus
(cut)

posterior
tibial
artery
(cut)

base of
fifth
metatarsal

tendon of
peroneus
brevis

tendon of
peroneus
longus

long
plantar
ligament

tibial
nerve
(cut)

flexor
hallucis
longus
(cut)

FIGURE 8-24. (A) The tendons of the peroneus longus and the tibialis posterior lie deep in the sole of the foot. The long plantar ligament has been preserved. *continued*

A

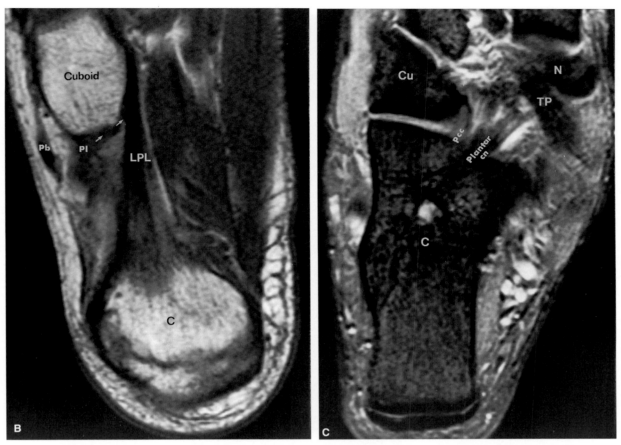

FIGURE 8-24. *Continued.* (**B**) T1-weighted axial image showing the long plantar ligament (LPL) and the course of the peroneus longus (pl) tendon as it passes along the inferior surface of the cuboid within an osseous groove (*arrow*). An inferior extension of the long plantar ligament creates a tunnel for the passage of the peroneus longus (pl) tendon proximal to its insertion on the base of the first metatarsal and medial cuneiform. pb, peroneus brevis tendon; C, calcaneus. (**C**) T2* axial image displays the tibialis posterior (TP), the plantar calcaneonavicular ligament (Plantar cn), and the plantar calcaneocuboid ligament (Pcc). Cu, cuboid; C, calcaneus; N, navicular bone.

METATARSOPHALANGEAL AND INTERPHALANGEAL JOINTS OF THE FOOT.   The metatarsophalangeal joints are ball-and-socket articulations between the metatarsal head and the base of the proximal phalanx and the fibrocartilaginous plantar plate (Figs. 8-28 through 8-30). The interphalangeal joints are hinge joints that permit flexion and extension (see Figs. 8-28 and 8-31).

Normal Magnetic Resonance Appearance of the Ankle and Foot

Axial Images

In the axial plane, the low signal intensity bands of the anterior and posterior inferior tibiofibular ligaments are demonstrated at the level of the tibial plafond (Fig. 8-32). The inferior extensor retinaculum is identified anterior to and at its attachment to the medial malleolus, and represents the upper limb of this Y-shaped band of deep fascia. On axial images through the tibiotalar joint, the tendons of the tibialis anterior, extensor hallucis longus, extensor digitorum longus, and peroneus tertius muscles occupy the anterior compartments in a medial-to-lateral direction. The peroneus brevis muscle and tendon and the more lateral peroneus longus tendon are located posterior to the lateral malleolus. The tendons of the tibialis posterior, flexor digitorum longus, and flexor hallucis longus can be identified posteriorly, running from a medial position posterior to the medial malleolus to a lateral position posterior to the tibial plafond and talar dome. Posterior and medial to the greater saphenous vein, the anterior tibionavicular fibers of the deltoid ligament blend with the low signal cortex of the anterior surface of the medial malleolus.

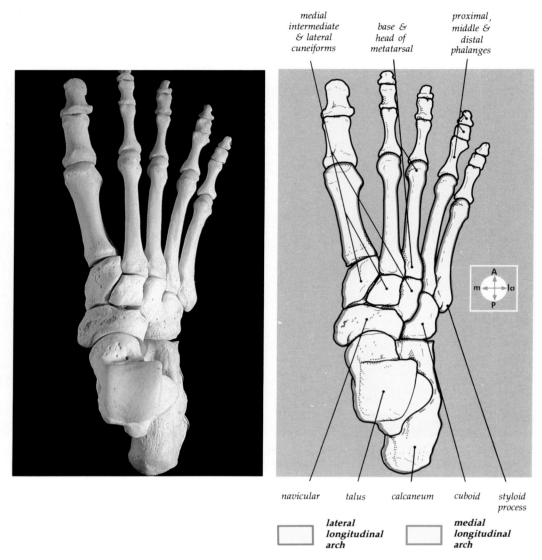

FIGURE 8-25. The dorsal aspect of the bones of the foot shows the medial and lateral longitudinal arches.

The Achilles tendon is identified in cross section as a thick structure of low signal intensity with a convex posterior surface and a flattened anterior surface. The posterior Achilles tendon is formed by the convergence of the gastrocnemius, plantaris, and soleus muscles. The soleus muscle group that is present at the level of the distal tibia is not seen at the tibiotalar joint level. Sections through the level of the distal lateral malleolus demonstrate the anterior and posterior talofibular ligaments. Medially, the tibionavicular and tibiocalcaneal parts of the deltoid ligament are also shown at this level. The peroneal retinaculum can be seen coursing medial and posterior to the lateral malleolus. The interosseous talocalcaneal ligament is posterolateral to either the anterior talus or the talar head. The plantar calcaneonavicular ligament, or spring ligament, is located inferior to the lateral malleolus between the lateral talus and tibialis posterior tendon.

The calcaneofibular ligament is optimally seen with the foot in 40° of plantar flexion, and on neutral axial images it can be seen lateral to the posterior inferior talus and anterior and medial to the peroneus brevis tendon. The sural nerve, intermediate in signal intensity, is located posteromedial to the peroneus brevis muscle. The tibial nerve is medial to the flexor hallucis longus tendon and continues distally as the medial and lateral plantar nerves. The flexor retinaculum is superficial to the tendons of the deep muscles on the medial side of the ankle. In the foot, the tendons of the flexor hallucis brevis and longus muscles are seen posterior to the first metatarsal and cuneiform. The longitudinally oriented quadratus plantae and abductor hallucis muscles are medial to the calcaneus and cuboid. The peroneus longus tendon—a fourth-layer muscle of the sole of the foot—enters the foot by passing posterior to the lateral malleolus and can be

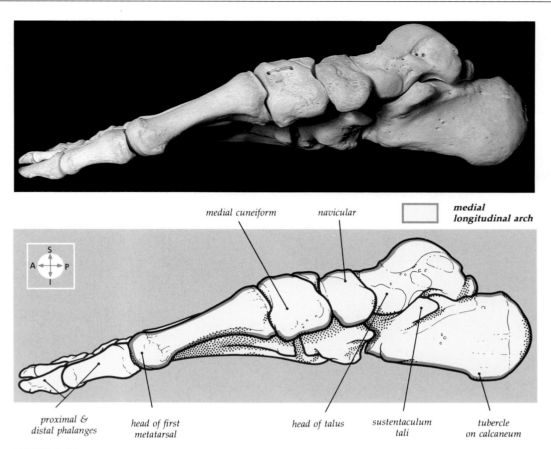

FIGURE 8-26. The medial aspect of the bones of the foot shows the medial longitudinal arch (blue).

seen obliquely crossing the foot to its insertion onto the base of the first metatarsal and medial cuneiform bone.

The anterior neurovascular bundle, composed of the anterior tibial artery and vein and deep peroneal nerve, is located posterior to the extensor tendons, whereas the posterior neurovascular bundle, composed of the posterior tibial artery, vein, and tibial nerve, is located posterior to the flexor digitorum and flexor hallucis longus tendons.

Sagittal Images

The long axis of the tendons crossing the ankle joint can be seen on sagittal planar images (Fig. 8-33).

MEDIAL SAGITTAL IMAGES. In the plane of the medial malleolus, the tibialis posterior and flexor digitorum longus tendons are directly posterior to the medial malleolus. The tibialis posterior tendon enters the foot by passing deep to the flexor retinaculum and superior to the sustentaculum tali to its insertion on the tuberosity of the navicular bone. The flexor digitorum longus tendon also enters the foot after passing posterior to the medial malleolus and deep to the flexor retinaculum. This tendon is divided into four segments

after crossing the flexor hallucis longus tendon, which contributes slips to the medial two divisions. These segments insert onto the bases of the distal phalanges. The quadratus plantae muscle inserts at the division of the flexor hallucis into four tendons. Distally, each tendon is an origin for the lumbrical muscles.

The deltoid ligament, composed of the tibiocalcaneal, tibionavicular, and anterior and posterior tibiotalar ligaments, appears as a wide band of low signal intensity radiating from the distal tibia (ie, medial malleolus) to the tuberosity of the navicular bone and the sustentaculum tali. The flexor hallucis longus tendon is located posterior to the tibialis posterior tendon and the flexor digitorum longus. It passes posterior to the medial malleolus, deep to the flexor retinaculum. The low signal intensity tendon hugs the posterior talar process and inferior surface of the sustentaculum tali proximal to its insertion onto the base of the distal phalanx of the great toe.

The plantar flexor digitorum brevis (a first-layer muscle of the sole of the foot) and the quadratus plantae (a second-layer muscle of the sole of the foot) are displayed on medial

text continues on page 496

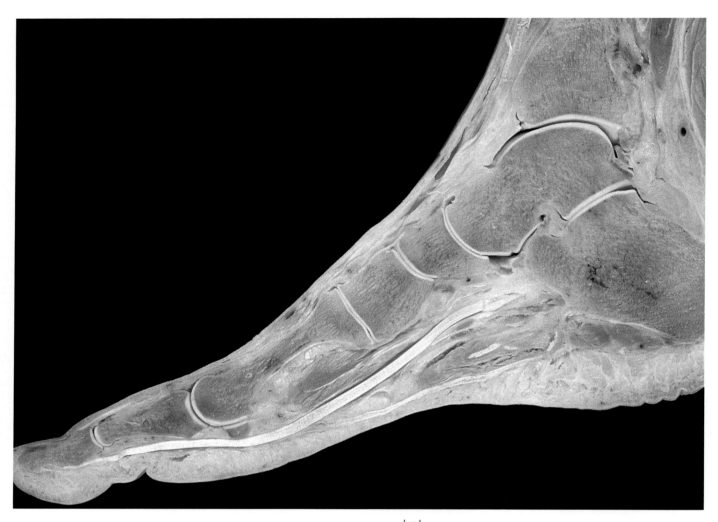

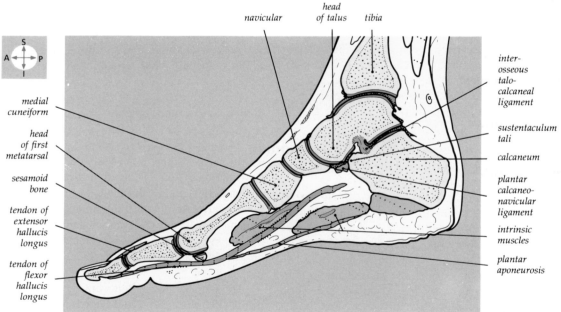

FIGURE 8-27. A sagittal section of the foot shows the medial longitudinal arch.

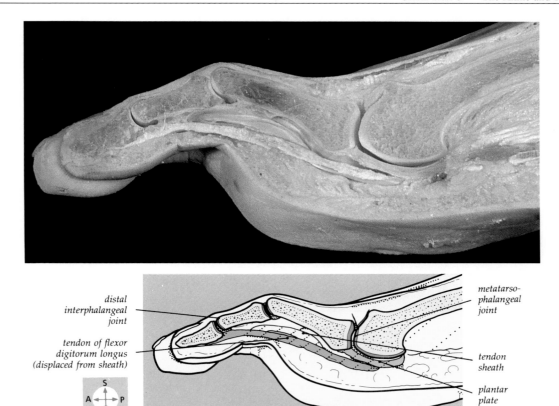

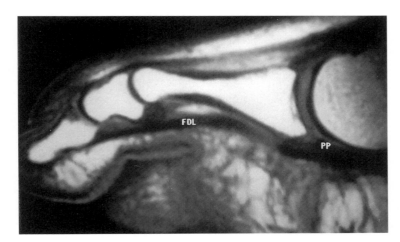

FIGURE 8-28. A sagittal section through the third toe shows the metatarsophalangeal and interphalangeal joints.

FIGURE 8-29. A T1-weighted sagittal image demonstrates the tendon of the flexor digitorum longus (FDL) and the plantar plate (PP).

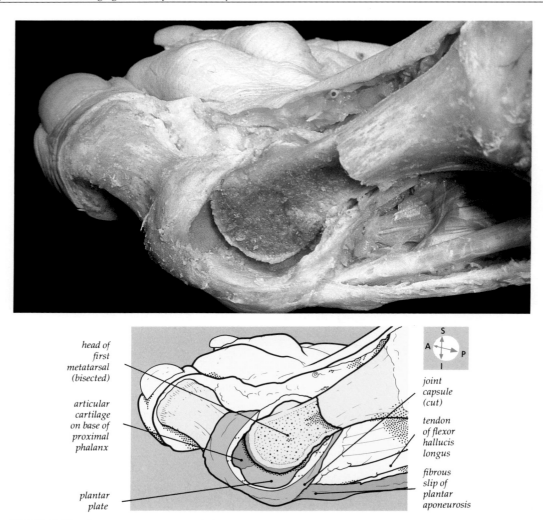

FIGURE 8-30. The internal features of the first metatarsophalangeal joint are revealed when part of the capsule and the distal part of the metatarsal bone are removed.

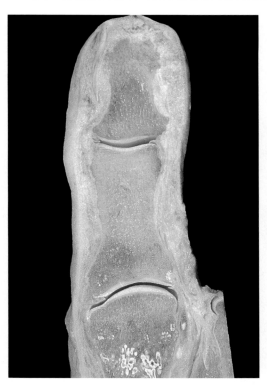

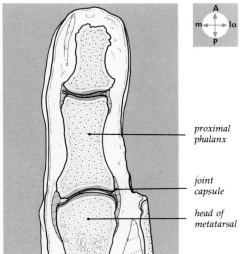

proximal
phalanx

joint
capsule

head of
metatarsal

FIGURE 8-31. A longitudinal section through the great toe shows its joints.

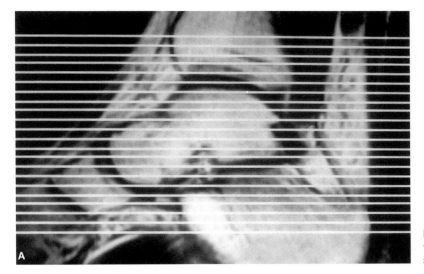

FIGURE 8-32. Normal axial MR anatomy. **(A)** This T1-weighted sagittal localizer was used to prescribe axial image locations from **(B)** superior to **(W)** inferior.

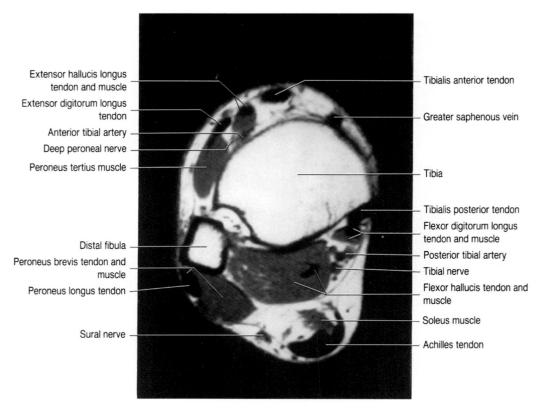

Extensor hallucis longus tendon and muscle

Extensor digitorum longus tendon

Anterior tibial artery

Deep peroneal nerve

Peroneus tertius muscle

Distal fibula

Peroneus brevis tendon and muscle

Peroneus longus tendon

Sural nerve

Tibialis anterior tendon

Greater saphenous vein

Tibia

Tibialis posterior tendon

Flexor digitorum longus tendon and muscle

Posterior tibial artery

Tibial nerve

Flexor hallucis tendon and muscle

Soleus muscle

Achilles tendon

FIGURE 8-32B.

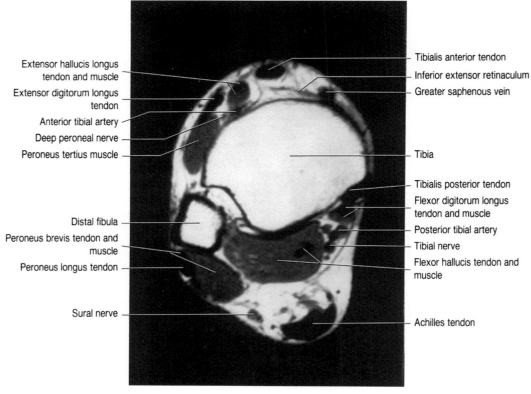

Extensor hallucis longus tendon and muscle

Extensor digitorum longus tendon

Anterior tibial artery

Deep peroneal nerve

Peroneus tertius muscle

Distal fibula

Peroneus brevis tendon and muscle

Peroneus longus tendon

Sural nerve

Tibialis anterior tendon

Inferior extensor retinaculum

Greater saphenous vein

Tibia

Tibialis posterior tendon

Flexor digitorum longus tendon and muscle

Posterior tibial artery

Tibial nerve

Flexor hallucis tendon and muscle

Achilles tendon

FIGURE 8-32C.

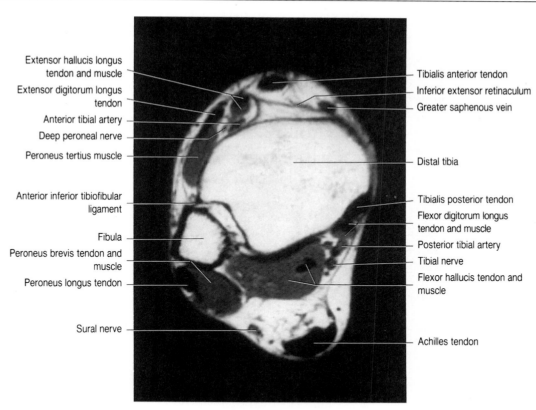

Extensor hallucis longus tendon and muscle
Extensor digitorum longus tendon
Anterior tibial artery
Deep peroneal nerve
Peroneus tertius muscle

Anterior inferior tibiofibular ligament

Fibula
Peroneus brevis tendon and muscle
Peroneus longus tendon

Sural nerve

Tibialis anterior tendon
Inferior extensor retinaculum
Greater saphenous vein

Distal tibia

Tibialis posterior tendon
Flexor digitorum longus tendon and muscle
Posterior tibial artery
Tibial nerve
Flexor hallucis tendon and muscle

Achilles tendon

FIGURE 8-32D.

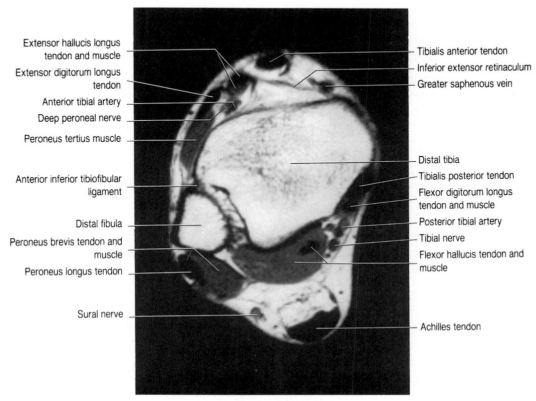

Extensor hallucis longus tendon and muscle
Extensor digitorum longus tendon
Anterior tibial artery
Deep peroneal nerve
Peroneus tertius muscle

Anterior inferior tibiofibular ligament

Distal fibula
Peroneus brevis tendon and muscle
Peroneus longus tendon

Sural nerve

Tibialis anterior tendon
Inferior extensor retinaculum
Greater saphenous vein

Distal tibia
Tibialis posterior tendon
Flexor digitorum longus tendon and muscle
Posterior tibial artery
Tibial nerve
Flexor hallucis tendon and muscle

Achilles tendon

FIGURE 8-32E.

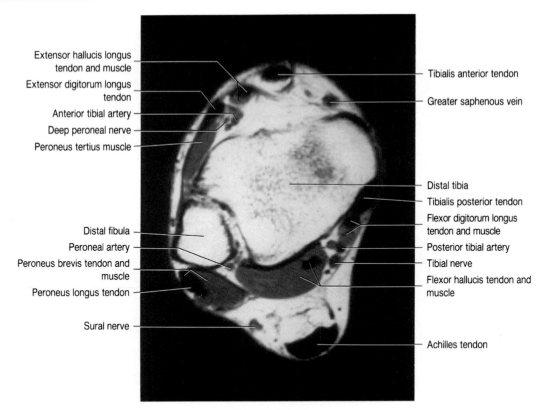

Extensor hallucis longus tendon and muscle

Extensor digitorum longus tendon

Anterior tibial artery

Deep peroneal nerve

Peroneus tertius muscle

Distal fibula

Peroneal artery

Peroneus brevis tendon and muscle

Peroneus longus tendon

Sural nerve

Tibialis anterior tendon

Greater saphenous vein

Distal tibia

Tibialis posterior tendon

Flexor digitorum longus tendon and muscle

Posterior tibial artery

Tibial nerve

Flexor hallucis tendon and muscle

Achilles tendon

FIGURE 8-32F.

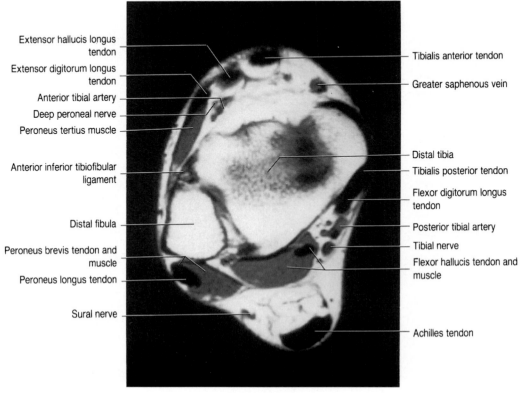

Extensor hallucis longus tendon

Extensor digitorum longus tendon

Anterior tibial artery

Deep peroneal nerve

Peroneus tertius muscle

Anterior inferior tibiofibular ligament

Distal fibula

Peroneus brevis tendon and muscle

Peroneus longus tendon

Sural nerve

Tibialis anterior tendon

Greater saphenous vein

Distal tibia

Tibialis posterior tendon

Flexor digitorum longus tendon

Posterior tibial artery

Tibial nerve

Flexor hallucis tendon and muscle

Achilles tendon

FIGURE 8-32G.

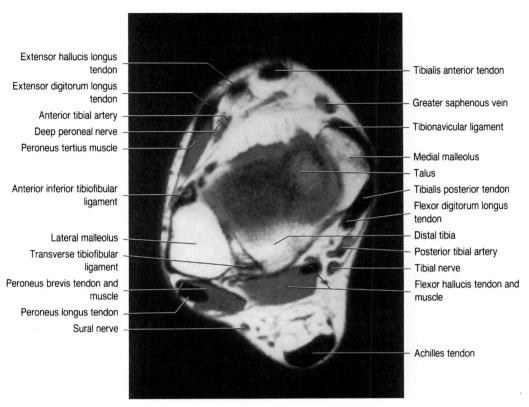

Extensor hallucis longus tendon
Extensor digitorum longus tendon
Anterior tibial artery
Deep peroneal nerve
Peroneus tertius muscle

Anterior inferior tibiofibular ligament

Lateral malleolus
Transverse tibiofibular ligament
Peroneus brevis tendon and muscle
Peroneus longus tendon
Sural nerve

Tibialis anterior tendon
Greater saphenous vein
Tibionavicular ligament
Medial malleolus
Talus
Tibialis posterior tendon
Flexor digitorum longus tendon
Distal tibia
Posterior tibial artery
Tibial nerve
Flexor hallucis tendon and muscle

Achilles tendon

FIGURE 8-32H.

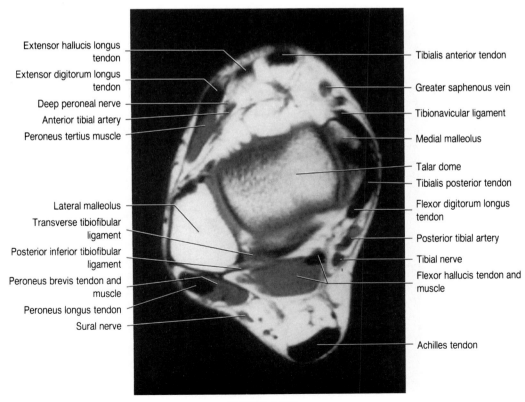

Extensor hallucis longus tendon
Extensor digitorum longus tendon
Deep peroneal nerve
Anterior tibial artery
Peroneus tertius muscle

Lateral malleolus
Transverse tibiofibular ligament
Posterior inferior tibiofibular ligament
Peroneus brevis tendon and muscle
Peroneus longus tendon
Sural nerve

Tibialis anterior tendon
Greater saphenous vein
Tibionavicular ligament
Medial malleolus
Talar dome
Tibialis posterior tendon
Flexor digitorum longus tendon
Posterior tibial artery
Tibial nerve
Flexor hallucis tendon and muscle

Achilles tendon

FIGURE 8-32I.

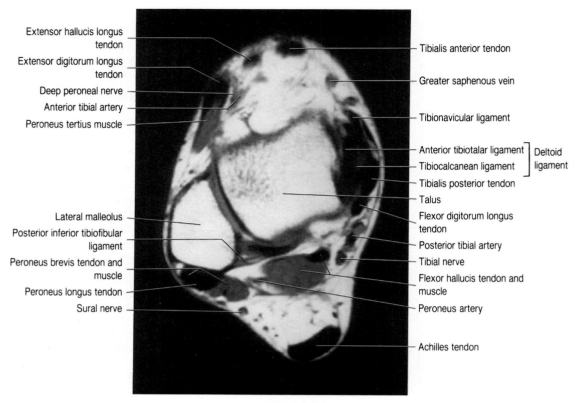

Extensor hallucis longus tendon
Extensor digitorum longus tendon
Deep peroneal nerve
Anterior tibial artery
Peroneus tertius muscle

Lateral malleolus
Posterior inferior tibiofibular ligament
Peroneus brevis tendon and muscle
Peroneus longus tendon
Sural nerve

Tibialis anterior tendon
Greater saphenous vein
Tibionavicular ligament
Anterior tibiotalar ligament ⎤ Deltoid
Tibiocalcanean ligament ⎦ ligament
Tibialis posterior tendon
Talus
Flexor digitorum longus tendon
Posterior tibial artery
Tibial nerve
Flexor hallucis tendon and muscle
Peroneus artery
Achilles tendon

FIGURE 8-32J.

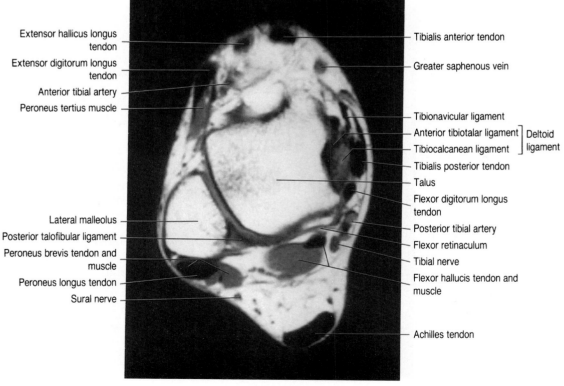

Extensor hallicus longus tendon
Extensor digitorum longus tendon
Anterior tibial artery
Peroneus tertius muscle

Lateral malleolus
Posterior talofibular ligament
Peroneus brevis tendon and muscle
Peroneus longus tendon
Sural nerve

Tibialis anterior tendon
Greater saphenous vein
Tibionavicular ligament
Anterior tibiotalar ligament ⎤ Deltoid
Tibiocalcanean ligament ⎦ ligament
Tibialis posterior tendon
Talus
Flexor digitorum longus tendon
Posterior tibial artery
Flexor retinaculum
Tibial nerve
Flexor hallucis tendon and muscle
Achilles tendon

FIGURE 8-32K.

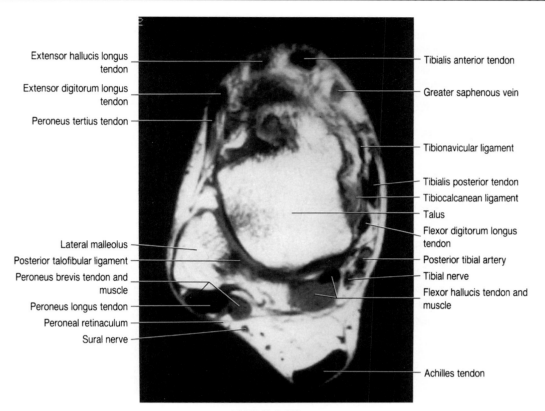

Extensor hallucis longus tendon
Extensor digitorum longus tendon
Peroneus tertius tendon

Lateral malleolus
Posterior talofibular ligament
Peroneus brevis tendon and muscle
Peroneus longus tendon
Peroneal retinaculum
Sural nerve

Tibialis anterior tendon
Greater saphenous vein

Tibionavicular ligament

Tibialis posterior tendon
Tibiocalcanean ligament
Talus
Flexor digitorum longus tendon
Posterior tibial artery
Tibial nerve
Flexor hallucis tendon and muscle

Achilles tendon

FIGURE 8-32L.

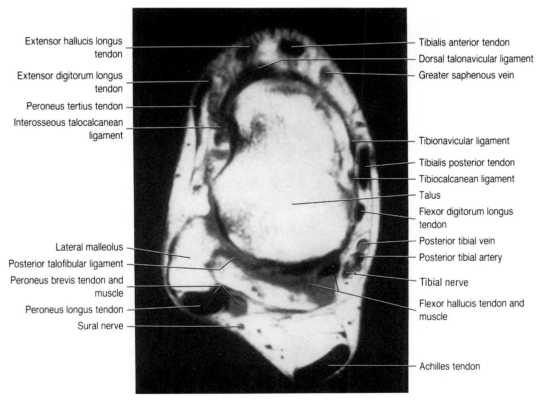

Extensor hallucis longus tendon
Extensor digitorum longus tendon
Peroneus tertius tendon
Interosseous talocalcanean ligament

Lateral malleolus
Posterior talofibular ligament
Peroneus brevis tendon and muscle
Peroneus longus tendon
Sural nerve

Tibialis anterior tendon
Dorsal talonavicular ligament
Greater saphenous vein

Tibionavicular ligament
Tibialis posterior tendon
Tibiocalcanean ligament
Talus
Flexor digitorum longus tendon
Posterior tibial vein
Posterior tibial artery
Tibial nerve
Flexor hallucis tendon and muscle

Achilles tendon

FIGURE 8-32M.

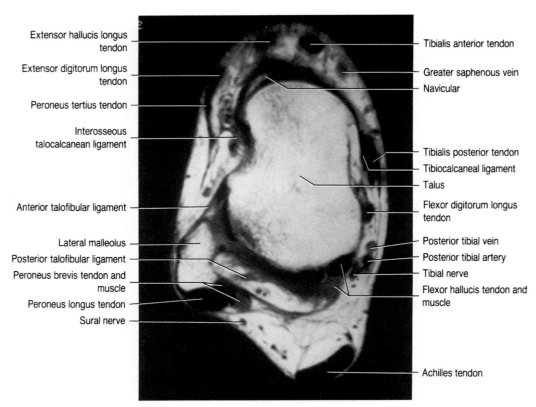

Extensor hallucis longus tendon
Extensor digitorum longus tendon
Peroneus tertius tendon
Interosseous talocalcanean ligament
Anterior talofibular ligament
Lateral malleolus
Posterior talofibular ligament
Peroneus brevis tendon and muscle
Peroneus longus tendon
Sural nerve

Tibialis anterior tendon
Greater saphenous vein
Navicular
Tibialis posterior tendon
Tibiocalcaneal ligament
Talus
Flexor digitorum longus tendon
Posterior tibial vein
Posterior tibial artery
Tibial nerve
Flexor hallucis tendon and muscle
Achilles tendon

FIGURE 8-32N.

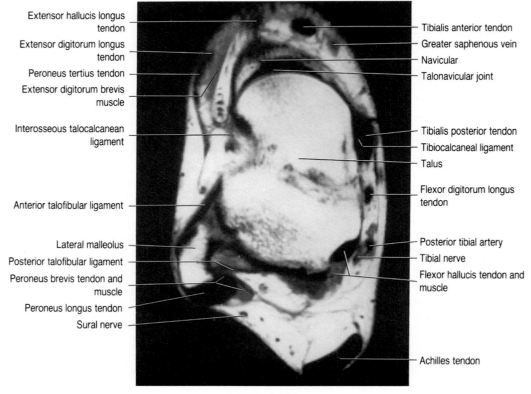

Extensor hallucis longus tendon
Extensor digitorum longus tendon
Peroneus tertius tendon
Extensor digitorum brevis muscle
Interosseous talocalcanean ligament
Anterior talofibular ligament
Lateral malleolus
Posterior talofibular ligament
Peroneus brevis tendon and muscle
Peroneus longus tendon
Sural nerve

Tibialis anterior tendon
Greater saphenous vein
Navicular
Talonavicular joint
Tibialis posterior tendon
Tibiocalcaneal ligament
Talus
Flexor digitorum longus tendon
Posterior tibial artery
Tibial nerve
Flexor hallucis tendon and muscle
Achilles tendon

FIGURE 8-32O.

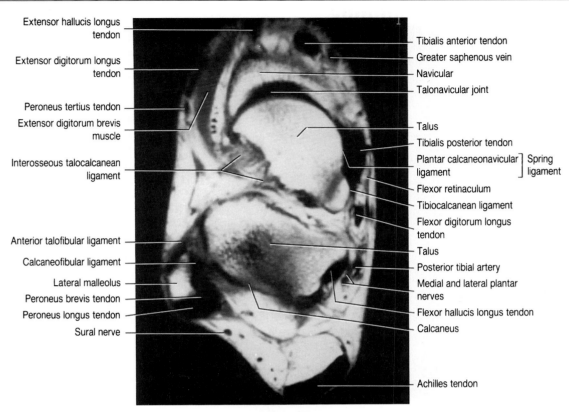

Extensor hallucis longus tendon

Extensor digitorum longus tendon

Peroneus tertius tendon

Extensor digitorum brevis muscle

Interosseous talocalcanean ligament

Anterior talofibular ligament

Calcaneofibular ligament

Lateral malleolus

Peroneus brevis tendon

Peroneus longus tendon

Sural nerve

Tibialis anterior tendon

Greater saphenous vein

Navicular

Talonavicular joint

Talus

Tibialis posterior tendon

Plantar calcaneonavicular ligament ⎤ Spring ligament ⎦

Flexor retinaculum

Tibiocalcanean ligament

Flexor digitorum longus tendon

Talus

Posterior tibial artery

Medial and lateral plantar nerves

Flexor hallucis longus tendon

Calcaneus

Achilles tendon

FIGURE 8-32P.

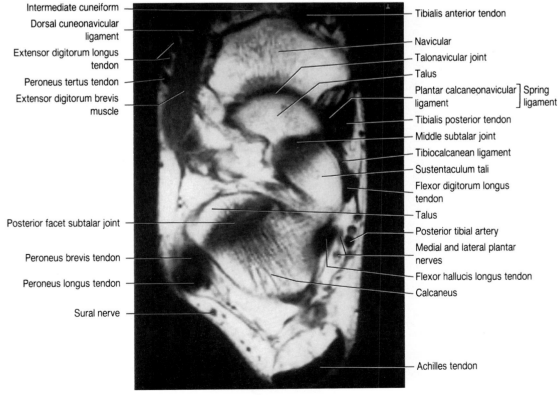

Intermediate cuneiform

Dorsal cuneonavicular ligament

Extensor digitorum longus tendon

Peroneus tertus tendon

Extensor digitorum brevis muscle

Posterior facet subtalar joint

Peroneus brevis tendon

Peroneus longus tendon

Sural nerve

Tibialis anterior tendon

Navicular

Talonavicular joint

Talus

Plantar calcaneonavicular ligament ⎤ Spring ligament ⎦

Tibialis posterior tendon

Middle subtalar joint

Tibiocalcanean ligament

Sustentaculum tali

Flexor digitorum longus tendon

Talus

Posterior tibial artery

Medial and lateral plantar nerves

Flexor hallucis longus tendon

Calcaneus

Achilles tendon

FIGURE 8-32Q.

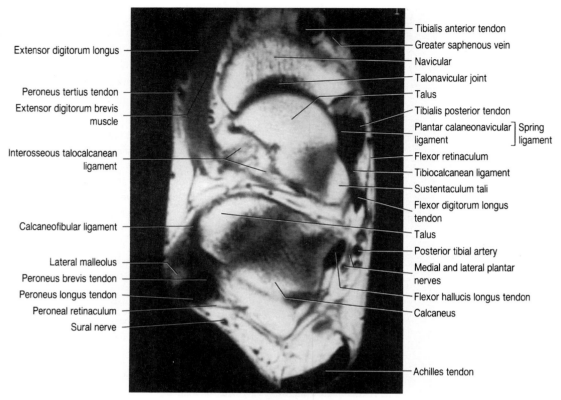

Extensor digitorum longus

Peroneus tertius tendon

Extensor digitorum brevis muscle

Interosseous talocalcanean ligament

Calcaneofibular ligament

Lateral malleolus
Peroneus brevis tendon
Peroneus longus tendon
Peroneal retinaculum
Sural nerve

Tibialis anterior tendon
Greater saphenous vein
Navicular
Talonavicular joint
Talus
Tibialis posterior tendon
Plantar calaneonavicular ligament ⎤ Spring
                                    ⎦ ligament
Flexor retinaculum
Tibiocalcanean ligament
Sustentaculum tali
Flexor digitorum longus tendon
Talus
Posterior tibial artery
Medial and lateral plantar nerves
Flexor hallucis longus tendon
Calcaneus

Achilles tendon

FIGURE 8-32R.

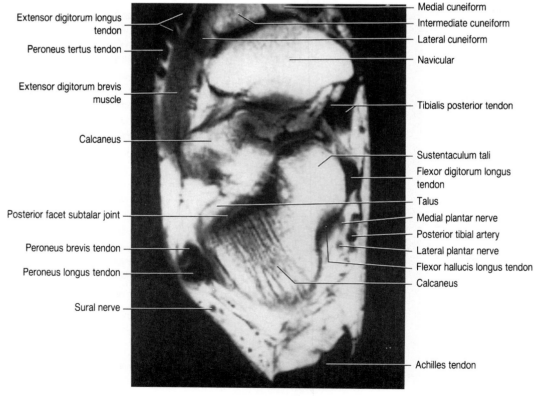

Extensor digitorum longus tendon

Peroneus tertus tendon

Extensor digitorum brevis muscle

Calcaneus

Posterior facet subtalar joint

Peroneus brevis tendon

Peroneus longus tendon

Sural nerve

Medial cuneiform
Intermediate cuneiform
Lateral cuneiform
Navicular

Tibialis posterior tendon

Sustentaculum tali
Flexor digitorum longus tendon
Talus
Medial plantar nerve
Posterior tibial artery
Lateral plantar nerve
Flexor hallucis longus tendon
Calcaneus

Achilles tendon

FIGURE 8-32S.

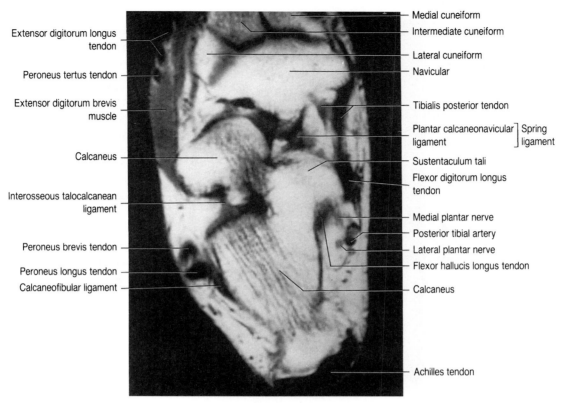

Extensor digitorum longus tendon

Peroneus tertus tendon

Extensor digitorum brevis muscle

Calcaneus

Interosseous talocalcanean ligament

Peroneus brevis tendon

Peroneus longus tendon

Calcaneofibular ligament

Medial cuneiform

Intermediate cuneiform

Lateral cuneiform

Navicular

Tibialis posterior tendon

Plantar calcaneonavicular ligament ⎤ Spring ligament

Sustentaculum tali

Flexor digitorum longus tendon

Medial plantar nerve

Posterior tibial artery

Lateral plantar nerve

Flexor hallucis longus tendon

Calcaneus

Achilles tendon

FIGURE 8-32T.

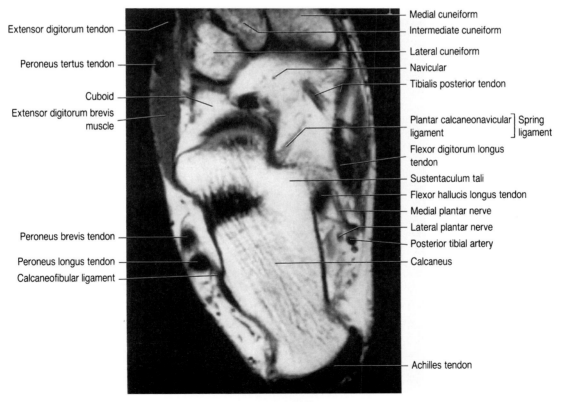

Extensor digitorum tendon

Peroneus tertus tendon

Cuboid

Extensor digitorum brevis muscle

Peroneus brevis tendon

Peroneus longus tendon

Calcaneofibular ligament

Medial cuneiform

Intermediate cuneiform

Lateral cuneiform

Navicular

Tibialis posterior tendon

Plantar calcaneonavicular ligament ⎤ Spring ligament

Flexor digitorum longus tendon

Sustentaculum tali

Flexor hallucis longus tendon

Medial plantar nerve

Lateral plantar nerve

Posterior tibial artery

Calcaneus

Achilles tendon

FIGURE 8-32U.

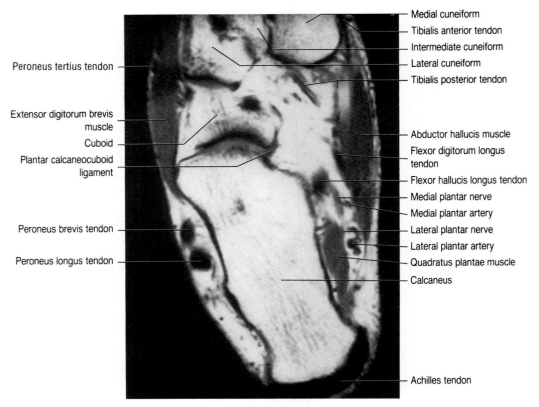

Medial cuneiform
Tibialis anterior tendon
Intermediate cuneiform
Lateral cuneiform
Tibialis posterior tendon

Peroneus tertius tendon

Extensor digitorum brevis muscle
Cuboid
Plantar calcaneocuboid ligament

Abductor hallucis muscle
Flexor digitorum longus tendon
Flexor hallucis longus tendon
Medial plantar nerve
Medial plantar artery

Peroneus brevis tendon
Peroneus longus tendon

Lateral plantar nerve
Lateral plantar artery
Quadratus plantae muscle
Calcaneus

Achilles tendon

FIGURE 8-32V.

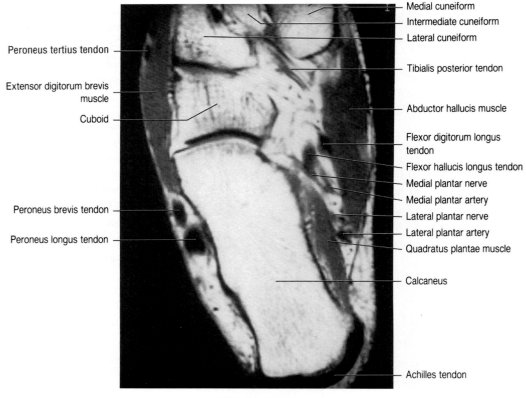

Medial cuneiform
Intermediate cuneiform
Lateral cuneiform

Peroneus tertius tendon

Extensor digitorum brevis muscle
Cuboid

Tibialis posterior tendon

Abductor hallucis muscle

Flexor digitorum longus tendon
Flexor hallucis longus tendon
Medial plantar nerve
Medial plantar artery

Peroneus brevis tendon
Peroneus longus tendon

Lateral plantar nerve
Lateral plantar artery
Quadratus plantae muscle

Calcaneus

Achilles tendon

FIGURE 8-32W.

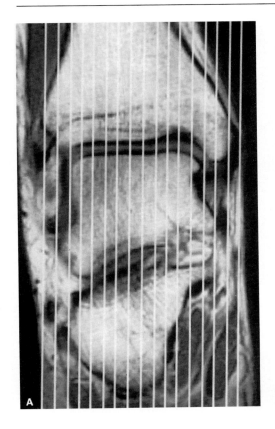

FIGURE 8-33. Normal sagittal MR anatomy. (**A**) This T1-weighted coronal localizer was used to prescribe sagittal images from (**B**) medial to (**R**) lateral.

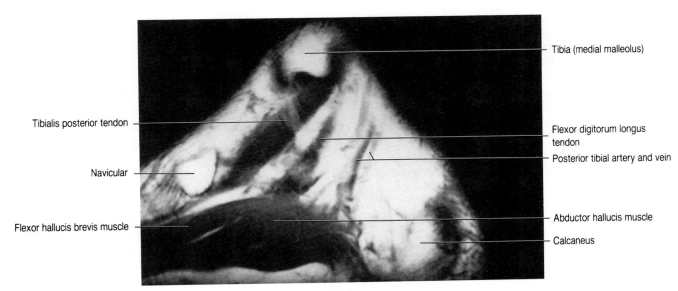

Tibia (medial malleolus)

Tibialis posterior tendon

Navicular

Flexor hallucis brevis muscle

Flexor digitorum longus tendon

Posterior tibial artery and vein

Abductor hallucis muscle

Calcaneus

FIGURE 8-33B.

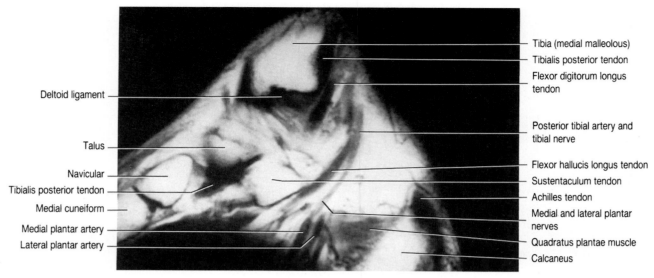

Deltoid ligament

Talus

Navicular

Tibialis posterior tendon

Medial cuneiform

Medial plantar artery

Lateral plantar artery

Tibia (medial malleolous)

Tibialis posterior tendon

Flexor digitorum longus tendon

Posterior tibial artery and tibial nerve

Flexor hallucis longus tendon

Sustentaculum tendon

Achilles tendon

Medial and lateral plantar nerves

Quadratus plantae muscle

Calcaneus

FIGURE 8-33C.

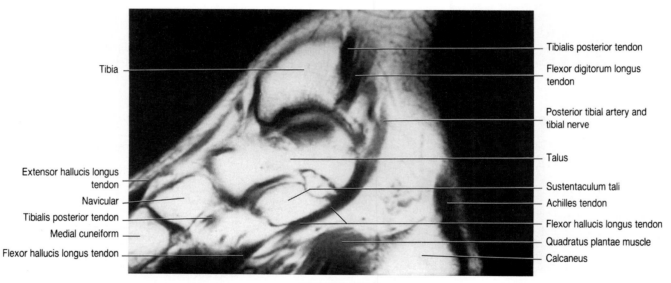

Tibia

Extensor hallucis longus tendon

Navicular

Tibialis posterior tendon

Medial cuneiform

Flexor hallucis longus tendon

Tibialis posterior tendon

Flexor digitorum longus tendon

Posterior tibial artery and tibial nerve

Talus

Sustentaculum tali

Achilles tendon

Flexor hallucis longus tendon

Quadratus plantae muscle

Calcaneus

FIGURE 8-33D.

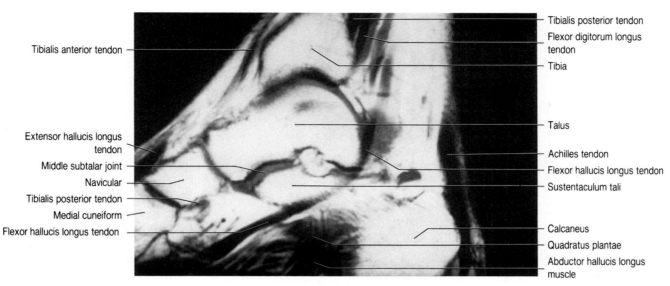

Tibialis anterior tendon

Extensor hallucis longus tendon
Middle subtalar joint
Navicular
Tibialis posterior tendon
Medial cuneiform
Flexor hallucis longus tendon

Tibialis posterior tendon
Flexor digitorum longus tendon
Tibia

Talus
Achilles tendon
Flexor hallucis longus tendon
Sustentaculum tali

Calcaneus
Quadratus plantae
Abductor hallucis longus muscle

FIGURE 8-33E.

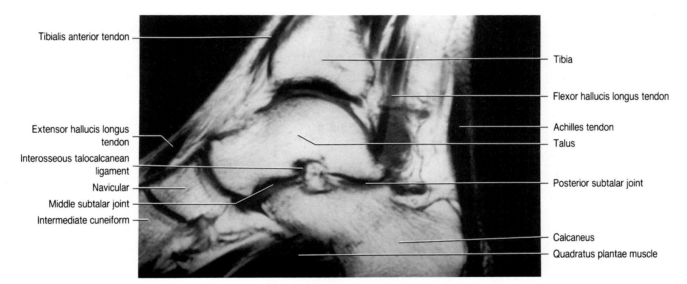

Tibialis anterior tendon

Extensor hallucis longus tendon
Interosseous talocalcanean ligament
Navicular
Middle subtalar joint
Intermediate cuneiform

Tibia

Flexor hallucis longus tendon

Achilles tendon
Talus

Posterior subtalar joint

Calcaneus
Quadratus plantae muscle

FIGURE 8-33F.

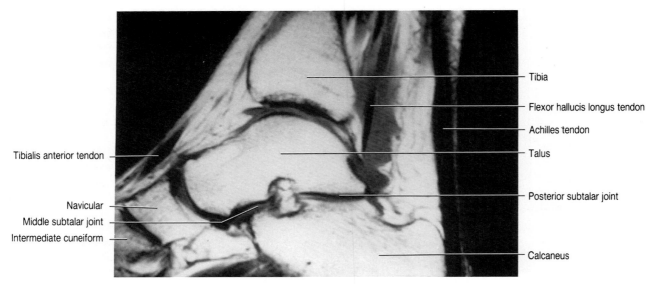

Tibialis anterior tendon —

Navicular —
Middle subtalar joint —
Intermediate cuneiform —

— Tibia
— Flexor hallucis longus tendon
— Achilles tendon
— Talus

— Posterior subtalar joint

— Calcaneus

FIGURE 8-33G.

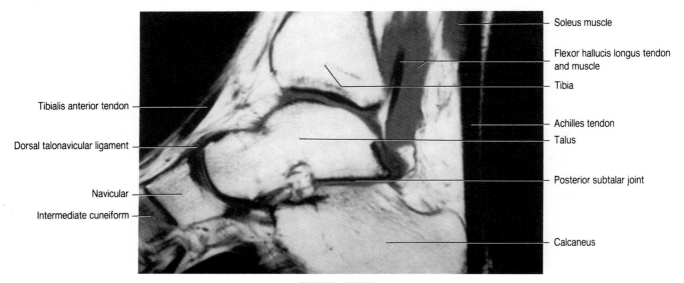

Tibialis anterior tendon —

Dorsal talonavicular ligament —

Navicular —
Intermediate cuneiform —

— Soleus muscle

— Flexor hallucis longus tendon and muscle
— Tibia

— Achilles tendon
— Talus

— Posterior subtalar joint

— Calcaneus

FIGURE 8-33H.

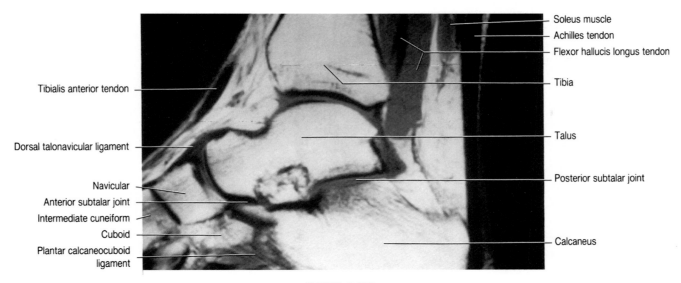

FIGURE 8-33I.

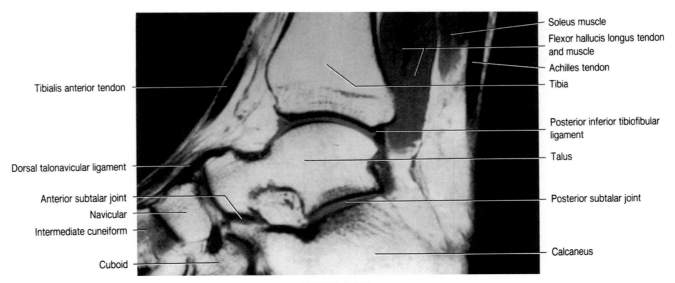

FIGURE 8-33J.

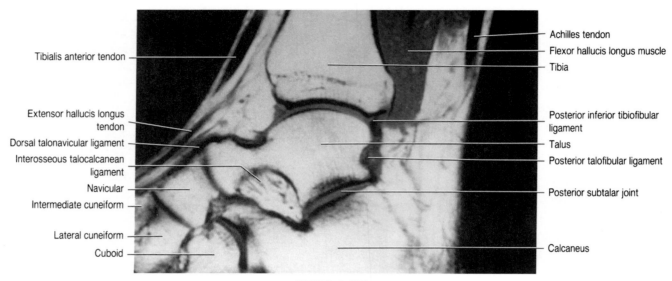

Tibialis anterior tendon

Extensor hallucis longus tendon

Dorsal talonavicular ligament

Interosseous talocalcanean ligament

Navicular

Intermediate cuneiform

Lateral cuneiform

Cuboid

Achilles tendon

Flexor hallucis longus muscle

Tibia

Posterior inferior tibiofibular ligament

Talus

Posterior talofibular ligament

Posterior subtalar joint

Calcaneus

FIGURE 8-33K.

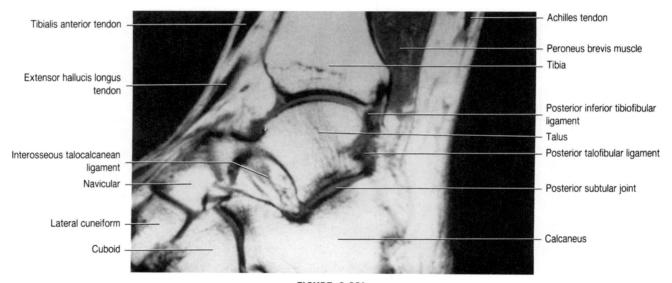

Tibialis anterior tendon

Extensor hallucis longus tendon

Interosseous talocalcanean ligament

Navicular

Lateral cuneiform

Cuboid

Achilles tendon

Peroneus brevis muscle

Tibia

Posterior inferior tibiofibular ligament

Talus

Posterior talofibular ligament

Posterior subtular joint

Calcaneus

FIGURE 8-33L.

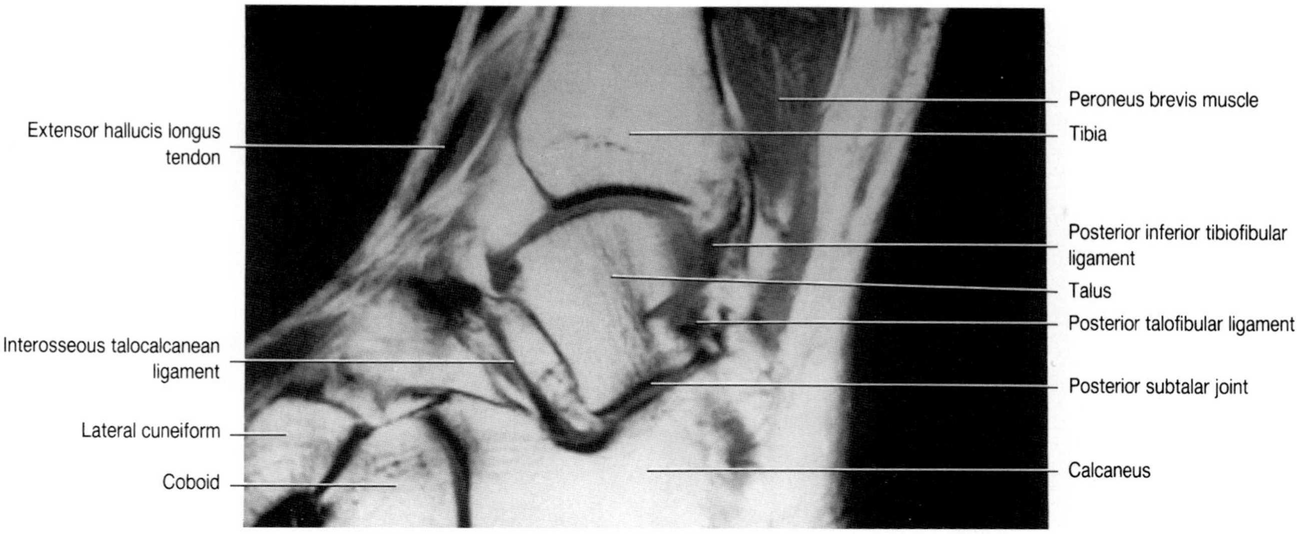

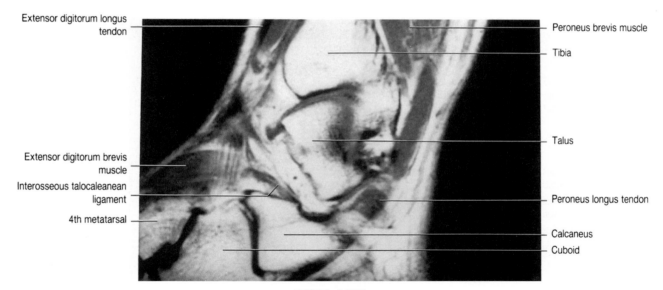

Extensor hallucis longus tendon

Interosseous talocalcanean ligament

Lateral cuneiform

Coboid

Peroneus brevis muscle

Tibia

Posterior inferior tibiofibular ligament

Talus

Posterior talofibular ligament

Posterior subtalar joint

Calcaneus

FIGURE 8-33M.

Extensor digitorum longus tendon

Extensor digitorum brevis muscle

Interosseous talocaleanean ligament

4th metatarsal

Peroneus brevis muscle

Tibia

Talus

Peroneus longus tendon

Calcaneus

Cuboid

FIGURE 8-33N.

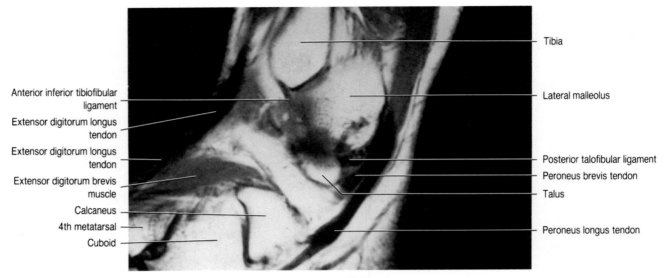

Tibia

Anterior inferior tibiofibular ligament

Lateral malleolus

Extensor digitorum longus tendon

Extensor digitorum longus tendon

Posterior talofibular ligament

Extensor digitorum brevis muscle

Peroneus brevis tendon

Talus

Calcaneus

4th metatarsal

Peroneus longus tendon

Cuboid

FIGURE 8-33O.

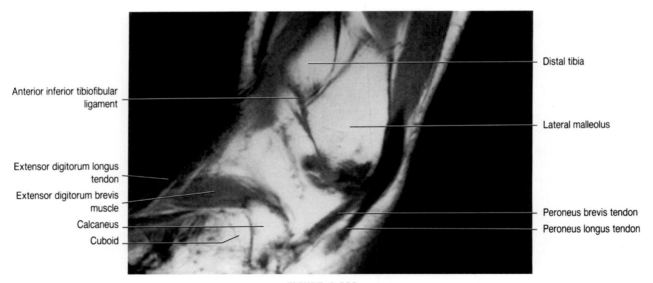

Distal tibia

Anterior inferior tibiofibular ligament

Lateral malleolus

Extensor digitorum longus tendon

Extensor digitorum brevis muscle

Peroneus brevis tendon

Calcaneus

Peroneus longus tendon

Cuboid

FIGURE 8-33P.

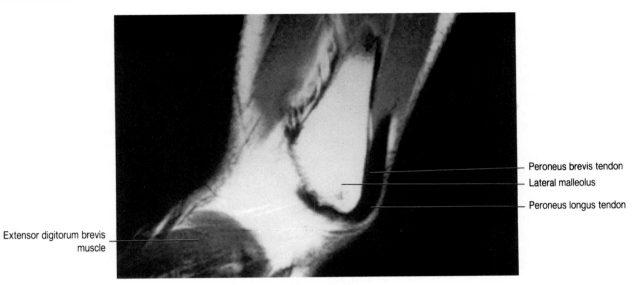

Extensor digitorum brevis muscle

Peroneus brevis tendon
Lateral malleolus
Peroneus longus tendon

FIGURE 8-33Q.

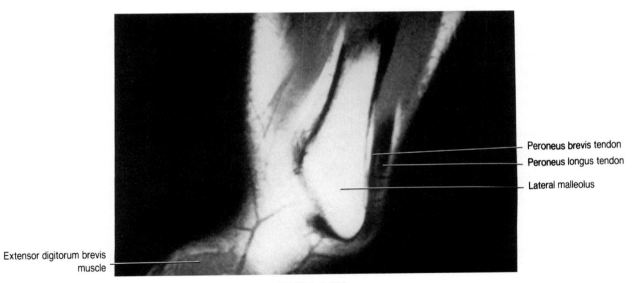

Extensor digitorum brevis muscle

Peroneus brevis tendon
Peroneus longus tendon
Lateral malleolus

FIGURE 8-33R.

sagittal images. The adductor hallucis (a first-layer muscle) inserts onto the medial proximal phalanx of the first toe and is seen between the first and second metatarsals on medial sagittal images. The tibialis anterior tendon crosses the dorsal surface of the talus before it inserts on the medial cuneiform bone and the bone of the first metatarsal.

MIDPLANE SAGITTAL IMAGES. The middle subtalar joint, the tarsal sinus, and the posterior subtalar joint are demonstrated on sagittal images medial to the midsagittal plane. The anterior subtalar joint is shown in the plane of the cuboid and calcaneocuboid joint. The peroneus longus, which extends anteriorly along the lateral inferior surface of the calcaneus and is inferior to the peroneal tubercle, enters the foot at the lateral inferior margin of the cuboid. The extensor hallucis longus tendon is identified along the dorsum of the foot and inserts onto the distal phalanx of the first toe. The interosseous talocalcaneal ligament, with its associated high signal intensity fat, is bordered anteriorly by the anterior process of the calcaneus and posteriorly by the lateral process of the talus. On T1-weighted sequences, the high signal intensity pre-Achilles fat pad is located directly anterior to the low spin density Achilles tendon.

LATERAL SAGITTAL IMAGES. In the plane of the fibula, the peroneus brevis and longus tendons pass posterior to the lateral malleolus. The peroneus brevis lies anterior to the peroneus longus tendon and is in direct contact with the lateral malleolus. The peroneus brevis can be followed to its insertion on the base of the fifth metatarsal bone. The peroneus longus tendon disappears inferior and medial to the peroneus brevis tendon and enters the cuboid sulcus; therefore, it appears shorter than the peroneus brevis tendon on lateral sagittal images.

Coronal Images

Figure 8-34 provides examples of coronal images in the ankle from posterior to anterior.

POSTERIOR CORONAL IMAGES. The thick, low signal intensity Achilles tendon is clearly displayed on posterior coronal images. Its attachment to the calcaneal tuberosity can also be observed on these images. The soleus muscle, with its inverted-V–shaped origin from the soleal line of the tibia and posterior fibula, contributes to the calcaneal tendon (or Achilles tendon), along with the gastrocnemius and plantaris. The peroneus brevis and flexor hallucis longus muscles are identified lateral to the soleus muscle, and the peroneal tendons are located inferior to the lateral malleolus. The flexor digitorum longus muscle and tendon cross superficially, in a medial-to-lateral direction, to the tibialis posterior in the distal calf. The tibialis posterior tendon is located medial to the posterior malleolus. The posterior talofibular and inferior tibiofibular ligaments are shown on coronal images at the level of the posterior malleolus and posterior process of the

talus. The plantar aponeurosis is superficial to the flexor digitorum brevis muscle, whereas the quadratus plantae muscle lies deep to this muscle.

MIDPLANE CORONAL IMAGES. The calcaneofibular ligament is best imaged at the level of the posterior subtalar joint and lateral malleolus. The lateral process of the talus can be seen in the same sections as the anterior lateral malleolus. The middle subtalar joint is formed by the sustentaculum tali and the inferior medial talar surface. This is the best plane for evaluating talocalcaneal coalitions. The peroneus brevis and longus tendons course laterally, superior and inferior, respectively, to the peroneal groove of the calcaneus.

ANTERIOR CORONAL IMAGES. The tibiotalar and tibiocalcaneal fibers of the deltoid ligament extend obliquely to the talus and vertically to the sustentaculum tali, respectively. The tibialis posterior tendon is medial to the deltoid ligament and superior to the sustentaculum tali, and can be used as a landmark. The flexor digitorum longus tendon enters the foot, having crossed superficially in a medial-to-lateral direction to both the tibialis posterior and the flexor hallucis longus tendons, which are parallel. The flexor digitorum longus tendon is located medial to the sustentaculum tali. The anterior compartment tendons (the tibialis anterior, the extensor hallucis longus, and the extensor digitorum longus) are displayed on the anterior surface of the distal tibia, medially and laterally. The anterior tibiotalar fibers of the deltoid ligament are also seen in the plane of the anterior tibia.

Anatomic Variants

A number of normal anatomic variants of the ankle as seen on MR images may be misleading. These have been characterized in studies of asymptomatic patients.[15] In the posterior tibiotalar joint, a low signal intensity cortical irregularity may mimic the appearance of osteonecrosis (Figs. 8-35 and 8-36). The posterior inferior tibiofibular ligament may be mistaken for a loose body in the posterior capsule on midsagittal images (see Fig. 8-36). Occasionally, the intact posterior talofibular ligament may appear as an attenuated structure with signal inhomogeneity. Less frequently, fluid in the peroneal tendon sheath may be confused with a longitudinal tendon tear. In one patient, axial planar images revealed marked asymmetry and hypertrophy of the peroneus brevis muscle and tendon as a normal anatomic variant (Fig. 8-37). An accessory soleus muscle is an anatomic variant that may present as a mass in the distal calf or medial ankle.[16] The tensor fasciae suralis represents an anomalous muscle and tendon that contributes to the Achilles tendon and originates from the semitendinosus muscle. It may be mistaken for a posterior thigh, popliteal, calf, or Achilles tendon mass or lesion. MR imaging demonstrates imaging characteristics of either muscle or tendon.[17] The peroneus quartus muscle

text continues on page 507

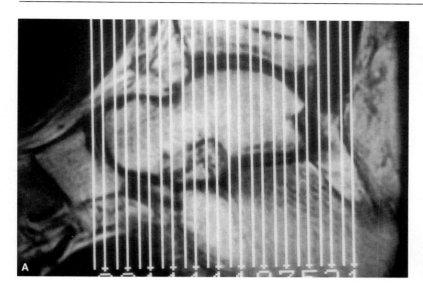

FIGURE 8-34. Normal coronal MR anatomy. (**A**) This T1-weighted sagittal localizer was used to prescribe coronal images from (**B**) posterior to (**U**) anterior.

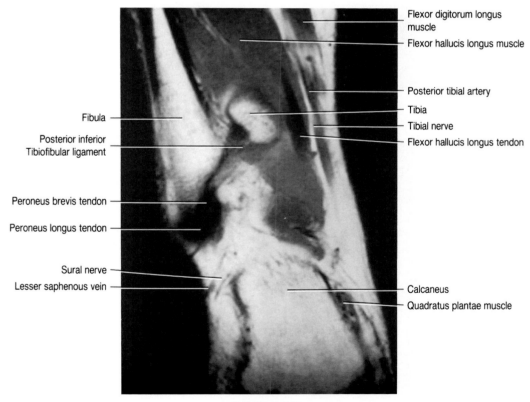

Flexor digitorum longus muscle

Flexor hallucis longus muscle

Posterior tibial artery

Tibia

Tibial nerve

Flexor hallucis longus tendon

Fibula

Posterior inferior Tibiofibular ligament

Peroneus brevis tendon

Peroneus longus tendon

Sural nerve

Lesser saphenous vein

Calcaneus

Quadratus plantae muscle

FIGURE 8-34B.

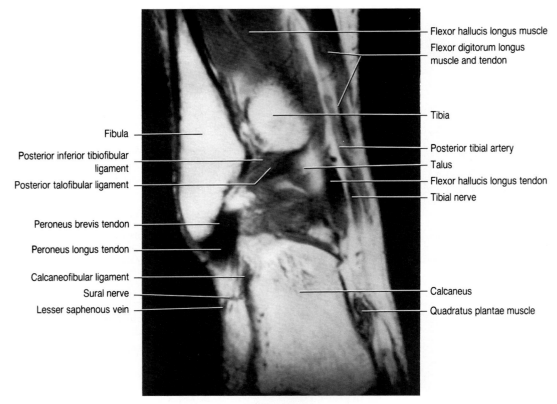

Flexor hallucis longus muscle

Flexor digitorum longus muscle and tendon

Tibia

Posterior tibial artery

Talus

Flexor hallucis longus tendon

Tibial nerve

Calcaneus

Quadratus plantae muscle

Fibula

Posterior inferior tibiofibular ligament

Posterior talofibular ligament

Peroneus brevis tendon

Peroneus longus tendon

Calcaneofibular ligament

Sural nerve

Lesser saphenous vein

FIGURE 8-34C.

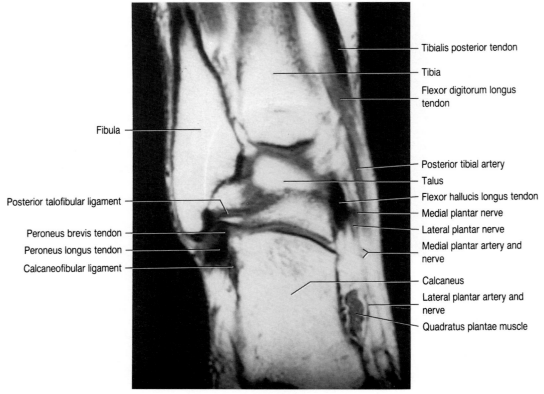

Tibialis posterior tendon

Tibia

Flexor digitorum longus tendon

Posterior tibial artery

Talus

Flexor hallucis longus tendon

Medial plantar nerve

Lateral plantar nerve

Medial plantar artery and nerve

Calcaneus

Lateral plantar artery and nerve

Quadratus plantae muscle

Fibula

Posterior talofibular ligament

Peroneus brevis tendon

Peroneus longus tendon

Calcaneofibular ligament

FIGURE 8-34D.

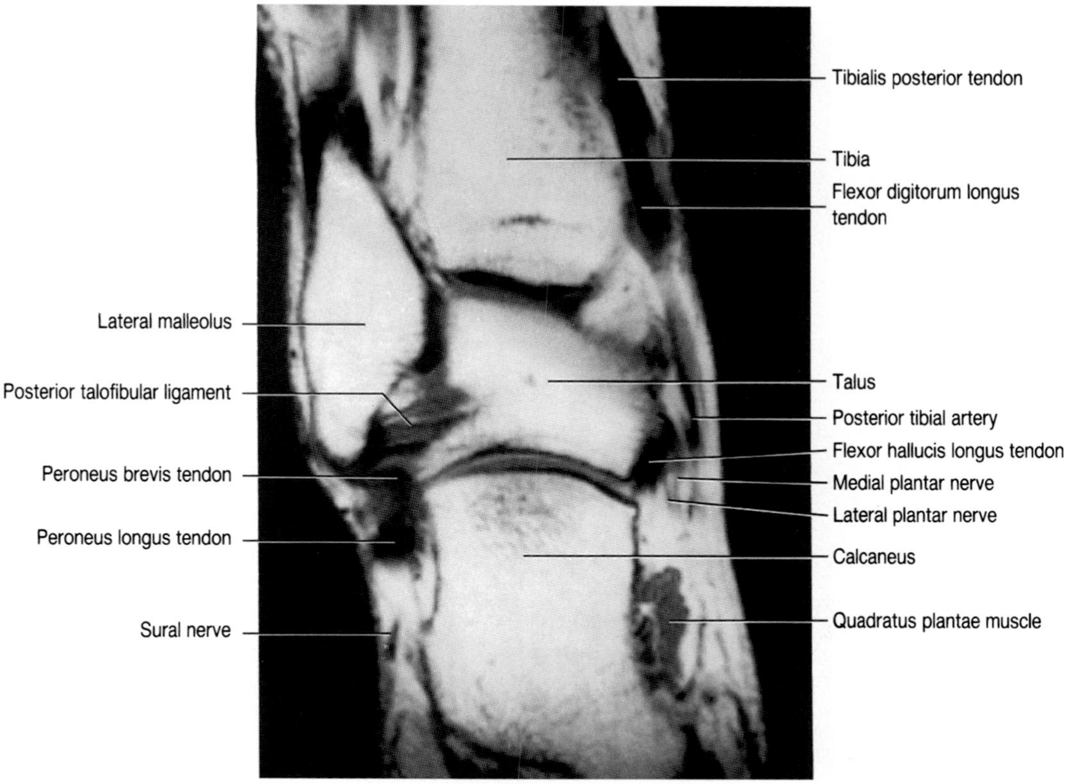

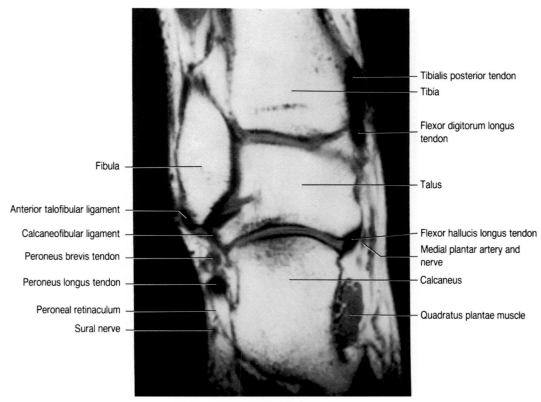

Lateral malleolus
Posterior talofibular ligament
Peroneus brevis tendon
Peroneus longus tendon
Sural nerve

Tibialis posterior tendon
Tibia
Flexor digitorum longus tendon
Talus
Posterior tibial artery
Flexor hallucis longus tendon
Medial plantar nerve
Lateral plantar nerve
Calcaneus
Quadratus plantae muscle

FIGURE 8-34E.

Fibula
Anterior talofibular ligament
Calcaneofibular ligament
Peroneus brevis tendon
Peroneus longus tendon
Peroneal retinaculum
Sural nerve

Tibialis posterior tendon
Tibia
Flexor digitorum longus tendon
Talus
Flexor hallucis longus tendon
Medial plantar artery and nerve
Calcaneus
Quadratus plantae muscle

FIGURE 8-34F.

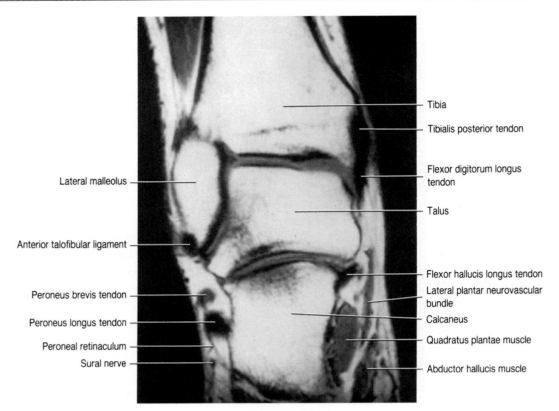

Lateral malleolus

Anterior talofibular ligament

Peroneus brevis tendon

Peroneus longus tendon

Peroneal retinaculum

Sural nerve

Tibia

Tibialis posterior tendon

Flexor digitorum longus tendon

Talus

Flexor hallucis longus tendon

Lateral plantar neurovascular bundle

Calcaneus

Quadratus plantae muscle

Abductor hallucis muscle

FIGURE 8-34G.

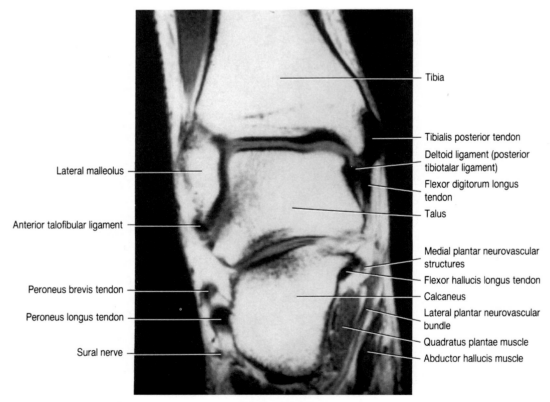

Lateral malleolus

Anterior talofibular ligament

Peroneus brevis tendon

Peroneus longus tendon

Sural nerve

Tibia

Tibialis posterior tendon

Deltoid ligament (posterior tibiotalar ligament)

Flexor digitorum longus tendon

Talus

Medial plantar neurovascular structures

Flexor hallucis longus tendon

Calcaneus

Lateral plantar neurovascular bundle

Quadratus plantae muscle

Abductor hallucis muscle

FIGURE 8-34H.

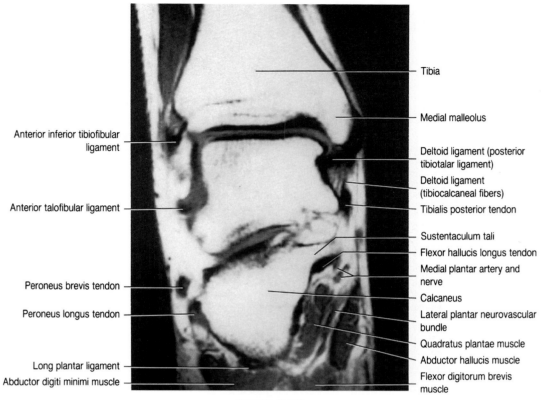

Anterior inferior tibiofibular ligament

Anterior talofibular ligament

Peroneus brevis tendon

Peroneus longus tendon

Long plantar ligament
Abductor digiti minimi muscle

Tibia

Medial malleolus

Deltoid ligament (posterior tibiotalar ligament)
Deltoid ligament (tibiocalcaneal fibers)
Tibialis posterior tendon

Sustentaculum tali
Flexor hallucis longus tendon
Medial plantar artery and nerve
Calcaneus
Lateral plantar neurovascular bundle
Quadratus plantae muscle
Abductor hallucis muscle
Flexor digitorum brevis muscle

FIGURE 8-34I.

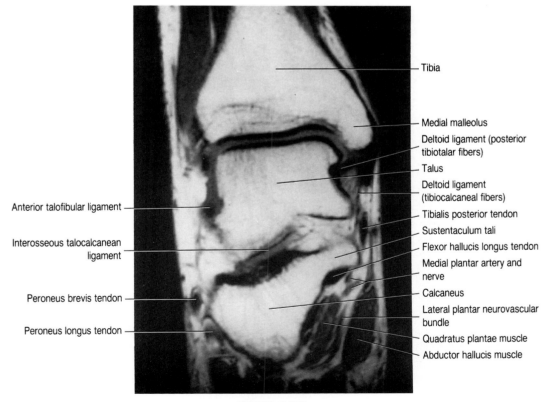

Anterior talofibular ligament

Interosseous talocalcanean ligament

Peroneus brevis tendon

Peroneus longus tendon

Tibia

Medial malleolus
Deltoid ligament (posterior tibiotalar fibers)
Talus
Deltoid ligament (tibiocalcaneal fibers)
Tibialis posterior tendon
Sustentaculum tali
Flexor hallucis longus tendon
Medial plantar artery and nerve
Calcaneus
Lateral plantar neurovascular bundle
Quadratus plantae muscle
Abductor hallucis muscle

FIGURE 8-34J.

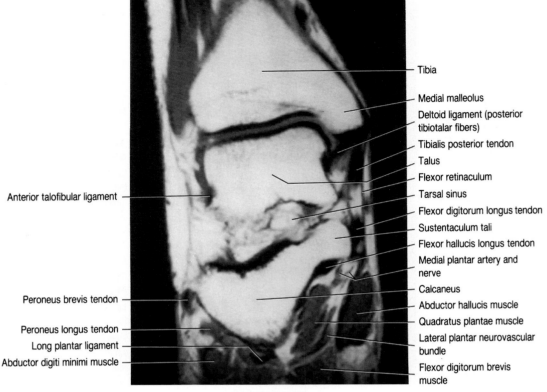

Tibia

Medial malleolus

Deltoid ligament (posterior tibiotalar fibers)

Tibialis posterior tendon

Talus

Flexor retinaculum

Tarsal sinus

Flexor digitorum longus tendon

Sustentaculum tali

Flexor hallucis longus tendon

Medial plantar artery and nerve

Calcaneus

Abductor hallucis muscle

Quadratus plantae muscle

Lateral plantar neurovascular bundle

Flexor digitorum brevis muscle

Anterior talofibular ligament

Peroneus brevis tendon

Peroneus longus tendon

Long plantar ligament

Abductor digiti minimi muscle

FIGURE 8-34K.

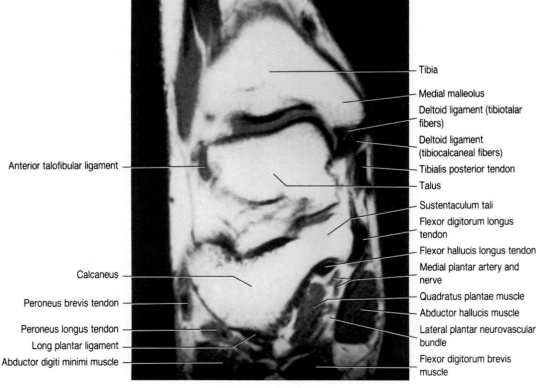

Tibia

Medial malleolus

Deltoid ligament (tibiotalar fibers)

Deltoid ligament (tibiocalcaneal fibers)

Tibialis posterior tendon

Talus

Sustentaculum tali

Flexor digitorum longus tendon

Flexor hallucis longus tendon

Medial plantar artery and nerve

Quadratus plantae muscle

Abductor hallucis muscle

Lateral plantar neurovascular bundle

Flexor digitorum brevis muscle

Anterior talofibular ligament

Calcaneus

Peroneus brevis tendon

Peroneus longus tendon

Long plantar ligament

Abductor digiti minimi muscle

FIGURE 8-34L.

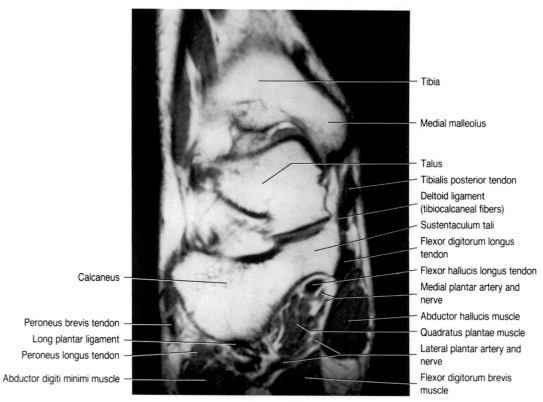

Tibia

Medial malleolus

Talus

Tibialis posterior tendon

Deltoid ligament
(tibiocalcaneal fibers)

Sustentaculum tali

Flexor digitorum longus
tendon

Flexor hallucis longus tendon

Medial plantar artery and
nerve

Abductor hallucis muscle

Quadratus plantae muscle

Lateral plantar artery and
nerve

Flexor digitorum brevis
muscle

Calcaneus

Peroneus brevis tendon

Long plantar ligament

Peroneus longus tendon

Abductor digiti minimi muscle

FIGURE 8-34M.

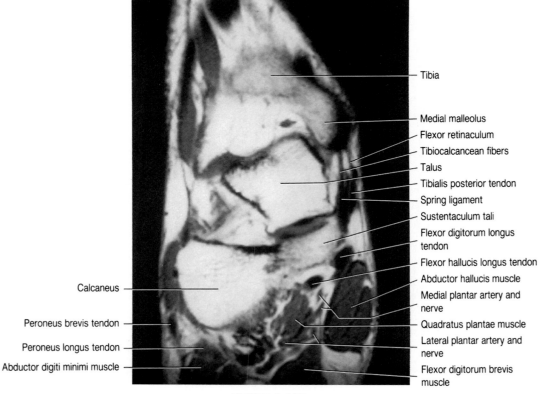

Tibia

Medial malleolus

Flexor retinaculum

Tibiocalcancean fibers

Talus

Tibialis posterior tendon

Spring ligament

Sustentaculum tali

Flexor digitorum longus
tendon

Flexor hallucis longus tendon

Abductor hallucis muscle

Medial plantar artery and
nerve

Quadratus plantae muscle

Lateral plantar artery and
nerve

Flexor digitorum brevis
muscle

Calcaneus

Peroneus brevis tendon

Peroneus longus tendon

Abductor digiti minimi muscle

FIGURE 8-34N.

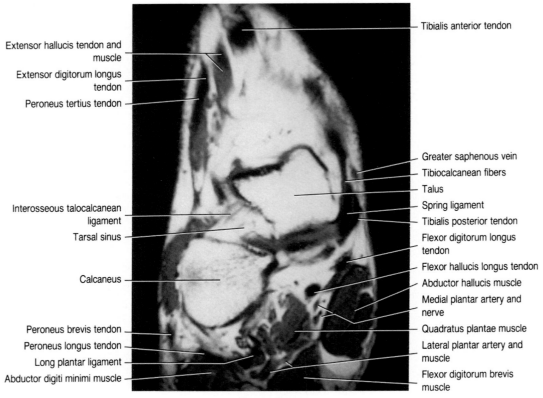

Extensor hallucis tendon and muscle

Extensor digitorum longus tendon

Peroneus tertius tendon

Interosseous talocalcanean ligament

Tarsal sinus

Calcaneus

Peroneus brevis tendon

Peroneus longus tendon

Long plantar ligament

Abductor digiti minimi muscle

Tibialis anterior tendon

Greater saphenous vein

Tibiocalcanean fibers

Talus

Spring ligament

Tibialis posterior tendon

Flexor digitorum longus tendon

Flexor hallucis longus tendon

Abductor hallucis muscle

Medial plantar artery and nerve

Quadratus plantae muscle

Lateral plantar artery and muscle

Flexor digitorum brevis muscle

FIGURE 8-34O.

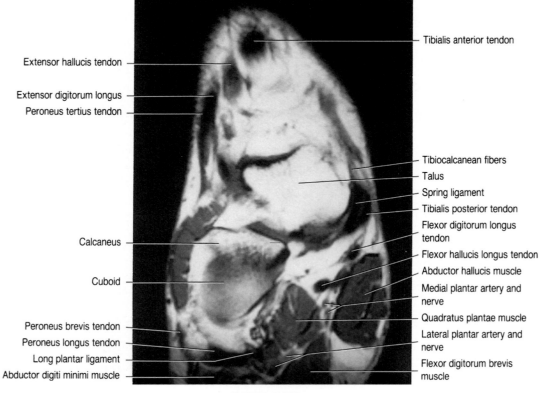

Extensor hallucis tendon

Extensor digitorum longus

Peroneus tertius tendon

Calcaneus

Cuboid

Peroneus brevis tendon

Peroneus longus tendon

Long plantar ligament

Abductor digiti minimi muscle

Tibialis anterior tendon

Tibiocalcanean fibers

Talus

Spring ligament

Tibialis posterior tendon

Flexor digitorum longus tendon

Flexor hallucis longus tendon

Abductor hallucis muscle

Medial plantar artery and nerve

Quadratus plantae muscle

Lateral plantar artery and nerve

Flexor digitorum brevis muscle

FIGURE 8-34P.

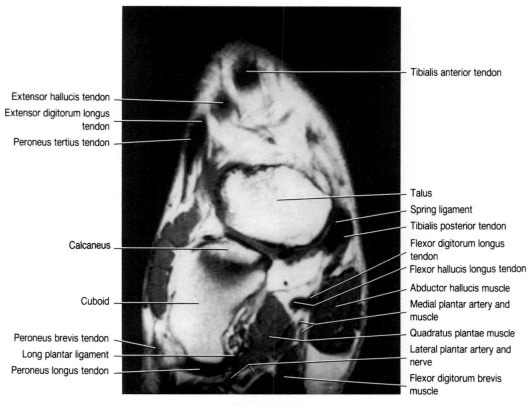

Tibialis anterior tendon

Extensor hallucis tendon
Extensor digitorum longus tendon
Peroneus tertius tendon

Talus
Spring ligament
Tibialis posterior tendon
Flexor digitorum longus tendon
Flexor hallucis longus tendon
Abductor hallucis muscle
Medial plantar artery and muscle
Quadratus plantae muscle
Lateral plantar artery and nerve
Flexor digitorum brevis muscle

Calcaneus

Cuboid

Peroneus brevis tendon
Long plantar ligament
Peroneus longus tendon

FIGURE 8-34Q.

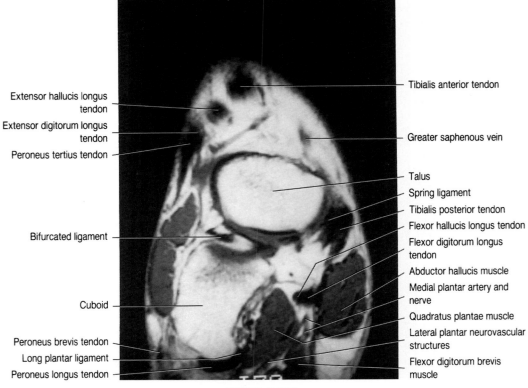

Tibialis anterior tendon

Extensor hallucis longus tendon
Extensor digitorum longus tendon
Peroneus tertius tendon

Greater saphenous vein

Talus
Spring ligament
Tibialis posterior tendon
Flexor hallucis longus tendon
Flexor digitorum longus tendon
Abductor hallucis muscle
Medial plantar artery and nerve
Quadratus plantae muscle
Lateral plantar neurovascular structures
Flexor digitorum brevis muscle

Bifurcated ligament

Cuboid

Peroneus brevis tendon
Long plantar ligament
Peroneus longus tendon

FIGURE 8-34R.

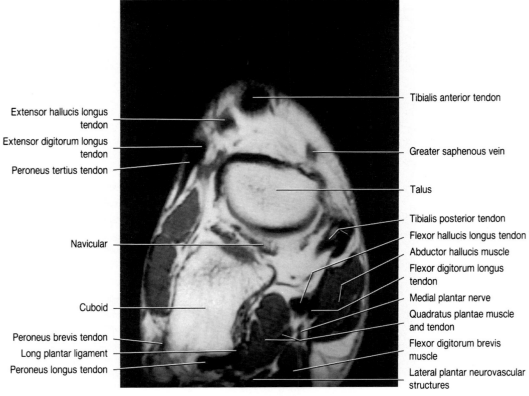

Extensor hallucis longus tendon

Extensor digitorum longus tendon

Peroneus tertius tendon

Navicular

Cuboid

Peroneus brevis tendon

Long plantar ligament

Peroneus longus tendon

Tibialis anterior tendon

Greater saphenous vein

Talus

Tibialis posterior tendon

Flexor hallucis longus tendon

Abductor hallucis muscle

Flexor digitorum longus tendon

Medial plantar nerve

Quadratus plantae muscle and tendon

Flexor digitorum brevis muscle

Lateral plantar neurovascular structures

FIGURE 8-34S.

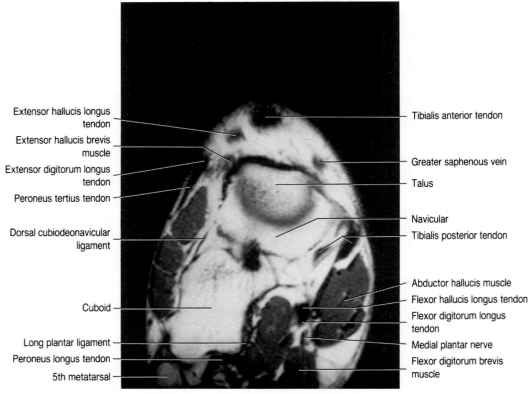

Extensor hallucis longus tendon

Extensor hallucis brevis muscle

Extensor digitorum longus tendon

Peroneus tertius tendon

Dorsal cubiodeonavicular ligament

Cuboid

Long plantar ligament

Peroneus longus tendon

5th metatarsal

Tibialis anterior tendon

Greater saphenous vein

Talus

Navicular

Tibialis posterior tendon

Abductor hallucis muscle

Flexor hallucis longus tendon

Flexor digitorum longus tendon

Medial plantar nerve

Flexor digitorum brevis muscle

FIGURE 8-34T.

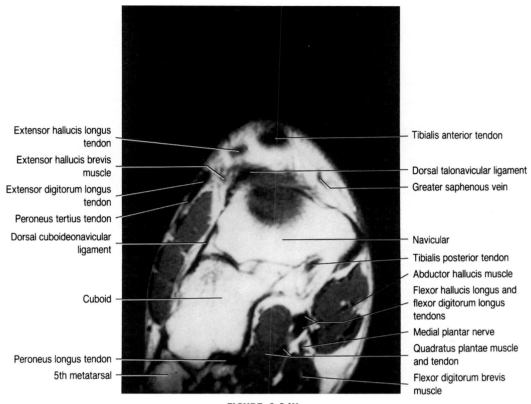

Extensor hallucis longus tendon

Extensor hallucis brevis muscle

Extensor digitorum longus tendon

Peroneus tertius tendon

Dorsal cuboideonavicular ligament

Cuboid

Peroneus longus tendon

5th metatarsal

Tibialis anterior tendon

Dorsal talonavicular ligament

Greater saphenous vein

Navicular

Tibialis posterior tendon

Abductor hallucis muscle

Flexor hallucis longus and flexor digitorum longus tendons

Medial plantar nerve

Quadratus plantae muscle and tendon

Flexor digitorum brevis muscle

FIGURE 8-34U.

is present in 13% to 22% of individuals. This anatomic variant originates from the peroneus brevis muscle and inserts onto the peroneal tubercle of the calcaneus.[18]

The orientation of a tendon relative to the main magnetic field (B_0) affects its MR appearance. When the orientation approximates the ''magic angle'' of 55°, the collagen may demonstrate intermediate signal intensity with loss of the normal low spin-density characteristics.[18] The magic angle effect is prominent on short TE spin-echo or gradient-echo images. T2-weighted images minimize the magic angle signal intensity. On sagittal images, the peroneus longus tendon and flexor hallucis longus tendon are commonly affected and often display intermediate signal intensity in their midportions. Changes in ankle position can be used to confirm that the tendon is normal, by altering its orientation relative to the main magnetic field.

Most ankle ligaments, including the anterior talofibular, the calcaneofibular, and the superficial deltoid, show uniform

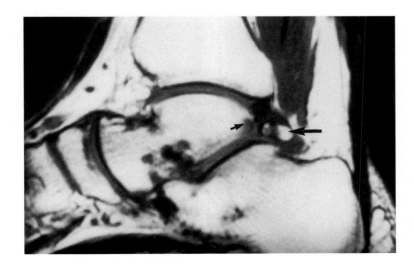

FIGURE 8-35. The low signal intensity irregular posterior talar cortex (*small black arrow*) is a normal variant. Normal fat signal intensity is present in the os trigonum (*large black arrow*) (T1-weighted sagittal image).

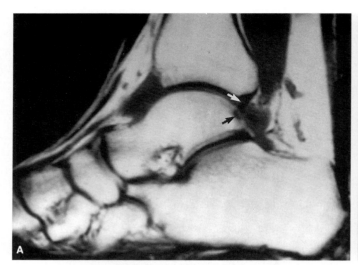
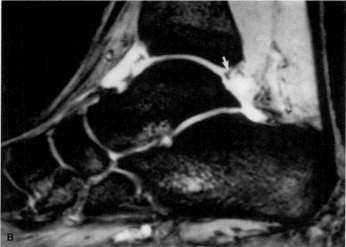

FIGURE 8-36. **(A)** A T1-weighted sagittal image demonstrates focal low signal intensity irregularity mimicking an osteochondral lesion of the posterior talar cortex (*black arrow*). The low signal intensity posterior inferior tibiofibular ligament is located posterior to the tibiotalar joint and is not a loose body (*white arrow*). **(B)** A T2*-weighted sagittal image shows the posterior inferior tibiofibular ligament (*white arrow*) in contrast to a high signal intensity joint effusion.

low signal intensity on all pulse sequences. A mixed or striated signal intensity, however, can be seen in the posterior talofibular, posterior inferior tibiofibular, deep deltoid, and interosseous talocalcaneal ligaments.

Normally, the sesamoid bones within the peroneus longus (os peroneum) or the distal tibialis posterior demonstrate hyperintensity on T1-weighted images, secondary to fatty marrow. This finding should not be mistaken for tendon degeneration or tear. Accessory bones, including the os tibi-

ale externum (an accessory navicular bone medial to the navicular) and the os trigonum (located posterior to the talus and occurring approximately 10% of the time), represent commonly seen secondary ossification centers. These are normal variants that may be misinterpreted as a fracture or loose body.[18]

Small fluid collections in the ankle joint, including the tibiotalar and subtalar joints as well as the ankle tendon sheath, are common in asymptomatic individuals.[19] Rela-

FIGURE 8-37. Asymmetric hypertrophy of the peroneus brevis muscle can occur as a normal anatomic variant (*black arrows*). The contralateral, normal-sized peroneus brevis muscle is shown for comparison (*open arrow*). Associated Achilles tendinitis demonstrates a central area of intermediate signal intensity within an enlarged, low-signal intensity tendon (*white arrow*) on a T1-weighted axial image.

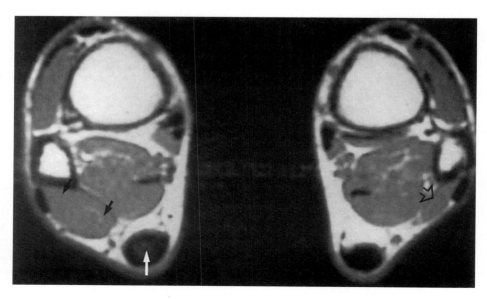

tively larger amounts of fluid, however, are usually associated with the flexor hallucis longus tendon. Fluid is not commonly seen in the extensor tendons. The amount of fluid in normal or asymptomatic and symptomatic patients may be similar in volume and distribution.

PATHOLOGY OF THE ANKLE AND FOOT

Osteochondral Lesions

Osteochondral lesion of the talus (OLT) is the accepted term for a variety of disorders including transchondral fracture, osteochondral fracture, osteochondritis dissecans, and talar dome fracture. Osteochondral lesions of the medial and lateral talar dome involve the articular cartilage and subchondral bone, and have a high association with antecedent trauma (eg, torsional impaction).

Etiology

Trauma remains the best accepted theory for the etiology of OLT, which is thought to represent the chronic phase of a compressed or avulsed talar dome fracture.[13] Direct trauma or repetitive microtrauma may contribute to the development of this lesion in individuals predisposed to talar dome ischemia. An osteonecrotic process leads to subchondral fracture and collapse. The influx of synovial fluid into the fracture site along with increased joint pressure may prevent healing.

Diagnosis and Staging

Since conventional radiographs are not sensitive to early lesions, immobilization and surgery may be delayed, resulting in arthritis in 50% of cases. MR imaging of the talar dome is more accurate than CT scanning and complements diagnostic arthroscopic examination of the tibiotalar joint in early diagnosis (Fig. 8-38).

Forced inversion and dorsiflexion produces lateral lesions (ie, impingement between the lateral margin of the talar dome and the fibular styloid) (Fig. 8-39), which usually occur in the mid- to anterior aspect of the talar dome. Forced inversion and plantar flexion with external rotation of the tibia causes medial lesions (ie, impact between the posteromedial tibia and medial talar margin) (Fig. 8-40). The medial and lateral surfaces of the talus are involved in approximately 60% and 40% osteochondral lesions of the talus, respectively. Medial lesions, usually cup shaped and deeper than lateral lesions, are not as strongly associated with a history of antecedent trauma as are lateral lesions, which tend to be wafer shaped and thin.

If the collateral ligament fails to rupture because articular surfaces are in direct contact, pain may be minimal. More severe injuries are accompanied by ligamentous tearing. Berndt and Harty[20] have developed a four-part staging system for characterizing osteochondral lesions of the talus based on plain radiographs. In stage I, there is a subchondral compression fracture of the talus with no ligamentous sprain. Radiograph results are negative, and lesions in this stage may be painless. Stage II lesions involve a partially detached osteochondral fragment with a hinge or flap of articular cartilage. A T2- or T2*-weighted image may be necessary to identify the osteochondral fragment. In stage III lesions, a complete nondisplaced fracture remains within the bony crater. Stage IV lesions are characterized by detachment with a loose osteochondral fragment. Although lesions in stages II to IV are themselves painless, they may be associated with a painful sprain or rupture of the collateral ankle ligaments.

In order to improve on the correlation between arthro-

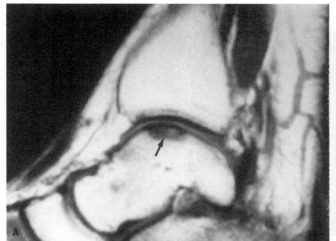
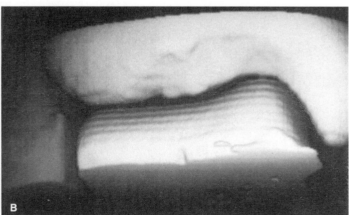

FIGURE 8-38. **(A)** A T1-weighted sagittal image shows a stage I osteochondral lesion with a low signal intensity compression fracture (*arrow*) of the talus. **(B)** Preservation of the tibiotalar joint surfaces can be seen on a 3D CT image.

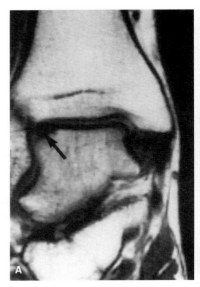
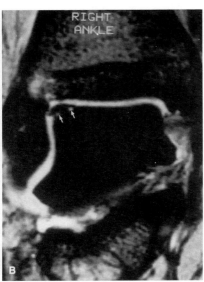

FIGURE 8-39. A stage III osteochondral lesion of the lateral talar dome is seen on (**A**) T1-weighted (*black arrow*) and (**B**) T2*-weighted (*white arrows*) coronal images. High signal intensity joint fluid undermines the osteochondral fracture on the T2*-weighted image. In the development of the osteochondral lesion, if the shear stress is greater than the strength of the subchondral bone but less than that of cartilage, the overlying articular cartilage surface may remain intact. Both the articular cartilage surface and bone will fail if the shear stress is greater than the strength of both cartilage and bone, as shown in this case. A complete lesion or fracture of articular cartilage and bone may be associated with displacement of the fragment from its bed.

scopic and conventional radiographic findings, another classification system, based on CT findings, was developed by Ferkel and Sgaglione.[21] CT is performed in the direct axial and coronal planes at 1.5 mm, in association with sagittal reformations. (CT scans are performed for a known diagnosis of OLT, whereas MR imaging is preferred in patients with ankle pain of unknown etiology.) The CT classification progresses from stage I to stage IV. In stage I there is a cystic lesion of the talar dome with an intact roof. In stage IIA there is a cystic lesion with communication to the talar dome surface, and in stage IIB there is an open articular surface lesion with an overlying nondisplaced fragment. In stage III there is a nondisplaced lesion with lucency, and in stage IV there is a displaced fragment. Both CT and MR

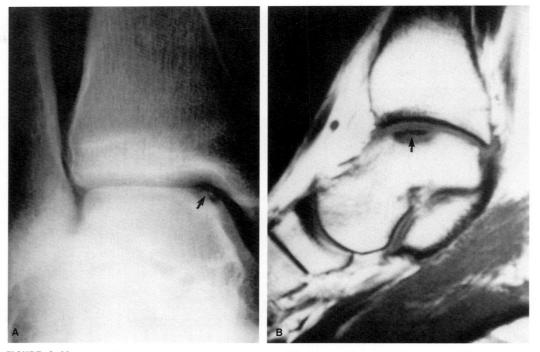

FIGURE 8-40. Stage III osteochondral lesion (*arrow*) with a complete nondisplaced osteochondral fragment shown on (**A**) an anteroposterior radiograph and (**B**) a T1-weighted sagittal image. The osteochondral fragment demonstrates low signal intensity sclerosis.

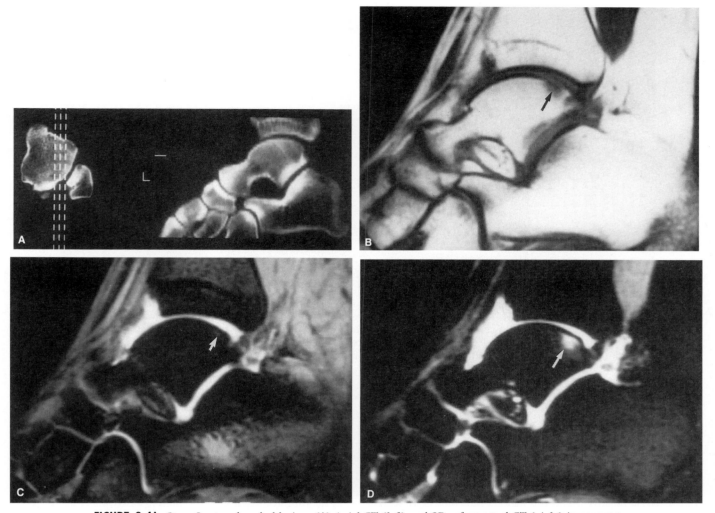

FIGURE 8-41. Stage I osteochondral lesion. **(A)** Axial CT (*left*) and 2D reformatted CT (*right*) images are negative for an osteochondral lesion. **(B)** The low signal intensity posterolateral osteochondral lesion is revealed on a T1-weighted sagittal image (*arrow*). **(C)** Minimal signal abnormality is seen on a T2*-weighted sagittal image (*arrow*). **(D)** The hyperintense osteochondral lesion is more accurately displayed on a short TI inversion recovery image (*arrow*). Note that the area of increased signal intensity is greater than that seen on T1 and T2*-weighted sagittal images.

imaging provide more information about the size and location of the lesion than does conventional radiography.

MR imaging can also be used to stage OLT, and it has the advantage of detecting radiographically occult lesions that in certain cases may not be evident on CT. In a direct comparison of CT with MR imaging, Anderson and colleagues[22] found that, compared with MR imaging, CT did not detect stage I lesions in 4 of 24 patients. The following proposed four-stage classification of OLT lesions is based on MR findings:

- Stage I: subchondral trabecular compression (radiograph results are negative with positive bone scan findings, and marrow edema is seen on MR imaging; Fig. 8-41)

- Stage IIA: subchondral cyst (Figs. 8-42 and 8-43)
- Stage IIB: incomplete separation of the fragment (Figs. 8-44 and 8-45)
- Stage III: fluid around an undetached, undisplaced fragment (Figs. 8-46 and 8-47)
- Stage IV: a displaced fragment (Fig. 8-48)

An arthroscopic classification of OLT has been proposed by Pritsch and colleagues,[23] based on categorizing the appearance of the overlying cartilage into three grades: (1) intact, firm, shiny articular cartilage; (2) intact but soft cartilage; and (3) frayed cartilage.[23] Another arthroscopic staging system was developed by Cheng and

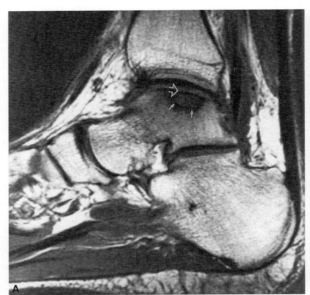
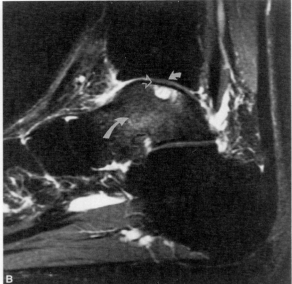

FIGURE 8-42. A subchondral cyst is hypointense on sagittal T1-weighted image (**A**) and hyperintense on sagittal STIR image (**B**). Focal inhomogeneity of overlying talar dome articular cartilage (*small curved arrow*) and associated talar bone marrow edema (*large curved arrow*) are best demonstrated on the STIR image. However, the rim of hypointense subchondral sclerosis (*small straight arrows*) is best appreciated on the T1-weighted image (**A**). There is congruity without disruption of the subchondral plate (*open arrow*) as assessed in the sagittal plane.

others[24] after reviewing 100 consecutive ankle arthroscopies (Table 8-1).

MR Appearance

As mentioned, results of x-rays in the early stages of OLT may be negative, and the lesions may not be detected until a necrotic focus is observed.[22] Necrosis is characterized by increased bone density in the necrotic focus and surrounding demineralization secondary to increased vascularization. In addition, it is not possible to assess the integrity of hyaline articular cartilage surfaces in osteocartilaginous defects with conventional radiographs or CT scans. With MR imaging, however, tibiotalar anatomy can be displayed in the coronal, axial, or sagittal planes to identify the talar defect and the presence of an avulsed body fragment. Subchondral marrow and articular cartilage surfaces are uniquely demonstrated on MR images.

The hyaline articular cartilage surface of the talar dome demonstrates intermediate signal intensity on T1- and T2-weighted images, low to intermediate signal intensity on fat-suppressed T2-weighted fast spin-echo images, and high signal intensity on T2*-weighted images. A detached cortical fragment, on the other hand, remains low in signal intensity. Adherent hyaline articular cartilage, reparative fibrocartilage, and associated fibrous tissue demonstrate intermediate signal intensity. On T1-weighted images, the bony defect of the talus demonstrates low or intermediate signal intensity, depending on the degree of synovial fluid

and fibrous tissue, respectively. On T2-weighted images, synovial fluid contents generate increased signal intensity. Peripheral areas of low signal intensity within the subchondral bone on T1- and T2-weighted images have been correlated with reactive bone sclerosis on plain radiographs. On STIR (including fast spin-echo STIR) and fat-suppressed T2-weighted fast spin-echo sequences, larger areas of adjacent subchondral talar marrow edema or hyperemia are hyperintense compared with the low signal intensity observed on T1-weighted images. These subchondral changes should not be misinterpreted and do not indicate that the overlying osteochondral lesion is more extensive or more aggressive than the focal and smaller superficially located lesion. In contrast to avascular necrosis (AVN) of the talus, the marrow hyperemia associated with the osteochondral lesion is usually less extensive and directly radiates from the lesion. Early AVN of the talus may be seen in association with a more diffuse hyperemia or edema of the entire talar head and body.

Abnormalities of the articular surface include regions of cartilage thinning, bowing, nodularity, or disruption.[25] The accumulation of high intensity joint fluid at or undermining the cartilage surface indicates small fissures or breaks.

On sagittal or coronal images, a focal, upward bowing of the hyaline cartilage overlying the bony defect may be demonstrated (see Fig. 8-47). The cartilage may be deformed or bowed without disruption, and it frequently shows softening at surgery. A postsurgical fibrocartilaginous scar can

text continues on page 517

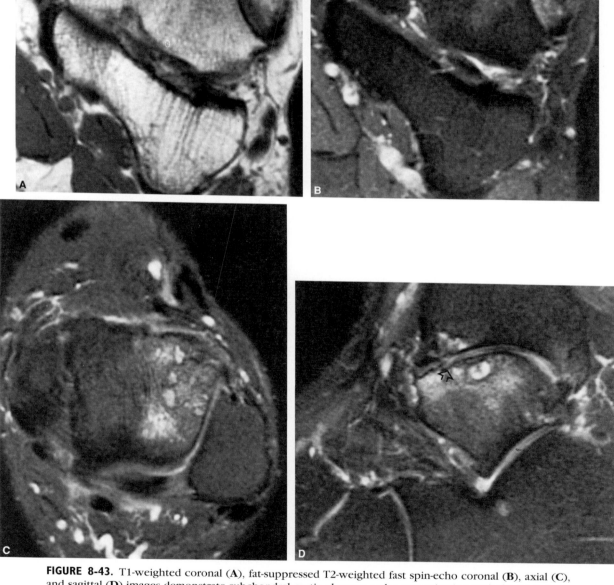

FIGURE 8-43. T1-weighted coronal (**A**), fat-suppressed T2-weighted fast spin-echo coronal (**B**), axial (**C**), and sagittal (**D**) images demonstrate subchondral cystic changes and communication with the talar dome surface (*straight arrow*). There is focal hyperintensity in denuded overlying articular cartilage (*curved arrow*). The cystic fluid contents and larger area of adjacent subchondral marrow are hyperintense on fat-suppressed T2-weighted fast spin-echo images. The axial image displays the anterior-to-posterior extent of the lesion, and its lateral location and multicystic morphology. Flattening and initial collapse of the anteromedial talar articular surface (*open arrow*) is best identified on the sagittal image.

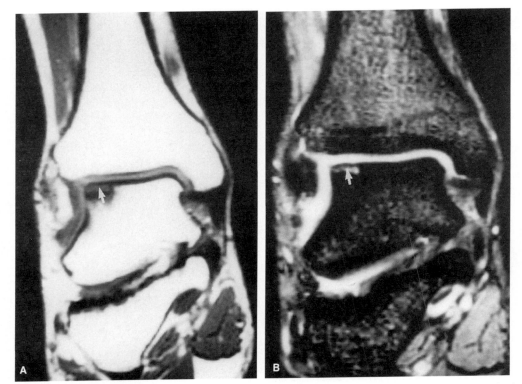

FIGURE 8-44. A stage II lesion with a partial osteochondral fracture (*arrow*) involving the lateral talar dome can be seen on (**A**) T1-weighted and (**B**) T2*-weighted coronal images. The hyperintense fluid undermines the lateral aspect of the osteochondral lesion on the T2*-weighted image.

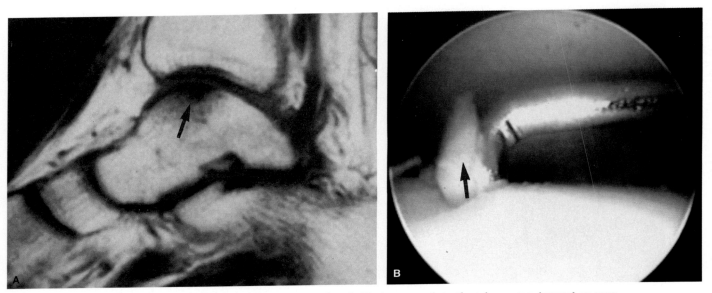

FIGURE 8-45. (**A**) A low signal intensity osteochondral lesion extends to the talar cortex (*arrow*) as seen on a T1-weighted sagittal image. (**B**) The partially detached cartilaginous flap (*arrow*) is mobilized during arthroscopy of the tibiotalar joint.

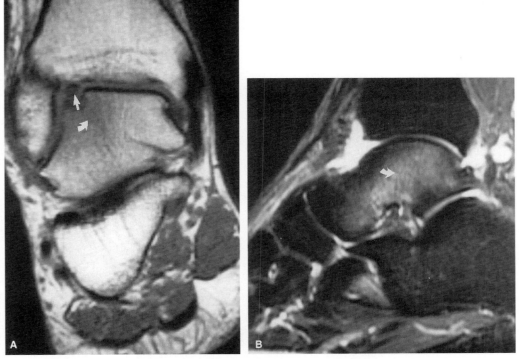

FIGURE 8-46. (A) A T1-weighted coronal image shows a stage III osteochondral lesion with a low signal intensity, complete, nondisplaced osteochondral fracture (*straight arrow*). Note the associated diffuse low signal intensity subchondral talar marrow edema (*curved arrow*). (B) High signal intensity talar edema (*curved arrow*) is displayed on a short TI inversion recovery sagittal image. Tibiotalar joint effusion distends the anterior and posterior capsules.

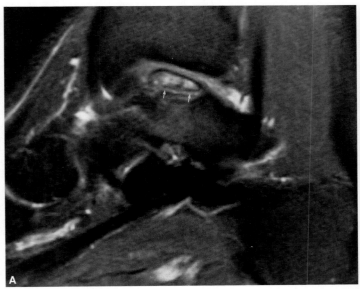

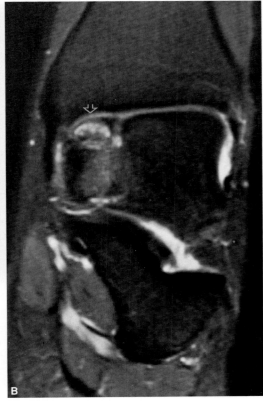

FIGURE 8-47. Stage III osteochondral lesion with an unattached, non-displaced fragment circumferentially surrounded by hyperintense joint fluid (*small arrows*). The fragment itself and adjacent talar subchondral bone exhibit hyperintense bone marrow edema. There is upward convex bowing of the medial talar hyaline articular cartilage (*open arrow*). Fat-suppressed T2-weighted fast spin-echo sagittal (**A**) and coronal (**B**) images.

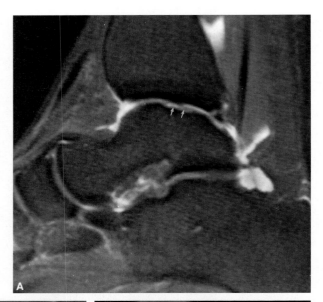

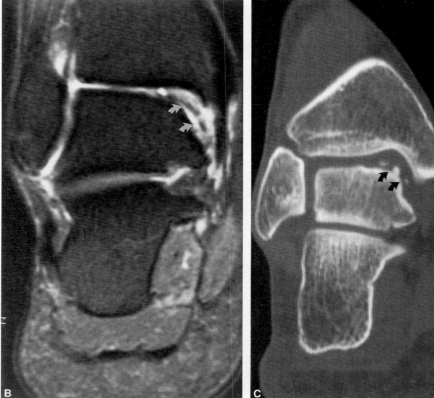

FIGURE 8-48. (**A**) A fat-suppressed T2-weighted fast spin-echo sagittal image shows a stage IV osteochondral lesion with focal articular surface flattening, loss of articular cartilage, and an irregular contour of the subchondral bone (*arrows*). A corresponding fat-suppressed T2-weighted fast spin-echo coronal image (**B**) and a coronal CT scan (**C**) identify displaced medial talar dome fragments associated with the adjacent segment abnormal subchondral bone. The chronicity of this lesion is confirmed by lack of associated marrow signal intensity changes.

TABLE 8-1
Surgical Grade Based on Articular Cartilage Findings

Grade	Arthroscopic Appearance
A	Smooth and intact, but soft or ballotable
B	Rough surface
C	Fibrillations/fissures
D	Flap present or bone exposed
E	Loose, undisplaced fragment
F	Displaced fragment

appear as an intermediate-intensity, focal area of thickening, bridging a cartilaginous defect. T2*-weighted images are useful for identification of small areas of cartilage disruption. However, fat-suppressed T2-weighted fast spin-echo and STIR images are more sensitive[26] (Fig. 8-49). The articular cartilage surface and bone are both involved in a complete lesion when the shear stress is greater than the ultimate strength of both articular cartilage and bone.[26] MR imaging identifies both the presence of undermining fluid and fragment displacement (see Fig. 8-39). Fluid transgressing articular cartilage and subchondral bone edema can be identified routinely on fat-suppressed T2-weighted fast spin-echo and STIR images with greater sensitivity than with corresponding T2- or T2*-weighted images. De Smet and colleagues[27] have correlated the stability of the osteochondral fragment with signal intensity on T2-weighted images. They found an irregular high signal intensity zone at the fragment-talar interface in partially attached fragments, whereas a complete ring of fluid signal intensity surrounding the lesion occurred in unattached fragments. Granulation tissue may also produce a high signal intensity band at the fragment-subchondral bone interface, which should not be misinterpreted as articular cartilage violation.

Intravenous MR contrast may help to evaluate the congruity of the articular cartilage surface and to enhance subchondral hyperemia and synovial tissue hypertrophy. Intraarticular contrast (MR arthrography) with fat-suppression is used to directly evaluate the flow of contrast over the articular cartilage surface of the talar dome. This is useful in identifying unstable and free fragments.

Value of MR Imaging

Although conventional radiographs are still the first choice for initial evaluation of patients with suspected osteochondral defects, MR imaging offers the ability to assess both the talar defect and the integrity of overlying cartilage surfaces. MR depiction of an intact articular surface, for example, may guide the decision about therapy in the direction of more conservative treatments, such as drilling, and obviate the need for surgical excision and curettage. Although the ultimate treatment decision in an osteochondral

lesion is determined at surgery, preoperative MR imaging can help to determine whether the lesion is loose or not.

Treatment

Treatment protocols for osteochondral lesions of the talus vary, depending on the stage of the lesion and whether it is acute or chronic in nature. Immobilization with conservative treatment may be used in chronic stage I and II lesions and in some stage III lesions. Generally, however, stage III or IV lesions require free fragment excision, curettage, drilling, or abrasion arthroplasty. A drilled or abraded base permits fibrocartilaginous ingrowth in lesions with a nonreplaceable fragment. Complications—including locking of the joint, which occurs with larger bone fragments; degenerative arthritis, which is more likely to occur with lateral, often symptomatic, lesions; and nonunion of the fracture—often lead to traumatic osteoarthritis.

Arthroscopic treatment of talar dome fractures has relatively low morbidity and complication rates.[28] Cystic areas are bone grafted if cartilage is intact; otherwise, the cyst is corrected with drilling or abrasion of the base. Arthroscopic treatment for acute osteochondral lesions of the talus is different from that for chronic lesions. Acute lesions may require the use of CT or MR imaging to identify the lesion and characterize the size, morphology, and stage. In displaced

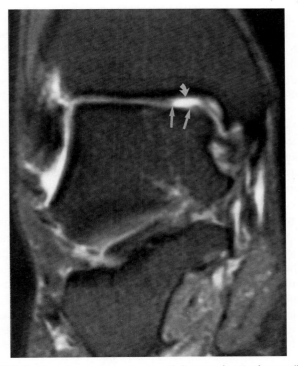

FIGURE 8-49. A focal discontinuity of disrupted articular cartilage in a medial osteochondral lesion can be seen on this fat-suppressed T2-weighted fast spin-echo coronal image. The edges of the unaffected talar articular cartilage surfaces are indicated (*arrows*). Hyperintense fluid fills the articular cartilage defect (*curved arrow*).

lesions, arthroscopy is performed with possible open pinning or removal of the osteochondral lesion. Acute lesions are palpated with a small joint probe. The chondral fragment is then assessed to determine whether or not there is enough bone to permit healing, if reattachment with absorbable pins, K-wires, or screws is undertaken. Primary chondral lesions without attached bone are excised, with debridement and drilling or abrading of the base. Loose fragments are either fixated with absorbable pins, K-wires, or screws, or they are excised with drilling of the base. Displaced lesions are excised, and the base is drilled or abraded if it cannot be reattached.

Injuries to the Tendons

A variety of studies have confirmed the usefulness of MR imaging in the evaluation of tendinous and ligamentous structures about the ankle. Intact tendons and ligaments demonstrate low signal intensity on all pulsing sequences. The thicker tendons of the ankle can be studied in multiple planes, although smaller ligamentous bands may be seen in only one orthogonal plane.

Achilles Tendon Rupture

The Achilles tendon, the largest tendon in the body, is formed by the confluence of the gastrocnemius and soleus muscle complexes. Injuries to this tendon secondary to athletic activity are frequent in middle-aged men.[29,30] In patients with disorders such as rheumatoid arthritis, systemic lupus erythematosus, diabetes mellitus, and gout, there may be a predisposition to disruption of the Achilles tendon because of already weakened connective tissue and collagen fibers. The Achilles tendon is most susceptible to rupture 2 to 6 cm superior to the os calcis. Acute rupture is associated with forced dorsiflexion of the foot against a contracting force generated by the triceps surae group. Rupture of the contracted musculotendinous unit may occur secondary to direct trauma.

DIAGNOSIS. With clinical examination alone, rupture of the Achilles tendon is missed in up to 25% of cases, perhaps because the other tendons of the posterior calf maintain plantar flexion and allow a tendinous gap to be missed on clinical examination. Clinical assessment by the Thompsen test is performed in the prone position. In Achilles tendon rupture, squeezing the calf does not produce the normal response of plantar flexion. This represents a positive Thompsen test.

Lateral radiography and xerography have not been effective in identifying abnormalities in the Achilles tendon. Although tendon thickening in inflammation and discontinuities in tears have been observed with some success using real time ultrasonography, this technique is limited in soft-tissue contrast discrimination, FOV, and by the inability to accurately evaluate both adjacent soft-tissue and bony structures.

MR IMAGING TECHNIQUE. The Achilles tendon can be demonstrated on sagittal, axial, and thin section coronal MR images.[31] A routine examination of the tendon uses a 14 to 16 cm FOV and sections 3 to 4 mm thick. A T1-weighted sequence is performed in the sagittal plane through the Achilles tendon. T2*-weighted, fat-suppressed T2-weighted fast spin-echo, or STIR images show associated hemorrhage or edema in the intratendinous or peritendinous soft-tissue structures. Fat-suppressed T2-weighted fast spin-echo or STIR axial sequences reveal fluid, hemorrhage, or inflammatory tendon changes and evaluate the integrity of other tendons and ligaments supporting the ankle. Thin section (3 mm) coronal images display the width of the Achilles tendon and the condition of disrupted tendon fibers.

MR APPEARANCE. The normal Achilles tendon demonstrates uniform low signal intensity. Axial images show the tendon in cross section with a mildly flattened anterior surface and a convex posterior surface. In ruptures of the Achilles tendon, the relationship of the proximal and distal portions of the torn tendon can be seen on MR studies either before or after application of a plaster cast (Fig. 8-50). High signal intensity fat may be interposed at the tear site in complete tendinous disruptions with discontinuity (Fig. 8-51). Fraying or corkscrewing of the tendon edges is frequently associated with proximal tendon retraction (Fig. 8-52). In the absence of overlapping tendon edges, no tendon fibers can be seen at the tear site on axial images. In one study, preoperative MR imaging findings, including tendon morphology, orientation of torn fibers, and measurement of tendon diastases, all correlated with surgical findings during tendon repair.[32] Associated hemorrhage within peritendinous soft tissues is also revealed on axial or sagittal MR images. Subacute hemorrhage generates high signal intensity on T1-weighted images. Areas of edema or inflammation demonstrate increased signal intensity on T2- or T2*-weighted images. A musculotendinous junction tear involves disruption of muscle fibers, although on gross examination the tendon appears intact.

TREATMENT. In making a decision about conservative management of Achilles tendon tear, principally serial casting, MR imaging has become invaluable for documenting the degree of apposition of the disrupted proximal and distal tendon fragments. Retracted tendon sections are less likely to heal with conservative management, and MR evaluation allows early identification of these patients, who are candidates for surgical intervention (Fig. 8-53). Fibrous bridging also appears to be more tenuous with increased tendon separation. A bulbous contour may be demonstrated in the proliferating ends of a torn Achilles tendon, and it increases with greater tendon diastases. Fibrous healing, with approxima-

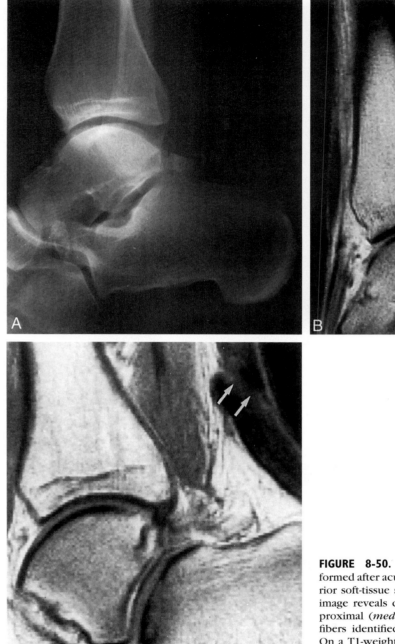

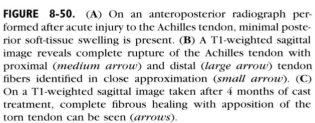

FIGURE 8-50. (**A**) On an anteroposterior radiograph performed after acute injury to the Achilles tendon, minimal posterior soft-tissue swelling is present. (**B**) A T1-weighted sagittal image reveals complete rupture of the Achilles tendon with proximal (*medium arrow*) and distal (*large arrow*) tendon fibers identified in close approximation (*small arrow*). (**C**) On a T1-weighted sagittal image taken after 4 months of cast treatment, complete fibrous healing with apposition of the torn tendon can be seen (*arrows*).

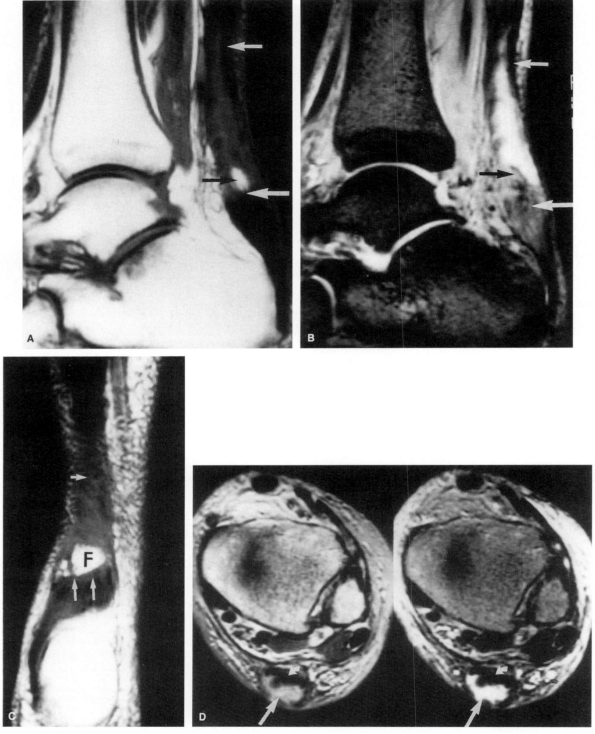

FIGURE 8-51. A complete Achilles tendon tear with a large tendinous gap (*white arrows*). Interposed fat demonstrates (**A**) bright signal intensity on a T1-weighted sagittal image and (**B**) intermediate signal intensity on a T2*-weighted image. (**C**) On a 3 mm T1-weighted posterior coronal image, the proximal (*single arrow*) and distal (*double arrow*) tendon edges are indicated with interposed high signal intensity fat (**F**). (**D**) On intermediate weighted (*left*) and T2-weighted (*right*) axial images, a high signal intensity hemorrhagic tear site (*straight arrows*) with unattached low signal intensity anterior tendon fibers (*curved arrows*) is revealed at the level of the distal tibia.

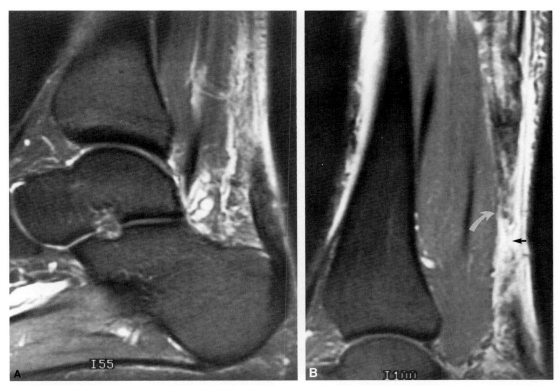

FIGURE 8-52. Complete Achilles tendon tear with proximal tendon retraction (*curved arrow*) on a fat-suppressed T2-weighted fast spin-echo sagittal image obtained at the level of (**A**) the distal tendon and (**B**) the proximal tendon ends. Hyperintense edema and hemorrhage are shown at the tear site and gap (*straight arrow*). It was not possible to assess the degree of proximal tendon retraction without repositioning the surface coil.

tion of torn fibers, can be evaluated with MR imaging performed at monthly intervals. The healing of conservatively or surgically managed tendons may be associated with intratendinous fluid spaces, studied at 3 and 6 months by Dillon and colleagues.[33] Over time, decreased signal intensity was found in the areas of successful healing. By 12 months, these areas demonstrated low signal intensity within a widened tendon. Caution must be exercised in interpreting MR images obtained in the first 2 months postoperatively; Achilles tendon pathology should not be overread as retear, poor healing, or failed surgical repair.[34]

The Achilles tendon and overlying skin are relatively avascular and may become infected after surgery with implanted material or autogenous tendon. The incidence of complications with surgical repair is reported to be 20%. Rerupture of the Achilles tendon is significantly higher in patients who undergo nonsurgical treatment than in those who have had surgical repair. Surgery is the preferred treatment for any patient who has a rerupture of the Achilles tendon treated conservatively, and possibly should be the primarily treatment choice for any patient who is active and athletic.[35] Chronic thickening of the Achilles tendon or residual inflammatory changes are demonstrated on axial and sagittal MR images. After repair with strands of a polymer of lactic acid (PLA), T1-weighted images show a thickened

fusiform tendon with moderate signal intensity streaks[36] (Fig. 8-54). Changes in signal intensity are attributed to the PLA implant and surrounding collagenogenic response.

MR imaging may be most useful in Achilles tendon rupture in the selection of patients best suited for conservative therapy, thereby improving the present statistics for rerupture (10% with conservative treatment compared with 4% with surgical treatment).[37,38] Retear of a primary repaired tendon shows residual suture artifact (Fig. 8-55).

Partial Tears of the Achilles Tendon

Partial tendon tears can be defined on MR images in the sagittal and axial planes. Linear or focal regions of increased signal and thickening of fibers without a tendinous gap are characteristic of partial tears of the Achilles tendon (Figs. 8-56 through 8-58). Without inflammatory reaction, tendinitis—a common affliction among joggers—can be recognized by a thickening of the tendon complex. Incomplete tears may also be present with partial continuity of a portion of tendon fibers on at least one sagittal image. Longitudinal splits in chronic Achilles tendinitis which are low to intermediate in signal intensity on long TR/TE images may be seen in association with a superimposed acute partial tear. The acute partial tear is hyperintense on long TR/TE images.

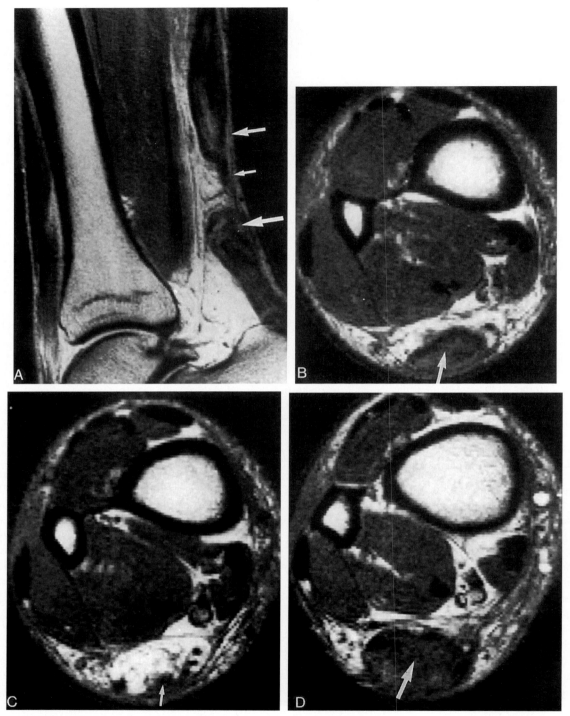

FIGURE 8-53. (**A**) T1-weighted sagittal and corresponding (**B**) superior, (**C**) mid-, and (**D**) inferior axial images demonstrate a healing Achilles tendon with an enlarged proximal end (*medium arrow*), tenuous union (*small arrow*), and bulbous distal tendon (*large arrow*). These signs indicate suboptimal Achilles tendon union.

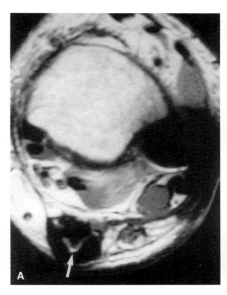
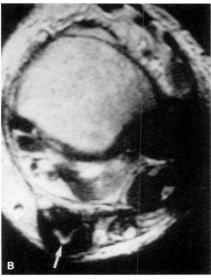

FIGURE 8-54. A postoperative high signal intensity suture artifact (*arrows*) is seen on (**A**) intermediate weighted and (**B**) T2-weighted axial images of a thickened Achilles tendon.

Achilles Tendinitis

The Achilles tendon does not have a true tendon synovial sheath. Inflammatory conditions are thus classified as tendinitis, paratendinitis, and peritendinitis. Tendinitis represents intrinsic or intrasubstance inflammation of the Achilles tendon. Paratendinitis shows inflammatory changes about the Achilles tendon, and peritendinitis involves inflammation of the peritenon. An irregular pre-Achilles fat pad may be seen with peritendinitis or paratendinitis with or without abnormal Achilles tendon morphology (Fig. 8-59).

Overuse of the calf muscles may lead to tendinitis, paratendinitis, or peritendinitis. In stenosing tenosynovitis, chronic inflammation of the peritenon is found. Partial tearing, intrasubstance cysts from chronic partial tears, or nodules may also be identified. New collagen formation and associated fibrillation, nodularity, degeneration, and discoloration contribute to constriction of the peritenon.

MR findings in Achilles tendinitis (Fig. 8-60) include

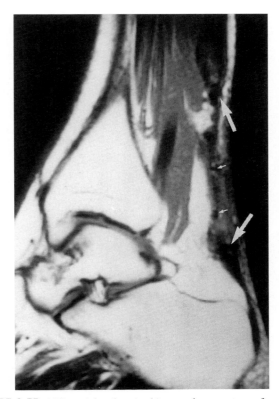

FIGURE 8-55. A T1-weighted sagittal image shows retear of an Achilles tendon repair with postoperative suture artifact (*small arrows*) and tendon discontinuity (*large arrows*).

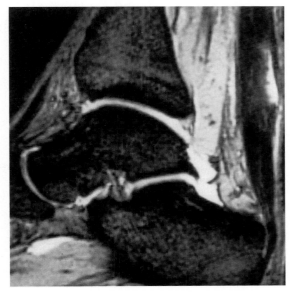

FIGURE 8-56. A partial tear of the posterior aspect of the Achilles tendon is seen on a T2*-weighted sagittal image. High signal intensity fluid is demonstrated in the longitudinally oriented tear. Associated diffuse thickening of the tendon is present.

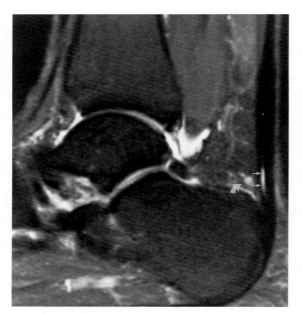

FIGURE 8-57. Linear hyperintense partial tear (*straight arrow*) of the distal Achilles tendon on a fat-suppressed T2-weighted fast spin-echo sagittal image. There is associated mild tendon thickening and mild edema (*curved arrow*) superficial to the distal Achilles tendon.

focal or fusiform thickening of the Achilles tendon (Fig. 8-61) and diffuse or linear low to intermediate signal intensity on T2-weighted, fat-suppressed T2-weighted fast spin-echo, or STIR images. T2* sequences demonstrate an increased hyperintensity (relative to other pulse sequences) in areas of tendon degeneration (Fig. 8-62). Fat-suppressed T2-weighted fast spin-echo sequences not as sensitive to intrasubstance signal intensity as T2*-weighted or STIR techniques are. Inflammatory changes may coexist with mucinous or myxoid degeneration, which may or may not demonstrate similar increases in signal intensity on T2-weighted images. Anterior convexity of the enlarged tendon may also be revealed on sagittal images, and proximal extension of fluid in the retrocalcaneal bursa may also be seen. It may be difficult to distinguish areas of chronic tendinitis from intrasubstance tendon tears without documenting either discontinuity in tendon fibers or discrete hyperintense signal intensity on T2-weighted or STIR images with partial tears (Fig. 8-63). Chronic Achilles tendinitis is seen with widening of the tendon diameter or contours. This may be focal or diffuse. Intrasubstance increased signal intensity may not be evident in uncomplicated (not associated with partial tears) chronic lesions. Adhesions between the peritenon and Achilles tendon are associated with chronic peritendinitis. A healed Achilles tendon tear displays thickening without associated increased signal intensity.

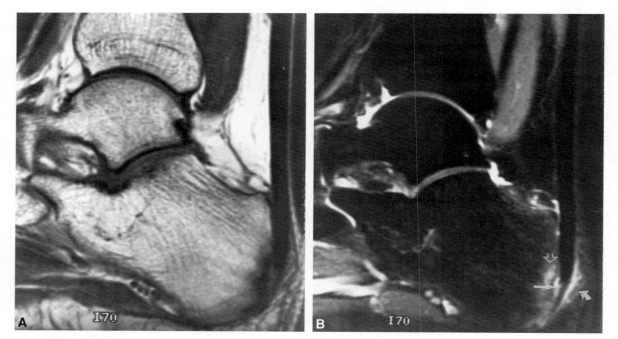

FIGURE 8-58. Partial tear of the distal attachment of the Achilles tendon (*arrow*) on (**A**) T1-weighted and (**B**) STIR sagittal images. Subcutaneous tissue edema is present posterior to the os calcis attachment of the Achilles tendon (*curved arrow*). Posterior calcaneal erosions and marrow edema (*open arrow*) are appreciated on the STIR sequence (**B**).

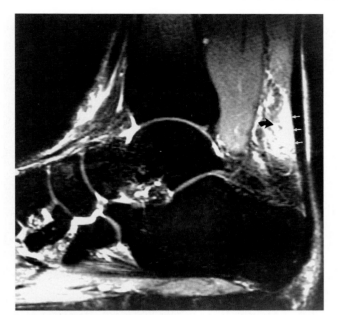

FIGURE 8-59. A STIR sagittal image displays hyperintense Achilles peritendinitis and paratendinitis involving the pre-Achilles fat pad (*curved arrow*) and peritenon (*straight arrow*) anterior to the anterior surface of a morphologically normal hypointense Achilles tendon.

If treatment by immobilization is not successful, stripping and excision of the thickened peritenon and granulation tissue are performed. The use of steroids may weaken the tendon and produce rupture. In gout, deposition of tophaceous material may also lead to spontaneous rupture of the Achilles tendon (Fig. 8-64). Tophi appear similar to nodular myxoid-like degeneration and demonstrate intermediate and increased signal inhomogeneity on T2-weighted, T2*-weighted, or STIR images. Xanthomas of the Achilles tendon have been shown to produce infiltrative lesions with diffuse tendon thickening and enlarged soft-tissue components (masses)[39–41] (Fig. 8-65). Bilaterality of these lesions is common. Xanthomas enhance with intravenous gadolinium administration. The soft-tissue component displays hyperintense inhomogeneity on fat-suppressed T2-weighted fast spin-echo images.

Tibialis Posterior Injuries

DIAGNOSIS.   Rupture of the tibialis posterior tendon (posterior tibial tendon [PTT]), which may occur spontaneously, is usually associated with prior synovitis, steroid injection, or trauma. Chronic tibialis posterior tendon rupture usually occurs in middle-aged women in their fifth or sixth decades. Clinically, a unilateral flatfoot deformity develops, often with no history of trauma.[42] There is intrinsic

text continues on page 530

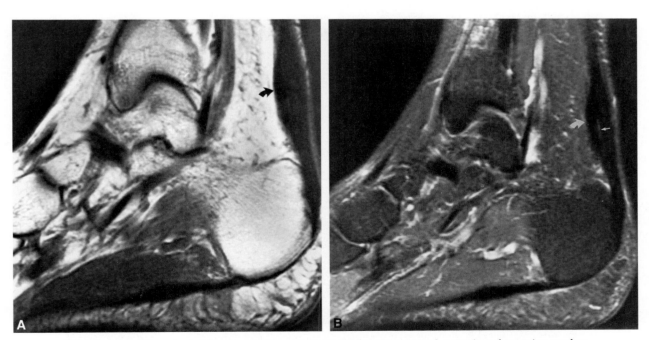

FIGURE 8-60. Chronic Achilles tendinitis with focal thickening (*curved arrow*) and anterior tendon convexity on (**A**) T1-weighted and (**B**) fat-suppressed T2-weighted fast spin-echo sagittal images. There is minimal-weighted intratendinous increased signal intensity on the fat-suppressed T2-weighted fast spin-echo image (*straight arrow*).

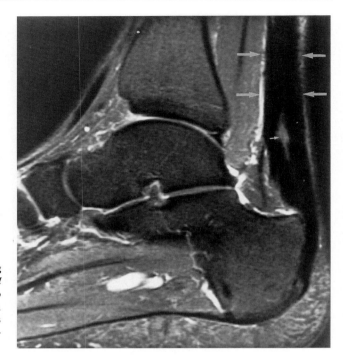

FIGURE 8-61. Chronic Achilles tendinitis with diffuse tendon thickening throughout its length (*large arrow*). Central linear hyperintensity (*small arrow*) is demonstrated on this fat-suppressed T2-weighted fast spin-echo sagittal image. Chronic tendinitis may be difficult to differentiate from chronic tendinitis associated with an acute partial tear of the Achilles tendon. In chronic tendinitis, longitudinal tendon splits and mucoid tendon degeneration coexist.

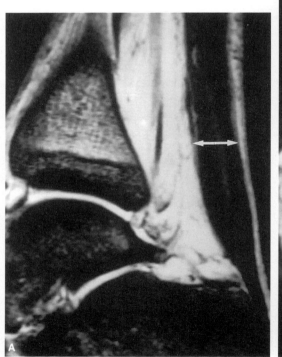

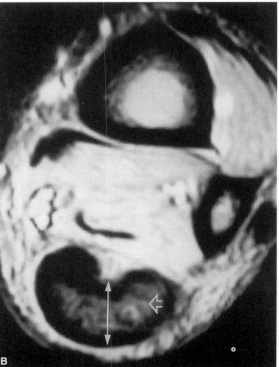

FIGURE 8-62. **(A)** A T2*-weighted sagittal image shows Achilles tendinitis with abnormal tendon thickening (*double-headed arrow*) and convexity to the anterior tendon margin. **(B)** A T2*-weighted axial image demonstrates high signal intensity tendinitis (*open arrow*) and diffuse thickening (*double headed arrows*) without tendon discontinuity. Since it does not have a true synovial sheath, the Achilles tendon responds to inflammation with tendon thickening and intrasubstance signal change. The paratenon, or loose connective tissue anterior to the Achilles tendon, may show associated edematous changes.

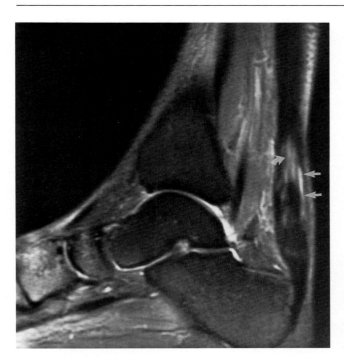

FIGURE 8-63. Chronic Achilles tendinitis with superimposed acute partial tear. Multiple areas of intrasubstance linear longitudinal hyperintensity are present within a widened tendon (*curved arrow*). A discrete posterior partial surface tear (*straight arrow*) demonstrates the greatest degree of increased signal intensity on this fat-suppressed T2-weighted fast spin-echo sagittal image. There is mild edema of soft tissue including the pre-Achilles fat pad anterior to the Achilles tendon.

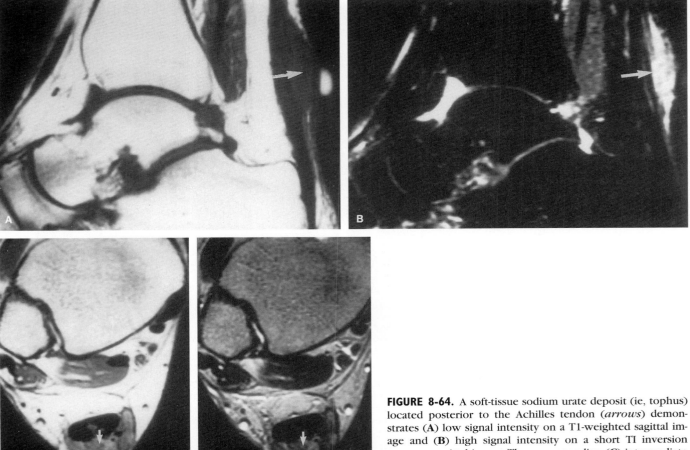

FIGURE 8-64. A soft-tissue sodium urate deposit (ie, tophus) located posterior to the Achilles tendon (*arrows*) demonstrates (**A**) low signal intensity on a T1-weighted sagittal image and (**B**) high signal intensity on a short TI inversion recovery sagittal image. The corresponding (**C**) intermediate weighted and (**D**) T2-weighted axial images show no significant increase in signal intensity in the gouty deposit.

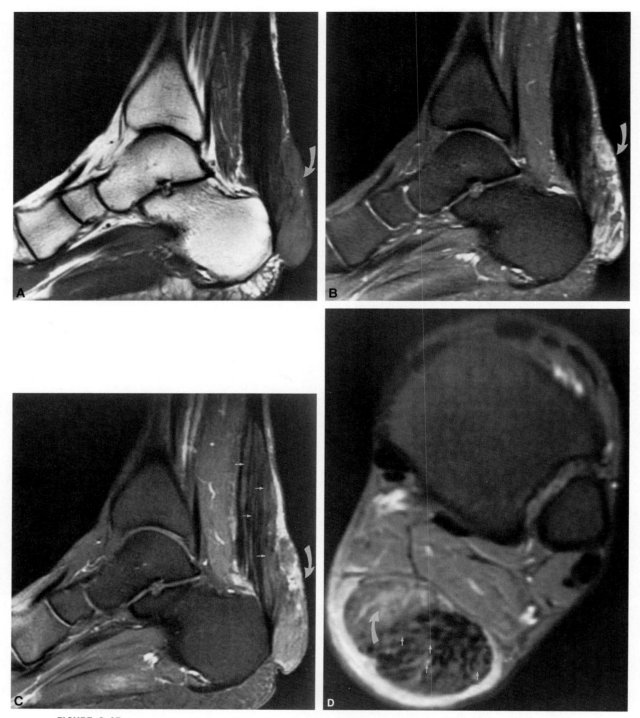

FIGURE 8-65. Xanthomas of the Achilles tendon with a large soft-tissue component (*curved arrow*) and diffuse infiltration of the Achilles tendon (*straight arrow*) on (**A**) sagittal T1-weighted images, (**B**) fat-suppressed T2-weighted fast spin-echo images, (**C**) fat-suppressed gadolinium enhanced T1-weighted images, and (**D**) axial fat-suppressed T2-weighted fast spin-echo images. Tendinous enhancement is demonstrated with intravenous gadolinium (**C, D**). The soft-tissue component posterior to the Achilles tendon is hyperintense on fat-suppressed T2-weighted fast spin-echo sequences (**B**) and demonstrates partial enhancement with intravenous contrast (**C**).

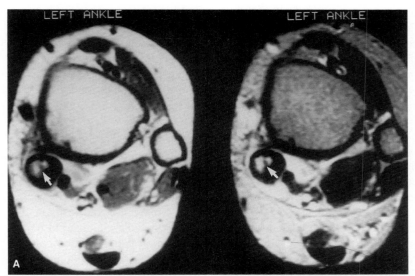

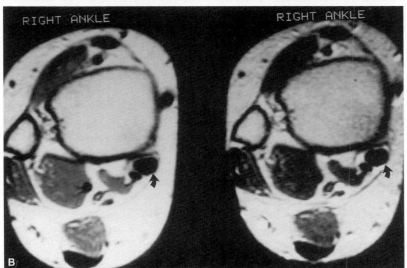

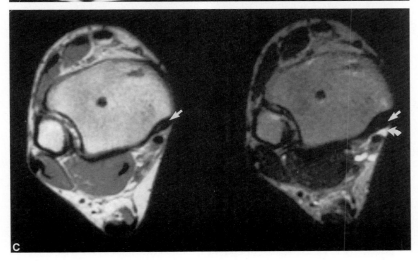

FIGURE 8-66. (**A**) A type I (ie, incomplete) tear of the tibialis posterior tendon is characterized by tendon thickening and central high signal intensity (*arrow*) on intermediate weighted (*left*) and T2-weighted (*right*) axial images of the left ankle. (**B**) Normal morphology, size, and low signal intensity of the tendon (*curved arrow*) of the uninjured right ankle is shown for comparison on intermediate weighted (*left*) and T2-weighted (*right*) axial images. (**C**) A type II lesion (partial tear) demonstrates associated tendon attenuation (*straight arrows*) and an adjacent hyperintense fluid signal intensity (*curved arrow*).

degeneration of the tendon, and the typical site of rupture is either at or within 6 cm proximal to its navicular insertion. Collapse of the medial longitudinal arch creates the characteristic flatfoot deformity with associated heel valgus, talar plantar flexion, and forefoot abduction.[43] Failure of calcaneal inversion with a valgus heel is observed on clinical examination when the patient stands on tiptoe. The clinical diagnosis is not straightforward, and in some cases as many as 43 months have elapsed between initial presentation and diagnosis.

Edema or soft-tissue thickening may be demonstrated inferior to the medial malleolus, although conventional radiographs do not demonstrate tendon pathology. Loss of a convex arch may be observed on weight-bearing views through the talonavicular or naviculocuneiform joint. Radiographs may also reveal a decreased calcaneal plantar angle, an increased lateral talometatarsal angle, an increased anterior talocalcaneal angle, and an increased lateral talocalcaneal angle.[43] Forefoot abduction is associated with lateral subluxation of the navicular at the talonavicular joint, which is shown on axial images through the midfoot. The presence of an accessory navicular bone is associated with both pes planus and tibialis posterior tendon dysfunction.

MR APPEARANCE. In complete tears, MR imaging demonstrates disruption of the tibialis posterior tendon with or without abnormal morphology of the ends of the tendon. Partial or chronic tears or a retracted tendon may present with enlargement. T2-weighted axial images that extend inferior to the medial malleolus should demonstrate the normal tibialis posterior tendon anterolateral to the flexor digitorum longus tendon.

Tibialis posterior tendon tears are classified into three types. Types I and II are partial tears; type I tears are charac-

terized by hypertrophy of the tendon, with heterogeneous signal intensity in vertical splits (Figs. 8-66 and 8-67), and type II tears are characterized by attenuated sections of tendon[44] (see Fig. 8-66C). Complete tears (ie, type III) are delineated by a tendinous gap (Fig. 8-68). In comparison with CT scans, and using surgical exploration as the gold standard, MR imaging is superior in detecting the spectrum of early partial tendon ruptures, longitudinal tearing, and the presence of synovial fluid.[45] Subtle areas of associated periostitis, however, are more readily delineated with CT.

The tendon hypertrophy seen in type I partial tears (Figs. 8-69 and 8-70), is best appreciated on axial images as an increased cross-sectional diameter. An increase in central intrasubstance signal intensity may also be seen on T1-weighted and often on fat-suppressed T2-weighted fast spin-echo or STIR images. In a common pattern of presentation associated with prominent or long segment longitudinal splits of the tibialis posterior in type I tears, there are three medial flexor tendons instead of two flexor tendons seen at or proximal to the level of the medial malleolus (Figs. 8-71 and 8-72). Proximal to the split, the tibialis posterior tendon is enlarged and seen as a single tendon (see Fig. 8-72).

The longitudinal splitting of the tibialis posterior tendon into two subtendons is also seen in type II tears of the tibialis posterior. Type II partial tears, in which the tibialis posterior tendon is attenuated or reduced in size, are usually identified at the level of the medial malleolus (see Fig. 8-66C). A nonconcentric reduction in tendon width may give the tibialis posterior tendon an elongated appearance, without any associated intrasubstance hyperintensity. In these type II tears, the two subtendons of the tibialis posterior are usually located proximal to the medial malleolus, and a single attenu-

text continues on page 534

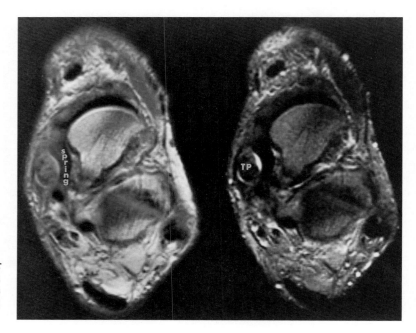

FIGURE 8-67. Type I tibialis posterior tendon (TP) tear with increased signal intensity within an enlarged tendon medial to the spring ligament, distal to the medial malleolus (fast spin-echo intermediate [*left*] and T2-weighted [*right*] axial images).

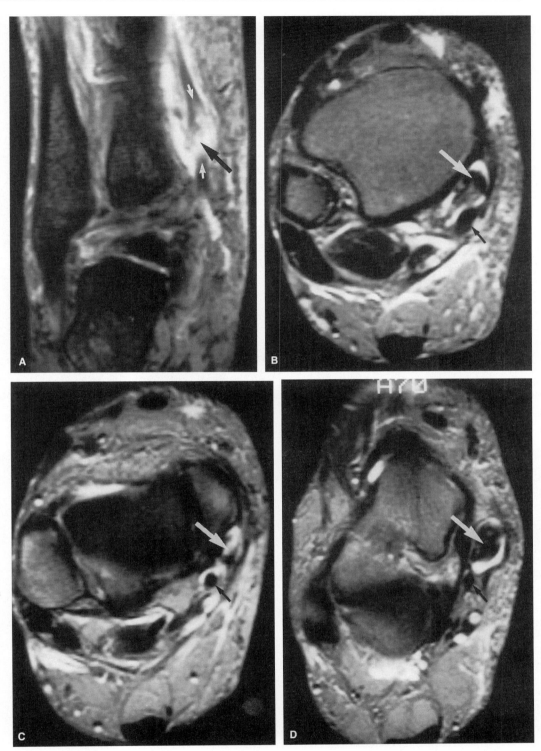

FIGURE 8-68. (**A**) A type III tibialis posterior tendon tear (*large black arrow*) shows a retracted proximal tendon (*white arrow oriented inferiorly*) and distal tendon segment (*white arrow oriented superiorly*) on a T2*-weighted posterior coronal image. Three separate T2-weighted axial images demonstrate tendon morphology (*large white arrows*) (**B**) proximal to the tear site, (**C**) at the tear site, and (**D**) distal to the tear site. Note the absence of the tibialis posterior tendon at the tear site and the low signal intensity thickened tendon proximal and distal to the area of disruption. The normal flexor digitorum longus tendon is indicated (*small black arrows*).

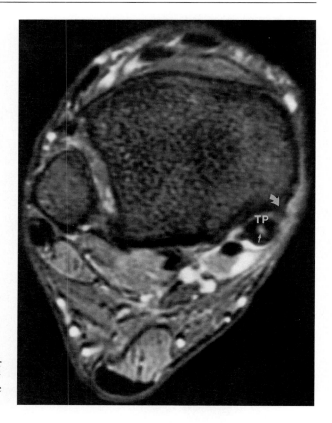

FIGURE 8-69. A T2*-weighted axial image displays a type I tibialis posterior (TP) tendon tear with enlarged cross sectional area and central hyperintensity (*straight arrow*). A small spur is identified on the posterior aspect of the medial malleolus (*curved arrow*).

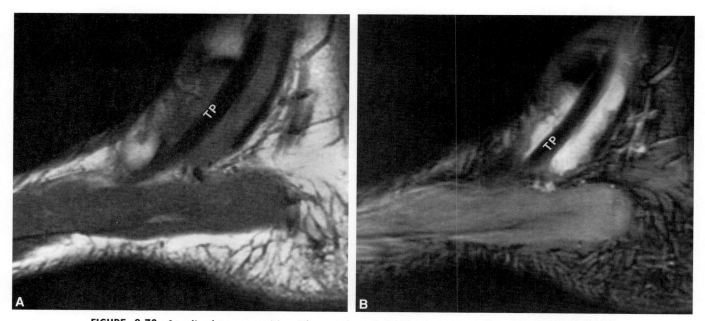

FIGURE 8-70. Localized tenosynovitis with an enlarged tibialis posterior tendon (TP). Intrasubstance longitudinal splits are not seen in the sagittal plane (T1 [**A**] and fat-suppressed T2-weighted fast spin-echo [**B**] sagittal images).

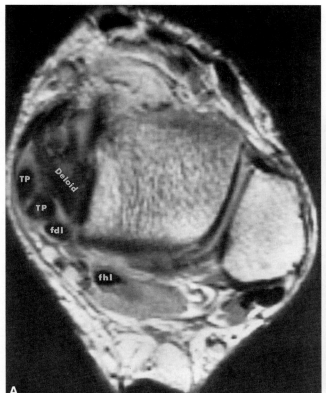

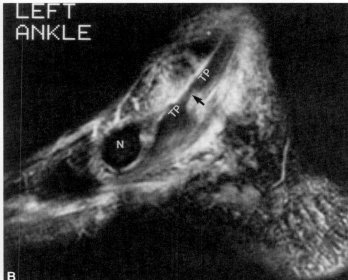

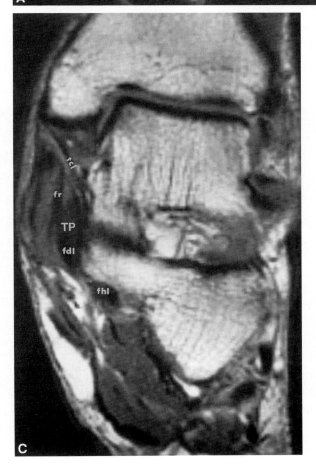

FIGURE 8-71. (**A**) A T1-weighted axial image depicts a longitudinal rupture of the tibialis posterior tendon resulting in two subtendons of the tibialis posterior (TP) at the level of the medial malleolus and deltoid ligament. Note that this split creates the appearance of four separate medial tendons. The two anterior medial tendons represent the anterior and posterior half of the tibialis posterior. (**B**) A T2*-weighted sagittal image identifies the attenuated portion of the tibialis posterior at the longitudinal tear site (*arrow*). (**C**) The relationship of the tibialis posterior (TP) to the adjacent medial structures on a corresponding T1-weighted coronal image. fdl, flexor digitorum longus tendon; fhl, flexor hallucis longus tendon; N, navicular bone; TP, tibialis posterior; tcl, tibiocalcaneal ligament; fr, flexor retinaculum.

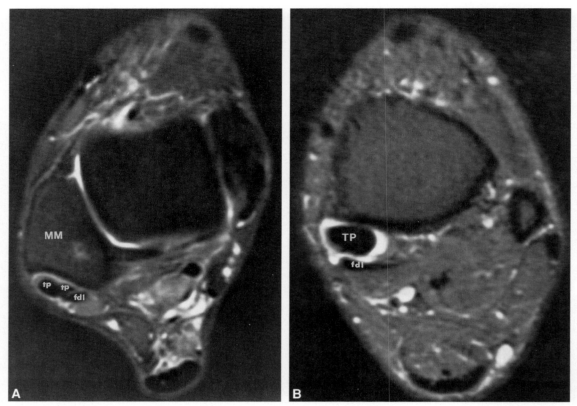

FIGURE 8-72. **(A)** A fat-suppressed T2-weighted fast spin-echo axial image showing a longitudinal tendon split with two sections of the tibialis posterior (tp) tendon identified posterior to the medial malleolus (MM). fdl, flexor digitorum longus tendon. **(B)** A fat-suppressed T2-weighted fast spin-echo axial image proximal to the medial malleolus shows gross enlargement of the tibialis posterior tendon (TP) relative to the normal flexor digitorum longus tendon (fdl). Hyperintense fluid surrounds the tibialis posterior.

ated tibialis posterior tendon is identified at the level of the medial malleolus. A medial malleolus periostitis or spur may contribute to the spectrum of tendon degeneration preceding rupture (see Fig. 8-69). The native tibialis posterior is seen directly posterior to the medial malleolus, and the torn or split fragment is seen posterior to the tendon. The normal flexor hallucis longus tendon is the most posterior and laterally positioned of the three tendons. Normally, only two tendons, the tibialis posterior and flexor digitorum longus, should be visualized medially.

Complete (or type III) tears of the tibialis posterior demonstrate a discontinuity on axial, coronal, and sagittal images (Fig. 8-73). Tendon retraction and a fluid-filled gap are present on T2 (fat-suppressed T2-weighted fast spin-echo), T2*, or STIR images. Additional, secondary, signs of tibialis posterior or PTT tear as reported by Schweitzer and colleagues[46] include the following: (1) prominence or hypertrophy of the medial tubercle of the navicular (sensitivity 89%, specificity 75%); (2) abnormalities of talonavicular alignment (sensitivity 82%, specificity 100%); and (3) presence of an accessory navicular (sensitivity 20%, specificity 100%). Normal talonavicular alignment can be determined by a line drawn through the long axis of the talus, which normally bisects

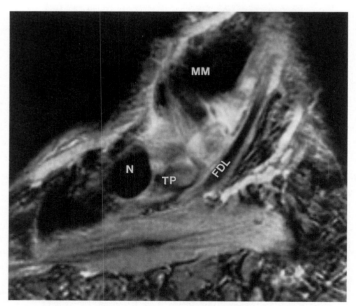

FIGURE 8-73. A complete tear of the tibialis posterior tendon (TP) with a stump of tissue identified adjacent to the navicular bone (N). No tendon is seen anterior to the flexor digitorum longus (FDL) on this fast spin-echo STIR sagittal image. MM, medial malleolus.

the navicular bone. Schweitzer and colleagues[46] additionally found that there is an overlap in the range of normal and abnormal distal tibialis posterior tendon size. There is also overlap in the range of intratendinous signal intensity in normal and torn tibialis posterior tendons. This overlap is primarily observed on T1-weighted images and is not observed on T2-weighted images. In clinical practice, tendon tears of the tibialis posterior are usually evident proximal to the navicular and diagnosis can be made without reliance on characterizing the bulbous configuration of the distal attachment.

Intrinsic degenerations usually demonstrate varying degrees of increased internal signal intensity with fusiform enlargement. Fluid in the tendon sheath, which demonstrates increased signal intensity on conventional T2, fat-suppressed T2-weighted fast spin-echo, and T2*-weighted images, may be observed in patients with tenosynovitis. Laxity or rupture of the plantar calcaneonavicular or spring ligament is associated with chronic dysfunction of the tibialis posterior tendon,[47] and may lead to a pes planovalgus deformity. The spring ligament normally functions as a stabilizer of the longitudinal arch of the foot. Traumatic dislocation of the tibialis posterior tendon is a rare injury attributed to forced dorsiflexion with inversion.

TREATMENT. Conservative treatment, which frequently fails, involves support of the medial longitudinal arch with orthoses. Surgical treatment consists of either osseous stabilization (ie, double or triple arthrodesis) with hindfoot arthrodesis, repair, or replacement of the ruptured tendon. A side-to-side anastomosis to the flexor digitorum longus or transfer of the flexor digitorum longus with suturing of its distal stump to the flexor hallucis longus may also be attempted. Treatment of chronic dislocation, which occurs anterior to the ruptured flexor retinaculum and flexor digitorum longus tendon, involves reconstruction of the flexor retinaculum and deepening of the groove around the medial malleolus, as described by Healy and coworkers[48].

Tibialis Anterior Tendon Injuries

Rupture of the tibialis anterior tendon can occur between the extensor retinaculum and the insertion onto the medial first cuneiform and adjacent base of the first metatarsal. Weakness of dorsiflexion, localized tenderness, and drop foot gait are observed on clinical evaluation.

Although spontaneous rupture of the tibialis anterior tendon is rare (usually seen in individuals older than 50 years of age), tibialis tendon ruptures may occur in athletes secondary to forced plantar flexion and ankle eversion.[49] Traumatic lacerations, related to the superficial and anterior location of this tendon, may also occur (Fig. 8-74). Tibialis anterior tendon injuries are best seen on oblique axial images oriented perpendicular to the tendon distal to the level of the medial

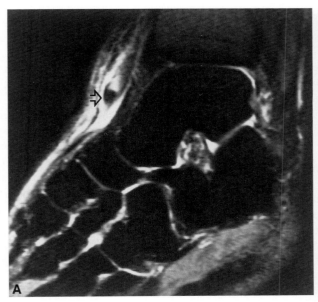
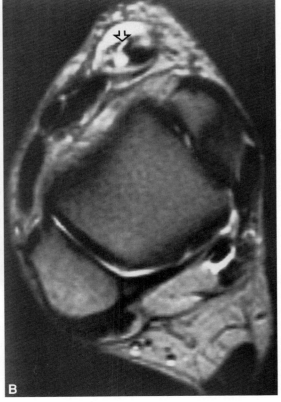

FIGURE 8-74. Traumatic laceration (*open arrow*) of the tibialis anterior tendon on (**A**) STIR sagittal and (**B**) T2-weighted axial images. Partial proximal tendon retraction is appreciated on the sagittal STIR sequence (**A**). Hyperintense fluid fills the area of the tendon gap.

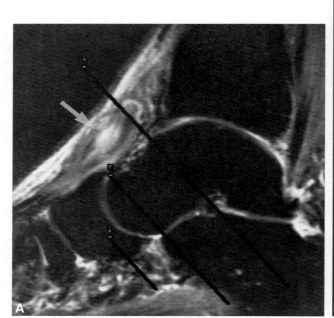

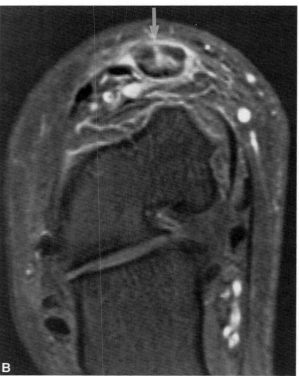

FIGURE 8-75. Partial tear of the tibialis anterior tendon (*arrow*) shown on (**A**) fast STIR sagittal and (**B**) gadolinium-enhanced fat-suppressed T1-weighted axial oblique images. The axial oblique prescriptions designated from the STIR sagittal image ensure that the axial images are acquired perpendicular to the long axis of the tendon. The gadolinium-contrast enhances the partial tear pattern within the tibialis anterior tendon (**B**, cross section).

malleolus.[50] In this locations, partial tears are less likely to be overread as complete ruptures because the tibialis anterior tendon changes its course and orientation at the level of the midfoot (Fig. 8-75). Inflammation of the synovial tendon sheath may be associated with tendon rupture, rheumatoid disease, or it may occur idiopathically.

Peroneal Tendon Abnormalities

The peroneal brevis and longus tendons share a common synovial sheath posterior to the lateral malleolus. The peroneal brevis is anterior to the peroneus longus tendon within the retromalleolar sulcus of the distal fibula.[49] Distally, the peroneus longus tendon is located along the lateral surface of the calcaneus, inferior to the peroneus brevis tendon and peroneal trochlea and superior to the calcaneal tubercle, which is the point of insertion of the calcaneofibular ligament. The peroneus longus tendon courses deep to the inferior peroneal retinaculum and occupies a groove and tunnel (created by the long plantar ligament) along the plantar surface of the cuboid. The peroneus brevis tendon can be seen superior to the peroneal trochlea in an osteoaponeurotic canal contributed to by the inferior peroneal retinaculum. There is a close relationship of the common peroneal tendon sheath and adjacent, more medially located, calcaneofibular liga-

ment. This intimate relationship is appreciated on axial MR images through the ankle joint.

The peroneal tendons may rupture secondary to trauma or laceration of the lateral aspect of the ankle. MR imaging defines the position of the peroneal tendons as well as fibular and retinacular anatomy.[45] Absence of the low signal intensity tendon within the peroneal tendon sheath may be observed on sagittal or axial images. The peroneal tendons are also involved in partial or complete dislocations. An absent or convex peroneal canal in the distal fibula may be a contributing factor. Dislocation of the tendon may be associated with stripping of the loosely attached superior peroneal retinaculum.

TENDON RUPTURE. Partial or complete tearing of the peroneal tendons usually occurs in association with an acute injury, rarely it occurs spontaneously.[49] An autopsy study by Sobel and coworkers[51] showed that 11% of specimens had varying degrees of attritional changes in the peroneus brevis tendon. The existence of preexisting tendon degeneration, prior to tendon rupture, is also suggested by McMaster's work,[52] which shows that intratendinous rupture is less common than failure of the musculotendinous unit at the insertion to bone, within the muscle or at the musculotendinous junction.[52] In rupture of the peroneus longus, there may be associated proximal migration of the os peroneum. This sesamoid is normally identified near the calcaneocuboid joint. Fracture of the os peroneum has also been seen with rupture of the peroneus longus.

MR imaging demonstrates longitudinal splits, hypertrophy, and fluid within partial tears of the peroneus brevis tendon. The peroneus brevis partial tears or longitudinal splits occur at the level of the lateral malleolus, and are associated with a sprain and superior peroneal retinacular or lateral ligament complex injury (Fig. 8-76). Identification of peroneus brevis involvement is important, in case the peroneus brevis is to be used in a lateral ligament reconstruction. Abrasion of the peroneus brevis from the calcaneofibular ligament or lateral cartilaginous ridge of the fibula is thought to be an initiating factor in the development of longitudinal tears.[53] Lateral ligament tears with associated laxity of the superior peroneal retinaculum may lead to peroneus brevis tendon splits and anterolateral subluxation of both peroneal tendons (Fig. 8-77). Complete rupture of a peroneal tendon should be confirmed on images obtained in more than one imaging plane. Reactive lateral calcaneal marrow edema at the attachment site of the inferior peroneal retinaculum (the peroneal tubercle) is associated with acute rupture of the peroneus brevis tendon (Fig. 8-78). Degeneration and intrasubstance longitudinal splits of the peroneus longus tendon may also be seen in association with tears of the peroneus brevis tendon (see Fig. 8-78). A complete tendon rupture of the peroneus longus is unusual. Peroneal tendon entrapment or impingement is associated with a fracture of the calcaneus in which lateral fragment displacement narrows the fibulocalcaneal space.[49]

Flexor Hallucis Longus Abnormalities

Tearing of the flexor hallucis longus has been demonstrated on axial MR images at the level of the musculotendinous junction[54] (Fig. 8-79). The flexor hallucis longus is a plantar flexor of the first toe and participates in plantar flexion and inversion of the foot (see Fig. 8-18C). Rupture of this tendon may be difficult to identify on clinical examination without the assistance of MR localization. A distal rupture requires coronal images performed through the distal foot in addition to routine axial images through the tibiotalar joint (Fig. 8-80).

Flexor hallucis longus injuries at the level of the medial malleolus are seen in dancers in conjunction with active plantar flexion mechanisms of injury. Hallux saltans refers to the development of a nodule or partial tear with triggering of the big toe. MR imaging normally demonstrates communication of fluid between the flexor hallucis longus tendon sheath and the tibiotalar joint. In addition to tendinitis, ballet dancers may have muscle strains at or near the musculotendinous junction (Fig. 8-81). Fat-suppressed T2-weighted fast spin-echo and STIR sequences are the most sensitive techniques in these injuries. In os trigonum syndrome (see the

section titled "os Trigonum Syndrome"), there is hypertrophy of the os trigonum, resulting in a partial tethering of the flexor hallucis longus tendon.[49] The os trigonum is identified as an ununited lateral tubercle in the posterior aspect of the talus in 10% of individuals.

The fibro-osseous tunnel of the flexor hallucis longus runs between the medial and lateral posterior talar tubercles. In dancers, posterior impingement or talar compression syndrome results from full weight-bearing in maximum ankle plantar flexion in demi pointe or full en pointe position.[55] This is accentuated in the presence of an os trigonum, laxity of the lateral ligaments, and/or soft-tissue entrapment between the posterior lip of the talus and the os calcis. A fixed tethering of the flexor hallucis longus tendon proximal to the flexor retinaculum produces a checkrein deformity with a flexion contracture of the interphalangeal joint of the hallux and an extension contracture of the first metatarsophalangeal joint.[49]

Other Tendon Injuries and Tenosynovitis

Tearing of muscle fibers of the flexor digitorum brevis or quadratus plantae at the level of the flexor digitorum longus tendons may present clinically as tenderness over the plantar aponeurosis (Fig. 8-82).

Tenosynovitis, either inflammatory or infectious, affects the tendons and synovial sheaths. The flexor hallucis longus tendon is susceptible to tendinitis and rupture where it passes through the tarsal tunnel. This injury is common in ballet dancers and presents with swelling and tenderness posterior to the medial malleolus. The flexor hallucis longus tendon is often referred to as the Achilles tendon of the foot in ballet dancers (see Fig. 8-81). Occasionally, tendinitis is found at Henry's knot under the base of the first metatarsal. This is where the flexor digitorum longus crosses over the flexor hallucis longus beneath the first metatarsal head between the sesamoids.[55] Flexor hallucis tendon pathology may be misdiagnosed as tendinitis of the tibialis posterior or flexor digitorum longus tendons. T2-weighted axial images show areas of increased fluid signal intensity in the tendon sheath. However, communication with the ankle joint also occurs in 10% to 20% of normal studies (Fig. 8-83). A low signal intensity tendon on scans with a long TR and TE excludes a partial tear.

Tenosynovitis may also involve the tibialis posterior and peroneal tendons (Fig. 8-84). Tibialis posterior tenosynovitis is associated with rheumatoid arthritis and planovalgus foot, and usually occurs in older patients. Peroneal tenosynovitis is associated with spastic flatfoot and is usually found in a younger patient population, often with a history of trauma. In acute tenosynovitis, findings include a synovial effusion without a thickened tendon or sheath. In chronic tenosynovitis, effusion is accompanied by a thickened tendon and synovial sheath. On T2-weighted images, synovial sheath thick-

text continues on page 544

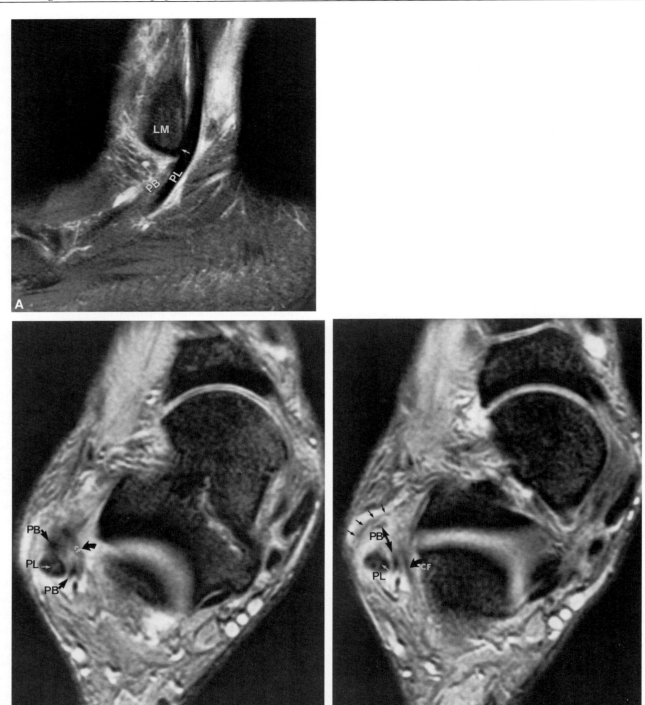

FIGURE 8-76. Split peroneal brevis tendon. **(A)** Attenuation and increased signal intensity can be seen within the peroneus brevis tendon anterior to the normal hypointense peroneus longus tendon. There is also mild anterolateral subluxation (*arrow*) of the peroneus longus tendon relative to the lateral malleolus (LM), the result of tearing of the superior peroneal retinaculum (fat-suppressed T2-weighted fast spin-echo sagittal image). PL, peroneal longus tendon; PB, peroneus brevis tendon; LM, lateral malleolus. **(B, C)** T2*-weighted axial images demonstrate the split and separation of the peroneus brevis tendon (*large straight arrows*), intrasubstance longitudinal splits within the peroneus longus tendon (*small white arrow*), torn superior retinaculum (*multiple small black arrows*), and intact calcaneofibular ligament (CF; *curved arrow*). Image **B** is superior to **C**.

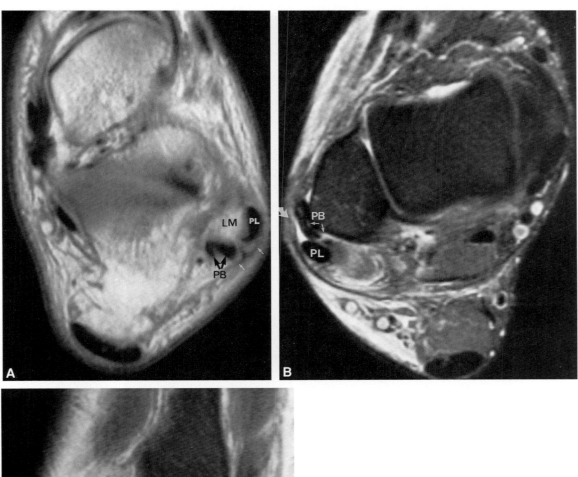

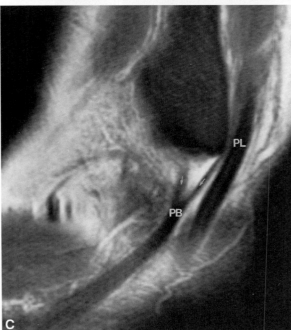

FIGURE 8-77. **(A)** Intermediate weighted axial image displaying anterolateral dislocation of the peroneus longus tendon (PL) and split of the peroneus brevis tendon (PB; *black arrows*), both associated with a torn superior peroneal retinaculum (*white arrows*). LM, lateral malleolus. **(B, C)** In a separate case there is anterolateral subluxation of the split (*small arrows*) peroneus brevis tendon (PB) associated with a torn superior peroneal retinaculum (*curved arrow*) and partial lateral subluxation of the peroneus longus tendon (PL) (**B**: fat-suppressed T2-weighted fast spin-echo axial image; **C**: fat-suppressed T2-weighted fast spin-echo sagittal image).

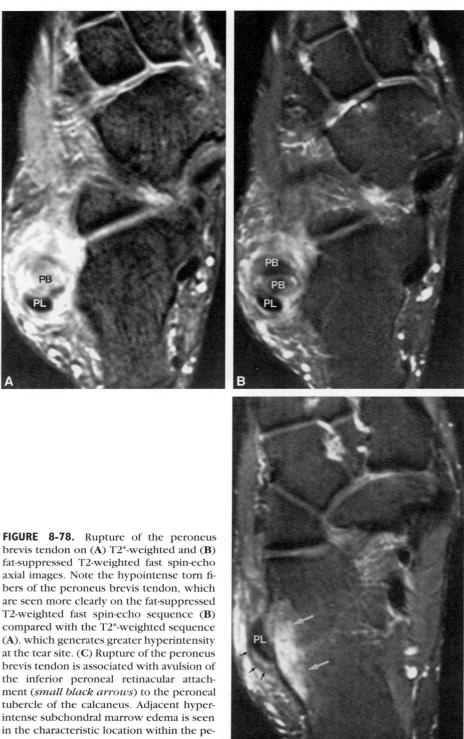

FIGURE 8-78. Rupture of the peroneus brevis tendon on (**A**) T2*-weighted and (**B**) fat-suppressed T2-weighted fast spin-echo axial images. Note the hypointense torn fibers of the peroneus brevis tendon, which are seen more clearly on the fat-suppressed T2-weighted fast spin-echo sequence (**B**) compared with the T2*-weighted sequence (**A**), which generates greater hyperintensity at the tear site. (**C**) Rupture of the peroneus brevis tendon is associated with avulsion of the inferior peroneal retinacular attachment (*small black arrows*) to the peroneal tubercle of the calcaneus. Adjacent hyperintense subchondral marrow edema is seen in the characteristic location within the peroneal tubercle (*large white arrows*). PL, peroneus longus tendon.

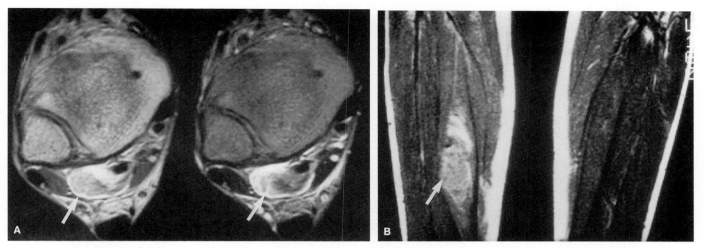

FIGURE 8-79. (A) A grade II (ie, partial) tear of the flexor hallucis longus muscle with high signal intensity hemorrhage (*arrow*) is seen on intermediate weighted (*left*) and T2-weighted (*right*) axial images. (B) The subacute hemorrhage (*arrow*) is bright on a T1-weighted coronal image.

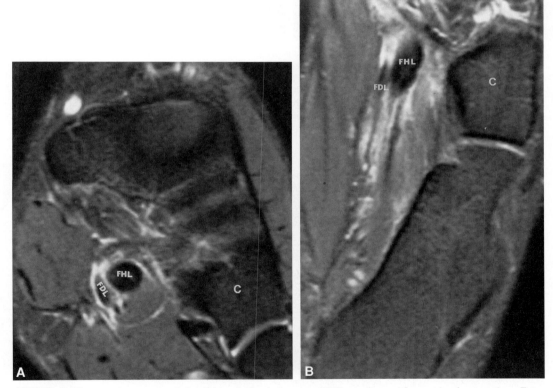

FIGURE 8-80. Distal rupture of the flexor hallucis longus (FHL) tendon with proximal retraction. Fat-5suppressed T2-weighted fast spin-echo coronal (**A**) and axial (**B**) images. The retracted flexor hallucis longus tendon is enlarged in cross sectional area relative to the normal adjacent flexor digitorum longus tendon (FDL). Associated soft-tissue edema is hyperintense on fat-suppressed T2-weighted fast spin-echo images. The flexor hallucis longus tendon normally inserts at the base of the distal phalanx of the first toe. C, cuboid.

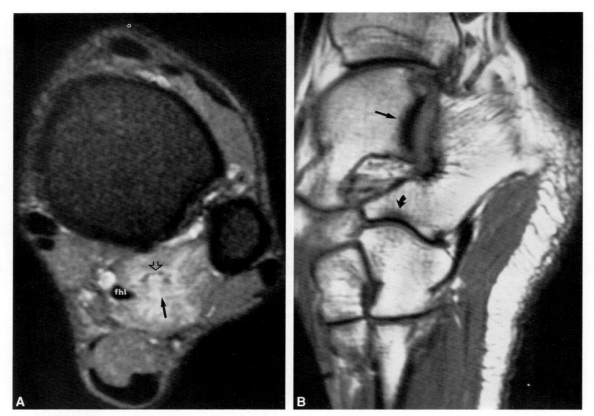

FIGURE 8-81. (**A**) Ballet dancer with flexor hallucis longus muscle strain proximal to the musculotendinous junction. Hyperintense edema (*straight arrow*) and focal hypointense hemorrhage (*open arrow*) are shown within the muscle of the flexor hallucis longus on a fat-suppressed T2-weighted fast spin-echo axial image. (**B**) Corresponding T1-weighted sagittal image, obtained with the patient in the en pointe position, demonstrates the redistribution of weight-bearing mechanical stress with subchondral sclerosis of the subtalar (*straight arrow*) and calcaneocuboid (*curved arrow*) joints.

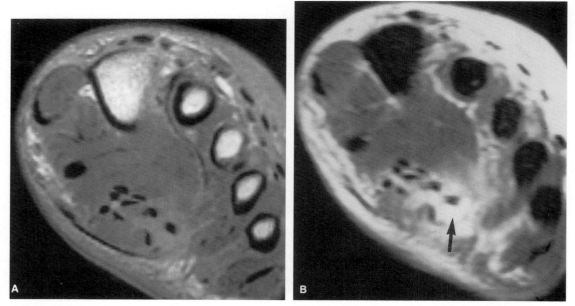

FIGURE 8-82. A grade I to II muscle tear with localized hemorrhage and edema involving the flexor digitorum brevis (*straight arrow*) and quadratus plantar muscle groups. Injury was caused by a windsurfing accident. Edema and hemorrhage are isointense compared with muscle on an intermediate weighted coronal image (**A**) and hyperintense on a short TI inversion recovery coronal image (**B**).

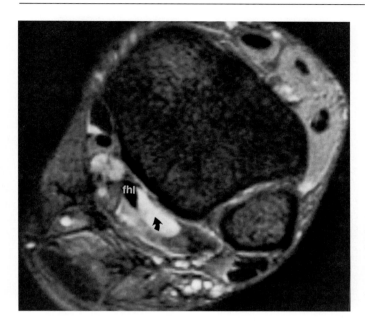

FIGURE 8-83. Flexor hallucis longus (fhl) tenosynovitis with hyperintense joint fluid within the flexor hallucis longus tendon sheath (*curved arrow*). Since the flexor hallucis longus tendon sheath normally communicates with the ankle joint in 20% of patients, the diagnosis of tenosynovitis requires either a disproportionate amount of fluid within the tendon sheath or an absence of an associated ankle joint effusion (T2*-weighted axial image).

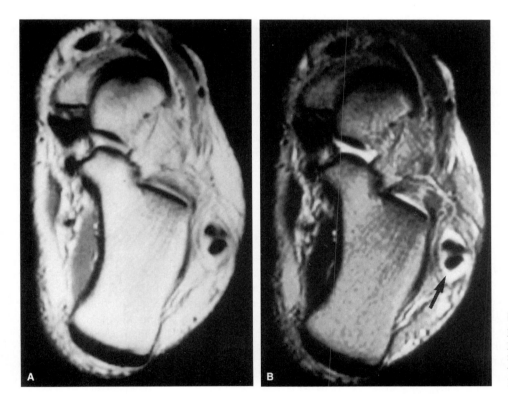

FIGURE 8-84. Longitudinal split of the peroneus brevis tendon with associated peroneal tenosynovitis is seen on (**A**) intermediate weighted and (**B**) T2-weighted axial images (*arrow*). Fluid is hyperintense on the T2-weighted image.

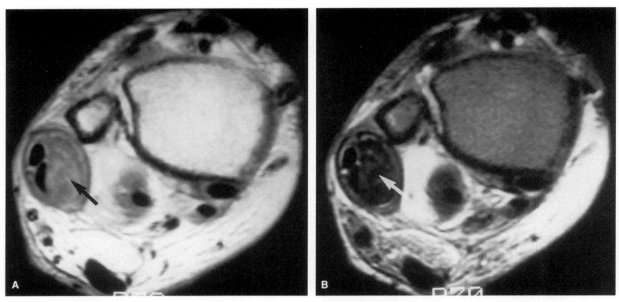

FIGURE 8-85. In chronic peroneal tenosynovitis, thickened low signal intensity synovium (*arrows*) encases the peroneus brevis and longus tendons. There is no increased signal intensity within synovial tissue on (**A**) intermediate weighted or (**B**) T2-weighted axial images.

ening demonstrates intermediate signal intensity (Fig. 8-85). Focal peroneus longus tendinosis may occur at the level of the distal calcaneus in association with an os peroneum as part of the painful os peroneum syndrome. Osteochondritis dissecans of the os peroneum may also contribute to painful syndromes. Thompson and Patterson[56] have reported on degenerative rupture of the peroneus longus distal to the os peroneum.

Ligamentous Injuries

Pathogenesis

Injuries to the ligaments about the ankle usually result from inversion and internal rotation of the foot combined with ankle plantar flexion.[57] Normally, when the foot is positioned in neutral or plantar flexion, the orientation of the anterior talofibular ligament is 45° to the horizontal, and it functions as a restraint to internal rotation[57] (Fig. 8-86). The vertically oriented calcaneofibular ligament (Fig. 8-87) primarily protects against varus force and offers little resistance to internal rotation. The anterior talofibular ligament is the weakest, and usually is the first ligament to rupture with forced inversion and plantar flexion.[58] Even when inversion and plantar flexion forces cause rupture of the calcaneofibular ligament, the posterior talofibular ligament may remain uninjured, except in severe ankle trauma with dislocation.[58]

If all three ligaments are ruptured, the ankle is unstable. With complete disruption of the anterior talofibular ligament, forward displacement of the talus in the ankle mortise is present. With sequential rupture of the anterior talofibular and calcaneofibular ligaments, there is medial tilting of the talus with progressive widening of the lateral joint space. The strong deltoid or medial collateral ligament (Fig. 8-88), which consists of the tibionavicular, anterior tibiotalar, tibiocalcaneal, and posterior tibiotalar ligaments, rarely ruptures. Avulsion fracture of the medial malleolus and disruption of the anterior inferior tibiofibular ligament are associated with abduction and laterally directed forces.[58]

Diagnosis

Ankle sprains are classified into three clinical grades.[57] In a grade I sprain, there is stretching or partial tearing of anterior talofibular ligament fibers. Grade II represents a moderate sprain associated with significant edema in which there is partial tearing of the anterior talofibular ligament with stretching of the calcaneofibular ligament. In a grade III injury, there is tearing of the anterior talofibular and calcaneofibular ligaments causing ankle instability.

MR Appearance

The normal ligamentous anatomy of the ankle is clearly demonstrated on MR images. Indications for the use of MR imaging in evaluation of patients with ligament sprains or ruptures, however, have not yet been established. MR imaging provides direct visualization of ankle ligaments, which is not possible with conventional radiographs, arthrography, or CT. Clinical assessment of ligament injury is frequently difficult because of concomitant soft-tissue swelling and

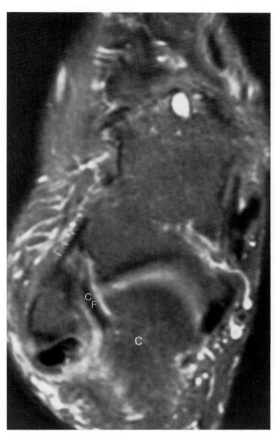

FIGURE 8-86. Fat-suppressed T2-weighted fast spin-echo axial image shows the relationship of the calcaneofibular ligament (CF) and the anterior talofibular ligament (*arrows*). The CF ligament originates from the lower segment of the anterior border of the lateral malleolus and courses inferiorly and slightly posteriorly to its insertion onto a small tubercle at the upper part of the lateral surface of the calcaneus (C). The anterior talofibular ligament originates from the anterior border of the lateral malleolus and courses obliquely anterior and medially to insert onto the talus immediately anterior to the lateral articular facet. The anterior talofibular ligament is intimately related to the talofibular joint capsule and is taut in plantar flexion.

joint effusion. Results of stress positioning with conventional radiographs may be variable, and the patient may require anesthesia to limit pain and guarding. Comparison views with the opposite ankle are also necessary. MR imaging is particularly useful in assessing the tibial plafond and talar dome. Subchondral and articular damage to the superior talar dome may occur with subluxation of the ankle (ie, talar displacement in plantar flexion) secondary to anterior talofibular ligament interruption.

Lateral Ligament Complex Injuries

The normal anatomy and pathologic changes affecting the anterior talofibular ligament are best displayed on axial or axial oblique planar images with T2, fat-suppressed T2-weighted fast spin-echo, or 3DFT T2*-weighted contrast and MR arthrography[59,60] (Fig. 8-89). 3DFT axial images with thin (1 to 2 mm) sections eliminate the need to dorsiflex the foot (to optimize visualization of the tibiofibular and talofibular ligaments) or to plantar flex the foot (to optimize visualization of the calcaneofibular ligament in the axial plane). At the level of the distal lateral malleolus, the anterior talofibular ligament is seen as a prominent, low signal intensity, 2 to 3 mm band, oriented anteromedially and extending to its talar attachment. Axial oblique images perpendicular to the talonavicular joint may be used to demonstrate anterior talofibular ligament fibers more parallel with the plane of section. Acute tears are associated with either partial ligamentous disruption, ligament laxity, or complete absence of the ligament. T2- or T2*-weighted images identify localized high signal intensity fluid or hemorrhage.[59] Anterior talofibular ligament tears are frequently associated with a capsular rupture and extravasation of joint fluid into the anterolateral soft tissues[61] (Fig. 8-90). Inversion mechanisms of injury are confirmed by the observation of a medial talar bone contusion in association with an acute tear of the anterior talofibular ligament (Fig. 8-91). An avulsed anterior talofibular ligament may be associated with a distal fibular avulsion fracture (Fig. 8-92). Chronically torn talofibular ligament fibers have

text continues on page 549

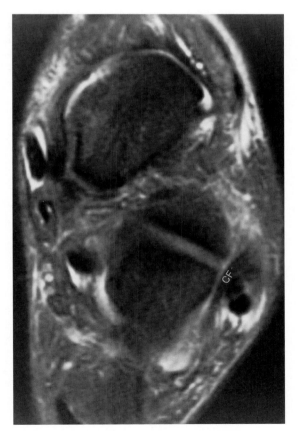

FIGURE 8-87. Fat-suppressed T2-weighted fast spin-echo axial image depicts the intact calcaneofibular ligament (CF), which is crossed superficially by the peroneal tendons and their sheaths.

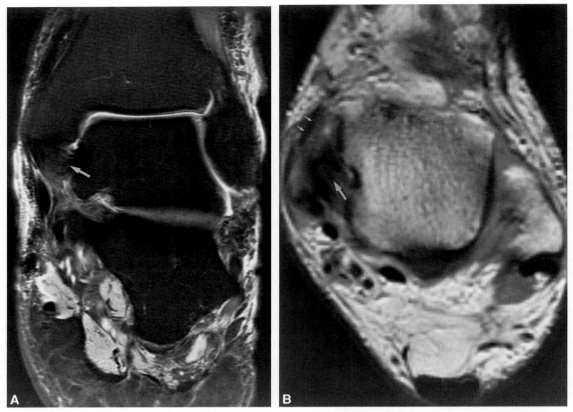

FIGURE 8-88. (**A**) Posterior tibiotalar fibers (*arrow*) of the deltoid ligament complex. The deltoid ligament provides stability to the medial aspect of the ankle (fat-suppressed T2-weighted fast spin-echo coronal image). (**B**) Anterior tibiotalar fibers of the deltoid ligament (*large arrow*) are seen deep to the tibialis posterior and flexor digitorum longus tendons. Tibionavicular fibers are also identified (*small arrows*) (T1-weighted axial image).

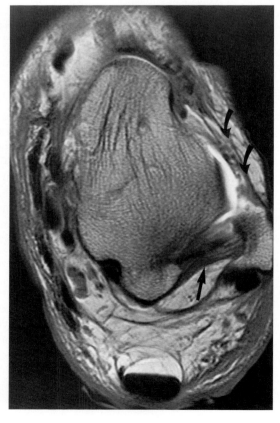

FIGURE 8-89. Complete tear with absence of the anterior talofibular ligament (*curved arrows*) on a T1-weighted axial MR arthrographic image. The posterior talofibular ligament (*straight arrow*) is intact.

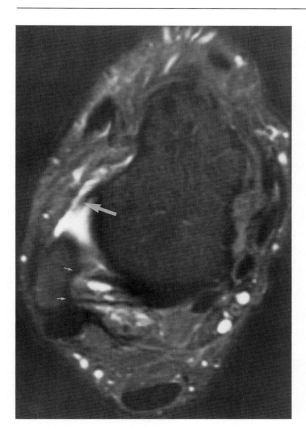

FIGURE 8-90. Complete tear of the anterior talofibular ligament (*large arrow*). There is anterolateral extension of fluid into the soft-tissues across the discontinuity in the anterior talofibular ligament. Note the fan-like insertion of the posterior talofibular ligament on the fibula at the deep malleolar fossa (*small arrows*) (fat-suppressed T2-weighted fast spin-echo axial image).

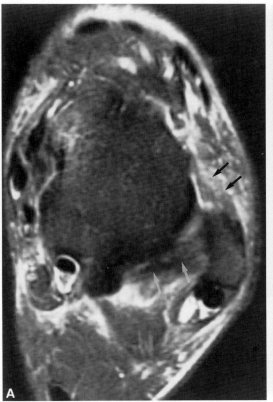

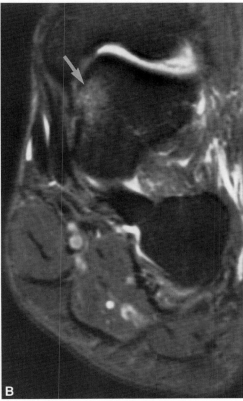

FIGURE 8-91. (**A**) Fat-suppressed T2-weighted fast spin-echo axial image shows acute rupture of the anterior talofibular ligament (*black arrows*) with intact posterior talofibular ligament. (**B**) Corresponding fat-suppressed T2-weighted fast spin-echo coronal image demonstrates medial talar subchondral bone contusion (*arrow*) associated with an inversion mechanism of injury.

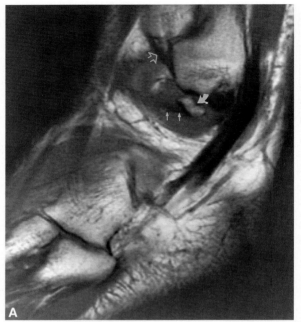

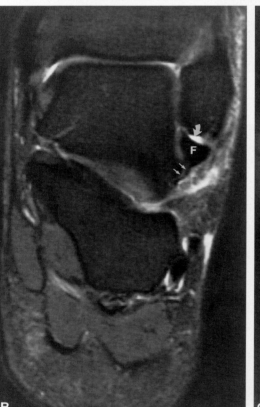

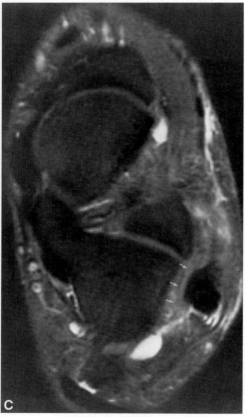

FIGURE 8-92. (A, B) Avulsed distal fibular fragment (*curve arrow*) at the level of the lateral malleolus with attached anterior talofibular ligament (*small straight arrows*) on T1-weighted sagittal (A) and fat-suppressed T2-weighted fast spin-echo coronal (B) images. Intact anterior inferior tibiofibular ligament (*open arrow*) is seen on the T1-weighted sagittal sequence (A). (C) Associated calcaneofibular ligament tear (*arrows*) is identified on a fat-suppressed T2-weighted fast spin-echo axial image.

been infrequently reported to form a meniscoid lesion, with tissue interposed between the talus and the fibula. Chronic or healed ligamentous disruptions show generalized thickening of the ligament (Fig. 8-93). MR arthrography (see Fig. 8-89) is more accurate and sensitive in diagnosing anterior talofibular ligament tears than noncontrast MR imaging or stress radiography.[62]

We have observed an association between anterior talofibular ligament tears and isolated subtalar joint arthrosis. Although chronic subtalar instability was traditionally thought to be associated with lateral ankle sprains, conventional radiographs alone are inadequate for displaying this anatomy.[57,63]

Calcaneofibular ligament tears, when associated with anterior talofibular ligament injuries, are best seen on coronal or axial plane images distal to and through the plane of the lateral malleolus[58] (Fig. 8-94). Posterior oblique (ie, anterior-superior to posterior-inferior) axial images, or axial images performed with the foot in plantar flexion, also display the calcaneofibular ligament fibers.[64] Axial images show the calcaneofibular ligament between the peroneal tendons and the lateral aspect of the calcaneus (anteromedial to the peroneal tendons) (see Fig. 8-86). The normal calcaneofibular liga-

ment is 2 to 3 mm thick and is visualized as a linear or cord-like low signal intensity structure.[61] Calcaneofibular ligament tears (Fig. 8-95) are associated with localized edema, peroneal retinacular thickening, tenosynovitis, and tendon subluxation. MR arthrography is very sensitive for the detection of anterior talofibular and calcaneofibular ligament tears, 100% and 90%, respectively.[62] Tearing of the calcaneofibular ligament may result in communication between the ankle joint and the peroneal tendon sheaths.[57]

Medial Ligament Complex Injuries

Both superficial and deep portions of the deltoid ligament can be identified on axial images. On these images, deltoid ligament injuries usually demonstrate inflammatory or edematous changes without complete ligament disruptions[65] (Fig. 8-96). On coronal plane images, however, it is often possible to identify associated avulsions of the medial malleolus and to separate tibiotalar from tibiocalcaneal fibers. Focal areas of increased signal intensity on T2, fat-suppressed T2-weighted fast spin-echo, or T2*-weighted images are more commonly seen than complete absence of the ligament.

In its normal configuration, the tibiotalar ligament dem-

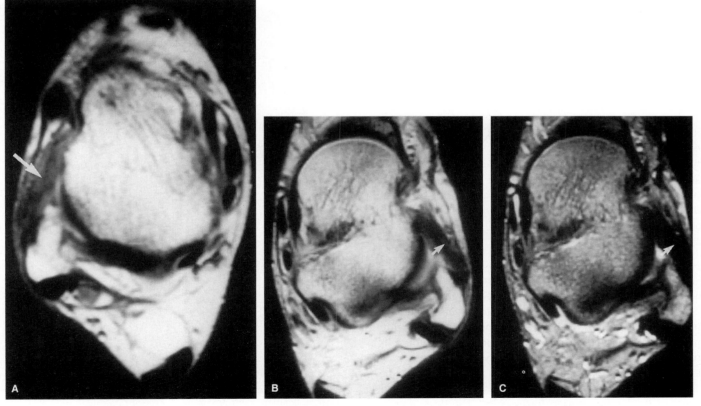

FIGURE 8-93. **(A)** A T1-weighted axial image shows a chronically thickened intermediate signal intensity anterior talofibular ligament (*arrow*). The normal thickness is 2 to 3 mm. Thickening is secondary to a previous inversion injury. A different patient shows a healed anterior talofibular ligament tear (*arrows*), which is seen as a low signal intensity thickened ligament on axial **(B)** intermediate weighted and **(C)** T2-weighted axial images.

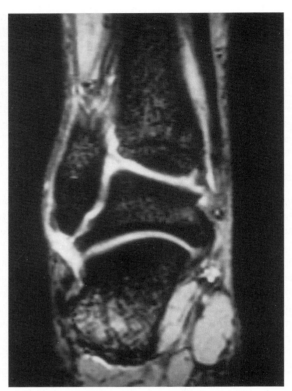

FIGURE 8-94. There is an absence of ligamentous fibers on this T2*-weighted coronal image of calcaneofibular ligament disruption.

onstrates separated fibers with interposed fatty tissue. This finding should not be mistaken for ligament disruption on T1-weighted images. Most injuries to the deltoid ligament are ligamentous sprains that appear as an amorphous increase in signal intensity on fat-suppressed T2-weighted fast spin-echo, T2*-weighted, or STIR images. Isolated deltoid ligament injuries are rare, and most deltoid injuries have associated lateral ligamentous pathology, a fibular fracture, and/or syndesmotic injuries.[66] Kinematic and stress positioning of the ankle may be effective in showing rupture, thinning, and lengthening of the ligament.

Syndesmosis Sprains

The clinical diagnosis of anterior inferior tibiofibular ligament injuries, which frequently occur in football and downhill skiing, may be difficult because acute swelling is uncommon in this setting of distal anterior tibiofibular syndesmotic pain. Therefore, identification of an intact or disrupted ligament on MR scans may be particularly useful in diagnosing and treating an ankle injury.

A sprain of syndesmosis ligaments can occur without a tibial or fibular fracture or diastasis.[36,67] The three key ligaments connecting the tibia and fibula are the anterior inferior tibiofibular (AITF) (Fig. 8-97), the posterior inferior tibiofibular (PITF) (Fig. 8-98), and the interosseous ligaments. The lower fibers of the interosseous membrane also contrib-

ute to the stability of the distal ankle syndesmosis. External rotation is thought to represent the primary mechanism of syndesmosis sprain. External rotation forces can result in disruption of the anterior inferior tibiofibular ligament, the interosseous ligament, and the interosseous membrane. Hyperdorsiflexion has also been implicated as a mechanism of injury.

Tears of the anterior inferior tibiofibular and posterior inferior tibiofibular ligaments are characterized by ligament thickening, irregularity (eg, a lobulated contour) or frank discontinuity (Fig. 8-99). Ligament thickening results in an increased AP dimension, usually seen in association with areas of increased signal intensity within the ligaments. Posterior inferior tibialis ligament rupture is uncommon. The normal appearance of the anterior inferior tibialis ligament is variable, and it may be visualized as a thick substantial ligament or a thin attenuated structure even in the absence of pathology. Interosseous membrane injuries are seen as a linear hyperintensity at the level of the distal tibia and fibula on heavily weighted T2, fat-suppressed T2-weighted fast

text continues on page 554

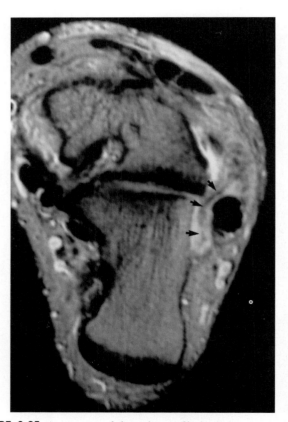

FIGURE 8-95. Acute tear of the calcaneofibular ligament as part of a lateral ligament complex injury (anterior talofibular and calcaneofibular ligaments). A lax ligament (*arrows*) surrounded by hyperintense edema is shown on this T2-weighted axial image. Partial tears or longitudinal splits of the peroneus brevis tendon may be seen in association with or develop secondary to severe lateral collateral injuries.

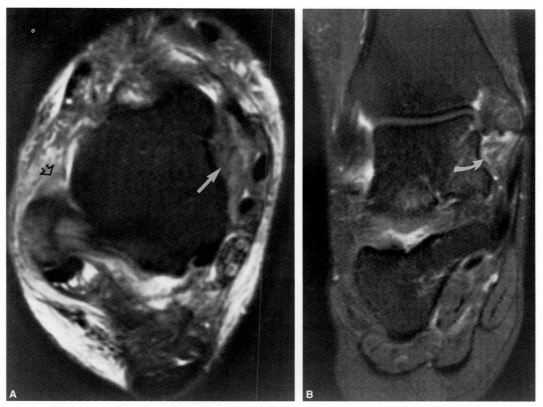

FIGURE 8-96. (A) Deltoid ligament sprain (*solid arrow*) with mild hyperintensity and inhomogeneity on a fat-suppressed T2-weighted fast spin-echo axial image. The anterior talofibular ligament is also torn (*open arrow*). **(B)** In a separate case, intravenous gadolinium enhancement demonstrates a deltoid ligament sprain involving posterior tibiotalar fibers (*curved arrow*).

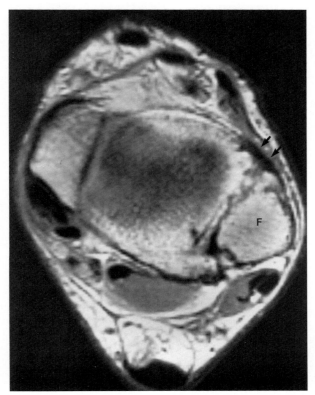

FIGURE 8-97. Normal anterior inferior tibiofibular ligament (*arrows*) on a T1-weighted axial image. A hypointense band extends from the anterior inferior aspect of the lateral malleolus to the anterolateral tubercle of the tibia. The accessory fascicle of the anterior inferior tibiofibular ligament can cause impingement across the lateral talar dome. F, fibula.

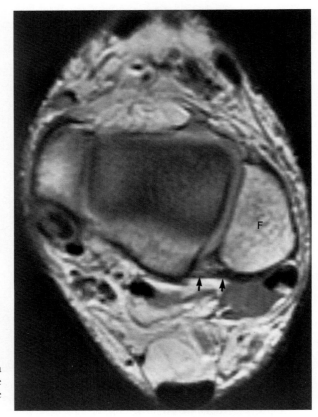

FIGURE 8-98. Normal posterior inferior tibiofibular ligament (*arrows*) on a T1-weighted axial image. Hypointense fibers are seen extending from the posterior aspect of the lateral malleolus to the posterolateral tibial tubercle medially.

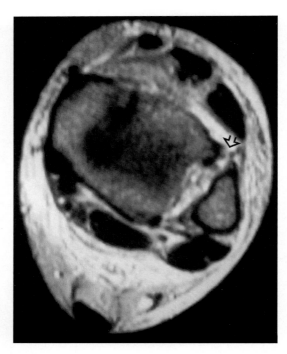

FIGURE 8-99. Torn anterior inferior tibiofibular ligament (*open arrow*) as a component of a syndesmotic sprain. Increased signal intensity in a widened syndesmosis is present on this T2-weighted axial image.

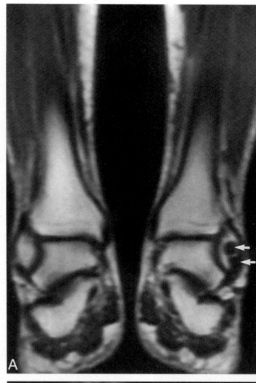

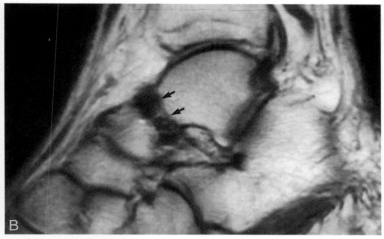

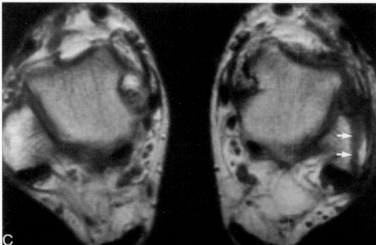

FIGURE 8-100. (**A–C**) Reconstruction of the anterior talofibular and the calcaneofibular ligaments. The peroneus brevis tendon is tunneled through the neck of the talus (*black arrows*) and the fibula (*white arrows*), as seen on T1-weighted (**A**) coronal, (**B**) sagittal, and (**C**) axial images. (**D, E**) In a separate case, the Evans technique is used to reconstruct only the calcaneofibular ligament, shown on T1-weighted (**D**) and fat-suppressed T2-weighted fast spin-echo (**E**) sagittal images. The peroneus brevis tendon is divided, mobilized, and placed in a fibular tunnel. Erosion of the bony tunnel and fluid (*straight arrow*) and longitudinal tear of the peroneus brevis tendon within the tunnel (*curved tunnel*) are demonstrated in this symptomatic patient.   *continued*

spin-echo, or STIR images. Low signal intensity foci in the interosseous membrane represent hemosiderin, fibrosis, or calcification.

Postoperative Findings

In lateral ankle reconstruction, the recommended surgical procedures attempt to either rebuild the lateral ligaments or use a peroneus brevis tendon tenodesis.[68,69] The mobilized peroneus brevis tendon, rerouted through the fibula, can be seen in patients with a Watson-Jones reconstruction of the lateral (ie, anterior talofibular and calcaneofibular) ligaments or in an Evans reconstruction of the calcaneofibular ligament (Fig. 8-100). In the Watson-Jones reconstruction, MR imaging identifies the reconstructed lateral ligaments and assesses the course of the peroneus brevis tendon through the tunnel in the neck of the talus. The status of the anterior talofibular ligament is also seen in other lateral ligament reconstructions (Fig. 8-101). The modified Bröstrom direct repair with imbrication technique repairs and reinforces the anterior talofibular ligament without sacrificing another musculotendinous unit. This technique is particularly useful in athletes and dancers.

Soft-Tissue Impingement

Chronic pain after an ankle sprain is commonly caused by soft-tissue impingement. Impingement syndromes include anterolateral, syndesmotic, and posterior impingement.[14,70]

ANTEROLATERAL IMPINGEMENT. Anterolateral impingement is the most common of the soft-tissue impingements because of its relationship to the inversion mechanism of most ankle sprains (Fig. 8-102). Wolin and associates[71] has described the "meniscoid" lesion as massive hyalinized connective tissue extending into the joint from the anterior inferior portion of the talofibular ligament. Although the meniscoid lesion is often discussed, the lesion itself is rarely seen. Impingement can occur at the anterior inferior tibiofibular ligament (Fig. 8-103), the lateral gutter, and the anterior talofibular ligament. Radiographic findings include calcification or heterotopic bone in the interosseous space (distal tibiofibular syndesmosis injury), ossicles distal to the lateral malleolus, and lateral talar dome (anterior talofibular ligament) injuries. In 30% to 40% of cases, it is possible to identify lateral gutter lesions on MR images. Some impingement lesions may require kinematic or dynamic imaging techniques. Arthroscopic findings indicate pathology usually limited to the syndesmosis and lateral gutter. Synovitis usually affects the anterior inferior tibiofibular and anterior talofibular ligaments. There is often lateral gutter fibrosis and associated chondromalacia of the talus and fibula. Less commonly, a meniscoid lesion is seen extending from the anterolateral aspect of the distal tibia toward the lateral gutter. Ferkel and colleagues attribute soft-tissue impingement primarily to chronic hypertrophy of the synovium without a mass of ligamentous tissue as the meniscoid lesion.[72] The meniscoid lesion is thus thought to represent an advanced form of anterolateral soft-tissue impingement.

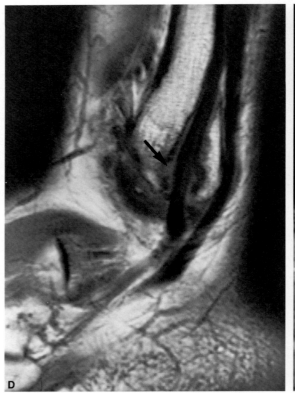
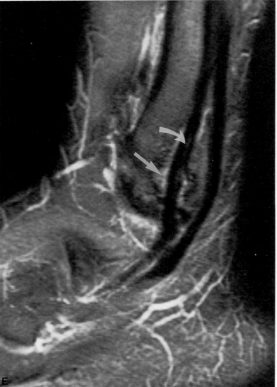

FIGURE 8-100. *Continued.*

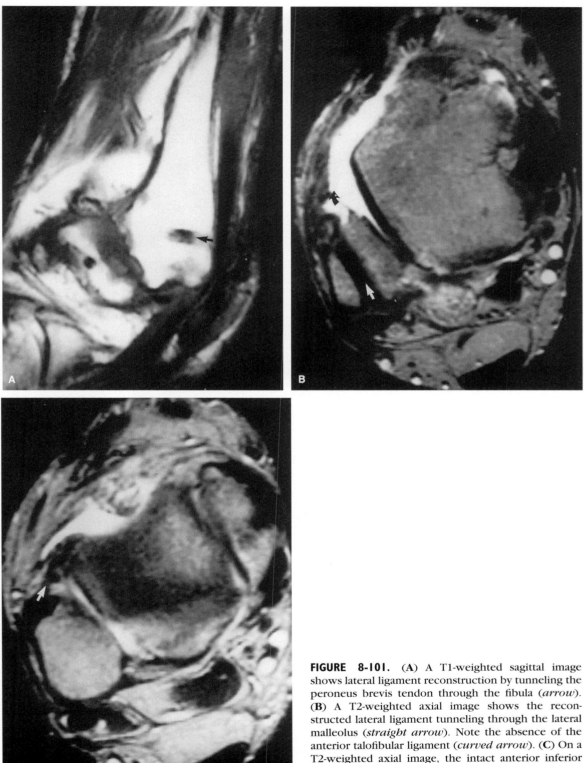

FIGURE 8-101. (A) A T1-weighted sagittal image shows lateral ligament reconstruction by tunneling the peroneus brevis tendon through the fibula (*arrow*). (B) A T2-weighted axial image shows the reconstructed lateral ligament tunneling through the lateral malleolus (*straight arrow*). Note the absence of the anterior talofibular ligament (*curved arrow*). (C) On a T2-weighted axial image, the intact anterior inferior tibiofibular ligament is seen at the level of the ankle joint (*arrow*).

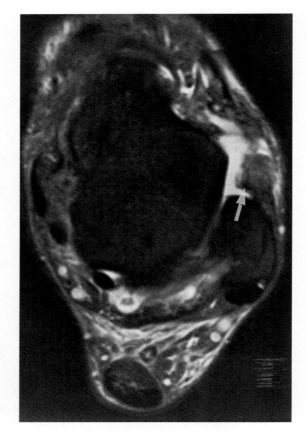

FIGURE 8-102. Enlargement of anterolateral soft tissue (*arrow*) at the site of anterior talofibular ligament disruption. Anterolateral impingement can occur at the anterior inferior tibiofibular ligament, the lateral gutter, and the anterior talofibular ligament. At arthroscopy, findings of anterolateral impingement include synovitis of the anterior inferior tibiofibular ligament and anterior talofibular ligament, as well as fibrosis of the lateral gutter (fat-suppressed T2-weighted fast spin-echo axial image).

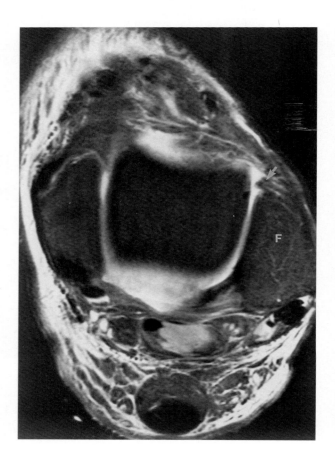

FIGURE 8-103. A thickened remnant of the anterior inferior tibiofibular ligament (syndesmotic ligament) may cause symptoms of anterolateral impingement (*arrow*) (fat-suppressed T2-weighted fast spin-echo axial arthrographic image). F, fibula.

SYNDESMOTIC IMPINGEMENT. Syndesmotic sprains include the anterior inferior tibiofibular ligament, the posterior inferior tibiofibular ligament (including its distal and deep component, the transverse ligament), and the interosseous membrane (Fig. 8-104). Arthroscopic findings include an inflamed synovium (and synovial nodules) and scarring which envelop the anterior inferior tibiofibular ligament and inferior articulation of the tibia and fibula. Synovitis of the anterior and posterior aspects of the syndesmotic ligament (anterior inferior tibiofibular ligament) may also be seen. Loose bodies, chondromalacia, and osteophytes are associated findings. A separate fascicle of the anterior inferior tibiofibular ligament may cause impingement by abrading against the lateral dome of the talus, particularly in an unstable ankle.

POSTERIOR IMPINGEMENT. Posterior impingement also usually occurs along the lateral side of the ankle and involves the posterior inferior tibiofibular ligament and the transverse

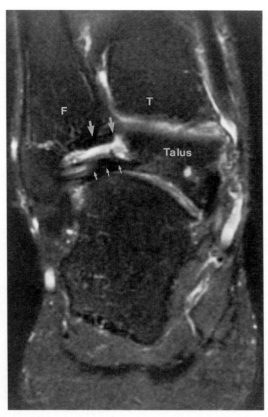

FIGURE 8-105. Potential posterior impingement sites include the posterior inferior tibiofibular ligament, the transverse tibiofibular ligament (*large arrows*), and the posterior talofibular ligament (*small arrows*). A tibial slip of the transverse tibiofibular ligament can also be an area of soft-tissue impingement (fat-suppressed T2-weighted coronal image). F, fibula; T, tibia.

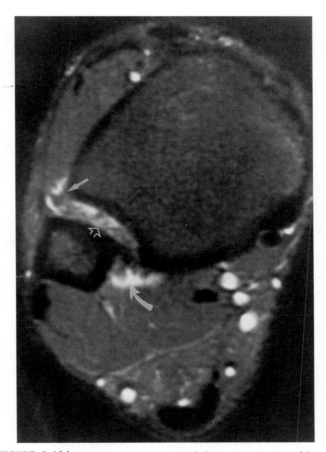

FIGURE 8-104. Syndesmotic sprain with hyperintense signal intensity along the distribution of the torn anterior inferior tibiofibular ligament (*straight arrow*), the partially torn posterior inferior tibiofibular ligament (*curved arrow*), and the interosseous membrane (*open arrow*). Syndesmotic sprains may be seen in up to 10% of all ankle injuries (fat-suppressed T2-weighted fast spin-echo axial image).

tibiofibular ligament (Fig. 8-105). Impingement is caused by hypertrophy or tear of the posterior inferior or transverse tibiofibular ligaments, by a tibial slip, or by a pathologic labrum on the posterior ankle joint.[14] Posterior impingement may coexist with anterolateral and syndesmosis impingement.

In studying the normal anatomy of the ankle, Rosenberg and coworkers[70] identified the posterior intermalleolar ligament, which may have a role in the development of posterior impingement, on 19% of MR images. It is seen on coronal T1- and T2-weighted images as a hypointense band traversing the posterior talofibular ligament and the inferior transverse ligament. The posterior impingement syndrome may be related to the meniscus-like shape and occasional extension of this ligament into the ankle joint.

Sinus Tarsi Syndrome

ANATOMY OF THE TARSAL SINUS AND CANAL. The tarsal canal and cone-shaped tarsal sinus are found between the posterior lateral subtalar joint and the anteriorly located talocalcaneonavicular or anterior subtalar joint.[73] The tarsal sinus and canal are visualized from posteromedial to anterolateral. The tarsal canal extends medially, posterior to the sustentaculum tali. The contents of the tarsal canal and sinus include fat, nerve endings, and arterial anastomoses with the posterior tibial and peroneal artery branches, and ligaments. The five distinct ligaments of the tarsal canal and sinus include the medial, intermediate, and lateral roots of the inferior extensor retinaculum, the cervical ligament, and the interosseous talocalcaneal ligament (Fig. 8-106).

CLINICAL AND IMAGING FINDINGS. The sinus tarsi syndrome is thought to represent a minor subtalar instability.[66] Pathologic changes have been described, including scarring and degenerative changes to the soft-tissue structures of the sinus tarsi. On clinical examination, there is lateral ankle pain and tenderness over the sinus tarsi with a frequent (70%)

of cases) history of prior inversion injury. There is no symptomatic instability. Conventional radiographs and stress views yield negative results. Findings in subtalar arthrography performed for the evaluation of sinus tarsi syndrome include the absence of normal subtalar joint microrecesses in the area of the interosseous and cervical ligaments, with cutoff of contrast at the interosseous ligament. This finding, however, has not been validated on MR scans of the tarsal sinus and canal, on which the absence of anterior microrecesses of the posterior subtalar joint may be a normal finding.[73]

Klein and Spreitzer[73] found MR abnormalities of the sinus tarsi, including tears of the tarsal sinus and tarsal canal ligaments, associated with lateral collateral ligament tears. Other findings in the sinus tarsi syndrome include diffuse infiltration by fibrosis (low signal intensity on T1- and T2-

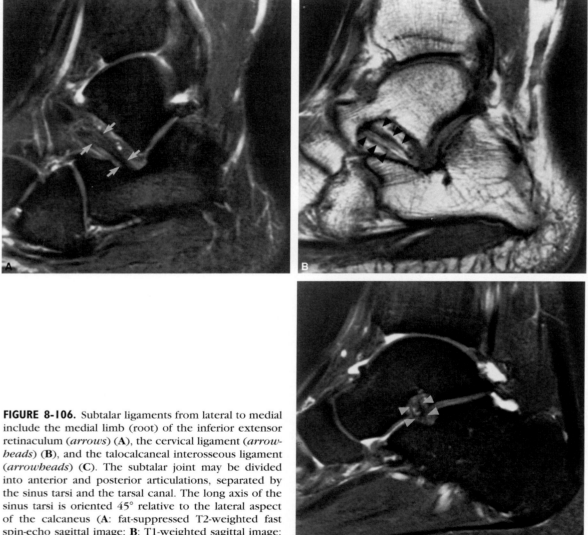

FIGURE 8-106. Subtalar ligaments from lateral to medial include the medial limb (root) of the inferior extensor retinaculum (*arrows*) (**A**), the cervical ligament (*arrowheads*) (**B**), and the talocalcaneal interosseous ligament (*arrowheads*) (**C**). The subtalar joint may be divided into anterior and posterior articulations, separated by the sinus tarsi and the tarsal canal. The long axis of the sinus tarsi is oriented 45° relative to the lateral aspect of the calcaneus (**A**: fat-suppressed T2-weighted fast spin-echo sagittal image; **B**: T1-weighted sagittal image; **C**: fat-suppressed T2-weighted fast spin-echo sagittal image).

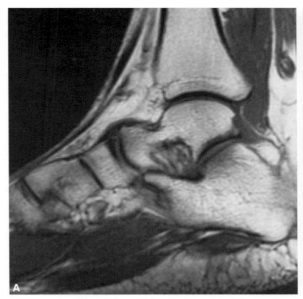

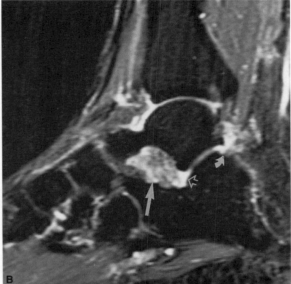

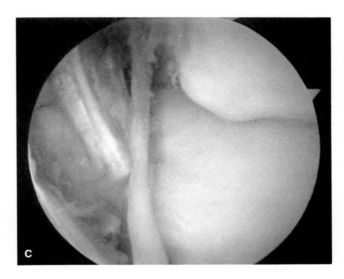

FIGURE 8-107. Edema with multiple small fluid collections of the sinus tarsi are hypointense on T1-weighted (**A**) and hyperintense (large straight arrow) on STIR (**B**) images. The cervical ligament is poorly defined. Hyperintense fluid is identified in the normal anterior microrecesses (*open arrow*) and posterior recess (*curved arrow*) at the level of the posterior facet of the subtalar joint. (**C**) Sinus tarsi syndrome in a separate patient. This arthroscopic view of the subtalar joint of the left ankle displays synovitis and scar bands that surround a damaged interosseous ligament. The sinus tarsi is to the left and the talocalcaneal articulation is to the right.

weighted images), diffuse infiltration with synovitis (low signal intensity on T1-weighted images and increased signal intensity on T2-weighted images) (Fig. 8-107), and multiple synovial cystic fluid collections (hyperintense on T2-weighted images). Posterior tibial tendon tears may be found in association with the sinus tarsi syndrome. Klein and Spreitzer also reported that 60% of patients with an abnormal tarsal sinus and canal were clinically diagnosed as having sinus tarsi syndrome.[73]

Fractures

Ankle Fractures

The classification of ankle fractures by the Lauge-Hansen system is based on the position of the foot and the direction of the injuring force.[74] Four categories of fracture are

recognized: (1) supination-external rotation injuries, (2) supination-adduction injuries, (3) pronation-external rotation injuries, (4) pronation-abduction injuries.[75]

MR imaging complements conventional radiographic and CT evaluation of these injuries, allowing more specific demonstration of trabecular and soft-tissue ligamentous lesions. For example, conventional radiographs rely on the positive predictive value of an ankle joint effusion to suggest the presence of an occult fracture (effusions greater than 13 mm have a positive predictive value of 82%). With MR imaging, however, the fracture can be visualized directly.[76] A more common mechanism of injury is the supination-external rotation mechanism, in which the injury progresses through four stages:

- Stage 1: anterior inferior tibiofibular ligament rupture
- Stage 2: oblique spiral fracture of the lateral malleolus (Fig. 8-108)

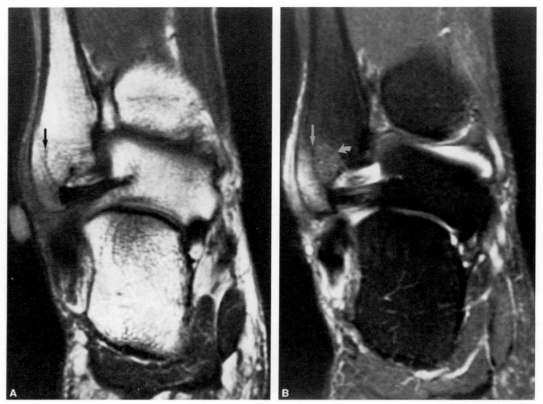

FIGURE 8-108. An oblique nondisplaced spiral fracture (*straight arrow*) of the distal fibula below the level of the tibial plafond is associated with adjacent marrow edema (*curved arrow*), which is hypointense on T1-weighted coronal images (**A**) and hyperintense on fat-suppressed T2-weighted fast spin-echo coronal images (**B**).

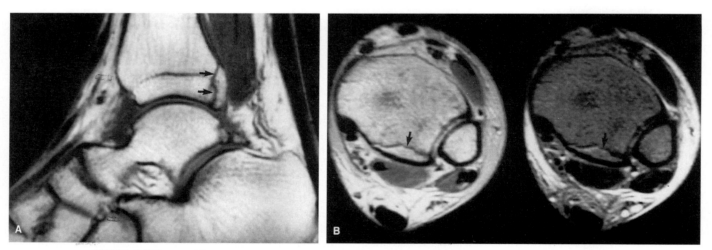

FIGURE 8-109. An old posterior malleolar fracture (*arrows*) with a sclerotic low signal intensity segment is identified on (**A**) T1-weighted sagittal and (**B**) T2-weighted axial images. Continuity of the tibial plafond and the posterior tibial cortex indicate a united fracture.

- Stage 3: a posterior lip or margin fracture of the tibia (Fig. 8-109)
- Stage 4: avulsion fracture of the medial malleolus or deltoid ligament rupture.

The pronation-external rotation injury starts with fracture of the medial malleolus and progresses clockwise through injuries similar to those outlined for supination-external rotation fractures. In supination-external rotation injuries, fracture of the fibula usually occurs within 2.5 cm of the ankle mortise. In pronation-external rotation injuries, the fracture is usually 8 to 9 cm proximal to the tip of the lateral malleolus (more than 2.5 cm from the ankle joint). Adduction forces usually result in horizontal transverse fractures of the lateral malleolus and vertical oblique fracture of the medial malleolus, whereas abduction forces produce a horizontal fracture of the medial malleolus and an oblique distal fibular fracture.[57,75]

Tibial pilon (plafond) fractures occur secondary to vertical loading. There is cancellous bone compression above the tibial plafond[77] and a stable comminuted fracture of the distal tibia, which may be associated with a fracture of the fibula. The pilon fracture extends into the tibiotalar joint (Fig. 8-110) and incongruity of the joint surfaces may result in the late complication of posttraumatic arthritis.

LeFort's fracture is an isolated vertical fracture of the medial aspect of the distal fibula (lateral malleolus).[78] This avulsion fracture corresponds to the insertion site of the anterior inferior tibiofibular ligament. An external rotation force is the mechanism of injury. Although radiographic evaluation is usually satisfactory, MR imaging can be used to differentiate an avulsion of the anterior inferior tibiofibular ligament from an avulsion injury of the lateral malleolus corresponding to the anterior talofibular ligament attachment.

Epiphyseal Fractures

NORMAL MR APPEARANCE. The normal MR pattern of distal tibial and fibular epiphyseal ossification and physeal closure has been described by Chung and Jaramillo.[79] It is important to understand these normal patterns in order to appreciate physeal and epiphyseal injuries. For example, prior to closure the normal tibial physis shows an anteromedial undulation (Kump hump), which may be mistaken for premature physeal closure (Fig. 8-111). In addition, on T2-weighted images the cartilaginous epiphysis has a lower signal intensity than the physis. T2-weighted images are useful in differentiating the epiphysis from the physeal articular cartilage before complete ossification of the epiphysis. The ossific nucleus is most conspicuous on T2*-weighted images and is seen as a low signal intensity area surrounded by a relatively hyperintense articular cartilage. The physis is best visualized on gradient-echo and fat-suppressed T2-weighted spin-echo images, especially when ossification of the epiphysis is almost complete. Distal epiphyseal ossification and physeal closure begin anteromedially, and occur earlier than in the fibula.

SPECIFIC PATTERNS OF EPIPHYSEAL INJURIES. The Salter-Harris (SH) classification describes injuries to the physis (growth plate). The most common epiphyseal injury is a lateral malleolus SH type I fracture, which is through the growth plate[77] (Fig. 8-112). SH type II fractures extend through the physis and metaphysis, and SH type II displaced fractures of the tibial epiphysis are usually associated with a greenstick fracture of the fibula, which occurs with eversion and external rotation injuries. SH type III fractures extend through the physis and into the epiphysis. SH type IV fractures involve the physis, metaphysis, and epiphysis. In SH type V injuries, there is compression across the physis. Medial malleolar fractures are usually SH type III or IV, and are associated with growth disturbance.

A Tillaux fracture is caused by an external rotation force that avulses the anterolateral portion of the epiphysis producing an SH type III injury.[77] There is usually rotational instability of the ankle.

The triplane fracture is a complex fracture of the distal tibial epiphysis that features a SH type IV injury in the coronal plane medially, a SH type II injury in the coronal plane laterally, and a SH type III injury in the sagittal plane laterally.[77,80]

Medial Tibial Stress Syndrome

The medial tibial stress syndrome has been ascribed to stress fractures, the deep posterior compartment syndrome, and to shin splints.[66] It is thought to be caused by a stress

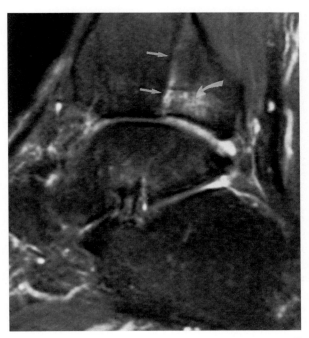

FIGURE 8-110. Vertical intraarticular fracture of the distal tibia or pilon fracture with minimal displacement and incongruity of the tibial plafond. The fracture line (*straight arrow*) and adjacent hyperintense subchondral bone marrow edema (*curved arrow*) are shown on a fat-suppressed T2-weighted fast spin-echo sagittal image.

text continues on page 564

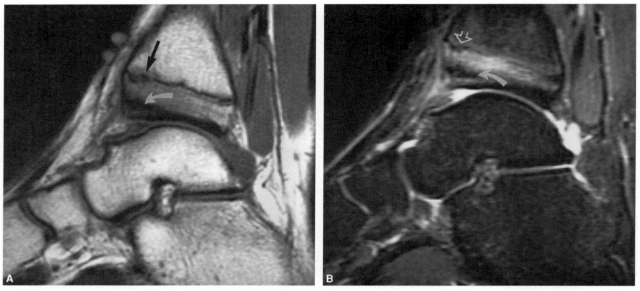

FIGURE 8-111. (A) Normal appearance of the Kump hump with irregularity of the anteromedial distal tibial physis (*straight arrow*). Discontinuity or irregularity where the physis is curved and thin may be mistaken for physeal closure. In addition, this patient has a nondisplaced epiphyseal fracture (*curved arrow*) with associated adjacent bone marrow edema (T1-weighted sagittal image). (B) Corresponding fat-suppressed T2-weighted fast spin-echo sagittal image shows a normal open physis (*open arrow*) over the Kump hump as well as the anterior epiphyseal fracture (*curved arrow*) and adjacent marrow edema.

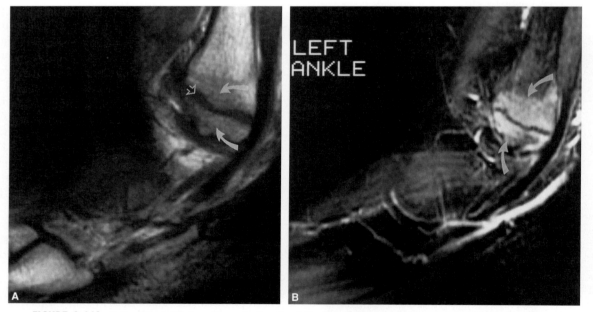

FIGURE 8-112. Salter-Harris I injury through the distal fibular physis (*open arrow*). There is bone marrow edema (*arrows*) involving the adjacent metaphysis and epiphysis symmetrically on either side of the physis (**A**: T1-weighted sagittal image; **B**: fast spin-echo STIR sagittal image).

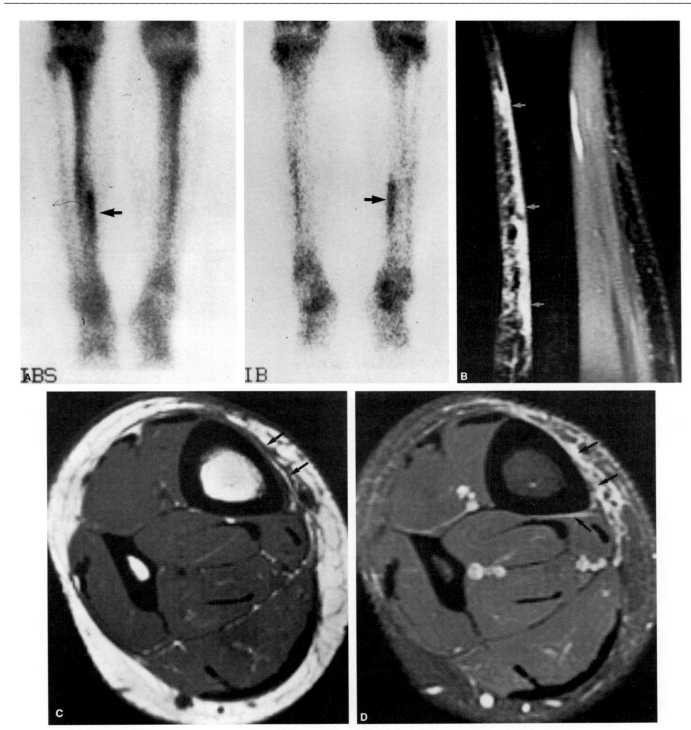

FIGURE 8-113. Medial tibial stress syndrome. **(A)** Positive (*arrow*) radionuclide bone scan. Corresponding anteromedial and posteromedial tibial periosteal edema (*arrows*) on a STIR sagittal image **(B)**, a T1-weighted axial image **(C)**, and a fat-suppressed T2-weighted fast spin-echo axial image **(D)**. No cortical or marrow abnormality was demonstrated. Conventional radiographs were normal in this patient. Periosteal edema is hyperintense on the STIR sequence **(B)** and the fat-suppressed T2-weighted fast spin-echo sequence **(D)**.

reaction of the fascia, periosteum, and/or bone along the posteromedial tibia. Pain and tenderness is present along the medial aspect of the mid- to distal tibia, and symptoms are exacerbated by exercise and decreased by rest. Beck and Osternig,[81] performing cadaveric dissections, studied the structures that attach to the tibia at the site of symptoms of medial tibial stress syndrome.[81] They found that the soleus, the flexor digitorum longus, and the deep crural fascia attached more frequently at the site corresponding to the symptoms of the medial tibial stress syndrome. The tibialis posterior was not found to attach in this area. Previously, it had been thought that periostitis underneath the tibialis posterior muscle was a contributing factor in this syndrome. These findings suggest that the soleus, through its postero-medial tibial aponeurotic insertion, is a major contributor to traction-induced medial tibial stress syndrome. The soleus muscle is supposed to cause muscle traction-induced periostitis of the distal one half to one third of the medial border of the tibia. Surgical findings in shin splints include avulsion of the tibial periosteum by the soleus.[82]

The early changes of medial tibial stress syndrome are not appreciated on conventional radiography and require bone scans or MR imaging for detection.[83] Fredericson and colleages[84] have proposed a MR rating system to ensure accuracy when correlating MR findings with clinical symptoms and scintigraphy.[84] In this system, grade I changes of periosteal edema demonstrate mild to moderate increased signal intensity on T2-weighted images (Fig. 8-113), and

marrow is normal on T1- and T2-weighted images. A grade II injury demonstrates moderate to severe periosteal edema and associated marrow edema, both hyperintense on T2-weighted images (Fig. 8-114). Grade III injuries display marrow edema on both T1 and T2 (hyperintensity weighted) images. A fracture line can be seen in grade IV injuries. Periostitis or shin splints corresponds to a grade I stress injury. The bone marrow edema in grades II and III represents a more severe injury along a spectrum that could lead to a defined fracture. Fat-suppressed MR imaging is helpful in the identification of these early changes, similar to our experience in using the STIR or fat-suppressed T2-weighted fast spin-echo sequences to identify early periosteal edema and muscle reaction. It is interesting to note that Fredericson's work shows periosteal edema at the origin of the tibialis posterior, the flexor digitorum longus, and the soleus muscles, without the predominant involvement of any one particular muscle group.

Fractures of the Foot

CALCANEUS. Calcaneal fractures are divided into intraarticular and extraarticular types according to the involvement or extension of the fracture into the subtalar joint.[75,85] Extraarticular fractures that do not involve the subtalar joint include fractures of the tuberosity, the anterior process (Fig. 8-115), the sustentaculum tali, or the body.[75] Intraarticular fractures, which are more common, are classified by Essex-

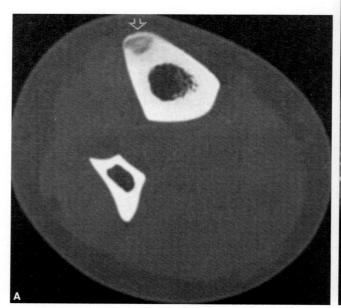
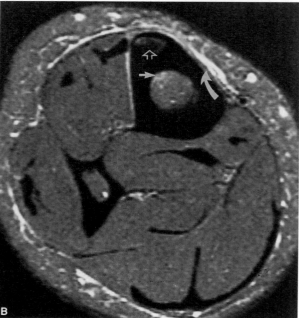

FIGURE 8-114. Medial tibial stress syndrome in a sprinter. **(A)** Axial CT scan shows intracortical cystic reaction (*open arrow*) with remodeling of repeated cortical stress fractures. **(B)** Corresponding fat-suppressed T2-weighted fast spin-echo axial image demonstrates hyperintense signal intensity within the bone marrow (*straight arrow*), intracortical cystic area (*open arrow*), and medial periosteum (*curved arrow*).

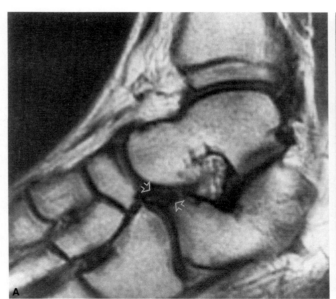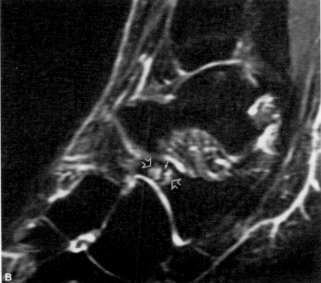

FIGURE 8-115. Anterior process fracture of the lateral calcaneus is associated with reactive bone marrow edema (*open arrows*) which is hypointense on T1-weighted (**A**) and hyperintense on STIR (**B**) sagittal images. The hypointense fracture line (*small solid arrow*) is best seen on the STIR sequence (**B**). Anterior process fractures may be difficult to detect on conventional radiographs.

Lopresti into two categories, a tongue-type injury and a depression-type injury, based on the secondary fracture pattern seen in association with the primary or oblique fracture segment.[75] The tongue-type fracture is transverse and extends to the posterior tuberosity. The depression-type fracture has a secondary fracture line that runs from the body of the calcaneus directly posterior to the subtalar joint (Fig. 8-116). Both MR imaging and CT are useful in demonstrating joint alignment, fragment displacement, and involvement of the subtalar joint. Prognosis is better for extraarticular fractures that do not involve the subtalar joint.[85] MR imaging is sensitive to the hyperemia, morphology, and location of calcaneal stress fractures. STIR and fat-suppressed T2-weighted fast spin-echo sequences are used to identify these areas of hyperintensity. T1-weighted images may be unremarkable.

TALUS.   Since the ankle mortise protects the talus from direct injury, talar fractures usually result from transmitted forces.[75] Fractures of the talus may involve the neck (Fig. 8-117), the body (Fig. 8-118), the head, and the posterior and lateral processes (Fig. 8-119). Fractures of the lateral process of the talus are a recently recognized complication of snowboarding, associated with dorsiflexion and inversion injuries.[86] AVN is a known complication of talar neck fractures, and with MR imaging it is possible to assess adjacent bone marrow for signs of this process and to demonstrate nondisplaced fracture morphology.[86] The articular cartilage surfaces can

also be directly evaluated on MR studies. MR imaging has also been used to identify talar insufficiency fractures.[87] In addition to demonstrating talar stress fractures in the classic location (paralleling the talonavicular articulation at the level of the talar neck), MR imaging depicts these other fracture locations. These fractures involve vertically and horizontally oriented insufficiency fractures of the medial aspect of the posteroinferior talus, and transverse or horizontal fractures of the talar body parallel to the tibiotalar joint.

NAVICULAR AND CUNEIFORM FRACTURES.   Navicular fractures are characterized by ligamentous capsular avulsions and fractures of the tuberosity and body.[75] CT is effective for detecting navicular stress fractures and for performing follow-up examinations.[88] CT fracture patterns all include involvement of the central third of the proximal dorsal margin of the navicular. Most stress fractures are characterized as partial and linear. In nonunion, persistence of a fracture gap cam be seen. Medullary cysts and cortical notching may persist even after fracture healing. Sagittal plane MR images are particularly useful for identification of fractures involving one or both cortices (Fig. 8-120). Axial images, however, may be required to display fracture lines that are parallel with the sagittal plane. When present, diffuse edema demonstrates hyperintensity on STIR or fat-suppressed T2-weighted fast spin-echo sequences. Although AVN is not common, MR imaging is also helpful in demonstrating subchondral sclero-

text continues on page 568

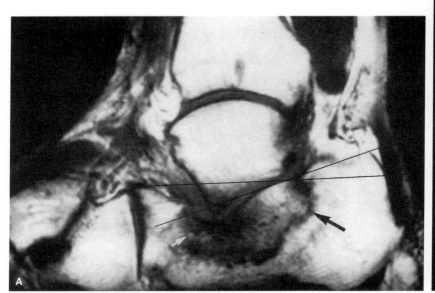
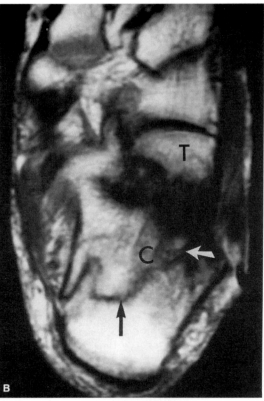

FIGURE 8-116. (A) A T1-weighted sagittal image shows a joint-depression type intraarticular calcaneal fracture with a secondary fracture line (*black arrow*) exiting the body posterior to the subtalar joint. The primary fracture component is more anterior (*white arrow*) relative to the secondary fracture line. Depression of the fracture fragment causes a decrease in Bohler's angle (*crossed lines*), which is normally between 20° and 40°. (B) A T1-weighted axial image shows subtalar joint extension (*white arrow*) of a calcaneal fracture (*black arrow*). C, calcaneus; T, talus.

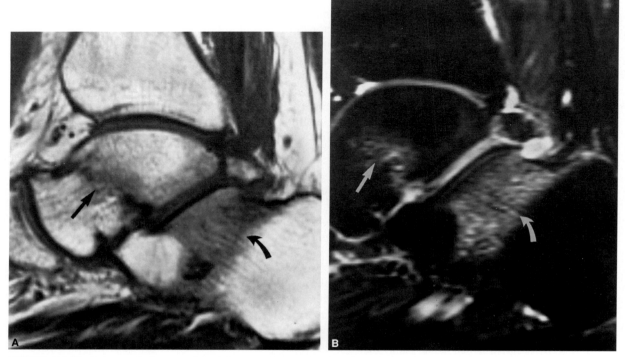

FIGURE 8-117. Talar neck fracture (*straight arrow*) associated with wide band of calcaneal trabecular stress injury (*curved arrow*). Talar fracture and calcaneal trabecular microfracture are hypointense on T1-weighted sagittal image (**A**) and hyperintense on STIR sagittal image (**B**).

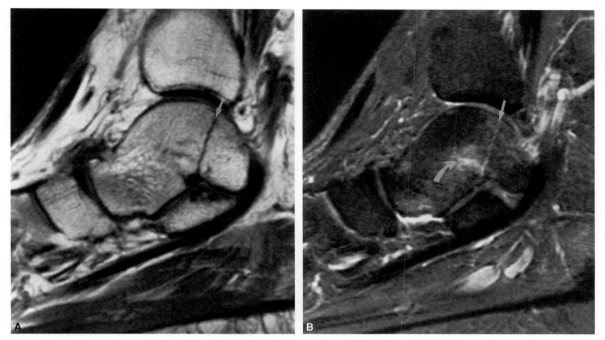

FIGURE 8-118. A coronal shearing fracture (*straight arrow*) of the talar body with subtalar joint extension is shown on T1-weighted (**A**) and fat-suppressed T2-weighted fast spin-echo (**B**) sagittal images. Bone marrow edema (*curved arrow*) is hyperintense on the fat-suppressed T2-weighted fast spin-echo sagittal image (**B**). Talar dome articular congruity is maintained in this nondisplaced fracture.

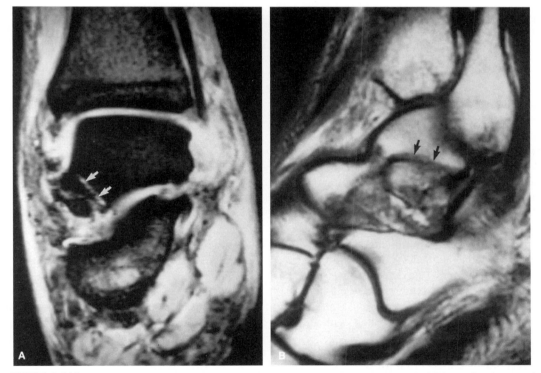

FIGURE 8-119. A fracture of the lateral process of the talus (*arrows*) is seen on (**A**) T2*-weighted coronal and (**B**) T1-weighted sagittal images. This fracture involves the posterior aspect of the subtalar joint.

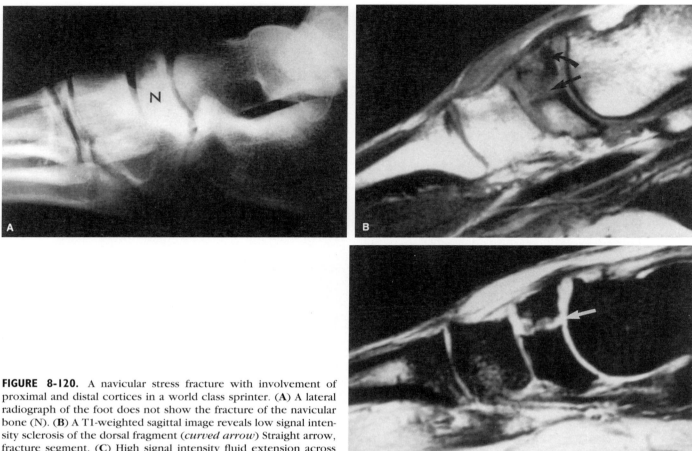

FIGURE 8-120. A navicular stress fracture with involvement of proximal and distal cortices in a world class sprinter. (**A**) A lateral radiograph of the foot does not show the fracture of the navicular bone (N). (**B**) A T1-weighted sagittal image reveals low signal intensity sclerosis of the dorsal fragment (*curved arrow*) Straight arrow, fracture segment. (**C**) High signal intensity fluid extension across the fracture site is revealed on a T2*-weighted sagittal image (*arrow*).

sis prior to the appearance of increased radiographic density. A navicular stress fracture should be differentiated from the symptomatic accessory tarsal navicular bone.[89] In the latter, the normal variant of the medially located accessory tarsal navicular bone may develop a bone marrow edema pattern on fat-suppressed T2-weighted images in symptomatic patients with focal pain in the adjacent navicular tuberosity (Fig. 8-121). This hyperemia or edema pattern is associated with chronic stress or osteonecrosis and can be seen adjacent to the synchondrosis with a diffuse nonlinear hyperintensity. The accessory navicular bone is located posterior to the posteromedial tuberosity of the tarsal navicular in 4% to 21% of the population. The pattern of bone marrow edema just described is not seen in asymptomatic patients. Cuneiform fractures are less common and are associated with direct trauma.

TARSOMETATARSAL OR LISFRANC FRACTURES. The homolateral and divergent types of Lisfranc fractures are best evaluated by standard radiographs or coronal reformatted 1.5 mm CT scans (Fig. 8-122). The medial border of the middle or intermediate cuneiform and the lateral border of the medial cuneiform should be in line with or directly congruent with their respective metatarsals. In these injuries the role of MR imaging may be limited to evaluating soft-tissue and capsular structures when radiographic or CT examination results are negative. In our experience with Lisfranc injuries, MR imaging has proved to be more sensitive than CT in identifying the extent of posttraumatic marrow hyperemia and the number of bones of the tarsus affected, but thin section (1.5 mm) CT scans in both the coronal and axial planes are more accurate in identifying small osseous corner or chip fragments in the cuneiforms and base of the metatarsals (see Fig. 8-122).

METATARSAL STRESS FRACTURES AND SESAMOID INJURIES.
MR imaging and CT have been used for early diagnosis of metatarsal stress fractures prior to positive findings with conventional radiography. Ballet dancers are particularly prone to developing stress injuries involving the base of the second and third metatarsals (Fig. 8-123). Harrington and colleagues[90] have described overuse ballet injuries involving the base of the second metatarsal and the adjacent Lisfranc

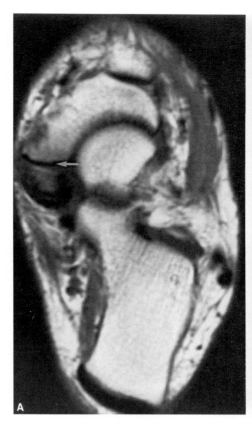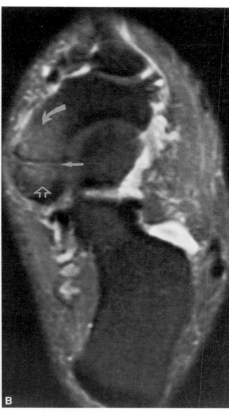

FIGURE 8-121. A symptomatic accessory tarsal navicular bone (os naviculare externum) with bone marrow edema of the accessory navicular bone (*open arrow*) and navicular tuberosity (*curved arrow*). Marrow changes are hypointense on T1-weighted axial image (**A**) and hyperintense on fat-suppressed T2-weighted fast spin-echo axial image (**B**). Marrow hyperintensity is located immediately adjacent to the synchondrosis (*straight arrow*).

joint.[90] With MR imaging it is possible to distinguish synovitis of the Lisfranc joint from a stress fracture at the base of the second metatarsal. We have also seen degenerative joint changes on MR images in cases with negative conventional radiographs.[91] Arthrosis of the calcaneocuboid joint, the first metatarsophalangeal joint, as well as the ankle and subtalar joints demonstrates low signal intensity on T1- and T2-weighted images, respectively, showing changes of sclerosis. Although sometimes positive in these cases, technetium (methylene diphosphonate [99mTC-MDP]) scintigraphy may not be specific for fracture as opposed to degenerative arthrosis. STIR and fat-suppressed T2-weighted fast spin-echo protocols demonstrate marrow hyperemia in recurrent injuries in the presence of negative or unchanged radiographs or CT evaluations. Cast immobilization or non–weight-bearing is necessary in dancers who have significant pain. Additional abnormalities of the plantar plate of the foot (extending from the distal metatarsal neck to the plantar aspect of the proximal phalangeal base) and metatarsal sesamoids can also be detected and characterized on MR studies.[92,93] Sesamoid fractures are usually transverse and involve the tibial sesamoid (Fig. 8-124). The fracture site is irregular and may be associated with soft-tissue swelling. Bipartite sesamoid bone morphology is more common than a complete sesamoid bone

fracture (Fig. 8-125). The bipartite cleft is transverse, smooth and round, with sclerotic cortical edges without callus.

Os Trigonum Syndrome

As discussed earlier, the posterior bony impingement or talar compression is a condition seen with injuries in dancers. This syndrome may be associated with an os trigonum or posterior trigonal process[55] (Fig. 8-126). The os trigonum syndrome is characterized by symptoms caused by pathology of the lateral tubercle of the posterior talar process,[94] and includes various descriptions including posterior ankle impingement, talar compression syndrome, posterior ankle impingement, and posterior tibiotalar impingement syndrome. Pain is associated with disruption of the cartilaginous synchondrosis between the os trigonum and the lateral tubercle secondary to repetitive microtrauma and chronic inflammation (see Fig. 8-126B). Trigonal process fracture, flexor hallucis longus tenosynovitis, posterior tibiotalar bony impingement, and intraarticular loose bodies are considered additional etiologies. Clinically there is chronic pain, stiffness, tenderness, and soft-tissue swelling in the posterior ankle. Activities involving extreme plantar flexion including

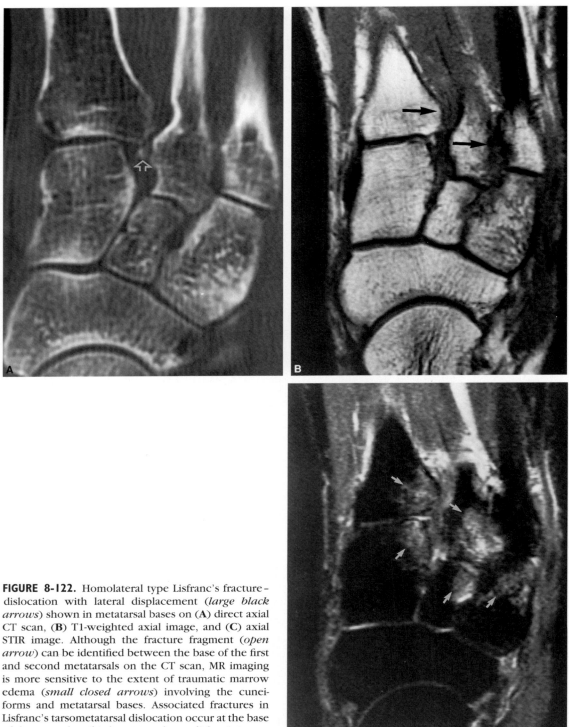

FIGURE 8-122. Homolateral type Lisfranc's fracture–dislocation with lateral displacement (*large black arrows*) shown in metatarsal bases on (**A**) direct axial CT scan, (**B**) T1-weighted axial image, and (**C**) axial STIR image. Although the fracture fragment (*open arrow*) can be identified between the base of the first and second metatarsals on the CT scan, MR imaging is more sensitive to the extent of traumatic marrow edema (*small closed arrows*) involving the cuneiforms and metatarsal bases. Associated fractures in Lisfranc's tarsometatarsal dislocation occur at the base of the second or third metatarsals, medial or intermediate cuneiforms, or the navicular bone.

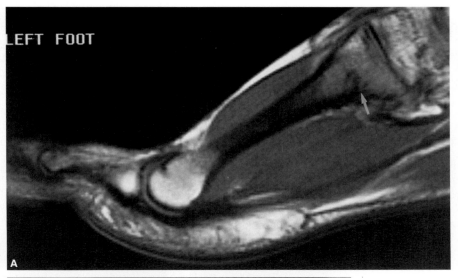

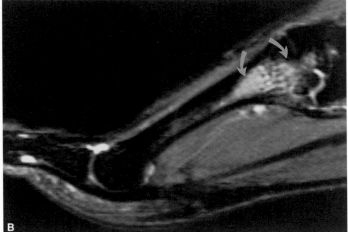

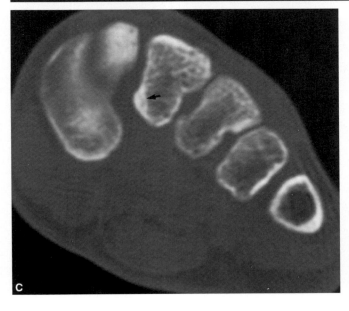

FIGURE 8-123. (A) Second metatarsal base stress fracture in a ballet dancer is shown with hypointense linear stress fracture (*straight white arrow*) on T1-weighted image. (B) STIR sagittal images display associated hyperintense bone marrow edema (*curved arrows*). (C) Corresponding direct coronal CT demonstrates subtle medial cortical sclerosis (*black arrow*) along the plantar aspect of the second metatarsal base.

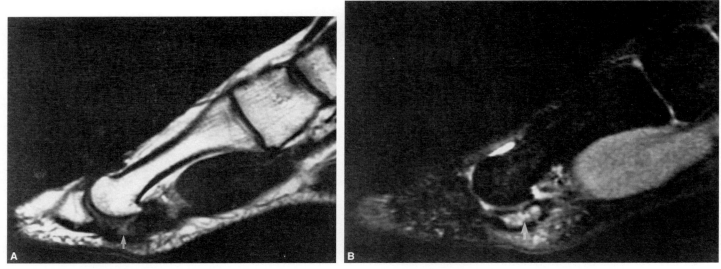

FIGURE 8-124. Tibial sesamoid fracture. Sesamoid edema (*arrow*) is inhomogeneous on the T1-weighted sagittal image (**A**) and hyperintense on the STIR sagittal image (**B**).

ballet, soccer, football, and downhill running may result in compression and entrapment of synovial and capsular tissue against the posterior tibia, causing soft-tissue thickening, fibrosis, and sometimes the development of associated flexor hallucis longus tenosynovitis. In 7% to 14% of patients, it remains unfused as a separate ossicle. MR imaging or CT may not be able to distinguish between a chronic ununited fracture of the lateral tubercle (Shepherd's fracture) and the unfused os trigonum. The flexor hallucis longus tendon is medial to the os trigonum in the sulcus between the smaller medial tubercle and the larger lateral tubercle. This relation-ship is seen on axial MR images. Isolated tenosynovitis of the flexor hallucis longus tendon sheath may not be associated with a corresponding effusion in the tibiotalar joint. A disruption of the cartilaginous synchondrosis is seen with hyperintense fluid between the os trigonum and lateral talar process on T2-weighted images. Degenerative cystic chang-es exist at the synchondrosis or between the os trigonum and calcaneus. Failed conservative treatment and rehabilitation is usually followed by simple surgical excision. Clinical con-firmation of the diagnosis is often provided by relief of symptoms following the injection of a local anesthetic.[95]

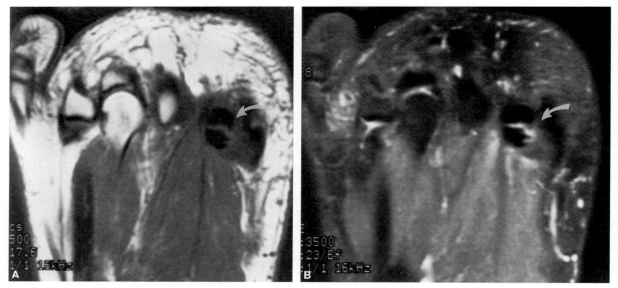

FIGURE 8-125. Bipartite fibular sesamoid with osteochondritis. The bipartite sesamoid is enlarged with smooth edges (*curved arrow*). Osteochondritis demonstrates hypointensity on both (**A**) T1-weighted and (**B**) fat-suppressed T2-weighted fast spin-echo axial images.

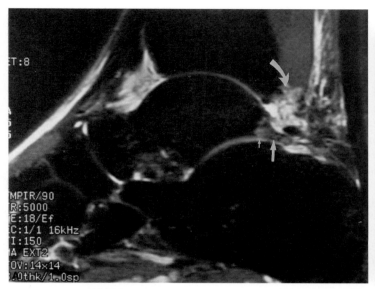
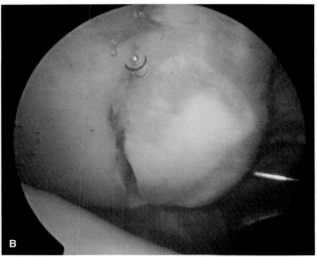

FIGURE 8-126. (A) Hyperintensity of the os trigonum (*large straight arrow*) to the level of the synchondrosis (*small straight arrow*) on a fast STIR sagittal image. Synovitis (*curved arrow*) is shown adjacent and posterior to the os trigonum. The os trigonum represents a congenital nonunion of the lateral tubercle of the posterior process of the talus. (B) Subtalar arthroscopy of the left ankle in a patient with a painful os trigonum. Notice the separation between the os trigonum and the posterior aspect of the talus. The calcaneus is inferior and the flexor hallucis longus neurovascular bundle are just medial to the os trigonum.

Compartment Syndrome

Acute compartment syndrome is associated with fracture or severe trauma. Chronic compartment syndrome is the result of elevated compartment pressures with the development of muscle and nerve ischemia.[66] Noncompliant fascial compartments, increased muscle bulk (secondary to contraction, and intracellular and extracellular fluid accumulation), and muscle microtears contribute to increased pressures and associated venous and lymphatic compromise. Chronic compartment syndrome is seen most frequently in runners with symptoms of pain during exercise with or without neurologic symptoms. Bilateral and asymmetric involvement is common. The anterior and deep posterior compartments are more commonly involved than the lateral and superficial posterior compartments. There may be a history of a recent stress fracture. Muscle herniations through fascial defects may be identified following exercise, although herniations can also cause chronic leg pain in the absence of compartment syndrome. Wick catheter measurements show that preexercise compartment pressures are greater than or equal to 15 mm of Hg, 1 minute postexercise pressures are greater than or equal to 30 mm of Hg, and 5 minute postexercise pressures are greater than or equal to 20 mm Hg.[66] MR techniques using axial STIR or fat-suppressed T2-weighted fast spin-echo sequences are sensitive to early changes of muscle compartment edema, which is seen as an infiltrative or feather-like pattern of hyperintensity (Fig. 8-127). Bulging and hyperintensity may also be seen in the adjacent fascia.

Acute compartment syndrome of the foot, with elevation of tissue fluid pressure within a closed space, has also been reported following trauma. It is usually associated with calcaneal fracture[96] but may also follow crush injuries, even in the absence of severe fracture.[97] Although MR imaging can be used to confirm clinical findings and identify a compart-

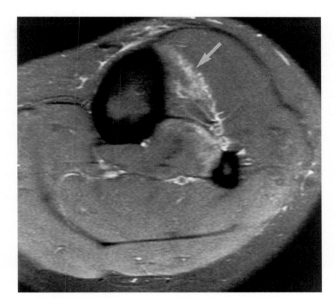

FIGURE 8-127. Symptoms referred to the anterior compartment correlated with hyperintense muscle edema along the distribution of the tibialis anterior muscle group (*arrow*) (fat-suppressed T2-weighted fast spin-echo axial image).

ment hematoma, appropriate treatment with fasciotomy should not be postponed to obtain such studies.

Gastrocnemius-Soleus Strain

Strain or rupture of the gastrocnemius-soleus muscle complex is a common sports injury seen in racquet sports, basketball, running or skiing.[66] There may be an associated plantaris muscle rupture at the myotendinous junction.[98] Because of the paucity of reported cases in the surgical literature, the association between the rupture of the plantaris muscle and the clinical presentation of tennis leg has not been fully appreciated. A sharp sudden calf pain is frequently followed by swelling and ecchymosis. This injury occurs during knee extension with the ankle dorsiflexed while in the crouched position. There is impaired gait locomotion and difficulty with the toe-off portion of the stance phase. The calf hemorrhage can be associated with aching and cramping pain for several weeks. Although there may be a palpable knot or defect on physical examination, surgical treatment is not indicated. Conservative management with a brace or crutches is used in the acute stages.

MR findings in myotendinous junction rupture of the plantaris muscle include hemorrhage (intermuscular hematoma) between the medial head of the gastrocnemius muscle and soleus muscle (Fig. 8-128). The retracted tendon of the plantaris and associated hemorrhage may produce a condensed mass of intermediate signal intensity blood and tissue within the plane of the hematoma. Distal axial images at the level of the ankle joint demonstrate a curvilinear fluid collection in the expected location of the plantaris tendon contribution to the medial aspect of the Achilles tendon. Fat-suppressed T2-weighted and STIR images are the most sensitive sequences for detection of hemorrhage and associated intramuscular strain, and should be performed from the level of the proximal tibia to the ankle joint distally. Plantaris injuries can occur as an isolated finding or be associated with partial tear of the gastrocnemius or popliteus muscle. The hematoma is greatest in acute injury. The plantaris tendon is absent in 7% to 10% of the population and does not require repair. In fact, the plantaris tendon is frequently used as an autograft for ligament reconstructions. More proximal plantar muscle strains at the level of the knee joint have been associated with anterior cruciate ligament and posterolateral corner injuries. In complete ruptures of the plantaris, the proximal retracted muscle may be identified between the popliteus tendon and lateral head of the gastrocnemius muscle at the level of the knee. A posterior compartment syndrome could result from swelling and hematoma associated with complete rupture of the plantaris or tear of the gastrocnemius-soleus muscle complex.

Tarsal Coalition

Tarsal coalition represents either a congenital or acquired fibrous, cartilaginous, or bony fusion of the tarsal bones.[99] Calcaneonavicular coalition is the most common type, reported in 53% of cases; talocalcaneal coalitions represent

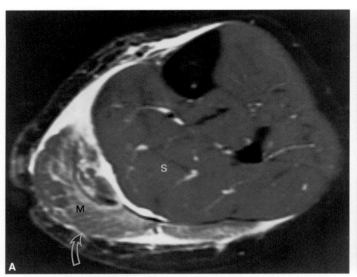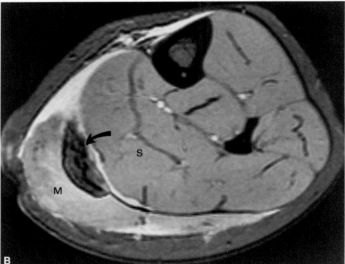

FIGURE 8-128. Acute rupture of the plantaris with intermuscular hemorrhage (*solid curved arrow*) identified in the plane between the soleus (S) and medial head of the gastrocnemius muscle (M) groups. (**A**) Hemorrhage is isointense to hyperintense on a fat-suppressed T2-weighted fast spin-echo axial image. (**B**) On a T2*-weighted axial image the hemorrhage demonstrates hypointensity (magnetic susceptibility effect). Edema of the medial head of the gastrocnemius muscle (*open curved arrow*) is best demonstrated on the fat-suppressed T2-weighted fast spin-echo sequence (**A**).

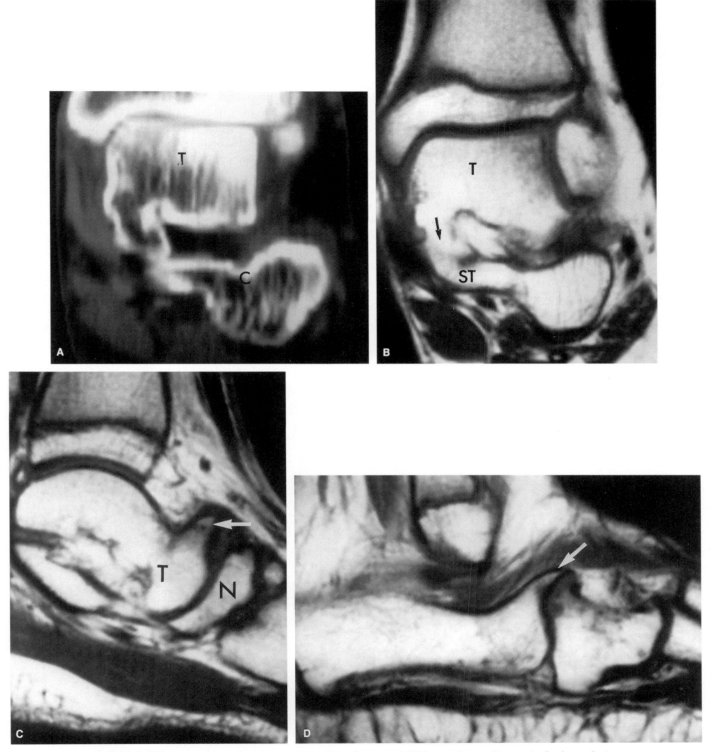

FIGURE 8-129. Talocalcaneal coalition. (**A**) A 2D reformatted CT image is not diagnostic for bony fusion between the talus (T) and calcaneus (C). (**B**) On the corresponding 3 mm T1-weighted coronal image there is continuity (*arrow*) of marrow fat from the tali (T) through the sustentaculum tali (ST). T1-weighted sagittal images show secondary signs of talocalcaneal coalition with talar beaking (**C,** *arrow*) and degenerative changes at the calcaneal cuboid joint (**D,** *arrow*). N, navicular bone; T, talus.

37%.[100] Talonavicular and calcaneocuboid types are infrequent. Although coalitions are present at birth, radiographic detection is difficult because ossification of the fibrous or cartilaginous connection does not occur until the second decade.[99] Tarsal coalition may also be associated with a painful pes planus or flatfoot in a child or adolescent.[100] Forefoot abduction and hindfoot valgus can result in tension in the peroneal muscles and tendons (ie, peroneal spastic flatfoot).

CT scanning with 1.5 mm sections has been used to complement specialized radiographic studies (AP, lateral, 45° lateral oblique, and 45° views) to better distinguish the facets and coalitions. CT scans performed in the direct axial and coronal planes as well as sagittal reformations are recommended. CT demonstrates fibrous coalitions indirectly, by displaying irregular or roughened cortical surfaces. However, CT is limited in that direct multiplanar scanning is not possible and reformatted sagittal and coronal scans must be performed. The close proximity of the sustentaculum tali and talus may produce a pseudocoalition on coronal reformations in talocalcaneal coalitions (Fig. 8-129).

We have used coronal, sagittal, and axial 3 mm T1-weighted MR images to successfully identify the continuity of marrow signal intensity in bony coalitions. Fibrous tissue maintains low signal intensity on T1-, T2-, and T2*-weighted images. Three-dimensional volume acquisitions allow greater operator control in designating optimal planes for reformatting suspected coalitions. Secondary signs of calcaneonavicular coalition include hypoplasia of the head of the talus and abnormal close approximation of the navicular bone and the calcaneus, with irregularity of opposing cortical surfaces (Fig. 8-130). Secondary signs of a talocalcaneal coalition are talar beaking adjacent to the talonavicular articulation, a broadening lateral talar process, and a ball-and-socket ankle joint.[99] The normal talar ridge should not be confused with talar beaking. Talocalcaneal coalitions usually occur through the sustentaculum tali in the middle facet. In symptomatic patients, adjacent subchondral hyperemia may be seen on fat-suppressed T2-weighted fast spin-echo or STIR sequences in selected cases of fibrous coalitions across the sustentaculum tali (Fig. 8-131). Direct sagittal MR images have also demonstrated contour irregularities in the middle facet in patients with fibrous coalitions. Wechsler and colleagues[101] have also demonstrated subchondral hyperintensity, thought to be secondary to altered biomechanics, in calcaneonavicular coali-

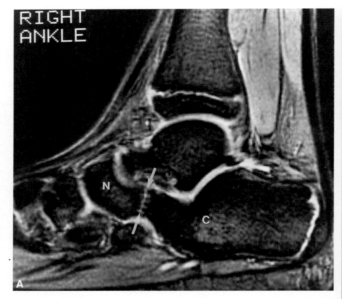

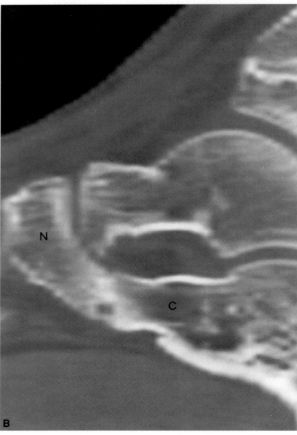

FIGURE 8-130. Fibrous calcaneonavicular coalition (*arrows*) displayed on a T2*-weighted sagittal image (**A**) and a corresponding 2D reformatted CT sagittal image (**B**). The MR image demonstrates the lack of complete solid bony continuity between the calcaneus and navicular bone more accurately than the CT scan. N, navicular bone; C, calcaneus.

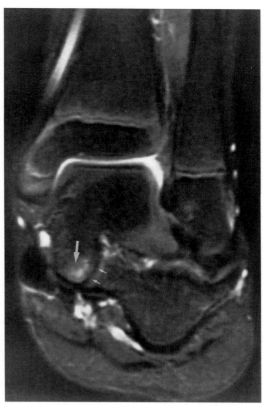

FIGURE 8-131. Symptomatic fibrocartilaginous talocalcaneal coalition (*small arrows*) with subchondral bone marrow edema (*large arrow*) identified on the talar side of the middle facet (fat-suppressed T2-weighted fast spin-echo coronal image).

tions.[101] A potential pitfall of MR imaging is mistaking proliferative low signal intensity synovitis for fibrous coalition.

Clubfoot

Talipes equinovarus or congenital clubfoot deformity involves forefoot plantar flexion with inversion of the heel and forefoot. The plantar aspect of the foot faces medially, and the calcaneus is turned in a plantar direction. Three-dimensional CT renderings are preferable to MR imaging for characterization of complex spatial deformities, because orthogonal or oblique images are difficult to interpret since key structures pass in and out of the plane of section (Fig. 8-132). In addition, three-dimensional displays reveal the following abnormalities[102]:

- A medially and inferiorly displaced navicular bone with an associated wedge deformity of the cuneiforms and cuboid
- A medially displaced anterior calcaneus
- A cavus deformity
- Medially curved metatarsals
- Flattening of the talar dome
- Hypertrophy of the talar head
- Internal tibial torsion.

MR imaging is being used to study Achilles tendon lengthening techniques in spastic equinus foot,[103] and to evaluate postoperative residual deformities when surgery fails.

Congenital Vertical Talus

In congenital convex pes valgus (congenital vertical talus), the talocalcaneal angle is abnormally increased, in contrast to clubfoot where the long axis of the talus and calcaneus

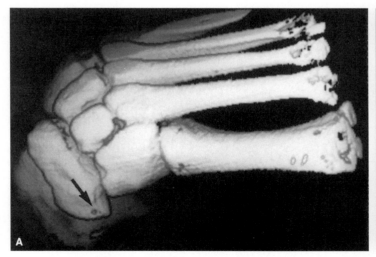
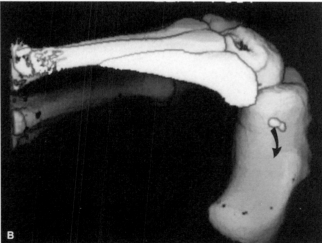

FIGURE 8-132. (A, B) Three-dimensional CT images show talipes equinovarus with inferomedial displacement of the navicular bone (*straight arrow*), a high arch or cavus deformity (*curved arrow*), inversion and adduction of the forefoot, and medial curving of the metatarsals.

are parallel.[104] Congenital vertical talus, in which there is rigid dorsal dislocation of the navicular onto the talar head and neck, represents the most severe form of congenital flatfoot. MR imaging has been used in a limited application to demonstrate not only the dorsal displacement of the navicular, but also to characterize the talar articular cartilage, which may extend across the entire surface of the abnormal joint. Abnormalities of the extrinsic and intrinsic muscles can also be assessed on MR images.

Tarsal Tunnel Syndrome

Tarsal tunnel syndrome is an entrapment or compression neuropathy of the posterior tibial nerve as it passes through the fibro-osseous tunnel deep to the flexor retinaculum and posterior and inferior to the medial malleolus.[58] The neurovascular bundle is located between the compartments containing the flexor digitorum longus and the flexor hallucis longus tendons. Within 1 cm of the medial malleolus, the posterior tibial nerve trifurcates into the medial and lateral plantar nerves and sensory calcaneal branches.[100]

Symptoms of tarsal tunnel syndrome are pain, sensory deficits of the sole of the foot and toes, and intrinsic muscle weakness. Etiologies of compression neuropathy in this region include lipomas, varicose veins, ganglia (Fig. 8-133), neurilemmomas, scarring, tenosynovitis, and accessory muscles.[100,105] Common surgical findings are entrapment of the flexor retinaculum or fibrous origin of the abductor hallucis muscle, tenosynovitis, and posttraumatic (ie, postfracture) fibrosis.[106,107] MR findings in the tarsal tunnel syndrome, including a ganglion cyst originating from the flexor hallucis longus tendon sheath, posttraumatic fibrosis, and neuroma, have been documented with surgical correlation.[108] The anatomy of the tarsal tunnel is effectively displayed on MR images, including the posterior tibial nerve and its branches.[109]

Comparison with the opposite ankle may be useful when a space-occupying lesion is not identified. If conservative treatment is not successful, surgical decompression is performed, with division of the retinaculum and mobilization of the medial and lateral plantar nerves and the fibrous origin of the abductor hallucis.[106] Clinical results of tarsal tunnel decompression reported by Pieffer and Cracchiolo,[110] however, suggest that unless a specific lesion is identified near or within the tarsal tunnel preoperatively, subsequent surgical decompression of the posterior tibial nerve may not be successful. They found that surgical decompression in patients with a history of previous surgical treatment for pain in the foot, plantar fasciitis, or for systemic inflammatory disease

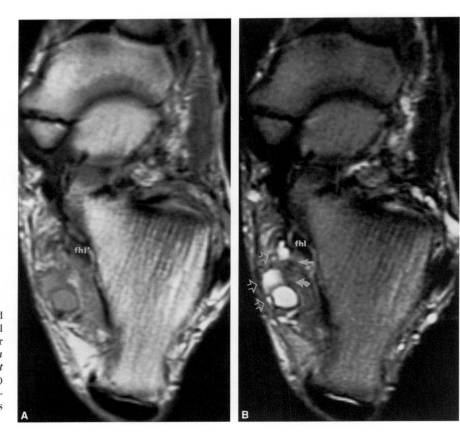

FIGURE 8-133. (**A**) Intermediate weighted and (**B**) T2-weighted axial images display the tarsal tunnel syndrome secondary to neurovascular compression by a septated ganglion (*open arrows*) at the level of the medial (*straight arrow*) and lateral plantar (*curved arrow*) nerves. The ganglion is hyperintense on T2-weighted image (**B**). fhl, flexor hallucis longus tendon.

did not show favorable results compared with patients with space-occupying lesions.[110]

Morton's Neuroma

Morton's neuroma is a metatarsalgia that involves localized enlargement of the interdigital nerve and begins between the third and fourth metatarsal heads. The lateral branch of the medial plantar nerve to the third interspace is usually involved. The second and fourth interspaces are also occasionally involved.[111] This condition occurs more frequently in women 40 to 60 years of age. Plantar foot pain and tenderness in the involved interspace is characteristic.

Histologic findings include deposition of eosinophilic material and degeneration of nerve fibers, attributed to entrapment neuropathy.[111] Frequently, no palpable mass is clinically apparent, and MR coronal or sagittal T1- and T2-weighted images have been used to identify these lesions.[112] Forefoot imaging can be performed using smaller FOVs (8 to 10 cm) to provide for increased spatial resolution defining musculotendinous and neurovascular structures.[113] T1- and T2-weighted images usually demonstrate a low to intermediate signal intensity mass arising between the plantar aspects of the involved metatarsal heads. Fibrosis of the epineurium and perineurium may contribute to the intermediate signal intensity on T2-weighted images. However, we have observed greater increases in signal intensity on T2*-weighted, STIR (Fig. 8-134) and fat-suppressed T2-weighted fast spin-echo (Fig. 8-135) images. This is in contrast to a conventional neuroma or neurofibroma, which displays bright signal intensity on both T2- and T2*-weighted images. Fat-suppressed contrast enhanced MR imaging is the most sensitive technique, however, providing high contrast images for depicting Morton's neuroma[114] (Fig. 8-136). This technique displays lesion hyperintensity in cases where conventional T2-weighted images either fail to demonstrate the lesion or show the lesion with decreased conspicuity. Surgical treatment involves excision of the neuroma or swelling proximal to the site of digital nerve bifurcations.[111]

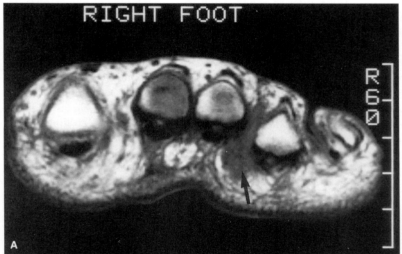

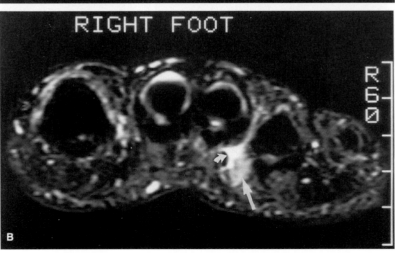

FIGURE 8-134. Morton's neuroma (*straight arrow*), located between the third and fourth metatarsal heads, is isointense with adjacent inflammation on a T1-weighted coronal image (**A**), and is mildly hyperintense on a short TI inversion recovery coronal image (**B**). Inflammatory soft-tissue edema demonstrates greater hyperintensity (*curved arrow*) than reactive connective-tissue proliferation and associated nerve degeneration. STIR protocols are more sensitive for Morton's neuroma than either T1 or T2-weighted images.

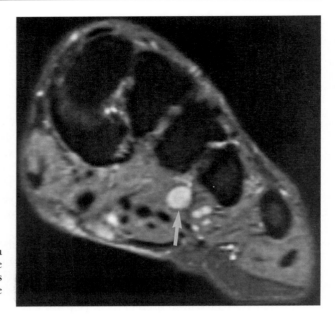

FIGURE 8-135. Morton's neuroma. Interdigital or Morton's neuroma (*arrow*) located between the third and fourth metatarsals is hyperintense on a fat-suppressed T2-weighted fast spin-echo coronal image. Morton's neuroma represents a degenerative, fibrosing process associated with the plantar digital nerve.

Avascular Necrosis of the Talus

Avascular necrosis of the body of the talus is seen with talar neck fractures associated with subtalar joint disruption.[115] The major talar blood supply is from the tarsal canal artery, a branch of the posterior tibial artery, which extends through the medial aspect of the tarsal canal. There are anastomoses between the tarsal canal artery and branches of the dorsal pedis and peroneal arteries, which enter the lateral aspect of the tarsal canal at the base of the tarsal sinus to form a rich vascular arcade to supply the body of the talus. Talar injuries with subtalar dislocation are associated with a 40% to 50% rate of AVN of the talus. During reduction, operative preser-

vation of a small deltoid branch of the tarsal canal artery proximal to where it enters the tarsal canal can reduce the risk of AVN. On MR images, AVN of the talus may demonstrate a diffuse pattern of involvement (Fig. 8-137), similar in morphology to bone infarcts seen in other locations (Fig. 8-138).

The MR appearance of nontraumatic AVN of the talus is similar to that seen in AVN of the distal femoral condyle of the knee. Early in the disease, a small low signal intensity focus corresponds to the necrotic lesion as seen in the superior talar dome. This, however, is frequently overshadowed by an extreme pattern of diffuse bone marrow edema throughout the entire talus (Fig. 8-139). This hyperemia or

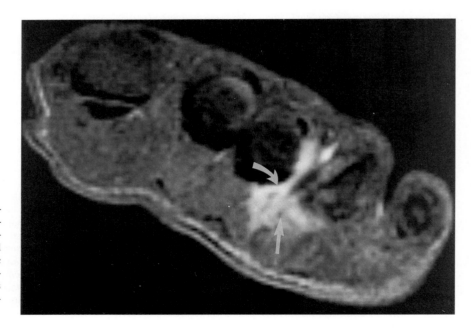

FIGURE 8-136. Recurrence of a Morton's neuroma (*straight arrow*) identified on a intravenous gadolinium-enhanced fat-suppressed T1-weighted coronal image. Irregularly marginated hyperintensity can be identified between the plantar aspects of the third and fourth metatarsals. Reactive inflammatory soft-tissue changes also demonstrate hyperintensity on gadolinium-enhanced image (*curved arrow*).

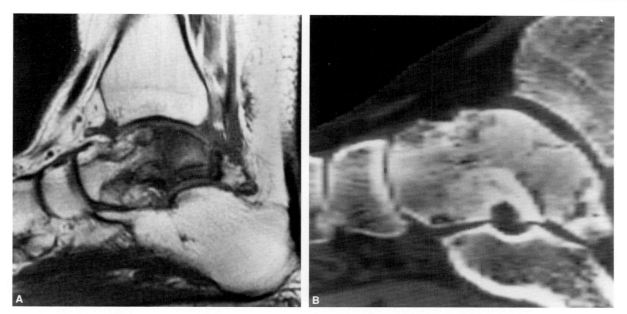

FIGURE 8-137. Talar osteonecrosis in a patient with old history of trauma. (**A**) T1-weighted sagittal image demonstrates diffuse talar involvement with areas of decreased signal intensity adjacent to marrow fat signal intensity. (**B**) Corresponding 2D reformatted sagittal CT scan shows diffuse talar sclerosis.

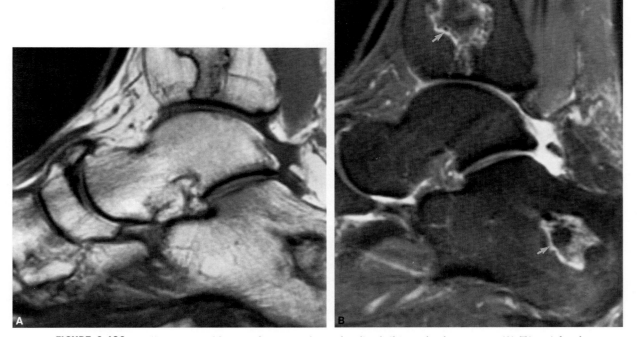

FIGURE 8-138. Well-marginated bone infarcts involving the distal tibia and calcaneus on (**A**) T1-weighted and (**B**) fat-suppressed T2-weighted fast spin-echo sagittal images. Peripheral hyperintensity (*arrows*) is appreciated on the fat-suppressed T2-weighted fast spin-echo sequence (**B**).

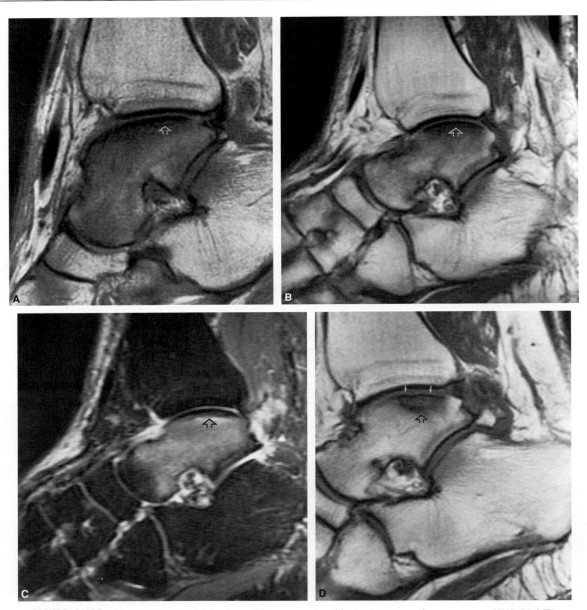

FIGURE 8-139. Osteonecrosis of the talus with an associated bone marrow edema pattern. **(A)** Initial T1-weighted sagittal image demonstrates diffuse hypointense talar bone marrow edema. A subtle focus of osteonecrosis (*open arrow*) is seen in the superior talar dome. Follow-up MR imaging within 1 year shows partial resolution of bone marrow edema on a T1-weighted sagittal image **(B)**, although diffuse talar edema is still detected on the STIR sequence **(C)**. The superior focus of osteonecrosis (*arrow*) is better defined on these follow up images. **(D)** Comparison with the opposite ankle shows a more discrete focus of osteonecrosis (*arrow*) with complete resolution of previously documented bone marrow edema. There are initial changes of subarticular collapse (*small arrows*).

bone marrow edema is low in signal intensity on T1-weighted images and hyperintense on fat-suppressed T2-weighted fast spin-echo or STIR images. Caution should be taken not to mistake this pattern of bone marrow edema for infection, tumor, or reflex sympathetic dystrophy (RSD). Bone biopsy is not required. Within twelve months, the bone marrow edema shows partial resolution, leaving behind a persistent, well-defined focus of osteonecrosis. In contrast to the bone marrow edema pattern in the hip, which may proceed the development of AVN, it is less common to see diffuse marrow talar edema without an associated focus of AVN. The morphology of this early AVN, however, may be less well-demarcated and smaller prior to the resolution of associated marrow edema. Bilaterality and asynchrony of involvement is not uncommon in the talus with AVN. Follow-up MR examination within twelve months can be used to document resolution of bone marrow edema. Acute symptoms with ankle pain are frequently significantly relieved with the resolution of marrow edema. Partial or decreased weightbearing is usually recommended at the onset of symptoms.

Freiberg's Infraction

In Freiberg's infraction, osteochondrosis of the second metatarsal head prior to closure of the epiphyseal plate occurs during the second decade of life. AVN of the metatarsal epiphysis is attributed to repetitive trauma with microfracture at the metaphyseal physeal junction.[58] Deformity of the metatarsal head, shaft hypertrophy, and secondary osteoarthritis of the metatarsophalangeal joint result from repeated weight-bearing trauma.

In a patient with a normal or widened joint space, MR imaging allows early identification of Freiberg's infraction by demonstrating the low signal intensity changes of subchondral sclerosis that occur prior to radiographic signs of increased density and fragmentation of the epiphysis. Sub-

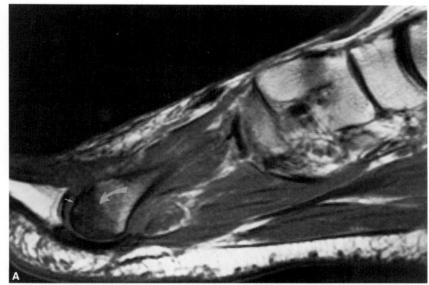

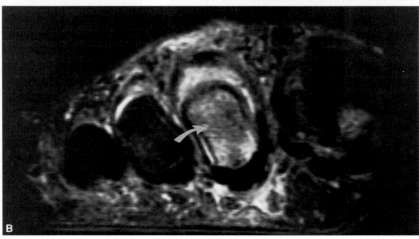

FIGURE 8-140. Freiberg's infraction (*curved arrow*) with osteonecrosis of the second metatarsal head is hypointense on a T1-weighted sagittal image (**A**) and hyperintense on STIR coronal image (**B**). Early flattening of the metatarsal head is appreciated on the T1-weighted sagittal image (*small arrows*).

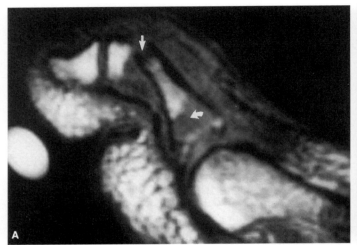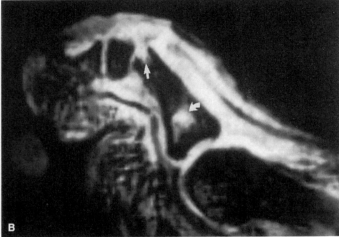

FIGURE 8-141. A neuropathic fracture of the distal aspect of the proximal phalanx (*straight arrows*) is seen on (**A**) T1-weighted and (**B**) T2*-weighted sagittal images. Note the irregular cortical edge and subluxation at the proximal metaphalangeal joint. Abnormal marrow hyperemia is seen in the proximal aspect of phalanx (*curved arrows*).

chondral marrow hyperemia can be shown on STIR (Fig. 8-140) and fat-suppressed T2-weighted fast spin-echo sequences. An undiagnosed stress fracture can also be excluded using T1-weighted and STIR images. The increased signal intensity of the articular cartilage surface is best shown on fat-suppressed T2-weighted fast spin-echo images. Irregularity and flattening of the epiphysis with spurring are more advanced changes, as are loss of joint space and low signal intensity metatarsal shaft hypertrophy. Treatment is at first directed at unloading weight-bearing forces, before consideration is given to surgical management.

Neuropathic Foot in Diabetes Mellitus

A Charcot or neuropathic joint may develop secondary to underlying neuropathic processes, commonly diabetes associated with repetitive microtrauma. The end result is articular cartilage and bone fragmentation, disintegration and dislocation of the involved joint, and new bone formation[116] (Fig. 8-141). The ankle and midfoot, including the metatarsophalangeal and midtarsal joints, are frequently involved in diabetic neuropathy. Clinically, differential diagnosis includes superimposed or associated infection. When there is extensive involvement of all midtarsal joints and pathologic fractures, the cause is likely to be neuropathic involvement.[111] Soft-tissue changes in diabetes mellitus include subaponeurotic edema, cellulitis, abscess, sinus tracts, ulcers, and tenosynovitis (acute and chronic). When there is central compartment fluid in the foot, it may be associated with infections affecting the second through fourth metatarsal heads. Medial or lateral dissections may also be associated with the central compartment and corresponding medial or lateral compartment fluid collections, respectively.[117]

MR imaging is sensitive to underlying marrow hyperemia in the ankle, subtalar, midtarsal, and metatarsophalangeal joints (Figs. 8-142 and 8-143). Areas that demonstrate diffuse or patchy low signal intensity on T1-weighted images show increased signal intensity on T2-weighted, T2*-weighted, fat-suppressed T2-weighted fast spin-echo, and STIR images. Early destructive changes, such as periarticular fractures and associated soft-tissue reactions, are frequently detected with MR imaging.[118] Collapse of the mid-metatarsus along the weightbearing axis of the foot is commonly seen as a deformity associated with neuroarthropathy. A more localized region or focus of increased subchondral or medullary signal intensity may be associated with osteomyelitis (Fig. 8-144). Osteomyelitis-related bone changes may be in direct communication with an open ulcer, decreasing the likelihood of a focal neuropathic process. In RSD, the marrow signal alteration is more periarticular. STIR contrast is required to demonstrate any significant marrow hyperintensity.

Yeh and colleagues[119] studied osteomyelitis in diabetic patients and reported a higher sensitivity and specificity with MR imaging than with ^{99m}TC-MDP bone scans.[119] Wang and associates[120] compared MR findings using T1-weighted and STIR images with histologic reports and found MR imaging to have a sensitivity rate of 99%, a specificity rate of 81%, and an accuracy rate of 94%.[120] Chemical-shift imaging may be used to assess the water content of the sural nerve—a technique that may help to identify patients with acute neuropathic changes.[121] Morrison and colleagues[122] reported that MR studies were useful and cost effective in the evaluation of osteomyelitis in the feet of diabetics.[122] Sensitivity and specificity for the diagnosis of osteomyelitis in nondiabetics were 82% and 80%, respectively, and in diabetics 89% and 94%, respectively. MR imaging also improved de-

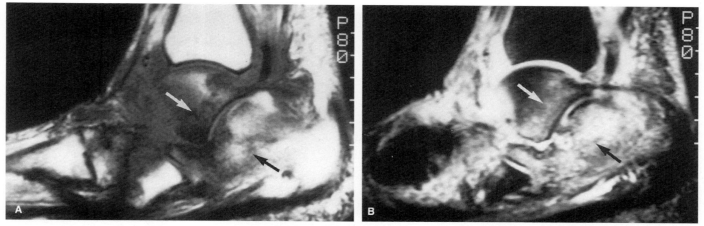

FIGURE 8-142. Neuropathic hyperemic marrow changes in diabetes mellitus are characterized by (**A**) low signal intensity areas within the talus (*white arrow*) and calcaneus (*black arrow*) on a T1-weighted sagittal image and (**B**) relative hyperintensity (*arrows*) on a short TI inversion recovery sagittal image. The differentiation between neuroarthropathy and osteomyelitis may be more difficult with STIR contrast. Neuropathic marrow changes, however, usually do not produce similar increases in signal intensity on T2 or T2*-weighted images when compared with STIR protocols. In osteomyelitis, affected marrow spaces produce increased signal intensity on T2, T2*, and STIR weighted images.

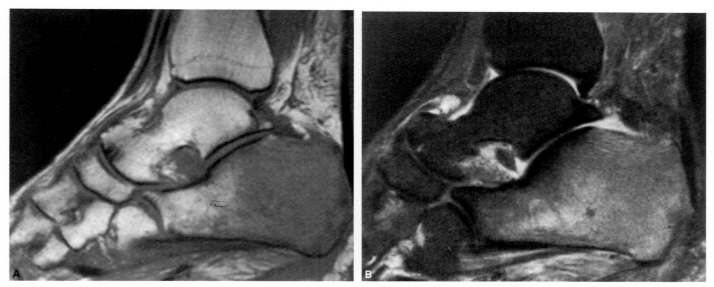

FIGURE 8-143. Neuropathic marrow edema of the calcaneus is hypointense on T1-weighted sagittal images (**A**) and hyperintense on fat-suppressed T2-weighted fast spin-echo sagittal images (**B**). Although similar marrow signal changes may occur in osteomyelitis, in this case no cortical erosion, abscess, or sinus tract was identified.

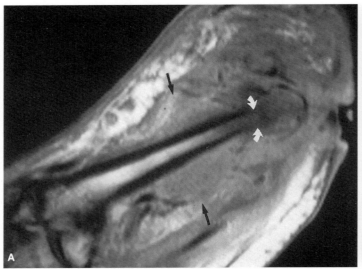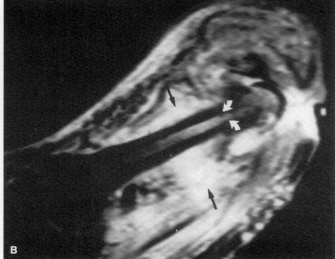

FIGURE 8-144. Osteomyelitis of the distal metatarsal in a diabetic patient. **(A)** A T1-weighted sagittal image shows a low signal intensity soft-tissue mass (*straight black arrows*) and hyperemia (*curved white arrows*) with associated loss of normal medullary fat signal intensity. **(B)** With short TI inversion recovery contrast, the hyperintense soft-tissue infection (*straight black arrows*) and marrow involvement (*curved white arrows*) are evident. Attenuation of distal cortices is best seen on the T1-weighted image.

lineation of the extent of infection, allowing limited surgical resection. MR accuracy increased with fat-suppressed intravenous contrast-enhanced studies. Since intravenous MR contrast may demonstrate enhancement in both osteomyelitis and neuropathic joints, it is important to identify other findings associated with osteomyelitis, including cortical interruption, a rim enhancing abscess within the marrow cavity, a sequestrum, an osseous to skin sinus tract extension, or cellulitis adjacent to an osseous erosion or abnormality.

Infection

Early detection and treatment of osteomyelitis and joint sepsis are critical in preserving joint function before cartilage breakdown and local or hematogenous spread occurs.[123] Changes on conventional radiographs are frequently nonspecific, with effusion (ie, capsular distention) or disruption of soft-tissue planes as the only findings. Often, there is no evidence of cortical destruction until marrow involvement is extensive, possibly up to 10 to 14 days after initial infection.

MR imaging is useful in the early detection of musculoskeletal infections. Although applications in the ankle and foot are preliminary, new clinical indications are being developed. The capability to detect skip lesions; to obtain high soft-tissue contrast in a multiplanar format; and to evaluate marrow, cartilage, and cortex separately shows great potential for the further use of MR imaging for detection and monitoring of infection targeting the foot and ankle.

Infection causes an alteration in the ratio of free water to bound water that prolongs T1 and T2 tissue relaxation times. As a result, infected regions demonstrate low signal intensity on T1-weighted images and high signal intensity on T2-weighted images. Although this provides the basis for diagnostic sensitivity, neoplastic tissues undergo similar TI and T2 relaxation changes. Therefore, secondary characteristics such as location, distribution, extent, and morphology of signal intensity assume an important role in improving diagnostic specificity.

Osteomyelitis

Early osteomyelitis (see ''Neuropathic Foot in Diabetes Mellitus'') demonstrates low signal intensity on T1-weighted images and high signal intensity on T2, fat-suppressed T2-weighted fast spin-echo or STIR weighted images. Acute and chronic osteomyelitis have been studied in the calcaneus, the cuboid, the metatarsals, and the distal tibia and fibula.[124] On T2-weighted sequences in the acute or subacute phase, a diffuse or patchy increase of signal intensity in the medullary bone indicates marrow involvement. A peripheral rim of low signal intensity, representing reactive bone, may demarcate the focus over time. Alterations in signal intensity may also be seen at sites of cortical transgression, periosteal reaction, soft-tissue masses, and sequestrae.

Staphylococcal osteomyelitis of the distal tibial metaphysis may present with a stellate pattern of signal change that mimics the MR appearance of a stress fracture. On T2-weighted images, infected material in serpiginous tracts is seen as linear segments of high signal intensity. Infectious soft-tissue and osseous involvement are successfully identified using a combination of T1-, T2-, T2*-weighted, and STIR protocols.[125] Fat-suppressed contrast-enhanced MR imaging is significantly more sensitive than scintigraphy and more specific than nonenhanced MR imaging in the diagnosis of osteomyelitis.[126] Osteomyelitis of the talus is frequently in the differential diagnosis of limping in children.[127] MR imaging defines the metaphyseal-equivalent locations of the talus at risk for infection both proximally and distally (Fig. 8-145). Fat-suppressed T2-weighted fast spin-echo or STIR techniques are required to increase sensitivity for areas adjacent to cartilage and that border the physeal plates, areas commonly involved in hematogenous osteomyelitis.

Reflex Sympathetic Dystrophy

Magnetic resonance imaging using fat-suppressed T2-weighted sequences, fat-suppressed contrast-enhanced sequences, and STIR images have increased the sensitivity for detecting soft-tissue and osseous abnormalities in RSD. Schweitzer and coworkers[128] have shown skin thickening and presence of soft-tissue edema in stage I RSD, skin thickening and thinning without soft-tissue edema in stage II RSD, and muscle atrophy in stage III RSD.[128] We have used STIR and fat-suppressed T2-weighted fast spin-echo sequences as primary techniques for identification of subchondral hyperemia in either a subarticular distribution or in a more atypical diffuse punctate pattern of hyperintensity (Fig. 8-146). This corresponds to CT changes of osteopenia and focal lucencies. T1-weighted and conventional T2- and T2*-weighted techniques may not be sensitive to the bone marrow edema of RSD.

Plantar Fibromatosis

Plantar fibromatosis is characterized by the development of fibrous nodules in the plantar aponeurosis similar to Dupuytren's contracture of the palmar aponeurosis.[58,129] Single or multiple nodules in thickened plantar fascia are found in non–weight-bearing surfaces of the foot, with lesions frequently identified in the longitudinal arch.[111] Histologic findings include proliferating fibroblasts and an acellular collagenous stroma.[58]

The nodules demonstrate low signal intensity on sagittal or coronal T1- and T2-weighted images. The increased collagen content of the plantar fibromas may explain their relative low signal intensity characteristics on T2-weighted sequences. Central areas of intermediate to increased signal intensity may be seen on T2*-weighted or STIR images[130] (Fig. 8-147). The lesions studied by Morrison and coworkers[130] showed

infiltrative upper margins, and 15% of developed deep to the plantar aponeurosis.[130] Adjacent inflammatory edema is usually not present in plantar fibromatosis. The differential diagnosis includes a ganglion, neurofibroma, or fibrosarcoma, and in most cases can be made by the presence of increased signal intensity on T2-weighted images.

Plantar Fasciitis

Inflammation of the plantar aponeurosis may be associated with a calcaneal spur, inflammatory changes, or thickening of the plantar aponeurosis adjacent to the calcaneus. On MR studies, it frequently demonstrates hyperintense signal intensity changes on T2-weighted, T2*-weighted, STIR and fat-suppressed T2-weighted fast spin-echo images (Fig. 8-148). T1-weighted sagittal images display the low signal intensity fascia in contrast to high signal intensity superficial fat. Subcutaneous edema may be seen both superficial and deep to the plantar fascia. Pain in the area of the medial tuberosity of the calcaneus is exacerbated with activity.[131] The pain of plantar fasciitis (the subcalcaneal pain syndrome) is related to microtrauma of the plantar fascia adjacent to its attachment leading to attempted repair and chronic inflammation (Fig. 8-149). Nerve entrapment or irritation of the medial calcaneal nerve and/or of the nerve to the abductor digiti quinti off the lateral plantar nerve have also been proposed as causes of pain. A heel spur (plantar calcaneal enthesophyte) is identified in 50% of cases of plantar fasciitis (Fig. 8-150).

Arthritis

To date, most experience with MR imaging of ankle arthritis has been restricted to cases of osteoarthritis and post-traumatic arthritis, and to infectious and hemophiliac arthropathies.[132]

In osteoarthritis, including cases of posttraumatic etiology, thinning of the tibiotalar and subtalar hyaline cartilage surfaces can be appreciated on coronal and sagittal T1-weighted images. Identification of loose bodies may require T2-weighted imaging to create contrast with the surrounding synovial fluid, which demonstrates high signal intensity on T2-weighted sequences (Fig. 8-151). Osteophytic spurs with marrow contents are seen as areas of bright signal intensity, isointense with fat, with a cortical rim of low signal intensity (ie, anterior tibial border). Cortical and subchondral irregularities can be seen in association with denuded articular cartilage. A calcaneal enthesophyte and adjacent subchondral marrow edema may be seen in the seronegative arthritides (Fig. 8-152).

The presence of an acute or chronic joint effusion of low signal intensity on T1-weighted images can also be

text continues on page 590

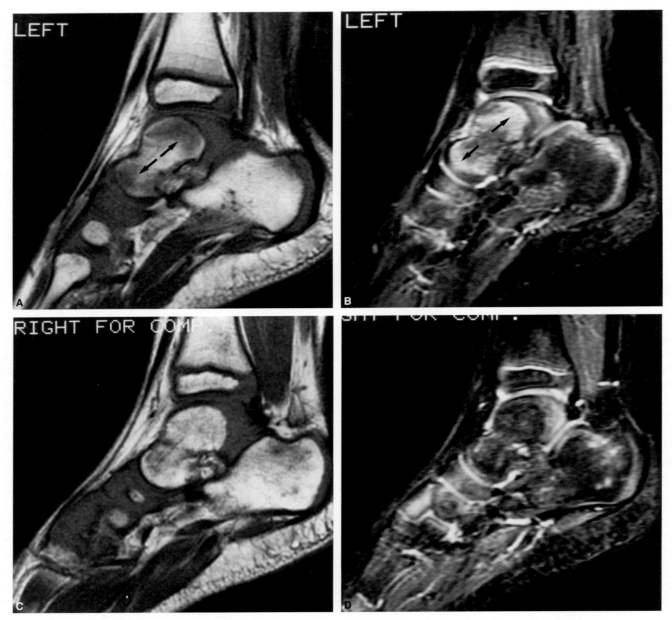

FIGURE 8-145. (A, B) Osteomyelitis of the left talus with involved metaphyseal-equivalent locations (*arrows*) of the talus. There is hypointense signal intensity on T1-weighted sagittal images (A) and hyperintense signal intensity on STIR sagittal images (B). In comparison, the right talus displays normal marrow signal characteristics on T1-weighted (C) and STIR (D) images.

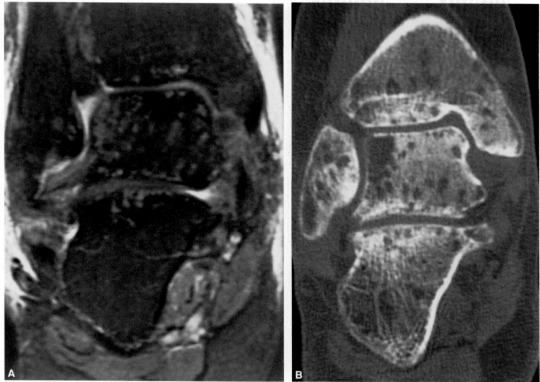

FIGURE 8-146. Reflex sympathetic dystrophy. (**A**) There are hyperintense foci distributed throughout the talus, subarticular portions of the calcaneus, the distal tibia, and the fibula on this fat-suppressed T2-weighted fast spin-echo coronal image. (**B**) A corresponding direct coronal CT image identifies discrete lucencies with focal loss of bone density.

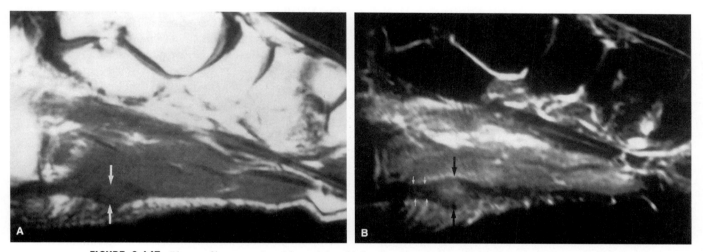

FIGURE 8-147. Plantar fibromatosis with nodular thickening (*large arrows*) in plantar aponeurosis. (**A**) Low signal intensity is seen on a T1-weighted sagittal image and (**B**) central increased signal intensity is seen in an area of proliferating fibroblasts on a short TI inversion recovery sagittal image. The normal thickness of an adjacent plantar aponeurosis is shown (*small arrows*).

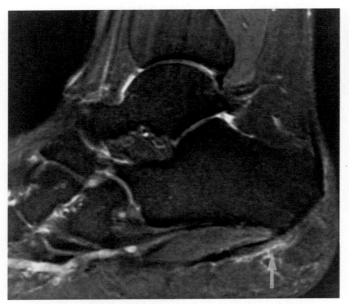

FIGURE 8-148. Plantar fasciitis (*arrow*) with hyperintensity involving the calcaneal attachment of the plantar aponeurosis and adjacent plantar soft tissue on a fat-suppressed T2-weighted fast spin-echo sagittal image.

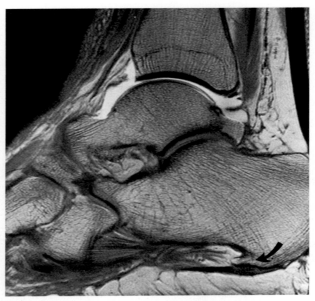

FIGURE 8-150. Plantar calcaneal enthesophyte (*curved arrow*) associated with mild thickening of the os calcis attachment of the plantar fascia (T1-weighted sagittal MR arthrogram).

determined with MR scans. Subchondral or juxtaarticular cysts, which possess gelatinous synovial fluid, demonstrate increased signal intensity with progressive T2 weighting (Fig. 8-153). MR imaging is particularly useful in assessing subtalar joint arthrosis displaying the anterior, middle, and posterior facets separately. Sub-

chondral and metaphyseal infarcts may coexist with joint-space narrowing and arthrosis. STIR images are more sensitive than T2*-weighted images in documenting subchondral fluid through fissured articular cartilage. We have not routinely used MR imaging to document uncomplicated osteoarthritis or hallux valgus.

On MR images, hemophilic arthropathy is indicated by low signal intensity synovial hypertrophy with paramagnetic hemosiderin deposits. On gradient-echo images, hyaline cartilage demonstrates high signal intensity, permitting identification of subtle cartilage irregularities.[132]

Ganglions

Ganglions arise from tendon sheaths, tibiotalar joints, or subtalar joints, They may or may not be septated, and demonstrate uniform low signal intensity on T1-weighted images and high signal intensity on T2-, T2*-weighted and STIR images (Fig. 8-154). Posterior subtalar joint ganglions may be mistaken for effusion with capsular distention. Giant cell tumor of the tendon sheath about the ankle appears as a heterogeneous mass on gradient-echo images with low signal intensity hemosiderin deposits. The intense vascularity of these lesions may demonstrate enhancement on dynamic perfusion imaging with a MR paramagnetic contrast agent.[133] Further experience with inflammatory and noninflammatory arthritides is required before routine use of MR imaging of the ankle and foot is indicated.

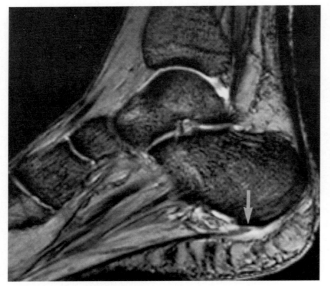

FIGURE 8-149. Detached plantar aponeurosis (*arrow*). Inflammatory edema and fluid are hyperintense on T2* gradient-echo sagittal images.

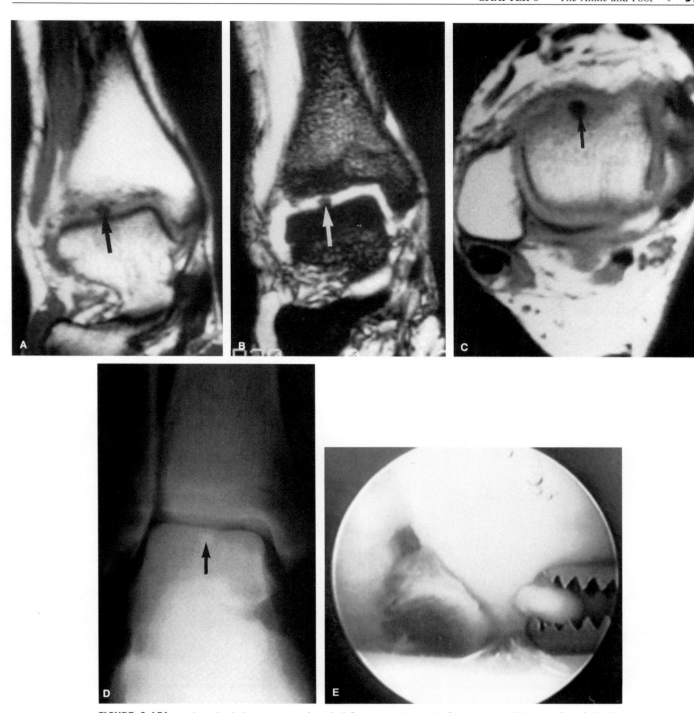

FIGURE 8-151. A detached, loose, osteochondral fragment (*arrows*) from a stage IV osteochondral talar dome lesion. The loose body can be seen on (**A**) a T1-weighted coronal image, (**B**) a T2*-weighted coronal image, (**C**) a T1-weighted axial image, (**D**) an anteroposterior radiograph, and (**E**) the corresponding arthroscopic photograph.

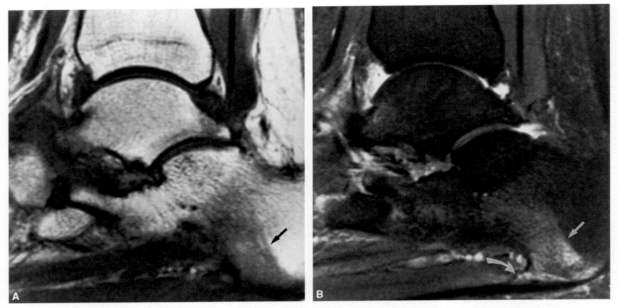

FIGURE 8-152. Seronegative arthritis with painful heel correlated with calcaneal enthesophyte (*straight arrow*). The band-like region of marrow edema (*curved arrow*) is hypointense on T1-weighted sagittal image (**A**) and hyperintense on fat-suppressed T2-weighted fast spin-echo sagittal image (**B**).

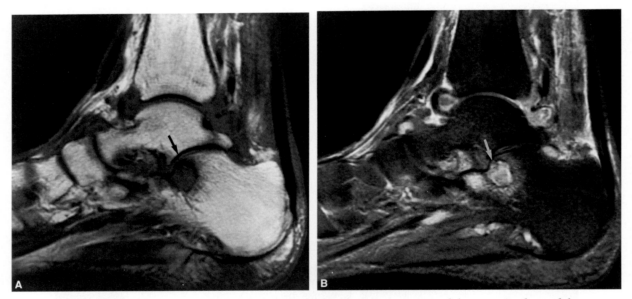

FIGURE 8-153. Degenerative subchondral cyst involving the anterior aspect of the posterior facet of the subtalar joint on (**A**) T1-weighted sagittal image and (**B**) fat-suppressed T2-weighted fast spin-echo sagittal image. The cyst and adjacent marrow are hyperintense on the fat-suppressed T2-weighted fast spin-echo sequence (**B**). Patient also has a tibiotalar joint effusion with capsular distension and synovitis.

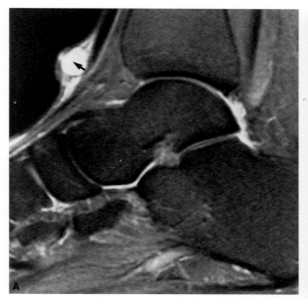

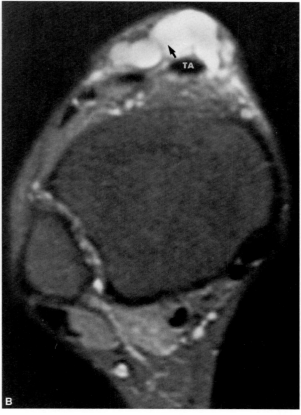

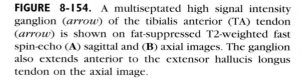

FIGURE 8-154. A multiseptated high signal intensity ganglion (*arrow*) of the tibialis anterior (TA) tendon (*arrow*) is shown on fat-suppressed T2-weighted fast spin-echo (**A**) sagittal and (**B**) axial images. The ganglion also extends anterior to the extensor hallucis longus tendon on the axial image.

References

1. Yousem DM, Scott WW Jr. The foot and ankle. In: Scott WW, et al, eds. Computed tomography of the musculoskeletal system. New York: Churchill Livingstone, 1987:113.

2. Crim JR, et al. Magnetic resonance imaging of the hindfoot. Foot Ankle 1989;10:1.

3. Rubin DA, Towers JD, Britton CA. MR imaging of the foot: utility of complex oblique imaging planes. AJR 1996;166:1079.

4. Kneeland JB, et al. MR imaging of the normal ankle: correlation with anatomic sections. AJR 1988;151:117.

5. Preidler KW, Wang Y, Brossman J, et al. Tarsometatarsal joint: anatomic details on MR images. Radiology 1996;199:733.

6. Sartoris DJ, Resnick D. Cross-sectional imaging of the foot: test of anatomical knowledge. J Foot Surg 1988;27:374.

7. Kingston S. Magnetic resonance imaging of the ankle and foot. Clin Sports Med 1988;7:15.

8. Noto AM, et al. MR imaging of the ankle: normal variants. Radiology 1989;170:121.

9. Aerts P, Disler DG. Abnormalities of the foot and ankle: MR findings. AJR 1995;165:119.

10. Beltran J. MR techniques and practical applications. Magnetic resonance imaging of the ankle and foot. Orthopedics 1994;17:1075

11. Kerr R, et al. Magnetic resonance imaging of foot and ankle trauma. Orthop Clin North Am 1990;21:591.

12. Klein MA. Reformatted three-dimensional fourier transform gradient-recalled echo MR imaging of the ankle: spectrum of normal and abnormal findings. AJR 1993:161:831.

13. Ferkel RD. The foot and ankle. In: Whipple TL, ed. Arthroscopic surgery. Philadelphia: Lippincott-Raven:85.

14. Ferkel RD, Scranton PE. Arthroscopy of the ankle and foot. J Bone Joint Surg [Am] 1993;75A:1233.

15. Noto AM. MR imaging of the ankle. Normal variants. Radiology 1987;165:148.

16. Ekstrom JE, et al. MR imaging of accessory soleus muscle. J Comput Assist Tomogr 1990;14:239.

17. Chason DP, Schultz SM, Fleckenstein JL. Tensor fasciae suralis: depiction on MR images. AJR 1995;165:1220.

18. Link SC, Erickson SJ, Timins ME. MR imaging of the ankle and foot: normal structures and anatomic variants that may simulate disease. AJR 1993;161:607.

19. Schweitzer ME, VanLeersum M, Ehrlich SS, Wapner K. Fluid in normal and abnormal ankle joints: amount and distribution as seen on MR images. AJR 1994;162:111.

20. Berndt A, Harty M. Transchondral fractures (osteochondritis dissecans) of the talus. J Bone Joint Surg [Am] 1959;41:988.

21. Ferkel RD, Sgaglione NA. Arthroscopic treatment of osteochondral lesions of the talus: long-term results. Orthop Trans 1993–1994;17:1011.

22. Anderson IF, et al. Osteochondral fractures of the dome of the talus. J Bone Joint Surg [Am] 1989;71:1143.

23. Pritsch M, Horoshouski H, Farine I. Arthroscopic treatment of osteochondral lesions of the talus. J Bone Joint Surg [Am] 1986;68A:862.

24. Cheng MS, Ferkel RD, Applegate GR. Osteochondral lesions of the talus: a radiologic and surgical comparison. Presented at the Annual Meeting of the Academy of Orthopaedic Surgeons, New Orleans, February 1995.

25. Yulish BS, et al. MR imaging of osteochondral lesions of the talus. J Comput Assist Tomogr 1987;1:296.

26. Stauffer RN. Intraarticular ankle problems. In: Evarts CM, ed. Surgery of the musculoskeletal system, vol 3. New York: Churchill Livingstone, 1983.

27. De Smet AA, et al. Value of MR imaging in staging osteochondral lesions of the talus (oseochondritis dissecans): results in patients. AJR 1990;154:555.

28. Alexander AH, et al. Arthroscopic technique in talar dome fracture. Surg Rounds Orthop 1990:27.

29. Hattrup SJ, Johnson KA. A review of ruptures of the Achilles tendon. Foot Ankle 1985;6:34.

30. Willis CA, et al. Achilles tendon rupture: a review of the literature comparing surgical versus nonsurgical treatment. Clin Orthop 1986;207:156.

31. Quinn SF, et al. Achilles tendon: MR imaging at l.5 T. Radiology 1987;164:767.

32. Keene JS, et al. Magnetic resonance imaging of Achilles tendon ruptures. Am J Sports Med 1989; 17:333.

33. Dillon E, Pope C, Barber V, et al. Achilles tendon healing: 12-month follow up with MR imaging. Radiology 1990;177P:306.

34. Mink JH. Ligaments of the ankle. In, Deutsch AL, Mink JH, Kerr R, eds. MRI of the foot and ankle. New York: Raven Press, 1992:173.

35. Cetti R, Christensen SE, Ejsted R, et al. Operative versus nonoperative treatment of Achilles tendon rupture: a prospective randomized study and review. Am J Sports Med 1993;21:791.

36. Liem MD, et al. Repair of Achilles tendon ruptures with polylactic acid implant: assessment with MR imaging. AJR 1991;156:769.

37. Alanen A. Magnetic resonance imaging of hematomas in a 0.02T magnetic field. Acta Radiol (Diagn) 1986;27:589.

38. Kellam JF, et al. Review of the operative treatment of Achilles tendon rupture. Clin Orthop 1985;201:80.

39. Bude RO, Adler RS, Bassett DR. Diagnosis of Achilles tendon xanthoma in patients with heterozygous familial hypercholesterolemia: MR vs. sonography. AJR 1994;162:913.

40. Koivunen-Niemela T, Komu M, Viikari J, Alanen A. MRI and MRS of human tendon xanthoma at 1.5 T: an in vivo study. MAGMA 1994;2:121.

41. Dussault RG, Kaplan PA, Roederer G. MR imaging of Achilles tendon in patients with familial hyperlipidemia: comparison with plain films, physical examination, and patients with traumatic tendon lesions. AJR 1995;164:403.

42. Downey DJ, et al. Tibialis posterior tendon rupture: a cause of rheumatoid flat foot. Arthritis Rheum 1988;31:441.

43. Karasick D, Schweitzer ME. Tear of the posterior tibial tendon causing asymmetric flatfoot: radiologic findings. AJR 1993;161:1237.

44. Rosenberg ZS. Chronic tears of the posterior tibial tendon: a correlative study of CT, MR imaging, and surgical exploration. Radiology 1987;165P:149.

45. Rosenberg ZS, et al. Rupture of posterior tibial tendon: CT and MR imaging with surgical correlation. Radiology 1988;169:229.

46. Schweitzer ME, Caccese R, Karasick D, Wapner KL. Posterior tibial tendon tears: utility of secondary signs for MR imaging diagnosis. Radiology 1993;188:655.

47. Rule J, Yao L, Seeger LL. Spring ligament of the ankle: normal MR anatomy. AJR 1993;161:1241.

48. Healy WA III, Starkweather KD, Gruber MA. Chronic dislocation of the posterior tibial tendon: a case report. Am J Sports Med 1995;23:776.

49. Resnick D (ed). Internal derangements of joints. In: Diagnosis of Bone and Joint Disorders, 3rd ed, vol 5. Philadelphia: WB Saunders, 1995.

50. Khoury NJ, El-Khoury GY, Saltzman CL, et al. Rupture of the anterior tibial tendon: diagnosis by MR imaging. AJR 1996;167:351.

51. Sobel M, Bohne WHO, Levy ME. Longitudinal attrition of the peroneus brevis tendon in the fibular groove: an anatomic study. Foot Ankle 1990;11:124.

52. McMaster PE. Tendon and muscle ruptures: clinical and experimental studies on the causes and location of subcutaneous ruptures. J Bone Joint Surg 1933;15:705.

53. Meyer AW: Further evidences of attrition in the human body. Am J Anat 1924;34:241.

54. Berquist TH, et al. Musculoskeletal trauma. In: Berquist TH, et al,

55. eds. Magnetic resonance of the musculoskeletal system. New York: Raven Press, 1987:127.

55. Hamilton WG. Foot and ankle injuries in dancers. St Louis: CV Mosby, 1993:1241.

56. Thompson FM, Patterson AH. Rupture of the peroneus longus tendon: report of thee cases. J Bone Joint Surg [Am] 1989;71:293.

57. Berquist TH. Imaging of orthopaedic trauma and surgery. Philadelphia: WB Saunders, 1986:408.

58. Turek SL. The foot and ankle. In: Turek SL, ed. Orthopaedics: principles and their application, 4th ed. Philadelphia: JB Lippincott, 1984:1407.

59. Rijke, et al. MRI of lateral ankle ligament injuries. Am J Sports Med 1993;21:527.

60. Marder RA. Current methods for the evaluation of ankle ligament injuries 1994. J Bone Joint Surg [Am] 1994;76A:1103.

61. Deutsch AL, Mink JH, Kerr R. MRI of the foot and ankle. New York: Raven Press, 1992.

62. Chandnani VP, Harper MT, Ficke Jr, Gagliardi JA. Chronic ankle instability: evaluation with MR arthrography, MR imaging and stress radiography. Radiology 1994;192:189.

63. Brantigan JW, et al. instability of the subtalar joint. J Bone Joint Surg [Am] 1977;59:321.

64. Erickson SJ, et al. MR imaging of the lateral collateral ligament of the ankle. AJR 1991;156:131.

65. Klein MA. MR imaging of the ankle: normal and abnormal findings in the medial collateral ligament. AJR 1994;162:377.

66. Clanton TO, Schon LC. Athletic injuries to the soft tissues of the foot and ankle. In: Mann RA, Coughlin MJ, eds. Surgery of the foot and ankle, 6th ed, vol 2. St Louis: CV Mosby 1993:1095.

67. Ogilvie-Harris DJ, Reed SC. Disruption of the ankle syndesmosis: diagnosis and treatment by arthroscopic surgery. Arthroscopy 1994;10:561.

68. Colville MR. Reconstruction of the lateral ankle ligaments. J Bone Joint Surg [Am] 1994;76A:1092.

69. Liu SH, Baker CL. Comparison of lateral ankle ligamentous reconstruction procedures. Am J Sports Med 1994;22:313.

70. Rosenberg ZS, Cheung YY, Bertran J, et al. Posterior intermalleolar ligament of the ankle: normal anatomy and MR imaging features. AJR 1995;165:387.

71. Wolin I, Glassman F, Sideman S. Internal derangement of the talofibular component of the ankle. Surg Gynecol Obstet 1950;91:1993.

72. Liu SH, Raskin A, Osti L, Baber C. Arthroscopic treatment of anterolateral ankle impingement. Arthroscopy 1994;10:215.

73. Klein MA, Spreitzer AM. MR imaging of the tarsal sinus and canal: normal anatomy, pathologic findings, and features of the sinus tarsi syndrome. Radiology 1993;186:233.

74. Michelson JD. Current concepts review: fractures about the ankle. J Bone Joint Surg [Am] 1995;74A:142.

75. Levin PE. Traumatic injury to the lower limb in adults. In: Dee R, eds. Principles of orthopaedic practice. New York: McGraw-Hill, 1989:1209.

76. Clark TW, Janzen DL, Ho K, et al. Detection of radiographically occult ankle fractures following acute trauma: positive predictive value of an ankle effusion. AJR 1995;164:1185.

77. Chapman MN. Fractures and fracture-dislocations of the ankle. In: Mann RA, Coughlin MJ, eds. Surgery of the foot and ankle, 6th ed, vol 2. St Louis: CV Mosby, 1993:1439.

78. Roberts CS. Le Fort's fracture. Surgical Rounds for Orthopaedics 1989:58.

79. Chung T, Jaramillo D. Normal maturing distal tibia and fibula: changes with age at MR imaging. Radiology 1995;194:227.

80. Whipple TL, Martin DR, McIntyre LF, Meyers JF. Arthroscopic treatment of triplane fractures of the ankle. Arthroscopy 1993;9:456.

81. Beck BR, Osternig LR. Medial tibial stress syndrome: the location of muscles in the leg in relation to symptoms. J Bone Joint Surg [Am] 1994;76A:1057.

82. Detmer DE. Chronic shin splints: classification and management of medial tibial stress syndrome. Sports Med 1986;3:436.

83. Batt ME. Shin splints: a review of terminology. Clin J Sports Med 1995;5:53.

84. Fredericson M, Bergman G, Hoffman KL, Dillingham MS. Tibial stress reaction in runners: correlation of clinical symptoms and scintigraphy with a new magnetic resonance imaging grading system. Am J Sports Med 1995;23:472.

85. Johnson EE. Intraarticular fractures of the calcaneus: diagnosis and surgical management. Orthopedics 1990;13:1091.

86. McCrory P, Bladin C. Fractures of the lateral process of the talus: a clinical review ''Snowboarder's Ankle.'' Clin J Sport Med 1996; 6:124.

87. Umans H, Pavlov H. Insufficiency fracture of the talus: diagnosis with MR imaging. Radiology 1995;197:439.

88. Kiss ZS, Khan KM, Fuller PJ. Stress fractures of the tarsal navicular bone: CT findings in 55 cases. AJR 1993;160:111.

89. Miller TT, Staron RB, Feldman F, et al. The symptomatic accessory tarsal navicular bone: assessment with MR imaging. Radiology 1995;195:849.

90. Harrington T, Crichton KJ, Anderson IF. Overuse ballet injury of the base of the second metatarsal: a diagnostic problem. Am J Sports Med 1993;21:591.

91. Van Dijk CN, Lim LSL, Poortman A, et al. Degenerative joint disease in female ballet dancers. Am J Sports Med 1995;23:295.

92. Yao L, Do HM, Cracchiolo A, Farahanic K. Plantar plate of the foot: findings on conventional arthrography and MR imaging. AJR 1994;163:641.

93. Taylor JAM, Sartoris DJ, Huang GS, Resnick DL. Painful conditions affecting the first metatarsal sesamoid bones. Radiographics 1993;13:817.

94. Karasick D, Schweitzer ME. The os trigonum syndrome: imaging features. AJR 1996;166:125

95. Marotta JJ, Micheli LJ. Os trigonum impingement in dancers. Am J Sports Med 1992;20:23.

96. Myerson M. Soft-tissue trauma: acute and chronic management. In: Mann RA, Coughlin MJ eds. Surgery of the foot and ankle, 6th ed, vol 2. St Louis: CV Mosby 1993;1367.

97. Silas SI, Herzenberg JE, Myerson MS, Sponseller PD. Compartment syndrome of the foot in children. J Bone Joint Surg [Am] 1995: 77A:356.

98. Helms CA, Fritz RC, Garvin GJ. Plantaris muscle injury: evaluation with MR imaging. Radiology 1995;195:201.

99. Kricun ME. Congenital foot deformities. In: Kricun ME, ed. Imaging of the foot and ankle. Rockville: Aspen Publications, 1988:47.

100. Gruber MA, et al. Congenital and developmental abnormalities of the foot in children. In: Dee R, ed. Principles of orthopaedic practice. New York: McGraw-Hill, 1989:1138.

101. Wechsler RJ, Schweitzer ME, Deely DM, Horn D. Tarsal coalition: depiction and characterization with CT and MR imaging. Radiology 1994;193:447.

102. Turek SL: Congenital deformities. In: Turek SL, ed. Orthopaedics: principles and their application, 4th ed. Philadelphia: JB Lippincott, 1984:283.

103. Villani C, et al. Nuclear magnetic resonance as a contribution to the choice of technique in lengthening the Achilles tendon in a spastic equinus foot. Ital J Orthop Traumatol 1989;15:103.

104. Drennan JC. Congenital vertical talus. J Bone Joint Surg [Am] 1995;77A:1916.

105. Sammarco GJ, Conti SF. Tarsal tunnel syndrome caused by an anomalous muscle. J Bone Joint Surg [Am] 1994;76A:1306.

106. Misoul C. Nerve injuries and entrapment syndromes of the lower extremity. In: Dee R, ed. Principles of orthopaedic practice. New York: McGraw-Hill, 1989:1420.

107. Takakura Y, et al. Tarsal tunnel syndrome. J Bone joint Surg [Am] 1991;73:125.

108. Erickson SJ, et al. MR imaging of the tarsal tunnel and related spaces: normal and abnormal findings with anatomic correlation. AJR 1990;155:323.

109. Zeiss J, et al. Normal magnetic resonance anatomy of the tarsal tunnel. Foot Ankle 1990;10:214.

110. Pfeiffer WH, Cracchiolo A. Clinical results after tarsal tunnel decompression. J Bone Joint Surg [Am] 1994;76A:1222.

111. Dee R. Miscellaneous disorders of the foot. In: Dee R, ed. Principles of orthopaedic practice. New York: McGraw-Hill, 1989:1431.

112. Sartoris DJ, et al. Magnetic resonance images. Interdigital or Morton's neuroma. J Foot Surg 1989;28:78.

113. Erickson SJ, Rosengarten JL. MR imaging of the forefoot: normal anatomic findings. AJR 1993;160:565.

114. Terk MR, Kwong PK, Suthar M, et al. Morton neuroma: evaluation with MR imaging performed with contrast enhancement and fat suppression. Radiology 1993;189:239.

115. Johnston JO. Tumors and metabolic diseases of the foot. In: Mann RA, Coughlin MJ eds. Surgery of the foot and ankle, 6th ed, vol 2. St Louis: CV Mosby 1993:991.

116. Forrester DM. Arthritis. In: Kricun ME, ed. Imaging of the foot and ankle. Rockville: Aspen Publications, 1988:129.

117. Goodwin DW, Salonen DC, Yu JS, et al. Plantar compartments of the foot: MR appearance in cadavers and diabetic patients. Radiology 1995;196:623.

118. Sartoris DJ, et al. Magnetic resonance imaging of tendons in the foot and ankle. J Foot Surg 1989;28:370.

119. Yeh WT, et al. Osteomyelitis of the foot in diabetic patients: evaluation with plain film. ^{99m}Tc-MDP bone scintigraphy, and MR imaging. AJR 1989;152:795.

120. Wang A, et al. MRI and diabetic foot infections. Magn Reson Imaging 1990;8:805.

121. Griffey RH, et al. Correlation of magnetic resonance imaging and nerve conduction for the early detection of diabetic neuropathy in humans. In: Abstracts of the Meeting of the Society of Magnetic Resonance in Medicine, New York City, August 17, 1987:125.

122. Morrison WB, Schweitzer ME, Wapner KL, et al. Osteomyelitis in feet of diabetics: clinical accuracy. surgical utility, and cost-effectiveness of MR imaging. Radiology 1995;196:557.

123. Tang JSH, et al. Musculoskeletal infection of the extremities: evaluation with MR imaging. Radiology 1988;166:205.

124. Berquist TH. Musculoskeletal infection. In: Berquist TH, et al, eds. Magnetic resonance of the musculoskeletal system. New York: Raven Press, 1987:109.

125. Harms SE, Greenway G. Musculoskeletal system. In: Stark DD, Bradley WG, eds. Magnetic resonance imaging. St Louis: CV Mosby, 1988:1323.

126. Morrison WB, Schweitzer ME, Bock GW, Mitchell DG. Diagnosis of osteomyelitis: utility of fat-suppressed contrast-enhanced MR images. Radiology 1993;189:251.

127. Grattan-Smith JD, Wagner ML, Barnes DA. Osteomyelitis of the talus: an unusual cause of limping in childhood. AJR 1991;156:785.

128. Schweitzer ME, Mandel S, Schwartzman RJ, Knobler RL. Reflex sympathetic dystrophy revisited: MR imaging findings before and after infusion of contrast material. Radiology 1995;195:211.

129. Lee TH, Wapner KL, Hecht PJ. Current concepts review: plantar fibromatosis. J Bone Joint Surg [Am] 1993;75A:1080.

130. Morrison WB, Schweitzer ME, Wapner KL, Lackman RD. Plantar fibromatosis: a benign aggressive neoplasm with a characteristic appearance on MR images. Radiology 1994:193:841.

131. Bordelon RL. Heel pain. In: Mann RA, Coughlin MJ, eds. Surgery of the foot and ankle. St Louis: CV Mosby 1993:837.

132. Beltran J, et al. Ankle: surface coil MR imaging at 1.5 T. Radiology 1986;161:203.

133. Narra VR, Shirkhoda A, Shetty AN, et al. Giant cell tumor of the tendon sheath in the ankle: MRI with pathologic correlation. J Magn Reson Imaging 1995;5:781.

Magnetic Resonance Imaging in Orthopaedics & Sports Medicine, Second Edition,
edited by David W. Stoller. Lippincott-Raven Publishers, Philadelphia, © 1997.

Chapter 9

The Shoulder

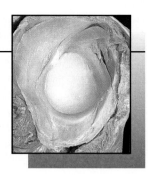

David W. Stoller
Eugene M. Wolf

Conventional radiographic techniques demonstrate the osseous structure of the shoulder girdle, but provide only limited evaluation of soft-tissue anatomy including the rotator cuff, the ligamentous attachments of the glenoid labrum capsule, and the subacromial space. Routine radiographs do not allow direct visualization of the rotator cuff tendons, their defects and abnormalities, and their relationship to their undersurface of the acromion and the acromioclavicular (AC) joint. As a result, impingement disorders are difficult to characterize on plain film radiographic studies.

With single and double contrast arthrography, the extension of contrast into the subacromial-subdeltoid bursa, superior and lateral to the greater tuberosity, depicts complete tears of the rotator cuff.[1] Arthrography is limited in assessing the size and morphology of cuff tears, and is even less well suited for displaying partial tears, especially those involving the superior bursal surface of the supraspinatus tendon. Arthrography cannot assess the degree of retraction of the cuff tendons or the status of cuff musculature.

Contrast computed arthrotomography has been used to visualize the glenoid labrum and capsule through the intraarticular injection of air and contrast material[2-4] (Fig. 9-1). Limited soft-tissue contrast and spatial resolution in reformatted scans restrict the usefulness of this technique for routine assessment of the rotator cuff and subacromial space in impingement disorders.

Ultrasonography has been used to visualize the subacromial-subdeltoid bursa and areas of increased echogenicity in the rotator cuff.[5-12] This technique is operator dependent, however, and poorly delineates the individual tendons of the rotator cuff. Vick and colleagues report a low sensitivity (67%) and accuracy rate (85%) for sonographic detection of rotator cuff tears.[13] Conflicting results have been reported for the usefulness of ultrasonography in its ability to differentiate partial and full thickness tears.[10,11]

Magnetic resonance (MR) imaging of the rotator cuff provides direct coronal oblique images parallel with the course of the supraspinatus tendon as localized on axial plane images[14-28] (Fig. 9-2). Axial plane images through the glenohumeral joint display capsular and labral anatomy. Sagittal oblique images demonstrate acromial anatomy, display the coracoacromial and coracohumeral ligaments, and show the relationships of the capsulolabral complex. Two- and three-dimensional (3D) gradient-echo images provide axial coverage from the AC joint through the glenohumeral joint. Contrast enhancement with intraarticular gadolinium diethylenetriamine pentacetic acid (Gd-DTPA) improves diagnostic conspicuity in partial articular surface tears of the rotator cuff, helps distinguish severe tendinitis from rotator cuff tears, and better defines the capsulolabral anatomy of the glenohumeral joint.[20,21,23,29] T1-weighted Gd-DTPA images also minimize the effect of magnetic susceptibility that is seen with gradient-echo images in the postoperative cuff. With or without gadolinium enhancement, MR imaging affords visualization of both soft-tissue and osseous pathology, which is not possible with conventional arthrography or computed tomography (CT) (Fig. 9-3).

IMAGING PROTOCOLS FOR THE SHOULDER

Improvements in surface coil design, with development of custom-curved coils that conform to the shoulder apex and coils mounted with a fixed platform (free of transmitted respiratory artifact), have resulted in more uniform signal intensity than was possible with a planar circular coil placed posterior to the shoulder (Fig. 9-4). Quadrature and phased array coils permit the acquisition of high resolution images of both the rotator cuff and the glenohumeral joint and capsule. Off-axis (offset) capability is required to eliminate the requirement for positioning the shoulder isocenter with respect to the magnet. Also, direct coronal oblique images replace the need to bolster the affected shoulder to align the supraspinatus tendon parallel with the coronal imaging plane. The entire length of the supraspinatus muscle and tendon are shown in the coronal oblique plane. Direct coro-

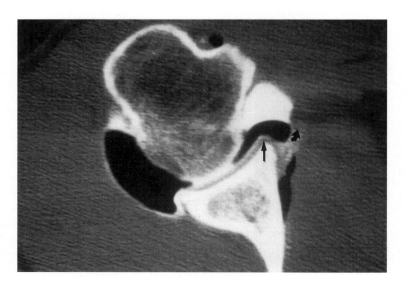

FIGURE 9-1. The anterior labrum (*straight arrows*) and middle glenohumeral ligament (*curved arrow*) can be seen on an air contrast CT study.

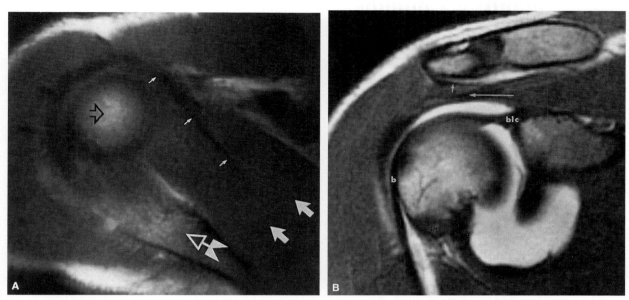

FIGURE 9-2. Localization of the supraspinatus tendon. (**A**) A T1-weighted superior axial image demonstrates an intact supraspinatus muscle (*large white arrows*) and low signal intensity tendon (*small white arrows*). The humeral head (*open black arrow*) and acromion (*flagged white arrow*) are also shown. (**B**) A T1-weighted coronal oblique MR arthrogram shows the continuity between the supraspinatus muscle and tendon (*long white arrow*), biceps labral complex (blc), biceps tendon (b) and coracoacromial ligament (*small white arrow*).

nal images result in foreshortening of the supraspinatus muscle and falsely give the appearance of a discontinuity between the supraspinatus muscle and tendon.

The shoulder and arm (placed alongside and parallel to the body) are positioned in either neutral or neutral-to-mild external rotation with the patient in the supine position. Internal rotation causes the anterior capsular structures to appear more lax and less sharply defined, and may make analysis in this position more difficult. Most patients cannot tolerate

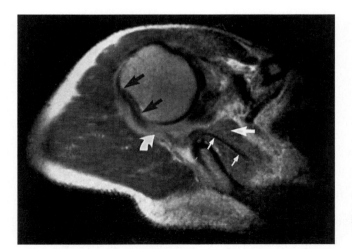

FIGURE 9-3. A rotator cuff tear (*large white arrow*) and a Hill-Sachs fracture (*black arrows*) are displayed on an axial image through the shoulder. The low signal intensity supraspinatus tendon displays loss of continuity (*small white arrows*). Intermediate signal intensity joint effusion (*curved white arrow*) is present.

the position of extreme or full external rotation, resulting in muscle spasms producing motion artifacts. Also, the position of exaggerated external rotation makes it more difficult to follow the course of the biceps tendon, which is located more laterally, near the supraspinatus tendon attachment, in this position. Bicipital tendon fluid could be mistaken for a rotator cuff in this position.[30] The neutral position of the arm is indicated by the thumbs-up position of the extended hand.

Routine shoulder evaluations are performed with a T1-weighted axial localizer to identify the anatomic area of the AC joint through the glenohumeral joint. T1-weighted axial images demonstrate the normal high signal intensity of bony glenoid marrow fat, which may be useful in identifying osseous Bankart lesions. The low-signal-intensity tendon of the supraspinatus muscle is identified on axial images between the AC joint and the superior aspect of the glenohumeral joint. The coronal oblique plane is parallel to the supraspinatus tendon in this location. The tendon, and not the muscle of the supraspinatus (the tendon and muscle frequently have different degrees of obliquity), is used to prescribe coronal oblique images. Accurate cuff diagnosis may be limited if this technique is not carefully followed by the technologist.

Coronal oblique images are obtained with a combination of T1, fat-suppressed T2-weighted fast spin-echo, and T2-weighted fast spin-echo sequences (Fig. 9-5), at 3 to 4 mm slice thickness, with a 256 (frequency) × 256 or 192 (phase) imaging matrix and a 12 to 14 cm field of view (FOV). Alternatively, a conventional spin-echo sequence with proton density and T2-weighted contrast can be used to evaluate the rotator cuff. Fat-suppressed T2-weighted fast spin-echo

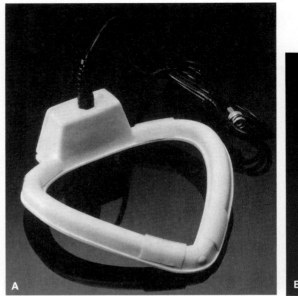
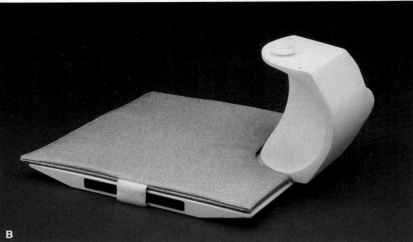

FIGURE 9-4. Surface coils from (**A**) General Electric (Milwaukee, WI) and (**B**) MRI Devices (Waukesha, WI) conform to the curved shoulder girdle. The fixed platform base in **B** minimizes transmitted respiratory motion from the patient to the coil.

images are more sensitive to subacromial bursal fluid than non–fat-suppressed T2-weighted fast spin-echo or conventional T2-weighted images. Image blurring with T2-weighted fast spin-echo techniques can be reduced by keeping the echo train short and using a higher resolution matrix and longer TE values. To maximize signal-to-noise in fat-suppressed T2-weighted fast spin-echo images, TE values are usually between 40 and 50 msec and TRs are between

3000 and 4000 msec. These parameters provide adequate coverage and maximum signal-to-noise. We do not use T2*-weighted coronal oblique images to evaluate the rotator cuff. Although gradient-echo techniques adequately demonstrate bursal and articular cuff outlines, areas of increased signal intensity may be seen in both cuff degeneration and tears, making the distinction between tendinopathy or tendinosis and rotator cuff tear difficult. We do use 1 to 3 mm 3D

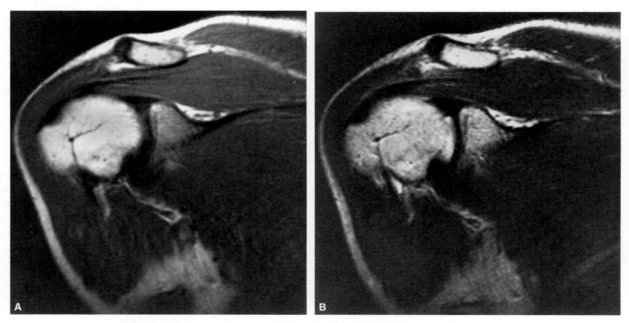

FIGURE 9-5. Comparison of (**A**) T1, (**B**) T2-weighted fast spin-echo. *continued*

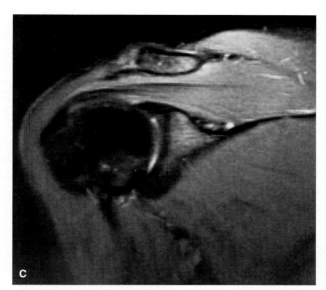

FIGURE 9-5. *Continued.* **(C)** fat-suppressed T2-weighted fast spin-echo coronal oblique images through the rotator cuff. Of these sequences, the fat-suppressed T2-weighted fast spin-echo image is the most sensitive to small amounts of fluid and marrow and soft-tissue pathology.

Fourier transform (3DFT) T2*-weighted axial images to evaluate the glenohumeral capsule and labrum, however. Gradient-echo images provide superior contrast between fluid and the low signal intensity labrum, while still allowing characterization of labral degeneration, tears, and avulsions.[31] Magnetic susceptibility artifacts (signal void) are prominent in gradient-echo techniques, especially when evaluating the postoperative shoulder. This susceptibility may be useful in identifying loose bodies or foci of calcific tendinitis.

Axial images, obtained with a 10 to 14 cm FOV, are also included in the evaluation of the shoulder. T1 spin-echo axial images are obtained as for the initial localizer. An optional axial fat-suppressed T2-weighted fast spin-echo sequence is useful to increase sensitivity to subacromial fluid as well as to help identify paraglenoid cysts, spinoglenoid notch ganglion cysts, and muscle pathology. Fast spin-echo sequences are less sensitive to internal labral signal intensity in the spectrum of degenerations or tears. They are, however, superior for the demonstration of labral morphology in cases of avulsions. We have not found the second echo of a conventional T2-weighted sequence to provide enough tissue contrast for the evaluation of the glenoid labrum in relationship to adjacent soft-tissue structures and fluid.

Sagittal oblique plane images, conventional T2-weighted or T2-weighted fast spin-echo, have become important in evaluating the conjoined insertion of the supraspinatus and infraspinatus tendons and in characterizing the anteroposterior size and location of rotator cuff tears initially detected or suspected from coronal plane images. For example, tears of the supraspinatus tendon located in a far anterior position are frequently easier to identify on sagittal oblique images, which do not have the partial volume effect seen on anterior coronal oblique images. The coracoacromial arch, including the rotator cuff and glenohumeral joint capsule relationships, is also displayed in the sagittal oblique plane.

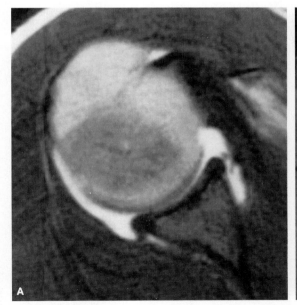
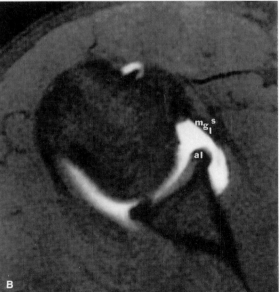

FIGURE 9-6. Intraarticular gadolinium contrast in the glenohumeral joint on **(A)** T1-weighted and **(B)** fat-suppressed T1-weighted axial images. Note the superior contrast resolution among the labrum, capsular structures, and gadolinium on the fat-suppression image. al, anterior labrum; mgl, middle glenohumeral ligament; s, subscapularis tendon.

T1-weighted contrast in the sagittal oblique plane is inadequate to characterize rotator cuff tears. Optionally, a 3DFT sagittal sequence with thin sections and gradient-echo contrast can be used. The addition of fat-suppression to a T2-weighted fast spin-echo sequence improves visualization of the biceps, labral, and inferior glenohumeral ligament complexes (IGLCs) on sagittal oblique images.

MR arthrography with intraarticular contrast is performed using either a paramagnetic contrast agent such as Gd-DTPA (Fig. 9-6) or saline to facilitate capsular distention and improve contrast between fluid and the rotator cuff and glenohumeral joint capsule. MR arthrog-

raphy with gadolinium is performed with a preinjection T2-weighted fast spin-echo coronal oblique and T2*-weighted axial sequence. This permits identification of a bursal surface tear or intrasubstance degenerative cuff changes. T2* axial images may demonstrate a ganglion or cyst, which does not directly communicate with the joint, and thus may not be appreciated on postintraarticular paramagnetic contrast injection T1-weighted images. Preinjection images also document preexisting fluid secondary to an effusion or hemorrhage. Fluid in the subacromial-subdeltoid bursa may be secondary to impingement or may be caused by a rotator cuff, which

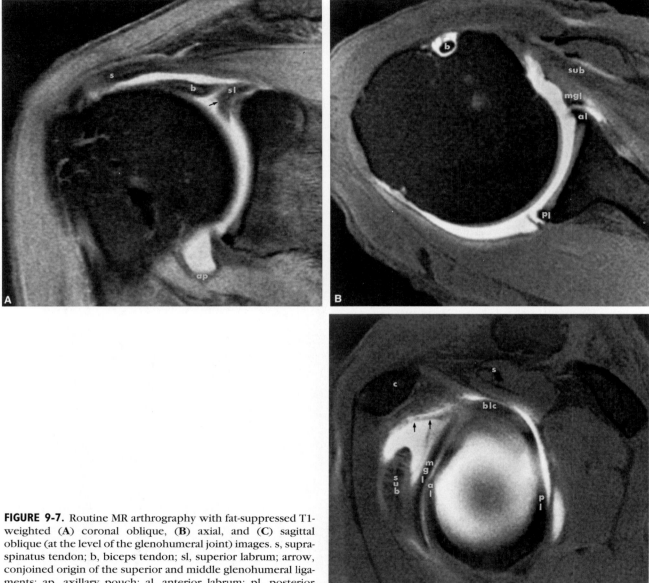

FIGURE 9-7. Routine MR arthrography with fat-suppressed T1-weighted **(A)** coronal oblique, **(B)** axial, and **(C)** sagittal oblique (at the level of the glenohumeral joint) images. s, supraspinatus tendon; b, biceps tendon; sl, superior labrum; arrow, conjoined origin of the superior and middle glenohumeral ligaments; ap, axillary pouch; al, anterior labrum; pl, posterior labrum; mgl, middle glenohumeral ligament; sub, subscapularis tendon; c, coracoid; blc, biceps labral complex; small arrows, superior glenohumeral ligament.

allows direct communication between the glenohumeral joint and subacromial-subdeltoid bursa. The finding of fluid within the shoulder joint may eliminate or obviate the need to perform an intraarticular injection.

A routine MR arthrography protocol uses fat-suppressed T1-weighted images at a 3 mm slice thickness in all three planes (coronal oblique, axial, and sagittal oblique) postinjection (Fig. 9-7). Fat-suppression helps to avoid mistaking areas of normal fat from high signal intensity contrast, increasing the conspicuity of the paramagnetic contrast agent. The entire labral complex is displayed on a single 3 mm sagittal oblique image. The gadolinium is diluted (0.4 cc into 100 cc of saline) and approximately 12 to 16 cc is then injected into the joint.[32] The injection of a nondiluted paramagnetic contrast agent produces an unacceptable susceptibility artifact and may serve as a synovial irritant. Although not presently FDA approved for intraarticular use, many academic and private centers use and have accepted this technique to improve the accuracy of specific shoulder evaluations. Verbal and written informed consent is usually obtained from the patient for this procedure. Since lack of access to fluoroscopy may make MR arthrography difficult in certain outpatient centers, an alternative option is to use intraarticular saline, which does not require a patient consent form and can potentially be performed

without fluoroscopy. The intraarticular injection of saline can be administered via a posterior approach. Saline MR arthrography requires T2 (conventional or fatsuppressed T2-weighted fast spin-echo) and T2*-weighted sequences. T1-weighted images are not adequate for visualizing capsular fluid in the saline arthrograms. MR arthrography outlines the anatomy of the glenoid labrum, identifies partial articular or full thickness tears of the rotator cuff, and demonstrates glenohumeral capsular ligaments not adequately appreciated in the nondistended joint capsule.

In a specialized technique developed for evaluating glenohumeral anterior instability and multidirectional instability, the arm is placed in abduction to tighten the inferior glenohumeral ligament labral complex (IGLLC; Fig. 9-8). This technique evaluates tears or laxity of the anterior band of the inferior glenohumeral ligament (IGL). O'Brien and colleagues[33] have reclassified the bands of the IGL into anterior and posterior, and the band formerly termed superior is now referred to as the anterior band.

On axial images, the brachial plexus can be identified adjacent to the subclavian vessels, which are used as landmarks for off-axis coronal images (Figs. 9-9 and 9-10). Axial STIR (including fast STIR techniques) or conventional T2-weighted images of both upper extremi-

text continues on page 606

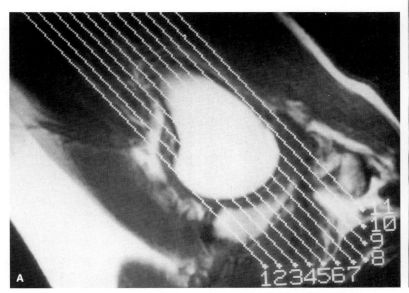

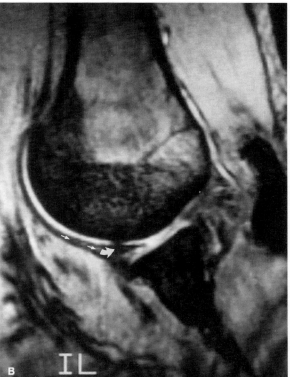

FIGURE 9-8. Functional anatomy of the inferior glenohumeral joint (IGL). (**A**) A coronal localizer obtained with the arm placed in 90° of abduction (ie, the position of function of the IGL) and external rotation. (**B**) The corresponding axial image through the glenohumeral joint shows a taut IGL (*small straight arrows*) and intact anterior labrum (*curved arrow*).

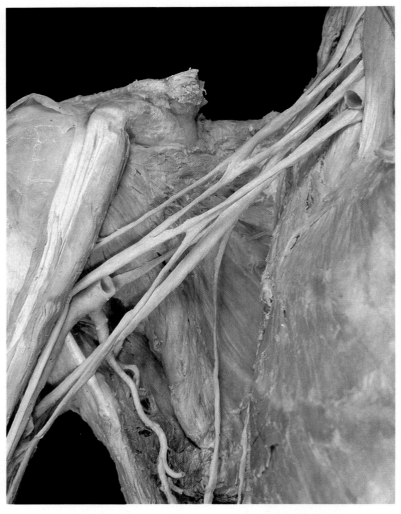

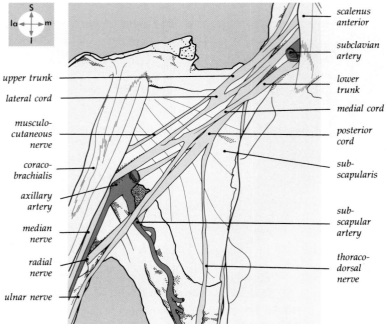

FIGURE 9-9. The components of the brachial plexus. The veins and most of the axillary artery have been removed.

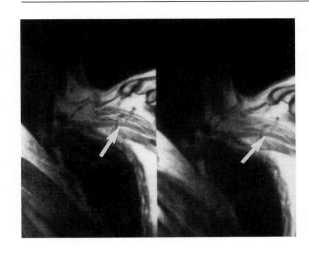

FIGURE 9-10. T1-weighted coronal oblique images through the trunk and cords of the brachial plexus (*arrows*).

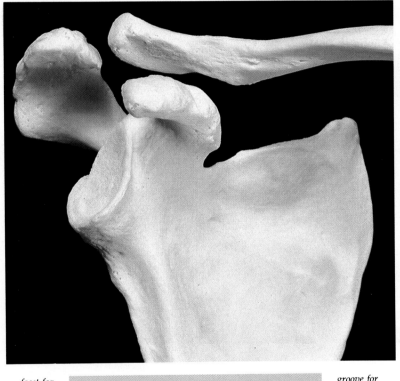

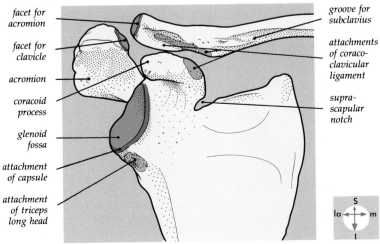

facet for acromion
facet for clavicle
acromion
coracoid process
glenoid fossa
attachment of capsule
attachment of triceps long head

groove for subclavius
attachments of coraco-clavicular ligament
supra-scapular notch

FIGURE 9-11. An oblique anterior view of the scapula and lateral part of the clavicle. The bones have been separated to show the articular surfaces of the acromioclavicular joint and the sites of attachment of the coracoclavicular ligament.

ties are obtained to demonstrate any extrinsic effacement of the brachial plexus (from either soft-tissue or osseous encroachment) or secondary increased signal intensity from the area of trauma.

NORMAL ANATOMY OF THE SHOULDER

Shoulder girdle articulations include the glenohumeral joint, the AC joint, the scapulothoracic joint, and the sternoclavicular joint (Fig. 9-11). The humeral head articulates with the relatively shallow glenoid fossa of the scapula and is dependent on muscular, ligamentous, and labral integrity for its stability (Fig. 9-12).

Osteology of the Shoulder

The clavicle connects the axial and appendicular skeletons of the upper extremity.[34] It is S-shaped in configuration, with a convex anterior border medially and a concave anterior border laterally. It is flattened and narrowed laterally, and has a thicker cylindrical configuration medially. Medially, the clavicle articulates with the sternoclavicular joint and laterally with the AC joint. The surfaces of the sternoclavicular joint are covered by fibrocartilage, and a fibrocartilaginous articular disk divides the joint into separate recesses.[35]

The scapula consists of the scapular body, the scapular spine, the scapular neck, the acromion, the glenoid fossa, and the coracoid process.[34] The subscapular fossa

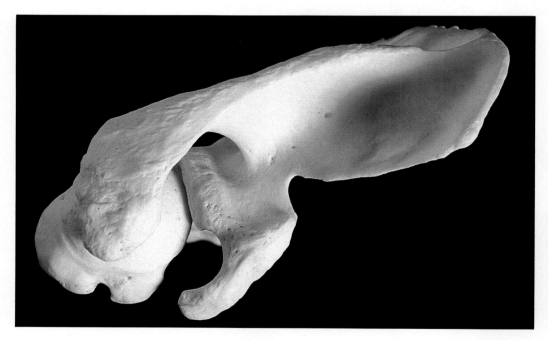

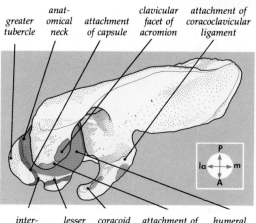

FIGURE 9-12. A superior view of the scapula and the upper end of the humerus. The acromion and the coracoacromial ligament prevent upward displacement of the numeral head.

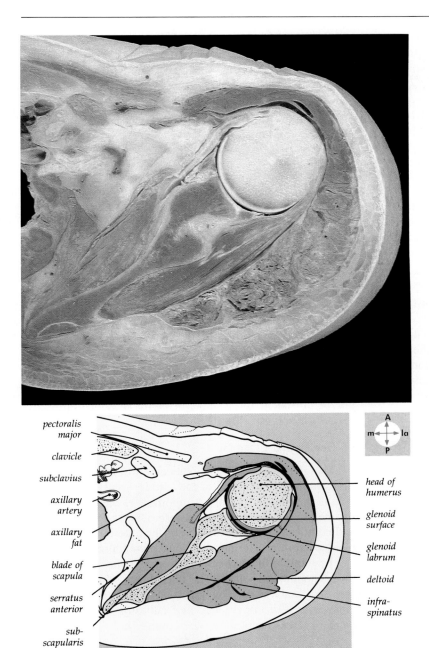

pectoralis major

clavicle

subclavius

axillary artery

axillary fat

blade of scapula

serratus anterior

sub-scapularis

head of humerus

glenoid surface

glenoid labrum

deltoid

infra-spinatus

FIGURE 9-13. A transverse section at the level of the humeral head shows the relations of the glenohumeral joint.

represents the costal concave surface of the scapula. The dorsal convex surface of the scapula is separated into a supraspinous and infraspinous fossa divided by the spine of the scapula. The suprascapular nerve is located in the supraspinous or spinoglenoid notch, at the superior border of the supraspinous fossa. Compression of the suprascapular nerve by a ganglion or entrapment, secondary to thickening of the suprascapular ligament, occurs in this location. The tip of the coracoid projects anterior and lateral to the glenoid, with its origin superior and medial on the scapular neck. The coracoid is an important surgical landmark because neurovascular structures travel along its inferomedial surface. The acromion, classified into three types according to its morphology, is either type 1 (a flat or straight undersurface with a high angle of inclination), type 2 (a curved arc and decreased angle of inclination), or type 3 (hooked anteriorly with a decreased angle of inclination) (see Shoulder Impingement Sydrome Etiology). The angle of inclination is formed by the intersection of a line drawn from the posteroinferior aspect of the acromion and the anterior margin of the acromion with a line formed by the posteroinferior aspect of the acromion and the inferior tip of the coracoid process. At the lateral angle of the scapula is the glenoid cavity (glenoid fossa) with its su-praglenoid and infraglenoid tuberosities. The glenoid version angle varies and may contribute to instability patterns of the shoulder.

The proximal humerus consists of the head, anatomic neck, and the greater and lesser tuberosities. The intertuber-cular or bicipital groove is located between the greater and lesser tuberosities along the anterior surface of the humerus. A decrease in the height of the medial wall of the lesser tuberosity and the presence of a supratubercular ridge of bone projecting from the superolateral aspect of the lesser tuberosity may predispose to instability of the biceps tendon within the groove, but dislocation or subluxation of the bi-ceps tendon is extremely rare in the absence of a massive rotator cuff tear.

Glenohumeral Joint and Capsular Gross Anatomy

The anatomic configuration of the glenohumeral joint (Fig. 9-13) allows a greater range of motion than any other joint in the body. Glenohumeral motion depends on the congruity of the humeral head, the glenoid, the rotator cuff mechanism, and the deltoid muscle. Glenohumeral joint version or hu-meral retroversion projects the axis of the humeral head joint surfaces 25° to 40° from the coronal plane, whereas the glenoid surface is retroverted 4° to 12° with respect to the scapula.[36] The glenoid labrum, wedge-shaped in cross sec-tion, is a ring of fibrous tissue with transitional fibrocartilage attached to the margin of the glenoid cavity.[37] Labral tissue deepens the depression of the glenoid fossa and enlarges the glenohumeral socket contact area (Figs. 9-14 and 9-15).

Glenoid Labrum

The glenoid labrum is the fibrous attachment of the gle-nohumeral ligaments and capsule to the glenoid rim[38] (Fig. 9-16). The labrum is ovoid, conforming to the essentially kidney-shaped glenoid rim. The normal glenoid labrum is 3 mm high and 4 mm wide, but its size, shape, and configura-tion vary considerably.

The anterior glenoid labrum provides the major area of attachment for the anterior band of the IGL.[33] The middle glenohumeral ligament (MGL) is considerably more vari-able, but may also contribute fibers to the more superior aspects of the anterior glenoid labrum as it approaches the biceps tendon.

Above the epiphyseal line (ie, the junction of the upper and middle thirds of the glenoid body fossa), the attachment of the glenoid labrum is variable. The superior labrum does have a role in the stability of the glenohumeral joint and functions in conjunction with the biceps tendon (Figs. 9-17 and 9-18), with which it is contiguous (the biceps labral complex [BLC]). Inferior to the epiphyseal line the labrum is continuous with the glenoid articular cartilage and serves as the insertion site for the IGL. It is the superior and antero-

superior portion of the labrum that can be variably attached to the glenoid.[39] There are three different types of attachment of the biceps labral complex (BLC) to the glenoid (Fig. 9-19):

- Type 1: The BLC is firmly adherent to the superior pole of the glenoid (see Fig. 9-19A). There is no sublabral foramen in the anterosuperior quadrant.
- Type 2: The BLC is attached several millimeters medial to the sagittal plane of the glenoid (see Fig. 9-19B). The superior pole of the glenoid continues its hyaline cartilage surface medially under the labrum. This configuration has a small sulcus at the superior pole of the glenoid that may be continuous with a subla-bral foramen and communicate with the subscapularis bursa.
- Type 3: In type 3 BLC the labrum is very meniscoid in shape (see Fig. 9-19C) and has a large sulcus that projects under the labrum and over the cartilaginous pole of the glenoid.

Rodosky and coworkers[40] have demonstrated that tension placed on the biceps tendon stabilizes the humeral head. Although significant lesions of the BLC have been noted in traumatic dislocations, an incomplete or meniscoid attach-ment of the superior labrum may represent a variation of normal anatomy. The type 3 BLC attaches primarily to the supraglenoid tubercle, creating a synovial lined sulcus at the superior aspect of the glenoid.[39,41] This normal sulcus should not be mistaken for a superior-labral-anterior-to-posterior (SLAP) lesion (see Slap Tears).

Glenohumeral Ligaments

The glenohumeral ligaments (superior, middle, and infe-rior) are thickened bands of the anterior joint capsule.[38] The IGL is the largest and most important of the glenohumeral ligaments. Its anterior and posterior bands are attached to and contribute to the formation of the anterior and posterior glenoid labrum. The normally lax glenohumeral ligaments can be thought of as check reins on extremes of motion for the glenohumeral joint.[36] The importance of joint compres-sion and stabilization by the rotator cuff, as well as the maintenance of congruency and adhesion of the glenohu-meral surfaces, cannot be over emphasized.

INFERIOR GLENOHUMERAL LIGAMENT. The IGL consists of anterior and posterior bands and an axillary pouch that attaches to the inferior two thirds of the entire circumference of the glenoid by means of the labrum[33] (Figs. 9-20 through 9-23). The IGL is lax in the adducted position. As it tightens with increasing abduction, the anterior and posterior bands move superiorly with respect to the humeral head. At 90° of abduction, the IGL is the primary restraint for anterior and posterior dislocations.[42] The axillary pouch is located between the anterior and posterior bands and, like the ante-rior and posterior bands, is lax with the arm by the patient's side in the adducted position. The axillary pouch extends inferior to the body of the glenohumeral joint as a redun-dancy of thickened capsular tissue best visualized on coronal oblique images.

text continues on page 615

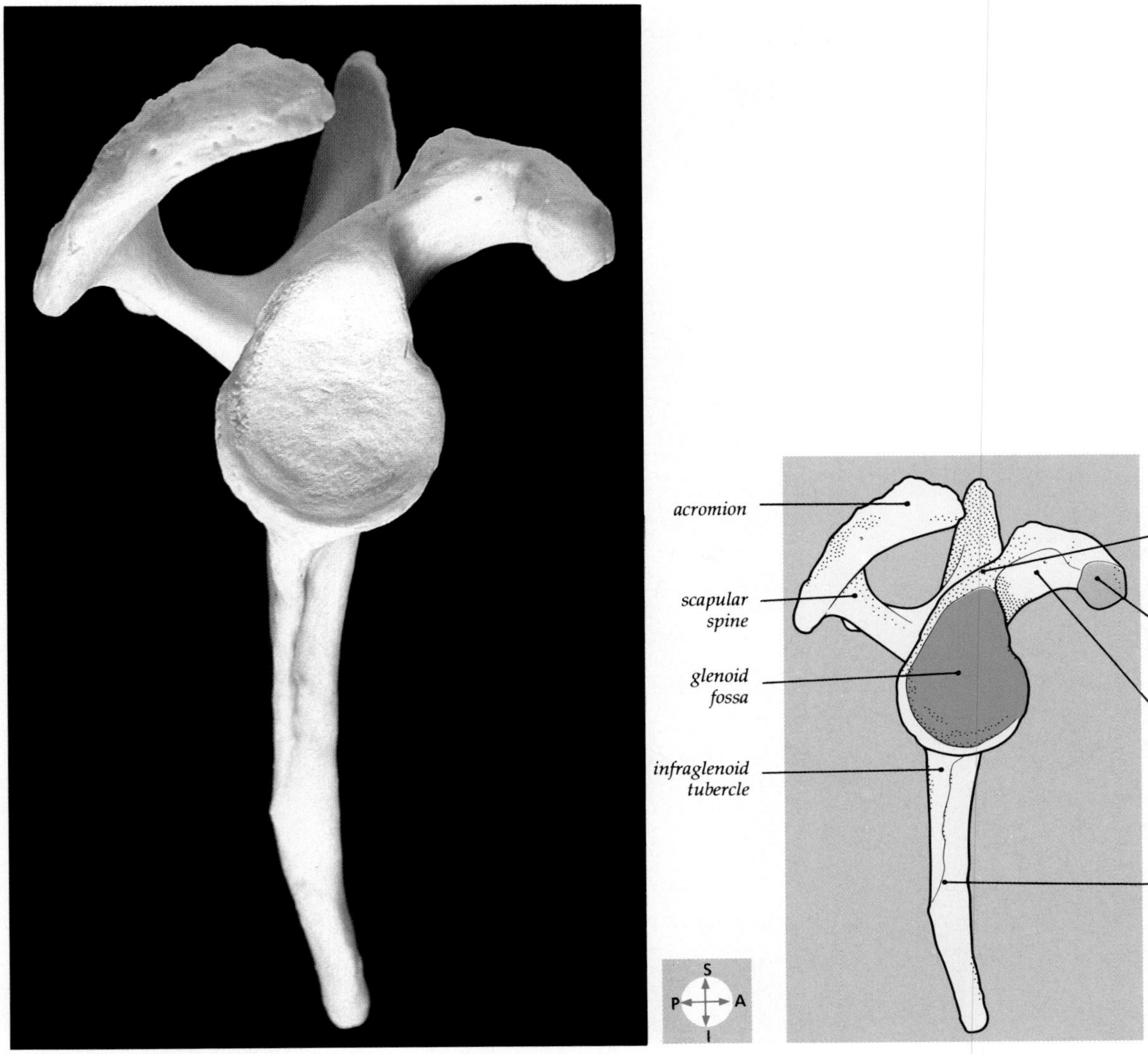

FIGURE 9-14. The lateral aspect of the scapula shows the pear-shaped glenoid fossa. The positions of the supraspinatus, infraspinatus, and subscapular fossae are shown.

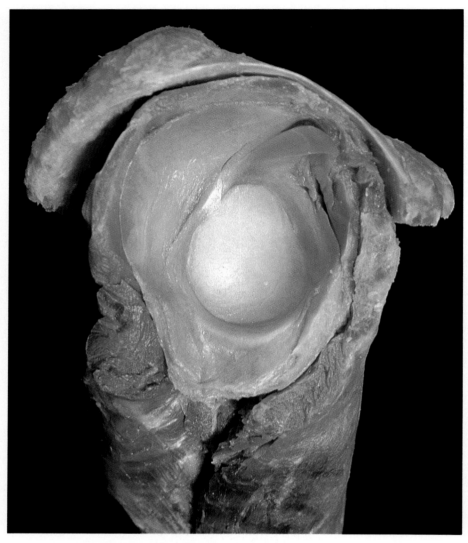

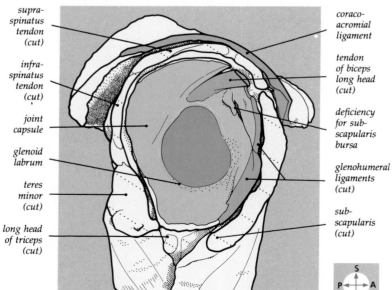

supra-
spinatus
tendon
(cut)

infra-
spinatus
tendon
(cut)

joint
capsule

glenoid
labrum

teres
minor
(cut)

long head
of triceps
(cut)

coraco-
acromial
ligament

tendon
of biceps
long head
(cut)

deficiency
for sub-
scapularis
bursa

glenohumeral
ligaments
(cut)

sub-
scapularis
(cut)

FIGURE 9-15. The scapular component of a disarticulated shoulder joint. The relations and internal features of the joint are seen.

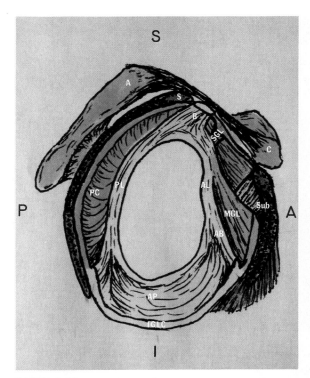

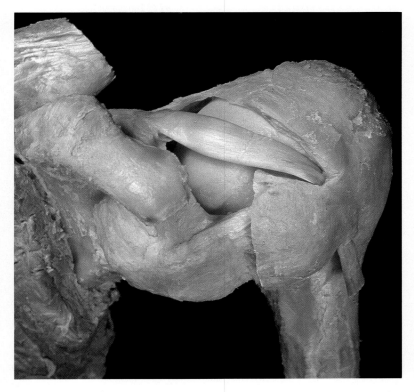

FIGURE 9-16. Glenohumeral capsular anatomy. A, acromion; AB, anterior band of inferior glenohumeral ligament; AL, anterior labrum; AP, axillary pouch of inferior glenohumeral ligament; B, biceps tendon; C, coracoid; IGLC, inferior glenohumeral ligament complex; MGL, middle glenohumeral ligament; PC, posterior capsule; PL, posterior labrum; S, supraspinatus tendon; SGL, superior glenohumeral ligament; Sub, subscapularis tendon.

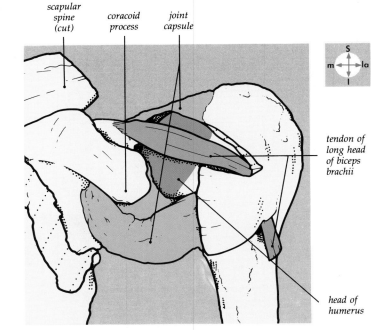

FIGURE 9-17. **(A)** Removal of part of the shoulder joint capsule reveals the intracapsular but extrasynovial tendon of the long head of the biceps brachii. **(B)** Corresponding anterior coronal oblique fat-suppressed MR arthrogram shows the course of the long head of the biceps tendon (bt).   continued

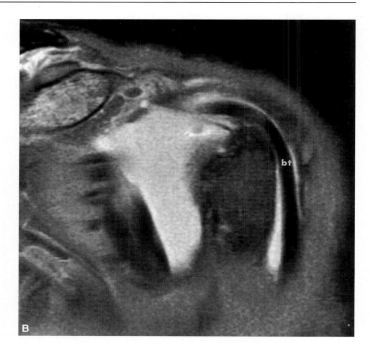

FIGURE 9-17. *Continued*

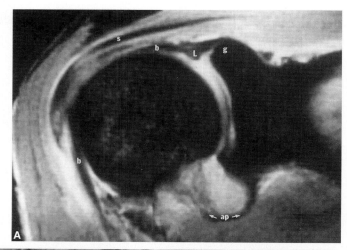

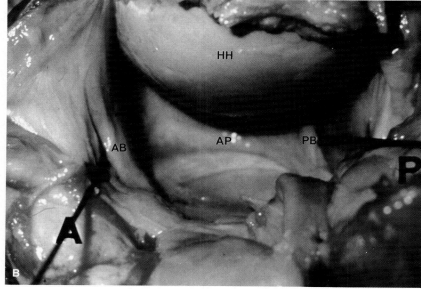

FIGURE 9-18. (**A**) The biceps origin can be located on a T2*-weighted coronal oblique image. The glenoid origin of the long head of the biceps (b) is shown, as are the attachment to the anterior labrum (l) and superior glenoid (g). The biceps courses laterally and exits the joint between the supraspinatus (s) and subscapularis tendons. The axillary pouch (ap) of the inferior glenohumeral ligament is indicated. The tendon of the long head of the biceps enters the intertubercular groove under the transverse ligament. (**B**) Gross dissection demonstrates the anterior band (AB) and posterior band (PB) of the inferior glenohumeral ligament complex. This surgical view is from the perspective of viewing inferiorly into the axillary pouch. Anterior (A), Posterior (P) and humeral head (HH) are indicated. Both the biceps tendon and posterior band contribute to the posterior labrum.

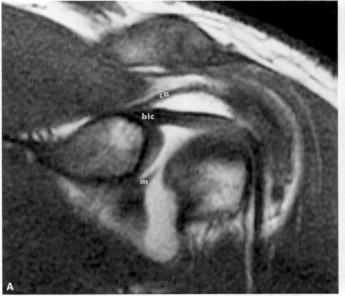

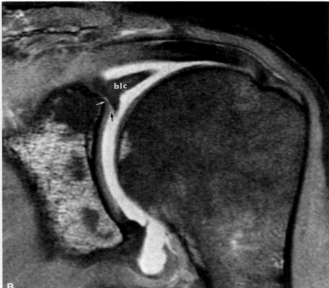

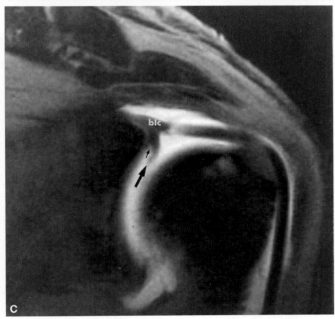

FIGURE 9-19. Biceps labral complex (blc) attachments. (**A**) In type 1, the biceps labral complex (blc) is firmly attached to the superior pole of the glenoid. m, middle glenohumeral ligament; ca, coracoacromial ligament. (**B**) In type 2, the biceps is attached to the superior labrum lateral to the superior glenoid. A fluid-filled sublabral sulcus (*black arrow*) is formed at the superior pole of the glenoid. Intermediate signal intensity cartilage (*white arrow*) of the glenoid extends medially over the superior glenoid surface. (**C**) Meniscoid labrum (*large arrow*) associated with a large sulcus (*small arrow*) which extends underneath the meniscoid superior labrum. (**A** through **C**: fat-suppressed T1-weighted coronal oblique MR arthrography images.)

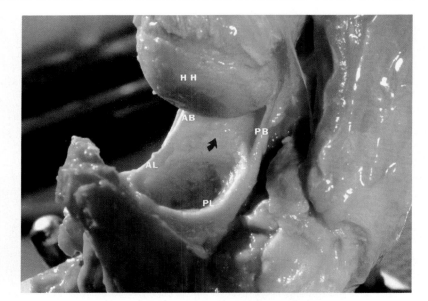

FIGURE 9-20. A gross shoulder specimen illustrates the structure of the inferior glenohumeral ligament (IGL) complex. With abduction of the humerus, the IGL structures are more prominent and taut in position. Coronal oblique MR images routinely show the lax axillary pouch of the IGL when the humerus is in the adducted position. Curved arrow, axillary pouch; AB, anterior band; AL, anterior labrum; HH, humeral head; PB, posterior band; PL, posterior labrum.

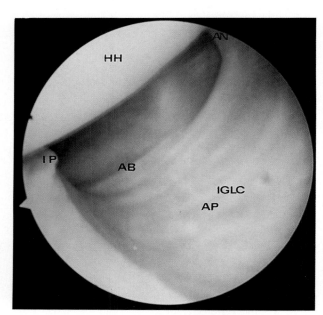

FIGURE 9-21. The inferior glenohumeral ligaent complex. An arthroscopic photograph shows the anterior band (AB) and axillary pouch (AP) components of the inferior glenohumeral ligament (IGL) complex. The inferior pole of the glenoid (IP) and the anatomic neck attachments of the IGL complex (AN) are shown as viewed from the axillary pouch. HH, humeral head.

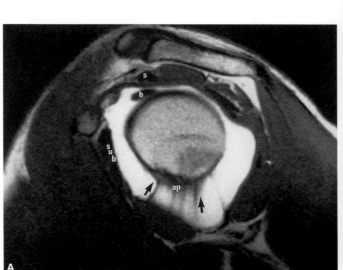

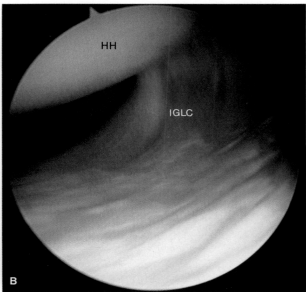

FIGURE 9-22. (**A**) The axillary pouch of the inferior glenohumeral ligament is seen on an enhanced T1-weighted sagittal image. Arrows and ap, axillary pouch of inferior glenohumeral ligament; b, biceps tendon; s, supraspinatus tendon; sub, subscapularis tendon. (**B**) Arthroscopic photograph of the axillary pouch of the inferior glenohumeral ligament complex (IGLC). Humeral head (HH) is indicated.

The inferior glenohumeral ligament complex (IGLC) originates from either the glenoid labrum or glenoid neck and inserts into the humeral neck at the periphery of the articular margin.[39] In the right shoulder, the origin of the anterior band is located near the 3 o'clock (2 to 4 o'clock) position on the glenoid, and the origin of the posterior band is near the 9 o'clock (7 to 9 o'clock) position. The anterior band forms the anterior labrum at the medial attachment of the IGL to the glenoid. Because of the important role of the IGLC in forming the anterior labrum, this relationship has also been referred to as the inferior glenohumeral ligament complex, or IGLLC. The posterior band contributes to the formation of the posterior labrum. The IGLC inserts onto the anatomic neck of the humerus in one of two configurations: as a collar-like attachment, or as a V-shaped attachment.[33,41] The IGLC functions as a hammock, cradling the humeral head with increasing abduction. Different portions of the complex support the humeral head both anteriorly and posteriorly during 90° of abduction with internal and external rotation. With internal rotation of the abducted arm, the posterior band of the IGLC fans out and supports the humeral head posteriorly with the anterior band moving under the humeral head. When the abducted arm is in external rotation, the anterior band of the IGLC fans out and supports the humeral head anteriorly, while the posterior band stabilizes the joint inferiorly. Thus, the IGLC has a role in anterior-posterior and superior-inferior stability, as represented by the function of its two bands and intervening axillary pouch. The IGLC and its components (anterior band, axillary pouch, and posterior band) have been shown to be histologically present in all specimens studied by O'Brien and colleagues.[33] As discussed earlier, the anterior and posterior bands can be

accentuated through external and internal rotation of the arm, respectively.

MIDDLE GLENOHUMERAL LIGAMENT. The MGL attaches to the anterior aspect of the anatomic neck of the humerus, medial to the lesser tuberosity[38] (Fig. 9-24). It arises from the glenoid by way of the labrum and scapular neck. This structure can be identified between the subscapularis tendon (ie, it passes across the subscapularis tendon) and the anterior labrum or anterior band of the IGL (Figs. 9-25 and 9-26). The foramen of Weitbrecht is located between the superior and middle glenohumeral ligaments, and the foramen of Rouviere is located between the middle and inferior glenohumeral ligaments (see Fig. 9-26). Of the three glenohumeral ligaments, the MGL demonstrates the greatest variation in size and thickness.[39] Wall and O'Brien[41] found that it was absent in up to 27% of specimens. This is consistent with the work of De Palma,[43] who originally described a poorly defined or absent MGL in 30% of shoulders studied. The MGL, which may be present as thin ligamentous tissue or appear cord-like and as thick as the biceps tendon, has a role in the stability of the shoulder joint from 0° to 45° of abduction.[39] Along with the subscapularis tendon and the superior part of the IGL, the MGL contributes to anterior stability at 45° of abduction.[44] In the lower and middle ranges of abduction, the MGL limits external rotation. The MGL has been shown to have a secondary role in anterior stability of the shoulder in 90° of abduction when the anterior band of the IGL is cut.[45] Inferior translation of the abducted and externally rotated shoulder was limited as a secondary restraint function of the MGL. The MGL demonstrates a more

text continues on page 620

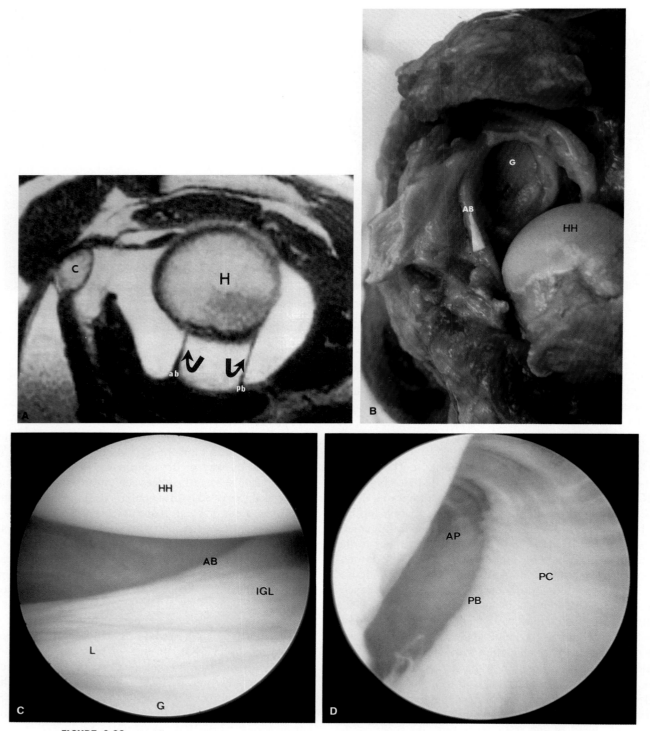

FIGURE 9-23. **(A)** The anterior band (ab) and posterior band (pb) of the inferior glenohumeral ligament (*curved arrows*) extend from the glenoid origin to the humeral attachment, as seen on an enhanced T1-weighted sagittal oblique image. C, coracoid; H, humeral head. **(B)** On a gross shoulder specimen, the superior course of the anterior band (AB) of the inferior glenohumeral ligament is identified (*triangular marker*). Glenoid (G) and humeral head (HH) are identified. **(C)** Arthroscopic photograph of the anterior band (AB) of the inferior glenohumeral ligament (IGL). HH, humeral head; L, labrum; G, glenoid. **(D)** Arthroscopic photograph of the posterior band (PB) of the IGL. AP, axillary pouch; PC, posterior capsule.

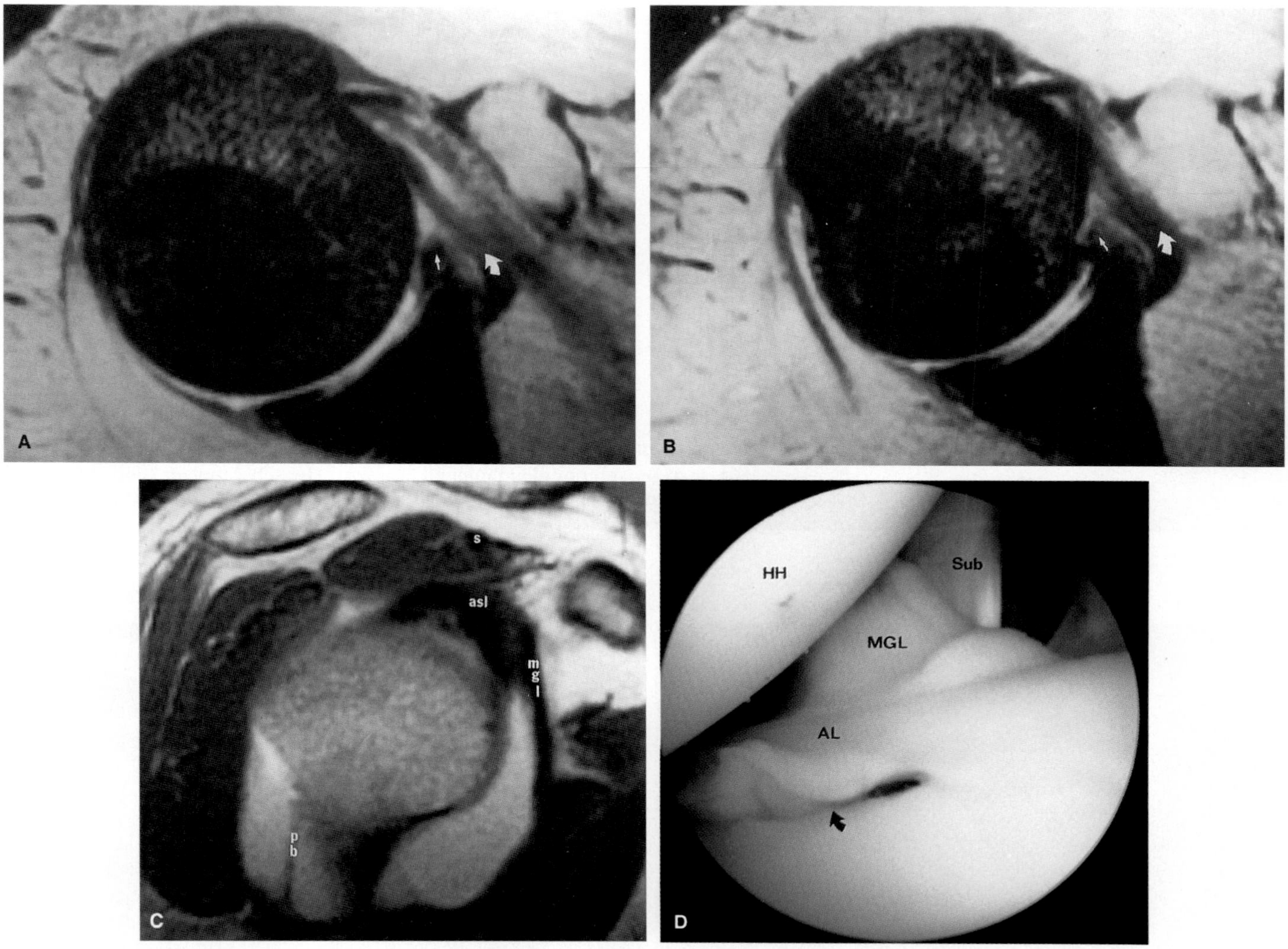

FIGURE 9-24. T2*-weighted axial images at (**A**) and below (**B**) the level of the subscapularis show the normal middle glenohumeral ligament (MGL; *curved arrows*), its medial origin from the glenoid and neck of the scapula, and its attachment to the lesser tuberosity. Small straight arrows, anterior labrum. (**C**) An enhanced T1-weighted sagittal oblique image shows the attachment of the MGL (mgl) to the anterior superior glenoid labrum (asl). The MGL arises from the labrum below the superior glenohumeral ligament and from the neck of the scapula. The humeral attachment of the MGL is located medial to the lesser tuberosity. The MGL may arise only from the labrum or may have no attachment to it as normal anatomic variants. pb, posterior band of IGL; s, supraspinatus tendon. (**D**) Arthroscopic view of the middle glenohumeral ligament (MGL) anterior to the anterior labrum (AL) and posterior to the subscapularis tendon (Sub). An anterior superior quadrant sublabral foramen (*curved arrow*) exists as a normal variant. HH, humeral head.

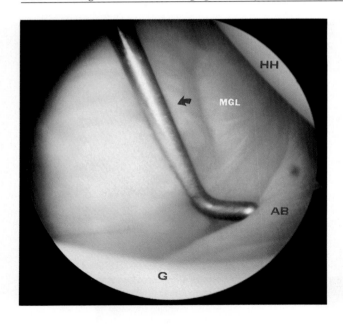

FIGURE 9-25. An arthroscopic photograph shows the anterior band (AB) of the inferior glenohumeral ligament. The subscapularis tendon (*arrow*) is located beneath the middle glenohumeral ligament (MGL) and is not directly seen. G, glenoid; HH, humeral head.

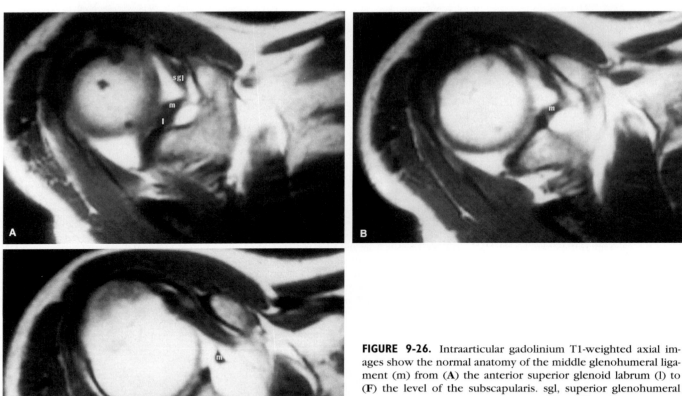

FIGURE 9-26. Intraarticular gadolinium T1-weighted axial images show the normal anatomy of the middle glenohumeral ligament (m) from (**A**) the anterior superior glenoid labrum (l) to (**F**) the level of the subscapularis. sgl, superior glenohumeral ligament. (**G**) On a fat-suppressed T1-weighted sagittal oblique arthrogram, the normal foramen of Weitbrecht (*solid curved arrow*) is shown between the middle glenohumeral ligament (mgl) and the superior glenohumeral ligament. The foramen of Rouviere (*open curved arrow*) is located between the middle glenohumeral ligament (mgl) and the inferior glenohumeral ligament (IGL). *continued*

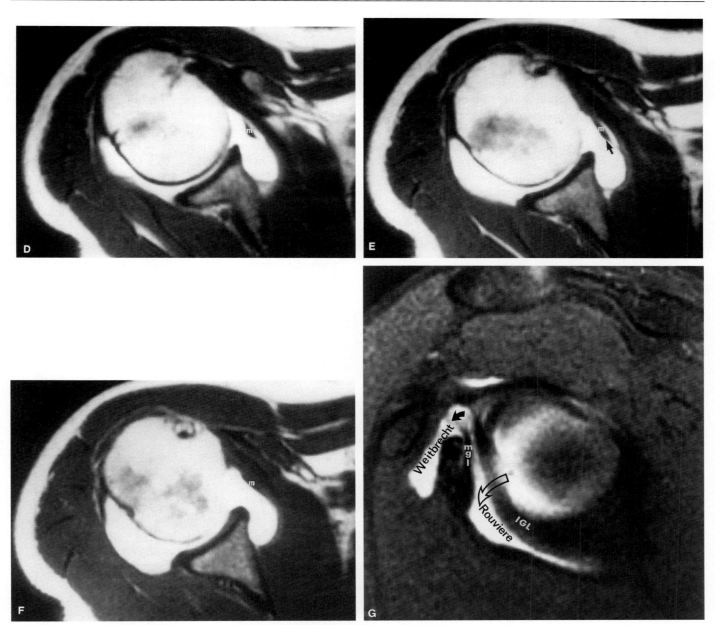

FIGURE 9-26. *Continued*

vertical orientation with internal rotation and horizontal orientation (elongation of the MGL) with external rotation of the shoulder.

SUPERIOR GLENOHUMERAL LIGAMENT. The SGL is the smallest and least understood of the glenohumeral capsular structures.[38] The SGL originates from the upper pole of the glenoid cavity and base of the coracoid process, and is attached to the MGL, to the biceps tendon, and to the labrum (see Figs. 9-7C and 9-27). It inserts just superior to the lesser tuberosity in the region of the bicipital groove.[39] A normal foramen or opening exists between the SGL and MGL, allowing communication with the subscapularis bursa.[46] The SGL has been reported to be present in 90%

to 97% of shoulder studies.[33,47] The size of the SGL varies, ranging from a thin thread-like thickening of the capsule to a more substantial ligament. The SGL is closely related to the extraarticular coracohumeral ligament. The coracohumeral ligament originates in the lateral aspect of the coracoid and inserts on the greater tuberosity. The SGL and the coracohumeral ligament contribute to the stabilization of the glenohumeral joint and prevent posterior and inferior translation of the humeral head. Warner and colleagues showed that the SGL was well-developed in 50% of shoulders.[48] When present and well formed (developed), the SGL represents the primary capsuloligamentous restraint to inferior translation of the unloaded, abducted shoulder joint.[39,48]

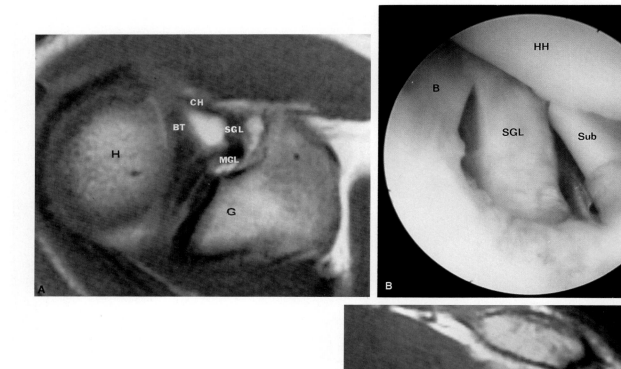

FIGURE 9-27. **(A)** The superior glenohumeral ligament (SGL) is seen on an enhanced T1-weighted axial image above the level of the coracoid. The extraarticular coracohumeral ligament (CH) and intraarticular SGL are closely related. The middle portion of the CH crosses the SGL. The SGL is oriented perpendicular to the middle glenohumeral ligament (MGL) as shown. BT, biceps tendon; G, glenoid; H, humeral head. **(B)** Arthroscopic photograph (posterior view) showing the lateral location of the biceps (B) relative to the superior glenohumeral ligament (SGL). HH, humeral head; Sub, subscapularis tendon. **(C)** The horizontal course of the coracohumeral ligament (CH) from the coracoid to the greater tuberosity is shown on an anterior T1-weighted coronal oblique image.

Other Capsuloligamentous Structures

Coracohumeral Ligament

The coracohumeral ligament, which originates on the lateral aspect of the base of the coracoid inferior to the origin of the coracoacromial ligament (see Fig. 9-27C), courses in a horizontal or transverse direction to its insertion on the greater tuberosity on the lateral aspect of the bicipital groove.[39] At the anterior superior aspect of the shoulder, the coracohumeral ligament overlies and is superficial to the SGL. The coracohumeral ligament has been reported to contribute, along with the SGL, to the restraint of inferior translation in external rotation in the abducted shoulder. However, Cooper and coworkers[49] have characterized it as a folded portion of the glenohumeral joint capsule in the interval between the subscapularis and supraspinatus, without contribution to glenohumeral joint stability.[49]

Posterior Capsule

The posterior capsule includes the capsule posterior to the biceps tendon and superior to the posterior band of the IGL. This represents the thinnest portion of the capsule. The posterior capsule has a role in limiting both the posterior and anterior translation of the glenohumeral joint.[39,50] With an intact anterior capsule, posterior dislocation does not occur even with division of the posterior capsule.

Rotator Cuff and Long Head of the Biceps

The supraspinatus, infraspinatus, teres minor, and subscapularis muscles constitute the rotator cuff (Figs. 9-28 through 9-30). Their primary function is to centralize the humeral head, limiting superior translation during abduction. The supraspinatus, infraspinatus, and teres minor ten-

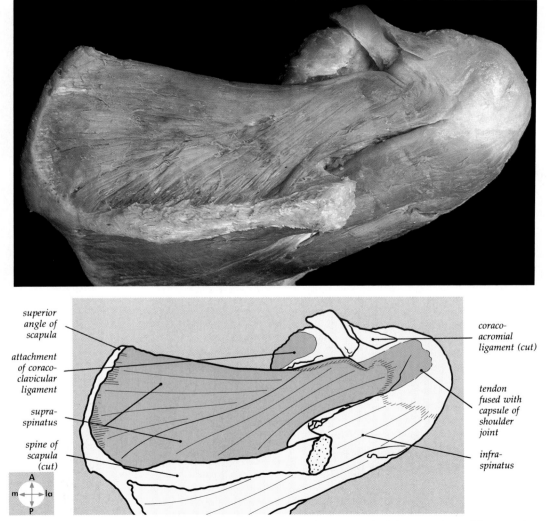

FIGURE 9-28. A superior view of the supraspinatus tendon after removal of the acromion of the scapula.

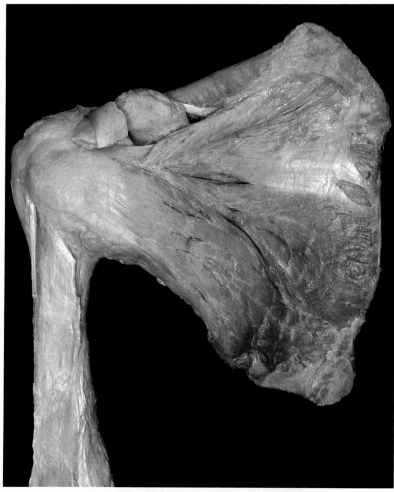

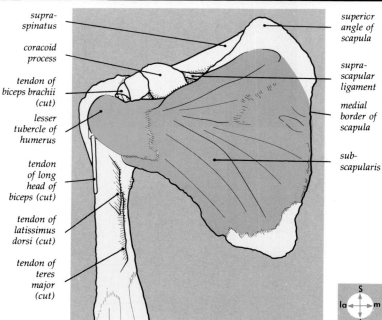

supra-
spinatus

coracoid
process

tendon of
biceps brachii
(cut)

lesser
tubercle of
humerus

tendon
of long
head of
biceps (cut)

tendon of
latissimus
dorsi (cut)

tendon of
teres
major
(cut)

superior
angle of
scapula

supra-
scapular
ligament

medial
border
of scapula

sub-
scapularis

FIGURE 9-29. An anterior view of the subscapularis. The attachment of the serratus anterior to the medial border of the scapula has been excised.

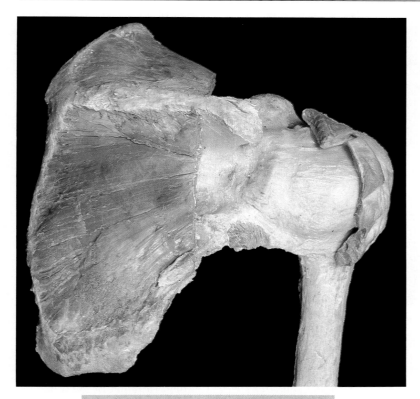

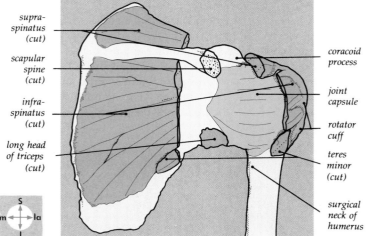

supra-
spinatus
(cut)

scapular
spine
(cut)

infra-
spinatus
(cut)

long head
of triceps
(cut)

coracoid
process

joint
capsule

rotator
cuff

teres
minor
(cut)

surgical
neck of
humerus

FIGURE 9-30. The posterior aspect of the shoulder joint. The acromion and parts of the rotator cuff muscles have been excised to reveal the joint capsule.

dons insert on the greater tuberosity, whereas the subscapularis tendon inserts on the lesser tuberosity. The subscapularis tendon lies on the anterior aspect of the anterior capsule of the glenohumeral joint, and its superior portion is intraarticular.[38] The subscapularis bursa lies between the subscapularis tendon and the scapula. The subscapularis muscle may be the cause of recurrent instability as it becomes attenuated from repeated episodes of dislocations.[34] The rotator cuff interval is located between the superior aspect of the subscapularis tendon and the inferior aspect of the supraspinatus tendon. This interval con-

tains the coracohumeral ligament and the SGL. The rotator interval lesion has been attributed to a possible deficiency of the SGL. Surgical closure of the interval appears to eliminate excessive inferior translation.[39]

The triangular space through which the scapular circumflex vessels travel is formed by the teres major, the lower border of the teres minor, and the long head of the triceps. Lateral to the triangular space, the quadrilateral space (through which the axillary nerve and posterior humeral circumflex artery travel) is formed by the lower border of the teres minor, the upper border of the teres major, the lateral

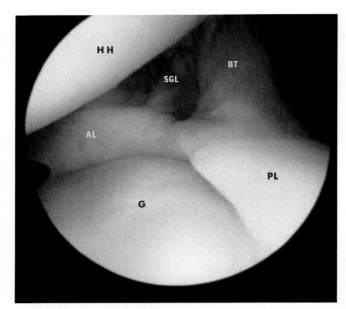

FIGURE 9-31. The biceps tendon (BT) contributes to the superior anterior labrum (AL) and the superior posterior labrum (PL) in the biceps lateral complex. One component of the long head of the BT attaches to the supraglenoid tubercle. Extraarticular fibers attach to the lateral edge of the base of the coracoid process. The intraarticular portion of the long head of the BT is oriented at an approximate right angle to the surface of the glenoid (G). HH, numeral head; SGL, superior glenohumeral ligament.

border of the long head of the biceps, and the medial border of the humerus.[34]

The long head of the biceps tendon attaches to the supraglenoid tubercle, and exits the joint in the bicipital groove in the hiatus between the subscapularis and supraspinatus tendons.[38]

Fibers of the biceps contribute to the posterior and anterior superior labrum (Figs. 9-31 and 9-32). The long head of the biceps, with the BLC, centralizes and stabilizes the joint, as does the rotator cuff. The biceps tendon has a synovial sheath as an extension of the synovial lining of the glenohumeral joint.

Coracoacromial Arch

Coracoacromial Ligament

The coracoacromial ligament is the key structure of the coracoacromial arch, and plays an important role in the spectrum of impingement disorders of the shoulder (Fig. 9-33). This ligament is a triangular band of two fascicles, which originates from the lateral aspect of the coracoid and attaches to the anterior, lateral, and inferior surfaces of the acromion. The coracoacromial arch stabilizes the humeral head and prevents superior ascent. The subacromial bursa is located between the acromion, the coracoacromial ligament, and the rotator cuff.[34] The bursa runs from the AC joint medially, under the anterior third of the acromion and coracoacromial ligament, to a line that extends approximately 4 cm anterior and lateral to the anterolateral margins of acromion. Anterior acromial spurs, caused by chronic irritation of the humerus against this ligamentous structure, can form within the acromial portion of the coracoacromial ligament.[36] Frequently, anterior acromial spurs are identified adjacent to the acromial attachment of the coracoacromial ligament. The normal low signal intensity acromial attachment of the coracoacromial ligament is frequently mistaken for an anterior acromial spur on coronal oblique MR images. The additive thickness of the coracoacromial ligament and the inferior acromial cortex

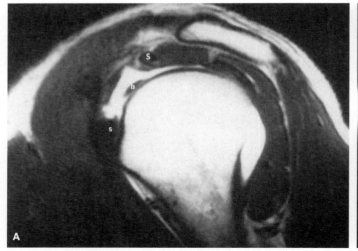

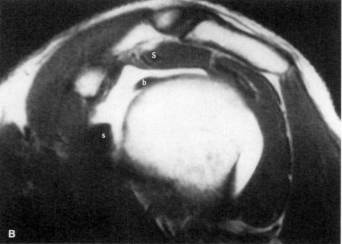

FIGURE 9-32. Intraarticular gadolinium-enhanced MR images show the normal biceps lateral complex (blc) from **(A)** lateral through **(E)** medial. Arrows and ap, axillary pouch of IGL; al, anterior labrum; b, biceps tendon; ch, coracohumeral ligament; mgl, middle glenohumeral ligament; S, supraspinatus tendon; s, subscapularis tendon. **(F)** A corresponding T2*-weighted coronal image. S, supraspinatus tendon. **(G)** A corresponding anteroposterior arthrogram and **(H)** enhanced T1-weighted coronal oblique image. AP, axillary pouch; b, biceps tendon; l, labrum; S, supraspinatus tendon. *continued*

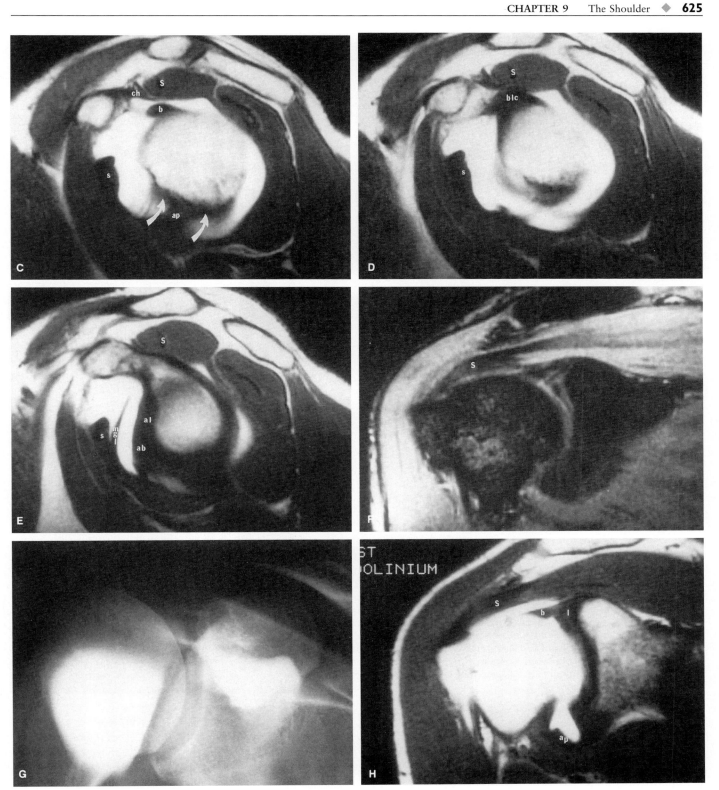

FIGURE 9-32. *Continued*

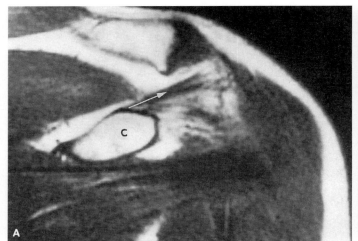

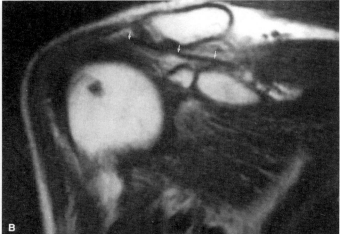

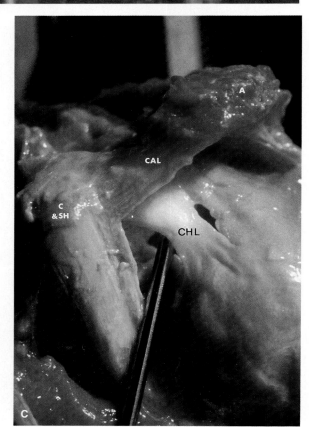

FIGURE 9-33. **(A)** Intact, low signal intensity coracoacromial ligament (*arrow*) with a broad inferior acromial attachment on a T1-weighted coronal oblique image. C, coracoid. **(B)** Narrowing of the subacromial space with buffering of the superior ascent of the humeral head by the coracoacromial ligament (*arrows*) on a T1-weighted coronal oblique image. Development of a subacromial spur is associated with chronic impingement of the greater tuberosity on the coracoacromial ligament. **(C)** Gross specimen highlighting the anatomy of the coracohumeral ligament (CHL) and coracoacromial ligament (CAL). The coracobrachialis (C), short head of the biceps (SH), and acromion (A) are indicated.

produce this pseudospur (Fig. 9-34). In acromioplasty performed for chronic impingement, the coracoacromial ligament is resected, and the anterior inferior margin of the acromion is resected.

The Acromioclavicular Joint

The AC joint is a synovial joint with articular surfaces covered by fibrocartilage like the sternoclavicular joint.[51] The articular capsule is reinforced by superior and inferior AC ligaments. The articular surfaces are separated by a wedge-shaped articular disc. The coracoclavicular ligament, with its conoid and trapezoid components, provides major stability to the joint (see Fig. 9-11). The coracoclavicular ligament assists in controlling vertical stability, and the AC ligament restrains posterior translation of the clavicle.[34]

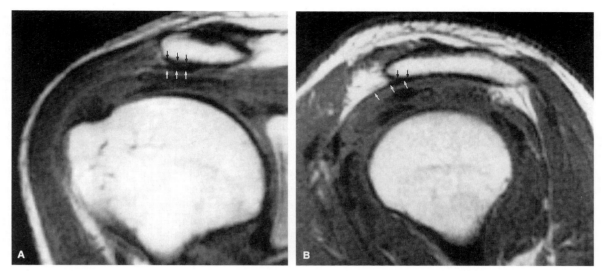

FIGURE 9-34. Pseudospur. The normal broad attachment of the coracoacromial ligament to the inferior surface of the acromion is shown on (**A**) T1-weighted coronal oblique and (**B**) sagittal oblique images. The low signal intensity acromial cortex (*black arrows*) and adjacent coracoacromial ligament and lateral slip of the deltoid attachment (*white arrows*) give the false impression of a small subacromial spur in the coronal plane, which should not be misinterpreted as impingement. Unnecessary acromioplasties may be performed on patients with a normal coracoacromial ligament attachment and no associated acromial spurs.

Subacromial Bursa

The subacromial bursa extends under the acromion and coracoacromial ligament. Laterally, the bursa lies over the superior surface of the supraspinatus and infraspinatus tendons and extends beyond the lateral and anterior aspects of the acromion, under the deltoid. The bursa serves as a gliding mechanism between the rotator cuff and coracoacromial arch.[52] Although communication exists between the subacromial and subcoracoid bursae, there may be no communication between the subcoracoid and subscapularis bursae[53,54] (Figs. 9-35 and 9-36). Therefore,

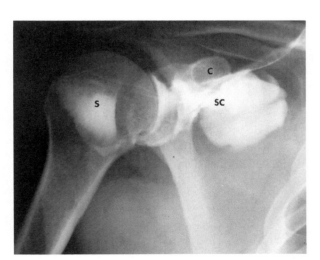

FIGURE 9-35. After separate contrast injections into the subcoracoid (SC) and subscapularis bursa (S), the subacromial bursa are seen to communicate, whereas no communication occurs between the subacromial and subscapularis bursae. C, coracoid.

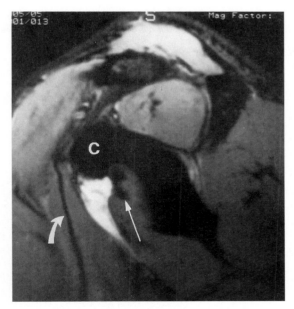

FIGURE 9-36. T2*-weighted sagittal oblique gadopentetate-saline subcoracoid bursagram demonstrates filling of the subcoracoid bursa anterior to the subscapularis tendon (*straight arrow*) and posterior to the conjoined tendon of the coracobrachialis and short head of the biceps (*curved arrow*). C, coracoid.

an inadvertent MR contrast injection or saline injection to the subcoracoid bursa does not allow visualization of capsular structures because the subscapularis bursa is not distended. In this situation, gadolinium contrast in the subacromial bursa is not related to rotator cuff pathology. When obliterated, the peribursal fat plane has been used as an ancillary sign of shoulder disease. Fibrous bands may be found within the subacromial bursa.[38]

MAGNETIC RESONANCE APPEARANCE OF THE SHOULDER

Axial Images

On superior axial images, the normal oblique course of the supraspinatus muscle is displayed with intermediate signal intensity (Fig. 9-37). The supraspinatus tendon, from its

insertion on the capsule and greater tuberosity posterior to the bicipital groove, to the supraspinatus fossa of the scapula, is displayed with low signal intensity. The supraspinatus muscle appears intermediate in signal intensity on T2-weighted and fat-suppressed T2-weighted fast spin-echo images, demonstrating low signal intensity within its tendinous fibers. High signal intensity marrow fat is present in the acromion, seen lateral to and parallel with the supraspinatus muscle. In the adducted position, the tendon of the supraspinatus projects lateral to the acromion. At the level of the superior coracoid process, the long axis of the infraspinatus originates from the posteroinferior surface of the scapula, crosses the glenohumeral joint posterior to the supraspinatus, and inserts on the lateral aspect of the greater tuberosity. As it approaches the greater tuberosity postero-

text continues on page 637

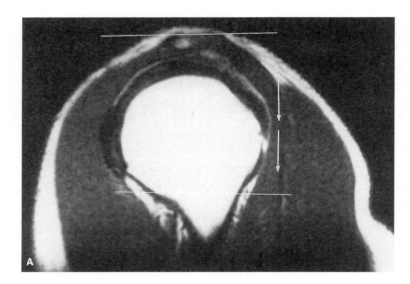

FIGURE 9-37. Normal axial MR anatomy. (**A**) This sagittal oblique localizer was used to graphically prescribe 18 axial T1-weighted image locations from (**B**) superior to (**S**) inferior.

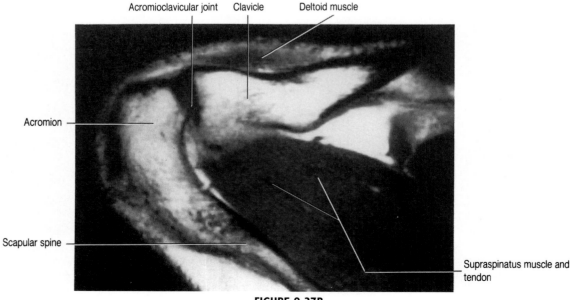

Acromioclavicular joint   Clavicle   Deltoid muscle

Acromion

Scapular spine

Supraspinatus muscle and tendon

FIGURE 9-37B.

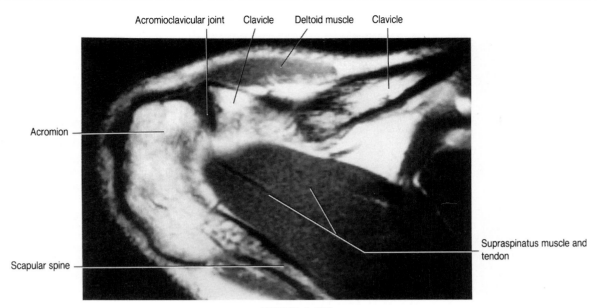

Acromioclavicular joint   Clavicle   Deltoid muscle   Clavicle

Acromion

Scapular spine

Supraspinatus muscle and tendon

FIGURE 9-37C.

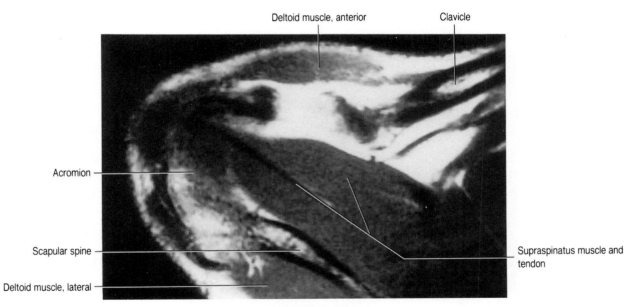

Deltoid muscle, anterior   Clavicle

Acromion

Scapular spine

Deltoid muscle, lateral

Supraspinatus muscle and tendon

FIGURE 9-37D.

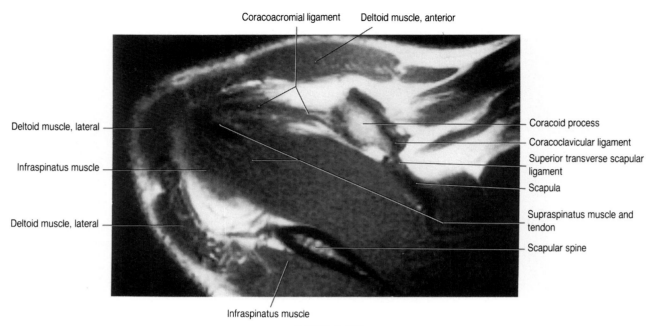

Coracoacromial ligament   Deltoid muscle, anterior

Deltoid muscle, lateral

Infraspinatus muscle

Deltoid muscle, lateral

Coracoid process

Coracoclavicular ligament

Superior transverse scapular ligament

Scapula

Supraspinatus muscle and tendon

Scapular spine

Infraspinatus muscle

FIGURE 9-37E.

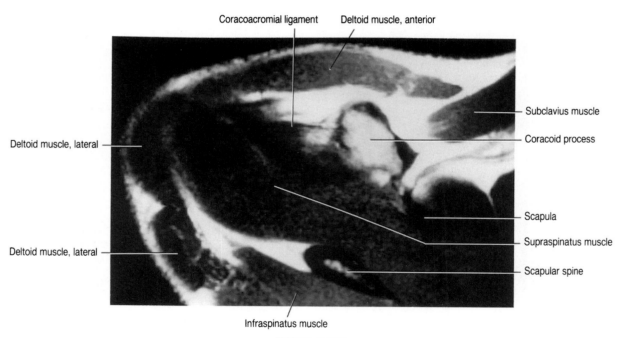

Coracoacromial ligament   Deltoid muscle, anterior

Deltoid muscle, lateral

Deltoid muscle, lateral

Subclavius muscle

Coracoid process

Scapula

Supraspinatus muscle

Scapular spine

Infraspinatus muscle

FIGURE 9-37F.

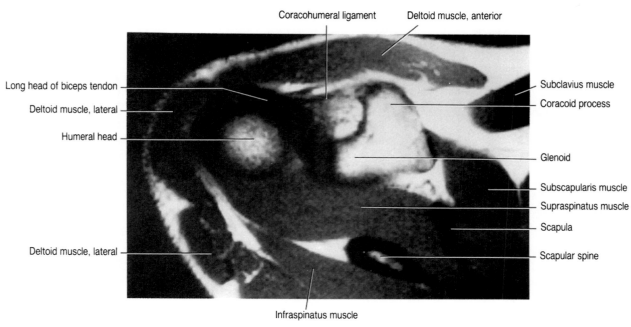

Coracohumeral ligament   Deltoid muscle, anterior

Long head of biceps tendon

Deltoid muscle, lateral

Humeral head

Subclavius muscle

Coracoid process

Glenoid

Subscapularis muscle

Supraspinatus muscle

Scapula

Deltoid muscle, lateral

Scapular spine

Infraspinatus muscle

FIGURE 9-37G.

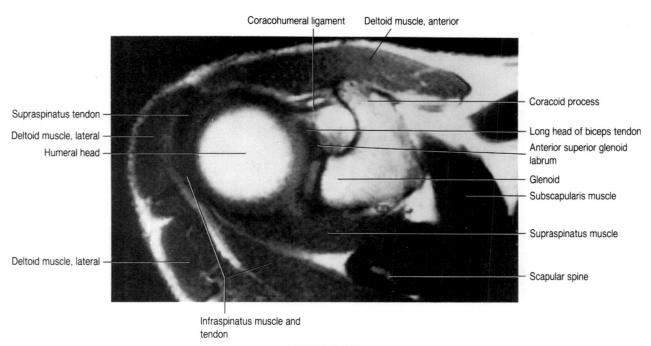

Coracohumeral ligament   Deltoid muscle, anterior

Supraspinatus tendon

Deltoid muscle, lateral

Humeral head

Coracoid process

Long head of biceps tendon

Anterior superior glenoid labrum

Glenoid

Subscapularis muscle

Supraspinatus muscle

Deltoid muscle, lateral

Scapular spine

Infraspinatus muscle and tendon

FIGURE 9-37H.

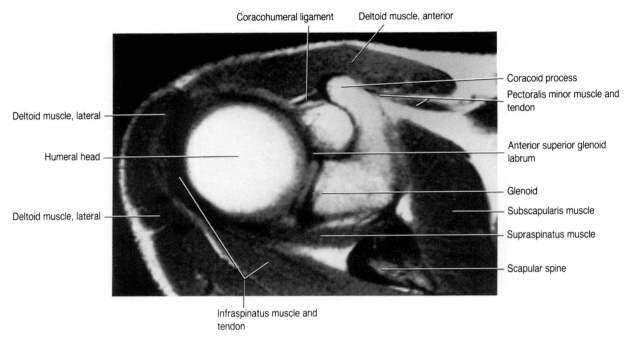

Coracohumeral ligament · Deltoid muscle, anterior

Deltoid muscle, lateral

Humeral head

Deltoid muscle, lateral

Coracoid process

Pectoralis minor muscle and tendon

Anterior superior glenoid labrum

Glenoid

Subscapularis muscle

Supraspinatus muscle

Scapular spine

Infraspinatus muscle and tendon

FIGURE 9-37I.

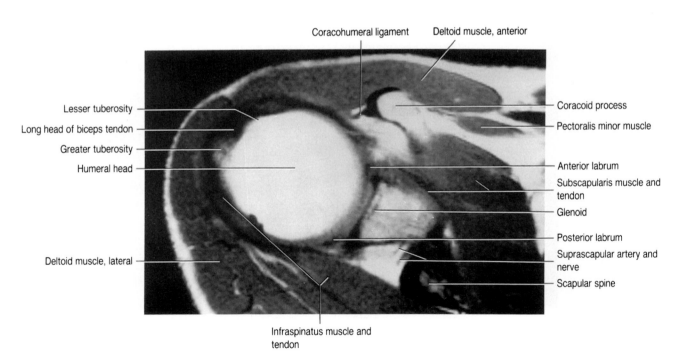

Coracohumeral ligament · Deltoid muscle, anterior

Lesser tuberosity

Long head of biceps tendon

Greater tuberosity

Humeral head

Deltoid muscle, lateral

Coracoid process

Pectoralis minor muscle

Anterior labrum

Subscapularis muscle and tendon

Glenoid

Posterior labrum

Suprascapular artery and nerve

Scapular spine

Infraspinatus muscle and tendon

FIGURE 9-37J.

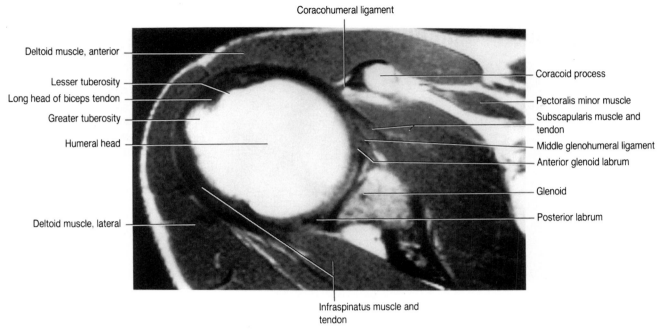

Coracohumeral ligament

Deltoid muscle, anterior

Lesser tuberosity

Long head of biceps tendon

Greater tuberosity

Humeral head

Deltoid muscle, lateral

Coracoid process

Pectoralis minor muscle

Subscapularis muscle and tendon

Middle glenohumeral ligament

Anterior glenoid labrum

Glenoid

Posterior labrum

Infraspinatus muscle and tendon

FIGURE 9-37K.

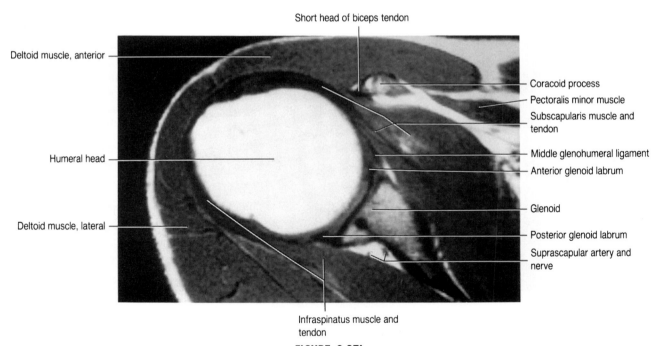

Short head of biceps tendon

Deltoid muscle, anterior

Humeral head

Deltoid muscle, lateral

Coracoid process

Pectoralis minor muscle

Subscapularis muscle and tendon

Middle glenohumeral ligament

Anterior glenoid labrum

Glenoid

Posterior glenoid labrum

Suprascapular artery and nerve

Infraspinatus muscle and tendon

FIGURE 9-37L.

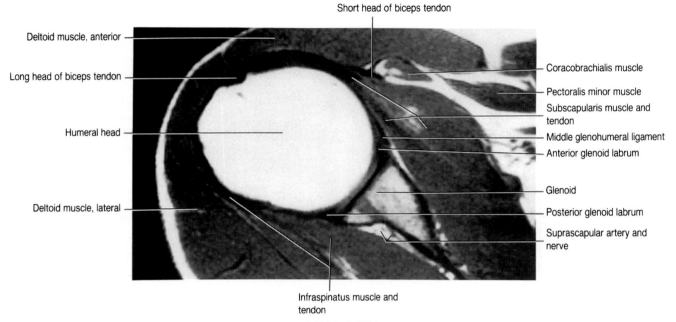

Deltoid muscle, anterior

Long head of biceps tendon

Humeral head

Deltoid muscle, lateral

Short head of biceps tendon

Coracobrachialis muscle

Pectoralis minor muscle

Subscapularis muscle and tendon

Middle glenohumeral ligament

Anterior glenoid labrum

Glenoid

Posterior glenoid labrum

Suprascapular artery and nerve

Infraspinatus muscle and tendon

FIGURE 9-37M.

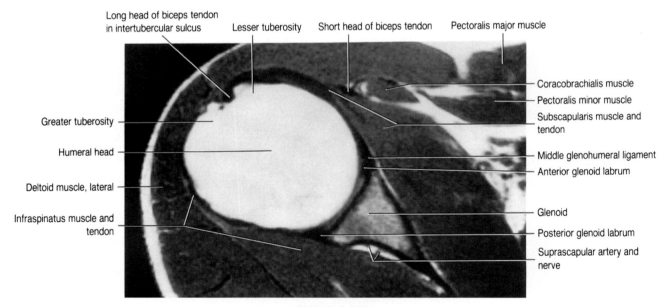

Long head of biceps tendon in intertubercular sulcus

Lesser tuberosity

Short head of biceps tendon

Pectoralis major muscle

Greater tuberosity

Humeral head

Deltoid muscle, lateral

Infraspinatus muscle and tendon

Coracobrachialis muscle

Pectoralis minor muscle

Subscapularis muscle and tendon

Middle glenohumeral ligament

Anterior glenoid labrum

Glenoid

Posterior glenoid labrum

Suprascapular artery and nerve

FIGURE 9-37N.

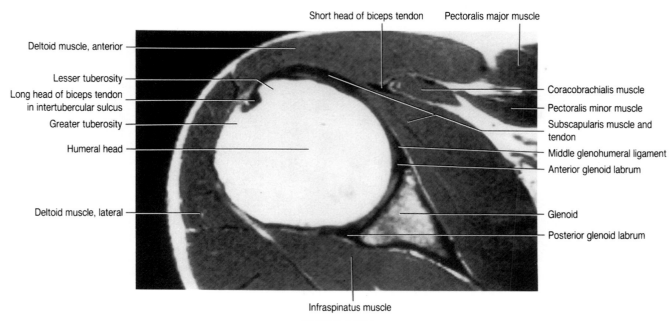

Deltoid muscle, anterior

Lesser tuberosity

Long head of biceps tendon
in intertubercular sulcus

Greater tuberosity

Humeral head

Deltoid muscle, lateral

Short head of biceps tendon

Pectoralis major muscle

Coracobrachialis muscle

Pectoralis minor muscle

Subscapularis muscle and
tendon

Middle glenohumeral ligament

Anterior glenoid labrum

Glenoid

Posterior glenoid labrum

Infraspinatus muscle

FIGURE 9-37O.

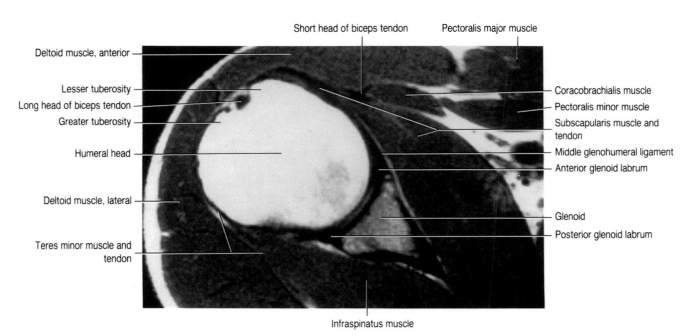

Deltoid muscle, anterior

Lesser tuberosity

Long head of biceps tendon

Greater tuberosity

Humeral head

Deltoid muscle, lateral

Teres minor muscle and
tendon

Short head of biceps tendon

Pectoralis major muscle

Coracobrachialis muscle

Pectoralis minor muscle

Subscapularis muscle and
tendon

Middle glenohumeral ligament

Anterior glenoid labrum

Glenoid

Posterior glenoid labrum

Infraspinatus muscle

FIGURE 9-37P.

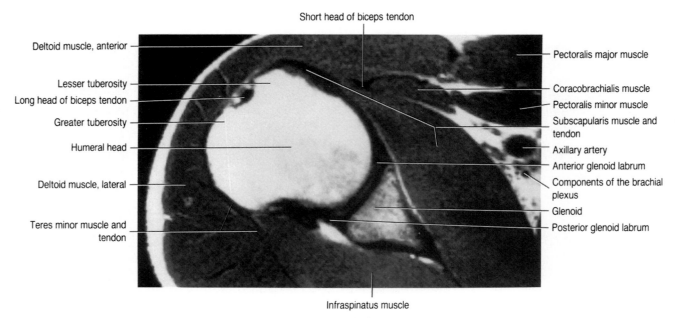

Short head of biceps tendon

Deltoid muscle, anterior

Lesser tuberosity
Long head of biceps tendon
Greater tuberosity
Humeral head

Deltoid muscle, lateral

Teres minor muscle and
tendon

Pectoralis major muscle

Coracobrachialis muscle
Pectoralis minor muscle
Subscapularis muscle and
tendon
Axillary artery
Anterior glenoid labrum
Components of the brachial
plexus
Glenoid
Posterior glenoid labrum

Infraspinatus muscle

FIGURE 9-37Q.

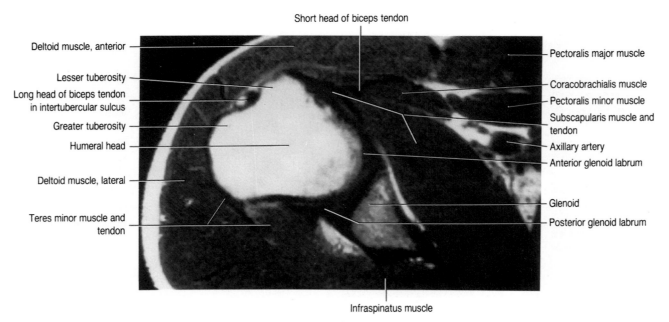

Short head of biceps tendon

Deltoid muscle, anterior

Lesser tuberosity
Long head of biceps tendon
in intertubercular sulcus
Greater tuberosity
Humeral head

Deltoid muscle, lateral

Teres minor muscle and
tendon

Pectoralis major muscle

Coracobrachialis muscle
Pectoralis minor muscle
Subscapularis muscle and
tendon
Axillary artery
Anterior glenoid labrum

Glenoid
Posterior glenoid labrum

Infraspinatus muscle

FIGURE 9-37R.

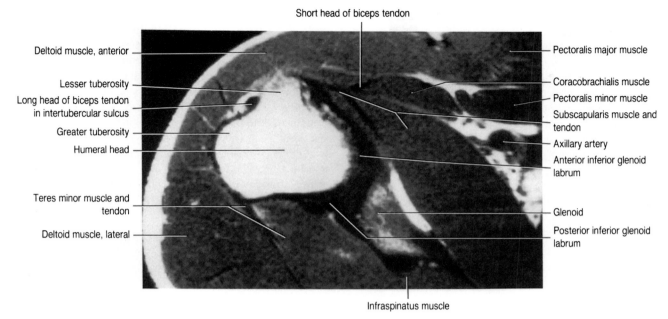

Short head of biceps tendon

Deltoid muscle, anterior

Lesser tuberosity

Long head of biceps tendon in intertubercular sulcus

Greater tuberosity

Humeral head

Teres minor muscle and tendon

Deltoid muscle, lateral

Pectoralis major muscle

Coracobrachialis muscle

Pectoralis minor muscle

Subscapularis muscle and tendon

Axillary artery

Anterior inferior glenoid labrum

Glenoid

Posterior inferior glenoid labrum

Infraspinatus muscle

FIGURE 9-37S.

laterally, the low signal intensity supraspinatus tendon merges with the low signal intensity cortex of the humerus. The spine of the scapula separates the supraspinatus and infraspinatus muscles. The teres minor is posterolateral to the infraspinatus, originating at the axillary border of the scapula and inserting on the inferior facet of the greater tuberosity.

In cross section, the tendon of the long head of the biceps is seen as a low signal intensity structure within the bicipital groove and is sometimes associated with a small amount of high signal intensity fat. The suprascapular artery and nerve are located posterior and medial to the superior glenoid rim. The dark, low signal intensity labrum is located at the level of the glenohumeral articulation, inferior to the coracoid. Normally, the anterior and posterior labrum have well-defined triangular shapes. The posterior labrum may be smaller and more rounded than the anterior labrum. With internal rotation, however, the anterior labrum appears to be larger than the posterior labrum. Glenohumeral articular cartilage follows the concave shape of the glenoid cavity, and demonstrates intermediate signal intensity on T1-weighted images and bright signal intensity on T2*-weighted images. Articular cartilage of the glenoid margin of the anterior labrum may be mistaken for a tear. Articular cartilage of the glenohumeral joint is better evaluated on fat-suppressed T2-weighted fast spin-echo sequences. Antero-medial to the glenoid, the subscapularis muscle arises from the subscapularis fossa and inserts on the lesser tuberosity. The low signal intensity subscapularis can then be identified anterior to the apex of the anterior glenoid labrum. The subscapularis tendon is present at the level of the middle and superior glenohumeral joint. The MGL is identified as a low signal intensity thin band or cord anterior to the anterior

labrum, and the anterior band of the IGL is between the anterior labrum and the subscapularis tendon. The MGL may be closely applied to the anterior aspect of the anterior labrum or plastered against the subscapularis tendon, indistinguishable from the low signal intensity subscapularis without the benefit of intraarticular contrast. The SGL is identified at the level of the coracoid and the biceps tendon.

With the arm abducted by the patient's side, axial images through the inferior glenohumeral joint display the IGL as a lax structure. The axillary pouch of the IGL is identified inferior to the level of the bony glenoid and requires axial sections that extend inferior to the glenohumeral joint. The subacromial-subdeltoid bursa and the deltoid muscle can be identified between the rotator cuff and the acromion.

Coronal Images

In rotator cuff evaluations, supraspinatus tendon anatomy is best displayed on coronal planar images (Fig. 9-38). On anterior and midcoronal oblique images, the supraspinatus muscle and its central tendon are seen in continuity. The low density supraspinatus tendon is defined at its insertion on the greater tuberosity. The subacromial bursa is interposed between the rotator cuff and the acromion. A fibrofatty layer lies between the acromion, the AC joint, and the superior bursal layer.

On anterior coronal images, the subscapularis muscle fibers and multitendinous fibers can be identified where they converge on the lesser tuberosity. Anterior coronal oblique images display the coracohumeral and coracoacromial ligaments as thin black structures. In a neutral position and with internal rotation of the humeral head, the long head of the biceps tendon is seen in the bicipital groove on anterior coronal oblique images. The long head of the biceps enters the capsule inferior to the supraspinatus tendon and can be traced to its insertion on the superior rim of the glenoid at the BLC. The coracoclavicular ligaments are also displayed on anterior coronal oblique images. The anatomy of the AC articulation is best displayed at the level of the supraspinatus tendon. When present, AC joint fluid may represent an asymptomatic manifestation of osteoarthritis.[55] The inferior glenoid labrum and axillary pouch are clearly demonstrated on these oblique images. Subscapularis bursal fluid may extend inferior and medial to the inferior glenoid on anterior coronal images.

On midcoronal images, the muscle belly of the supraspinatus extends laterally beyond the glenoid before its central tendon reaches the musculotendinous junction of the rotator cuff. The

axillary pouch of the IGL, with its attachment to the anatomic neck of the humerus and the inferior pole of the glenoid, can also be seen on these images. It is not unusual to see variable amounts of fluid in the axillary pouch in the presence of a joint effusion. Otherwise, the axillary pouch is collapsed. The presence of a glenohumeral joint effusion is associated with osteoarthritis and rotator cuff disease.[56] The axillary pouch can be followed from anterior to posterior on coronal oblique images through the shoulder.

On midcoronal to posterior coronal sections, there is a subtle transition between the supraspinatus and the conjoined insertion of the infraspinatus tendon. Posterior to the AC joint, the supra-

text continues on page 646

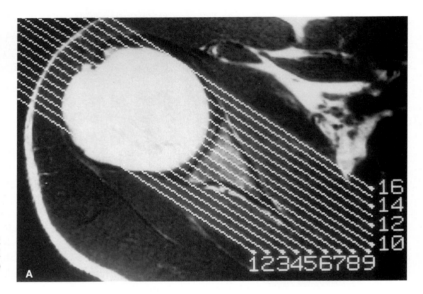

FIGURE 9-38. Normal coronal MR anatomy. **(A)** This axial localizer was used to graphically prescribe 16 coronal oblique T1-weighted image locations from **(B)** anterior to **(Q)** posterior.

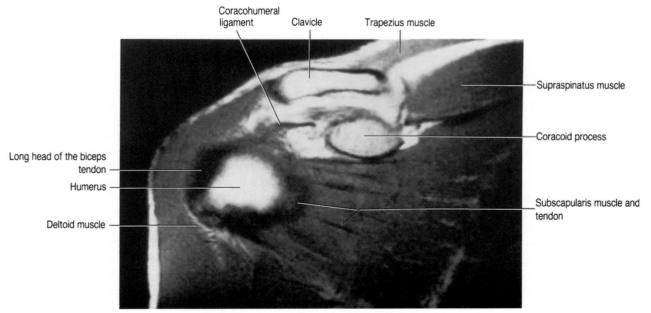

FIGURE 9-38B.

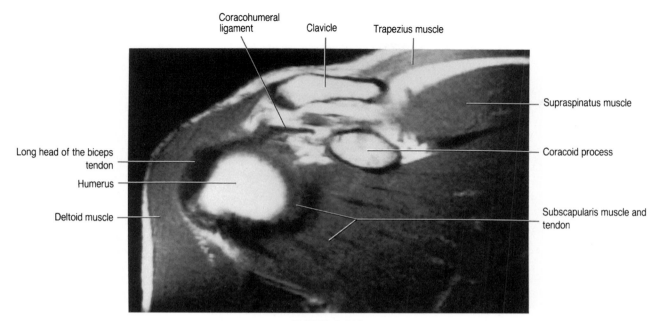

FIGURE 9-38C.

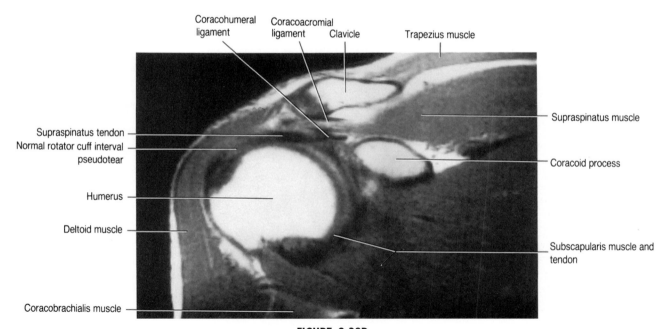

FIGURE 9-38D.

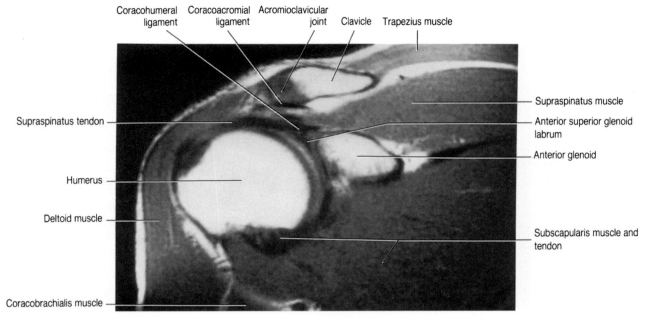

FIGURE 9-38E.

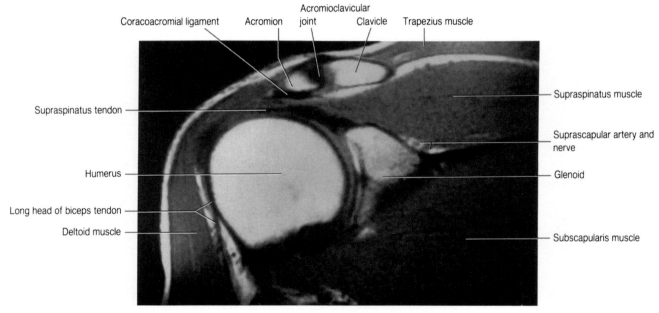

FIGURE 9-38F.

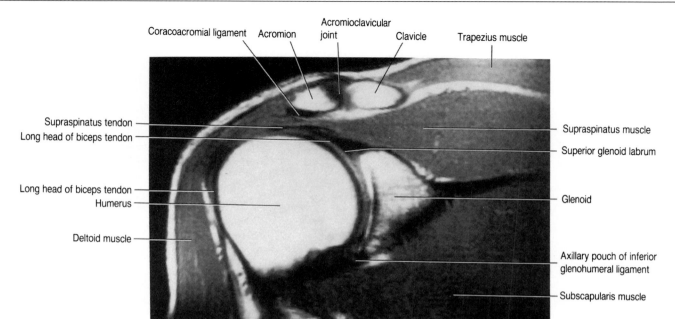

Coracoacromial ligament   Acromion   Acromioclavicular joint   Clavicle   Trapezius muscle

Supraspinatus tendon
Long head of biceps tendon

Long head of biceps tendon
Humerus

Deltoid muscle

Supraspinatus muscle
Superior glenoid labrum

Glenoid

Axillary pouch of inferior glenohumeral ligament

Subscapularis muscle

FIGURE 9-38G.

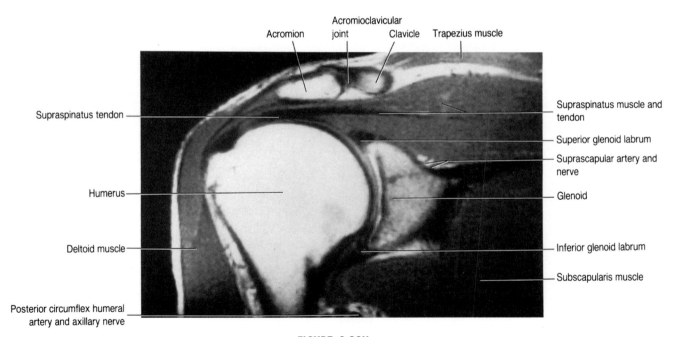

Acromion   Acromioclavicular joint   Clavicle   Trapezius muscle

Supraspinatus tendon

Humerus

Deltoid muscle

Posterior circumflex humeral artery and axillary nerve

Supraspinatus muscle and tendon
Superior glenoid labrum
Suprascapular artery and nerve
Glenoid

Inferior glenoid labrum
Subscapularis muscle

FIGURE 9-38H.

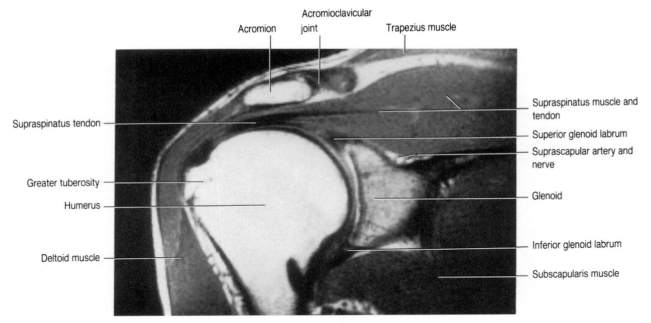

FIGURE 9-38I.

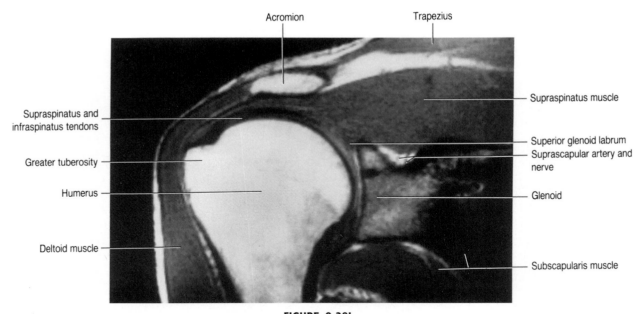

FIGURE 9-38J.

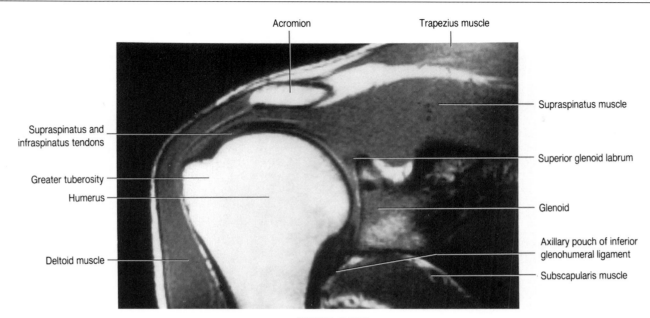

Acromion Trapezius muscle

Supraspinatus muscle

Supraspinatus and infraspinatus tendons

Superior glenoid labrum

Greater tuberosity

Humerus

Glenoid

Axillary pouch of inferior glenohumeral ligament

Deltoid muscle

Subscapularis muscle

FIGURE 9-38K.

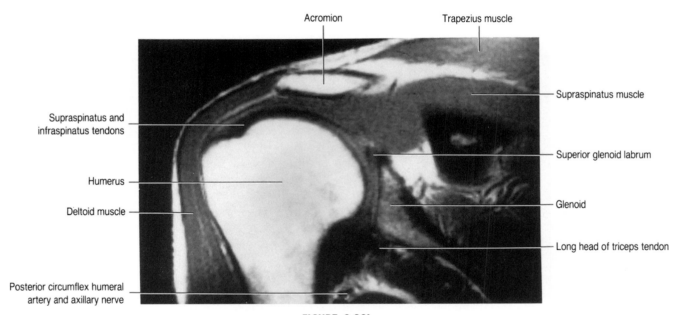

Acromion Trapezius muscle

Supraspinatus muscle

Supraspinatus and infraspinatus tendons

Superior glenoid labrum

Humerus

Deltoid muscle

Glenoid

Long head of triceps tendon

Posterior circumflex humeral artery and axillary nerve

FIGURE 9-38L.

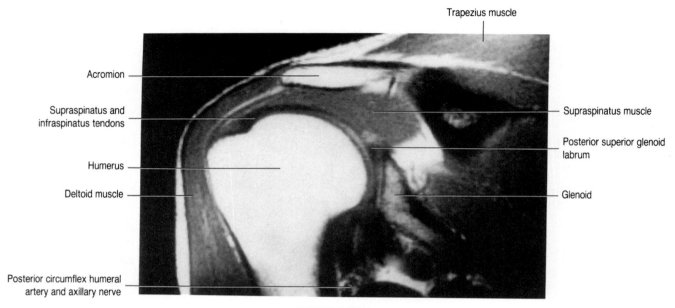

FIGURE 9-38M.

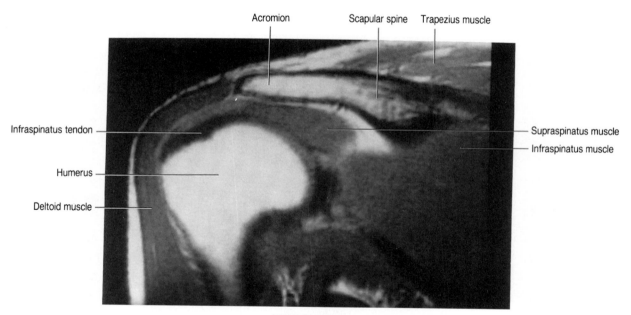

FIGURE 9-38N.

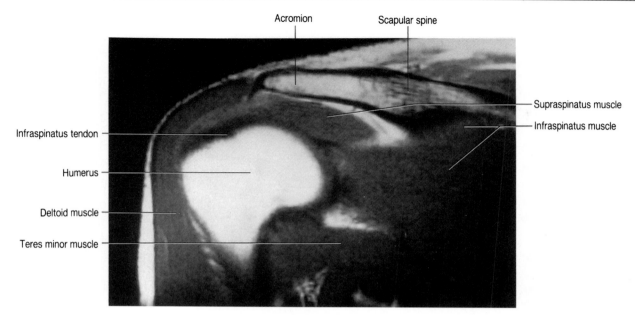

FIGURE 9-38O.

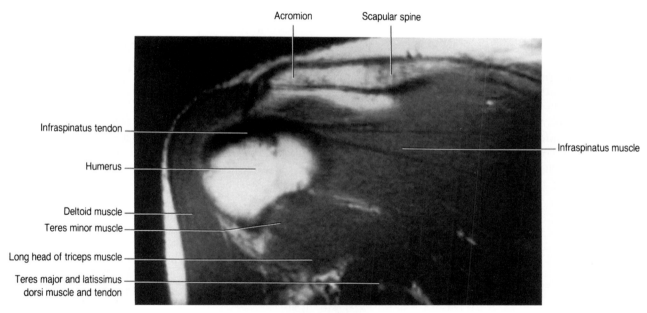

FIGURE 9-38P.

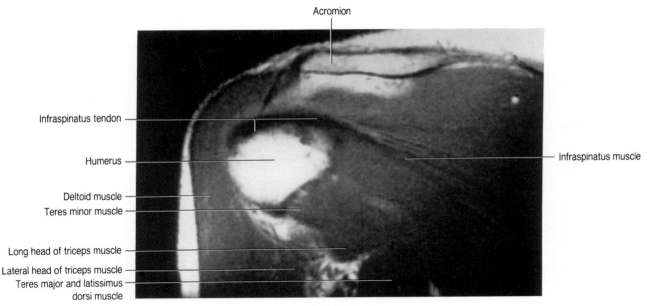

FIGURE 9-38Q.

spinatus tendon forms a conjoined attachment to the greater tuberosity with the infraspinatus tendon. On the more posterior sections, the infraspinatus tendon may be mistaken for the supraspinatus tendon, which may be out of the plane of section. Humeral head articular cartilage, intermediate in signal intensity on T1-weighted images, is interposed between the low signal intensity supraspinatus tendon superiorly and the cortex inferiorly. The posterior circumflex humeral artery and the axillary nerve are identified medial to the coracobrachialis, the latissimus dorsi, and the teres major muscles and tendons. The teres minor muscles and tendons are shown on more posterior coronal oblique images at the level of the scapular spine where the teres minor attaches to the greater tuberosity.

Sagittal Images

The muscle groups of the deltoid, supraspinatus, infraspinatus, teres minor, teres major, subscapularis, and coracobrachialis are defined on sagittal plane MR images (Fig. 9-39). On midsagittal and lateral sagittal images, the supraspinatus, infraspinatus, and

text continues on page 654

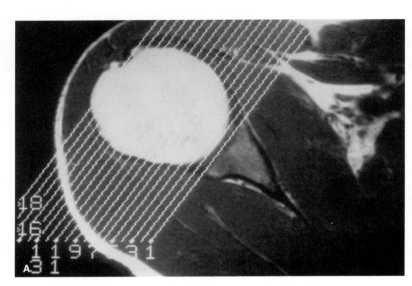

FIGURE 9-39. Normal sagittal MR anatomy. **(A)** This axial localizer was used to graphically prescribe 14 sagittal oblique T1-weighted image locations from **(B)** medial to **(O)** lateral.

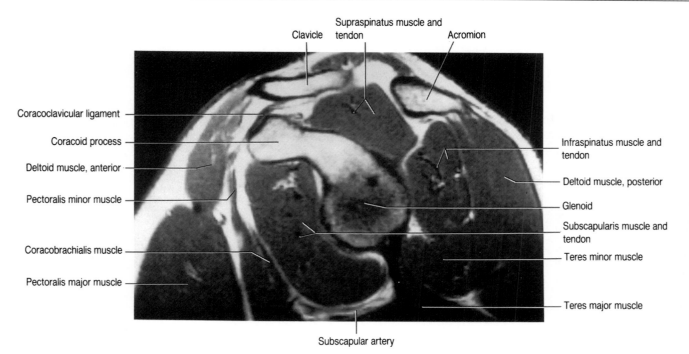

Clavicle

Supraspinatus muscle and
tendon

Acromion

Coracoclavicular ligament

Coracoid process

Deltoid muscle, anterior

Pectoralis minor muscle

Coracobrachialis muscle

Pectoralis major muscle

Infraspinatus muscle and
tendon

Deltoid muscle, posterior

Glenoid

Subscapularis muscle and
tendon

Teres minor muscle

Teres major muscle

Subscapular artery

FIGURE 9-39B.

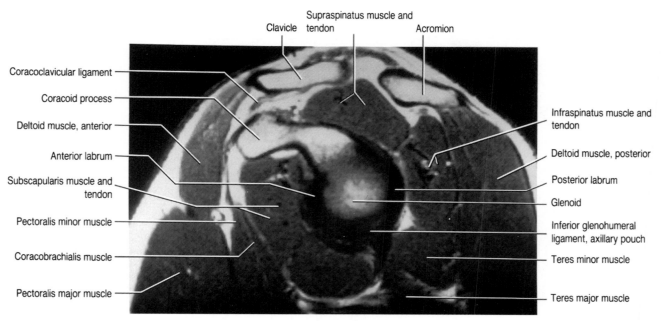

Clavicle

Supraspinatus muscle and
tendon

Acromion

Coracoclavicular ligament

Coracoid process

Deltoid muscle, anterior

Anterior labrum

Subscapularis muscle and
tendon

Pectoralis minor muscle

Coracobrachialis muscle

Pectoralis major muscle

Infraspinatus muscle and
tendon

Deltoid muscle, posterior

Posterior labrum

Glenoid

Inferior glenohumeral
ligament, axillary pouch

Teres minor muscle

Teres major muscle

FIGURE 9-39C.

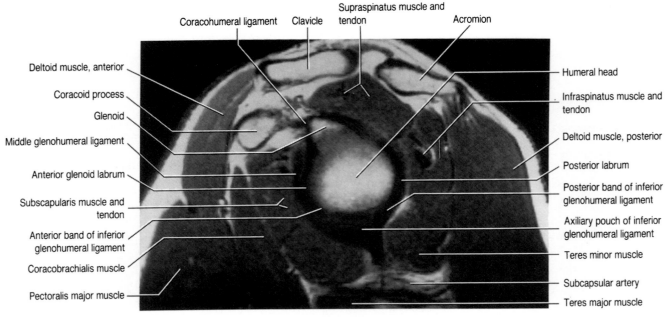

Coracohumeral ligament   Clavicle   Supraspinatus muscle and tendon   Acromion

Deltoid muscle, anterior

Coracoid process

Glenoid

Middle glenohumeral ligament

Anterior glenoid labrum

Subscapularis muscle and tendon

Anterior band of inferior glenohumeral ligament

Coracobrachialis muscle

Pectoralis major muscle

Humeral head

Infraspinatus muscle and tendon

Deltoid muscle, posterior

Posterior labrum

Posterior band of inferior glenohumeral ligament

Axillary pouch of inferior glenohumeral ligament

Teres minor muscle

Subcapsular artery

Teres major muscle

FIGURE 9-39D.

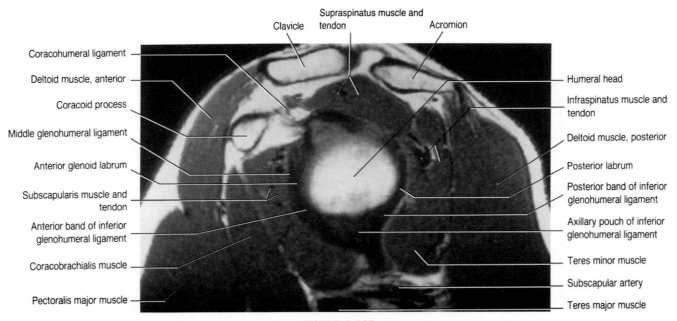

Clavicle   Supraspinatus muscle and tendon   Acromion

Coracohumeral ligament

Deltoid muscle, anterior

Coracoid process

Middle glenohumeral ligament

Anterior glenoid labrum

Subscapularis muscle and tendon

Anterior band of inferior glenohumeral ligament

Coracobrachialis muscle

Pectoralis major muscle

Humeral head

Infraspinatus muscle and tendon

Deltoid muscle, posterior

Posterior labrum

Posterior band of inferior glenohumeral ligament

Axillary pouch of inferior glenohumeral ligament

Teres minor muscle

Subscapular artery

Teres major muscle

FIGURE 9-39E.

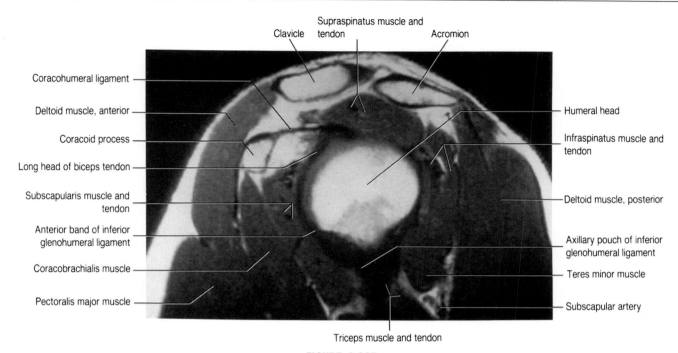

Clavicle

Supraspinatus muscle and
tendon

Acromion

Coracohumeral ligament

Deltoid muscle, anterior

Coracoid process

Long head of biceps tendon

Subscapularis muscle and
tendon

Anterior band of inferior
glenohumeral ligament

Coracobrachialis muscle

Pectoralis major muscle

Humeral head

Infraspinatus muscle and
tendon

Deltoid muscle, posterior

Axillary pouch of inferior
glenohumeral ligament

Teres minor muscle

Subscapular artery

Triceps muscle and tendon

FIGURE 9-39F.

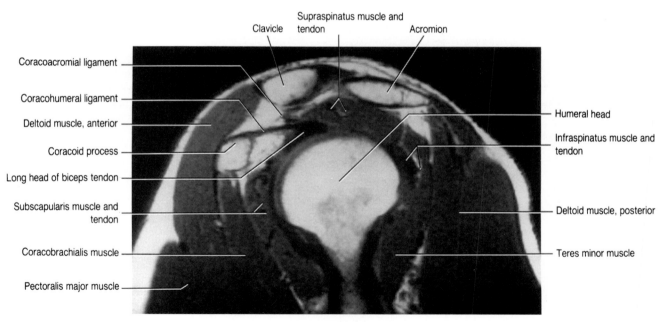

Clavicle

Supraspinatus muscle and
tendon

Acromion

Coracoacromial ligament

Coracohumeral ligament

Deltoid muscle, anterior

Coracoid process

Long head of biceps tendon

Subscapularis muscle and
tendon

Coracobrachialis muscle

Pectoralis major muscle

Humeral head

Infraspinatus muscle and
tendon

Deltoid muscle, posterior

Teres minor muscle

FIGURE 9-39G.

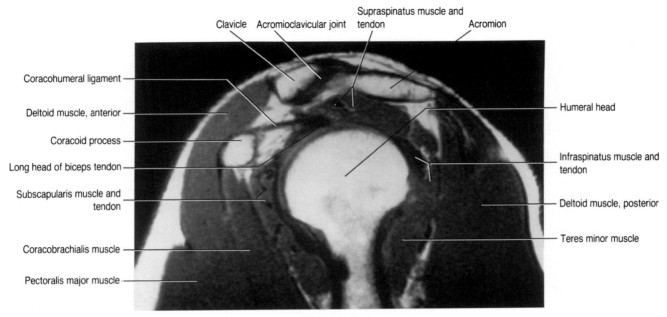

FIGURE 9-39H.

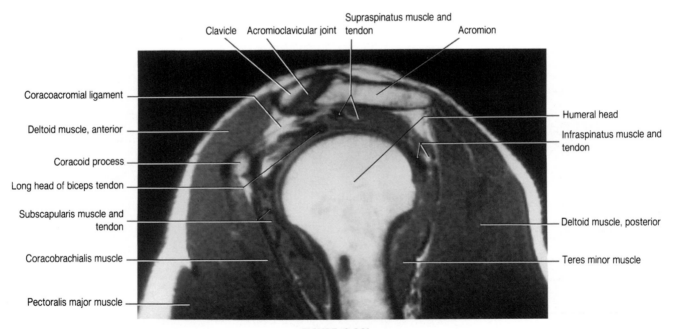

FIGURE 9-39I.

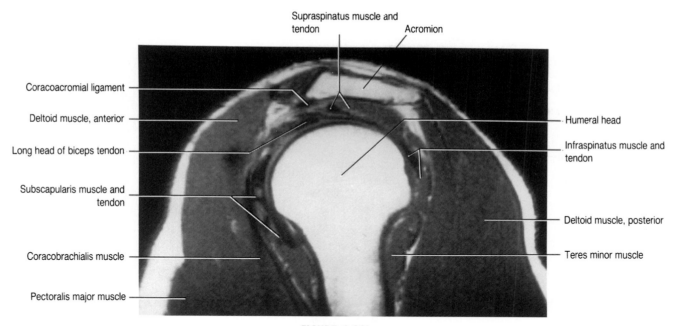

Supraspinatus muscle and tendon

Acromion

Coracoacromial ligament

Deltoid muscle, anterior

Long head of biceps tendon

Subscapularis muscle and tendon

Coracobrachialis muscle

Pectoralis major muscle

Humeral head

Infraspinatus muscle and tendon

Deltoid muscle, posterior

Teres minor muscle

FIGURE 9-39J.

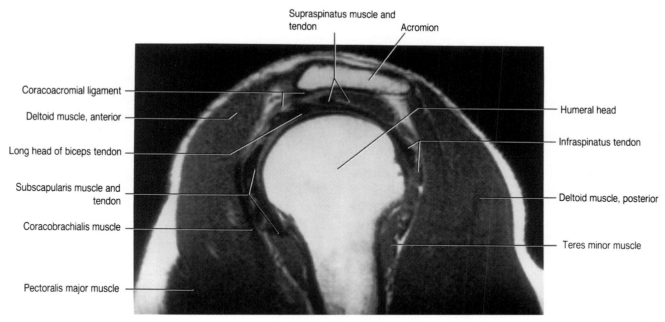

Supraspinatus muscle and tendon

Acromion

Coracoacromial ligament

Deltoid muscle, anterior

Long head of biceps tendon

Subscapularis muscle and tendon

Coracobrachialis muscle

Pectoralis major muscle

Humeral head

Infraspinatus tendon

Deltoid muscle, posterior

Teres minor muscle

FIGURE 9-39K.

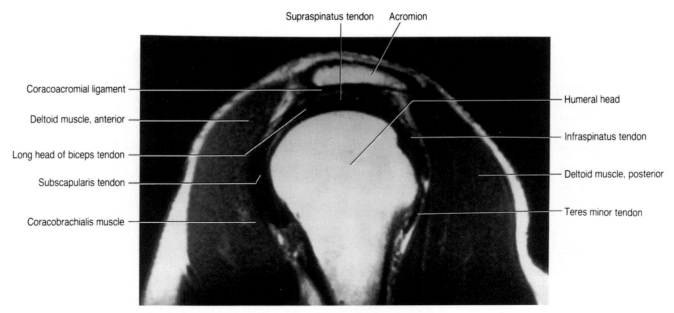

FIGURE 9-39L.

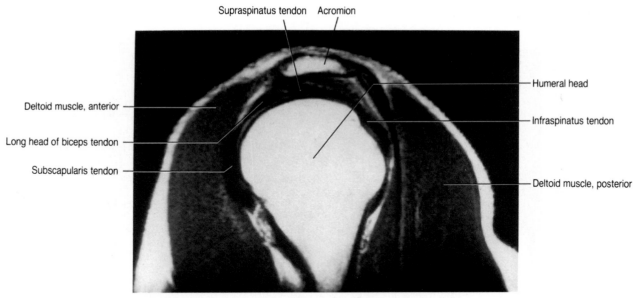

FIGURE 9-39M.

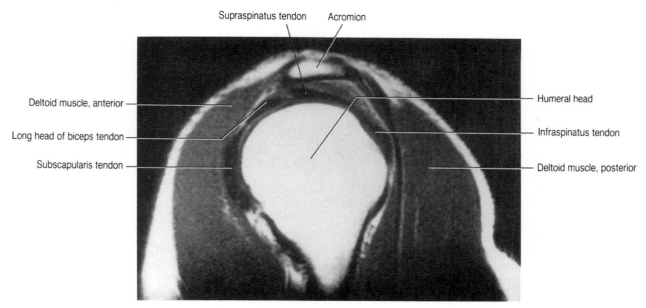

Supraspinatus tendon   Acromion

Deltoid muscle, anterior

Long head of biceps tendon

Subscapularis tendon

Humeral head

Infraspinatus tendon

Deltoid muscle, posterior

FIGURE 9-39N.

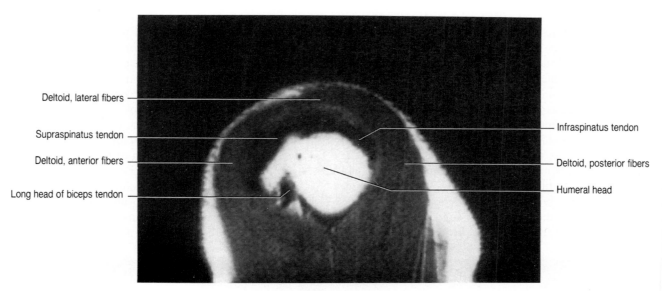

Deltoid, lateral fibers

Supraspinatus tendon

Deltoid, anterior fibers

Long head of biceps tendon

Infraspinatus tendon

Deltoid, posterior fibers

Humeral head

FIGURE 9-39O.

the conjoined cuff tendons demonstrate low signal intensity between the acromion and the superior articular surfaces of the humeral head. The thickened tendon seen in the anterior half of the sagittal images is the supraspinatus component, whereas the flatter tendon that arches over the posterior half of the humeral head is the infraspinatus component. The long head of the biceps tendon is identified anterior and inferior to the supraspinatus tendon on lateral sagittal images, and can be followed to its attachment to the BLC at the level of the glenohumeral joint. Toward the glenoid, the coracoacromial ligament is seen as a low signal intensity band that arches over the anterior aspect of the rotator cuff from the acromion and coracoid. Medial sagittal sections display the clavicle and AC joint in profile. The oblique transversely oriented physis is also delineated on sagittal images. Marrow inhomogeneity, seen frequently as red-to-yellow marrow conversion, may not be complete distal to the physis in the metadiaphyseal region.[57]

The low signal intensity glenoid labrum is also defined on sagittal images that transsect the glenohumeral joint. The anterior band of the IGL can be seen extending anterior and superior, to become the anterior labrum. The MGL is seen anterior to the anterior labrum. The subscapularis tendon is located anterior to the MGL. This relationship is constant, even though the MGL may be variable in size and shape. The MGL may also be absent. The axillary pouch extends between the anterior and posterior bands of the IGL.

Medial sagittal images demonstrate the coracoclavicular ligaments. The low spin density tendon of the supraspinatus is identified in the anterior portion of the supraspinatus muscle. The pectoralis minor and coracobrachialis muscles are anterior to the coracoid process. The axillary artery, vein, and brachial plexus are anterior to the subscapularis muscle, deep to the pectoralis minor. The subscapularis muscle and tendon are anterior to the capsule of the glenohumeral joint. The long head of the biceps tendon enters the joint capsule superiorly, anterior and inferior to the supraspinatus tendon. The SGL lies anterior to the humeral head and glenoid, and

inferior to the long head of the biceps tendon. The MGL is anterior to the medial humeral head or lateral glenoid. The thick inferior glenoid labrum is seen as a low signal intensity structure along the inferior aspect of the glenoid.

PATHOLOGY OF THE SHOULDER

Shoulder Impingement Syndrome

Pathogenesis

Degenerative changes develop where the tendinous fibers of the rotator cuff attach to the greater tuberosity, most often in the area of the insertion of the supraspinatus tendon. This tendon—anatomically confined, under tension, and compressed between bony structures at both its inferior and superior surfaces—is at risk for acute injury and chronic wear. Bursal inflammation and tendinitis produced by the compression may cause pain and lead to disuse atrophy of the supraspinatus and infraspinatus in the subacromial space. A hooked type 3 acromion with weakness leads to loss of the centralizing forces of these muscles, and increased compression can be a further negative factor. The chronic compressive and irritative forces cause changes in the coracoacromial ligament, producing an anterior spur that may contribute to further impingement in the subacromial space (Fig. 9-40).

The pathogenesis of rotator cuff tears includes acute trauma, chronic impingement, or both.[58-62] Some controversy exists as to whether chronic mechanical impingement precedes the development of complete rotator cuff lesions or whether primary degeneration of the cuff (Fig. 9-41) results in tears leading to chronic impingement syndrome.

There is an important relationship among the rotator cuff, the long head of the biceps, the subacromial bursa, the AC joint, the acromion, and the humeral head in the spectrum of impingement disorders.[52,63] The most common location

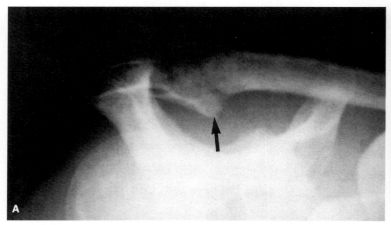
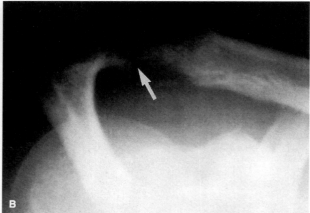

FIGURE 9-40. The outlet view (ie, lateral view of the scapula) shows the anterior acromial spur encroaching upon the supraspinatus outlet prior to acromioplasty (**A,** *black arrow*) and after acromioplasty (**B,** *white arrow*).

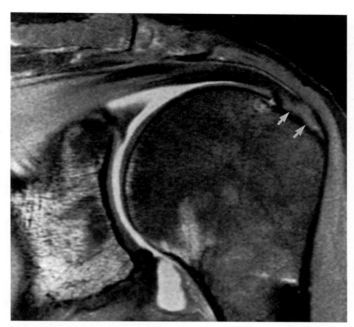

FIGURE 9-41. Rotator cuff tendinitis with intermediate signal intensity tendon degeneration (*arrows*) involving the distal cuff. No acromial spur or acromioclavicular osteophyte are present in this shoulder. Fat-suppressed T2-weighted fast spin-echo coronal oblique MR arthrogram.

for impingement is between the anterior one third of the acromion and the underlying tendons. Painful impingement syndrome is the most common presenting picture in rotator cuff lesions. The importance of the lateral edge of the acromion has been minimized, and the posterior portion of the acromion is no longer thought to be implicated in impingement. A decrease in the subacromial space secondary to anatomic or pathologic changes is usually associated with a large tear that has compromised the centralizing ability of the cuff, allowing proximal humeral migration.[64]

Etiology

A variety of causes has been proposed in the painful shoulder impingement syndrome, including hypovascularity in the supraspinatus tendon, mechanical wear, acute trauma, or repetitive microtrauma from overuse (this latter is especially common in athletes who use a throwing motion or work activities that emphasize over-hand motions).[65,66]

Factors that contribute to bony supraspinatus outlet compromise include anterior acromial spurs, the shape of the acromion (eg, curved or overhanging edge), the slope of the acromion (eg, flat or decreased angle), and the morphology of the AC joint (eg, hypertrophic bone, callus formation).[52,67,68] Less frequent mechanisms of impingement (not outlet impingement) include prominence of the greater tuberosity (eg, fracture, malunion, or nonunion); loss of humeral head depressors,[69] as seen in rotator cuff tears and biceps

tendon rupture; loss of the glenohumeral joint fulcrum function from articular surface destruction or ligamentous laxity; impaired scapular rotation from trapezius paralysis or AC joint disruption; lesions of the acromion, including an unfused anterior acromial epiphysis (apophysis); fracture malunion or nonunion; and subacromial bursal thickening (chronic bursitis or cuff thickening in calcific tendinitis). The shape of the acromion (acromial morphology), as seen on sagittal oblique MR images or on the outlet view on plain film radiographs, is also thought to be a factor in the etiology of impingement syndrome. Acromial morphology has been classified into three different types by Bigliani and associates[67] (Fig. 9-42). The type 1 acromion has a flat undersurface; the type 2 acromion has a smooth, curved, inferior surface; and the type 3 acromion has an anterior hook or beak. It is the type 3 acromion that is thought to be associated with a greater predisposition to rotator cuff tears (ie, tears involving the critical zone immediately proximal to the greater tuberosity insertion of the supraspinatus tendon). In the clinical series of Morrison and Bigliani,[70] 80% of patients with rotator cuff tears had type 3 acromions. Fukuda and colleagues[71] showed that the site of bursal-sided partial cuff tears corresponds to anterior inferior acromial impingement, and correlates with histological changes of degeneration.[71] This supports Neer's hypothesis that the majority of rotator cuff tears are caused by mechanical impingement leading to tendinitis, fibrosis, bursal surface pathology (partial tear), and eventual full thickness cuff tears.[62,72]

Neer has developed a three-stage classification system for impingement.[62] In this system, subacromial impingement is presented as a mechanical process of progressive wear (ie, a pretear impingement lesion) that causes 95% of rotator cuff tears.[58–60,62] The degeneration, thinning, and full thickness tears of the supraspinatus may extend to involve the long head of the biceps and infraspinatus tendons.

In stage 1 of Neer's classification, tendon edema and hemorrhage are present. Stage 2 is characterized by fibrosis and tendinitis. No radiographic findings or reversible changes are found in stage 1 or stage 2 impingement. In stage 3, a partial or complete rupture or tear of the rotator cuff is found, often in association with anterior acromial spurring or greater tuberosity excrescence. When present, radiographic changes include greater tuberosity sclerosis and hypertrophic bone formation. Bursal thickening, fibrosis, and partial tears of the superficial rotator cuff may be present.

Rotator cuff tendons examined at surgery display areas appearing gray, dull, edematous, and friable.[72] Degenerative changes, including angiofibroblastic hyperplasia without inflammatory cells, can be seen on correlative histologic examination. Because leukocyte infiltration of the rotator cuff tendons is rare, the tendinitis or inflammation of the cuff (especially in the later stages of rotator cuff pathology) as described in Neer's classification has not been adequately documented.[64]

Arthroscopic visualization of the rotator cuff from the articular and bursal surfaces has given us new perspectives

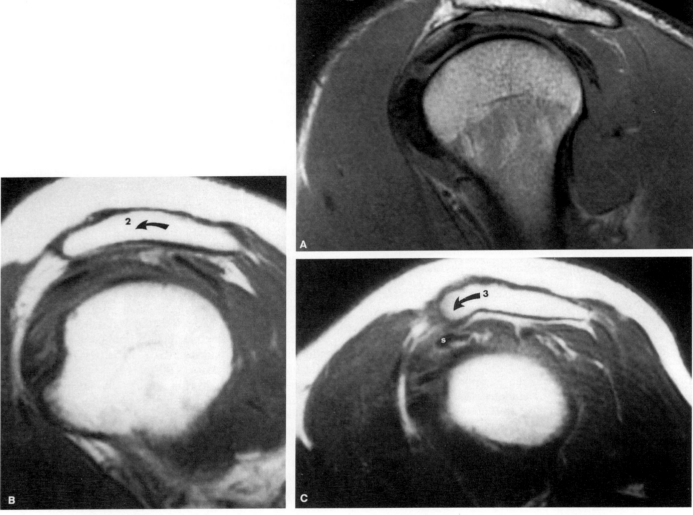

FIGURE 9-42. Acromial shapes. **(A)** Type 1 acromion (1) is predominantly flat in the sagittal oblique plane. **(B)** Type 2 acromion (2) demonstrates a mild symmetric curve or arc relative to the humeral head (*arrow*). **(C)** Type 3 acromion (3) with anterior hook morphology narrows the acromiohumeral distance (*arrow*). s, supraspinatus tendon. Type 3 acromion is thought to be associated with critical zone tears of the rotator cuff immediately proximal to the greater tuberosity insertion of the supraspinatus tendon.

on the progression of this disease process. We now have the advantage of a complete diagnostic arthroscopic evaluation of the entire glenohumeral joint to look for articular damage, labral tears, biceps labral lesions, and loose bodies, as well as articular surface tears of the rotator cuff. Similarly, we can inspect the subacromial space for ''kissing'' erosive lesions of the coracoacromial ligament and rotator cuff. The bursal view allows better evaluation of the extent and amenability to repair of full thickness rotator cuff tears. Thus, the progressive stages of impingement might be more accurately described as follows:

- Type 1: Rotator cuff degeneration or tendinosis without visible tears of either surface
- Type 2: Rotator cuff degeneration or tendinosis with partial thickness tears of either articular or bursal surfaces
- Type 3: Complete thickness rotator cuff tears of varying size, complexity, and functional compromise.

Most rotator cuff tears do not begin at the bursal surface of the tendon, as tears secondary to impingement had originally been described. Partial tears of the rotator cuff involving the articular surface of the rotator cuff adjacent to the tendon insertion, in fact, are more commonly seen.[64,73] Articular cuff lesions may be the result of tensile strength failure from overuse, whereas bursal cuff lesions are more closely associated with impingement.[73,74] Because a direct mechanical cause of impingement is frequently not found in patients with suspected impingement syndrome, intrinsic tendon degeneration (degenerative tendinopathy), and not mechanical impingement, may be the primary pathology in the development of most rotator cuff disorders.[72] Rotator cuff tendinitis has been attributed to repeated eccentric tensile overload of the rotator cuff tendons. Nirschl found acromial spurs in only 10% of patients referred for surgery for rotator cuff tendinitis.[75] Rotator cuff degeneration has also been observed in the absence of anteroinferior acromial spurs.[74] Ozaki and colleagues[68] found that bursal-sided and full thickness rotator cuff tears correlated with degenerative changes of the coracoacromial ligament and anterior third of the inferior acromion. Articular surface partial tears, however, were associated with normal acromial morphology and histology. Most tears of the rotator cuff were thus attributed to degenerative lesions that were associated with increasing age, and the acromial changes present were secondary. Athletes may demonstrate both degenerative rotator cuff tendinitis and primary mechanical impingement.[73]

Relative rotator cuff hypovascularity in the critical zone of the supraspinatus (the distal 1 cm) may be associated with tendon degeneration or may exacerbate changes associated with mechanical impingement.[72] The area of avascularity may be dependent on arm position, with decreased vascular perfusion when the arm is in the abducted position and normal perfusion with the arm adducted.[66]

In the Neer classification system of well-defined stages of impingement (edema, hemorrhage, fibrosis, and tendinitis leading to spur formation), cuff tear may be more correctly viewed as part of a progression of tendon degeneration leading to tendinopathy, with the subsequent development of a partial or complete rotator cuff tear and associated secondary changes.

Magnetic Resonance Appearance

The spectrum of MR changes in shoulder impingement have been characterized and documented.[20,37,58,76,77] Rotator cuff disease is evaluated on the basis of tendon morphology and changes in the observed signal intensity within the specific cuff tendons. In addition, pathologic processes in the coracoacromial arch—including the acromion, the AC joint, and the subacromial-subdeltoid bursa—may be identified in the spectrum of findings in impingement lesions.

SUBACROMIAL-SUBDELTOID BURSITIS.   The changes in the subacromial bursa are generally thought to be secondary to tendon degeneration or tendinopathy as part of impingement[78,79] (Fig. 9-43). Normally, the subacromial-subdeltoid bursa is small, with a flat and noninflamed synovial lining.[80] Identification of this structure, and of signal intensity within the peribursal fat, can be used to describe subacromial bursitis on MR images.[58,81] Bursal inflammation is seen as decreased signal intensity—or loss of peribursal fat—on T1-weighted images and increased signal intensity—from associated fluid, inflammation, or bursal proliferative disease—on conventional T2 or fat-suppressed T2-weighted fast spin-echo sequences (Fig. 9-44). Although the changes of subacromial bursal inflammation are usually associated with tendinitis or cuff tear, the finding of small amounts of subacromial bursal fluid may be seen without abnormal cuff

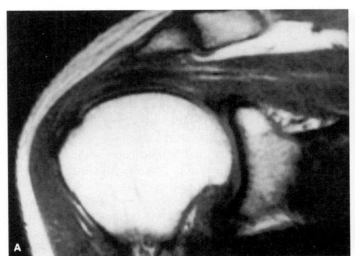
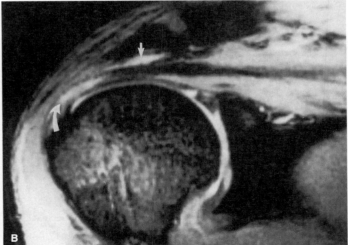

FIGURE 9-43. **(A)** T1-weighted and **(B)** T2*-weighted coronal oblique images show bursal surface inflammation (*curved arrow*) of the supraspinatus tendon without tear at arthroscopy. There is a small amount of subacromial-subdeltoid bursal fluid (*straight arrow*) in the absence of a rotator cuff tear.

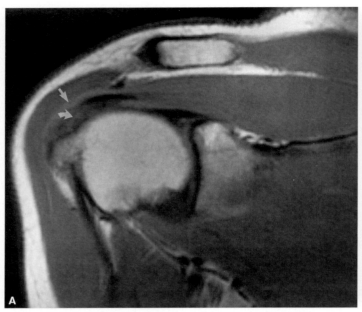

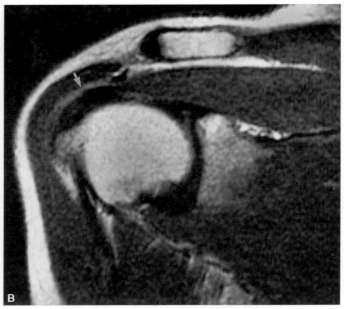

FIGURE 9-44. Subacromial-subdeltoid bursal thickening and hyperintensity (*straight arrow*) associated with supraspinatus tendon degeneration (*curved arrow*). (**A**) Intermediate- and (**B**) T2-weighted coronal oblique images. Tendon degeneration does not show any further increase in signal intensity with T2 weighting (**B**).

morphology or signal intensity alterations (Fig. 9-45). Low signal intensity within a thickened subacromial bursa on T1- and T2-weighted images indicates a proliferative process in chronic bursitis, also associated with rotator cuff disease.[82]

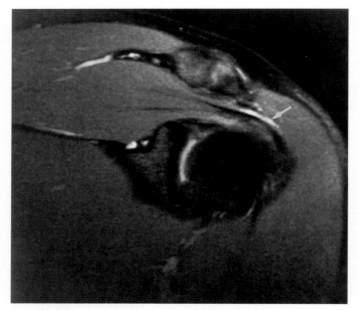

FIGURE 9-45. Subacromial bursal fluid (*arrow*) associated with normal hypointense supraspinatus tendon on a fat-suppressed T2-weighted fast spin-echo coronal oblique image. Increased signal intensity involving the distal clavicle and adjacent acromion represent degenerative AC joint disease.

Subacromial bursal thickening occurs in Neer's stage 2 impingement, although the subacromial bursa may not show any surgical signs of scarring in chronic impingement.[64,83] In our experience, the presence or absence of subacromial fat is a variable finding in asymptomatic volunteers and in the various stages of impingement. Fat-suppressed T2-weighted fast spin-echo images are more sensitive than conventional T2 or non–fat-suppressed T2-weighted fast spin-echo sequences in identifying small amounts of subacromial bursal fluid on coronal oblique or axial images. The subacromial bursa may be distended with fluid in both partial and complete rotator cuff tears. It is unusual to see a fluid-filled bursa in the presence of a normal cuff.

ROTATOR CUFF DEGENERATION AND PITFALLS. The normal rotator cuff tendons display low signal intensity on T1, conventional T2, T2-weighted fast spin-echo, fat-suppressed T2-weighted fast spin-echo, STIR, and T2* gradient-echo sequences. Areas of intermediate signal intensity or signal inhomogeneity, especially in the distal extent of the supraspinatus tendon on T1 and proton density weighted images, can be seen in both cadaver cuffs and asymptomatic volunteers.[84,85] These changes have been variously attributed to a "magic-angle phenomenon," partial volume averaging of the distinct components of the supraspinatus muscle and tendon, or to histologic degeneration (eosinophilic, fibrillar and mucoid).[86]

In the magic-angle phenomenon, tendon orientation at the magic-angle of 55° to B_0 contributes to increased signal intensity in the supraspinatus tendon on short TR/TE sequences.[87] These signal effects may also be seen on gradient-echo and fat-suppressed images. The routine use of T2-weighted images and observation of cuff morphology should minimize misinterpretation of these affected segments of the rotator cuff. It may be difficult, however, to distinguish between a "magic-angle effect" and early changes of cuff degeneration.

A partial volume averaging effect of tendon, muscle, connective tissue, or fat has not been accepted as an explanation of areas of intermediate signal intensity within the asymptomatic cuff on short TR/TE weighted images with the shoulder in a neutral position or in external rotation. Persistent cuff signal intensity has been shown independent of different imaging orientations along the axis of the supraspinatus tendon and muscle.[88] Interposed muscle has not been described in or near cuff insertions.[89,90]

The pseudogap is a zone of increased signal intensity seen adjacent to the supraspinatus tendon attachment in asymptomatic subjects. The pseudogap has been attributed to distinct portions of the supraspinatus muscle,[88] including the anterior fusiform portion, containing the dominant tendon of the supraspinatus, and a strap-like posterior portion. The orientation of the tendon differs from the main muscle by 10°. The pseudogap signal is not related to fat and is thought to represent a focal difference in tissue relaxation parameters.

In cuff tendon degeneration, there are areas of intermediate signal intensity on T1 and proton density weighted images, which display intermediate to high signal intensity on T2*, fat-suppressed T2-weighted fast spin-echo, and STIR sequences in both asymptomatic and symptomatic patients. On heavily weighted T2 or T2-weighted fast spin-echo images, however, these regions of altered signal intensity are diminished or remain unchanged.

IMPINGEMENT LESIONS OF THE ROTATOR CUFF. MR findings in degeneration and partial tears may overlap, and tendon pathology must be evaluated on the basis of bursal, intrasubstance, and articular surface morphology, and on signal intensity changes on T1, proton density, T2, or T2-weighted fast spin-echo sequences. Evaluation is best accomplished with coronal oblique and sagittal oblique planar images. The axial plane may be used secondarily, to evaluate specific sites or locations of abnormal tendon signal intensity.

In rotator cuff degeneration, there is intermediate signal intensity in cuff degeneration on T1 or proton density weighted images, with no increase in signal intensity on T2 or T2-weighted fast spin-echo images (Fig. 9-46). Fat-suppressed T2-weighted fast spin-echo sequences (TEs of 40 to 50 msec) are sensitive to changes of degeneration, and, in the absence of a partial or complete rotator cuff tear, display areas or regions of hyperintensity. T2* gradient-echo images in either the coronal oblique or sagittal oblique plane are not routinely used in the evaluation of the rotator cuff, because these images produce signal intensity, which may

be difficult to distinguish from that seen in degenerations and partial tears (see Fig. 9-43). Changes of tendon degeneration are seen as an age-related phenomenon in older patients and in normal asymptomatic volunteers. More severe changes of degeneration may be characterized by intermediate to increased signal intensity on short TE or T1 and proton density weighted images, which persist without further increase in signal intensity on T2-weighted images. These tendons may appear gray on long TE sequences. Increased signal intensity on short and long TE images (conventional T2 and fast spin-echo T2), with a further increase in signal intensity between T1 or proton density and T2-weighted images, is associated with a partial or full thickness tear. Differentiating severe tendinitis and partial tears may require careful attention to the continuity of the bursal and articular surfaces of the cuff as well as the increased signal intensity observed on both short and long TE images. Secondary findings of musculotendinous retraction and atrophy of the supraspinatus muscle are seen with complete cuff tears. Low signal intensity may be identified on T1- and T2-weighted images in areas of severe degeneration or tear obliterated by scar tissue or tendon remnants.[91]

The signal intensity changes described in degeneration are the result of macromolecular collagen changes.[73] In the normal tendon, there is no significant molecular motion of water, which is tightly bound to collagen macromolecules. Damage to collagen fibers is associated with an increase in absorbed water. The increased amount of absorbed water increases T2 relaxation times, resulting in hyperintensity from water molecules on short TE images. In severe degeneration and tears, there is a greater amount of free water within tendon defects, resulting in a long T2 and high signal intensity on long TE or T2-weighted spin-echo images. The increased signal intensity detected on T2-weighted sequences reflects significant macromolecular disruption, as would be seen in severe tendon degeneration or tears.

These imaging characteristics are used by Seeger and coworkers[58] in their classification of impingement lesions. In this system, impingement lesions are grouped into several types based on coronal plane MR images.[58] Type 1 impingement is characterized by the presence of subacromial bursitis, and signal intensity in the supraspinatus may remain normal. Isolated subacromial bursitis is an infrequent finding on MR images; however, it is usually associated with tendinitis. This is substantiated by postmortem and histologic studies in the surgical literature.[92–96] In Seeger's type 2 impingement, the supraspinatus tendon demonstrates increased signal intensity on T1-weighted images. Increased signal intensity on T2-weighted images is considered a type 2b change, and may represent a partial tear. Type 3 impingement is characterized by a complete tear of the rotator cuff, with or without supraspinatus retraction. Complete tears exist only in type 3 impingement, and in this classification system high signal intensity of the supraspinatus tendon on conventional T2-weighted images is considered pathognomonic for a tear.

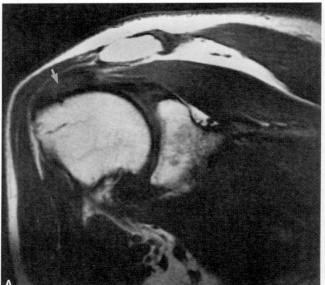

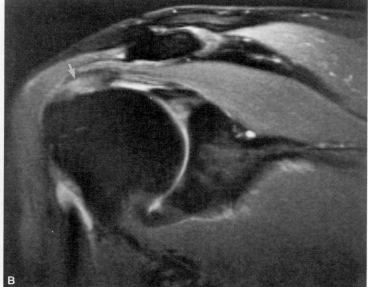

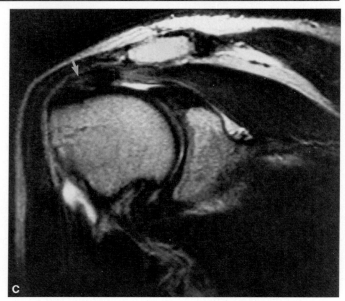

FIGURE 9-46. Rotator cuff degeneration (*arrow*) displays intermediate tendon signal intensity on a T1-weighted image (**A**), hyperintensity on a fat-suppressed T2-weighted fast spin-echo image (**B**), and intermediate signal intensity on a T2-weighted fast spin-echo image (**C**). Note that although cuff degeneration demonstrates increased signal intensity with the addition of fat-suppression, T2-weighted fast spin-echo images without fat-suppression and T1-weighted sequences show similar signal intensity. (**A** through **C**: coronal oblique images.)

In Zlatkin's grading system (grades 0 to 3) for characterization of the rotator cuff tendons, tendinitis with normal morphology (grade 1) is differentiated from tendinitis or tendon degeneration with abnormal morphology (grade 2).[22] Associated tendinous enlargement, which may be seen in the more acute stages of impingement, is still considered normal morphology (normal tendon outlines). In both grade 1 and grade 2 tendons, there is increased signal intensity on T1-weighted and proton density weighted images, without any further increase in signal intensity on T2-weighted images. A grade 3 tendon demonstrates both morphologic changes (a tendinous defect) and signal intensity changes (increased signal intensity on T2-weighted images). This increased signal intensity is related to corresponding T1-weighted (short TR/TE) and proton density weighted (long

TR/short TE) images, and is seen within the tendon defect as bright signal intensity from fluid. A grade 3 tendon represents a rotator cuff tear. Because Zlatkin specifically uses the term "degeneration" to designate surface morphologic changes (ie, thinning or irregularity) of the tendon, separate from histologic findings of degeneration, a grade 2 tendon with abnormal morphology by definition may represent tendinitis with superficial tendon degeneration or a partial rotator cuff tear. Thus, a rotator cuff tear may exhibit abnormal morphology (attenuation) but not increased signal intensity on T2-weighted images. In addition, the association of small amounts of fluid in the subacromial bursa or loss of the subacromial-subdeltoid fat plane on T1-weighted images, are not reliable secondary signs for distinguishing between degeneration and tears. The increased sensitivity of T2* gradient-echo images in detecting increases in tendon signal intensity may be secondary to increased proton density or prolonged T1 or T2 values. Careful evaluation of bursal and articular surfaces is necessary to identify the possible development of a partial tear.

Histologically, the inflammation and mucoid degeneration, seen on tendon biopsy specimens, is thought to correlate with increased signal intensity on T1 and proton density weighted images.[77] Both Raffi and colleagues and Kjellin and colleagues propose that areas of increased signal intensity in the supraspinatus tendon on proton density weighted images represent degeneration (eosinophilic, fibrillar, and mucoid) and scarring, and not active inflammation.[84,91] This is consistent with the fact that leukocytic infiltration of the rotator cuff tendons is rare. These studies support our observations of increased signal intensity in the supraspinatus tendon in some asymptomatic patients on short TR/TE, proton density, and T2*-weighted images.[85,97]

Raffi and colleagues suggest that tendinous enlargement associated with homogeneous or nonhomogeneous increased signal intensity is a more specific finding in symptomatic shoulders with tendinitis.[91] Tendinous enlargement, or the increased signal intensity of tendon degeneration, may also characterize the reparative process and healing of an interstitial tear.

It would seem that the common usage of the term tendinitis, which implies active inflammation, without histologic confirmation, may be imprecise in characterizing tendon signal intensity alterations. Kjellin and coworkers suggest the use of the term tendinosis or tendinopathy in such cases.[84]

In arthroscopic correlations of MR imaging and findings, degenerative tendon wear may be identified on the bursal or articular surface of the rotator cuff. Not all cuff tears are initiated on the bursal surface as a result of impingement. Most tears begin in the articular surface of the rotator cuff, adjacent to the tendon insertion on the greater tuberosity. In early impingement (pretear tendinitis), there is relative preservation of articular bursal tendon surface outlines. In addition, arthroscopic evaluation of impingement sometimes reveals tendon wear (degeneration with or without associated degenerative changes of the acromion and the coracoacromial ligament proximally) and not active inflammation.

Because the term tendinosis is not widely accepted, we characterize an area of increased signal intensity on intermediate weighted images without an increase in signal intensity on T2-weighted images as tendon degeneration. Impingement is a clinical diagnosis, not a radiologic or MR diagnosis.[98] The tendon findings or osseous changes seen in the impingement syndrome may be identified and described on MR images when patients are referred for study to determine whether these findings, in conjunction with the patient's clinical presentation, are consistent with impingement syndrome.

There are several pitfalls to be avoided in the interpretation of MR findings. For instance, although the subacromial peribursal fat plane is usually preserved on T1-weighted images in the early stages of impingement, it may be effaced by bursal surface inflammation in the absence of a rotator cuff tear.[58] Another pitfall is the appearance of an area of increased signal intensity on T2-weighted (long TR/long TE) sequences caused by the injection of long-acting steroids and local anesthetics used in the diagnosis and treatment of impingement. Prior use of this technique should be taken into consideration in order to decrease false-positive diagnoses.[61]

In addition to articular and bursal tendon degeneration, intrasubstance degeneration may also be associated with intrasubstance partial tears. Although intrasubstance cuff pathology can be identified on MR images, these changes are usually not confirmed on arthroscopic surface evaluations. Conventional and Gd-DTPA–enhanced MR imaging are also negative for intrasubstance degeneration and tear.

Arthroscopic Classification of Impingement

Arthroscopy allows identification of all structures involved in the impingement syndrome and determination of the cause and effect of the pathology in each case. Arthroscopic classification also allows more precise communication among clinicians, which has contributed to the development of a well-defined approach to treatment. In one proposed classification system, type 1 impingement, as seen on arthroscopy, is characterized by signs of tendon wear or degeneration on the articular or bursal surface, with associated fraying or irregularity of either articular or bursal structures (Figs. 9-47 and 9-48). Type 1 impingement is subdivided into type 1a (articular) or type 1b (bursal). Type 1 also includes any signs of wear or degeneration of any of

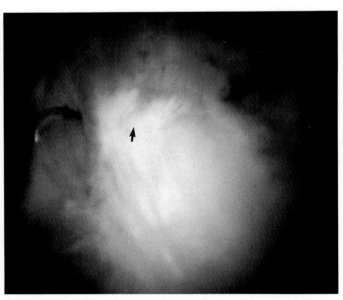

FIGURE 9-47. Arthroscopic view of coracoacromial ligament erosion in subacromial impingement.

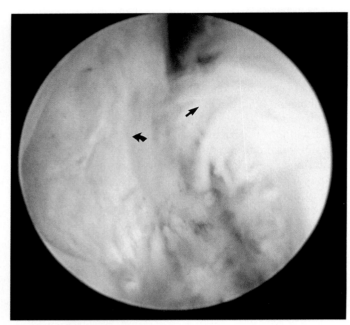

FIGURE 9-48. Arthroscopic bursal view of the frayed surface (*straight arrow*) of the cuff in impingement. The coracoacromial ligament attachment is shown (*curved arrow*).

the structures in the bursa (eg, coracoacromial ligament erosion or fraying).

In addition to articular (type 1a) and bursal (type 1b) tendon degeneration, intrasubstance degeneration, which we refer to as type 1c, may be associated with intrasubstance partial tears (Fig. 9-49). Such intrasubstance degeneration is

not detected and cannot be confirmed on arthroscopic surface evaluations. Conventional and gadolinium-enhanced MR imaging are negative in type 1 impingement.

In arthroscopic type 2 impingement, in addition to tendon wear or degeneration, there are partial thickness tears—of the articular surface in type 2a or the bursal surface in type 2b. Type 2 impingement lesions are also characterized on MR images as partial articular (type 2a) or bursal (type 2b) tears (Figs. 9-50 and 9-51). In the presence of a surface tear, it may be difficult and redundant to classify associated intrasubstance changes, whether secondary to degeneration or intrasubstance tearing. Cadaveric histopathologic studies have shown that partial tears may originate from regions of tendon degeneration without associated inflammation, as discussed earlier.[84] Coronal oblique MR images show increased signal intensity in the distal supraspinatus tendon on T1, intermediate, T2, T2*, and T2-weighted fast spin-echo images. Increased signal intensity fluid within the bursal or articular surface of the cuff is characteristic of this lesion. Small amounts of fluid may be seen in the subacromial bursa, especially in bursal surface type 2b lesions, in the absence of a full thickness or complete tear. In addition to a partial thickness tear, in type 2 impingement associated tendon thinning and fraying may be present. Well-defined, linear, high signal intensity on T2-weighted images, or an area of increased signal intensity on long TR/TE images, that does not extend to either the articular or bursal surfaces and may represent intrasubstance partial tears. Morphologic tendon changes, such as tendon irregularities or thinning, help support this diagnosis.

Arthroscopic type 3 impingement is characterized by a full thickness tear of the rotator cuff. Without retraction of the cuff, the tear is classified as a type 3a; with retraction

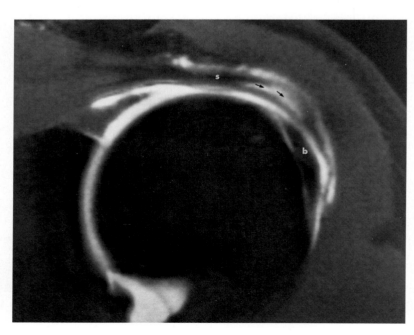

FIGURE 9-49. Surgically confirmed intrasubstance tear (*arrows*) with intact bursal and articular cuff surfaces on a fat-suppressed T1-weighted coronal oblique MR arthrogram. The biceps tendon (b) and supraspinatus (s) tendons are identified.

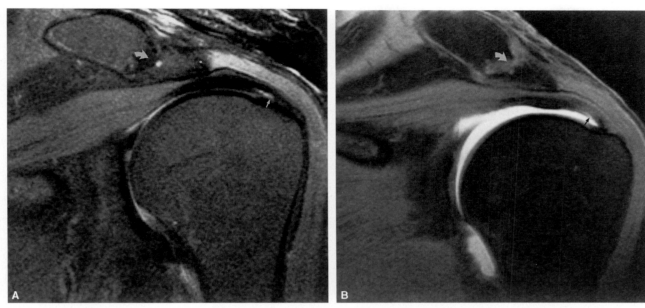

FIGURE 9-50. Partial articular surface tear (*straight arrow*) is hyperintense on fat-suppressed T2-weighted fast spin-echo coronal oblique image (**A**) with inferior surface irregularity confirmed on fat-suppressed T2-weighted coronal oblique arthroscopic image (**B**). Associated degenerative acromioclavicular joint changes are shown (*curved arrow*).

of the cuff, it is classified as a type 3b. In type 3 impingement, MR imaging depicts a complete tear of the rotator cuff (ie, type 3a), or with proximal tendon retraction (ie, type 3b) (Fig. 9-52). Without demonstration of a defined defect, retraction of the muscle belly, or extension of fluid

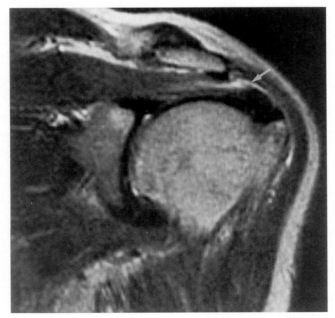

FIGURE 9-51. Partial bursal surface tear of the supraspinatus (*arrow*) with increased signal intensity on T2-weighted fast spin-echo coronal oblique image.

across the supraspinatus tendon into the subacromial-subdeltoid bursa, a complete tear cannot be unequivocally diagnosed. Increased signal intensity within the tendon on T2-weighted images in the presence of normal tendon morphology is not diagnostic of a rotator cuff tear. Therefore, the presence of small amounts of fluid within the subacromial-subdeltoid bursa should not be used as a primary sign of rotator cuff tear, unless associated with a direct communication of fluid from the glenohumeral joint into the subacromial-subdeltoid bursa.

Osseous Findings in Impingement

ACROMION. When present, an anterior acromial spur can be identified on MR images and acromial morphology and slope (potential risk factors for anterior acromial impingement) can be characterized. An anterior acromial spur, or enthesophyte, extends from the anteroinferior surface of the acromion in a medial and inferior direction (Fig. 9-53). These spurs may be seen on anteroposterior (outlet view) radiographs. They arise in or adjacent to the acromial attachment to the coracoacromial ligament, and are thought to represent traction osteophytes.[52] Acromial spurs containing marrow fat demonstrate high signal intensity on T1-weighted images. They may, however, blend with the adjacent acromial cortex on T2*-weighted images, obscuring their identification. Anterior acromial spurs are intermediate in signal intensity and may be overlooked on conventional T2 and T2-weighted fast spin-echo sequences. The anterior and inferior location of the spur is best shown on sagittal oblique images. Larger spurs are evident on coronal oblique images. Spurs

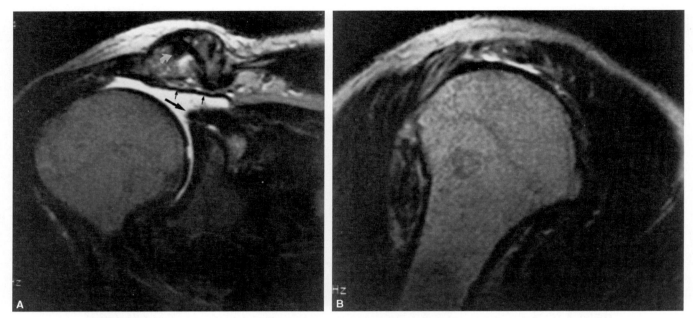

FIGURE 9-52. Complete rotator cuff tear with retraction (*large straight arrow*) to the level of the glenoid on T2-weighted fast spin-echo coronal (**A**) and sagittal oblique (**B**) images. Acromioclavicular joint arthrosis (*curved arrow*) with hypertrophy and inferior spurring is seen. Narrowing of the supraspinatus outlet is associated with a complete rotator cuff tear. There is free communication of fluid between the glenohumeral joint and subacromial-subdeltoid bursa. Cuff tissue is absent on the sagittal oblique image (**B**). The coracoacromial ligament is identified inferior to the AC joint and acromion (*small straight arrow*).

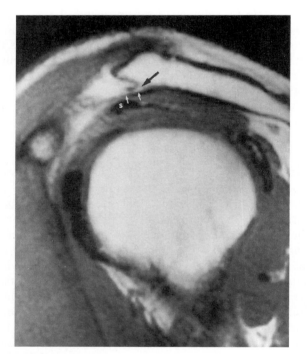

FIGURE 9-53. An anterior acromial spur (*black arrow*) effaces the proximal coracoacromial ligament (*white arrows*). Fatty marrow signal intensity is shown in the acromial spur. s, supraspinatus tendon.

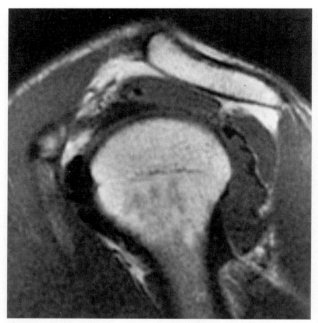

FIGURE 9-54. Type 4 acromion with convex inferior surface on a T1-weighted sagittal oblique image.

are composed of primary cortical bone and are low in signal intensity on all pulse sequences. It is important not to misinterpret the normal inferior acromial attachment of the coracoacromial ligament or lateral deltoid attachment as an acromial spur. An area of suspected cortical thickening on the inferior acromial surface, as identified on coronal oblique images, should be verified on corresponding sagittal oblique images.

Bigliani's classification of the shape of the acromion into three types (see Shoulder Impingement Syndrome, Etiology) can be adapted from his original radiographic description to characterization on MR imaging[67] (see Fig. 9-42). A type I acromion has a flat or straight inferior surface. Type II demonstrates a smooth, curved inferior surface that approximately parallels the superior humeral head in the sagittal oblique plane. Type III has an anterior inferior hook. The acromiohumeral distance is narrowed relative to the remainder of the acromion at the site of the hook. Type I and II acromions are more common than type III in the general population. The type III acromion is associated with a greater predisposition to association with rotator cuff tears (ie, tears involving the critical zone immediately proximal to the greater tuberosity insertion on the supraspinatus tendon). A true hook, however, is rare in incidence and represents a variant in the development of the preacromial epiphysis. The influence of the hook is related to the slope of its attached acromion.[99] A type IV acromion (Fig. 9-54) has recently been described by Vanarthos and Mono[99] and includes an acromion with an undersurface that is convex near its distal end. This type was found in 7% of the patient population studied by MR imaging in 30 patients. The significance of this acromial shape still needs to be validated with respect to the incidence of rotator cuff disease. The MR appearance of the acromial arch shape is sensitive to the MR section selected on oblique sagittal MR images.[100] For example, more medial sections closer to the AC joint may falsely produce the shape of a hooked anterior acromion, which has a flat undersurface on more peripheral sagittal oblique images. MR imaging should not be used as a substitute for the supraspinatus outlet view.[15,100]

The slope of the acromion can be assessed on sagittal oblique images. A line drawn tangent to the acromial surface can be used to estimate narrowing of the supraspinatus outlet by a decrease or flattening of the acromial angle.[101] A flat angle is associated with a higher incidence of impingement in rotator cuff tears in cadavers.

An anterior downsloping acromion (Fig. 9-55) is present when the anterior inferior cortex of the acromion is more inferiorly located relative to its posterior cortex as assessed in the sagittal oblique plane. The normal acromion is usually shown as nearly horizontal in its lateral aspect on sagittal oblique images. As discussed in the case of the flat or decreased acromial angle, an anterior downsloping acromion is thought to be associated with an increased risk for anterior acromial impingement.[101]

A lateral downsloping of the acromion, which narrows the acromiohumeral distance, can be appreciated on coronal oblique images (Fig. 9-56). The inferior surface of the distal acromion is inferior or caudally located, relative to the inferior surface of the more proximal aspect of the acromion, which is adjacent to the AC joint. This lateral downsloping of the acromion may be associated with impingement of

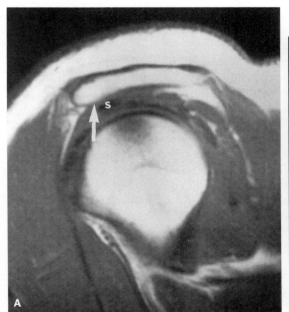
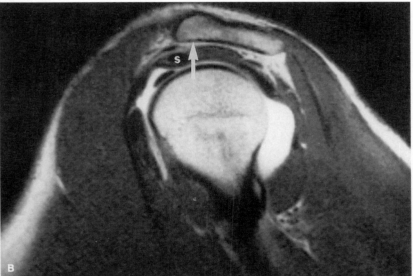

FIGURE 9-55. Acromial slope. **(A)** A T1-weighted sagittal oblique image demonstrates the anterior downsloped acromion (*arrow*) with the anterior inferior cortex projecting inferior to the posterior aspect of the acromion. The relative encroachment on the supraspinatus outlet may lead to impingement. **(B)** An enhanced T1-weighted sagittal oblique image shows a normally sloped acromion (*arrow*) with the anterior inferior cortex projecting superior to the posterior aspect of the acromion. S, supraspinatus tendon.

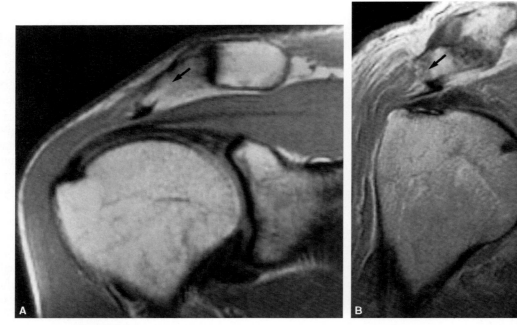

FIGURE 9-56. (A, B) Two separate cases of lateral downslope (*arrow*) of the acromion on T1-weighted coronal oblique images.

the supraspinatus tendon near its attachment to the greater tuberosity. The acromion may also appear inferiorly offset relative to the distal clavicle, even in the presence of a normal acromial slope (Fig. 9-57).

Acromial erosion and eburnation are chronic osseous changes of impingement that occur on the undersurface of the anterior third of the acromion (Fig. 9-58). This irregularity on the inferior surface of the acromion is identified on

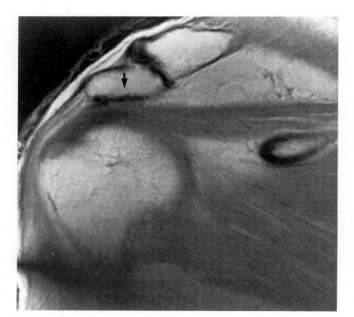

FIGURE 9-57. Inferior offset (*arrow*) of acromion despite normal lateral acromial slope (T1-weighted coronal oblique image).

both coronal and sagittal oblique images and may contribute to the further progression of rotator cuff disease.

An os acromiale may also be linked to the development of impingement and rotator cuff tears[102] (Fig. 9-59). Four types of os acromiale have been described (preacromial, meso-acromial, meta-acromial, and basiacromial). A movable unfused segment of the acromion may result in impingement. Attempts at epiphysiodesis may result in considerable morbidity with mixed results. Arthroscopic excision of even the largest of os acromiale, however, does not produce any deltoid defects or weakness of elevation.

The os acromiale is visualized in all imaging planes and should not be mistaken for the AC joint. Axial images best display the morphology and size of the os acromiale unfused segment. Osteophytic lipping at the margins of the acromial gap may cause direct impingement on the rotator cuff, and contraction of the deltoid muscle, secondary to the downward pull on the os acromiale, has also been implicated in impingement. An unstable os acromiale is also associated with aromioclavicular joint degeneration.

We have observed increased signal intensity in adjacent portions of the acromial marrow on either side of the fusion defect on both STIR and fat-suppressed T2-weighted fast spin-echo sequences (Fig. 9-60). This hyperintensity may correlate with degenerative changes or instability in symptomatic patients. It is important that impingement not be solely attributed to an os acromiale, because arthroscopic decompression of the os acromiale in patients with shoulder impingement have shown subsequent development of recurrent symptoms.[103] All causes of impingement syndrome, including os acromiale, should be carefully evaluated preoperatively and correlated with patients' symptoms.

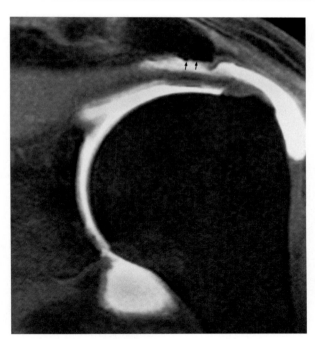

FIGURE 9-58. An irregular inferior acromial surface (*arrow*) is outlined by subacromial-subdeltoid bursal fluid on a fat-suppressed T1-weighted coronal oblique MR arthrogram.

Acromioclavicular Joint Disease and Impingement

Arthrosis of the AC joint, including callus and osteophytes, can contribute to impingement (Fig. 9-61). The AC joint may encroach on the supraspinatus outlet and cause an extrinsic effect on the bursal surface of the musculotendinous junction of the supraspinatus (Fig. 9-62). MR imaging is more accurate than conventional radiography in demonstrating the morphology and degree of AC joint enlargement and its relationship to soft-tissue structures under the coracoacromial arch (the rotator cuff). The portion of the cuff inferior to the AC joint is not as rigidly confined as the critical zone of the supraspinatus, which is more frequently affected by pathologic impingement at the location of the anterior inferior acromion. Even when the contour of the supraspinatus muscle or tendon is deformed by the AC joint, patients may be asymptomatic.

Although AC joint arthrosis may be described by the radiologist, the diagnosis of impingement remains a clinical one. Marginal osteophytes of the AC joint may precede the presence of anterior acromial erosion. The MR characteristics of degenerative changes in the AC joint may be evaluated in all three imaging planes. The coronal oblique and sagittal oblique planes are more useful in showing the relationship of the callus and osteophyte to the subacromial space and bursal cuff surface. Low signal intensity sclerosis, erosions, subchondral cysts, and marrow hyperemia (bright signal on T2, STIR, and fat-suppressed T2-weighted fast spin-echo sequences) are characteristic.

Humeral Head Changes

Degenerative cysts and sclerosis of the greater tuberosity can be seen in on MR scans in shoulder impingement. Squaring and sclerosis of the greater tuberosity are best seen on coronal and sagittal oblique images (Fig. 9-63). Glenohumeral joint degeneration and rotator cuff tears represent the end stage in the spectrum of impingement.[65,104] Loss of the acromiohumeral distance is also a finding in the later stages

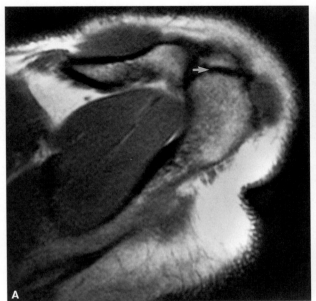
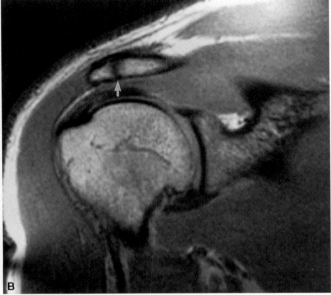

FIGURE 9-59. Asymptomatic os acromiale without associated marrow changes on T1-weighted axial (**A**) and coronal oblique (**B**) images.

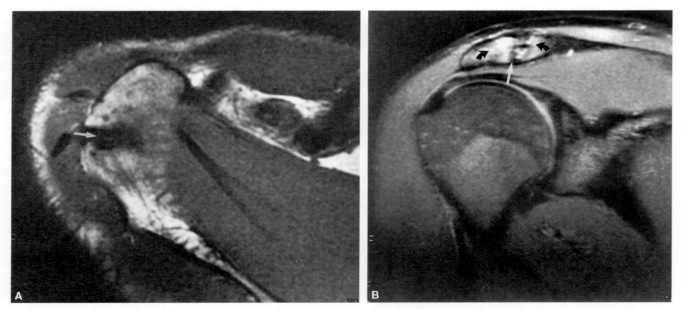

FIGURE 9-60. Symptomatic os acromiale with hyperintense bone marrow edema (*curved arrow*) in adjacent portions of the unfused (*straight arrow*) acromial apophysis. T1-weighted axial (**A**) and fat-suppressed T2-weighted fast spin-echo coronal oblique (**B**) images.

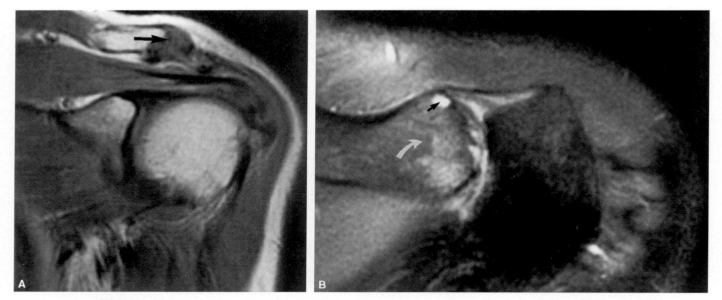

FIGURE 9-61. Degenerative acromioclavicular joint changes with subchondral sclerosis (*large straight arrow*), erosions (*small straight arrow*), and degenerative subchondral marrow edema (*curved arrow*) primarily involving the distal clavicle. (**A**: T1-weighted coronal oblique image; **B**: fat-suppressed T2-weighted fast spin-echo axial image.)

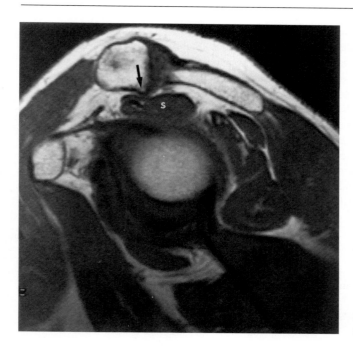

FIGURE 9-62. Acromioclavicular joint arthrosis (*arrow*) with secondary narrowing of the supraspinatus outlet. S, supraspinatus muscle.

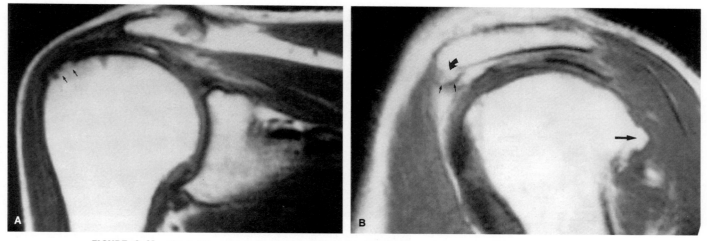

FIGURE 9-63. (**A**) A T1-weighted coronal oblique image shows early osseous evidence of impingement with osteophytic squaring of the greater tuberosity at the insertion site of the supraspinatus tendon (*arrows*). (**B**) A T1-weighted sagittal oblique image shows later changes of bony impingement with an anterior acromial spur (*curved arrow*) and humeral osteophyte (*large straight arrow*). The low signal intensity cortex of the acromial osteophyte is indicated (*small straight arrows*). The anterior acromiohumeral distance is narrowed.

of impingement. Rounding of the greater tuberosity also occurs in advanced impingement and is usually associated with corresponding changes of bone erosion or sclerosis on the inferior acromial surface.

The Coracoacromial Ligament

The coracoacromial ligament has a trapezoid shape and attaches to the undersurface of the acromion in a broad or wide insertion. It varies in thickness from 2 to 5.6 mm,[105] and twists in a helical orientation inferiorly to its narrower coracoid insertion. Arthroscopically, the coracoacromial ligament may present in a plane almost perpendicular to the anterior aspect of the supraspinatus tendon as viewed from above. Variation in the size of the coracoacromial ligament may explain the MR observation of ligament hypertrophy. The variable size and thickness of the wide portion of the ligament, inferior to the acromion, may contribute to narrowing of the supraspinatus outlet. Arthroscopic

findings of impingement include erosive changes in the acromial attachment of the coracoacromial ligament (see Fig. 9-47). Edelson and Luchs have shown enthesopathic transformations of the coracoacromial ligament into bone at its acromial insertion in cadaveric specimens.[106] These various enthesopathic bone changes can produce different configurations of the hooks and spurs on the inferior surface of the acromion (see Fig. 9-53). Although the coracoacromial ligament attachment can be detached from the overlying anterior deltoid muscle, the coracoacromial ligament blends with the deltoid muscle fascia along the lateral acromion, demarcating the anterior from the middle deltoid fibers.

Coracoid Impingement

Coracohumeral impingement is thought to occur secondary to narrowing of the space between the coracoid process and the humeral head (Figs. 9-64 and 9-65). The narrowing may be

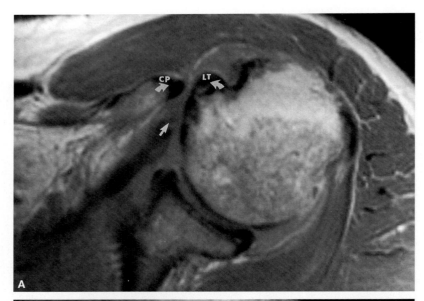

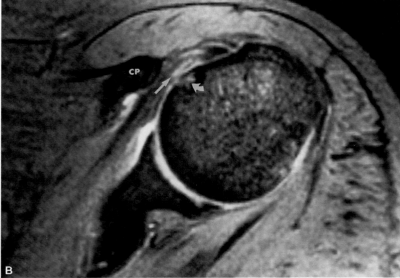

FIGURE 9-64. Coracoid impingement with narrowing (*curved arrows*) between the coracoid process (CP) and humeral head. Associated subscapularis tendon degeneration (*straight arrow*) and subchondral cystic change of the anteromedial humeral head (*curved arrow*) are shown on (**A**) T1- and (**B**) T2*-weighted axial images. LT, lesser tuberosity.

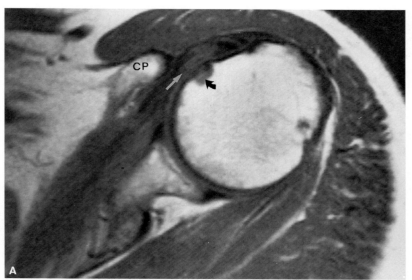

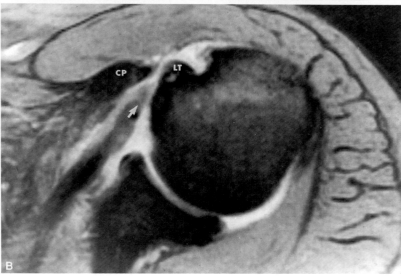

FIGURE 9-65. Coracohumeral impingement with rup-tured subscapularis tendon (*straight arrow*) and hypoin-tense subchondral sclerosis (*curved arrow*) of the cora-coid process (CP) and lesser tuberosity (LT) on (**A**) T1- and (**B**) T2*-weighted axial images. The distance be-tween the coracoid and the lesser tuberosity is less than 11 mm.

most evident in the position of internal rotation. Bonutti and colleagues[107] reported that the normal interval between the cora-coid process and the lesser tuberosity is greater than 11 mm in internal rotation as assessed on axial images.[107] Coracohumeral impingement is thought to be associated with interval measure-ments less than 11 mm. MR findings of impingement may include signal inhomogeneity as well as thickening and fluid within the subcoracoid bursa.[107] This type of impingement, which may encroach on the subscapularis, does not involve the supraspinatus tendon or cause outlet impingement.[36]

Posterior Superior Glenoid Impingement

Posterior superior glenoid impingement is a recently recog-nized mechanism of injury producing repetitive impingement of the inferior surface of the rotator cuff in the athlete who uses a throwing motion[108] (Fig. 9-66). Jobe[108] found that damage to more than one of the five structures at risk from this mechanism of injury—including (1) the superior labrum, (2) the rotator cuff tendon, (3) the greater tuberosity, (4) the IGL or labrum, and (5) the superior bony glenoid—resulted in posterior superior glenoid impingement.[108]This mechanism of injury represents su-perior or posterior-superior angulation in the position of abduc-tion and external rotation (the position of throwing). As a result, compression stresses occur in the superior glenoid labrum, the articular surface of the rotator cuff, the greater tuberosity, and the bony superior glenoid. The IGL is loaded in tension because it limits abduction in external rotation of the glenohumeral joint.

MR arthrography, performed with the arm positioned in abduction and external rotation, is the modality of choice for demonstration of associated cuff and labral pathology in posterior superior glenoid impingement.[109]

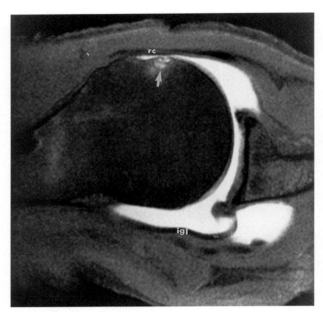

FIGURE 9-66. Posterior superior glenoid impingement. Osseous erosion (*arrow*) adjacent to the greater tuberosity is seen with the shoulder positioned in external rotation and abduction on this fat-suppressed T1-weighted MR arthrogram. The structures involved in posterior superior glenoid impingement include the greater tuberosity, rotator cuff (rc) including the articular surface, the superior labrum, the inferior glenohumeral ligament (igl), the labral complex, and the superior glenoid bone. Areas of humeral head osseous erosion often correspond to a contact area with an abnormal frayed labrum.

Treatment of Impingement Disorders

Treatment for the different types of impingement disorders depends on the age and activity level of the patient.[52,65] In general, most patients are treated with conservative therapy for a period of 6 months prior to surgical intervention.

CONSERVATIVE TREATMENT. In the acute phase, analgesics, nonsteroidal antiinflammatory drugs (NSAIDs), and steroid injection are the most effective forms of treatment. In less acute situations, conservative therapy may also include physical therapy, in particular, strengthening of the rotator cuff musculature with abduction and external rotation exercises. Internal rotation exercises for the subscapularis are also recommended. Subacromial bursal injections of various steroid antiinflammatory agents are effective, but the effect is often ephemeral, and steroids may be associated with painful postinjection flares. These flares can last as long as 48 hours and can produce significant distress. Repeated injections of steroids in and about the rotator cuff tendons may have a destructive effect. In general, not more than two or three injections should be used in this area during a 12-month period. Oral NSAIDs may prove to be effective when combined with a reduced activity level. Regardless of the specific treatment, more than 6 months of pain or dramatically decreased activity and sleep levels are often unacceptable to the patient. Therefore, if pain reduction through conservative measures is not achieved, an arthroscopic approach is warranted.

ACROMIOPLASTY. Arthroscopic subacromial decompression (ASD) is now the method of choice for the treatment of chronic outlet impingement. It is rapidly replacing open acromioplasty[52,65] because it does not violate the deltoid and overlying deltotrapezial fascia. Arthroscopic anterior acromioplasty, as part of ASD, is indicated for alleviation of pain secondary to the impingement of the anterior inferior surface of the acromion. In ASD, the coracoacromial ligament is detached from the anterior inferior acromial surface, and inflamed or frayed cuff tissue is debrided. A burr is used to perform the anterior acromioplasty.

Patients with early impingement, demonstrating degenerative irregularities of the articular bursal surface of the rotator cuff, are treated by ASD only. Arthroscopic findings usually include not only fraying of the articular or bursal surface, but also evidence of fraying of the coracoacromial ligament as it attaches to the anterior and lateral borders of the anterior inferior surface of the acromion. Kissing lesions are irregularities of the bursal surfaces of the cuff found opposite irregularities or fraying of the coracoacromial ligament. Subacromial decompression produces good to excellent results in 85% of patients followed for a minimum of 2 years.

Patients with partial thickness tears involving either the articular or bursal surfaces of the rotator cuff are also treated with subacromial decompression and debridement of the partial thickness tear. Results of treatment of these lesions depend on the extent of the rotator cuff tear: the deeper and more extensive the cleavage planes, the larger the flap of cuff produced by the tear, the greater the likelihood that a simple subacromial decompression will be insufficient and either an arthroscopic or an open repair of the more significantly damaged partially torn cuff will be necessary. Nonetheless, a good number of these patients respond positively to subacromial decompression alone, and because of its minimal morbidity, this procedure can be tried prior to reconstructive procedures.

Full thickness lesions of the rotator cuff are more difficult treatment dilemmas. In general, patients with full thickness tears of the rotator cuff require an open procedure, although arthroscopic-assisted rotator cuff repairs, and even purely arthroscopic repairs, are possible. The present standard of care is a deltoid-splitting approach, without significant detachment of the deltoid from the acromial edge, to close the tear following an ASD.

The information provided by MR imaging is helpful in preoperative planning. If MR images show a small tear with minimal retraction, a less invasive, arthroscopic approach can be used. If MR images show significant retraction of the tendon to the level of the superior pole of the glenoid, a more extensive approach is necessary.

In patients with severe tendon retraction and MR evidence of fiber changes (eg, fibrosis or atrophy), the prognosis for cuff repair is less optimistic, and the cuff may be irreparable. These patients may be best served with a simple ASD.

For patients with evidence of rotator cuff arthropathy with proximal humeral migration, the likelihood of a successful repair is remote. These patients are often older and their main complaint is pain; therefore, ASD alone produces satisfactory results (ie, pain relief) in approximately 50% of cases.

ASSOCIATED ARTHROSCOPIC PROCEDURES. During subacromial decompression, the entire glenohumeral joint is evaluated, and associated lesions are often noted and appropriate procedures undertaken. Resection of the coracoacromial ligament is always performed in addition to the acromioplasty.

Patients with significant degenerative changes in the AC joint need additional preoperative diagnostic tests, particularly local injections of lidocaine (Xylocaine), to distinguish between pain emanating from a degenerative AC joint and impingement pain produced by spurs. If joint pain is associated with impingement pain, it is necessary to perform an arthroscopic Mumford procedure (ie, resection of the distal 2 cm of the clavicle) at the same time as the ASD. If a degenerative prominence of the AC joint is producing extrinsic compression of the muscle belly of the supraspinatus, it can also be removed by resecting the distal clavicle.

The biceps tendon, a component of the rotator cuff, must also be arthroscopically evaluated intraoperatively. The tendon is pulled into the joint so that the part of the tendon that lies within the bicipital groove can be assessed. If it is significantly frayed or attenuated, it is resected from its insertion at the glenohumeral tubercle, a deltoid-splitting incision is made, and a tenodesis is performed in the bicipital groove (Fig. 9-67).

Rotator Cuff Tears

No two rotator cuff tears are alike, making their evaluation and treatment protocols complicated. The tears can be characterized as either partial or complete.[59,60] Partial tears may involve the articular or bursal surfaces in varying degrees of depth and extension into the tendon. Intratendinous lesions may not communicate with either bursal or articular surfaces. Complete rotator cuff tears, which extend through the entire thickness of the rotator cuff, allow direct communication between the subacromial bursa and the glenohumeral joint. A massive rotator cuff tear involves at least two of the rotator cuff tendons. MR images, particularly in the

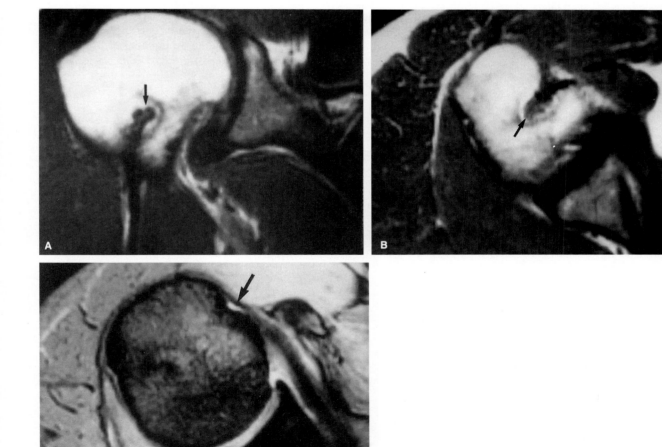

FIGURE 9-67. T1-weighted (**A**) coronal oblique and (**B**) axial images show biceps tenodesis (*arrow*). (**C**) The corresponding T2*-weighted axial image shows an absence of the biceps tendon in the bicipital groove (*arrow*).

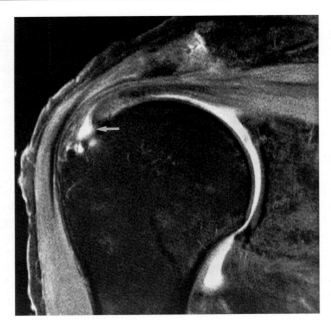

FIGURE 9-68. Partial articular surface tear (*arrow*) involving the conjoined portion of the rotator cuff. The bursal surface is intact and no fluid is identified in the subacromial-subdeltoid bursa. The tear is hyperintense on this fat-suppressed T2-weighted fast spin-echo coronal oblique image.

coronal and sagittal oblique planes, are able to demonstrate partial rotator cuff tears that escape arthrographic detection.[110] In middle-aged and older patients, traumatic tears from a single episode are more commonly found, as are tears associated with acute dislocations.[51]

Partial Tears

Using MR imaging characteristics, partial rotator cuff tears can be classified as either partial articular (Fig. 9-68) or bursal (Fig. 9-69) surface lesions. Cadaveric histopathologic studies have shown that partial tears may originate from regions of tendon degeneration. Partial articular surface tears occur more frequently than partial bursal surface or intrasubstance tears.[111] Partial or incomplete tears are thought to be twice as common as complete or full thickness tears of the rotator cuff.[86] On coronal oblique MR images, partial tears demonstrate low to intermediate signal intensity on T1-weighted images, intermediate to high signal intensity on proton density weighted images, and bright signal intensity on conventional T2, T2-weighted fast spin-echo, and fat-suppressed T2-weighted fast spin-echo sequences. Because severe degeneration and partial tears demonstrate similar regions of increased signal intensity on T2*-weighted images, we do not advocate the routine use of gradient-echo sequences for the detection of rotator cuff disease.

Increased signal intensity due to tracking of fluid within the bursal or articular surface of the cuff is characteristic of

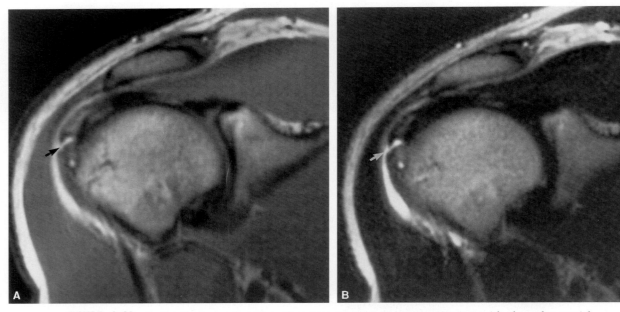

FIGURE 9-69. Partial thickness bursal surface tear (*arrow*) in communication with the subacromial-subdeltoid bursa. Fluid is hyperintense on (**A**) intermediate-weighted and (**B**) T2-weighted fast spin-echo coronal oblique images.

partial tears on T2 spin-echo or T2-weighted fast spin-echo sequences. Because fat-suppression increases the conspicuity of fluid in the subacromial bursa and in a tear site, the addition of fat-suppression to the T2-weighted fast spin-echo sequence can be useful. T2*-weighted images may also show fluid, which displays higher signal intensity than associated degeneration. Identification of bursal or articular surface defects on these images requires careful evaluation of tendon morphology. Small amounts of fluid may be seen in the subacromial bursa, especially in bursal surface lesions, in the absence of a full thickness or complete tear. In addition to a partial thickness tear, there may be associated tendon thinning and fraying. Well-defined linear high signal intensity changes on T2 spin-echo or T2-weighted fast spin-echo images, which do not extend to either the articular or bursal surfaces, may represent an intrasubstance partial tear.

Partial thickness tears are characterized by increased signal intensity extending to either the bursal or articular surfaces on coronal oblique or sagittal oblique T2-weighted images, or fast spin-echo images perpendicular to the long axis of the tendon. Alternatively, a partial tear may be associated with a more linearly oriented area of degeneration or an intrasubstance tear parallel to the long axis of the supraspinatus or infraspinatus tendons. Some partial thickness tears are seen in association with an attenuated or thickened cuff and surface morphologic irregularities with variable changes in tendon signal intensity[86] (Fig. 9-70). These tears may be difficult to evaluate without an intraarticular paramagnetic MR contrast agent or saline to improve visualization of tendon contours. Fat-suppression techniques, used in conjunction with T2-weighted fast spin-echo imaging, and STIR techniques may be more sensitive to fluid signal intensity within small partial tears than conventional spin-echo T2-weighted sequences.

Because of the T1 shortening effects of gadolinium, MR arthrography with intraarticular Gd-DTPA administration is useful in highlighting small, partial tears involving the articular surface (Fig. 9-71). Partial articular surface tears not seen on conventional arthrograms may be identified using MR arthrography, especially in areas of granulation tissue in chronic tears. Tears are bright on T1-weighted postinjection images.[112] The addition of fat-suppression improves the visualization of the hyperintense fluid while suppressing the normal bright signal from fat.[113] This technique helps to avoid mistaking areas of fat, especially linear streaks of fat, for gadolinium contrast extending into a partial tear site. The detection of partial articular surface tears can also be improved by using MR arthrography with the arm positioned in abduction and external rotation.[114]

In patients with tendinosis or tendon degeneration alone, there is no extension of contrast on postinjection images, and the supraspinatus tendon can be seen to be intact. In addition, intraarticular contrast is not helpful in the identification of partial bursal surface tears and does not enhance intrasubstance tears. A preliminary T2-weighted spin-echo or T2-weighted fast spin-echo sequence is performed to evaluate these areas. Intravenous use of an MR contrast agent may prove to be helpful in enhancing synovium and granulation tissue in partial bursal surface tears.

Since MR arthrography is not routinely used in uncomplicated evaluations of the rotator cuff, the detection of partial tears can also be optimized by using fat-suppression in conjunction with conventional or fast spin-echo T2-weighted sequences without the use of intraarticular contrast.

Full Thickness Tears

Complete (full thickness) tears of the rotator cuff, with or without proximal retraction, can be depicted clearly with MR imaging.[113,115–120]

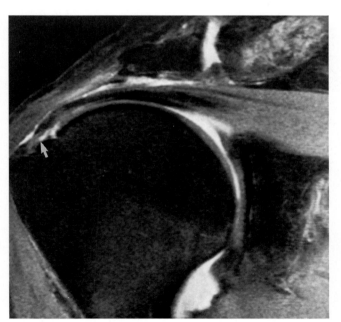

FIGURE 9-70. Partial tear with abnormal attenuation (*arrow*) of the distal conjoined supraspinatus and infraspinatus cuff tendons. Fluid is hyperintense and cuff degeneration is intermediate in signal intensity. There is no direct communication of fluid between the glenohumeral joint and subacromial-subdeltoid bursa on this fat-suppressed T2-weighted fast spin-echo coronal oblique image.

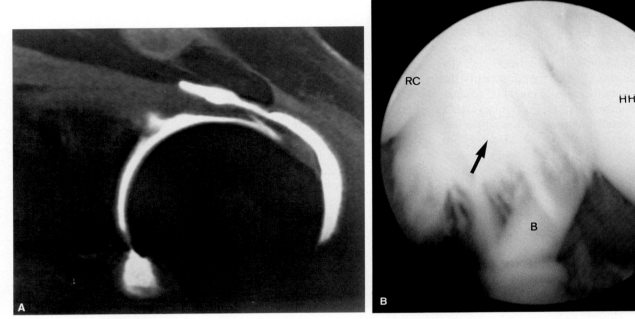

FIGURE 9-71. (A) Partial thickness articular surface tear (*arrow*) of the rotator cuff on fat-suppressed T1-weighted MR coronal oblique arthrogram. The hyperintense tear involves the undersurface of the conjoined supraspinatus and infraspinatus tendons. (B) Arthroscopy shows fraying (*arrow*) in partial articular surface tear. RC, intact rotator cuff; B, biceps tendon; HH, humeral head.

PRIMARY SIGNS. One of the primary signs of a full thickness rotator cuff tear is visualization of a tendon defect (Fig. 9-72). This defect, or tendinous gap, is seen as an interruption or loss of continuity of the normally low signal intensity tendon. Joint fluid or granulation tissue at the cuff tear site are seen as areas of intermediate to increased signal intensity on T1-weighted and proton density weighted images. On T2 spin-echo, T2-weighted fast spin-echo, and fat-suppression T2-weighted fast spin-echo sequences, these areas demonstrate markedly increased signal intensity. T1 and proton density weighted images are sensitive to changes in signal intensity in cuff tendons, but in comparison with T2-weighted images, these sequences are particularly limited in demonstrating small or partial cuff tears. T1-weighted images are, however, useful in demonstrating associated fatty atrophy in the supraspinatus muscle or alterations in the AC joint with osteophytes and

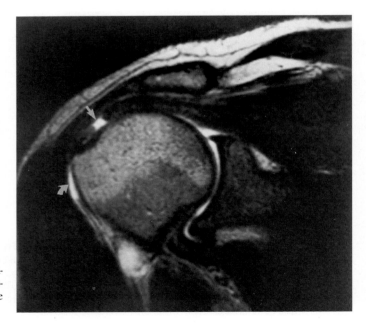

FIGURE 9-72. Full thickness supraspinatus tendon tear with hyperintense fluid gap (*straight arrow*) on T2-weighted fast spin-echo coronal oblique image. A small amount of fluid is identified lateral to the greater tuberosity (*curved arrow*).

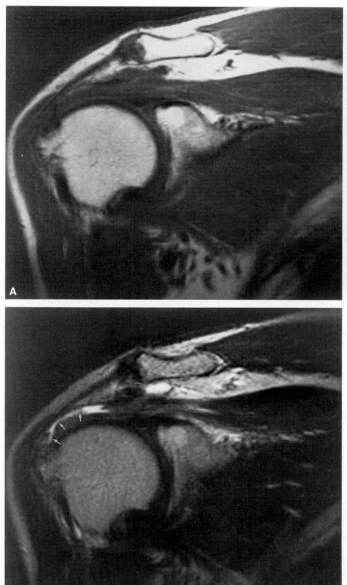

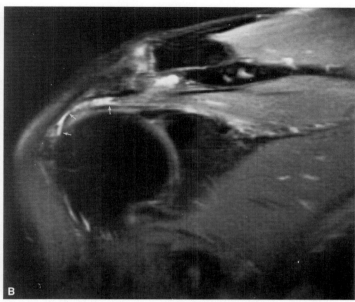

FIGURE 9-73. Full thickness rotator cuff tear (*arrows*) with direct linear extension of fluid between the glenohumeral joint and subacromial-subdeltoid bursa across the supraspinatus tendon. Note the horizontal tear plane indicated by the path of fluid through the torn cuff. (**A**: T1-weighted coronal oblique image; **B**: fat-suppressed T2-weighted fast spin-echo coronal oblique image; **C**: T2-weighted fast spin-echo coronal oblique image.)

subchondral sclerosis. A complete tear cannot be unequivocally diagnosed without visualization of either a defined tendon defect or indication of direct communication between the glenohumeral joint and the subacromial bursa (ie, extension of the joint line, by even a small amount, across the cuff tendons into the subacromial-subdeltoid bursa) (Fig. 9-73). T2 spin-echo or fast spin-echo sagittal oblique images provide additional information, allowing identification of articular and bursal surface extension and the location and size of the tear in the anteroposterior direction (Fig. 9-74).

Preoperative MR imaging studies provide important information about the size of the cuff tear, the degree of proximal or medial retraction, and the quality of the associated muscle tissue. Complete absence of the rotator cuff indicates a major tendinous disruption and is typical of rotator cuff arthropathy in which the proximal head is in direct contact with the undersurface of the acromion (Fig. 9-75). Involvement of the infraspinatus or subscapularis tendons may be seen in massive rotator cuff tears. Preoperative MR imaging can also identify associated muscle atrophy in chronic tears. Patients with complete tears complicated by cuff arthropathy, tendon retraction, and muscle atrophy may not be candidates for surgical repair (Fig. 9-76).

Retraction of the supraspinatus or infraspinatus tendons is best seen on coronal oblique images that demonstrate the

text continues on page 681

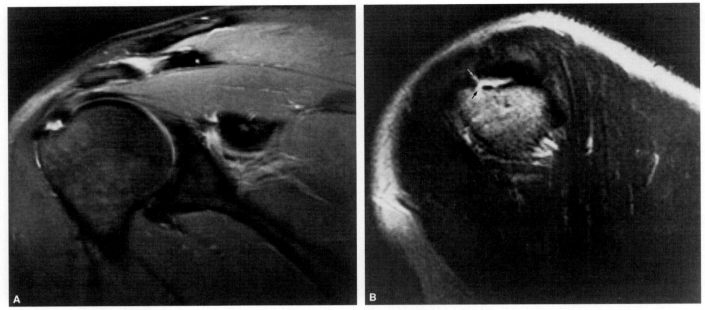

FIGURE 9-74. Full thickness rotator cuff tear on **(A)** fat-suppressed T2-weighted fast spin-echo coronal oblique image and **(B)** T2-weighted fast spin-echo sagittal oblique image. The sagittal image best demonstrates both bursal and articular surface extension (*arrows*) at the distal attachment of the supraspinatus tendon.

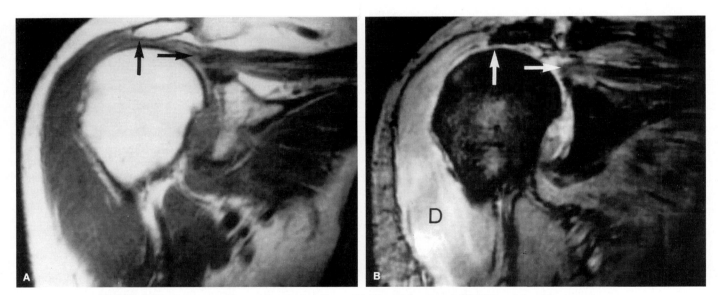

FIGURE 9-75. Rotator cuff tear. Coronal oblique **(A)** T1-weighted and **(B)** T2*-weighted images demonstrate a torn supraspinatus tendon retracted to the level of the glenoid (*horizontal arrows*). Superior ascent of the humeral head (*vertical arrows*) with decreased subacromial space is also seen. The supraspinatus muscle normally functions to prevent the ascent of the humeral head when the deltoid contracts. Deltoid muscle hemorrhage (D) is revealed on the T2*-weighted coronal oblique image.

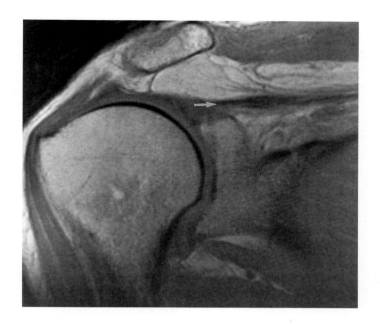

FIGURE 9-76. Chronic full thickness rotator cuff tear with severe supraspinatus muscle atrophy. Retracted tendon is identified at the level of the glenoid (*arrow*). (T1-weighted coronal oblique image.)

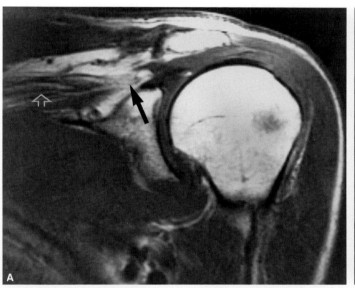

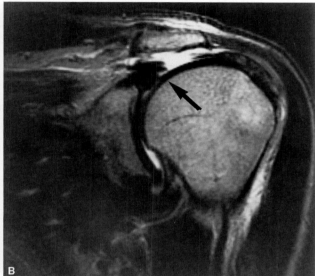

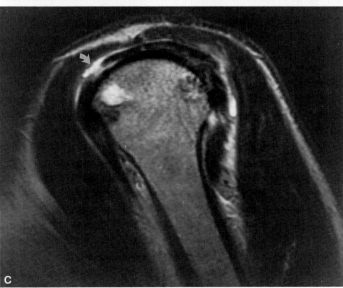

FIGURE 9-77. Full-thickness supraspinatus tendon tear with proximal retraction to the level of the glenoid (*straight arrow*) on (**A**) T1-weighted and (**B**) T2-weighted fast spin-echo coronal oblique images and (**C**) a T2-weighted fast spin-echo sagittal oblique image. The tear is proximal to the greater tuberosity attachment. Fatty atrophy (*curved arrow*) of the supraspinatus muscle (*open arrow*) is shown on the T1-weighted image (**A**), and fluid extension into the subacromial-subdeltoid bursa is demonstrated on the T2-weighted fast spin-echo coronal oblique (**B**) and sagittal oblique (**C**) scans. There is secondary superior ascent of the humeral head. Anterior involvement of the rotator cuff (the supraspinatus contribution) is evident on the sagittal oblique image (*curved arrow*).

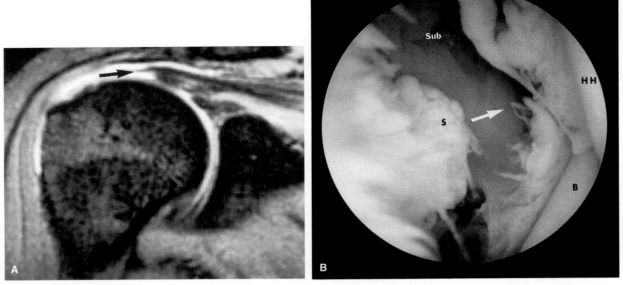

FIGURE 9-78. Rotator cuff tear. **(A)** A T2*-weighted image shows complete tear of the supraspinatus tendon with proximal retraction (*arrow*). Glenohumeral joint fluid communicates with the subacromial-subdeltoid bursa. The retracted tendon edge is clearly depicted. **(B)** The corresponding arthroscopic view shows the articular surface of the avulsed supraspinatus tendon (S; *arrow*). B, biceps tendon; HH, humeral head; Sub, subacromial space.

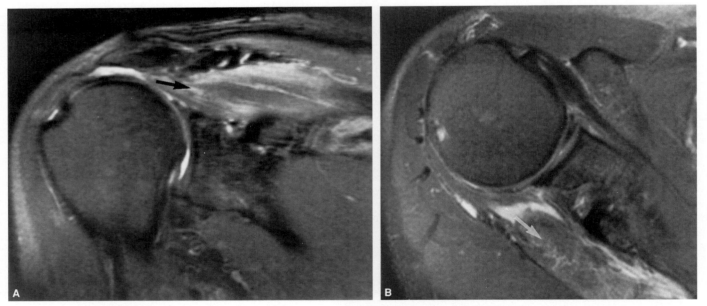

FIGURE 9-79. Full-thickness infraspinatus tendon tear with proximal retraction (*straight arrow*). Muscle edema and hemorrhage is hyperintense on fat-suppressed T2-weighted fast spin-echo coronal oblique **(A)** and axial **(B)** images. An infraspinatus tendon tear can occur as part of a massive rotator cuff tear.

medial and lateral extension of the cuff tear (Figs. 9-77 through 9-79). The retracted cuff tendon may be seen as far medially as the level of the bony glenoid rim. The retracted cuff margins may be thickened in response to healing or attenuated in more chronic tears. The uninvolved areas of the tendon adjacent to the tear site may demonstrate changes of degeneration or partial thickness tear. Less frequently, the remaining tendon demonstrates normal signal intensity or morphology. T2-weighted sagittal oblique images are used to identify the anteroposterior extent of the cuff tear (see Fig. 9-77). Subscapularis and infraspinatus tendon tears are evaluated on both sagittal oblique and axial plane images. The tendinous gap and high signal intensity fluid seen in large supraspinatus tendon tears can be shown on axial images superior to the glenohumeral joint.

SECONDARY SIGNS.   Secondary signs of rotator cuff tears can be used in conjunction with the primary assessment of changes in tendon signal intensity and morphology to help in the diagnosis of cuff tears.

Subacromial-subdeltoid bursal fluid should be readily identifiable, especially when there is a large volume of articular and bursal fluid associated with a complete tear. However, fluid in the subacromial bursa may also be present in impingement or in a partial bursal surface tear without communication with the glenohumeral joint. Subacromial-subdeltoid bursal fluid is also seen in asymptomatic individuals and in cases of isolated bursitis.[86]

Retraction of the supraspinatus musculotendinous junction is another secondary sign that may be seen in full thickness cuff tears. This finding is not observed with small cuff tears. The normal location of the supraspinatus musculotendinous junction is at approximately the 12 o'clock position, superior to the center of the humeral head. The location of this junction may vary within a 30° radius (15° either medial or lateral to the 12 o'clock position).[85] The location of the musculotendinous junction may change with the position of the arm in internal or external rotation. Although this finding, even without a defined cuff defect, may indicate an increased probability for a tear, it is still a secondary finding.

Tears with granulation tissue or hypertrophied synovium may not demonstrate bright signal intensity on T2 (spin-echo or fast spin-echo) weighted images. However, these low signal intensity cuff tears (Fig. 9-80) may be identified by careful evaluation of tendon contour abnormalities and associated secondary signs of cuff disease. Although signal intensity in complete subacute and chronic tears is bright on T2*-weighted gradient-echo images, particularly in the absence of associated glenohumeral joint effusion, the accuracy of T2*-weighted images in the diagnosis of cuff tears has not been determined and the sequence may result in a higher rate of false positive interpretations of cuff tears. Conventional T2 or the combination of fat-suppressed T2-weighted fast spin-echo and T2-weighted fast spin-echo sequences, improve the characterization of tear morphology. The exclusive use of fat-

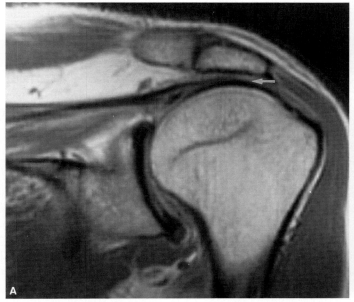
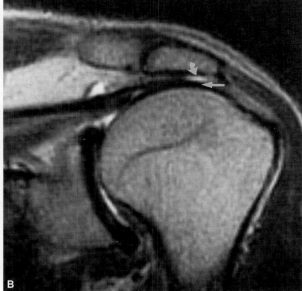

FIGURE 9-80. Chronic "low signal intensity" rotator cuff tear with low signal intensity scar and granulation tissue at the tear site (*straight arrow*). Minimal fluid (*curved arrow*) is present in the subacromial bursa. There is retraction of the musculotendinous junction and mild supraspinatus muscle atrophy. (**A:** intermediate-weighted coronal oblique image; **B:** T2-weighted spin-echo coronal oblique image.)

suppressed T2-weighted fast spin-echo images, however, may produce a false positive result because areas of degeneration may be misinterpreted as hyperintense partial tears. The fat-suppressed T2-weighted fast spin-echo sequence is used in conjunction with either a conventional T2 spin-echo or non–fat-suppressed T2-weighted fast spin-echo sequence.

Changes in subacromial and subdeltoid peribursal fat may also be considered secondary signs of cuff pathology. Because peribursal fat may be replaced by either low signal intensity granulation tissue or scar or bright signal intensity fluid, which is often limited to the site of the cuff tear, we use this abnormality as a secondary to tertiary sign when a cuff tear is not clearly visualized.

Fatty atrophy of the rotator cuff muscle is usually associated with more chronic complete tears (see Fig. 9-76). Fatty replacement is best demonstrated on T1-weighted images, which display high signal intensity (equal to fat) horizontal streaks parallel to the long axis of the supraspinatus (see Fig. 9-77). The changes of supraspinatus muscle atrophy are not conspicuous on gradient-echo, fat-suppressed T2-weighted fast spin-echo, or STIR sequences.

Alterations in the peribursal fat plane and proximal musculotendinous junction are present in up to 92% of complete tears. With the use of fat-suppression techniques, Mirowitz[121] has shown that many of the established secondary criteria for diagnosis of rotator cuff tears, including obliteration of the subacromial-subdeltoid fat plane and fluid in the subacromial-subdeltoid bursa, are routinely found in asymptomatic populations.[121]

According to Neer's classification, 95% of all rotator cuff tears are impingement tears caused by outlet impingement.[59] Together, traumatic tears and rotator interval tears account for only 5% of all cuff tears. MR imaging confirms the gross anatomic finding that most tears of the supraspinatus involve its anterior attachment to the greater tuberosity. In critical zone tears (tears immediately proximal to the greater tuberosity insertion of the supraspinatus tendon), a small remnant of tendon may be still attached to the greater tuberosity. In patients older than 40 years of age, rotator cuff tendon tears are frequently associated with acute glenohumeral dislocations. Infrequent traumatic tears in younger individuals may avulse a segment of the greater tuberosity.

The size of a rotator cuff tear can be determined by the measuring its long diameter in centimeters. A small cuff tear measures less than 1 cm, medium cuff tears measure 1 to 3 cm, a large cuff tear is 3 to 5 cm, and a massive tear is greater than 5 cm. The number of tendons involved, and their level of retraction, is of more clinical significance than size, however.

Rotator Interval Tears

The rotator interval is the space between the supraspinatus and superior border of the subscapularis tendons (Fig. 9-81). Since there is no tendon in this location, the

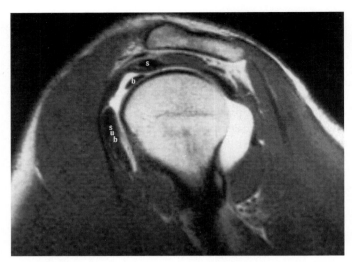

FIGURE 9-81. An intact rotator interval between the supraspinatus tendon (s) and subscapularis tendon (sub). The coracohumeral ligament is located on the anterior edge of the interval, whereas the long head of the biceps is located deep in the posterior aspect of the rotator interval. b, biceps tendon.

interval is not a site for impingement or degenerative wear.[52] The rotator interval is formed from thin elastic, membranous tissue. This tissue is reinforced by the coracohumeral ligament and the SGL and capsule. Longitudinal interval tears, with or without extension to the subscapularis tendon, are often seen in association with acute glenohumeral dislocations, especially in patients older than 40 years of age. An interval tear may also be associated with anterior and multidirectional laxity, secondary to repetitive trauma in patients younger than 35 years of age.

T2-weighted images in the sagittal oblique plane may show the anterior extension of fluid across the rotator cuff interval. This finding may be more easily demonstrated by MR arthrography (Fig. 9-82). The diagnosis of an interval tear may be difficult if previous arthroscopic surgery has created a defect or communication across this thin interval.

Subscapularis Tendon Tears

Most subscapularis tendon tears occur in association with tears of the supraspinatus and infraspinatus tendons. Rarely, however, they may occur as an isolated injury[117] (Fig. 9-83). Although increased signal intensity on T2-weighted images can be observed on coronal oblique and sagittal oblique images through the subscapularis, it is the axial plane that is most important and specific for the evaluation of subscapularis tendon tears. Partial tears may be associated with thickening of the subscapularis tendon in conjunction with regions of fiber discontinuity. Complete detachment from the lesser tuberosity is associated with fluid signal intensity extending anterior to the retracted tendon. Associated biceps tendon abnormalities, including medial dislocation, may be present.

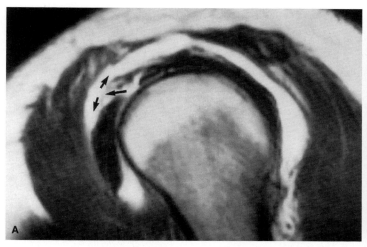
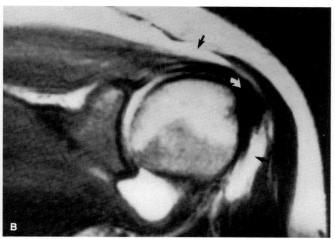

FIGURE 9-82. (A) A T1-weighted sagittal oblique image shows extension of intraarticular gadolinium contrast across the rotator interval (*arrows*) between the subscapularis and supraspinatus tendons, secondary to previous surgical release in entering the glenohumeral joint. (B) A T1-weighted coronal oblique image also demonstrates subacromial-subdeltoid gadolinium (*straight arrow*) with an intact supraspinatus tendon (*curved arrow*).

Teres Minor Tendon Tear

Tears of the teres minor tendon, either in association with massive cuff tears or as an isolated tear, are uncommon. Edema and atrophy of the teres minor (Fig. 9-84) may be associated with impingement or denervation of the axillary nerve in the quadrilateral space (the quadrilateral space syn-

drome).[122] These changes are best visualized on sagittal oblique images which show the infraspinatus in a superior position relative to the more inferiorly located teres minor muscle. MR signs of denervation include areas of hyperintensity on T2 or fat-suppressed images. Changes in fatty atrophy, however, do not show an increase in signal intensity on fat-suppressed T2-weighted or STIR images.

Magnetic Resonance Imaging Accuracy

According to reports by Zlatkin and colleagues,[22] MR sensitivity and specificity for imaging of partial and full thickness tears are 91% and 88%, respectively, with 89% accuracy. Preoperative assessment of the size of rotator cuff tear compares favorably with surgical findings in 95% of cases. In another study of arthroscopic or surgical correlation in complete cuff tears in 91 patients, MR imaging had a sensitivity of 100% and a specificity of 95%.[123] Burk and coworkers reported comparable findings (92%) for sensitivity of MR imaging and arthrography in the diagnosis of rotator cuff tears.[21] Raffi and colleagues, in their study of 37 documented full thickness tears, reported a sensitivity of 97% and specificity of 94%. Of 16 partial tears, 14 were diagnosed accurately with MR imaging.[91]

Fat saturation techniques improve the detection of both complete and partial rotator cuff tears when compared with conventional spin-echo techniques.[116] Fat-suppressed MR imaging, including fat-suppressed T2-weighted fast spin-echo, has been reported to have a combined accuracy rate of 93% (with a sensitivity of 84% and a specificity of 97%) in the detection of complete and partial tears of the rotator cuff.[115]

The addition of fat-suppression to MR arthrography increases sensitivity and specificity of this technique from 90% and 75%, respectively, to 100% for both sensitivity and specificity for the identification of full thickness and partial cuff

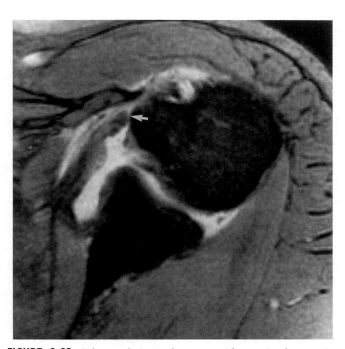

FIGURE 9-83. Subscapularis tendon tear with proximal retraction (*arrow*) to the level of the lesser tuberosity. There is free communication of fluid between the glenohumeral joint subscapularis bursa and the subcoracoid bursa anterior to the subscapularis tendon. (T2*-weighted axial image.)

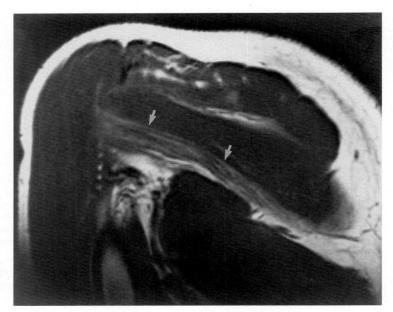

FIGURE 9-84. Isolated atrophy (*arrows*) of the teres minor shown as parallel streaks of fat signal intensity oriented along the long axis of the muscle on a T1-weighted coronal oblique image posterior to the humeral head.

tears.[113] Fat-suppressed images are also sensitive to the intra-tendinous imbibition of contrast material in regions of associated tendon swelling, fraying, and friability.

MR Findings in Asymptomatic Shoulders

In a study of 96 asymptomatic individuals, Sher and colleagues found tears of the rotator cuff in 34%.[124] The frequency of both full and partial thickness tears increases with age, and in asymptomatic individuals older than 60 years of age, 54% had a tear of the rotator cuff. Partial tears (24%) were more common than full thickness tears (4%) in younger individuals (40 to 60 years of age). Among 19- to 39-year-old patients, partial thickness tears were found in 4%, but no full thickness tears were found. Miniaci and coworkers found similar results, and reported no full thickness tears in 20 asymptomatic volunteers ranging in age from 17 to 49 with a mean age of 29.[125] It is clear that MR findings of rotator cuff disease must be considered in a clinical context and should never be used as the only basis for operative intervention.[124] Positive MR findings for a rotator cuff tear may not be concordant with a patient's symptoms or lack thereof.

Postoperative Rotator Cuff

Magnetic resonance imaging has also been used for postoperative evaluation of rotator cuff repairs. Because gradient-echo sequences frequently show increased magnetic susceptibility artifacts, the repair site may not be clearly visualized on the scans (Fig. 9-85). Conventional T1 and T2 spin-echo and fast spin-echo sequences minimize these low signal intensity artifacts, and allow visualization of increased signal intensity in cuff defects.

Postoperative MR arthrography, using a fat-suppressed short TR/TE T1-weighted sequence, also minimizes surgical artifacts (Fig. 9-86). Changes caused by acromioplasty, resection of the distal end of the clavicle and division of the coracoacromial ligament, are also displayed on MR images. There may be persistent changes from impingement (including tendon degeneration, partial tear, retear, a rough undersurface of the acromion, or residual AC joint callus or osteophytes), deltoid attachment instability, and nerve damage. The rotator cuff interval between the supraspinatus and subscapularis tendons may be interrupted at surgery, allowing communication of contrast with the subacromial-subdeltoid bursa, even though the rotator cuff repair is intact. The isolated findings of subacromial-subdeltoid fluid is not sufficient to diagnose a failed or retorn repair of the rotator cuff. Some retears may be associated with granulation tissue and adhesions, and may appear as a low signal intensity tear on T2-weighted images without associated fluid signal intensity at the tear site or in the subacromial-subdeltoid bursa. The presence of a gap or defined defect in the cuff associated with extension of fluid signal intensity on T2-weighted or fat-suppressed T2-weighted fast spin-echo sequences is diagnostic for a retorn repair. A retracted or nonvisualized section of the rotator cuff also represents a full thickness tear. Because rotator cuff contours may be irregular in the postsurgical cuff, the distinction between a partial thickness tear and an intact repair site may be difficult. Owen and coworkers[120] reported a 90% accuracy for the detection of full thickness tears in the postoperative shoulder.[120] Sagittal T2-weighted images are particularly useful in the evaluation of the anterior portion of the supraspinatus tendon. They minimize the partial volume effect of subacromial-subdeltoid fluid anteriorly, and demonstrate portions of the cuff that may be difficult to discern on coronal oblique images because of a micro-metallic or suture artifact.

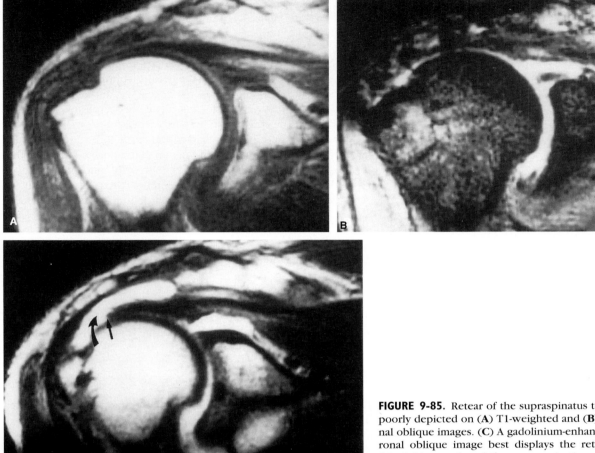

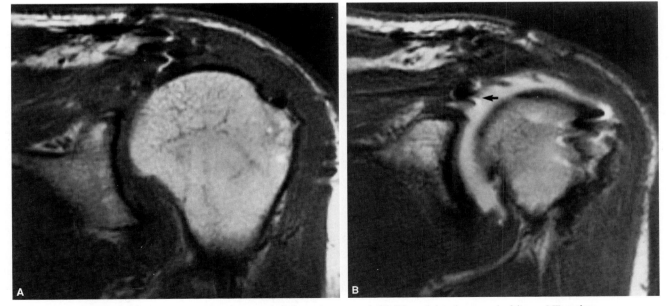

FIGURE 9-85. Retear of the supraspinatus tendon after repair is poorly depicted on (**A**) T1-weighted and (**B**) T2*-weighted coronal oblique images. (**C**) A gadolinium-enhanced T1-weighted coronal oblique image best displays the retracted tendon edge (*straight arrow*) and the communication of contrast with the subacromial bursa (*curved arrow*).

FIGURE 9-86. (**A**) T1-weighted coronal oblique image and (**B**) T1-weighted coronal oblique MR arthrogram of retorn supraspinatus tendon. The retear with retracted tendon edges (*arrow*) is best seen on the T1 coronal oblique MR arthrogram (**B**). Susceptibility artifact is identified overlying the greater tuberosity, and acromioplasty.

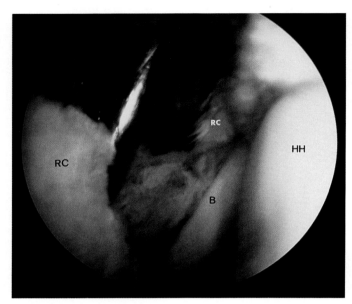

FIGURE 9-87. Arthroscopic photograph of a complete rotator cuff tear. Retracted rotator cuff (black RC) and stump of cuff tissue (white RC) are labeled. B, biceps tendon; HH, humeral head.

Surgical Management

Chronic impingement leads to complete rotator cuff tears. The repair procedure of choice begins with an ASD, followed by a deltoid-splitting approach to gain access to the torn cuff.[59] The supraspinatus most commonly tears at its insertion on the greater tuberosity (Fig. 9-87). Therefore,

primary repairs are fixed directly to the bone with drill holes or suture anchors. As mentioned earlier, a Mumford procedure may be performed when AC degeneration is evident.

The rotator cuff is usually repaired with nonabsorbable sutures used to reattach the avulsed tendon to a denuded bed of bone (Fig. 9-88). With the deltoid-splitting approach, drill holes in the acromion are not necessary, and proper subperiosteal reflection of the deltoid at the acromion permits a side-to-side closure. If extensive dissection of the deltoid from the acromion is carried out, drill holes are necessary to repair the deltoid, which is reflected during surgery. This approach has a higher rate of morbidity, and postoperative deltoid defects are more common. Most repairs can be achieved through a more limited deltoid-splitting approach.

Glenohumeral Joint Instability

The stability of the glenohumeral joint depends on the stabilizing musculotendinous structures of the rotator cuff as well as almost all the muscles of the shoulder girdle. The importance of the IGLLC and, particularly, the IGL, is discussed by Turkel and associates.[126]

Anterior Instability

The most common of all glenohumeral joint instabilities is anterior instability, particularly that produced by lesions of the IGLLC (Fig. 9-89). The anterior band of the IGLC, which forms the anterior labrum, has been shown by Turkel and coworkers to be the primary restraint to anterior transla-

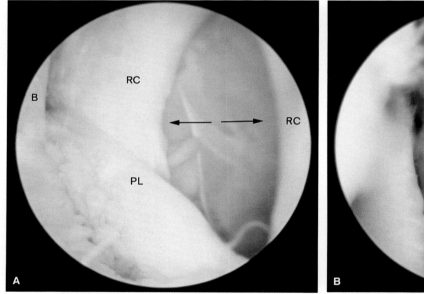

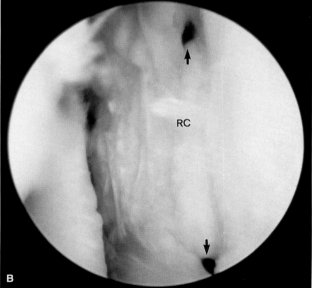

FIGURE 9-88. **(A)** Arthroscopic view of rotator cuff (RC) tear with tendinous gap identified (*arrows*). B, biceps edge; PL, posterior labrum. **(B)** Corresponding postoperative arthroscopic view of coapted and sutured (*arrows*) rotator cuff (RC).

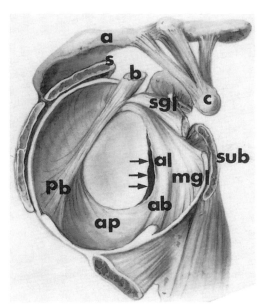

FIGURE 9-89. Anterior labrum avulsion from the anterior glenoid rim (*arrows*). a, acromion; ab, anterior band of inferior glenohumeral ligament; al, anterior labrum; ap, axillary pouch of inferior glenohumeral ligament; c, coracoid; pb, posterior band of inferior glenohumeral ligament; s, supraspinatus tendon; sgl, superior glenohumeral ligament; sub, subscapularis tendon; b, biceps tendon; mgl, middle glenohumeral ligament.

tion of the humeral head at 90° of abduction.[126] It is best demonstrated on sagittal oblique MR images and is routinely seen on MR arthrography in this plane.

Avulsion of the IGLLC from the glenoid rim, known as a Bankart lesion (Figs. 9-90 and 9-91), involves the detachment of the anterior labrum and the IGLC from the anterior glenoid rim. Rowe[127] has developed a classification system for Bankart lesions based on the detachment of the labrum and capsule from the anterior glenoid. A Bankart lesion can involve labral avulsion without a bony inferior glenoid rim fracture.

The IGL complex (Fig. 9-92) can also tear at its midportion or be avulsed from its humeral insertion. The humeral avulsion of the glenohumeral ligament (ie, HAGL lesion) can be demonstrated arthroscopically, and in some cases is solely responsible for shoulder instability[128] (Fig. 9-93). Pollock and Bigliani have shown that pathology or defects in the IGLLC are found at the humeral origin and within the substance of the ligament more commonly than was previously anticipated.[129] It is therefore important to evaluate the IGLLC from its humeral origin through its course to its labral insertion.

Measurement of IGL thickness by Pollock and Bigliani documents that the anterior band is the thickest region, followed by the anterior and posterior aspects of the axillary pouch.[129] Failure of the IGL can occur at the glenoid insertion site (40%), in the ligament substance (35%), and at the humeral insertion site (25%). Avulsions occur more frequently in the anterior band and the anterior aspect of the axillary pouch, whereas ligament substance tears are more common in the posterior aspect of the axillary pouch. Bankart avulsions represent failure of the IGL at the glenoid insertion (Fig. 9-94), and IGL capsule laxity represents intrasubstance ligament failure. The tensile properties of the IGL allow for significant stretching before failure; therefore, redundancy of the IGL may be as important as avulsions of the glenoid insertion at the IGL in producing glenohumeral instabilities.

text continues on page 693

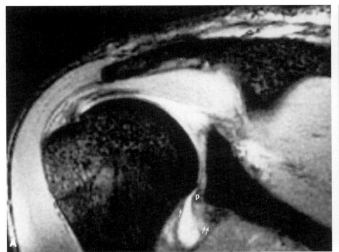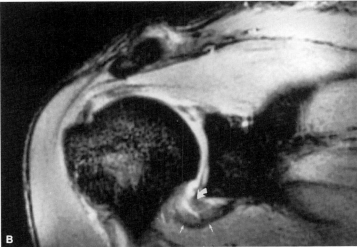

FIGURE 9-90. Avulsion of the anterior band of the inferior glenohumeral ligament (IGL). **(A)** A T2*-weighted posterior coronal image shows intact humeral (*single arrow*) and inferior glenoid pole attachments of the IGL (*double arrows*). p, posterior labrum. **(B)** A more anterior T2*-weighted coronal oblique image depicts the axillary pouch of the IGL (*straight arrows*) and the avulsed anterior inferior glenoid labrum (*curved arrow*).

continued

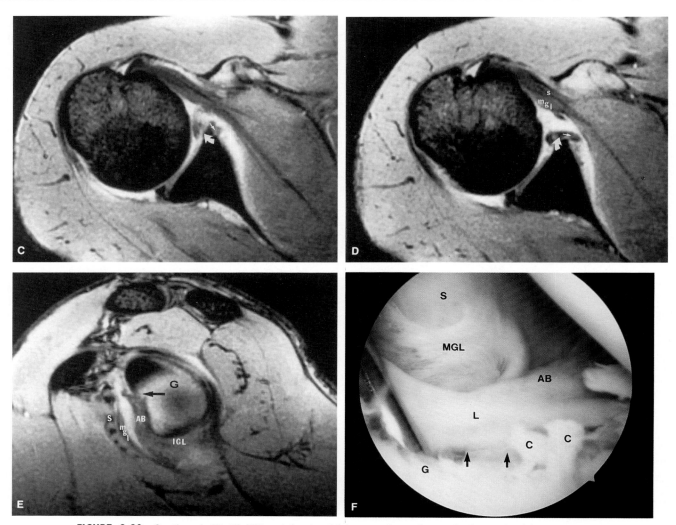

FIGURE 9-90. *Continued.* **(C, D)** T2*-weighted axial images show the avulsed anterior labrum (*curved arrow*) and the anterior band of the IGL (small straight arrow). mgl, middle glenohumeral ligament; s, subscapularis tendon. **(E)** A T2*-weighted sagittal oblique image shows the avulsed anterior band (AB; *arrows*) of the IGL. G, glenoid; mgl, middle glenohumeral ligament; S, subscapularis tendon. **(F)** The corresponding arthroscopic image shows the avulsed labrum (L; *arrows*) and anterior band (AB) of the IGL. C, articular cartilage debris; G, glenoid; MGL, middle glenohumeral ligament; S, subscapularis tendon.

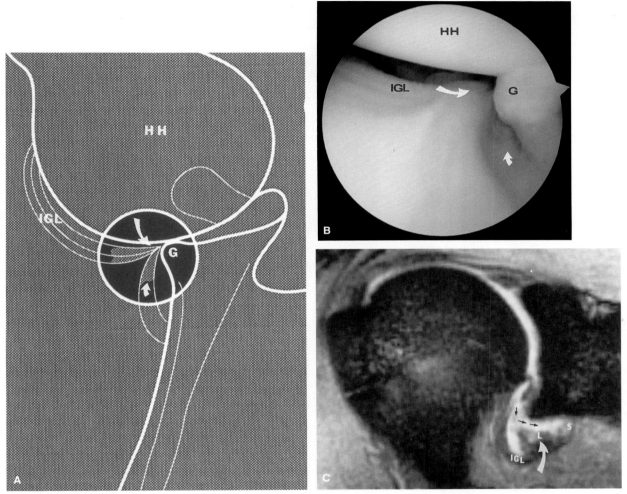

FIGURE 9-91. Bankart lesion. (**A**) A tear (*large curved arrow*) of the inferior glenoid and labral attachment of the inferior glenohumeral ligament (IGL) is present. Scarred muscle of the subscapularis is shown along the inferior glenoid neck (*small curved arrow*). The humeral head (HH) is subluxed inferiorly. G, glenoid. (**B**) The arthroscopic view from inferior to anterior is seen with the scope in the axillary pouch, oriented toward the anterior inferior pole of the glenoid. Note the avulsed labrum from glenoid rim (G) and torn inferior pole attachment (*large curved arrow*) of IGL. HH, humeral head. Scarred tearing of subscapularis muscle from scapular neck is also identified (*small curved arrow*). (**C**) Avulsed anterior glenoid labrum (L; *curved arrow*) and IGL attachment are shown on a T2*-weighted coronal oblique image. Fluid extension (*straight arrows*) is identified between the inferior glenoid neck, detached labrum, and subscapularis muscle (S).

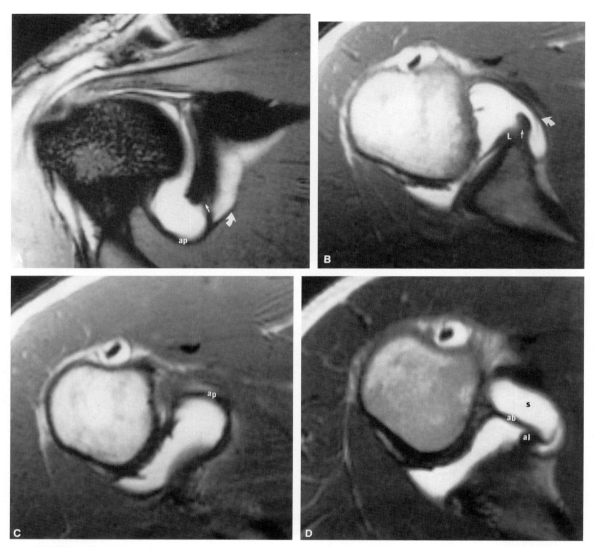

FIGURE 9-92. Inferior glenohumeral ligament lateral complex. **(A)** Enhanced T2*-weighted gradient-echo coronal oblique images demonstrate the normal inferior glenoid pole attachment of the axillary pouch (ap) of the inferior glenohumeral ligament (*straight arrow*). Note gadolinium contrast in normal inferior extension of subscapularis bursa (*curved arrow*). **(B)** An enhanced T1-weighted axial image displays subscapularis bursa (*curved arrow*) and glenoid origin (*straight arrow*) of the inferior glenohumeral ligament complex (IGLC). The IGLC may originate from the glenoid, the labrum (L), or the neck of the glenoid immediately adjacent to the labrum. There is no anterior lateral tear on this image. **(C)** An enhanced T1-weighted axial image below the level of the glenoid displays the normal axillary pouch (ap) of the inferior glenohumeral ligament. **(D)** An enhanced T1-weighted axial image in a different patient identifies the anterior band (ab) of the inferior glenohumeral ligament complex and its continuation as the anterior labrum (al). Gadolinium contrast is shown in the subscapularis bursa (s) anterior to the anterior band. There is no tear of the anterior inferior labrum.

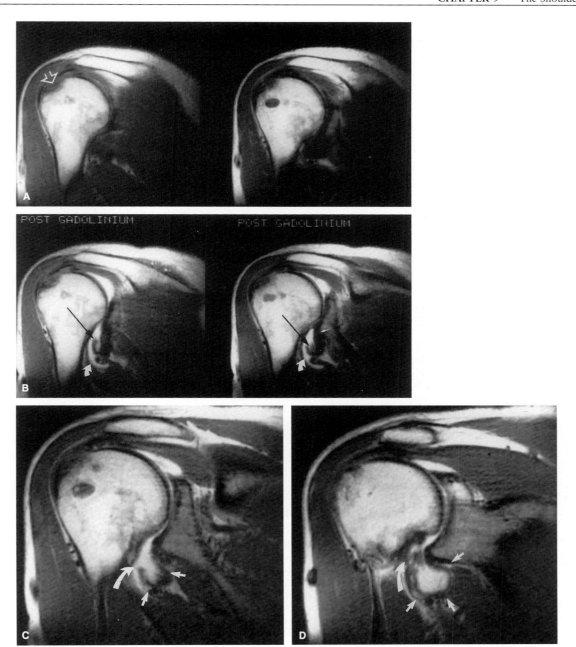

FIGURE 9-93. Humeral head avulsion of the glenohumeral ligament (HAGL lesion). T1-weighted coronal oblique images (**A**) before and (**B**) after intraarticular gadolinium administration are shown in a patient with a history of chronic anterior dislocation. A Hill-Sachs lesion is identified in the posterolateral humeral head (*open arrow*). The postgadolinium images document inferior extravasation of contrast (*curved white arrows*) through the avulsed insertion of the inferior glenohumeral ligament (IGL) to the anatomic neck of the humerus (long black arrows). This is diagnostic for the HAGL lesion. The IGL is also shown (*small white arrow*). (**C, D**) More anterior coronal oblique images display an abnormally capacious axillary pouch (*straight arrows*) secondary to avulsion of the IGL humeral insertion (*curved arrows*).

continued

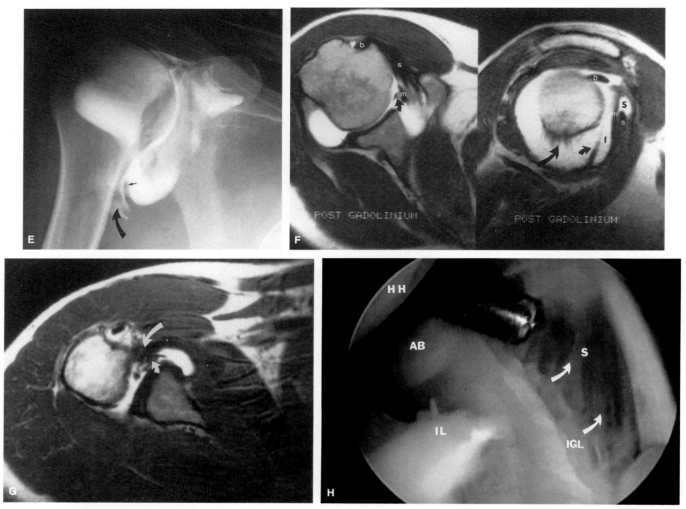

FIGURE 9-93. *Continued.* **(E)** The corresponding arthrogram confirms extravasation of contrast (*curved arrow*) through the tear in the IGL complex (*straight arrow*). **(F)** Enhanced axial (*left*) and sagittal oblique (*right*) images demonstrate abnormal anterior and lateral displacement of the anterior band of the IGL (*small curved arrow*). The sagittal oblique image shows a type 3 synovial recess with a superior subscapularis recess above the middle glenohumeral ligament (MGL, m) and an inferior subscapular recess below the MGL. Large curved arrow, axillary pouch of IGL; b, biceps tendon; S, superior subscapular recess; I, inferior subscapular recess; s, subscapularis tendon. **(G)** An inferior axial image shows an avulsed humeral attachment of the IGL (*large curved arrow*) and associated ligamentous and lateral fraying (*small curved arrow*). **(H)** An arthroscopic image also shows the avulsed humeral attachment of the IGL (*curved arrows*). AB, anterior band; HH, humeral head; IL, torn inferior labrum; S, subscapularis muscle.

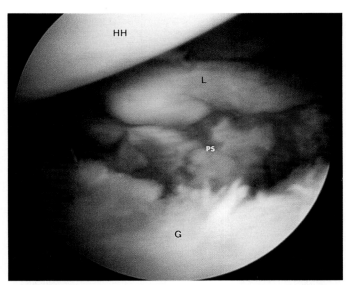

FIGURE 9-94. Arthroscopic view of an anterior labral (L) avulsion (Bankart avulsion) from the anterior inferior glenoid rim (G). Periosteal sleeve (PS) is shown between the avulsed labrum and glenoid. HH, humeral head.

Operative stabilization for anterior instability includes tightening of the anterior structures to limit external rotation (Magnuson-Stack and Putti-Platt procedures), coracoid transfer procedures (Bristow operation) to provide a bony block and a tenodesis effect to prevent anterior translation of the humeral head over the anterior glenoid rim, osteotomies of the glenoid or humerus, and reconstruction of the avulsed or stretched IGLC structures (Bankart procedure and its modifications). Arthroscopic stabilization procedures involve a capsular plication combined with reattachment of the IGLLC (arthroscopic Bankart repair)[130] (Fig. 9-95).

MR Findings in Anterior Instability

BANKART LESION. Magnetic resonance imaging demonstrates either the anterior labral avulsion (Fig. 9-96) or labral and anterior inferior glenoid rim fracture[131–134] (Fig. 9-97). Axial T1-weighted images show subchondral bone changes, including low signal intensity sclerosis or marrow hyperemia at the fracture site. T2*-weighted images are more useful in demonstrating the morphology of the labrum and associated tear pattern if present. Coronal oblique images show avulsion of the anterior inferior labrum and its relationship to the axillary pouch, which is lax when the arm is adducted. Sagittal oblique images define the size of the anterior inferior glenoid fracture (Fig. 9-98) and the extent of the labral tear (Fig. 9-99), both anterosuperiorly and superoinferiorly. The relationship of the anterior band of the IGL to the avulsed labrum is identified at the level of the glenoid fossa on sagittal oblique MR images. Medial displacement of the avulsed labrum, when it occurs, is secondary to medial and

inferior pull from the anterior band of the IGL. A linear area of hyperintensity is seen in the area of stretching or plastic deformation across the axillary pouch of the IGL. This is better visualized with the arm positioned in abduction and external rotation in order to tighten the IGLC.

It is important to differentiate between acute and chronic Bankart lesions (Fig. 9-100). In acute lesions, there is increased signal intensity in the subchondral bone of the glenoid on T2, fat-suppressed T2-weighted fast spin-echo, or STIR images. In athletes, there may be acute trauma superimposed on a chronic Bankart lesion that does not need to be clinically repaired. This is especially likely in high level amateur and professional athletes who perform despite a previous history of shoulder trauma or dislocation.

A Hill-Sachs posterolateral compression fracture can be seen in patients with subluxation and single or multiple episodes of dislocation[135] (see Figs. 9-96 and 9-98). This compression defect is identified on the posterolateral humeral head. There is a normal bare area of bone where the capsule attaches laterally to the anatomic neck of the humerus posteriorly. This bare area or normal flattening of the posterior aspect of the humeral head in its inferior portion should not be mistaken for a Hill-Sachs defect. Posterolateral bone contusions, without humeral head indentation, may also be identified on MR images.[136]

THE ALPSA LESION. The anterior labroligamentous periosteal sleeve avulsion (ALPSA) lesion (Fig. 9-101) represents an avulsion of the IGL through its anterior band attachment to the anterior labrum, similar to the Bankart lesion.[137] The ALPSA lesion differs from the Bankart lesion, however, in that the ALPSA lesion has an intact anterior scapular periosteum allowing the labroligamentous structures to displace medially and rotate inferiorly on the scapular neck. In the Bankart lesion, the anterior scapular periosteum ruptures, resulting in displacement of the labrum and attached ligaments anterior to the glenoid rim. After the ALPSA lesion heals, there may be recurrent anterior dislocations secondary to IGL incompetence. Arthroscopically, an ALPSA lesion is converted to a Bankart lesion to allow reconstruction of the anterior inferior structures of the capsule (capsulorrhaphy). Neviaser identified ALPSA lesions in 4 of 8 patients with primary anterior shoulder dislocations.[137] The mechanism of injury is the same for both the Bankart and ALPSA lesions.

On axial MR images, the anterior labrum with stripped periosteum can be seen to be displaced medially and rotated inferiorly on the neck of the glenoid (Fig. 9-101). Sagittal images at the level of the glenohumeral joint are used to identify medial displacement of the anterior band relative to the neck of the glenoid. In comparison, a Bankart lesion usually is shown with a space or gap between the anterior rim of the bony glenoid and displaced anterior glenoid. This gap is the result of rupture of the glenoid neck periosteum and is frequently filled with fluid signal intensity.

text continues on page 696

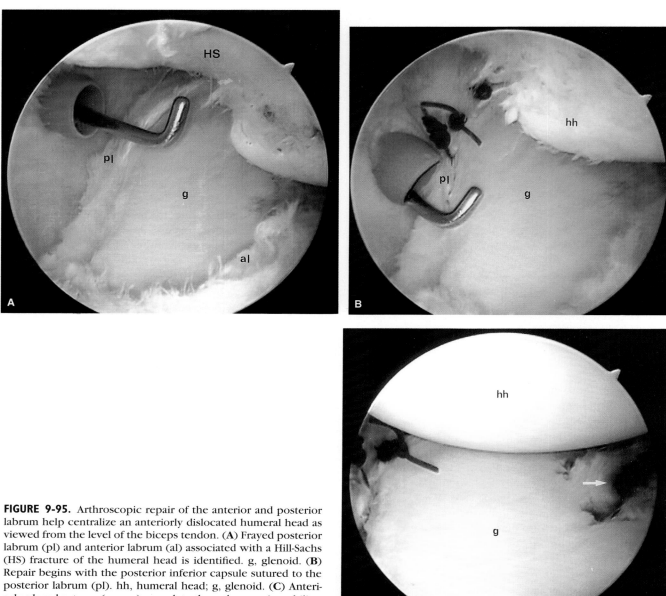

FIGURE 9-95. Arthroscopic repair of the anterior and posterior labrum help centralize an anteriorly dislocated humeral head as viewed from the level of the biceps tendon. (**A**) Frayed posterior labrum (pl) and anterior labrum (al) associated with a Hill-Sachs (HS) fracture of the humeral head is identified. g, glenoid. (**B**) Repair begins with the posterior inferior capsule sutured to the posterior labrum (pl). hh, humeral head; g, glenoid. (**C**) Anteriorly placed sutures (*arrow*) complete the arthroscopic stabilization centralizing the humeral head (hh) on the glenoid (g).

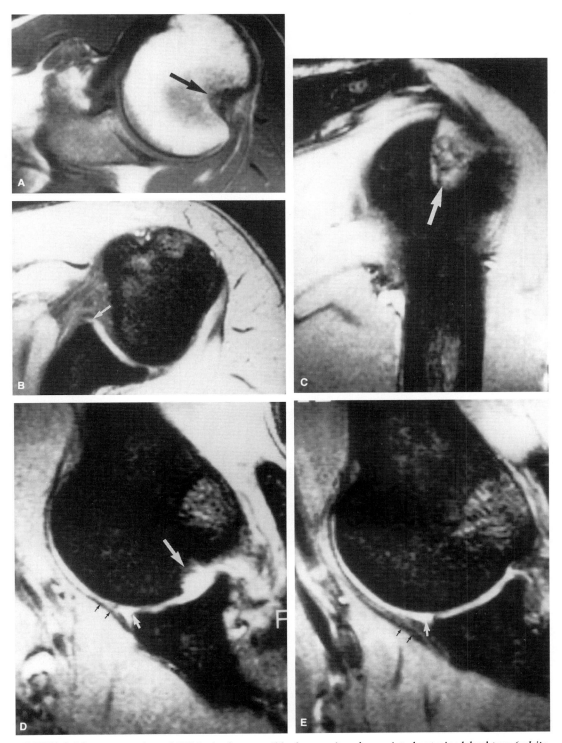

FIGURE 9-96. A posterolateral Hill-Sachs fracture (*black arrow*) and associated anterior labral tear (*white arrow*) are seen on axial (**A**) T1-weighted and (**B**) T2*-weighted images. (**C**) A posterolateral Hill-Sachs wedge-shaped impaction (*arrow*) is seen on a T2*-weighted coronal image. Corresponding T2*-weighted axial images with the arm in abduction and external rotation (**D** and **E**) show a Hill-Sachs lesion (*large white arrow*), an absence of the anterior labrum (*small white arrows*), and a taut inferior glenohumeral ligament (*small black arrows*).

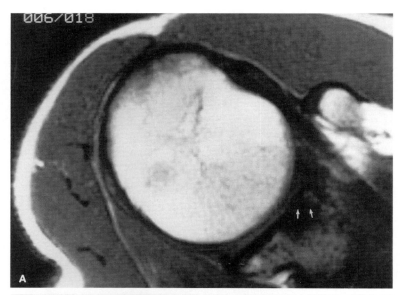

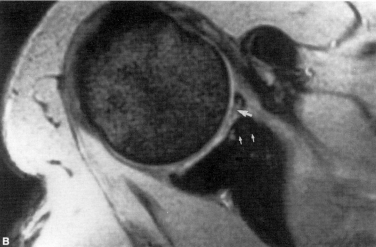

FIGURE 9-97. **(A)** A T1-weighted axial image shows an osseous Bankart lesion with fracture of the anterior inferior glenoid (*arrows*). **(B)** A linear tear of the anterior labrum (*large arrow*) can be seen. However, the osseous Bankart lesion (*small arrows*) demonstrates poor contrast on this T2*-weighted axial image.

THE GLAD LESION. As described by Neviaser,[138] the glenolabral articular disruption (GLAD) lesion results from a forced adduction injury occurring from the position of abduction and external rotation of the shoulder. There is a superficial anterior inferior labral tear, associated with an anterior inferior glenoid articular cartilage injury. There are no signs of clinical or surgical anterior instability. Identification of anterior inferior labral tears may require imaging of the shoulder with the arm positioned in external rotation and abduction. The use of intraarticular contrast helps to visualize small tears at the level of the anterior inferior glenoid rim. Articular cartilage lesions are best demonstrated with fat-suppressed T2-weighted fast spin-echo sequences or fat-suppressed MR arthrography at smaller FOVs (8 to 12 cm).

THE HAGL LESION. Humeral avulsion of the glenohumeral ligament, which causes anterior shoulder instability, is significantly less frequent than the classic Bankart lesion (see Fig. 9-93). Wolf and colleagues[128] identified HAGL lesions in 9.3% of 64 shoulders preoperatively evaluated by arthroscopy for anterior instability, and in 35% of the shoulders that were unstable without labral pathology at the level of the glenoid rim. Thus, the HAGL lesion may exist in patients with anterior instability with or without an associated anterior labral tear. The HAGL lesion is treated with surgical reattachment of the glenohumeral ligament to its humeral insertion.

Identification of the humeral detachment of the IGL on MR images (Fig. 9-102) usually requires the presence of a joint effusion or the use of MR arthrography. The axillary pouch is converted from a fluid-distended U-shaped structure to a J-shaped structure as the IGL drops inferiorly. The direct extension of fluid or contrast can be identified between the humerus and the avulsed IGL. On sagittal oblique images, the retracted or redundant IGL appears as a mass of low signal intensity tissue.

text continues on page 702

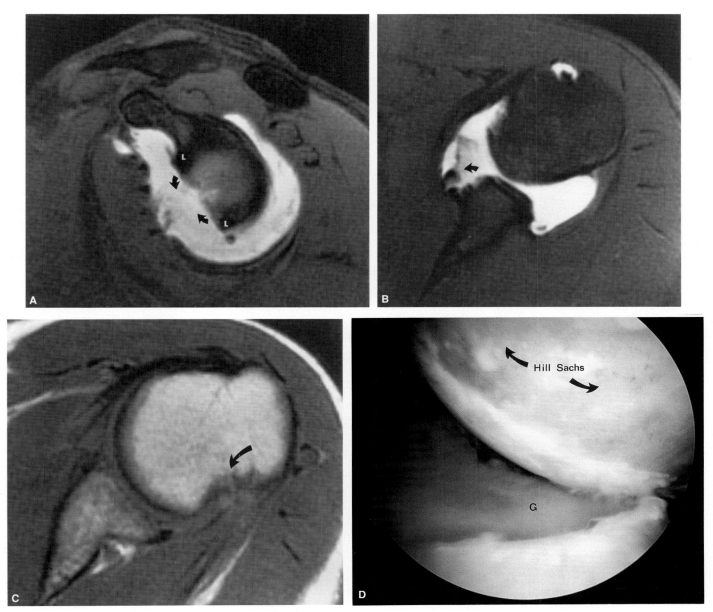

FIGURE 9-98. Bankart and Hill-Sachs lesions. Anterior inferior glenoid rim fracture and anterior labral (L) avulsion (*small curved arrows*) on fat-suppressed T1-weighted (**A**) sagittal oblique and (**B**) axial MR arthrograms. The extent of anterior inferior quadrant involvement with loss of bony and labral continuity is best shown on the sagittal oblique image (**A**). Corresponding (**C**) T1-weighted axial image and (**D**) arthroscopic photograph demonstrate the associated Hill-Sachs lesion (*curved arrow*) of the posterolateral humeral head. G, glenoid.

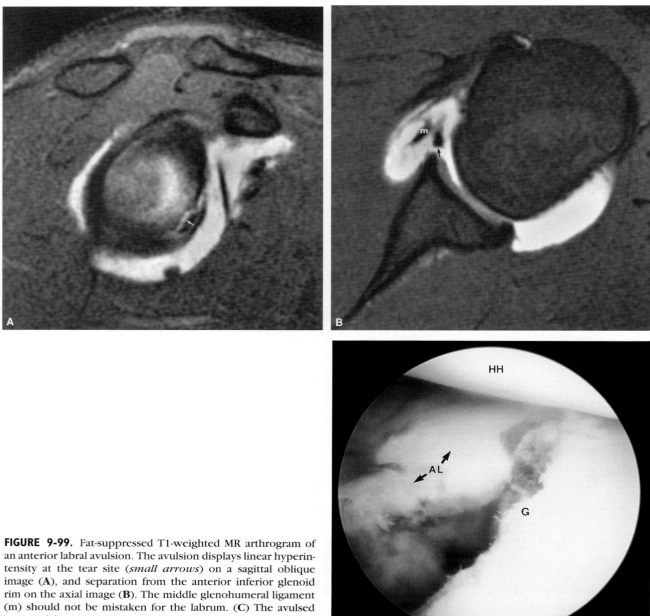

FIGURE 9-99. Fat-suppressed T1-weighted MR arthrogram of an anterior labral avulsion. The avulsion displays linear hyperintensity at the tear site (*small arrows*) on a sagittal oblique image (**A**), and separation from the anterior inferior glenoid rim on the axial image (**B**). The middle glenohumeral ligament (m) should not be mistaken for the labrum. (**C**) The avulsed anterior labrum (AL) is shown separated from the anterior glenoid (G) rim at arthroscopy. HH, humeral head.

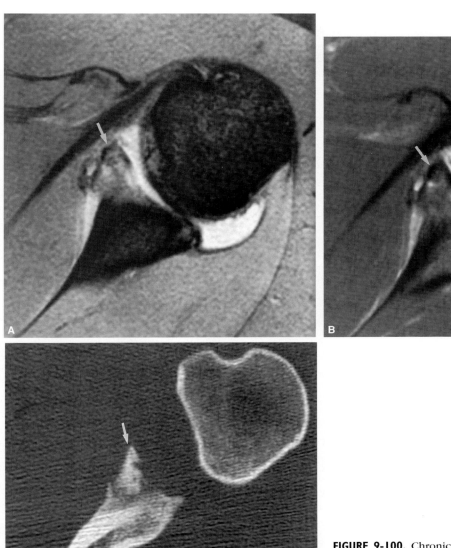

FIGURE 9-100. Chronic Bankart lesion (*arrow*) in an injured football player is seen on T2* (**A**), fat-suppressed T2-weighted fast spin-echo (**B**), and axial CT (**C**) images. On the fat-suppressed T2-weighted fast spin-echo image there is a lack of bone marrow edema at the fracture site or in adjacent glenoid subchondral bone marrow. Sclerotic changes are seen in the anterior inferior glenoid rim on corresponding CT scan (**C**).

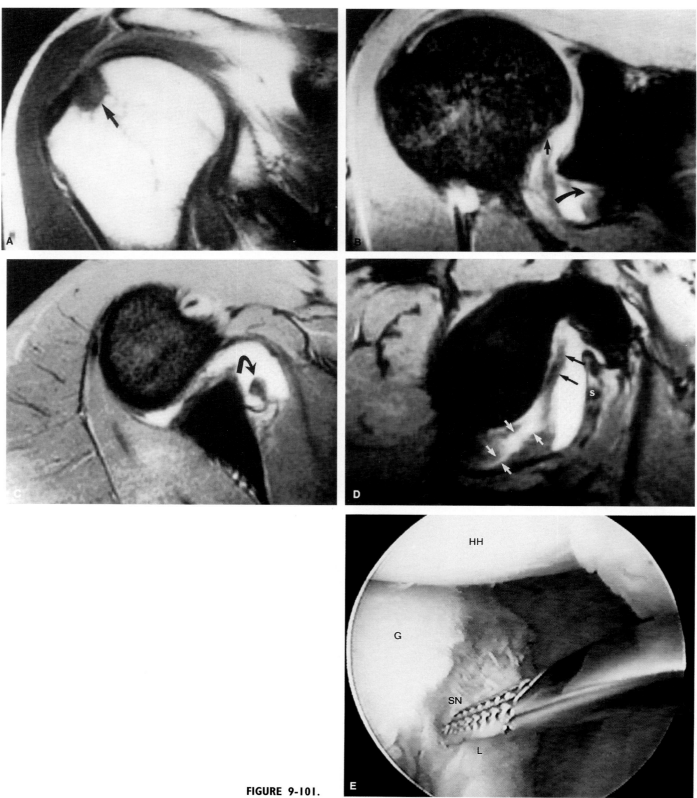

FIGURE 9-101.

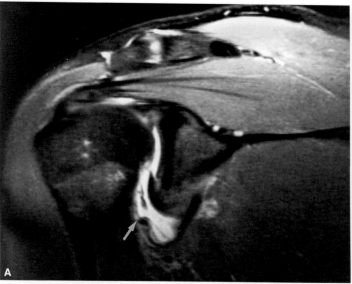

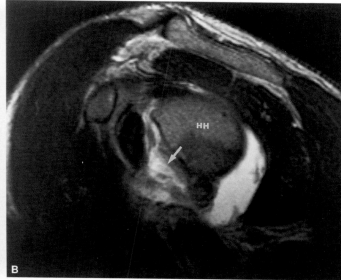

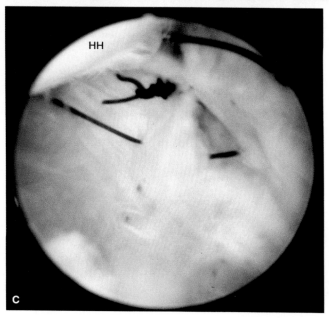

FIGURE 9-102. HAGL lesion with avulsion of the humeral attachment of the inferior glenohumeral ligament (*arrow*) on fat-suppressed T2-weighted fast spin-echo coronal oblique (**A**) and T2-weighted fast spin-echo sagittal oblique (**B**) images. Corresponding arthroscopic photograph (**C**) shows suturing with coaptation of the detached portion of the inferior glenohumeral ligament. HH, humeral head.

FIGURE 9-101. ALPSA lesion associated with a traumatic anterior dislocation. (**A**) A T1-weighted coronal oblique image shows a Hill-Sachs posterolateral compression fracture (*arrow*). (**B**) A T2*-weighted coronal oblique image demonstrates avulsion of the glenoid attachment of the inferior glenohumeral ligament (IGL; *curved arrow*), which results in a deformity of the axillary pouch. The humeral attachment of the IGL (*straight arrow*) is intact. (**C**) A T2*-weighted axial image shows the medial anterior displacement of the avulsed anterior band and labrum (*curved arrow*). (**D**) The avulsed and medially displaced anterior labrum (*black arrows*) is seen at the level of the coracoid on a sagittal T2*-weighted image. A tear of the axillary pouch and the lower portion of the anterior band is identified by a fluid-filled gap (*white arrows*). s, subscapularis tendon. (**E**) Arthroscopic view of the medial displaced labrum (L) avulsed from the glenoid (G) rim onto the scapular neck (SN). The anterior scapular periosteum is intact. HH, humeral head.

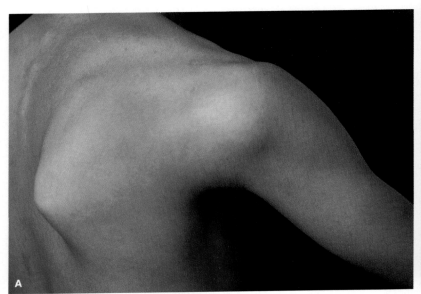
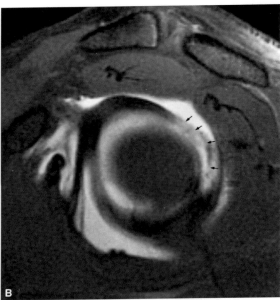

FIGURE 9-103. Posterior instability and labral tear. **(A)** Posterior instability with anterior rotation of the scapula post dislocation. **(B)** Fat-suppressed T1-weighted sagittal oblique MR arthrogram with posterior labral avulsion and discontinuity (*arrows*).

Posterior Instability

The posterior band of the IGLC is primarily responsible for capsuloligamentous restraint to posterior translation in 90° of abduction.[139,140] The anterior-superior capsule, or rotator interval capsule, has also been shown to be important in limiting posterior and inferior translation. Posterior dislocation occurred only with combined sectioning of the posterior capsule and anterior superior capsule.[141] The incidence of posterior instability has been reported to be between 2% and 4% of patients with shoulder instability (Fig. 9-103). Although relatively rare, it should be suspected in the presence of posterior labral disruption or fragmentation[142] (Figs. 9-104 and 9-105). A detailed examination with the patient under anesthesia (EUA) is critical in identifying this type of instability. Examination under anesthesia must be conducted in a lateral decubitus position with the patient's arm adducted, forward flexed, and in internal rotation. Stabilization of the scapula allows the examiner to appreciate the degree of posterior translation and relocation of the humeral head with abduction and external rotation. The results of the EUA, and the findings on diagnostic arthroscopy determine, the surgical procedure.

A reverse Bankart lesion, the association of a posterior labral tear with an anteromedial superior humeral head impaction (Fig. 9-106), may also be identified on MR images. The posterior labrum disruption is directly identified on axial or sagittal images. Axial images may display fluid undermining the base of a torn posterior labrum or show abnormal laxity (redundancy) of a torn posterior capsule. In posterior instability, the humeral head is often subluxed posteriorly relative to the glenoid fossa. In addition, MR arthrography demonstrates the posterior extension of contrast in the planes between the posterior labrum, the capsule, and the infraspinatus muscle.

Acute posterior dislocation may occur secondary to indi-

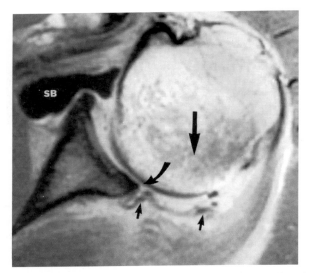

FIGURE 9-104. Traumatic posterior instability with complete fragmentation of the posterior labrum (*curved arrow*) and tearing of the posterior capsule (*small straight arrows*) in a football player. The humeral head is posteriorly subluxed relative to the glenoid (*large straight arrow*). This intermediate-weighted axial image was performed after air contrast CT arthrography. Low signal intensity air is shown in the subscapularis bursa (SB). There is also associated infraspinatus muscle-tendon disruption, demonstrated by increased signal intensity and irregularity of muscle fibers.

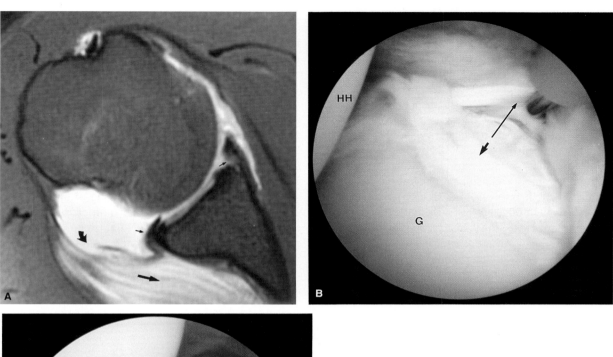

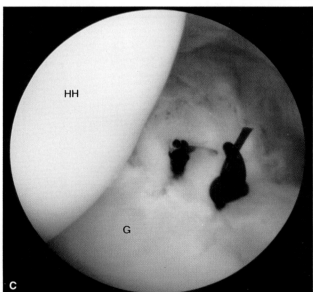

FIGURE 9-105. (A) Posterior capsular rupture (*curved arrow*) associated with tears of the anterior and posterior labrum (*small arrows*) and infraspinatus muscle (*large arrow*). Fat-suppressed T1-weighted axial MR arthrogram. (B, C) Arthroscopic suture repair of the posteroinferior labral tear (B, *arrows*) and anchored sutures reattaching the posterior labral tissue (C) are demonstrated. HH, humeral head; G, glenoid.

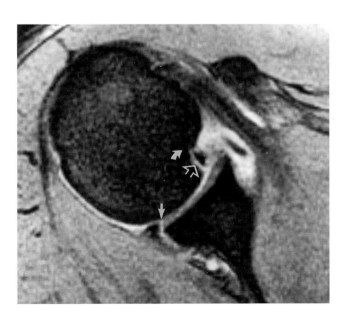

FIGURE 9-106. Reverse Bankart lesion with anteromedial humeral head impaction (*curved arrow*), anterior labral avulsion, and posterior labral tear. Fluid undermining the posterior labrum (*straight arrow*) and anterior fracture fragment (*open arrow*) are identified. (T2*-weighted axial image.)

rect forces (such as electric shock procedure), which produce adduction, flexion, and internal rotation. A fall on the outstretched hand with the arm abducted is another mechanism of injury in posterior instability. These same mechanisms, including a direct posterior force on an anteriorly flexed, abducted and internally rotated arm (eg, football pass blocking), may also produce acute posterior shoulder subluxation. Posterior instability may also occur as an operative complication in patients with multidirectional instability after a misdirected anterior capsular procedure.

With arthroscopy, it is possible to assess associated intraarticular lesions including labral tears, avulsions, and articular surface rotator cuff, SLAP, and biceps lesions.[141] The same arthroscopic capsulorrhaphy and anchor fixation can be used to treat posterior shoulder subluxations when there is a detachment of the posterior or superior capsule and/or

labrum. An open posterior capsular plication with capsular shift has a high success rate in the management of posterior shoulder instability.

THE BENNET LESION. The Bennet lesion, an extraarticular posterior ossification associated with posterior labral injury and posterior articular surface rotator cuff damage (Fig. 9-107), is believed to be the result of a posterior capsular avulsion secondary to traction of the posterior band of the IGL (during the deceleration phase of pitching, for example) or to the posterior subluxation that occurs during cocking of the arm.[143]

The crescentic extraarticular ossification, which extends from the posterior inferior medial glenoid posterior to the posterior labrum, can be demonstrated CT or MR scans. There may be associated reactive posterior inferior glenoid rim sclerosis. MR findings include low signal intensity calci-

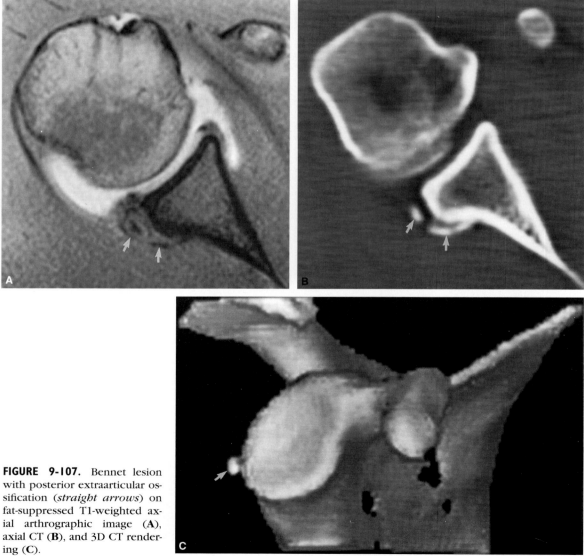

FIGURE 9-107. Bennet lesion with posterior extraarticular ossification (*straight arrows*) on fat-suppressed T1-weighted axial arthrographic image (**A**), axial CT (**B**), and 3D CT rendering (**C**).

fication, posterior humeral subluxation, and a posterior labral tear. Ferrari and colleagues[143] reported on a study of 7 elite baseball players, all of whom had an associated posterior labral tear on arthroscopic examination. The ossification cannot be identified arthroscopically because of its extraarticular location. The posterior labral tears are most frequent in the posterior superior quadrant of the glenoid labrum.

Multidirectional Instability

In true multidirectional instability of the glenohumeral joint, force applied distally in the upper extremity with the patient's arm abducted causes inferior subluxation of the humeral head. This produces a visible sulcus (ie, the sulcus sign) between the prominence of the acromion and the inferior subluxed humeral head.[144] In classic multidirectional instability, the ligament laxity is bilateral and atraumatic. The index of suspicion should be high in young patients, especially young female patients with generalized joint laxity and complaints referable to the shoulders. These patients are best treated with physical therapy. Specific muscle rehabilitation, with particular attention to the shoulder compressors, helps to provide stability to the lax joints.

No visible ligament labral lesions are seen in patients with true multidirectional instability of the glenohumeral joint. The capsular ligaments are redundant, and the labrum is often hypoplastic. Some patients with multidirectional laxity, however, present with unidirectional pathology and experience dislocation predominantly in only one direction. Intraarticular arthroscopic findings confirm the direction of the instability.

Labral Pathology

Normal Variations

SUBLABRAL FORAMEN.   There is considerable variation in the attachment and morphology of the glenoid labrum. The most significant variation is the relative attachment, or lack thereof, to the glenoid rim in the anterior superior quadrant above the epiphyseal line (Fig. 9-108). There is frequently a sublabral foramen between the labrum and the glenoid rim, which is often the cause for misinterpretation of anterior labral disruptions or tears (Figs. 9-109 and 9-110). Although the glenoid labrum in the superior one third of the glenoid above the epiphyseal line can be firmly fixed in its periphery, De Palma has shown that there is considerable variation in the anterior superior bursa and labral foramen of the complex.[43] Although the resulting differential bursal configurations produce MR images that appear to demonstrate superior and anterior labral tears, these are normal anatomic variations.

A normal anterosuperior sublabral foramen or hole has been reported in up to 11% of individuals.[41,145] The anterosuperior labrum is firmly attached to the glenoid rim in up to 88% of cases.[146] Cooper and coworkers reported the presence of a sublabral foramen as a normal variant in 17% of specimens.[147] Care must be taken not to mistake a sublabral foramen, which can vary in size from a few millimeters up to the entire anterosuperior quadrant above the level of the subscapularis tendon,[41] for a SLAP lesion or a Bankart lesion. Bright signal intensity fluid, which undermines the anterosuperior labrum, may be

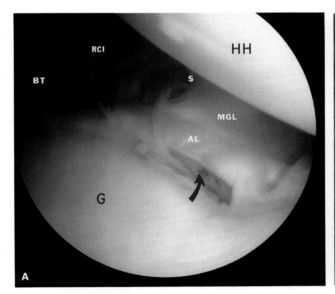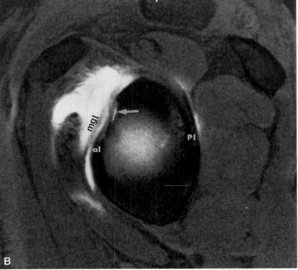

FIGURE 9-108. (A) An arthroscopic photograph of a normal anatomic variant of the sublabral foramen with a missing anterior labrum attachment above the epiphyseal line of the glenoid (*curved arrow*). AL, anterior labrum; BT, biceps tendon; G, glenoid; HH, humeral head; MGL, middle glenohumeral ligament; RCI, rotator cuff interval or Weitbrecht's foramen; S, subscapularis tendon. (B) Sublabral foramen (*arrow*) shown above the equator (above the anterior glenoid notch) on a fat-suppressed T1-weighted sagittal oblique MR arthrogram. Contrast extends between the anterosuperior labrum and the glenoid rim as a normal variant. mgl, middle glenohumeral ligament; al, anterior labrum; pl, posterior labrum).

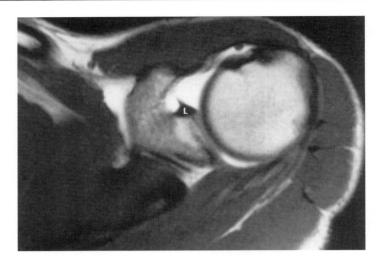

FIGURE 9-109. A normal adherent anterior superior glenoid labrum (L) as seen on an enhanced T1-weighted axial image.

overread as a SLAP lesion. In contrast to a Bankart lesion, the sublabral foramen is seen superior to the anterior glenoid notch or above the physeal line representing the superior one third of the glenoid. The Bankart lesion usually involves a labral tear or avulsion at or below the level of the subscapularis tendon on axial MR images. This is below the physeal line or equator. (The physeal line divides the bony glenoid into an upper one third and lower two thirds, corresponding to the two glenoid ossification centers. It is also referred to as the equator, as identified at the region of the anterior glenoid notch.[41]) Direct communication between the sublabral foramen and the subscapularis bursa can be seen on MR arthrography. Although a sublabral foramen may be seen with a type 2 or type 3 BLC, it is most often associated with a meniscoid superior labrum (ie, type 3 BLC).

THE BUFORD COMPLEX. The Buford complex (Fig. 9-111) consists of three elements: (1) a cord-like MGL, (2) a MGL that attaches directly to the superior labrum anterior to the biceps (at the base of the biceps anchor), and (3) an absent anterosuperior labrum[148,149] (see Fig. 9-111). Of 200 shoulder arthroscopies reviewed by Williams and Synder and their colleagues,[148,149] the Buford complex was found in 1.5%, and a sublabral foramen, located between the anterosuperior glenoid quadrant and the articular surface of the anterior glenoid, was found in 12%. In 75% of patients who demonstrated a sublabral foramen a cord-like MGL was present. This cord-like MGL attaches directly to the superior labrum. The additional finding of an absent antero-superior labrum placed patients into the subgroup diagnosed with the Buford complex.

Several key MR findings help to avoid misinterpretation of the absence of anterosuperior labral tissue as a sublabral foramen or a Bankart lesion. These findings include an absent anterior labrum at and above the level of the subscapularis tendon as assessed on axial images. A sublabral foramen can only exist in the presence of an anterior superior labrum. The anterior inferior glenoid labrum below the level of the subscapularis tendon is firmly attached to the glenoid with normal morphology.

A cord-like MGL must be identified anterior to the glenoid rim. There may be a remnant or hypoplastic anterosuperior labral tissue identified on axial images at the level of the subscapularis tendon (Fig. 9-112). It is easy to distinguish a Bankart lesion from the Buford complex because in the former the anterior inferior labrum is torn or avulsed and does not appear firmly attached to the anteroinferior glenoid rim.

The sagittal oblique plane demonstrates the course of the cord-like MGL attaching directly to the superior labrum at the anterior base of the biceps tendon. Although the Buford complex may be mistaken for a large sublabral foramen, a sublabral foramen or hole does not exist since there is no anterior superior labral tissue present. If this normal variant is not recognized and is mistakenly reattached to the glenoid neck, painful restriction of rotation and elevation can occur. It is important, however, to remember that a cord-like MGL with an associated sublabral hole beneath a normal anterior superior labrum is more common than a cord-like MGL in association with a deficient anterior superior labrum. Intraarticular MR arthrography can be used to improve visualization of the cord-like MGL distinct from the bare anterior glenoid rim. However, this complex can be recognized without the routine use of an MR contrast agent.

THE INFERIOR LABRUM. In general, the labrum is more firmly attached inferior to the epiphyseal line and is continuous with the cartilaginous surface of the glenoid. De Palma demonstrated that with increasing age and degeneration, separation of the fibrous labrum from the cartilaginous glenoid surface occurs throughout the periphery of the glenoid.[43] This is evident on arthroscopy in older patients. Subtle tears of the anterior inferior labrum are best demonstrated on MR scans performed with the shoulder abducted and in external rotation, which displays the IGL and IGLLC.

LABRAL TYPES. There are several normal variations in labral morphology. Initially, Detrisac and Johnson described five types[38]:

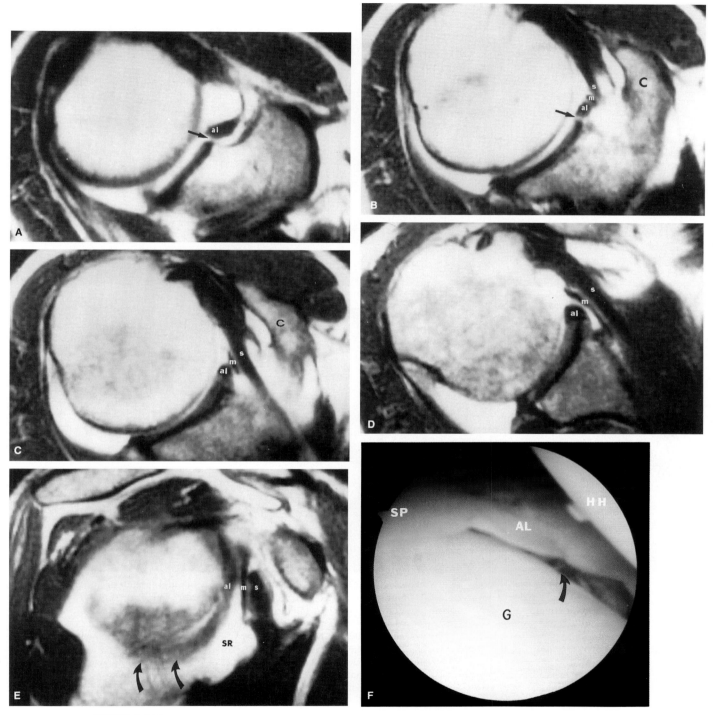

FIGURE 9-110. Sublabral foramen. (**A** through **D**) Enhanced T1-weighted axial images illustrate the normal anatomic relationship of subscapularis tendon (s), middle glenohumeral ligament (m), and anterior labrum (al) from anterior to posterior. Note the sublabral foramen (*arrow*) as a normal anatomic variant above (**A**) and at the level of (**B**) the superior coracoid (C). No foramen is present at the level of the inferior coracoid (**C**) or the subscapularis tendon (**D**). (**E**) The corresponding enhanced sagittal oblique image shows the subscapularis tendon (s), middle glenohumeral ligament (m), and anterior labrum (al). Curved arrows, axillary pouch of inferior glenohumeral ligament; SR, subscapularis recess inferior to middle glenohumeral ligament. (**F**) An arthroscopic image shows the sublabral foramen between the anterior superior labrum and glenoid rim (*curved arrow*). AL, anterior labrum; G, glenoid; SP, superior pole of the glenoid.

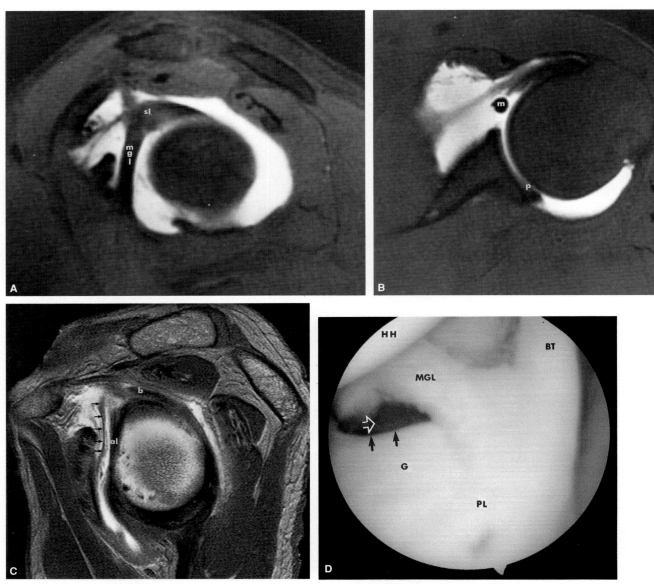

FIGURE 9-111. Buford complex. **(A)** Thick cord-like middle glenohumeral ligament (mgl) attaching directly to the superior labrum (sl) on fat-suppressed T1-weighted sagittal oblique arthrogram. **(B)** Corresponding fat-suppressed T1 axial image identifies cord-like middle glenohumeral ligament (m) with an absent anterior superior labrum as a normal variant. Note the posterior labrum (p) is present. **(C)** Normal anterior superior labrum (al), biceps (b), and middle glenohumeral ligament (*arrows*) in another patient shown for comparison. (T1-weighted sagittal oblique MR arthrogram.) **(D)** An arthroscopic view of cord-like MGL is shown in a Buford complex. The anterior superior glenoid edge (*black arrows*) shows an absence of the labrum as a normal variant in association with prominent MGL. The MGL originates from the anteromedial humeral neck and attaches medially on the glenoid (G) and the neck of the scapula. Open arrow, subscapularis recess; BT, biceps tendon; HH, humeral head; PL, posterior labrum.

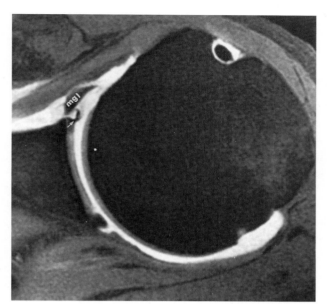

FIGURE 9-112. Buford complex showing cord-like middle glenohumeral ligament (mgl) and hypoplastic anterior labral tissue at the level of the subscapulis tendon (*arrow*). No anterior-superior labral tissue was present between the MGL attachment to the superior labrum and the midglenoid notch. The anterior inferior labrum below the level of the subscapularis was normal in this patient. (Fat-suppressed T1 axial MR arthrogram.)

1. A superior wedge labrum with the labrum firmly attached anteriorly, posteriorly, and inferiorly; separation (a sublabral foramen) between the glenoid and superior anterior labrum occurs as a normal variation (Fig. 9-113)
2. A posterior wedge-shaped labrum in which the superior labrum is smaller and more firmly attached to the superior glenoid (Fig. 9-114); the posterior labrum is wedge-shaped, overlaps the articular surface of the glenoid, and has a free central border

3. An anterior wedge labrum, which is characterized by a large anterior band of the IGL that replaces or covers a small anterior labrum (eg, the Buford complex)
4. A labrum with the characteristics of both a superior and anterior wedge labrum
5. A meniscal or meniscoid labrum, which has a circumferential free central margin with relatively symmetric anterior and posterior labral tissue on cross section above the epiphyseal line.

This classification was subsequently simplified into two labral types[149]:

1. A labrum that is attached to the glenoid in its periphery through a fibrocartilaginous transitional zone; above the physeal line or equator the labrum may be mobile along its central border with a meniscoid appearance.
2. A labrum that is entirely secured to the glenoid both peripherally and centrally.

Although a meniscoid-like labrum has been reported with a 10% incidence below the equator, the anterior inferior glenoid labrum is rarely visualized on MR images with fluid undermining its glenoid attachment.[146] We recommend classifying the labrum according to the three different types of attachment of the BLC, as discussed earlier.

Anterior labral anatomy has also been classified based on the relative contribution of the glenohumeral ligaments.[148] In this classification, a type 1 labrum (34%) is the IGL labrum. A type 2 labrum (11%) is the superior and MGL labrum. Type 3 (55%) represents the combined glenohumeral ligament labrum.

SYNOVIAL RECESSES.   The capsule can be categorized into one of six anatomic types as described by De Palma, based on the topographic arrangements of the synovial recesses with respect to the glenohumeral ligaments[33,43] (Fig. 9-115). MGL morphology determines the type of synovial recess

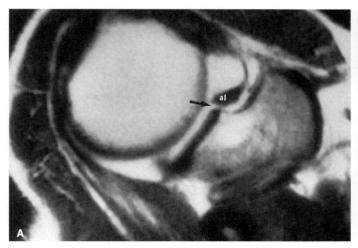

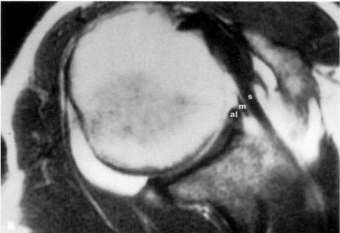

FIGURE 9-113. (**A, B**) Enhanced T1-weighted axial images show the superior wedge labrum with a firm attachment between the anterior labrum (al) and the glenoid articular surface at the level of the subscapularis tendon (s). No free central edge of the labrum is present. Normal separation of the labrum from the anterior superior glenoid rim creates a sublabral foramen (*arrow*). m, middle glenohumeral ligament.

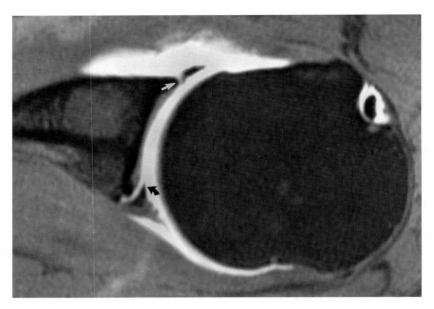

FIGURE 9-114. Posterior wedge labrum with superior labrum firmly attached to the anterior glenoid (*straight arrow*) and posterior labrum overlapping the glenoid articular surface with a free central edge (*curved arrow*). Fluid is seen partially undercutting the base of this normal posterior labrum. (Fat-suppressed T1-weighted axial MR arthrogram.)

present.[41] The six types of synovial recesses are best assessed on intraarticular gadolinium-enhanced sagittal oblique images in which the MGL and IGL can be identified (Figs. 9-116 and 9-117).

CORD-LIKE MGL. In almost two thirds of cases studied, the MGL is identified as a folded thickening of the anterior capsule between the anterior labrum and subscapularis tendon, inserting on the labrum or near the glenoid rim.[41,146] In 19% of cases, the MGL has a cord-like morphology, compared with the more normal sheet-like appearance of ligamentous tissue. An attenuated or thin variation of the MGL is observed in 5% of shoulders. The attenuated MGL is more frequently associated with a promi-

nent anterior band of the IGLC, thought to have a compensatory function. Complete absence of the MGL may be associated with a congenitally lax anterior capsule.

The cord-like MGL is best demonstrated on axial and sagittal MR images (Figs. 9-118 through 9-120). The thick and low signal intensity cord-like MGL may be mistaken for a detached anterior labrum above the epiphyseal line (Bankart lesion). The prominent MGL on multiple axial images, distinct from the normal anterior inferior glenoid labrum below the level of the subscapularis tendon, excludes the presence of a Bankart lesion. The direct course of the MGL as it crosses the superior border of the subscapularis is shown on sagittal images. The cord-like MGL can also

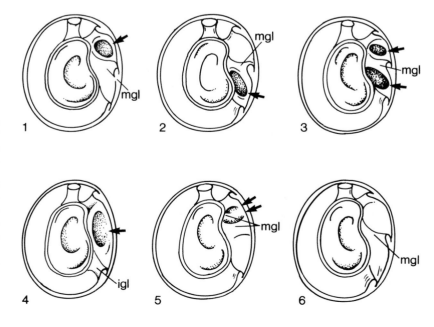

FIGURE 9-115. Six arrangements of synovial recesses (ie, joint capsule variations, *arrows*) are described by DePalma. Type 1: One synovial recess exists above the middle glenohumeral ligament. Type 2: One synovial recess exists below the middle glenohumeral ligament. Type 3: Two synovial recesses exist, with a superior subscapular recess above the middle glenohumeral ligament and an inferior subscapular recess below the middle glenohumeral ligament. Type 4: No middle glenohumeral ligament is present, and one large synovial recess exists above the inferior glenohumeral ligament. Type 5: The middle glenohumeral ligament exists as two small synovial folds. Type 6: Complete absence of synovial recesses. (From DePalma AF. Surgery of the shoulder. Philadelphia: JB Lippincott, 1983.)

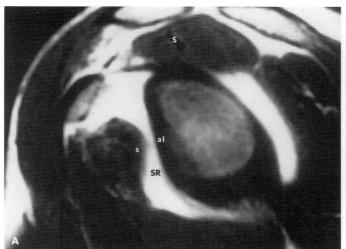

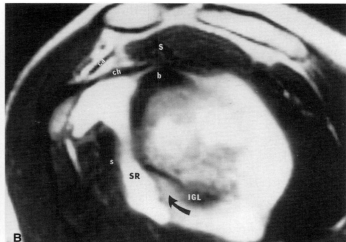

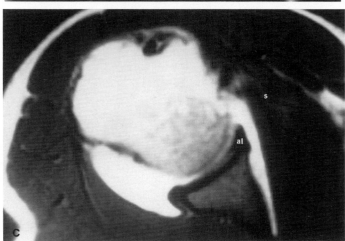

FIGURE 9-116. A single type 3 synovial recess. (**A, B**) Enhanced T1-weighted sagittal oblique images display absence of the middle glenohumeral ligament (MGL), resulting in one large synovial recess above the inferior glenohumeral ligament (IGL). Curved arrow, anterior band of IGL; al, anterior labrum; b, biceps tendon; ca, coracoacromial ligament; ch, coracohumeral ligament; S, supraspinatus tendon; SR, synovial recess; s, subscapularis tendon. (**C**) The corresponding enhanced T1-weighted axial image shows the anterior labrum (al) and subscapularis tendon (s) without the MGL interposed between them. Contrast outlines the normal subscapularis bursa. There is no type 3 capsule.

be identified as a distinct structure on sagittal images anterior to the anterior band and anterior labrum, and should not be misdiagnosed for a torn or avulsed anterior labrum. The filamentous extension or attachment may be identified between the cord-like MGL and the anterior labrum (see Figs. 9-119 and 9-120).

Biomechanics and Vascularity of the Labrum

The glenoid labrum provides approximately 50% of the total depth of the glenoid socket.[149,150] It also increases the glenoid surface in the vertical and horizontal planes to better accommodate the humeral head. The strength of the attachment between the fibrous labrum and the bony glenoid increases with age, and disruption of the labral glenoid connection (Bankart lesion) in cases of acute dislocations is more likely to occur in younger individuals (younger than 25 years of age).

In a cadaveric study by Karzel and coworkers,[151] the posteroinferior labrum was shown to absorb the majority of load in 90% of shoulder abduction with an applied compressive load.[149,151] This may explain why the posterior labrum is strong and usually more triangular in shape compared with the anterior labrum. Jobe demonstrated posterior superior labral impingement in cadaver shoulders in 70° of abduction and maximum external rotation.[108]

Vascularity in the superior and anterosuperior labrum segments is decreased in comparison with the posterosuperior and inferior segments. This decreased vascularity may be responsible for the development of superior labral degeneration with increasing age and may make the labrum more susceptible to the SLAP lesion.[147]

Labral Tears

The labrum can be arbitrarily divided into six areas: (1) the superior labrum; (2) the anterosuperior (superior to the mid-glenoid notch) labrum; (3) the anteroinferior labrum; (4) the inferior labrum; (5) the posteroinferior labrum, and (6) the posterosuperior labrum.[149] Labral tear patterns include degenerative lesions, flap tears, vertical split nondetached tears, bucket-handle tears, and SLAP lesions.[149]

text continues on page 715

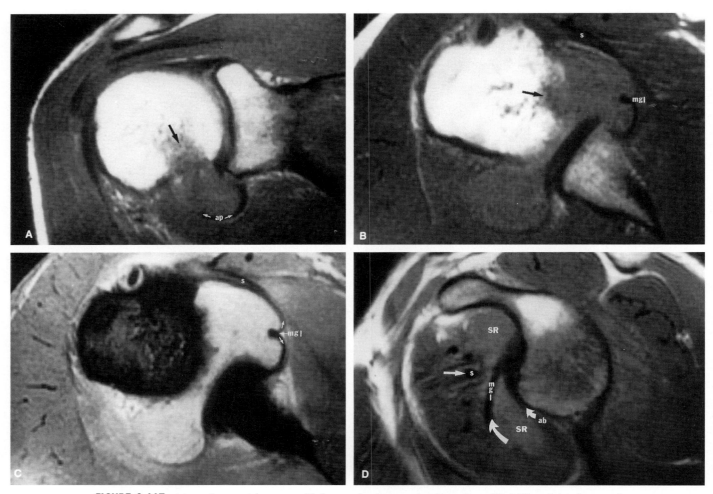

FIGURE 9-117. A type 3 synovial recess with hemorrhagic capsular distention. **(A)** A T1-weighted coronal oblique image shows the axillary pouch (ap; *white arrows*) and anteromedial humeral head contusion (*black arrow*). When associated with posterior dislocation, the impaction defect of the anteromedial humeral head is referred to as a reverse Hill-Sachs defect. **(B)** T1-weighted and **(C)** T2*-weighted axial images show capsular distention with a cord-like middle glenohumeral ligament (MGL, mgl; *white arrows*) and subscapularis tendon (s). Anteromedial humeral head contusion (*black arrow*) is also shown. The anterior labrum was intact at arthroscopy. **(D)** The corresponding T1-weighted sagittal oblique image shows the subscapularis tendon (s; *straight arrow*), the MGL (mgl; *large curved arrow*), and the anterior band of the IGL (ab; *small curved arrow*). Fluid can be seen in the synovial recesses (SR) above and below the MGL.

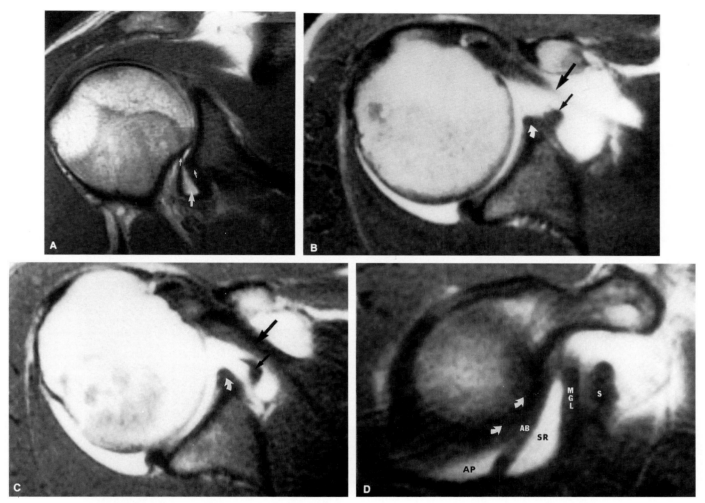

FIGURE 9-118. Cord-like middle glenohumeral ligament (MGL). **(A)** An enhanced coronal oblique T1-weighted image shows a normal axillary pouch distended with gadolinium (*large arrow*). The humeral and glenoid attachments of the inferior glenohumeral ligament (IGL; small arrows) are also shown. Enhanced T1-weighted axial images show a cord-like or hypertrophied MGL (small black arrows) that simulates an avulsion of the anterior labrum superior to **(B)** and at the midlevel of **(C)** the subscapularis tendon (large black arrows). The anterior labral morphology is normal (*curved white arrows*) superior to the subscapularis tendon. The MGL is closely applied to the anterior labrum. At the level of the subscapularis tendon, gadolinium contrast is seen in both the anterior and posterior surfaces of the MGL. **(D)** The corresponding enhanced T1-weighted sagittal image displays a normal anterior labrum (*curved arrows*) and anterior band of the IGL (AB). A thick, cord-like MGL and subscapularis tendon (S) can also be identified. Intraarticular gadolinium contrast is shown in the axillary pouch (AP) of the inferior glenohumeral ligament and in a synovial recess (SR) below the MGL. In the presence of a large synovial recess and cord-like MGL, the recess may be misinterpreted as a capsular rent and the ligament as a torn and displaced labrum.

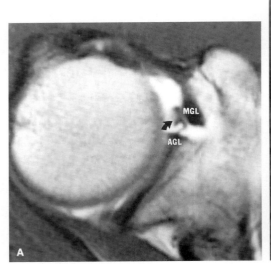

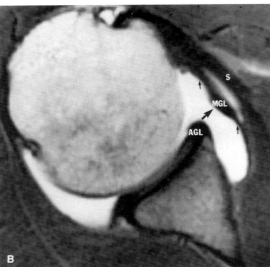

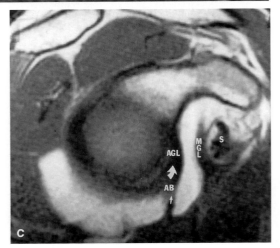

FIGURE 9-119. (A, B) Cord-like middle glenohumeral ligament (MGL) on T1-weighted enhanced axial images at the level of the coracoid (A) and inferior to the coracoid at the level of the subscapularis tendon (B). Curved arrow, filamentous attachment to cord-like MGL; large straight arrow, cord-like portion of MGL; small straight arrows, thin portion of MGL; AGL, anterior glenoid labrum. (C) The corresponding T1-weighted enhanced sagittal oblique image shows the relationship of the MGL to the anterior band of the IGL (AB; *straight arrow*), the anterior glenoid labrum (AGL; *curved arrow*), the middle glenohumeral ligament (MGL), and the subscapularis tendon (S). The MGL is located in the plane between the subscapularis tendon and the anterior band of the IGL or anterior glenoid labrum.

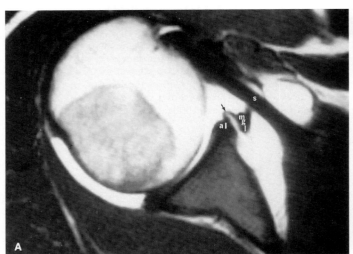

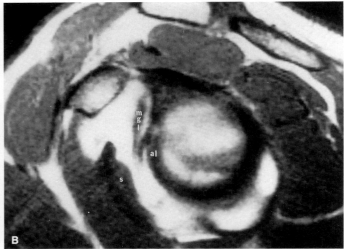

FIGURE 9-120. Pseudolabral tear. The cord-like middle glenohumeral ligament (MGL, mgl) simulates the appearance of a torn anterior labrum (al) on gadolinium-enhanced T1-weighted (A) axial and (B) sagittal oblique images. The filamentous attachments of the MGL to the anterior labrum (*black arrow*) and subscapularis tendons are shown.

DEGENERATIVE LABRUM. Degenerative lesions show a frayed labrum, probably as part of the spectrum of degenerative glenohumeral joint disease. De Palma and coworkers have described degenerative tears of the superior labrum associated with advancing age.[43,152] The degenerative roughened labrum may contribute to the process of joint degeneration by creating an abrasive articular interface in addition to humeral head chondromalacia. Treatment of degenerative labral tears is performed with arthroscopic resection of damaged tissue.

FLAP TEARS. Flap tears represent the most frequent labral tear pattern in acute or subacute injuries.[149] These tears may occur in any location, but are frequently identified in the posterosuperior segment of the labrum. Flap tears may occur secondary to chronic shear stress,[153] as seen in repetitive subluxation in throwing or overhead athletics. An unstable flap tear may cause mechanical symptoms of joint clicking, catching, and popping, and mimic instability. Treatment of these tears involves arthroscopic resection of the unstable tissue.

VERTICAL SPLIT AND BUCKET-HANDLE LABRAL TEARS. Vertical split labral tears are the least frequent labral tear pattern.[149] A complete vertical split labrum may be associated with a displaceable fragment and present as a bucket-handle tear. A vertical split labrum is seen in the meniscoid type labrum which is most commonly observed in the superior quadrant. A SLAP III lesion is a bucket handle tear of the superior labrum (see Slap Tears). Although a vertical split may occur in the anterior and posterior labrum, this tear pattern is unusual in the inferior labrum. Intraarticular compression from a fall on the outstretched arm or extensive humeral rotation associated with anterior or posterior labral compression are reported mechanisms of injury. Symptoms include pseudosubluxation with locking, catching, and popping. Associated clinical instability, however, is uncommon in this lesion. Treatment is directed at producing a stable meniscal rim by excision or repair of the tear.

SUPERIOR LABRAL TEARS. Anterosuperior labral tears with avulsion and fraying of the labrum have been described in high performance athletes who use a throwing motion.[154] There may be involvement of the biceps and associated partial rotator cuff tears. Traction by the long head of the biceps on the anterosuperior labrum occurs during the deceleration phase of throwing. Arthroscopic debridement is performed on the frayed labrum, cuff, and biceps tendon.

SLAP TEARS. Snyder and associates[155] have described SLAP (superior labrum from anterior-to-posterior, relative

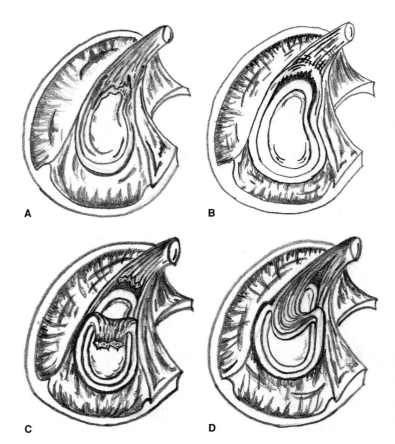

FIGURE 9-121. (**A**) SLAP type I lesion with frayed and degenerative superior labrum. (**B**) SLAP type II lesion with avulsion of the superior labrum and biceps anchor. (**C**) SLAP type III lesion with a bucket-handle tear through a meniscoid superior labrum and intact biceps anchor. (**D**) SLAP type IV lesion with a bucket-handle tear of the superior meniscoid labrum and extension into the biceps tendon.

to the biceps tendon anchor) lesions, which vary from simple fraying and fragmentation of the BLC, to a bucket-handle tear, to a tricorn bucket-handle tear in which one rim of the tear actually extends up into the biceps tendon, splitting it as the tear goes up toward the bicipital groove.[155] A fall on the outstretched abducted arm with associated superior joint compression and a proximal subluxation force is one proposed mechanism of injury.[149] A sudden contraction of the biceps tendon which avulses the superior labrum is another mechanism of injury. Less severe, repetitive stress acting through the biceps tendon may also produce SLAP lesions (Fig. 9-121). Instability of the glenohumeral joint has also been associated with SLAP lesions. SLAP tears are actually four distinct but related lesions. In type I lesions, there is a frayed and degenerative superior labrum with a normal (stable) biceps tendon anchor. Type II lesions have similar labral fraying, but have detachment of the superior labrum and biceps anchor, making them unstable (Fig. 9-122). A type II lesion may appear similar to the normal free edge of the meniscoid-like superior labrum. In the latter, the articular cartilage of the superior glenoid extends to the attachment of the labrum. In a type II SLAP lesion, however, there is usually a space or gap between the glenoid articular cartilage and attachment of the superior labrum and biceps anchor (Fig. 9-123). Displacement of the labrum from the superior glenoid of more than 3 to 4 mm is usually associated with an abnormal superior labrum and biceps anchor attachment (Fig. 9-124). A type II SLAP lesion may also be associated with anterior glenohumeral joint dislocation. Tearing of the superior labrum biceps anchor may contribute to anteroinferior capsule and labral stress in the development of anterior instability. Type III lesions involve a bucket-handle tear of

the superior labrum (a vertical tear through a meniscoid-like superior labrum) without extension into the biceps tendon (see Fig. 9-122). The biceps anchor is stable and the remaining labrum is intact. Type IV lesions also involve a bucket-handle tear associated with a meniscoid-type superior labrum, but in this case with extension into the biceps tendon (Fig. 9-125). The biceps anchor and the superior labrum are well attached. A partially torn biceps tendon may displace the superior labral flap into the joint. A complex SLAP lesion may consist of a combination of two or more types, usually type II and type IV.

Diagnosis and Treatment of SLAP Lesions. The clinical diagnosis of SLAP lesions may be difficult. Symptoms are often nonspecific and include pain associated with locking, snapping, and pseudosubluxation. Patient history may suggest a differential diagnosis that includes impingement syndrome, biceps tendinitis, or glenohumeral joint instability.

Treatment of SLAP lesions is based on the type of labral lesion present. A type I SLAP lesion is treated with arthroscopic debridement of the degenerative labrum. Treatment of a type II SLAP lesion (which involves detachment of the superior labrum and biceps anchor) addresses the avulsed labrum and reattachment of the detached biceps anchor to the superior glenoid. A suture anchor technique, for example, may be used for a type II SLAP tear. Since there is no involvement of the biceps anchor in a type III SLAP lesion (a bucket-handle tear and a meniscoid-type superior labrum) arthroscopic debridement of the loose labral fragment may be sufficient to relieve symptoms of catching and snapping. A type IV SLAP lesion, which also involves a bucket-handle tear associated with a meniscoid-type superior labrum, addi-

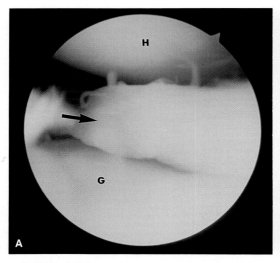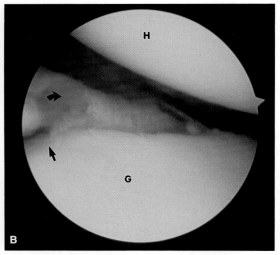

FIGURE 9-122. **(A)** An arthroscopically diagnosed bucket-handle superior labrum anterior to posterior SLAP type III lesion (*arrow*) involves the posterior superior glenoid labrum and extends anteriorly to the mid-glenoid notch, involving the glenoid attachment of the biceps tendon. G, glenoid; H, humerus. **(B)** Arthroscopic excision of the bucket-handle lateral tear reveals the anterior superior labrum (*curved arrow*) and the glenoid (G; *straight arrow*). H, humerus.

continued

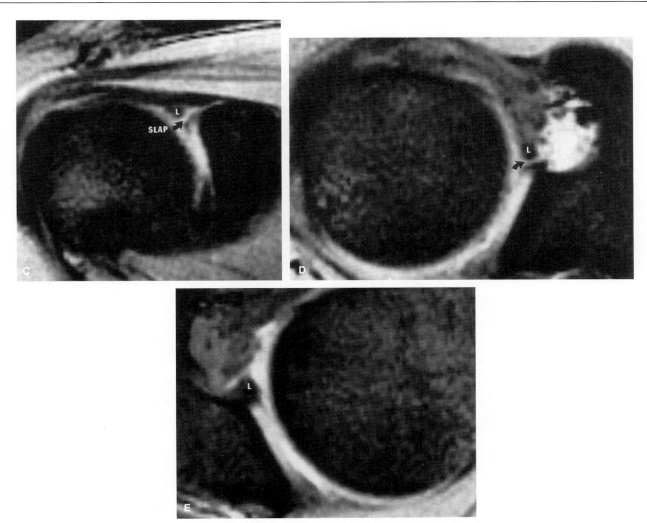

FIGURE 9-122. *Continued.* T2*-weighted coronal oblique (**C**) and axial (**D**) images in another patient show a SLAP type II lesion (*curved arrow*) that involves the anterior superior labrum (L) of the right shoulder. The avulsed labrum demonstrates linear high signal intensity that extends completely across the base of the labrum. Synovitis with effacement of fat lateral to the coracoid is noted. (**E**) A T2*-weighted axial image of the normal attachment of the anterior superior glenoid labrum (L) in the contralateral left shoulder is shown for comparison.

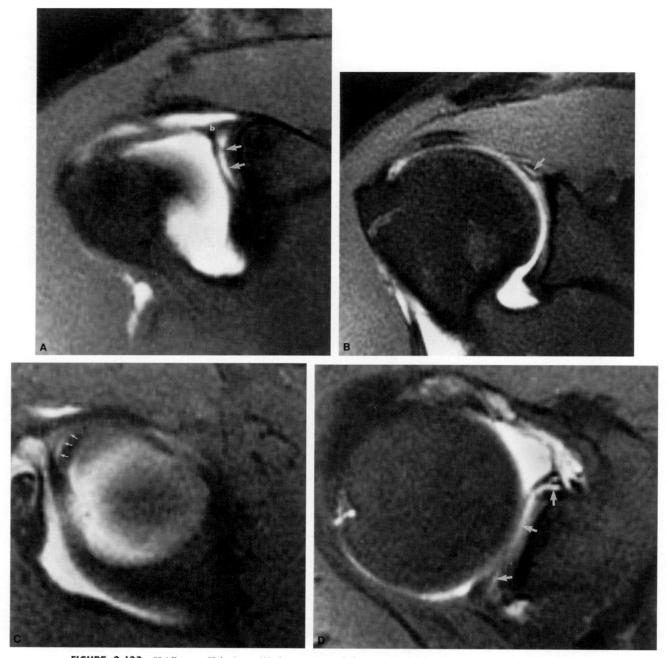

FIGURE 9-123. SLAP type II lesion. **(A)** Separation of the superior labrum and biceps anchor (b) from the underlying anterior glenoid rim. Hyperintense fluid (*arrows*) fills the detachment on fat-suppressed T1-weighted coronal oblique MR arthrogram. **(B)** Posterior extension of the tear is shown as a linear hyperintensity through the posterior superior labrum (*arrow*) on this fat-suppressed T1-weighted coronal oblique MR arthrogram. Corresponding fat-suppressed T1-weighted sagittal oblique **(C)** and axial **(D)** images display the avulsion (*arrows*) of the biceps labral complex **(C)** and anterior-to-posterior extension (*arrows*) of the superior labral tear **(D)**.

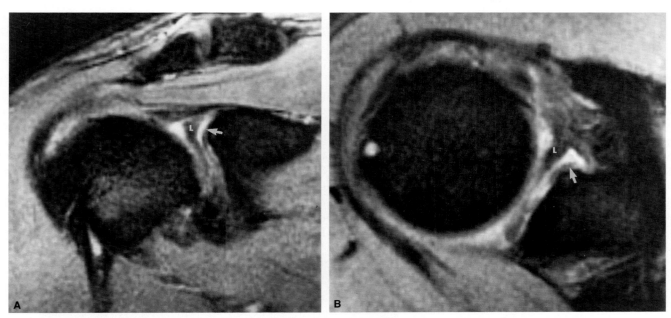

FIGURE 9-124. SLAP type II lesion with greater than 3 mm displacement of the superior labrum (*arrow*) and biceps anchor on T2* coronal oblique (**A**) and axial (**B**) images.

tionally extends into the biceps tendon. Treatment of type IV lesions ranges from resection of torn tissue to suture repair for bucket-handle tears associated with more extensive involvement of the biceps tendon.

MR APPEARANCE OF LABRAL TEARS. Magnetic resonance imaging has proved to be a sensitive, specific, and accurate modality for evaluating the glenoid labrum.[131–133,156–159] In

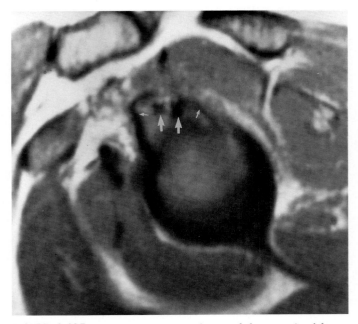

FIGURE 9-125. SLAP type IV vertical tear of the superior labrum producing a bucket-handle lesion (*small arrows*). Biceps tendon involvement is demonstrated (*large arrows*). (T1-weighted sagittal oblique image.)

MR studies of labral tears with surgical or arthroscopic correlation, sensitivity was reported to be 88% and specificity, 93%.[123,160] These statistics compare favorably with air-contrast CT arthrography,[161,162] and, in addition, MR imaging provides superior visualization of associated capsular structures and the IGL.[163] The glenoid labrum is routinely evaluated in all three imaging planes. Axial plane images, however, provide the most diagnostic information.

Routinely, axial images are obtained using T1 weighting, T2* weighting with a 2 mm 3DFT sequence, and fat-suppressed T2-weighted fast spin-echo sequences. When MR arthrography with a paramagnetic contrast agent is used, precontrast T1-weighted axial images; precontrast T2*-weighted axial images; and postcontrast T1-weighted fat-suppressed axial, sagittal, and coronal oblique images are obtained. When MR arthrography with saline is used, presaline T1 and T2* axial sequences and postsaline T2* and fat-suppressed T2-weighted fast spin-echo axial sequences are obtained.

Sagittal and coronal plane images are also routinely obtained to supplement axial images in the assessment of labral and capsulolabral abnormalities. The coronal oblique plane demonstrates the humeral and inferior glenoid attachment to the IGL and displays the anatomy of the BLC, especially in the diagnosis of superior labral tears (eg, SLAP lesions).[164] The sagittal oblique plane is used to view the relationship between the IGLLC and the anterior and posterior labrum relative to the anterior and posterior bands of the IGL. The anatomy and variation of the MGL and anterior labrum is frequently best visualized on sagittal oblique images. Complex labral tears and the location of the labral segments involved can be correlated between sagittal oblique and axial images.

The intact fibrous labrum demonstrates low signal intensity on all pulse sequences (T1, T2, T2*, and T2-weighted fast spin-echo). We have not found the radial MR sequence helpful in routine evaluations of the labrum.[165] The IGLLC and the anterior inferior glenoid labrum are also shown when scans are performed with the arm positioned in abduction and external rotation. The low signal intensity labrum circles the glenoid articular surface and is usually triangular in cross section on axial plane images. The peripheral attachment of the labrum joins the capsule and glenohumeral ligaments, creating the capsulolabral complex. This capsulolabral or labral ligamentous complex is best appreciated on sagittal oblique MR images on which the BLC and IGL labral anatomy are responsible for the formation of the superior one third and inferior two thirds of the glenoid labrum, respec-

tively. The central attachment of the labrum blends with the articular cartilage surface of the glenoid. A meniscoid appearance usually involves the superior labrum and is characterized by a free inner or central edge of the labrum.[149]

Loredo and colleagues[158] have correlated intralabral signal intensity with histology showing mucoid or eosinophilic degeneration of fibrovascular tissue.[158] An anterior sublabral band of intermediate signal intensity corresponds with a transition zone of fibrocartilage. These findings correlate with those of Detrisac and Johnson, which showed the labrum to be composed of bundles of fibrous tissue with a thin transition zone of fibrocartilage between the labrum and articular cartilage.[38] This thin transitional zone of fibrocartilage may be only a few cells in width and is variably visualized in Detrisac and Johnson's five types of variations of labral

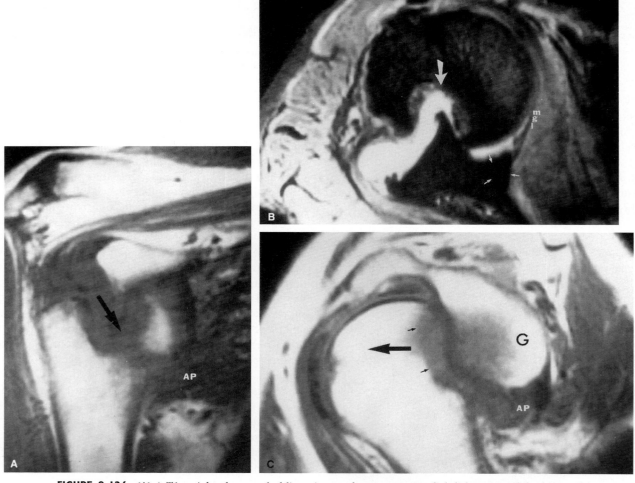

FIGURE 9-126. (**A**) A T1-weighted coronal oblique image shows anteromedial dislocation of the humeral head with a posterolateral Hill-Sachs fracture (*arrow*). Complete disruption of the axillary pouch (AP) of the inferior glenohumeral ligament has occurred. (**B**) A T2*-weighted axial image shows that the wedge-shaped impaction fracture (Hill-Sachs defect) was caused by the impact of the posterolateral humeral head on the anteroinferior glenoid rim (*large arrow*). Associated osseous fragmentation is identified along the anterior surface at the scapular neck (*small arrows*). The middle glenohumeral ligament (mgl) is intact. (**C**) A T1-weighted sagittal oblique image shows anterior dislocation (*large arrow*) of the humeral head relative to the anterior glenoid (G). The Hill-Sachs fracture (*small arrows*) and torn axillary pouch (AP) are shown.

anatomy. Without the use of MR arthrography with either intraarticular MR contrast or saline, this thin transitional cartilage may be overread as a sublabral foramen or potentially as a SLAP lesion.

A glenoid ovoid mass, or GLOM sign,[166] used by some as an indication of a labral tear, has not been used in our practice. In fact, a low signal intensity mass anterior to the glenoid rim may represent a cord-like MGL and should not be interpreted as a tear or avulsed anterior labrum.

Tears of the IGL are usually associated with traumatic dislocation or subluxation[38,167] (Fig. 9-126). Labral tissue may be interposed between the humeral head and glenoid rim, most often due to a labral tear with a relatively discoid and hypermobile biceps labral configuration. As the labrum becomes more meniscoid in shape, the likelihood of meniscal bucket-handle tears increases, and tissue may become interposed between the humeral head and glenoid surface. A posterolateral Hill-Sachs lesion and an anterior inferior glenoid rim fracture can be seen on MR images in all three imaging planes. Subacute or chronic bony Bankart lesions are best identified on T1-weighted axial images, which show low signal intensity sclerosis in contrast to higher signal intensity marrow fat.

Care must be taken not to over-diagnose SLAP lesions on MR images, especially in the case of SLAP type 1 and 2 tears. Superior labral degeneration in a SLAP 1 lesion may be difficult to appreciate. The degeneration and fraying display increased signal intensity in T2*-weighted images, and morphologic irregularities may be appreciated with MR arthrography with intraarticular contrast. There is no labral detachment in SLAP 1 lesions. In type 2 SLAP lesions, increased signal intensity, which undermines the superior labral base, may be seen on T2-weighted images or MR arthrography. This may communicate with a superior glenoid labral cyst. Separation of the superior labrum from the glenoid rim increases the specificity of diagnosing a type 2 lesion versus a sublabral foramen. A sublabral foramen is located more anteriorly within the anterior superior quadrant, in comparison to the more superior position of the SLAP lesion in the region of the BLC. Sagittal oblique images may be helpful in confirming fluid signal intensity crossing the base of the superior labrum or biceps anchor. Associated synovitis with effacement of fat may be seen between the coracoid and the anterior superior glenoid rim in acute or subacute SLAP lesions. A sublabral foramen should not demonstrate associated synovitis. We have observed intravenous MR contrast enhancement of synovial tissue and fat anterior to the superior labrum in cases of capsular strain without associated labral pathology. Sagittal images are particularly useful in identifying bucket-handle lesions or types 3 and 4 SLAP lesions with a bucket-handle tear. Extension of the tear into the biceps anchor (type 4) is also seen in the sagittal oblique plane. Displaced labral tissue in types 3 and 4 SLAP lesions is seen as low signal intensity fragments within the glenohumeral joint on both axial and coronal oblique images. A vacuum phenomenon, visualized as circular or linear areas of low signal intensity within the glenohumeral joint on

gradient-echo MR sequences, should not be misdiagnosed as a displaced labral fragment. This appearance is caused by intraarticular gas and is associated with positioning the arm in external rotation.[168]

Zlatkin and colleagues have devised a four category system of classification for abnormal labral signal intensity.[76,160] In type 1, there is increased signal intensity within the labrum, but there is no surface extension. Type 1 corresponds to internal labral degeneration without tear. In type 2, the blunted or frayed labrum demonstrates normal dark signal intensity. In type 3, T1-weighted or T2*-weighted images demonstrate increased signal intensity that extends to the surface, indicating a labral tear. In type 4, a labral tear is depicted by a combination of abnormal morphology with type 2 features and increased signal intensity extending to the surface of the labrum with type 3 features.

Large tears and detachments may demonstrate a more diffuse increase in signal intensity, whereas discrete tears maintain linear morphology.[159,163,169,170] It is not unusual, however, for avulsed labral tissue to demonstrate low signal intensity, especially in chronic injuries. Normal labral outlines, blunting, and avulsion of the labrum from the underlying bone are also seen. Articular cartilage, of intermediate signal intensity on T1- and T2-weighted images and increased signal intensity on T2*-weighted images, may undermine the base of anterior labral tissue and should not be mistaken for an oblique labral tear. Fluid undermining the anterior labrum below the level of the coracoid or subscapularis tendon is a pathologic finding that represents labral tearing. The normal sublabral foramen does not usually extend below the level of the coracoid process.

Linear tears and fragmentation of the posterior labrum are less common and can be seen in patients with posterior instability and recurrent posterior subluxation[171,172] (Fig. 9-127). Associated osseous findings include an impaction fracture or a defect on the anteromedial humeral head (reverse

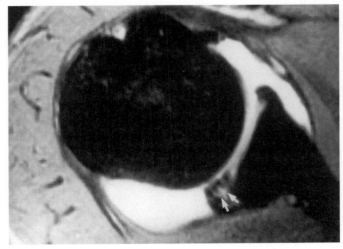

FIGURE 9-127. A T2*-weighted axial image shows multiple high signal intensity traumatic linear tears of the posterior labrum (*arrows*) in a baseball pitcher.

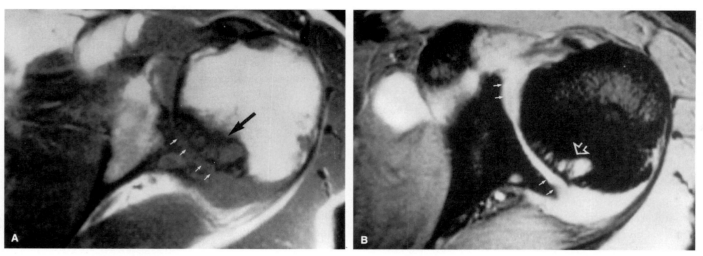

FIGURE 9-128. (**A**) T1-weighted and (**B**) T2*-weighted axial images show eccentric wear of the glenoid articular cartilage (*small arrows*). Subchondral degeneration sclerosis and cystic changes are seen in the posteriorly subluxed humeral head (*large arrow*). The posterior glenoid demonstrates decreased signal intensity in the posterior glenoid rim and is absent in the posterior labrum.

Bankart lesion), as well as fractures involving the posterior glenoid margin or lesser tuberosity.[76] Eccentric wear of the glenohumeral joint is frequently displayed as low signal intensity posterior glenoid subchondral sclerosis, which may be associated with fatty marrow conversion. The eccentric wear pattern may also be demonstrated by asymmetric attenuation of articular cartilage in the posterior aspect of the glenohumeral joint (Fig. 9-128).

Intraarticular gadolinium or saline distends the joint capsule and facilitates imaging of the glenohumeral ligaments.[29,131–133,156,157,173] Without knowledge of glenohumeral ligament anatomy, these structures may be mistaken for detached labral fragments. Gadolinium-enhanced MR imaging allows the spatial detection of avulsed labral tissue relative to the glenoid rim. Labral tears are usually highlighted on fat-suppressed T1-weighted images following intraarticular

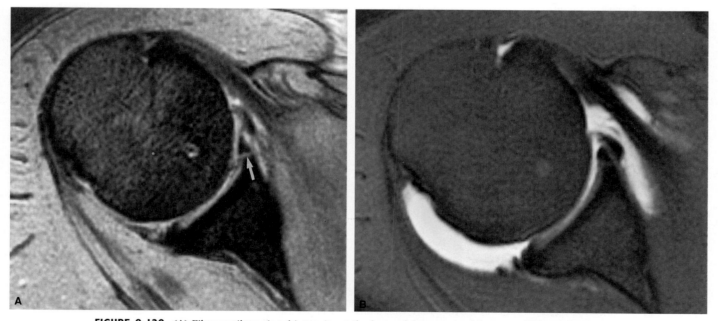

FIGURE 9-129. (**A**) Fibrocartilage signal intensity at the base of the anterior labrum on T2*-weighted axial image is shown not to represent a tear on corresponding fat-suppressed T1-weighted axial MR arthrographic image (**B**).

gadolinium administration. A synovial shelf in the subscapularis bursa is a normal finding sometimes seen on enhanced studies.[174] Normal intermediate signal intensity fibrocartilage at the base of the anterior labrum does not show extension of contrast with MR arthrography (Fig. 9-129).

Capsular Insertions

Zlatkin and colleagues identified three types of capsular insertions. Type 1 inserts near the anterior labrum, and types 2 and 3 insert more broadly or medially on the scapular neck.[175] These types of insertions represent normal variations in the size and morphology of the subscapularis recess, which are dependent on the rotation of the shoulder and are not the result of stripping of the capsule. With internal rotation, the recess is large and the capsule appears to insert more medially on the scapular neck (Fig. 9-130). It is unlikely that

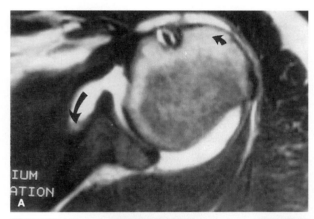

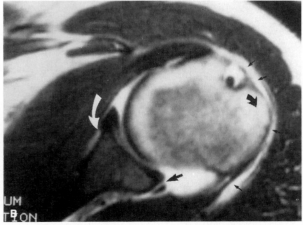

FIGURE 9-130. Normal variation in morphology of the subscapularis bursa is seen with (**A**) internal rotation and (**B**) external rotation on gadolinium-enhanced T1-weighted axial images. The subscapularis bursa has the appearance of a type 3 capsular insertion (*long black curved arrow*) in internal rotation (*short black curved arrow*) and a type 1 capsular insertion (*long curved white arrow*) in external rotation (*short black curved arrow*). Gadolinium contrast between the posterior band of the inferior glenohumeral ligament and the posterior labrum (*large straight black arrow*) and gadolinium contrast lateral to the humeral head in the subacromial bursa (*small straight black arrows*) are indicated.

the anterior pouch in a type 3 capsular insertion predisposes to anterior humeral subluxation or dislocation in a created potential space. However, in patients with a history of anterior dislocations there may be stretching of the capsular complex. However, on MR images it may be difficult to appreciate stretching of the IGL in the absence of tear or avulsion. Sperer and Wredmark,[176] using saline infusions and pressure/volume measurements during arthroscopic shoulder surgery, have shown that capsular elasticity and joint volume do not contribute to anterior shoulder instability.[176] Recurrent dislocations do not produce irreversible capsular distention.

Adhesive Capsulitis

Adhesive capsulitis is a clinical syndrome of pain and severely restricted joint motion (frozen shoulder), secondary to thickening and contraction of the joint capsule and synovium.[177] On arthrography, there is a decreased capacity to inject contrast material in a tight or resistant joint.[86] The subscapularis bursa and axillary pouch may be small and thickened. Emig and coworkers[177] reported that joint capsule and synovial thickness greater than 4 mm, as assessed at the level of the axillary recess, is a useful MR criterion for the diagnosis of adhesive capsulitis.[177] Articular fluid volumes are unreliable in the identification of adhesive capsulitis.

Calcific Tendinitis

Calcification of the rotator cuff most commonly occurs in the supraspinatus tendon but can occur in any of the tendons of the rotator cuff[178] (Fig. 9-131). The hydroxyapatite deposits can be seen in various views on conventional radiographs. Formation of calcific deposits in the tendinous portion of the rotator cuff is a degenerative process. The calcific build up can be extremely painful and act almost as an internal furuncle. Calcific tendinitis may exist in a subclinical or silent phase in which deposits are limited to the tendons of the rotator cuff (Fig. 9-132). In the mechanical or clinical phase, there may be elevation of the subacromial bursa as the foci of calcification increase in size.[179,180] Subbursal and intrabursal rupture may subsequently develop, with the extrusion of calcific deposits into the subacromial-subdeltoid bursa (Fig. 9-133).

Adhesive periarthritis is associated with adhesive bursitis as a complication of tendinous calcific deposits. Nodular deposits of calcium hydroxyapatite crystals demonstrate low signal intensity on all pulse sequences.[181] Bursitis, or an acute inflammatory reaction with the crystal deposits in a more semiliquid state, demonstrates a more heterogeneous hyperintensity with associated scattered foci of signal void on T2-, fast spin-echo T2-, or T2*-weighted images.[182] Treatment usually consists of a subacromial decompression, along with excision and removal of the calcific deposits by dissection and debridement.

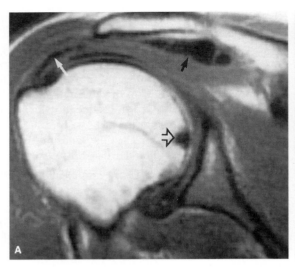

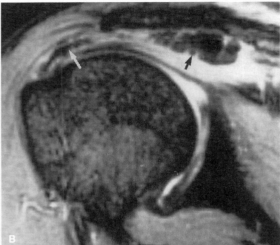

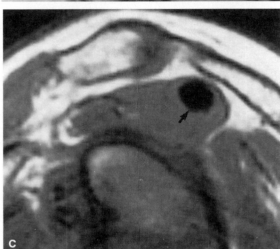

FIGURE 9-131. (A) T1-weighted coronal oblique, (B) T2*-weighted coronal oblique, and (C) T1-weighted sagittal oblique images show calcific tendinitis with low signal intensity calcium salt deposition in posterior supraspinatus muscle fibers (*black arrows*) and the infraspinatus tendon (*white arrow*). Infraspinatus involvement is best depicted on the T2*-weighted coronal oblique image. Calcific tendinitis may be related to local avascular changes and trauma. Calcium deposition may exist in a semiliquid form in the acute stage and as a more chalk-like deposit in the chronic stages. Rotator cuff pathology and calcific tendinitis may exist independently. As calcific tendinitis progresses from the silent phase to the mechanical phase, the subacromial bursa may be elevated, followed by subbursal and then intrabursal rupture associated with pain. Open arrow, subchondral sclerosis of the medial humeral head.)

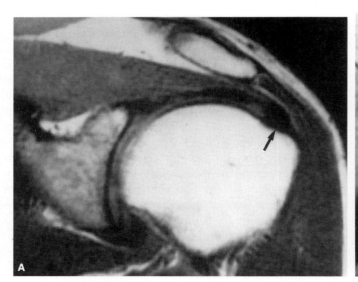

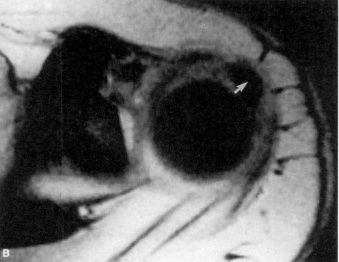

FIGURE 9-132. The subclinical or silent phase of periarticular calcium deposition (*arrows*) within the supraspinatus tendon is seen on (A) T1-weighted coronal oblique and (B) T2*-weighted axial images.

continued

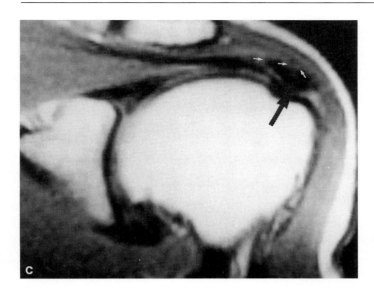

FIGURE 9-132. *Continued.* (**C**) A T1-weighted coronal image in a different patient shows a calcific deposit (*large arrow*) with elevation of the bursal floor (*small arrows*) in the mechanical phase prior to subbursal rupture.

Biceps Tenosynovitis and Related Pathology

Biceps tenosynovitis, or inflammation of the biceps tendon, is most frequently a degenerative process, with inflammation occurring in the bicipital groove. When located in the intraarticular or extraarticular portions of the tendon, it may be a result of trauma. MR images frequently display increased fluid, nonspecific for inflammation, in the bicipital synovial sheath.[183,184] Normally, communication exists between the joint capsule and the biceps tendon synovial sheath. Intrinsic hyperintensity or tendon thickening may be a more specific finding for biceps tendon inflammation (Fig. 9-134) than fluid in the bicipital synovial sheath. Fluid, however, may

be seen within the bicipital tendon sheath in the absence of fluid in the glenohumeral joint in cases of tenosynovitis. Tenosynovitis demonstrates low signal intensity on T1-weighted images and high signal intensity on T2- or fast spin-echo T2-weighted images.[185] Comparison with the opposite shoulder may be useful in assessing the significance of tendon inflammation. The Yergason test, in which forced supination produces pain in the biceps groove, is helpful in distinguishing biceps tendinitis from rotator cuff impingements. The biceps tendon lies within its groove, which makes it difficult to palpate; in fact, it is impossible to palpate the tendon in its intracapsular, intraarticular portion. The Yergason test is useful because it isolates the biceps tendon

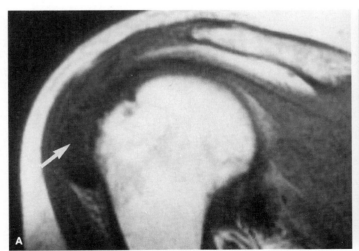

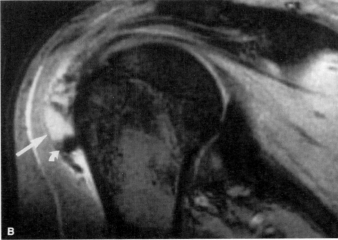

FIGURE 9-133. Low signal intensity bursal calcifications (*curved arrow*) and adjacent high signal intensity inflammatory fluid (*straight arrow*) are identified on posterior (**A**) T1-weighted and (**B**) T2*-weighted coronal oblique images in plane with the infraspinatus tendon. This finding represents the mechanical phase of calcific tendinitis with bursal extension.

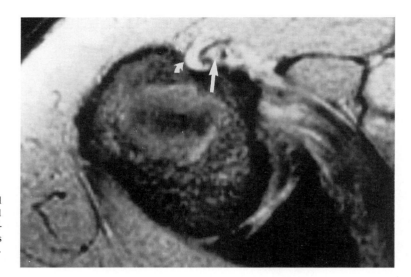

FIGURE 9-134. Bicipital tendinitis demonstrates high signal intensity on a T2*-weighted image and is centrally located within an enlarged biceps tendon (*straight arrow*). The finding of fluid in the biceps tendon sheath (*curved arrow*) is nonspecific, because the biceps tendon sheath normally communicates with the glenohumeral joint.

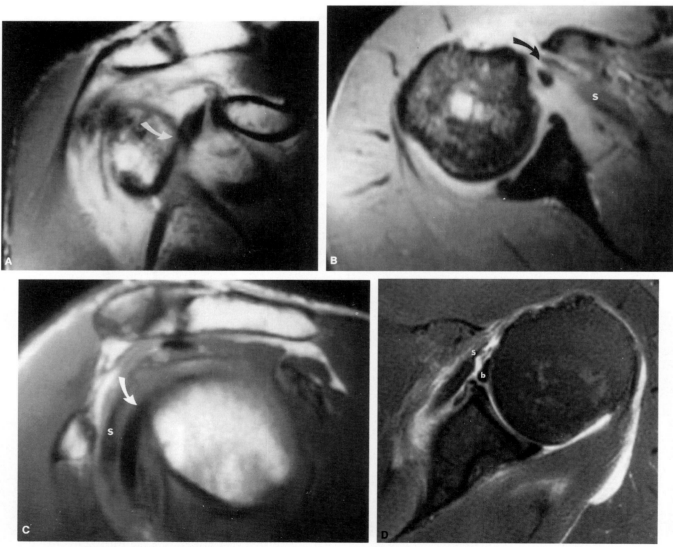

FIGURE 9-135. Dislocation of the tendon of the long head of the biceps medial to the bicipital groove (*curved arrow*) is seen on (**A**) T1-weighted coronal oblique, (**B**) T2*-weighted axial, and (**C**) T1-weighted sagittal oblique images. Degeneration and tearing of the insertion of the subscapularis tendon on the lesser tuberosity predispose the biceps to dislocate deep to the subscapularis tendon (S). There is complete rupture of the transverse ligament, which normally bridges the bicipital groove. In a separate case (**D**) the biceps tendon (b) is identified directly anterior to the anterior labrum on a fat-suppressed T2-weighted axial image. The torn and retracted subscapularis tendon (s) is shown.

and places it under stress without placing any stress on the infraspinatus, supraspinatus, or subscapularis tendons.

Biceps tenodesis in the bicipital groove is the treatment of choice in biceps tendinitis. If tenodesis is performed prior to rupture, the tendon and muscles are fixed under proper tension and the function of the biceps muscle as well as the long head of the biceps tendon is maintained. The contribution of the long head of the biceps tendon (through the BLC) to both superior and anterior stability of the glenohumeral joint is well documented,[186,187] and there is some concern that this fixation may compromise the stabilizing aspect of the glenohumeral ligament labral complex. However, since chronic biceps tendinitis generally occurs in older patients who are not prone to recurrent

instability, the use of biceps tenodesis is not usually contraindicated.

Biceps tendinitis and tenosynovitis are the earliest phases of biceps disease. Eventually, the biceps tendon may rupture and produce a classic "Popeye" muscle in the upper arm. Rupture of the long head of the biceps occurs in the bicipital groove. It is not approached surgically and is best treated conservatively.

Biceps subluxations, although rare, can be seen in disease processes in which loss of the integrity of the rotator cuff has occurred or in which the biceps tendon loses the support structures that maintain it in its groove (ie, the transverse ligament).[184] The long head of the biceps tendon attaches to the supraglenoid tubercle and contributes significantly to the

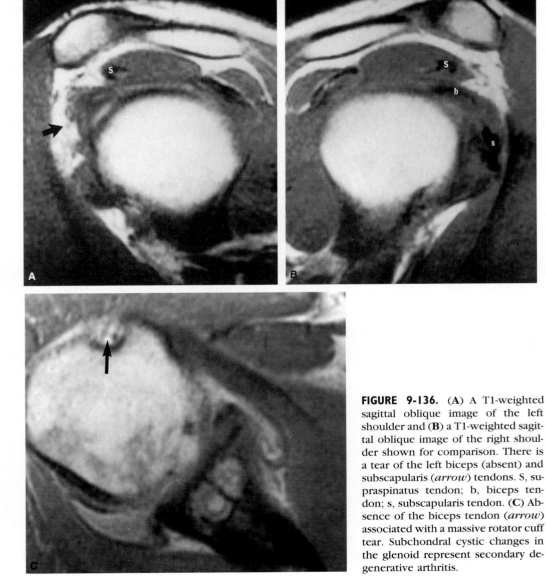

FIGURE 9-136. **(A)** A T1-weighted sagittal oblique image of the left shoulder and **(B)** a T1-weighted sagittal oblique image of the right shoulder shown for comparison. There is a tear of the left biceps (absent) and subscapularis (*arrow*) tendons. S, supraspinatus tendon; b, biceps tendon; s, subscapularis tendon. **(C)** Absence of the biceps tendon (*arrow*) associated with a massive rotator cuff tear. Subchondral cystic changes in the glenoid represent secondary degenerative arthritis.

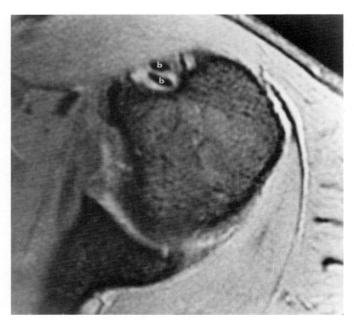

FIGURE 9-137. An asymptomatic bifid biceps tendon (b) not related to biceps labral complex pathology. There is no tear of the proximal biceps tendon.

superior and posterior labrum. Portions of the long head fibers also support and form the anterior labrum. Internal and external rotation views in the axial plane may be useful in identifying patients with subluxation of the biceps tendon.

The dislocated biceps tendon is usually identified medial to the bicipital groove and can be seen on anterior coronal oblique, axial, and sagittal oblique images[183,184,188,189] (Fig. 9-135). Associated findings may include a shallow bicipital

groove and tears of the coracohumeral ligament, subscapularis tendon, and supraspinatus tendon. The biceps tendon is located medial and anterior to the subscapularis tendon, with disruption of the transverse ligament, and an intact subscapularis. The biceps tendon dislocates beneath the subscapularis when there is associated tearing or degeneration of the subscapularis tendon insertion to the lesser tuberosity.

Biceps tendon rupture occurs at the top of the bicipital groove, usually occurs in patients older than 40 years of age, and is related to the spectrum of impingement. Pure musculotendinous junction ruptures are rare and are associated with violent trauma. Neer classifies ruptures of the long head of the biceps tendon into three types. Type 1 is tendon rupture without retraction. Type 2 is tendon rupture with partial recession, and type 3 is a self-attaching rupture without retraction.

Clinical diagnosis of a self-attaching long head rupture without retraction is difficult, and these types of injuries are usually identified at the time of rotator cuff repair. Absence of the biceps tendon on axial images through the bicipital groove or on sagittal images is diagnostic (Fig. 9-136). A bifid biceps tendon may be mistaken for a tear that splits the biceps tendon longitudinally (Fig. 9-137). A bifid biceps tendon is more likely to be visualized throughout all axial images in the glenohumeral joint and extends below the bony glenoid. A longitudinal split biceps tendon is more commonly restricted to a segment of the superior biceps tendon. Sagittal oblique MR images are used to confirm a normal BLC associated with a bifid biceps tendon. A bucket-handle tear of the labrum is not visualized in the presence of a normal BLC.

Fractures of the Proximal Humerus

Neer classifies upper humeral fractures into four parts: (1) those involving the anatomic neck of the humerus, (2) those involving

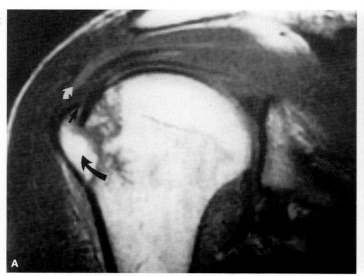
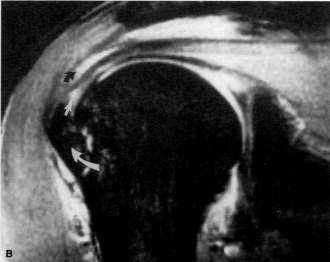

FIGURE 9-138. (**A**) T1-weighted and (**B**) T2*-weighted coronal oblique images show a greater tuberosity one-part fracture (*large curved arrows*) with an associated infraspinatus tendon tear (*straight arrow*). A small subacromial effusion is identified (*small curved arrows*).

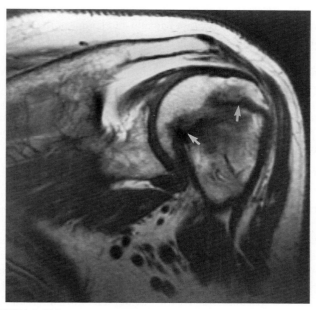

FIGURE 9-139. Fracture of the anatomical neck (*arrows*) with articular segment displacement on a T1-weighted coronal oblique image. Complications of this fracture include malunion or avascular necrosis.

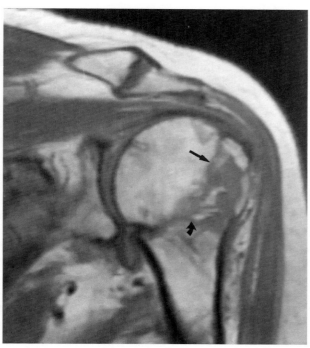

FIGURE 9-140. Surgical neck (*curved arrow*) and greater tuberosity fracture (*straight arrow*). Without displacement of one of the fragments, this injury is classified as a two-part fracture. In a three-part fracture there is a displaced greater tuberosity fracture and a displaced surgical neck fracture.

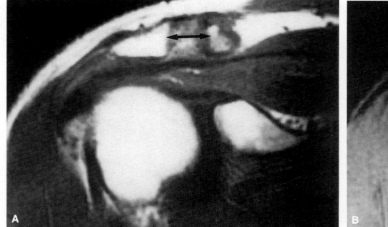
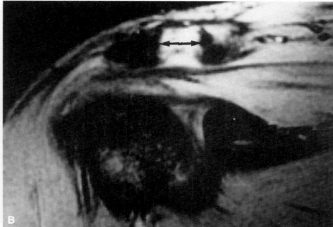

FIGURE 9-141. (**A**) T1-weighted and (**B**) T2*-weighted coronal oblique images show a type 2 (ie, moderate sprain) acromioclavicular separation (*double-headed arrows*) with widening of the acromioclavicular joint space to 10 mm. The normal acromioclavicular joint space is 3 to 8 mm.

the greater tuberosity, (3) those involving the lesser tuberosity, and (4) those involving the shaft or surgical neck of the humerus.[190]

A one-part fracture has either no displacement or angulation of any of the segments, or displacement and angulation are minimal (Fig. 9-138). A two-part fracture involves displacement of one segment (Fig. 9-139). A three-part fracture involves displacement of two segments with an associated unimpacted surgical neck fracture with rotatory displacement (Fig. 9-140). A four-part fracture is characterized by displacement of all four segments. Displacement is defined by fracture segment displacement of greater than 1 cm or angulation of more than 45°. Eight percent of proximal humeral fractures have minimal or no displacement and are held together by the rotator cuff, capsule, and periosteum. MR imaging is particularly useful in identifying one-part or non-displaced fractures not detected on conventional radiographs. MR images also display multiple fracture lines within any given segment. The axial plane is important in assessing the location of the humeral head in more complex fracture-dislocations and in determining involvement of the glenohumeral joint. STIR images are more sensitive than T2*-weighted protocols for the detection of areas of hemorrhage. Fat-suppressed T2-weighted fast spin-echo images can also be used to demonstrate areas of subchondral marrow hyperemia. T1-weighted images, however, adequately demonstrate the morphology of fracture segments and the continuity of articular cartilage surfaces.

Acromioclavicular Separations

There are three types of AC joint separations: type 1 is a sprain or incomplete tear of the AC joint capsule, type 2 is a complete tear of the AC joint capsule with intact coracocla-

vicular ligaments, and type 3 involves disruption of both the AC joint capsule and the coracoclavicular ligaments. Widening of the AC joint space to 1.0 to 1.5 cm and a 25% to 50% increase in coracoclavicular distance is associated with tearing of the AC joint capsule and sprain of the coracoclavicular ligament (Fig. 9-141). Widening of the AC joint to 1.5 cm or a 50% increase in the coracoclavicular distance correlates with coracoclavicular ligament disruption. Although the AC joint capsule and coracoclavicular ligaments can be directly assessed in the coronal and sagittal oblique planes, MR imaging is usually not indicated in AC joint separation unless the status of the rotator cuff and glenoid labrum are in question.

Arthritis

Degenerative osteoarthritis of the glenohumeral joint is relatively common. It is characterized by cartilage-space narrowing, hypertrophic bone formation, subchondral cysts, and associated soft-tissue abnormalities of the rotator cuff (Fig. 9-142). In rheumatoid disease, in contrast to osteoarthritis, joint space narrowing is more uniform and symmetric, without osteophytosis (Fig. 9-143). Rheumatoid erosions occur at the margins of the articular cartilage, including the greater tuberosity. Degenerative arthritis can be seen in younger patients, especially those who have had operative procedures for recurrent dislocation. Although the Bankart procedure and other capsular plication procedures prevent recurrent dislocation, they also significantly modify joint kinematics and may predispose the patient to degenerative joint disease. Secondary arthritis in younger patients eventually wears away the articular cartilage and produces significant joint incongruity, pain,

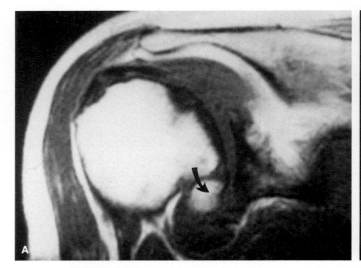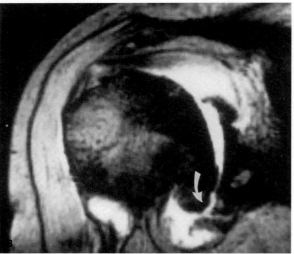

FIGURE 9-142. Advanced osteoarthritis can cause anterior and posterior osteophytosis (*large arrows; curved arrows*), denuded articular cartilage (*small arrows*), a macerated labrum, subchondral sclerosis, and cystic degeneration as seen on (**A**) a T1-weighted coronal oblique image; (**B**) a T2*-weighted coronal oblique image.

continued

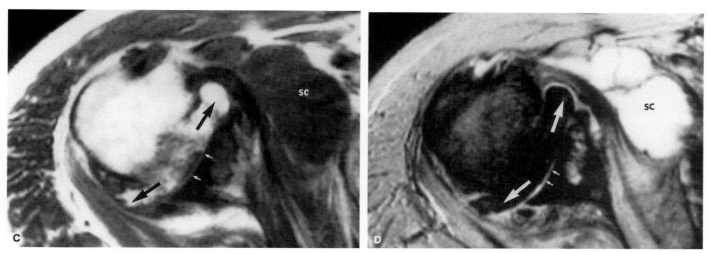

FIGURE 9-142. *Continued.* (**C**) a T1-weighted axial image; and (**D**) a T2*-weighted axial image. SC, subcoracoid fluid collection.

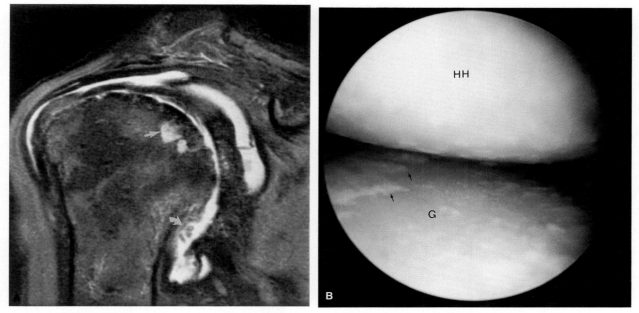

FIGURE 9-143. Rheumatoid arthritis and osteoarthritis. (**A**) Rheumatoid arthritis with concentric narrowing and loss of articular cartilage, erosive and subchondral cystic changes (*straight arrow*), chondral fragments (*curved arrow*), and superior migration of the humeral head are shown on a fat-suppressed T2-weighted fast spin-echo MR arthrographic image. (**B**) Arthroscopic photograph in a patient with osteoarthritis demonstrates denuded glenohumeral joint articular cartilage. Residual areas of articular cartilage are shown (*arrows*). HH, humeral head; G, glenoid.

and functional limitation. On T1-weighted images (Fig. 9-144), loose bodies demonstrate the low signal intensity of sclerosis, the intermediate signal intensity of articular cartilage, or the high signal intensity of fat marrow. Subchondral cysts with synovial fluid signal characteristics can be identified in either the distal clavicle or the acromial component of the AC joint as well as the glenohumeral joint (Fig. 9-145). Accurate assessment of humeral head articular cartilage thickness is somewhat limited on routine MR images, even with the benefit of intraarticular contrast. This may be secondary to the thinness of the articular cartilage.[191] Fat-suppressed fast spin-echo sequences combined with intraarticular contrast have shown the potential to differentiate both humeral head and glenoid articular cartilage surfaces (Fig. 9-146) and to identify specific sites of articular cartilage degeneration.

Avascular necrosis (AVN) of the humeral head can usually be differentiated from osteoarthritis by the restriction of subchondral low signal intensity ischemia (Fig. 9-147) to the humerus, without associated glenoid involvement (ie, sclerosis). AVN of the humeral head is associated with trauma, steroid use, sickle-cell disease, and alcoholism. The Neer classification for AVN of the humerus is similar to the Ficat staging for hip osteonecrosis.[192] In stage 1, which is asymptomatic, conventional radiographs produce negative results, whereas MR imaging results are positive for alterations in subchondral marrow. In stage 2 disease, which is

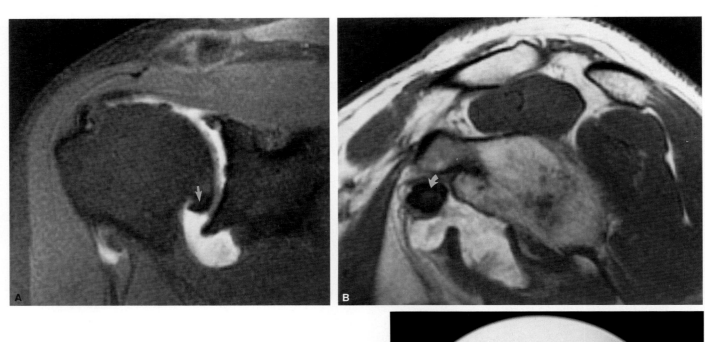

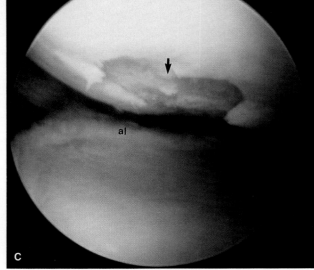

FIGURE 9-144. Fat-suppressed T2-weighted fast spin-echo coronal (**A**) and T1 sagittal oblique (**B**) images of degenerative osteoarthritis. Osteophytosis (**A**, *straight arrow*) and low signal intensity subcoracoid sclerotic loose body (**B**, *curved arrow*) are identified. (**C**) In a separate patient with osteoarthritis, the arthroscopic view identifies a humeral head chondral defect (*arrow*) as donor site for a loose body. al, anterior labrum.

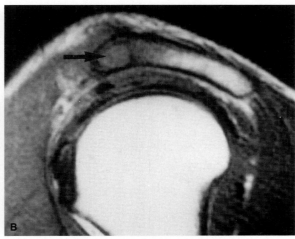

FIGURE 9-145. An acromial subchondral cyst (*arrow*) in the acromioclavicular joint. (**A**) T2*-weighted coronal oblique and (**B**) T1-weighted sagittal oblique images demonstrate a hooked type 3 acromion.

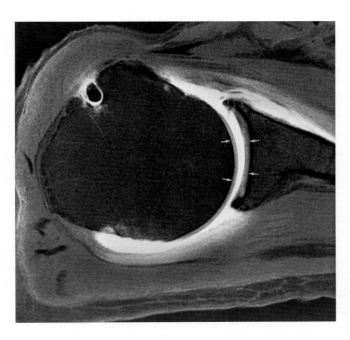

FIGURE 9-146. Fat-suppressed T2-weighted fast spin-echo axial image shows intact and congruous humeral head and glenoid articular cartilage surfaces (*arrows*), separate from the high signal intensity intraarticular contrast.

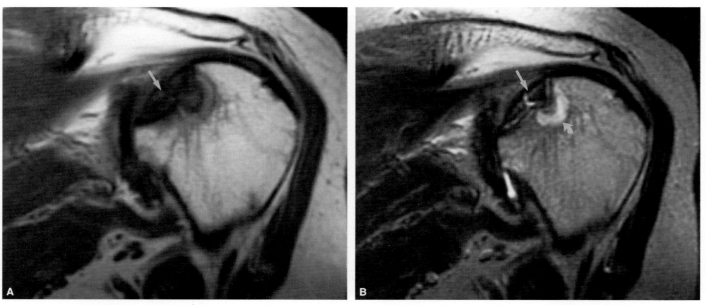

FIGURE 9-147. Avascular necrosis of the humeral head with hypointense necrotic segment (*straight arrow*) shown on T1 (**A**) and T2-weighted fast spin-echo (**B**) coronal oblique images. High signal intensity is also seen at the interface between necrotic and uninvolved marrow on the T2-weighted fast spin-echo image (**B**, *curved arrow*).

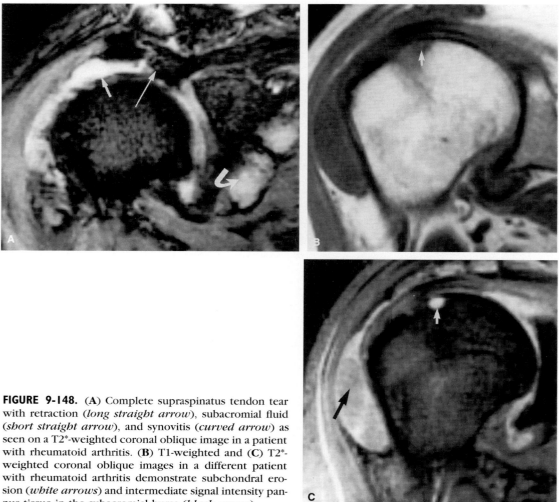

FIGURE 9-148. (**A**) Complete supraspinatus tendon tear with retraction (*long straight arrow*), subacromial fluid (*short straight arrow*), and synovitis (*curved arrow*) as seen on a T2*-weighted coronal oblique image in a patient with rheumatoid arthritis. (**B**) T1-weighted and (**C**) T2*-weighted coronal oblique images in a different patient with rheumatoid arthritis demonstrate subchondral erosion (*white arrows*) and intermediate signal intensity pannus tissue in the subacromial bursa (*black arrow*).

clinically characterized by pain, the humeral head retains its specific shape, although mild depression of the articular cartilage may be present in an area of subchondral bone. In stage 3 AVN, subchondral collapse or fracturing with overlying articular cartilage irregularity is seen. No involvement of the glenohumeral joint articular cartilage is found. Stage 4 disease leads to incongruity of the glenohumeral joint.

Rheumatoid disease of the shoulder, with its accompanying synovitis and aggressive synovial proliferation, targets the capsule of the rotator cuff and biceps tendon. On conventional T2-, fast spin-echo T2-, and T2*-weighted images, hyperplastic synovium demonstrates intermediate signal intensity and enhances with intravenous contrast. Disruptions of the rotator cuff with loss of subacromial space are frequently demonstrated (Fig. 9-148).

Paralabral Cysts

When synovial-filled ganglion cysts (sometimes called paralabral cysts because the term paralabral cyst better describes the relationship between the cyst and the glenoid labrum) involve the spinoglenoid notch, they can produce atrophy of the infraspinatus (Fig. 9-149) and/or the supraspinatus muscle (Fig. 9-150) secondary to suprascapular nerve entrapment.[193–195] Isolated infraspinatus atrophy is associated with more posteriorly located ganglion cysts and dorsal suprascapular nerve entrapment. Supraspinatus and infraspinatus muscle atrophy are seen in association with anteriorly located masses and proximal nerve entrapment. In the initial stage of suprascapular nerve compression, edematous changes in the infraspinatus muscle are characterized by low to intermediate signal intensity on T1-weighted images and hyperintensity on T2, fat-suppressed T2-weighted fast spin-echo, or gradient-echo T2*-weighted images. Chronic compression may lead to the development of fatty muscle atrophy.

Intramuscular hemorrhage may mimic the appearance of a synovial ganglion. There is a high correlation between paralabral cysts, which have a posterior location, and posterosuperior labral tears[194,196] (Fig. 9-151). These cysts may communicate and undermine the posterosuperior glenoid labrum, and they may extend medially in the spinoglenoid notch. Anterior inferior paralabral cysts may be identified in communication with tears of the anterior inferior glenoid labrum. These small tears of the anterior inferior glenoid labrum may not be appreciated on routine axial images and require the use of an abduction external rotation view to display the IGLLC. As discussed earlier, SLAP type II lesions may be visualized with fluid signal intensity communicating with a superiorly located paralabral cyst (Fig. 9-152). Anterior extension of a paralabral cyst through a labral tear can involve the subcoracoid space superior to the subscapularis bursa (Fig. 9-153).

text continues on page 738

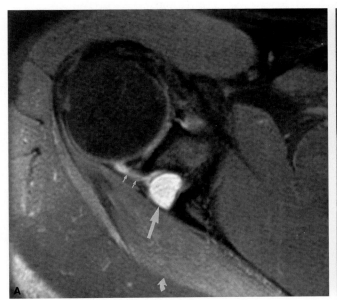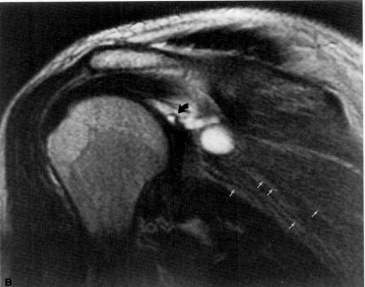

FIGURE 9-149. **(A)** Posteriorly located paralabral cyst (*large straight arrow*) of the spinoglenoid notch with the neck (*small straight arrows*) of the cyst communicating with the posterosuperior labral tear (as part of a SLAP type II lesion). (Fat-suppressed T2-weighted fast spin-echo axial image.) Denervation edema of the infraspinatus muscle is present (*curved arrow*) and is hyperintense relative to signal intensity in normal muscle. **(B)** Non fat-suppressed T2-weighted fast spin-echo coronal oblique image shows changes of both fatty atrophy and denervation within the infraspinatus muscle. The parallel streaks of linear increased signal intensity correspond to fatty atrophy (*small straight arrows*). The communication of the cyst (*curved arrow*) with the superior labral tear is also demonstrated.

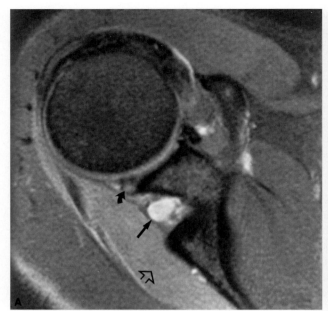

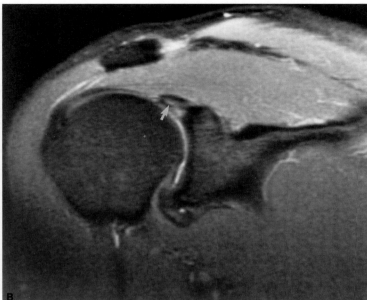

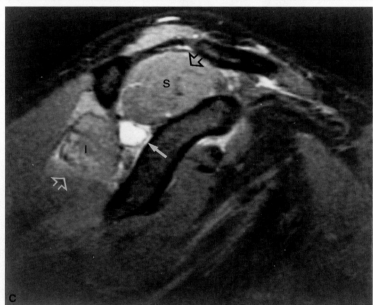

FIGURE 9-150. Paralabral cyst occupying the spinoglenoid notch associated with a SLAP type II labral tear. (**A**) T2* axial image displays the posterior location of the paralabral cyst in the spinoglenoid notch (*straight arrow*), a posterior labral tear (*curved arrow*), and denervation edema of the infraspinatus muscles (*open arrows*). (**B**) Fat-suppressed T2-weighted fast spin-echo coronal oblique image shows linear hyperintensity within the posterior superior labral tear (*arrow*). (**C**) Spinoglenoid notch cyst (*straight arrow*) with denervation of both the supraspinatus (S) and infraspinatus (I) muscles (*open arrows*) as seen on a fat-suppressed T2-weighted fast spin-echo sagittal image. Denervation changes in both muscles are secondary to previous anterior extension of the paralabral cyst, with affected muscular branches to the supraspinatus muscle at the level of the supraspinatus fossa. Isolated infraspinatus muscle involvement is a more common presentation of a spinoglenoid notch cyst.

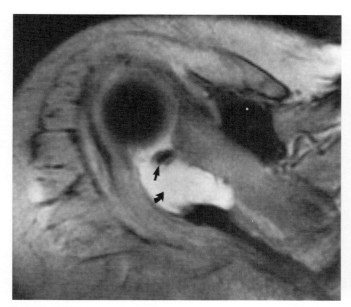

FIGURE 9-151. A bucket-handle tear of the posterior superior la-brum (*straight arrow*) associated with a paralabral cyst (*curved arrow*) as seen on a T2*-weighted axial image. This tear did not extend anteriorly to the biceps anchor.

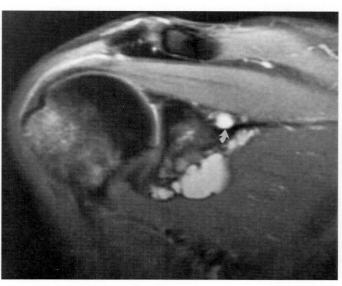

FIGURE 9-153. Paralabral cyst tracking anterior to the glenoid and extending into the suprascapular notch (*curved arrow*). The supra-scapular notch is located anterior to the spinoglenoid notch. (Fat-suppressed T2-weighted fast spin-echo coronal oblique image.)

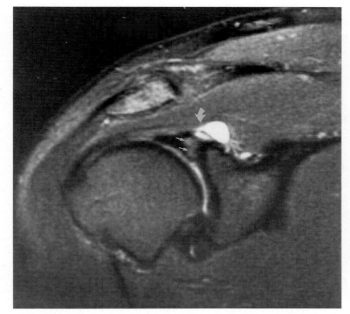

FIGURE 9-152. Direct communication between a SLAP type II lesion (*small arrows*) and a superiorly located paralabral cyst (*large arrow*) on a fat-suppressed T2-weighted fast spin-echo coronal oblique image.

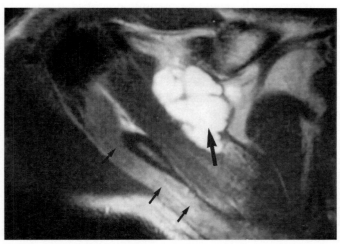

FIGURE 9-154. T2-weighted axial image shows a paralabral cyst (*large arrow*) associated with fatty atrophy and denervation (*small arrows*) of the infraspinatus muscle. The cyst presents anterior to the supraspinatus muscle within the suprascapular notch, although its point of origin was located more posteriorly, in the spinoglenoid notch. This patient had a SLAP type II lesion. Note that the supraspinatus muscle is unaffected.

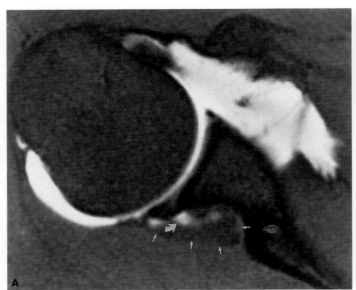
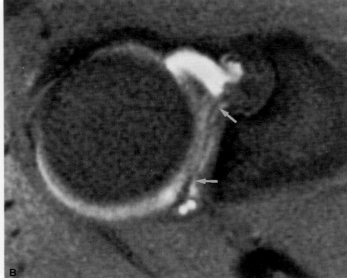

FIGURE 9-155. T1 fat-suppressed axial MR arthrograms of paralabral cyst. **(A)** Partial filling (*curved arrow*) of a spinoglenoid notch cyst (*small straight arrows*) with intraarticular contrast. **(B)** Communication of the cyst with a SLAP type II lesion. The superior labrum is torn from anterior to posterior (*arrows*) as assessed on the axial image through the most superior aspect of the glenohumeral joint.

The posterosuperior paralabral cyst is thus a common location for a cyst seen in association with a posterior capsulolabral injury, including SLAP lesions.[194,196] The location of these cysts should be carefully described. They usually involve the spinoglenoid notch, which is located posterior to the suprascapular notch and is the location for the suprascapular nerve after it turns around the lateral edge of the scapular spine.[194] The inappropriate use of the term suprascapular notch to describe the location of all superior paralabral cysts may result in surgical exploration that is far anterior to the correct location of the cyst within the spinoglenoid notch. Most superior paralabral cysts originate in the spinoglenoid notch. The spinoglenoid ligament (inferior transverse scapular ligament) is variably present and is located superior to the suprascapular nerve. Initial treatment of a paraglenoid cyst is conservative, progressing to cyst aspiration or surgical release of the suprascapular ligament in symptomatic patients. Cyst aspiration, which can be performed with CT guidance, may relieve some of the patient's symptoms, obviating the need for arthroscopy. The associated labral tear, however, may remain symptomatic.

In our experience, most paralabral cysts, including but not limited to posterosuperior cysts, communicate with a labral tear. The paralabral cyst may be confined to the spinoglenoid notch or it may demonstrate anterior extension into the suprascapular notch, as seen on anterior coronal oblique MR images or axial images with the cyst identified anterior to the supraspinatus muscle (Fig. 9-154). Superior and posterosuperior paralabral cysts are commonly seen in association with SLAP type II lesions and the associated labral tear is identified on both axial and coronal oblique T2-weighted images. Documentation of direct communica-tion of the paralabral cyst with the glenohumeral joint is possible with MR arthrography (Fig. 9-155). In retrospect, it is evident that the initial descriptions of suprascapular nerve entrapment and ganglion cysts did not appreciate the association with capsulolabral pathology, regardless of whether the patient was asymptomatic or symptomatic.[193]

Infection

A septic joint may be associated with effusion and joint debris. Osteomyelitis may be associated with bone marrow or subchondral involvement, both of which demonstrate low signal intensity on T1-weighted images and high signal intensity on conventional T2, fat-suppressed T2-weighted fast spin-echo, and STIR images.

References

1. Mink JH, Harris E, Rappaport M. Rotator cuff tears: evaluation using double contrast shoulder arthrography. Radiology 1985;157:621.
2. Rafii M, et al. Athlete shoulder injuries: CT arthrographic findings. Radiology 1987;162:559.
3. Rafii M, et al. CT arthrography of capsular structures of the shoulder. AJR 1986;146:361.
4. Resnick CS. The shoulder. In: Scott WW Jr, Majid D, Fishman EK, eds. Contemporary issues in computed tomography: CT of the musculoskeletal system. New York: Churchill Livingstone, 1987:139.
5. Middleton WE, et al. Sonographic detection of rotator cuff tears. AJR 1985;144:349.
6. Crass DR, Craig EV, Feinberg SB. Sonography of the post-operative rotator cuff. AJR 1986;146:561.

7. Mack LA, et al. US evaluation of the rotator cuff. Radiology 1985;157:205.

8. Van Holsbeeck M, Strouse PJ. Sonography of the shoulder: evaluation of the subacromial-subdeltoid bursa. AJR 1993;160:561.

9. Wiener SN, Seitz WH Jr. Sonography of the shoulder in patients with tears of the rotator cuff: accuracy and value for selecting surgical options. AJR 1993;160:103.

10. Paavolainen P, Ahovuo J. Ultrasonography and arthrography in the diagnosis of tears of the rotator cuff. J Bone Joint Surg [Am] 1994;76A:335.

11. Van Holsbeeck M, Kolowich PA, Eyler WR, Craig JG. Ultrasound depiction of partial-thickness tear of the rotator cuff. Radiology 1995;197:443.

12. Hollister MS, Mack LA, Patten RM, Winter TC. Association of sonographically detected subacromial/subdeltoid bursal effusion and intraarticular fluid with rotator cuff tear. AJR 1995;165:605.

13. Vick CW, et al. Rotator cuff tears: diagnosis with sonography. AJR 1990;154:121.

14. Middleton WD, et al. High resolution MR imaging of the normal rotator cuff. AJR 1987;148:559.

15. Middleton WD, et al. High resolution surface coil magnetic resonance imaging of the joints: anatomic correlation. Radiographics 1987; 7:645.

16. Kieft GJ, et al. Magnetic resonance imaging of glenohumeral joint diseases. Skeletal Radiol 1987;16:285.

17. Huber DJ, et al. MR imaging of the normal shoulder. Radiology 1986;158:405.

18. Seeger LL, et al. MR imaging of the normal shoulder: anatomic correlation. AJR 1987;148:83.

19. Kieft GJ, et al. Normal shoulder: MR imaging. Radiology 1986; 159:741.

20. Zlatkin MR, et al. Magnetic resonance imaging of the shoulder. Magn Reson Q 1989;5:3.

21. Burk DL Jr, et al. Rotator cuff tears: prospective comparison of the MR imaging with arthrography, sonography, and surgery. AJR 1989; 153:87.

22. Zlatkin MR, et al. Rotator cuff tears: diagnostic performance of MR imaging. Radiology 1989;172:223.

23. Seeger LL. Magnetic resonance imaging of the shoulder. Clin Orthop 1989;244:48.

24. Evancho AM, et al. MR imaging diagnosis of rotator cuff tears. AJR 1988;151:751.

25. Masciocchi C, et al. Magnetic resonance imaging of the shoulder: technique, anatomy, and clinical results. Radiol Med (Torino) 1989; 78:485.

26. Tsai NC, et al. Magnetic resonance imaging of the shoulder. Radiol Clin North Am 1990;28:279.

27. Holt RG, et al. Magnetic resonance imaging of the shoulder: rationale and current applications. Skeletal Radiol 1990;19:5.

28. Meter SJ, et al. MRI of the shoulder. Semin US CT MR 1990;11:253.

29. Palmer WE, Caslowitz PL, Chew FS. MR arthrography of the shoulder: normal intraarticular structures and common abnormalities. AJR 1995;164:141.

30. Davis SJ, Teresi LM, Bradley WG, et al. Effect of arm rotation on MR imaging of the rotator cuff. Radiology 1991;181:265.

31. McCauley TR, Pope CF, Jokl P. Normal and abnormal glenoid labrum: assessment with multiplanar gradient-echo MR imaging. Radiology 1992;183:35.

32. Recht MP, Kramer J, Petersilge CA, Yu J. Distribution of normal and abnormal fluid collections in the glenohumeral joint: implications for MR arthrography. JMRI 1994;4:173.

33. O'Brien SJ, et al. The anatomy and histology of the inferior glenohumeral ligament complex of the shoulder. Am J Sports Med 1990; 18:449.

34. Hurley JA. Anatomy of the shoulder. In: Nicholas JA, Hershman EB, eds. The upper extremity in sports medicine, 2nd ed. St Louis: Mosby Year Book 1995:23.

35. Klein MA, Miro PA, Spreitzer AM, Carrera GF. MR imaging of the normal sternoclavicular joint: spectrum of findings. AJR 1995; 165:391.

36. Neer CS. Shoulder reconstruction. Philadelphia: WB Saunders, 1990:1.

37. Moseley HF, et al. The anterior capsular mechanism in recurrent anterior dislocation of the shoulder. J Bone Joint Surg [Br] 1962;44:913.

38. Detrisac DJ, Johnson LL. Arthroscopic shoulder anatomy: pathologic and surgical implications. Thorofare, NJ: Slack, 1986.

39. Bowen MK, Warren RF. Ligamentous control of shoulder stability based on selective cutting and static translation experiments. Clin Sports Med 1991;10:757.

40. Rodosky MW, Harner CD, Fu FH. The role of the long head of the biceps muscle and superior glenoid labrum in anterior stability of the shoulder. Am J Sports Med 1994;22:121.

41. Wall MS, O'Brien SJ. Arthroscopic evaluation of the unstable shoulder. Clin Sports Med 1995;14:817.

42. Schwartz RE, et al. Capsular restraints to anterior-posterior motion of the shoulder. Trans Orthop Res Soc 1987;12:78.

43. DePalma AF. Surgery of the shoulder. Philadelphia: JB Lippincott, 1983.

44. Turkel SJ, Panio MW, Marshall JL, et al. Stabilizing mechanisms preventing anterior dislocation of the glenohumeral joint. J Bone Joint Surg [Br] 1981;67B:1208.

45. Schwartz RE, O'Brien SJ, Warren RF, et al. Capsular restraints to anterior-posterior motion of the abducted shoulder: a biomechanical study. Orthop Trans 1988;12:727.

46. Neer CS, et al. Inferior capsular shift for involuntary inferior and multidirectional instability of the shoulder: a preliminary report. J Bone Joint Sur [Am] 1980;62:897.

47. DePalma AF, Callery G, Bennett GA: Variational anatomy and degenerative lesions of the shoulder bone. Instruction course, American Academy of Orthopedic Surgery, vol 16, 1949:255.

48. Warner JP, Deng X, Warren RF, et al. Static capsuloligamentous restraints to superior-inferior translation of the glenohumeral joint. Presented at the Annual Meeting of the Orthopaedic Research Society, Anaheim, CA, 1991.

49. Cooper D, Warner JP, Deng X, et al. Anatomy and function of the coracohumeral ligament. Presented at the American Academy of Orthopaedic Surgeons, Anaheim, CA, 1991.

50. Ovesen J, Nielsen S: Anterior and posterior instability. Acta Orthop Scand 1986;57:324.

51. McMinn RMH. Last's anatomy: regional and applied, 8th ed. Edinburgh: Churchill Livingstone, 1990:53.

52. Neer CS. Shoulder reconstruction. Philadelphia: WB Saunders, 1990:41.

53. Naimark A, Baum A. Injection of the subcoracoid bursa: a cause of technical failure in shoulder arthrography. J Can Assoc Radiol 1989;40:170.

54. Horwitz TM, Tocantins LM. An anatomical study of the role of the long thoracic nerve and the related scapular bursae in the pathogenesis of local paralysis of the serratus anterior muscle. Anat Rec 1938;71:375.

55. Schweitzer ME, Magbalon MJ, Frieman BG, Ehrlich S. Acromioclavicular joint fluid: determination of clinical significance with MR imaging. Radiology 1994;192:205.

56. Schweitzer ME, Magbalon MJ, Fenlin JM, Frieman BG. Effusion criteria and clinical importance of glenohumeral joint fluid: MR imaging evaluation. Radiology 1995;194:821.

57. Richardson ML, Patten RM. Age-related changes in marrow distribution in the shoulder: MR imaging findings. Radiology 1994;192:209.

58. Seeger LH, et al. Shoulder impingement syndrome. MR findings in 53 shoulders. AJR 1988;150:343.

59. Brems J. Rotator cuff tear: evaluation and treatment. Orthopaedics 1988;11:69.

60. Ellman H. Shoulder arthroscopy: current indications and techniques. Orthopaedics 1988;11:45.

61. Kleft GJ, et al. Rotator cuff impingement syndrome: MR imaging. Radiology 1988;166:211.

62. Neer CS. Anterior acromioplasty for the chronic impingement syndrome: a preliminary report. J Bone Joint Surg [Am] 1972;54:41.

63. Neer CS, et al. Rupture of the long head of the biceps related to subacromial impingement. Orthop Trans 1977;1:111.

64. Uhthoff AK, Sarkar K. Classification and definition of tendinopathies. Clin Sports Med 1991;10:707.

65. Bigliani LU, Morrison DS. Subacromial impingement syndrome. In: Dee R, ed. Principles of orthopaedic practice. New York: McGraw-Hill, 1989:627.

66. Rathbun JB, Macnab I. The microvascular pattern of the rotator cuff. J Bone Joint Surg [Br] 1970;52:540.

67. Bigliani LU, et al. The morphology of the acromion and its relationship to rotator cuff tears. Orthop Trans 1986;10:216.

68. Ozaki J, et al. Tears of the rotator cuff of the shoulder associated with pathologic changes in the acromion. J Bone Joint Surg [Am] 1988;70:1224.

69. Sharkey NA, Marder RA. The rotator cuff opposes superior translation of the humeral head. Am J Sports Med 1995;23:270.

70. Morrison OS, Bigliani LU. The clinical significance of variations in acromial morphology. Orthop Trans 1987;11:234.

71. Fukuda H, Hamada K, Yamanaka K: Pathology and pathogenesis of bursal-side rotator cuff tears viewed from en bloc histologic sections. Clin Orthop 1990;254:75.

72. Miniaci A, Dowdy PA. Rotator cuff disorders. In: Hawkins RJ, Misamore GW, eds. Shoulder injuries in the athlete. New York: Churchill Livingstone, 1996:103.

73. Tyson LL, Crues J. Pathogenesis of rotator cuff disorders. In: Rafii M, ed. Magnetic resonance imaging. Magnetic Resonance Imaging Clin North Am 1993;1:37.

74. Ogata S, Uhthoff HK. Acromial enthesopathy and rotator cuff tear: a radiologic and histologic postmortem investigation of the coracoacromial arch. Clin Orthop 1990;254:39.

75. Nirschl RP. Rotator cuff tendinitis: basic concepts of pathoetiology. Instr Course Lecture 1989:38.

76. Zlatkin MB. MR imaging of the shoulder: current experience and future trends. In: Kressel, HY, Modic MT,Murphy WA, eds. Syllabus special course MR. Oak Brook, IL: RSNA Publications, 1990:255.

77. Kieft GJ, et al. Rotator cuff impingement syndrome. MR imaging. Radiology 1988;166:211.

78. Neer CS II, Welsh RP. The shoulder in sports. Orthop Clin North Am 1977;8:583.

79. Hawkins RJ, Kennedy JC. Impingement syndrome in athletes. Am J Sports Med 1980;8:151.

80. Johnson LL: Diagnostic and surgical arthroscopy of the shoulder. St Louis: Mosby Year Book, 1993:365.

81. Zlatkin MB, et al. The painful shoulder: MR imaging of the glenohumeral joint. J Comput Assist Tomogr 1988;12:995.

82. Rafii M. The shoulder. In: Firooznia HF, Golimbu C, Rafii M, et al, eds. MRI and CT of the musculoskeletal system. St Louis: Mosby Year Book, 1992:465.

83. Uhthoff HK, Sarkar K, Hammond DI. The subacromial bursa: a clinico-pathological study. In: Bateman JE, Welsh RP, eds. Surgery of the shoulder. Philadelphia: BC Decker, 1984:121.

84. Kjellin I, et al. Alterations in the supraspinatus tendon at MR imaging: correlation with histopathologic findings and cadavers. Radiology 1991;181:837.

85. Neumann CH, Holt RG, Steinback LS, et al. MR imaging of the shoulder: appearance of the supraspinatus tendon in asymptomatic volunteers. AJR 1992;158:1281.

86. Resnick D (ed). Internal derangements of joints. In: Diagnosis of bone and joint disorders, 3rd ed. Philadelphia: WB Saunders, 1995.

87. Timins ME, Erickson SJ, Estkowski LD, Carrera GF. Increased signal in the normal supraspinatus tendon on MR imaging: diagnostic pitfall caused by magic-angle effect. AJR 1995;165:109.

88. Vahlensieck M, Pollack M, Lang P, et al. Two segments of the supraspinous muscle: cause of high signal intensity at MR imaging? Radiology 1993;186:449.

89. Clark JM, Harryman DT. Tendons, ligaments, and capsule of the rotator cuff. J Bone Joint Surg [Am] 1992;74A:713.

90. Totterman SM, Miller RJ, Kwok E. MR imaging of the shoulder rotator cuff. In: Book of abstracts: Radiological Society of North America 1992. Chicago: Radiological Society of North America, 1992:240.

91. Rafii M, et al. Rotator cuff lesions: signal patterns at MR imaging. Radiology 1990;177:817.

92. Codman EA. The shoulder: rupture of the supraspinatus tendon and other lesions in or about the subacromial space. Boston: Thomas Todd, 1934.

93. Cotton RE, Rideout DF. Tears of the humeral rotator cuff: a radiological and pathological necropsy survey. J Bone Joint Surg [Br] 1964;46B:314.

94. McNab I, Hastings D. Rotator cuff tendinitis. Cal Med Assoc J 1968;99:91.

95. Skinner HA. Anatomical considerations relative to rupture of the supraspinatus tendon. J Bone Joint Surg [Am] 1937;18:137.

96. Strizak AM, Torrance LD, Jackson D, et al. Subacromial bursography: an anatomical and clinical study. J Bone Joint Surg 1982;64A:196.

97. Chandnani VP, Ho C, et al. MR findings in asymptomatic shoulders: a blind analysis using symptomatic shoulders as controls. Clin Imaging 1992;16:25.

98. Shellock FG, Stoller DW, Crues JV. MRI of the shoulder: a rational approach to the reporting of findings. JMRI 1996;6:268.

99. Vanarthos WJ, Mono JUV. Type 4 acromion: a new classification. Contemp Orthop 1995;30:227.

100. Peh CG, Farmer T, Totty W. Acromial arch shape: assessment with MR imaging. Radiology 1995;195:501.

101. Aoki M, Ishii S, Usui M. The slope of the acromion and rotator cuff impinement. Proc Am Shoulder Elbow Surg 1986.

102. Park JG, Lee JK, Phelps CT. Os acromiale associated with rotator cuff impingement: MR imaging of the shoulder. Radiology 1994;193:255.

103. Hutchinson MR, Veenstra MA. Arthroscopic decompression of shoulder impingement secondary to os acromiale. Arthroscopy 1993;9:28.

104. Neer CS, Craig EU, Fukuda H. Cuff-tear arthropathy. J Bone Joint Surg [Am] 1985;65:1232.

105. Gallino M, Battiston B, Annaratone G, Terragnoli F. Coracoacromial ligament: a comparative arthroscopic and anatomic study. Arthroscopy 1995;11:564.

106. Edelson JG, Luchs J. Aspects of coracoacromial ligament anatomy of interest to the arthroscopic surgeon. Arthroscopy 1995;11:715.

107. Bonutti PM, Norfray JF, Friedman RJ, Genez BM. Kinematic MRI of the shoulder. J Comput Assist Tomogr 1993;17:666.

108. Jobe CM. Posterior superior glenoid impingement: expanded spectrum. Arthroscopy 1995;11:530.

109. Tirman PFJ, Bost FW, Garvin GJ, et al. Posterosuperior glenoid impingement of the shoulder: findings at MR imaging and MR arthrography with arthroscopic correlation. Radiology 1994;193:431.

110. Morrison DS, et al. The use of magnetic resonance imaging in the diagnosis of rotator cuff tears. Orthopedics 1990;13:633.

111. Itoi E, Tabata S: Incomplete rotator cuff tears: results of operative treatment. Clin Orthop 1992;284:128.

112. Flannigan B, et al. MR arthrography of the shoulder. AJR 1990; 155:829.

113. Palmer WE, Brown JH, Rosenthal DI. Rotator cuff: evaluation with fat-suppressed MR arthrography. Radiology 1993;188:683.

114. Tirman PFJ, Bost FW, Steinbach LS, Mall JC. MR arthographic depiction of tears of the rotator cuff: benefit of abduction and external rotation of the arm. Radiology 1994;192:851.

115. Quinn SF, Sheley RC, Demlow TA, Szumowski J. Rotator cuff tendon

tears: evaluation with fat-suppressed MR imaging with arthroscopic correlation in 100 patients. Radiology 1995;195:497.

116. Reinus WR, Shady KL, Mirowitz SA, Totty WG. MR diagnosis of rotator cuff tears of the shoulder: value of using T2-weighted fat-saturated images. AJR 1995;164:1451.

117. Patten RM. Tears of the anterior portion of the rotator cuff (the subscapularis tendon): MR imaging findings. AJR 1994;162:351.

118. Hodler J, Kursunoglu-Brahme S, Snyder SJ, Cervella V. Rotator cuff disease: assessment with MR arthrography versus standard MR imaging in 36 patients with arthroscopic confirmation. Radiology 1992;182:431.

119. Robertson PL, Schweitzer ME, Mitchell DG, Schlessinger F. Rotator cuff disorders: interobserver and intraobserver variation in diagnosis with MR imaging. Radiology 1995;194:831.

120. Owen RS, Iannotti JP, Kneeland JB, Dalinka MK. Shoulder after surgery: MR imaging with surgical validation. Radiology 1993;186:443.

121. Mirowitz SA. Normal rotator cuff: MR imaging with conventional and fat-suppression techniques. Radiology 1991;180:735.

122. Linker CS, Helms CA, Fritz RC. Quadrilateral space syndrome: findings at MR imaging. Radiology 1993;188:675.

123. Iannotti JP, et al. Magnetic resonance imaging of the shoulder: sensitivity, specificity and predictive value. J Bone Joint Surg [Am] 1991;73:17.

124. Sher JS, Uribe JW, Posada A, et al. Abnormal findings on magnetic resonance imaging of asymptomatic shoulders. J Bone Joint Surg [Am] 1995;77A:10

125. Miniaci A, Dowdy PA, Willits KR, Vellet AD. Magnetic resonance imaging evaluation of the rotator cuff tendons in the asymptomatic shoulder. Am J Sports Med 1995;23142.

126. Turkel SJ, et al. Stabilizing mechanisms preventing anterior dislocation of the glenohumeral joint. J Bone Joint Surg [Am] 1981;63:1208.

127. Rowe C: Dislocations of the shoulder. In: Rowe C, ed. The shoulder. New York: Churchill Livingstone, 1988:165.

128. Wolf EM, Cheng JC, Dickson K. Humeral avulsion of glenohumeral ligaments as a cause of anterior shoulder instability. Arthroscopy 1995;11:600.

129. Pollock RG, Bigliani LU. The mechanical properties of the inferior glenohumeral ligamnet. Presented at the American Shoulder and Elbow Surgeons, 6th Opening Meeting. New Orleans, February 11, 1990.

130. Payne LZ, Altchek DW. The surgical treatment of anterior shoulder instability. Clin Sports Med 1995;14:863.

131. Chandnani VP, Yeager TD, DeBerardino T, Christensen K. Glenoid labral tears: prospective evaluation with MR imaging, MR arthrography, and CT arthrography. AJR 1993;161:1229.

132. Tirman PFJ, Stauffer AE, Crues JV III, Turner RM. Saline magnetic resonance arthrography in the evaluation of glenohumeral instability. Arthroscopy 9:550.

133. Palmer WE, Caslowitz PL. Anterior shoulder instability: diagnostic criteria determined from prospective analysis of 121 MR arthrograms. Radiology 1995;197:819.

134. Feller JF, Tirman PFJ, Steinbach LS, Zucconi F. Magnetic resonance imaging of the shoulder: review. Semin Roentgenol 1995;30:224.

135. Workman TL, Burkhard TK, Resnick D, et al. Hill-Sachs lesion: comparison of detection with MR imaging, radiography, and arthroscopy. Radiology 1992;185:847.

136. Richards RD, Sartoris DJ, Pathria MN, Resnick D. Hill-Sachs lesion and normal humeral groove: MR imaging features allowing their diffentiation. Radiology 1994;190:665.

137. Neviaser TJ. The anterior labroligamentous periosteal sleeve avulsion lesion: a cause of anterior instability of the shoulder. Arthroscopy 1993;9:17.

138. Neviaser TJ. The GLAD lesion: another cause of anterior shoulder pain. Arthroscopy 1993;9:22.

139. Schwartz R, O'Brien S, Warren RF. Capsular restraints to the abducted shoulder: a biomechanical study. Orthop Trans 1988;12:727.

140. Speer KP. Anatomy and pathomechanics of shoulder instability. Clin Sports Med 1995;14:751.

141. Murrell GA, Warren RF. The surgical treatment of posterior shoulder instability. Clin Sports Med 1995;14:903.

142. Schwartz E, et al. Posterior shoulder instability. Orthop Clin North Am 1987;18:409.

143. Ferrari JD, Ferrari DA, Coumas J, Pappas AM. Posterior ossification of the shoulder: the Bennett lesion. Etiology, diagnosis and treatment. J Sports Med 1994;22:171.

144. Neer CS. Shoulder reconstruction. Philadelphia: WB Saunders, 1990:273.

145. Snyder SJ: Diagnostic arthroscopy: normal anatomy and variations. In: Shoulder arthroscopy. New York: McGraw-Hill, 1994.

146. Morgan C, Rames RD, Snyder SJ. Anatomical variations of the glenohumeral ligaments. Presented at the Annual Meetings of the American Academy of Orthopedic Surgeons, Anaheim, CA, 1991.

147. Cooper DE, Arnoczky SP, O'Brien SJ, et al. Anatomy, histology and vascularity of the glenoid labrum: an anatomical study. J Bone Joint Surg [Am] 1992;74:46.

148. Williams MM, Snyder SJ, Buford D Jr. The Buford complex—the ''cord-like'' middle glenohumeral ligament and absent anterosuperior labrum complex: a normal anatomic capsulolabral variant. Arthroscopy 1994;10:241.

149. Williams MM, Karzel RP, Snyder SJ. Labral disorders. In: Hawkins RJ, Misamore GW, eds. Shoulder injuries in the athlete. New York: Churchill Livingstone, 1991:291.

150. Howell SM, Galinat BJ. The glenoid-labral socket: a constrained articular surface. Clin Orthop 1989;243:122.

151. Karzel R, Nuber G, Lautenschlager E. Contact stresses during compression loading of the glenohumeral joint: the role of the glenoid labrum. Proc Inst Med 1989;42:64.

152. DePalma AJ, White JB, Callery G. Degenerative lesions of the shoulder joint at various age groups which are compatible with good function. Intr Course Lect 1950;7:168.

153. Scarpinato DF, Bramhall JP, Andrews JR. Arthroscopic management of the throwing athlete's shoulder: indications, techniques and results. Clin Sports Med 1991;10:913.

154. Andrews JR, Carson WG, McLeod WD. Glenoid labrum tears related to the long head of the biceps. Am J Sports Med 1985;13:337.

155. Snyder SJ, et al. SLAP lesions of the shoulder. Arthroscopy 1990;6:274.

156. Palmer WE, Brown JH, Rosenthal DI. Labral-ligamentous complex of the shoulder: evaluation with MR arthrography. Radiology 1994;190:645.

157. Chandnani VP, Gagliardi JA, Murnane TG, Bradley YC. Glenohumeral ligaments and shoulder capsular mechanism: evaluation with MR arthrography. Radiology 1995;196:27.

158. Loredo R, Longo C, Salonen D, et al. Glenoid labrum: MR imaging with histologic correlation. Radiology 1995;196:33.

159. Gusmer PB, Potter HG, Schatz J, et al. Labral injuries: accuracy of detection with unenhanced MR imaging of the shoulder. Radiology 1996;200:519.

160. Zlatkin MB, et al. Evaluation of rotator cuff disease and glenohumeral instability with MR imaging: correlation with arthroscopy and arthrotomy in a large population of patients [abstr]. Magn Reson Imaging 1990;8(suppl 1):78.

161. Callaghan J, et al. A prospective comparison of double contrast computed tomography: CT, arthrography and arthroscopy of the shoulder. Am J Sports Med 1988;16:13.

162. Habibian A, et al. Comparison of conventional and computed arthrotomography with MR imaging in the evaluation of the shoulder. J Comput Tomogr 1989;13:968.

163. Kieft GJ, et al. MR imaging of recurrent anterior dislocation of the shoulder: comparison with CT arthrography. AJR 1988;150:1083.

164. Monu JUV, Pope Jr TL, Chabon SJ, Vanarthos WJ. MR diagnosis of superior labral anterior posterior (SLAP) injuries of the glenoid la-

brum: value of routine imaging without intraarticular injection of contrast material. AJR 1994;163:1425.

165. Munk P, et al. Glenoid labrum: preliminary work with use of radial-sequence MR imaging. Radiology 1989;73:751.

166. Legan JM, Burkhard TK, Goff WB II, et al. Tears of the glenoid labrum: MR imaging of 88 arthroscopically confirmed cases. Radiology 1991;179:241.

167. Caspari RB, et al. Shoulder arthroscopy: a review of the present state of the art. Contemp Orthop 1982;4:523.

168. Patten RM. Vacuum phenomenon: a potential pitfall in the interpretation of gradient-recalled-echo MR images of the shoulder. AJR 1994;162:1383.

169. Zlatkin MB, et al. The painful shoulder: MR imaging of the glenohumeral joint. J Comput Assist Tomogr 1988;12:995.

170. Seeger LL, et al. Shoulder instability: evaluation with MR imaging. Radiology 1988;168:685.

171. Hawkins RJ, Belle RM. Posterior instability of the shoulder. Instr Course Lect 1989;38:211.

172. Norwood LA, Terry GC. Shoulder posterior subluxation. Am J Sports Med 1984;12:25.

173. Kopka L, Funke M, Fischer V, Keating D. MR arthrography of the shoulder with gadopentetate dimeglumine: influence of concentration, iodinated contrast material, and time of signal intensity. AJR 1994;163:621.

174. Wilson AJ. Shoulder joint: arthrographic CT and long-term follow-up with surgical correlation. Radiology 1989;173:329.

175. Zlatkin MB, et al. Cross-sectional imaging of the capsular mechanism of the glenohumeral joint. AJR 1988;160:151.

176. Sperer A, Wredmark T. Capsular elasticity and joint volume in recurrent anterior shoulder instability. Arthroscopy 1994;10:598.

177. Emig EW, Schweitzer ME, Karisick D, Lubowitz J. Adhesive capsulitis of the shoulder: MR diagnosis. AJR 1995;164:1457.

178. Beltran J, et al. Tendons: high-field strength, surface coil MR imaging. Radiology 1987;162:735.

179. Hayes CW, et al. Calcium hydroxyapatite deposition disease. RadioGraphics 1990;10:1032.

180. Resnick D. Calcium hydroxyapatite crystal deposition disease. In: Resnick D, Niwayama G, eds. Diagnosis of bone and joint disorders, 2nd ed. Philadelphia: WB Saunders, 1988:1733.

181. Burk DL, et al. MR imaging of the shoulder: correlation with plain radiographs. AJR 1990;154:549.

182. Bigliani LU. Rheumatic and degenerative disorders. In: Dee R, ed. Principles of orthopaedic practice. New York: McGraw Hill, 1989:621.

183. Erickson SJ, Fitzgerald SW, Quinn SF, et al. Long bicipital tendon of the shoulder: normal anatomy and pathologic findings on MR imaging. AJR 1992;158:1091.

184. Tuckman GA. Abnormalities of the long head of the biceps tendon of the shoulder: MR imaging findings. AJR 1994;163:1183.

185. Kieft GJ, et al. Magnetic resonance imaging of the shoulder in patients with rheumatoid arthritis. Ann Rheum Dis 1990;49:7.

186. Rodosky MW, Harner CD, Fu FH. The role of the long head of the biceps muscle and superior glenoid labrum in anterior stability of the shoulder. AMJ Sports Med 1994;22:121.

187. Warner JJP, McMahon PJ. The role of the long head of the biceps brachii in superior stability of the glenohumeral joint. J Bone Joint Surg 1995:366.

188. Chan TW, et al. Biceps tendon dislocation evaluation with MR imaging. Radiology 1991;179:649.

189. Cervilla V, et al. Medial dislocation of the biceps brachii tendon: appearance at MR imaging. Radiology 1991;180:523.

190. Neer CS. Shoulder reconstruction. Philadelphia: WB Saunders, 1990:363.

191. Hodler J, Loredo RA, Longo C, et al. Assessment of articular cartilage thickness of the humeral head: MR anatomic correlation in cadavers. AJR 1995;165:615.

192. Neer CS. Shoulder reconstruction. Philadelphia: WB Saunders, 1990:194.

193. Fritz RC, Helms CA, Steinbach LS, Genant HK. Suprascapular nerve entrapment: evaluation with MR imaging. Radiology 1992;182:437.

194. Fehrman DA, Orwin JF, Jennings RM. Suprascapular nerve entrapment by ganglion cysts: a report of 6 cases with arthroscopic findings and review of the literature. Arthroscopy 1995;11:727.

195. Beltran J, Rosenberg ZS. Diagnosis of compressive and entrapment neuropathies of the upper extremity: value of MR imaging. AJR 1994;163:525.

196. Tirman PFJ, Feller JF, Janzen DL, et al. Association of glenoid labral cysts with labral tears and glenohumeral instability: radiologic findings and clinical significance. Radiology 1994;190:653.

Magnetic Resonance Imaging in Orthopaedics & Sports Medicine, Second Edition,
edited by David W. Stoller. Lippincott-Raven Publishers, Philadelphia, © 1997.

Chapter 10

The Elbow

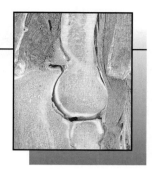

Russell C. Fritz
David W. Stoller

Magnetic resonance (MR) imaging provides clinically useful information in assessing the elbow joint. Superior depiction of muscles, ligaments, and tendons, as well as the ability to directly visualize nerves, bone marrow, and hyaline cartilage, are advantages of MR imaging relative to conventional imaging techniques. These features of MR imaging may help establish the cause of elbow pain by depicting accurately the presence and extent of bone and soft tissue pathology. Ongoing improvements in surface coil design and newer pulse sequences have resulted in higher quality MR images of the elbow that can be obtained more rapidly. Recent clinical experience has shown the utility of MR imaging in detecting and characterizing disorders of the elbow in a noninvasive fashion.[1–9]

The sequelae of medial traction and lateral compression from valgus stress include medial collateral ligament (MCL) injury, common flexor tendon pathology, medial traction spurs, ulnar neuropathy, and osteochondritis dissecans. These conditions, as well as lateral collateral ligament injury and lateral epicondylitis, may be characterized with MR im-

aging. MR imaging is also useful for identification of posttraumatic osseous abnormalities such as radiographically occult fractures, stress fractures, bone contusions, and apophyseal avulsions. MR imaging also can be used to assess cartilaginous extension of fractures in children. Intraarticular loose bodies can also be depicted with MR imaging, especially if fluid or contrast material is present within the elbow joint. Biceps and triceps tendon injuries can be diagnosed and characterized. MR imaging also can provide additional information regarding entrapment neuropathies, bursitis, arthropathies, and soft tissue masses about the elbow.

IMAGING TECHNIQUES AND PROTOCOLS FOR THE ELBOW

Extremity Coils and Patient Positioning

Typically, the elbow is scanned with the patient in a supine position with the arm at the side. A surface coil is essential for obtaining high-quality images (Fig. 10-1). Depending on

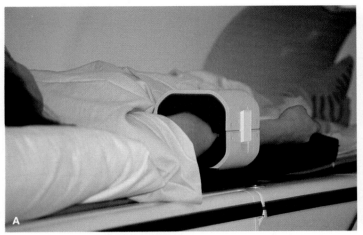
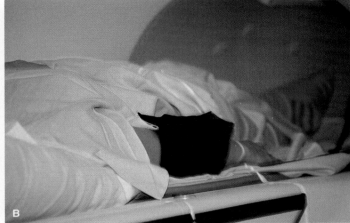
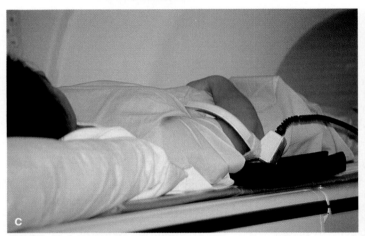
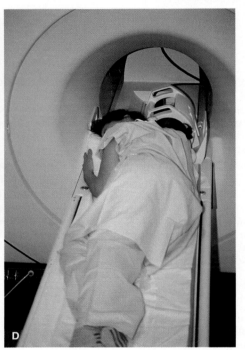

FIGURE 10-1. Surface coil options. (**A**) This wrist coil produces excellent elbow images in children and relatively small adults when a large field of view is not required. (**B**) This flexible coil is similar to a blood pressure cuff. Even large patients can be scanned in a supine position with this "low profile" coil design. (**C**) A shoulder coil used for patients who cannot fit into smaller coils because of inability to fully extend the elbow. (**D**) In high-field small bore magnets, larger patients may have to be scanned with the arm overhead. This position can be quite uncomfortable, requiring rapid scanning.

the size of the patient and the size of the surface coil relative to bore of the magnet, it may be necessary to scan the patient in a prone position with the arm extended overhead. In general, the prone position is less well tolerated and results in a greater number of motion-degraded studies. The elbow should be scanned in a comfortable position to avoid motion artifact. The elbow is typically extended and the wrist is placed in a neutral position. Patients who cannot extend the elbow are more difficult to position, and obtaining optimal imaging results requires more time and skill. Taping a vitamin E capsule or other marker to the skin at the site of tenderness or at the site of a palpable mass is useful to ensure that the area of interest has been included in the study, especially when there is no pathology identified on the images.

Pulse Parameters

Excellent images may be obtained with both midfield and high-field MR systems. Proton density and T2-weighted images are typically obtained in the axial and sagittal planes using spin-echo or fast spin-echo techniques. T1-weighted and short TI inversion recovery (STIR) sequences usually are obtained in the coronal plane. Although the STIR sequence has relatively poor signal-to-noise because of the suppression of signal from fat, pathology is often more conspicuous due to the effects of additive T1 and T2 contrast.

In general, axial images should extend from the distal humeral metaphysis to the radial tuberosity. The common flexor and extensor origins from the medial and lateral humeral epicondyles and the biceps insertion on the radial tuberosity are routinely imaged with this coverage. Images are usually obtained with 3 or 4 mm thick slices using a long TR sequence. Coronal images are angled parallel to a line through the humeral epicondyles on the axial images, and sagittal images are angled perpendicular to a line through the humeral epicondyles on the axial images.

The field of view on axial images should be as small as the signal of the surface coil and the size of the patient's elbow allow. The field of view selected on the coronal and sagittal sequences is usually larger than the field of view on the axial images, to include more of the anatomy about the elbow. This is especially important when imaging a ruptured biceps tendon that may retract to the normal superior margin of coverage. Slice thickness, interslice gap, and TR may be increased on axial sequences, just as the field of view is increased on coronal and sagittal sequences, as long as the surface coil provides adequate signal to image the entire length of the area of interest.

Additional sequences may be added or substituted, depending on the clinical problem being investigated. T2*-weighted gradient-echo sequences provide useful supplemental information for identifying loose bodies within the elbow. Gradient-echo volume sequences allow acquisition of multiple very thin axial images which may subsequently be reformatted in any plane using a computer workstation. In our experience, these volume sequences have not proven routinely useful, primarily because of their relatively poor soft tissue contrast compared with images obtained with the spin-echo technique. Fast spin-echo volume sequences may prove to be more useful than the currently available gradient-echo volume technique. In general, gradient-echo sequences are to be avoided after elbow surgery because magnetic susceptibility artifacts associated with micrometallic debris may obscure important findings and also may be mistaken for loose bodies. Artifact surrounding orthopaedic hardware is most prominent on gradient-echo sequences because of the lack of a 180° refocusing pulse, and is least prominent on fast spin-echo sequences due to the presence of multiple 180° pulses. If available, fast spin-echo and fast STIR sequences may be substituted for conventional T2-weighted spin-echo and conventional STIR sequences. These newer sequences allow greater flexibility in imaging the elbow while continuing to provide information that is comparable with that of conventional spin-echo and STIR sequences. The speed of fast spin-echo sequences may be used to obtain higher resolution T2-weighted images in the same amount of time as conventional spin-echo sequences or simply may be used to reduce the overall time of the examination. The ability to shorten the examination with fast spin-echo is useful when scanning claustrophobic patients or when scanning patients who become uncomfortable in the prone position with the arm overhead.

Fat suppression may be added to various pulse sequences to improve visualization of the hyaline articular cartilage.

Avoidance of chemical shift artifact at the interface of cortical bone and fat-containing marrow permits a more accurate depiction of the overlying hyaline cartilage. Fat-suppressed T1-weighted images are useful whenever gadolinium is administered, either intravenously or directly into the elbow joint as a dilute solution. Intravenous gadolinium may provide additional information in the assessment of neoplastic or inflammatory processes about the elbow. Articular injection of saline or dilute gadolinium may be useful in patients without a joint effusion to detect loose bodies, to determine if the capsule is disrupted, or to determine if an osteochondral fracture fragment is stable.

GROSS ANATOMY

A thorough understanding of the anatomy and function of the elbow is essential for accurate interpretation of MR images. The anatomic structures of the elbow are depicted reliably on MR images, and knowledge of the relative functional significance of these structures allows assessment of clinically important anatomy. Focusing on the relevant anatomic structures leads to more meaningful interpretation of the images and facilitates clinical problem solving.

Osseous and Articular Anatomy

The elbow is composed of three articulations contained within a common joint cavity. The articulation of the radius and ulna comprises the proximal radioulnar joint. The radial head rotates within the radial notch of the ulna, allowing supination and pronation distally. The capitellum also articulates with the radius and the trochlea articulates with trochlear notch of the ulna in a hinge fashion, allowing flexion and extension of the elbow joint (Fig. 10-2).

Humerus

The distal humerus consists of medial and lateral condyles as well as the articular surfaces of the trochlea and the capitellum. The trochlea is a pulley-like surface that articulates with the trochlear notch of the ulna. A continuous surface of articular cartilage covers the trochlea and forms an arc of about 300° to 330°. A trochlear groove courses from anterolateral to posteromedial, defining medial and lateral lips of the trochlea. The capitellum, also known as the capitulum, is an anteriorly directed sphere that articulates with a depression in the radial head. The trochleocapitellar groove articulates with the medial rim of the radial head throughout the arc of flexion and extension (Fig. 10-3). The crest at the trochlear margin of the trochleocapitellar groove and the adjacent medial rim of the radial head are common sites of early articular cartilage loss.[10]

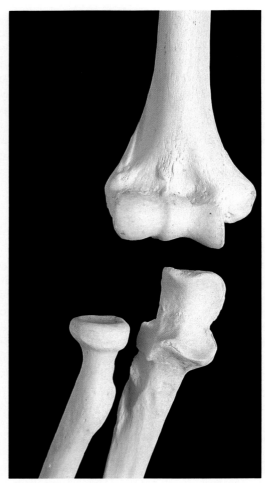

FIGURE 10-2. The bones that form the elbow and proximal radioulnar joints. The radial head articulates with the radial notch of the ulna and the capitellum. The trochlea articulates with the trochlear notch of the ulna. The trochlear notch is composed of the olecranon proximally and the coronoid distally.

The prominent medial epicondyle arises proximal to the trochlea and serves as the site of origin for the flexor-pronator muscle group via the common flexor tendon. The MCL also originates from the medial epicondyle. A groove or sulcus for the ulnar nerve is present at the posterior margin of the medial epicondyle. The lateral epicondyle is much less prominent than the medial epicondyle. The lateral epicondyle arises just proximal to the capitellum and serves as the site of origin for the extensor-supinator group and the lateral collateral ligament. The radial fossa of the humerus lies just proximal to the capitellum anteriorly and receives the radial head during flexion (see Fig. 10-3). The coronoid fossa lies just proximal to the trochlea and receives the coronoid process during flexion. Posteriorly, the olecranon fossa receives the tip of the olecranon during extension (Fig. 10-4). The olecranon and coronoid fossae are separated by a thin membrane of bone in about 90% of individuals. A supracondylar process of the humerus is found about 6 cm proximal to the medial epicondyle in 1% to 3% of individu-

als.[11] The supracondylar process may fracture and contribute to median and ulnar nerve entrapment.

Ulna

The proximal ulna is comprised of olecranon and coronoid processes that together form the articular surface of the trochlear notch. The trochlear notch is also known as the greater sigmoid notch or semilunar notch. The congruent articulation of the humeral trochlea and the trochlear notch of the ulna is largely responsible for the inherent bony stability of the elbow joint. This articulation allows for the hinge-like flexion and extension of the elbow. The trochlear notch is divided longitudinally into medial and lateral facets by a guiding ridge. In most individuals, the trochlear notch is also divided transversely by a bare area that is not covered by a continuous surface of articular cartilage (Fig. 10-5). Therefore, in most individuals there are four articular surfaces of the trochlear notch that articulate with the trochlea of the humerus. A fifth articular surface, known as the radial notch, arises just distal to the coronoid laterally and articulates with the radial head. This radial notch, also known as the lesser sigmoid notch, consists of an arc of about 70° and is oriented perpendicular to the greater sigmoid notch.

The triceps muscle and tendon attach to the posterosuperior nonarticular aspect of the olecranon (Fig. 10-6). The proximal tip of the olecranon is separated from the tendon by a subtendinous olecranon bursa. The brachialis muscle and tendon insert on the anterior nonarticular aspect of the coronoid and the ulnar tuberosity distally, at the level of the radial tuberosity. The anterior bundle of the MCL inserts at the medial margin of the coronoid process. A crest along the lateral aspect of the ulna is the site of the ulnar origin of the supinator muscle. A tubercle on the supinator crest serves as the insertion site for the ulnar part of the lateral collateral ligament, also known as the lateral ulnar collateral ligament (LUCL). The annular ligament arises from the posterior and anterior margins of the radial notch of the ulna (see Fig. 10-5).

Radius

The proximal radius is comprised of the radial head and neck as well as the radial tuberosity. The radial head has a central depression that articulates with the capitellum. Two thirds of the outer rim of the radial head is covered with hyaline cartilage and articulates with the radial notch of the ulna at the proximal radioulnar joint. The anterolateral one third of the radial circumference is normally devoid of articular cartilage and lacks strong subchondral bone. It is the portion of the radial head that is most commonly fractured. The radial tuberosity, at the distal margin of the radial neck, consists of an anterior surface for the bicipitoradial bursa and a posterior aspect where the biceps tendon attaches. The bicipitoradial bursa separates the biceps tendon from the radial tuberosity during full pronation.

text continues on page 752

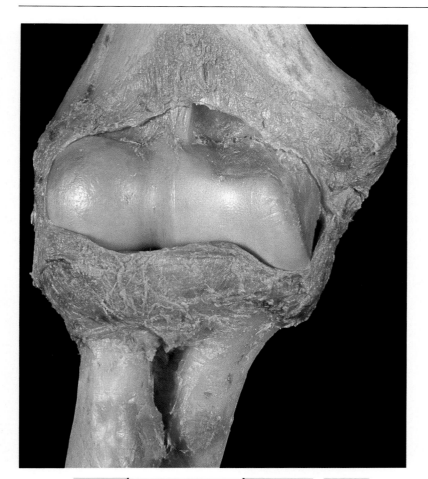

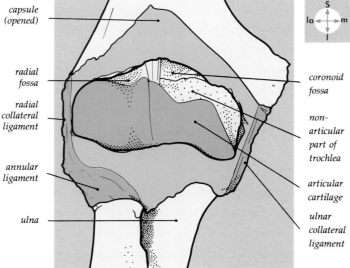

FIGURE 10-3. The anterior aspect of the extended elbow joint. The anterior capsule has been opened to expose the anterior articular surface. The capitellum and trochlea are separated by the trochleocapitellar groove that articulates with the medial rim of the radial head. The radial fossa of the humerus lies just proximal to the capitellum and receives the radial head during full flexion. The coronoid fossa lies just proximal to the trochlea and receives the coronoid process during full flexion. The anterior bundle of the medial collateral ligament is seen extending from the anteroinferior aspect of the medial epicondyle to the medial margin of the coronoid.

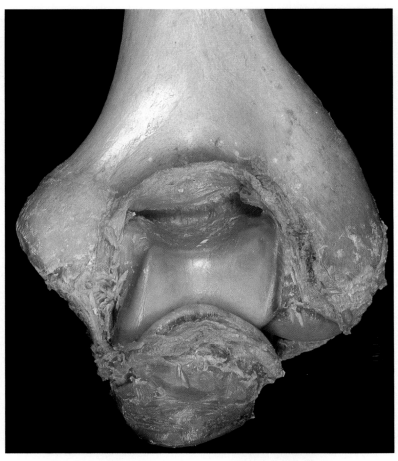

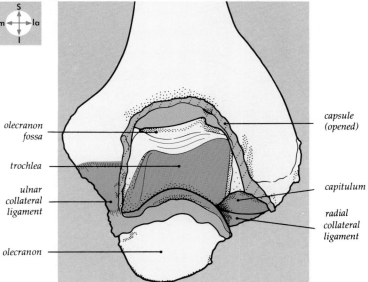

olecranon
fossa

trochlea

ulnar
collateral
ligament

olecranon

capsule
(opened)

capitulum

radial
collateral
ligament

FIGURE 10-4. The posterior aspect of the flexed elbow joint. The capsule has been opened to reveal the olecranon fossa that receives the olecranon during full extension. The posterior bundle of the medial collateral ligament is seen extending from the posteroinferior aspect of the medial epicondyle to the medial margin of the olecranon.

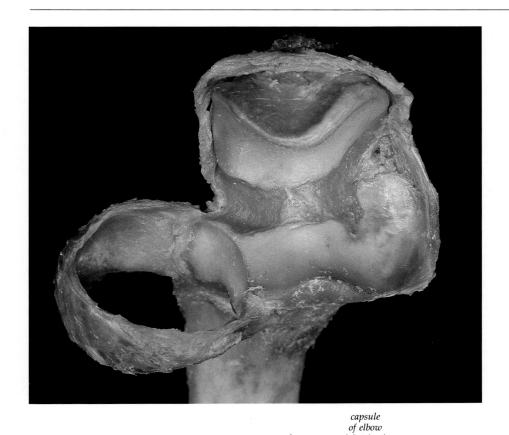

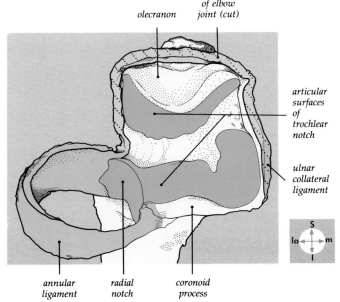

*capsule
of elbow
joint (cut)*

olecranon

*articular
surfaces
of
trochlear
notch*

*ulnar
collateral
ligament*

*annular
ligament*   *radial
notch*   *coronoid
process*

FIGURE 10-5. An anterior view of the proximal ulna with the humerus and radius removed shows the articular surfaces of the radial notch and the trochlear notch. The annular ligament extends from the anterior and posterior margins of the radial notch. A bare area that is normally devoid of articular cartilage extends transversely across the midportion of the trochlear notch.

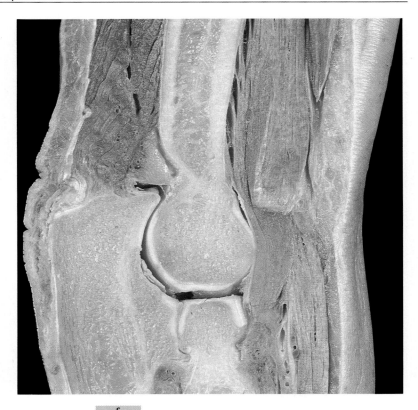

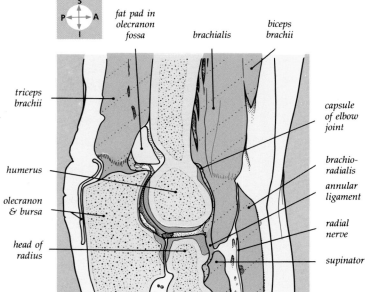

FIGURE 10-6. An oblique longitudinal section of the extended elbow and the proximal radioulnar joints shows the articular surfaces and relations of the joints. The triceps muscle and tendon are seen attaching to the olecranon. The posterior intracapsular fat pad is seen within the olecranon fossa.

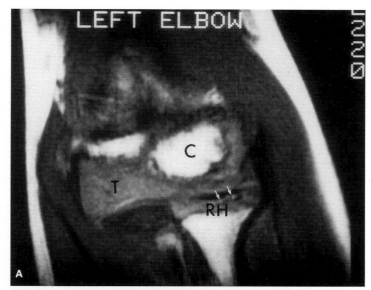

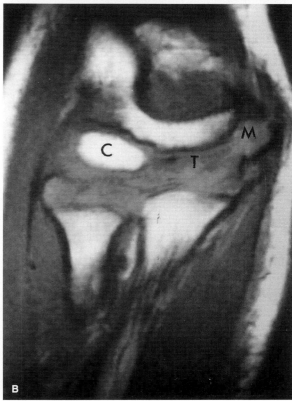

FIGURE 10-7. Epiphyseal maturation. **(A)** Ossification of the capitellum on a T1-weighted coronal image of the left elbow in a 5-year-old child. There is also early ossification (*arrows*) of the radial head (RH). The trochlea (T) remains unossified. **(B)** Ossification of the capitellum on a T1-weighted coronal image of the right elbow in a 2-year-old child. The radial head, trochlea, and medial epicondyle (M) remain unossified. The cartilaginous templates of the epiphyses are well seen.

Epiphyseal Maturation

The capitellum is the first of the six ossification centers about the elbow to appear radiographically. It generally becomes visible at 1 to 2 years of age (Fig. 10-7). The medial epicondyle appears next, at about 4 years of age. It is the last ossification center to fuse with the humerus. The medial epicondyle usually does not fuse with the humerus until age 15 or 16. The radial head ossifies shortly after the medial epicondyle, usually around 5 years of age. It often matures as one or more flat sclerotic centers which may, on radiographs, be mistaken for a fracture or avascular necrosis. At about 8 years of age the trochlea ossifies, sometimes in a multicentric fashion that on radiographs may be confused with fractures or osteochondrosis. MR imaging confirms the normal appearance of multiple trochlear ossification centers that contain high signal intensity yellow marrow on T1-weighted images. The olecranon ossifies at about 9 years of age, shortly after the trochlea and just before the lateral epicondyle. The lateral epicondyle appears at about 10 or 11 years of age and fuses at approximately age 14. It initially appears as a thin vertically oriented sliver that may be mistaken for an avulsion fracture.

Awareness of the normal orderly sequence of epiphyseal maturation about the elbow is important in recognizing a medial epicondyle that has been avulsed and trapped in the medial aspect of the joint. The trochlear ossification center is normally not seen radiographically before the appearance of the medial epicondyle. Therefore, the finding of an apparent trochlear ossification center (in a child 4 to 8 years of age) without visualization of the medial epicondyle suggests avulsion and displacement of the medial epicondyle.

Joint Capsule and Collateral Ligaments

The anterior and posterior portions of the joint capsule are relatively thin, whereas the medial and lateral portions are thickened to form the collateral ligaments. The fibers of the anterior capsule have a cruciate orientation which results in significant strength. The anterior capsule is normally lax in flexion and taut in extension. The synovial membrane lines the joint capsule. The normal capacity of the fully distended joint is 25 to 30 mL.[11] Intracapsular, but extrasynovial, fat pads normally occupy the coronoid fossa anteriorly and the olecranon fossa posteriorly (see Fig. 10-6). Displacement of these fat pads is a well known radiographic sign of an elbow effusion or hemarthrosis.

Medial Collateral Ligament Complex

The MCL complex consists of anterior and posterior bundles as well as an oblique band, which is also known as the transverse ligament. The posterior bundle and the

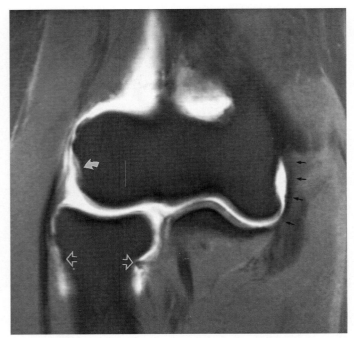

FIGURE 10-8. MR arthrography. A T1-weighted fat-suppressed coronal image obtained after intraarticular injection of dilute gadolinium reveals the normal anterior bundle of the medial collateral ligament attaching to the medial margin of the coronoid process (*small black arrows*). The inferior margin of the annular ligament (*open arrows*) is seen at the inferior margin of the radial head. Contrast extends through a defect in the lateral capsule, secondary to detachment of the radial collateral ligament and the extensor carpi radialis brevis tendon from the anterior aspect of the lateral epicondyle (*curved arrow*).

transverse ligament lie at the deep margin of the ulnar nerve and make up the floor of the cubital tunnel. The functionally important anterior bundle of the MCL extends from the inferior aspect of the medial epicondyle to the medial aspect of the coronoid process (see Fig. 10-3). The anterior bundle, which is clearly displayed on coronal images (Fig. 10-8), provides the primary constraint to valgus stress and commonly is damaged in throwing athletes[12–14] (Fig. 10-9).

Lateral Ligament Complex

The lateral ligament complex consists of the radial collateral ligament, the annular ligament, a variably present accessory lateral collateral ligament, and the lateral ulnar collateral ligament (LUCL).[15] The radial collateral ligament proper arises from the lateral epicondyle anteriorly and blends with the fibers of the annular ligament which surrounds the radial head. The annular ligament is the primary stabilizer of the proximal radioulnar joint and is evaluated best on axial images. The annular ligament is tapered distally to form a funnel about the radial head. The anterior fibers of the annular ligament become taut in supination whereas the posterior fibers become taut at the extreme of prona-

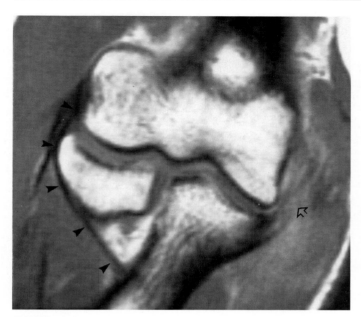

FIGURE 10-9. Primary ligamentous stabilizers of the elbow joint. A T1-weighted coronal image reveals a midsubstance rupture of the anterior bundle of the medial collateral ligament (*open arrow*). The normal lateral ulnar collateral ligament (*arrowheads*) is also well seen extending along the posterolateral aspect of the radial head from the lateral epicondyle to the lateral aspect of the ulna. The anterior bundle of the medial collateral ligament is the primary restraint to valgus stress, whereas the lateral ulnar collateral ligament is the primary restraint to varus stress and posterolateral rotatory stress.

tion. Disruption of the annular ligament results in proximal radio-ulnar joint instability. The accessory lateral collateral ligament is an inconstant structure that extends from the annular ligament to the supinator crest along the lateral aspect of the ulna. When present, it acts to further stabilize the annular ligament during varus stress. A more posterior bundle, known as the ulnar part of the lateral collateral ligament or the LUCL, arises from the lateral epicondyle and extends along the posterior aspect of the radius to insert on the tubercle of the supinator crest of the ulna. The LUCL has been demonstrated to be invariably present during anatomic dissection.[11] The LUCL acts as a sling or guy-wire that provides the primary ligamentous constraint to varus stress.[16–19] Disruption of the LUCL results in the recently recognized pivot shift phenomenon and posterolateral rotatory instability of the elbow.[16,20] Both the radial collateral ligament proper and the LUCL are clearly displayed on coronal images progressing from anterior to posterior. They should be considered separately because of the difference in functional significance of these structures (see Fig. 10-9).

Muscles and Tendons

The muscles of the elbow are divided into anterior, posterior, medial, and lateral compartments. The anterior compartment contains the biceps and brachialis muscles, which are evalu-

ated best on sagittal and axial images. The brachialis extends along the anterior joint capsule and inserts on the ulnar tuberosity. The biceps lies superficial to the brachialis and inserts on the radial tuberosity. The posterior compartment contains the triceps and anconeus muscles, and they are evaluated best on sagittal and axial images. The triceps inserts on the proximal aspect of the olecranon. The anconeus arises from the posterior aspect of the lateral epicondyle and inserts more distally on the olecranon. The anconeus provides dynamic support to the lateral collateral ligament in resisting varus stress. The medial and lateral compartment muscles are seen best on coronal and axial images. The medial compartment structures include the pronator teres and the flexors of the hand and wrist that arise from the medial epicondyle as the common flexor tendon. The common flexor tendon provides dynamic support to the MCL in resisting valgus stress. The lateral compartment structures include the supinator, the brachioradialis, the extensor carpi radialis longus, as well as the extensors of the hand and wrist that arise from the lateral epicondyle as the common extensor tendon.

Neurovascular Structures

The brachial artery and veins descend along the anteromedial aspect of the brachialis muscle in the arm. The brachial artery branches into the radial and ulnar arteries along the anteromedial aspect of the biceps tendon at the level of the radial head. The radial artery may have a more proximal origin in up to 15% of individuals. The ulnar, median, musculocutaneous, and radial nerves are subject to entrapment in the elbow region. These nerves normally are surrounded by fat and are seen best on axial images. Prominent veins may accompany the median or ulnar nerves and should not be mistaken for swollen, edematous nerves on T2-weighted or STIR sequences.

MAGNETIC RESONANCE ANATOMY

Axial Images

Representative axial images are shown in Figure 10-10. The biceps and brachialis muscles clearly depicted anteriorly. The biceps tendon can be followed to the radial tuberosity and the brachialis tendon can be followed to the ulnar tuberosity. The bicipital aponeurosis, also known as the lacertus fibrosus, appears as a thin black line that extends from the myotendinous junction of the biceps to the fascia overlying the flexor-pronator muscle group medially. The median nerve and the brachial artery and veins lie just deep to the lacertus fibrosus, at the level of the medial epicondyle. The low signal intensity common flexor and common extensor tendons can be seen arising from the medial and lateral epicondyles, respectively. The radial nerve is located between the brachialis and brachioradialis muscles, and the

text continues on page 762

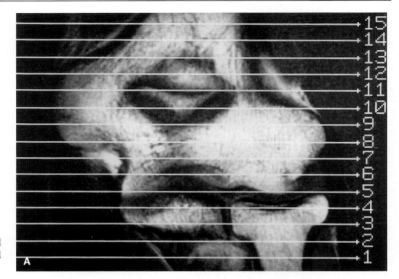

FIGURE 10-10. Normal axial MR anatomy. **(A)** This coronal image was used to graphically prescribe axial T1-weighted image locations that extend from proximal **(B)** to distal **(P)**.

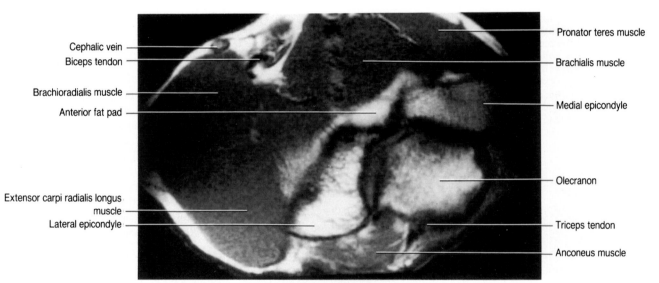

Cephalic vein

Biceps tendon

Brachioradialis muscle

Anterior fat pad

Extensor carpi radialis longus muscle

Lateral epicondyle

Pronator teres muscle

Brachialis muscle

Medial epicondyle

Olecranon

Triceps tendon

Anconeus muscle

FIGURE 10-10B.

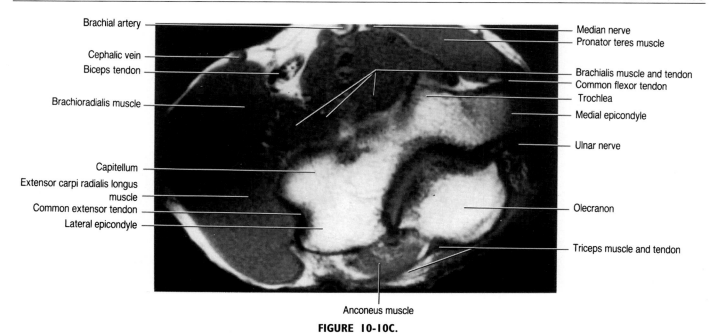

Brachial artery
Cephalic vein
Biceps tendon
Brachioradialis muscle
Capitellum
Extensor carpi radialis longus muscle
Common extensor tendon
Lateral epicondyle
Median nerve
Pronator teres muscle
Brachialis muscle and tendon
Common flexor tendon
Trochlea
Medial epicondyle
Ulnar nerve
Olecranon
Triceps muscle and tendon
Anconeus muscle

FIGURE 10-10C.

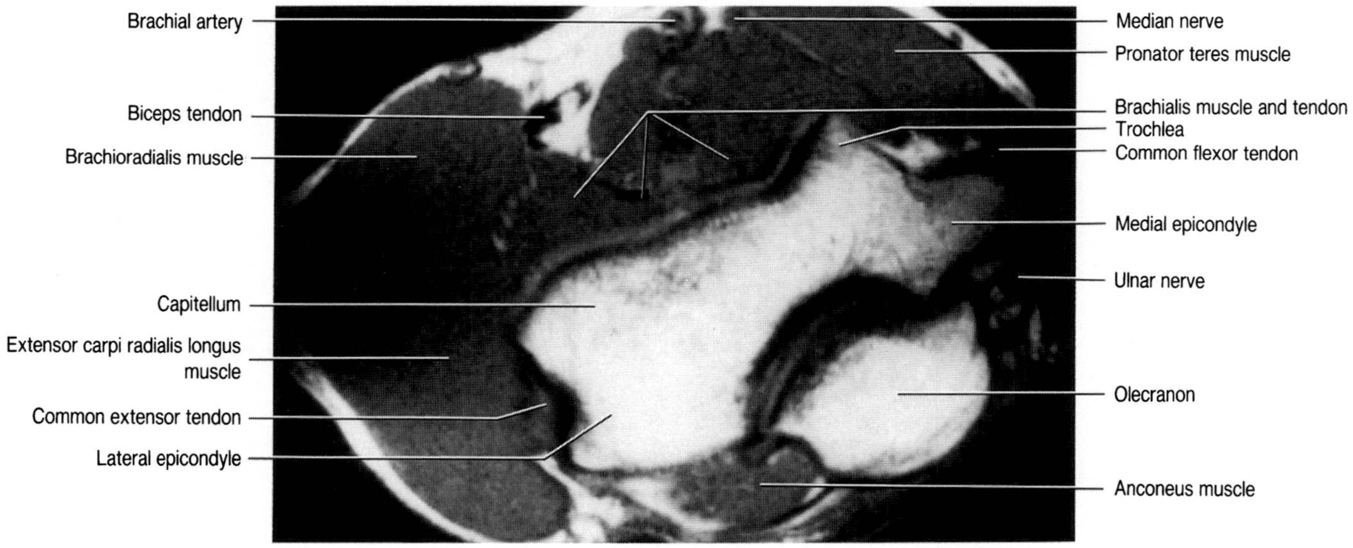

Brachial artery
Biceps tendon
Brachioradialis muscle
Capitellum
Extensor carpi radialis longus muscle
Common extensor tendon
Lateral epicondyle
Median nerve
Pronator teres muscle
Brachialis muscle and tendon
Trochlea
Common flexor tendon
Medial epicondyle
Ulnar nerve
Olecranon
Anconeus muscle

FIGURE 10-10D.

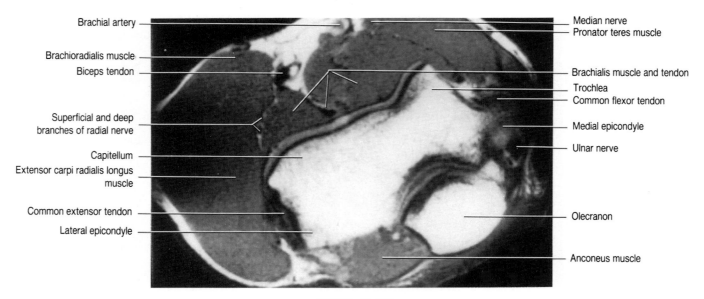

Brachial artery

Brachioradialis muscle
Biceps tendon

Superficial and deep
branches of radial nerve

Capitellum
Extensor carpi radialis longus
muscle

Common extensor tendon

Lateral epicondyle

Median nerve
Pronator teres muscle

Brachialis muscle and tendon
Trochlea
Common flexor tendon

Medial epicondyle

Ulnar nerve

Olecranon

Anconeus muscle

FIGURE 10-10E.

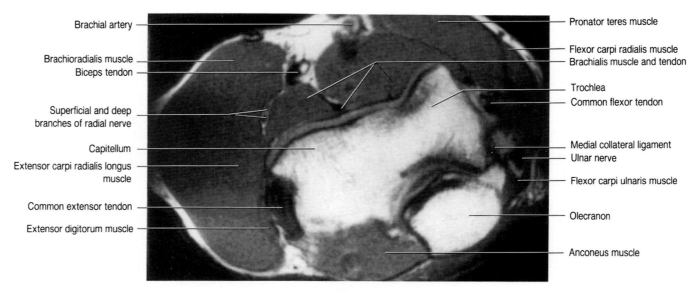

Brachial artery

Brachioradialis muscle
Biceps tendon

Superficial and deep
branches of radial nerve

Capitellum
Extensor carpi radialis longus
muscle

Common extensor tendon

Extensor digitorum muscle

Pronator teres muscle

Flexor carpi radialis muscle
Brachialis muscle and tendon

Trochlea
Common flexor tendon

Medial collateral ligament
Ulnar nerve

Flexor carpi ulnaris muscle

Olecranon

Anconeus muscle

FIGURE 10-10F.

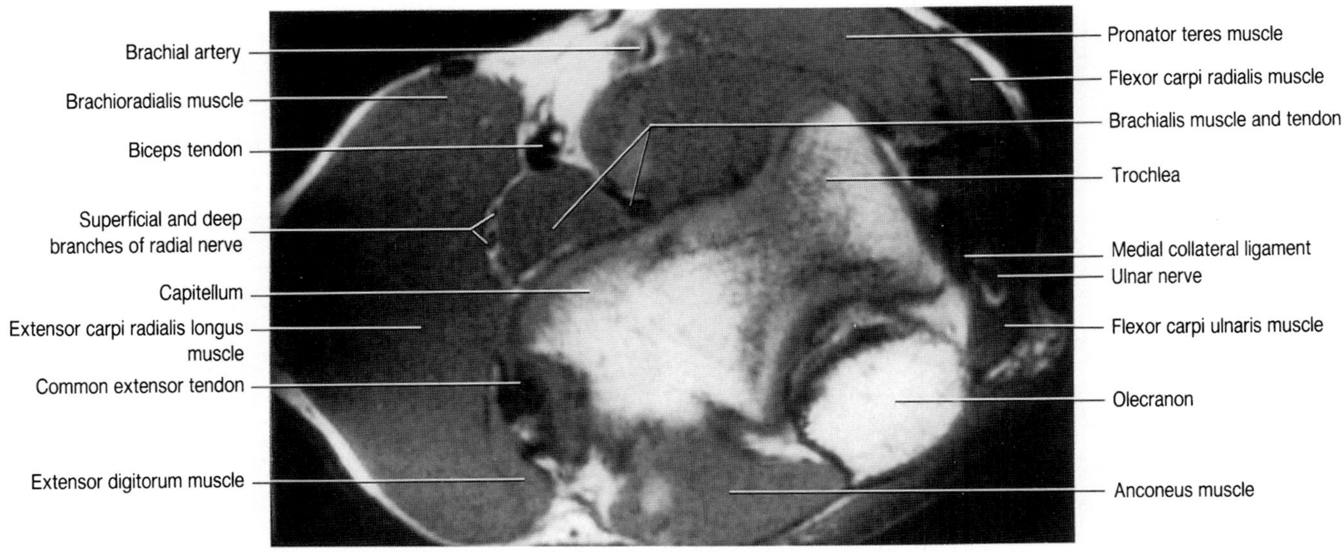

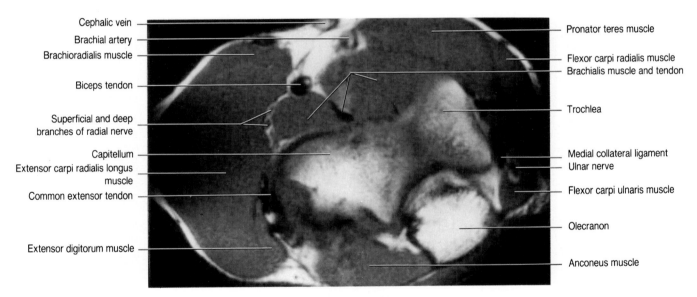

Brachial artery

Brachioradialis muscle

Biceps tendon

Superficial and deep
branches of radial nerve

Capitellum

Extensor carpi radialis longus
muscle

Common extensor tendon

Extensor digitorum muscle

Pronator teres muscle

Flexor carpi radialis muscle

Brachialis muscle and tendon

Trochlea

Medial collateral ligament

Ulnar nerve

Flexor carpi ulnaris muscle

Olecranon

Anconeus muscle

FIGURE 10-10G.

Cephalic vein

Brachial artery

Brachioradialis muscle

Biceps tendon

Superficial and deep
branches of radial nerve

Capitellum

Extensor carpi radialis longus
muscle

Common extensor tendon

Extensor digitorum muscle

Pronator teres muscle

Flexor carpi radialis muscle

Brachialis muscle and tendon

Trochlea

Medial collateral ligament

Ulnar nerve

Flexor carpi ulnaris muscle

Olecranon

Anconeus muscle

FIGURE 10-10H.

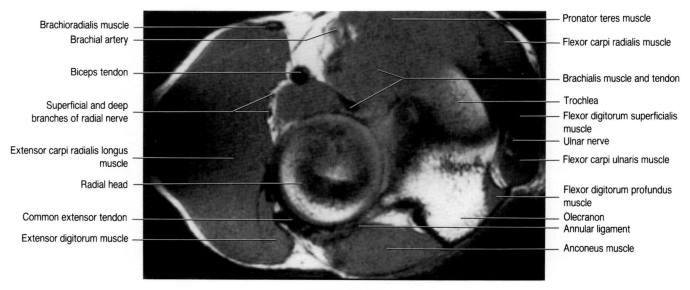

Brachioradialis muscle
Brachial artery

Biceps tendon

Superficial and deep
branches of radial nerve

Extensor carpi radialis longus
muscle

Radial head

Common extensor tendon

Extensor digitorum muscle

Pronator teres muscle
Flexor carpi radialis muscle

Brachialis muscle and tendon

Trochlea
Flexor digitorum superficialis
muscle
Ulnar nerve
Flexor carpi ulnaris muscle

Flexor digitorum profundus
muscle
Olecranon
Annular ligament
Anconeus muscle

FIGURE 10-10I.

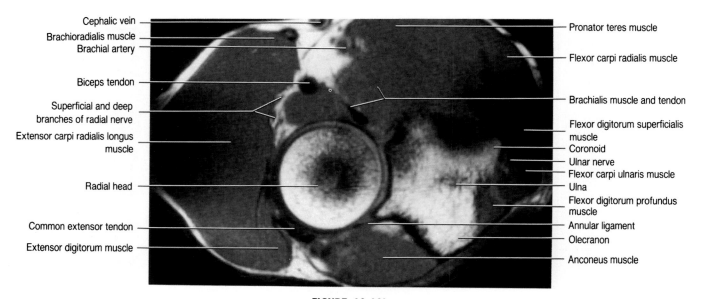

Cephalic vein
Brachioradialis muscle
Brachial artery

Biceps tendon

Superficial and deep
branches of radial nerve
Extensor carpi radialis longus
muscle

Radial head

Common extensor tendon

Extensor digitorum muscle

Pronator teres muscle

Flexor carpi radialis muscle

Brachialis muscle and tendon

Flexor digitorum superficialis
muscle
Coronoid
Ulnar nerve
Flexor carpi ulnaris muscle
Ulna
Flexor digitorum profundus
muscle
Annular ligament
Olecranon
Anconeus muscle

FIGURE 10-10J.

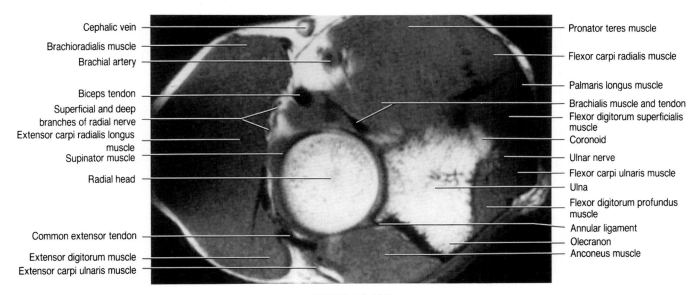

Cephalic vein — Pronator teres muscle
Brachioradialis muscle — Flexor carpi radialis muscle
Brachial artery — Palmaris longus muscle
Biceps tendon — Brachialis muscle and tendon
Superficial and deep branches of radial nerve — Flexor digitorum superficialis muscle
Extensor carpi radialis longus muscle — Coronoid
Supinator muscle — Ulnar nerve
Radial head — Flexor carpi ulnaris muscle
— Ulna
Flexor digitorum profundus muscle
Common extensor tendon — Annular ligament
Olecranon
Extensor digitorum muscle — Anconeus muscle
Extensor carpi ulnaris muscle

FIGURE 10-10K.

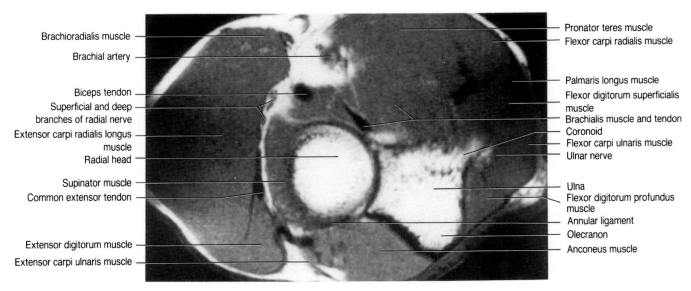

Brachioradialis muscle — Pronator teres muscle
Flexor carpi radialis muscle
Brachial artery — Palmaris longus muscle
Biceps tendon — Flexor digitorum superficialis muscle
Superficial and deep branches of radial nerve — Brachialis muscle and tendon
Extensor carpi radialis longus muscle — Coronoid
Flexor carpi ulnaris muscle
Radial head — Ulnar nerve
Supinator muscle — Ulna
Common extensor tendon — Flexor digitorum profundus muscle
Annular ligament
Olecranon
Extensor digitorum muscle — Anconeus muscle
Extensor carpi ulnaris muscle

FIGURE 10-10L.

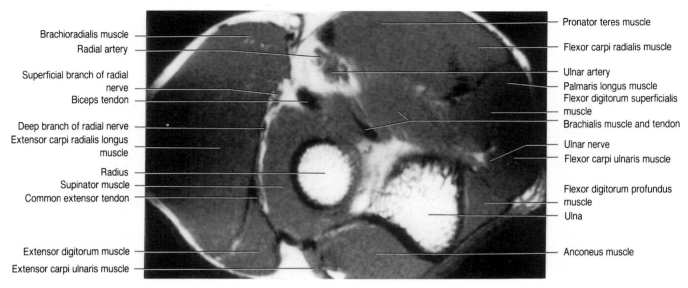

Brachioradialis muscle
Radial artery

Superficial branch of radial nerve
Biceps tendon

Deep branch of radial nerve
Extensor carpi radialis longus muscle

Radius
Supinator muscle
Common extensor tendon

Extensor digitorum muscle
Extensor carpi ulnaris muscle

Pronator teres muscle

Flexor carpi radialis muscle

Ulnar artery
Palmaris longus muscle
Flexor digitorum superficialis muscle
Brachialis muscle and tendon

Ulnar nerve
Flexor carpi ulnaris muscle

Flexor digitorum profundus muscle
Ulna

Anconeus muscle

FIGURE 10-10M.

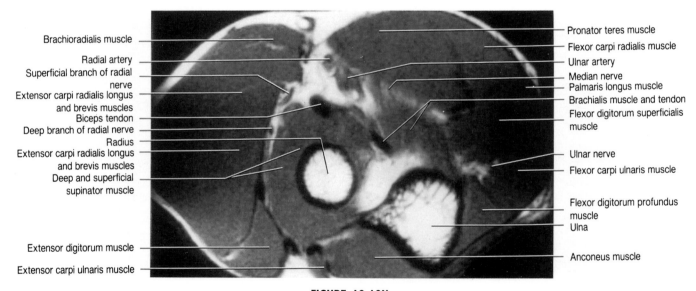

Brachioradialis muscle

Radial artery
Superficial branch of radial nerve
Extensor carpi radialis longus and brevis muscles
Biceps tendon
Deep branch of radial nerve
Radius
Extensor carpi radialis longus and brevis muscles
Deep and superficial supinator muscle

Extensor digitorum muscle
Extensor carpi ulnaris muscle

Pronator teres muscle
Flexor carpi radialis muscle
Ulnar artery
Median nerve
Palmaris longus muscle
Brachialis muscle and tendon
Flexor digitorum superficialis muscle

Ulnar nerve
Flexor carpi ulnaris muscle

Flexor digitorum profundus muscle
Ulna

Anconeus muscle

FIGURE 10-10N.

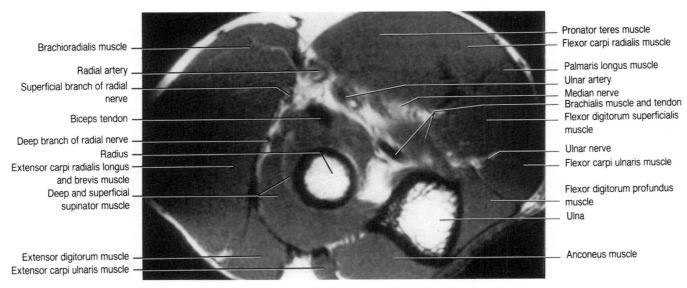

Brachioradialis muscle

Radial artery

Superficial branch of radial nerve

Biceps tendon

Deep branch of radial nerve

Radius

Extensor carpi radialis longus and brevis muscle

Deep and superficial supinator muscle

Extensor digitorum muscle

Extensor carpi ulnaris muscle

Pronator teres muscle

Flexor carpi radialis muscle

Palmaris longus muscle

Ulnar artery

Median nerve

Brachialis muscle and tendon

Flexor digitorum superficialis muscle

Ulnar nerve

Flexor carpi ulnaris muscle

Flexor digitorum profundus muscle

Ulna

Anconeus muscle

FIGURE 10-10O.

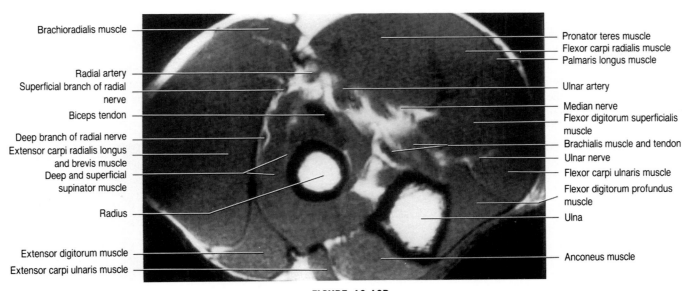

Brachioradialis muscle

Radial artery

Superficial branch of radial nerve

Biceps tendon

Deep branch of radial nerve

Extensor carpi radialis longus and brevis muscle

Deep and superficial supinator muscle

Radius

Extensor digitorum muscle

Extensor carpi ulnaris muscle

Pronator teres muscle

Flexor carpi radialis muscle

Palmaris longus muscle

Ulnar artery

Median nerve

Flexor digitorum superficialis muscle

Brachialis muscle and tendon

Ulnar nerve

Flexor carpi ulnaris muscle

Flexor digitorum profundus muscle

Ulna

Anconeus muscle

FIGURE 10-10P.

deep branch can be followed distally as it passes between the deep and the superficial heads of the supinator muscle. The annular ligament is a thin low signal intensity structure that lies just superficial to the articular cartilage of the radial head, which demonstrates intermediate signal intensity. The insertion of the lateral ulnar collateral ligament can be seen at the lateral margin of the ulna at the level of the radial neck. Further distally, the insertion of the anterior bundle of the MCL can be seen at the medial margin of the coronoid process, just anterior and lateral to the ulnar nerve. Posteriorly, the triceps tendon can be followed to the olecranon. The anconeus muscle is well seen posterolaterally, and the ulnar nerve and accompanying posterior ulnar recurrent artery and veins are seen posteromedially, deep to the cubital tunnel retinaculum at the level of the medial epicondyle. The ulnar nerve can be followed distally as it passes deep to the humeral and ulnar heads of the flexor carpi ulnaris muscle. The proximal radioulnar joint and the posterior compartment articulation between the olecranon and the olecranon fossa are also well seen. The usual site of osteochondritis dissecans—along the anterior aspect of the capitellum—is also well seen on axial images.

Sagittal Images

Representative sagittal images are shown in Figure 10-11. Laterally, the components of the common extensor tendon can be followed to the lateral epicondyle. Medially, the components of

the common flexor tendon can be seen extending proximally to the medial epicondyle. The intermediate signal intensity ulnar nerve is seen along the posterior margin of the medial epicondyle. Near the midline, the attachment of the triceps muscle and tendon to the olecranon can be seen. Normal obliteration of the subcutaneous fat is seen posterior to the olecranon at the site of the superficial olecranon bursa. The posterior and anterior fat pads can be seen along the margins of the distal humerus. The joint capsule appears as a thin, low signal intensity structure just superficial to the fat pads. The brachialis muscle lies just superficial to the anterior joint capsule, and can be followed distally to its insertion on the ulnar tuberosity. The biceps can be followed distally to its insertion on the radial tuberosity. The adjacent low signal intensity brachial and ulnar arteries should not be mistaken for the biceps tendon on sagittal images. The articulation of the radius and the capitellum, as well as the articulation between the trochlea and the trochlear notch, are also clearly demonstrated. The normal bare area of the ulna in the midportion of the trochlear notch should not be confused with an osteochondral defect. Similarly, the rough nonarticular area at the posterior margin of the capitellum should not be confused with an impaction fracture or osteochondral defect.

Coronal Images

Representative coronal images are shown in Figure 10-12. The components of the collateral ligaments and the common flexor and common extensor tendons that lie just superficial

text continues on page 775

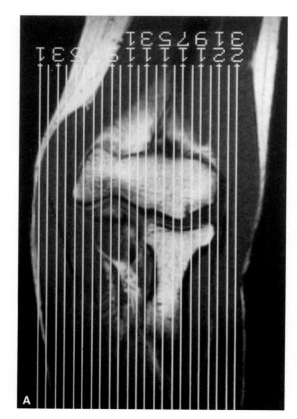

FIGURE 10-11. Normal sagittal MR anatomy. **(A)** This coronal image was used to graphically prescribe sagittal T1-weighted image locations that extend from medial **(B)** to lateral **(L)**.

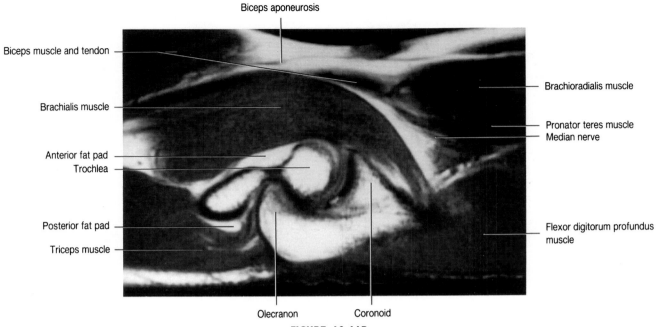

Biceps aponeurosis

Biceps muscle and tendon

Brachialis muscle

Anterior fat pad
Trochlea

Posterior fat pad

Triceps muscle

Brachioradialis muscle

Pronator teres muscle
Median nerve

Flexor digitorum profundus
muscle

Olecranon   Coronoid

FIGURE 10-11B.

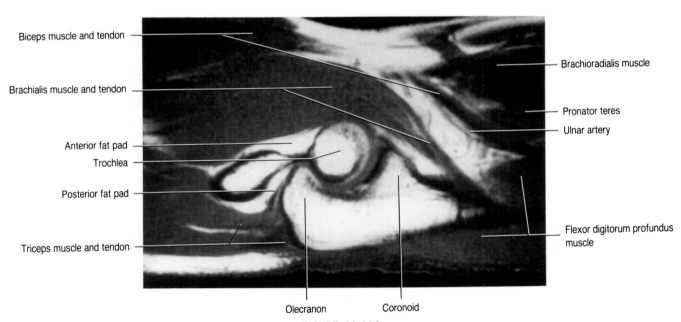

Biceps muscle and tendon

Brachialis muscle and tendon

Anterior fat pad
Trochlea

Posterior fat pad

Triceps muscle and tendon

Brachioradialis muscle

Pronator teres

Ulnar artery

Flexor digitorum profundus
muscle

Olecranon   Coronoid

FIGURE 10-11C.

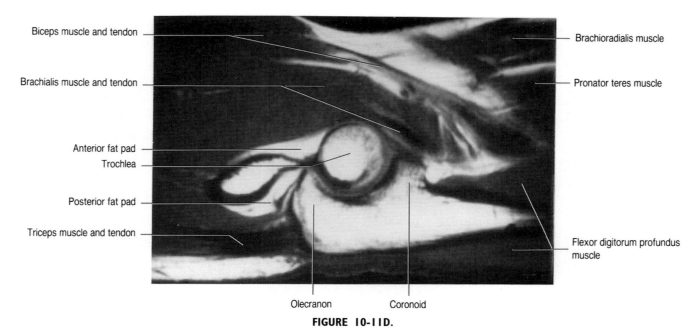

Biceps muscle and tendon

Brachialis muscle and tendon

Anterior fat pad

Trochlea

Posterior fat pad

Triceps muscle and tendon

Brachioradialis muscle

Pronator teres muscle

Flexor digitorum profundus muscle

Olecranon

Coronoid

FIGURE 10-11D.

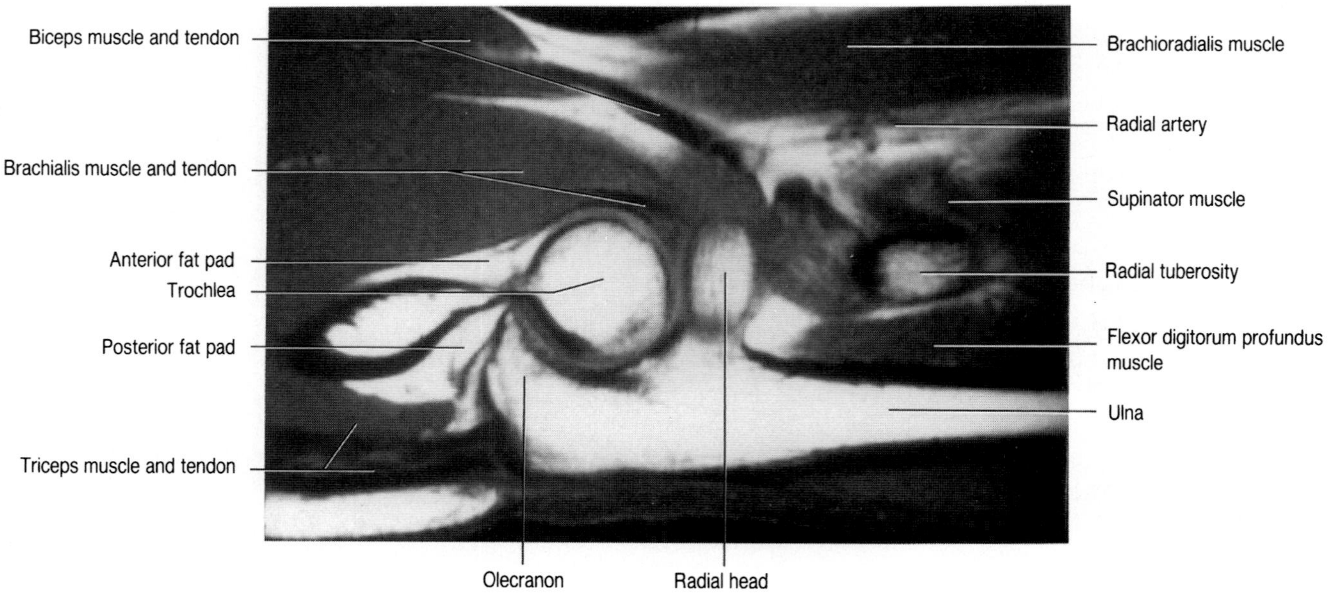

Biceps muscle and tendon

Brachialis muscle and tendon

Anterior fat pad

Trochlea

Posterior fat pad

Triceps muscle and tendon

Brachioradialis muscle

Radial artery

Supinator muscle

Radial tuberosity

Flexor digitorum profundus muscle

Ulna

Olecranon

Radial head

FIGURE 10-11E.

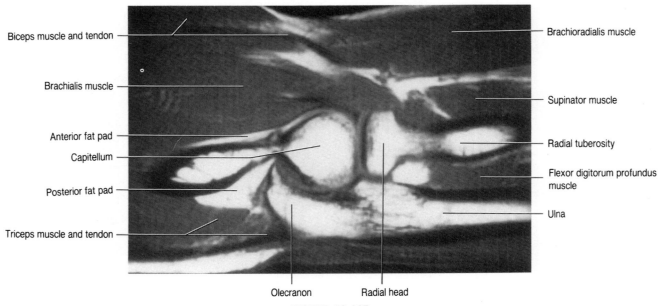

Biceps muscle and tendon

Brachialis muscle

Anterior fat pad

Capitellum

Posterior fat pad

Triceps muscle and tendon

Brachioradialis muscle

Supinator muscle

Radial tuberosity

Flexor digitorum profundus muscle

Ulna

Olecranon

Radial head

FIGURE 10-11F.

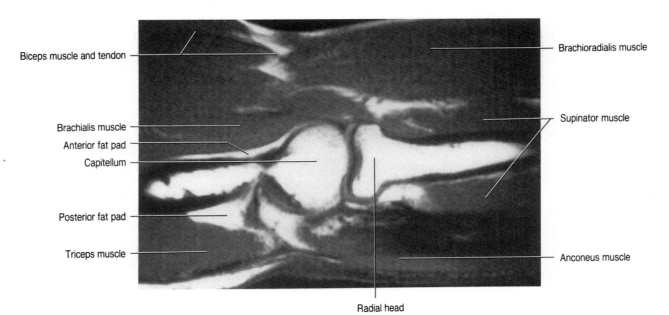

Biceps muscle and tendon

Brachialis muscle

Anterior fat pad

Capitellum

Posterior fat pad

Triceps muscle

Brachioradialis muscle

Supinator muscle

Anconeus muscle

Radial head

FIGURE 10-11G.

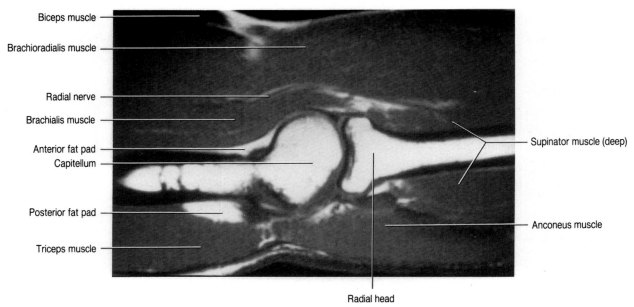

Biceps muscle

Brachioradialis muscle

Radial nerve

Brachialis muscle

Anterior fat pad

Capitellum

Posterior fat pad

Triceps muscle

Supinator muscle (deep)

Anconeus muscle

Radial head

FIGURE 10-11H.

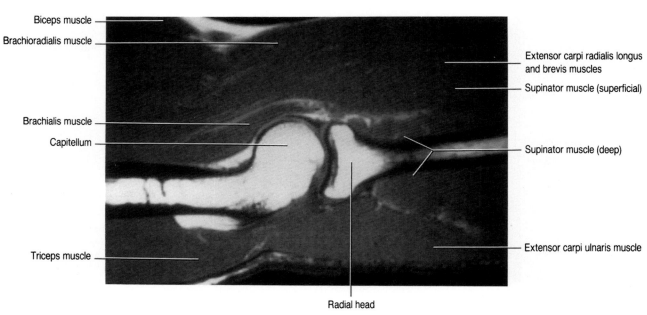

Biceps muscle

Brachioradialis muscle

Brachialis muscle

Capitellum

Triceps muscle

Extensor carpi radialis longus and brevis muscles

Supinator muscle (superficial)

Supinator muscle (deep)

Extensor carpi ulnaris muscle

Radial head

FIGURE 10-11I.

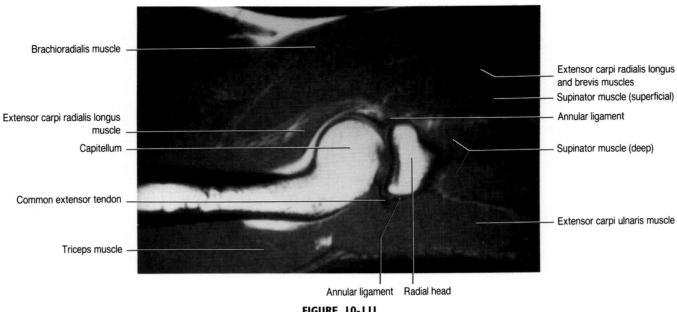

Brachioradialis muscle

Extensor carpi radialis longus
muscle

Capitellum

Common extensor tendon

Triceps muscle

Extensor carpi radialis longus
and brevis muscles

Supinator muscle (superficial)

Annular ligament

Supinator muscle (deep)

Extensor carpi ulnaris muscle

Annular ligament   Radial head

FIGURE 10-11J.

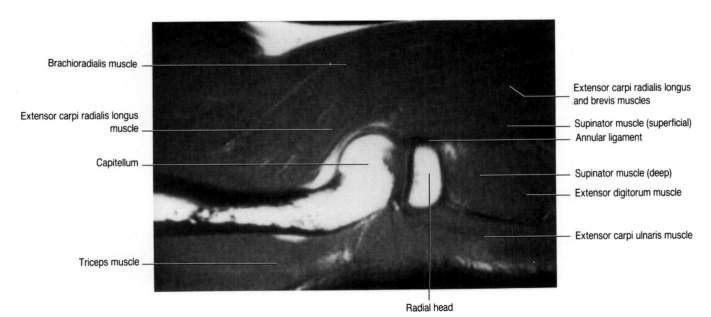

Brachioradialis muscle

Extensor carpi radialis longus
muscle

Capitellum

Triceps muscle

Extensor carpi radialis longus
and brevis muscles

Supinator muscle (superficial)

Annular ligament

Supinator muscle (deep)

Extensor digitorum muscle

Extensor carpi ulnaris muscle

Radial head

FIGURE 10-11K.

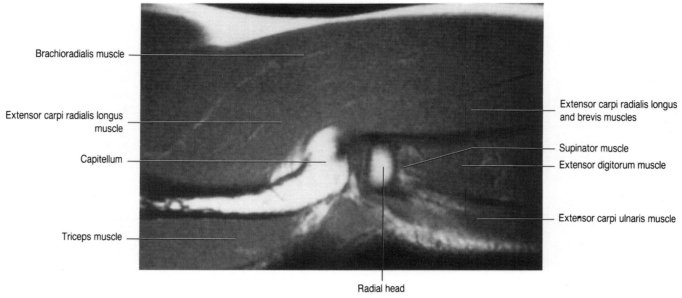

Brachioradialis muscle

Extensor carpi radialis longus muscle

Capitellum

Triceps muscle

Extensor carpi radialis longus and brevis muscles

Supinator muscle

Extensor digitorum muscle

Extensor carpi ulnaris muscle

Radial head

FIGURE 10-11L.

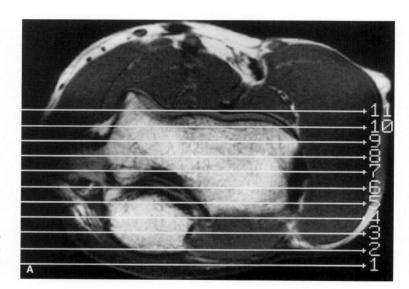

FIGURE 10-12. Normal coronal MR anatomy. **(A)** This coronal image was used to graphically prescribe coronal T1-weighted image locations that extend from posterior **(B)** to anterior **(K)**.

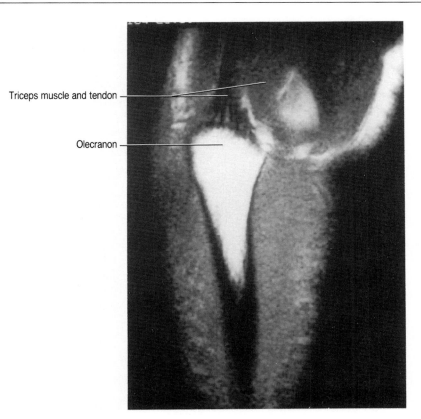

FIGURE 10-12B.

Triceps muscle and tendon

Olecranon

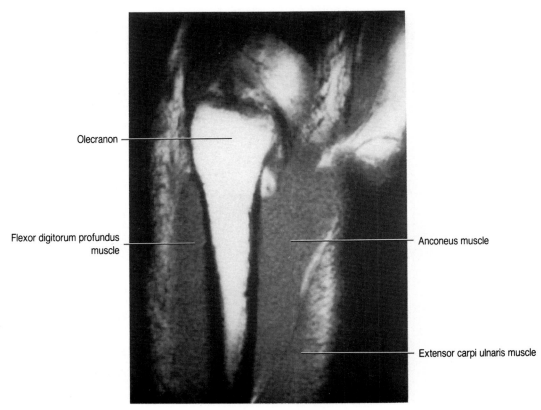

FIGURE 10-12C.

Olecranon

Flexor digitorum profundus muscle

Anconeus muscle

Extensor carpi ulnaris muscle

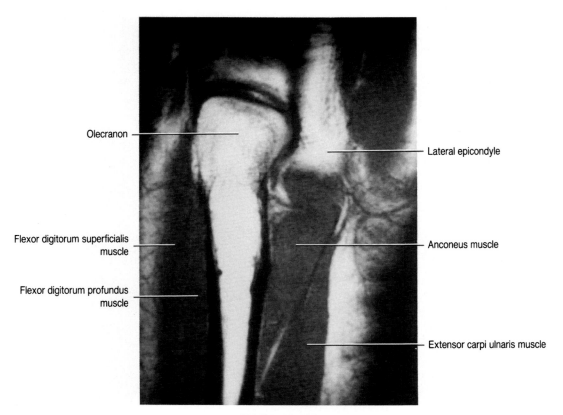

Olecranon

Lateral epicondyle

Flexor digitorum superficialis muscle

Anconeus muscle

Flexor digitorum profundus muscle

Extensor carpi ulnaris muscle

FIGURE 10-12D.

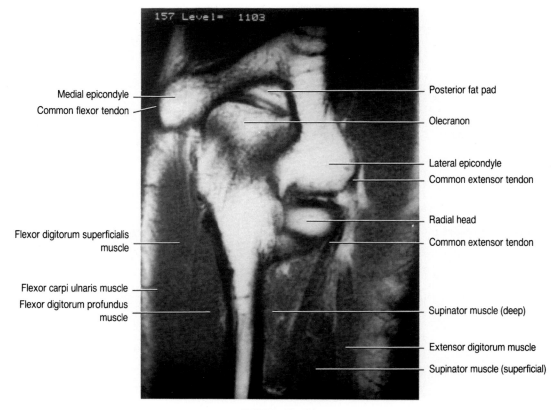

Medial epicondyle

Common flexor tendon

Posterior fat pad

Olecranon

Lateral epicondyle

Common extensor tendon

Radial head

Flexor digitorum superficialis muscle

Common extensor tendon

Flexor carpi ulnaris muscle

Flexor digitorum profundus muscle

Supinator muscle (deep)

Extensor digitorum muscle

Supinator muscle (superficial)

FIGURE 10-12E.

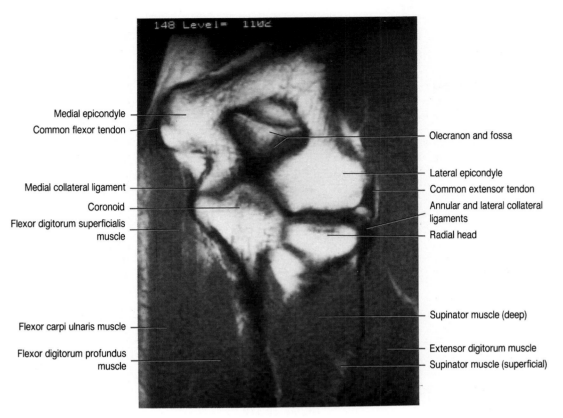

Medial epicondyle
Common flexor tendon

Medial collateral ligament
Coronoid
Flexor digitorum superficialis
muscle

Flexor carpi ulnaris muscle

Flexor digitorum profundus
muscle

Olecranon and fossa

Lateral epicondyle
Common extensor tendon
Annular and lateral collateral
ligaments
Radial head

Supinator muscle (deep)

Extensor digitorum muscle
Supinator muscle (superficial)

FIGURE 10-12F.

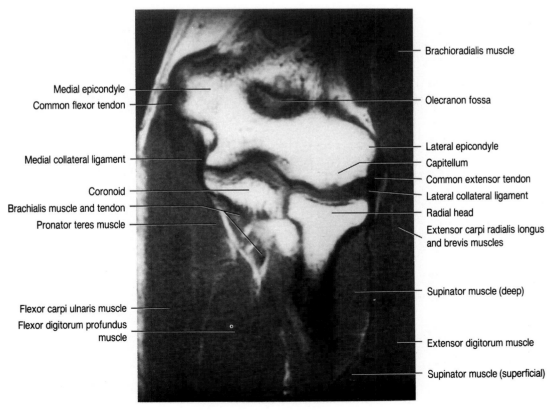

Medial epicondyle
Common flexor tendon

Medial collateral ligament

Coronoid
Brachialis muscle and tendon
Pronator teres muscle

Flexor carpi ulnaris muscle
Flexor digitorum profundus
muscle

Brachioradialis muscle

Olecranon fossa

Lateral epicondyle
Capitellum
Common extensor tendon
Lateral collateral ligament
Radial head
Extensor carpi radialis longus
and brevis muscles

Supinator muscle (deep)

Extensor digitorum muscle

Supinator muscle (superficial)

FIGURE 10-12G.

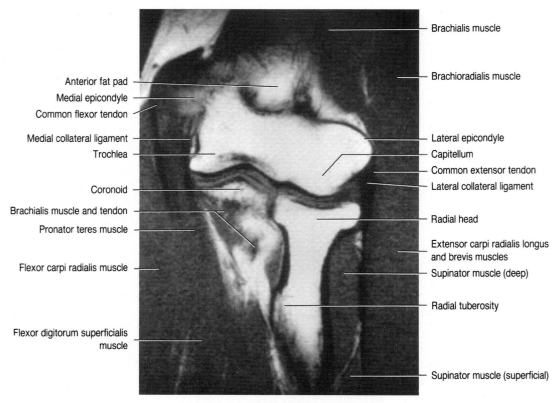

Brachialis muscle

Brachioradialis muscle

Anterior fat pad

Medial epicondyle

Common flexor tendon

Medial collateral ligament

Trochlea

Lateral epicondyle

Capitellum

Common extensor tendon

Lateral collateral ligament

Coronoid

Brachialis muscle and tendon

Pronator teres muscle

Radial head

Extensor carpi radialis longus and brevis muscles

Flexor carpi radialis muscle

Supinator muscle (deep)

Radial tuberosity

Flexor digitorum superficialis muscle

Supinator muscle (superficial)

FIGURE 10-12H.

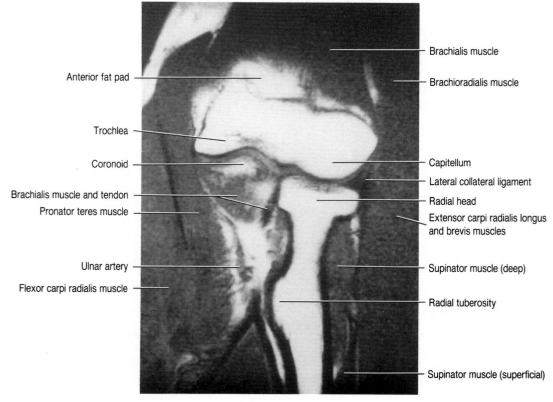

Brachialis muscle

Brachioradialis muscle

Anterior fat pad

Trochlea

Coronoid

Capitellum

Lateral collateral ligament

Brachialis muscle and tendon

Pronator teres muscle

Radial head

Extensor carpi radialis longus and brevis muscles

Ulnar artery

Flexor carpi radialis muscle

Supinator muscle (deep)

Radial tuberosity

Supinator muscle (superficial)

FIGURE 10-12I.

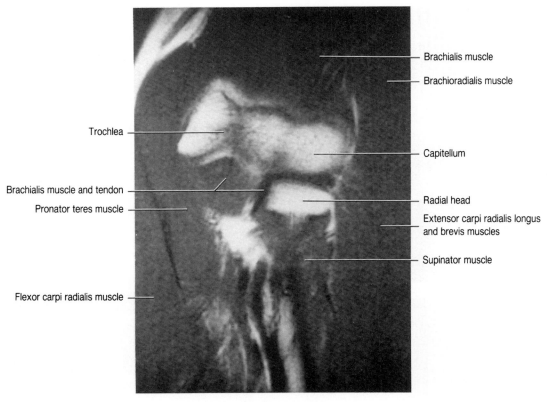

Brachialis muscle

Brachioradialis muscle

Trochlea

Capitellum

Brachialis muscle and tendon

Pronator teres muscle

Radial head

Extensor carpi radialis longus
and brevis muscles

Supinator muscle

Flexor carpi radialis muscle

FIGURE 10-12J.

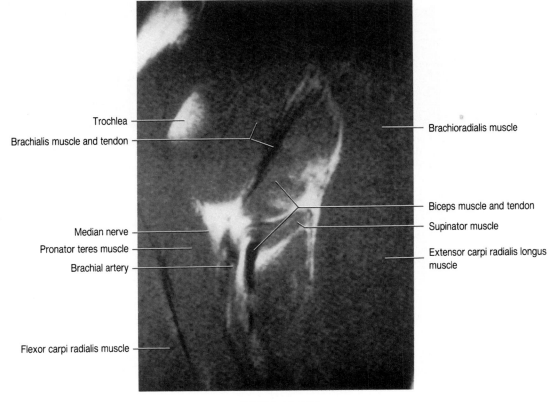

Trochlea

Brachialis muscle and tendon

Brachioradialis muscle

Median nerve

Pronator teres muscle

Brachial artery

Biceps muscle and tendon

Supinator muscle

Extensor carpi radialis longus
muscle

Flexor carpi radialis muscle

FIGURE 10-12K.

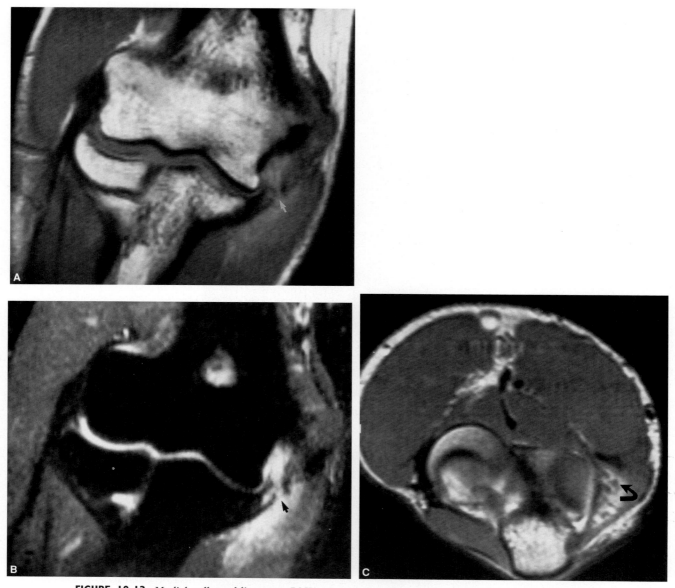

FIGURE 10-13. Medial collateral ligament (MCL) rupture. (**A**) T1-weighted and (**B**) STIR coronal images, as well as (**C**) a proton density axial image, reveal a midsubstance rupture of the anterior bundle of the MCL (*arrows*). A strain of the adjacent flexor digitorum superficialis muscle is also noted.

to the ligaments are clearly displayed. The anterior bundle of the MCL, extending from the inferior margin of the medial epicondyle to the medial anterior margin of the coronoid process, is especially well demarcated, as is the lateral ulnar collateral ligament, seen extending along the posterolateral aspect of the proximal radius to insert laterally on the tubercle of the supinator crest of the ulna. The anterior articulation between the trochlea and the coronoid, the proximal radioulnar joint, and the articulation between the radius and the capitellum are all well demonstrated. The rough nonarticular area at the posterior margin of the capitellum should not be mistaken for an osteochondral defect on coronal images through the posterior aspect of the radial head.

ELBOW PATHOLOGY

Medial Collateral Ligament Injury

Degeneration and tearing of the MCL, with or without concomitant injury of the common flexor tendon, commonly occurs in throwing athletes. Injury of these medial stabilizing structures is caused by chronic microtrauma from repetitive valgus stress during the acceleration phase of throwing.[21–23]

Acute injury of the MCL can be detected, localized, and graded with MR imaging. The status of the functionally important anterior bundle of the MCL complex may be assessed on axial and coronal images. Complete rupture of the anterior bundle of the MCL usually occurs as a sudden event. Acute ruptures of the MCL (Fig. 10-13) are clearly depicted with standard MR imaging. Partial detachment of the deep undersurface fibers of the anterior bundle (Fig. 10-14), which may also occur in pitchers with medial elbow pain, is more difficult to diagnose with standard MR imaging. These partial tears of the MCL characteristically spare the superficial fibers of the anterior bundle and are therefore not visible with an open surgical approach unless the ligament is incised to inspect the torn capsular fibers.[24,25] MR imaging, therefore, is particularly important in localizing these partial tears, which are treated with repair or reconstruction. Detection of these undersurface partial tears is improved when intraarticular contrast is administered and computed tomography (CT) arthrography (Fig. 10-15) or MR arthrography (Fig. 10-16) is used.[26] The capsular fibers of the anterior bundle of the MCL normally insert on the medial margin of the coronoid process (see Fig. 10-8). Undersurface partial tears of the anterior bundle are characterized by distal extension of fluid or contrast along the medial margin of the coronoid (see Figs. 10-14 through 10-16).[5,26]

Midsubstance MCL ruptures (see Fig. 10-13) can be differentiated from proximal avulsions (Fig. 10-17) and distal avulsions (Fig. 10-18). In one study of a large series of surgically treated throwing athletes,[12] midsubstance ruptures of the MCL were most common (87%), and distal (10%) and proximal (3%) avulsions were found less frequently. In

text continues on page 779

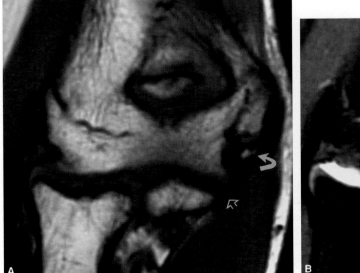
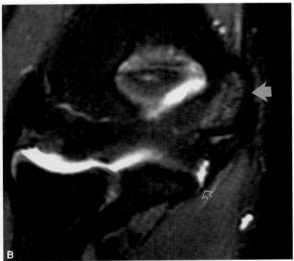

FIGURE 10-14. Proximal and distal tearing of the medial collateral ligament in a 16-year-old pitcher. T1-weighted (**A**) and STIR (**B**) coronal images reveal a small focus of heterotopic ossification (*curved arrows*) versus an old apophyseal avulsion fracture with fluid separating the anterior bundle of the medial collateral ligament from the medial epicondyle. There is increased signal within the medial epicondyle (*large arrow*) compatible with reactive marrow edema. Partial tearing of the distal attachment of the medial collateral ligament from the coronoid also is noted (*open arrows*).   *continued*

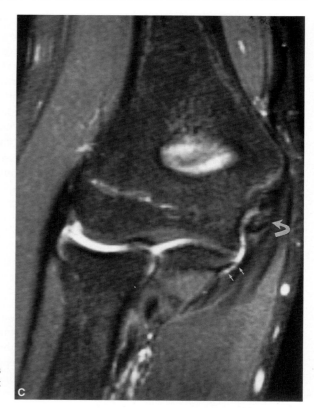

FIGURE 10-14. *Continued.* (**C**) A STIR coronal image further anteriorly reveals distal extension of fluid along the medial margin of the coronoid, consistent with an undersurface partial tear of the anterior bundle of the MCL.

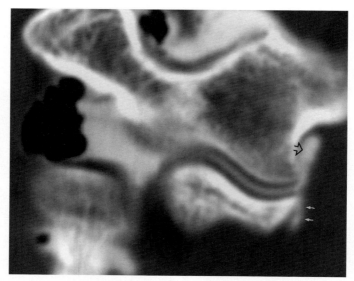

FIGURE 10-15. CT arthrography in a patient with partial detachment of the anterior bundle of the MCL from the coronoid process. Direct coronal CT was performed after intraarticular injection of radiographic contrast. There is leakage of contrast distal to the normal attachment of the anterior bundle of the MCL to the coronoid (*small arrows*). The contrast remains contained within the intact superficial layer of the ligament and capsule. The proximal extension of contrast (*open arrow*) beneath the MCL is normal. (Courtesy of Martin Schwartz, MD.)

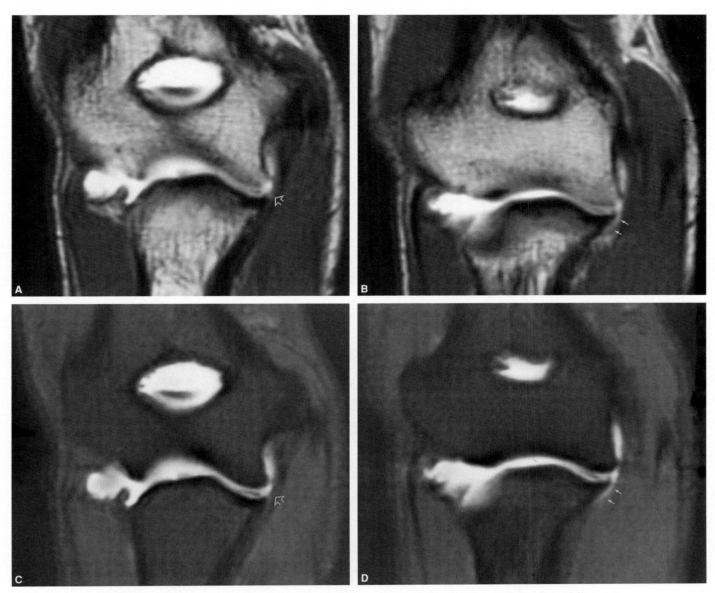

FIGURE 10-16. MR arthrography in a pitcher with partial detachment of the medial collateral ligament. T1-weighted (**A, B**) coronal images and T1-weighted fat-suppressed coronal images (**C, D**) reveal partial tearing of the anterior bundle of the MCL from the coronoid process (*open arrows*). (**D**) The distal extension of contrast, indicative of an undersurface partial tear, is more conspicuous with suppression of signal from adjacent fat.

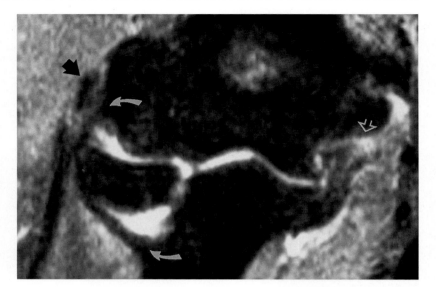

FIGURE 10-17. A 26-year-old pitcher with medial elbow pain. A STIR coronal image reveals thickening of the anterior bundle of the MCL with increased signal delineating the site of proximal detachment (*open arrow*). A focus of calcification is incidentally seen in the common extensor tendon due to tendinosis and previous steroid injections (*black arrow*). The normal lateral ulnar collateral ligament is also well seen (*curved arrows*).

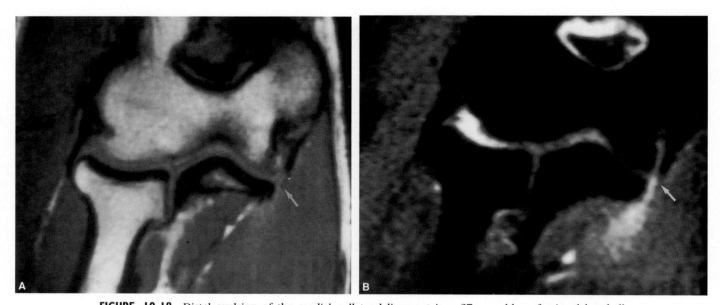

FIGURE 10-18. Distal avulsion of the medial collateral ligament in a 27-year-old professional baseball player. T1-weighted (**A**) and STIR (**B**) coronal images reveal complete detachment of the anterior bundle of the MCL from the coronoid (*arrows*).

other reports, midsubstance ruptures were not as commonly found.[27,28] Since the fibers of the flexor digitorum superficialis muscle blend with the anterior bundle of the MCL,[11,15,25] a strain of the flexor digitorum superficialis muscle commonly is seen when the MCL is injured (Fig. 10-19; see Fig. 10-13). In addition, ulnar traction spurs at the insertion of the MCL on the coronoid process (caused by repetitive valgus stress) have been found in 75% of professional baseball pitchers.[29] Chronic degeneration of the MCL is characterized by thickening of the ligament secondary to scarring, often accompanied by foci of calcification or heterotopic bone[12] (Fig. 10-20). The findings are similar to those seen after healing of MCL sprains in the knee, in which the development of heterotopic ossification has been termed the Pellegrini-Stieda phenomenon. Patients with symptomatic MCL insufficiency usually are treated with reconstruction using a palmaris tendon graft. Graft failure, although unusual, can be evaluated with MR imaging (Fig. 10-21). Lateral compartment bone contusions often are seen in association with acute MCL tears and may provide useful confirmation of recent lateral compartment impaction secondary to valgus instability (see Fig. 10-21).

A number of different conditions may occur secondary to the repeated valgus stress to the elbow that occurs with throwing. Medial tension overload typically produces extraarticular injury such as flexor/pronator strain, MCL sprain, ulnar traction spurring, and ulnar neuropathy. Lateral compression overload typically produces intraarticular injury such as osteochondritis dissecans of the capitellum or radial head, degenerative arthritis, and loose body formation. All of these related pathologic processes associated with repeated valgus stress can be assessed with MR imaging.[8,30] The additional information provided by MR imaging can be helpful in formulating a logical treatment plan, especially when surgery is being considered.

Rupture of the MCL is also commonly encountered as a result of posterior dislocation of the elbow.[31] After the shoulder, the elbow is the second most common joint to be dislocated.[32] The mechanism of posterior elbow dislocation usually involves falling on an outstretched arm. Typically there is rupture of the medial and lateral collateral ligaments as well as the anterior and posterior capsule during posterior elbow dislocation.[17] Associated rupture of the common extensor tendon or the common flexor tendon may also occur. The extent of injury secondary to elbow dislocation is well delineated with MR imaging.

Medial Epicondylitis

Medial epicondylitis—also known as golfer's elbow, pitcher's elbow, or medial tennis elbow—is less common than lateral epicondylitis.[33,34] It is caused by degeneration of the common flexor tendon secondary to overload of the flexor/pronator muscle group that arises from the medial epicondyle.[35-38] The spectrum of damage to the muscle-tendon unit that may be characterized with MR imaging includes muscle strain injury, tendon degeneration (tendinosis), and macroscopic tendon disruption.

MR imaging is useful for detecting and characterizing acute muscle injury as well as for following its resolution.[39-43] STIR sequences are the most sensitive for detecting muscle pathology (Fig. 10-22). The common flexor tendon and MCL should be evaluated carefully for associated tearing when there is evidence of medial muscle strain injury on MR images (Fig. 10-23). However, it should be noted that abnormal signal intensity within a muscle may simply be due to the effect of a therapeutic injection for epicondylitis, rather than an indication of muscle strain. Increased signal intensity on STIR and T2-weighted sequences may be seen after an intramuscular injection and may persist for as long as 1 month.[44] Ideally, therefore, steroid injections should be administered after MR imaging to avoid the confounding appearance of the injection on the structures about the elbow.

Although tears of a normal muscle-tendon unit may occur at the myotendinous junction[45] (Fig. 10-24), failure of a muscle-tendon unit through an area of tendinosis is a much more common clinical entity.[46] Tendon degeneration, or tendinosis, is common about the elbow,[33,38] and concurrent medial and lateral epicondylitis secondary to flexor and extensor tendinosis is not uncommon. With MR imaging, it is possible to determine if there is tendinosis (Fig. 10-25) (secondary to degeneration, microscopic partial tearing, and repair) versus macroscopic partial tearing or complete rupture (Fig. 10-26). This distinction is made by identifying fluid signal intensity delineating the presence or absence of tendon fibers on T2-weighted images. The appearance of medial and lateral epi-

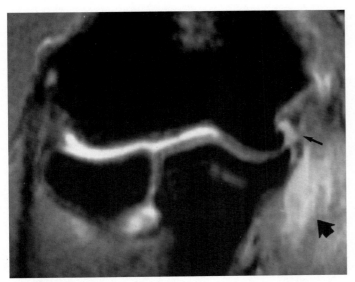

FIGURE 10-19. Medial collateral ligament (MCL) rupture. A STIR coronal image reveals a midsubstance rupture of the anterior bundle of the MCL (*small arrow*). A strain of the adjacent flexor digitorum superficialis muscle is also noted (*large arrow*).

text continues on page 783

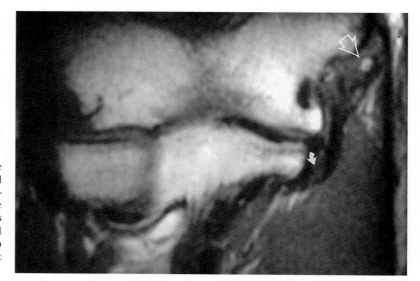

FIGURE 10-20. Degeneration and partial tearing of the medial collateral ligament in a 36-year-old professional baseball player. A T1-weighted coronal image reveals partial detachment of the medial collateral ligament from the medial margin of the coronoid process (*curved arrow*), as well as thickening and irregularity of the proximal medial collateral ligament. Heterotopic ossification (*open arrow*) is noted within the degenerated medial collateral ligament just distal to the medial epicondyle.

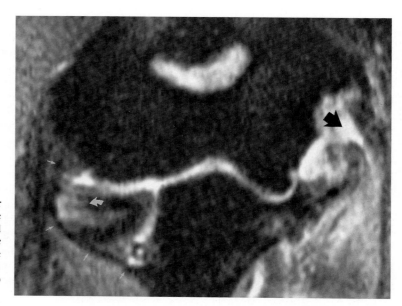

FIGURE 10-21. A 33-year-old professional baseball player after medial collateral ligament reconstruction with acute graft rupture. A STIR coronal image reveals increased signal and poor definition of a medial collateral ligament graft (*black arrow*). A contusion of the radial head (*curved arrow*) due to lateral impaction and valgus insufficiency is also noted. The normal lateral ulnar collateral ligament (*small arrows*) is well seen on this image.

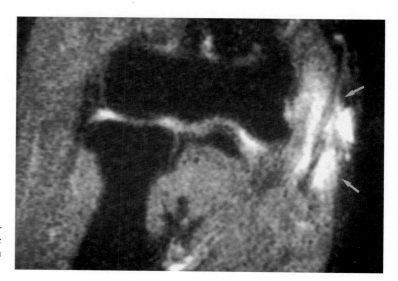

FIGURE 10-22. Muscle strain in a baseball player. A STIR coronal image reveals increased signal intensity throughout the pronator teres and adjacent flexors (*arrows*), compatible with a muscle strain injury.

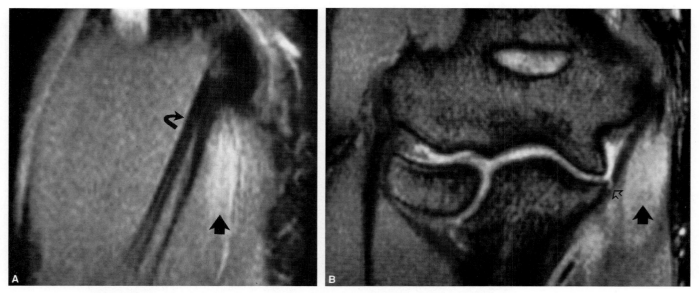

FIGURE 10-23. Muscle strain and partial tear of the medial collateral ligament (MCL). T2*-weighted sagittal (**A**) and coronal (**B**) images reveal increased signal within the flexor digitorum superficialis muscle (*large arrow*), as well as partial tearing of the anterior bundle of the MCL from the coronoid (*open arrow*). The common flexor tendon (*curved arrow*) is intact.

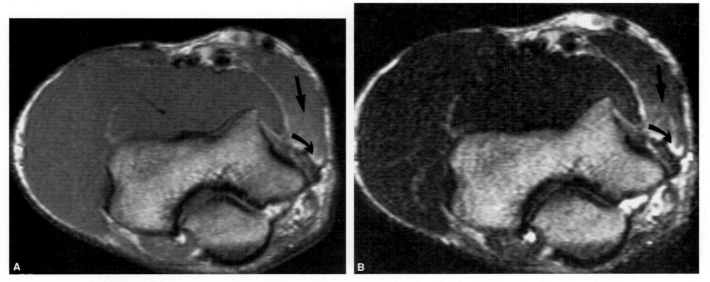

FIGURE 10-24. Acute muscle strain injury secondary to resisted supination. Proton density (**A**) and T2-weighted (**B**) axial images reveal increased signal within the pronator teres muscle (*large arrow*), as well as fluid delineating tearing of the muscle from the common flexor tendon (*curved arrow*).

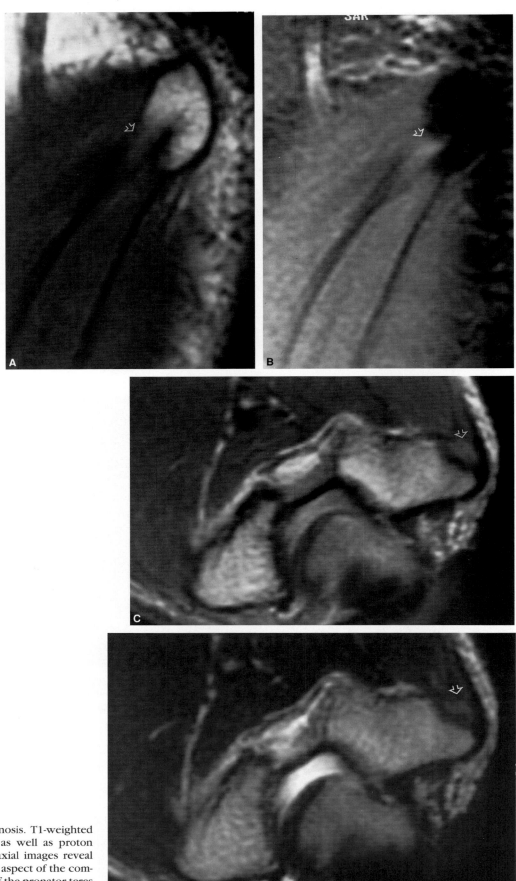

FIGURE 10-25. Degenerative tendinosis. T1-weighted (**A**) and STIR (**B**) sagittal images, as well as proton density (**C**) and T2-weighted (**D**) axial images reveal increased signal within the anterior aspect of the common flexor tendon at the junction of the pronator teres and flexor carpi radialis (*arrows*).

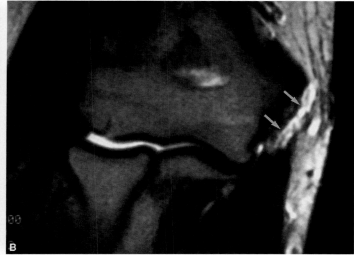

FIGURE 10-26. Rupture of the common flexor tendon in a 35-year-old softball player. T2-weighted sagittal (**A**) and coronal (**B**) images reveal fluid separating the central fibers of the common flexor tendon from the medial epicondyle (*arrows*).

condylitis about the elbow is similar to the appearance of other common degenerative tendinopathies that involve the attachment of tendons to bone. Similar MR criteria can be used to evaluate the common flexor and common extensor tendons in the elbow, the supraspinatus tendon in the shoulder, the patellar tendon in the knee, and the plantar fascia in the foot. In each of these conditions, there is degenerative tendinosis and a failed healing response that precedes rupture.[46-49]

Coronal, sagittal, and axial plane sequences are all useful for assessing the degree of tendon injury (see Figs. 10-24 through 10-26). MR imaging facilitates surgical planning by delineating and grading tears of the common flexor tendon as well as evaluating the underlying MCL and adjacent ulnar nerve. Ulnar neuritis commonly accompanies common flexor tendinosis and may be difficult to identify clinically. Patients with concomitant ulnar neuropathy have a significantly poorer prognosis after surgery than do patients with isolated medial epicondylitis.[50,51] Patients with coexisting ulnar neuritis and common flexor tendinosis (25% to 50% of patients undergoing surgery for medial epicondylitis) require transposition or decompression of the ulnar nerve in addition to debridement and repair of the abnormal flexor tendon.[35,37,50,51] The availability of improved preoperative information from MR studies may reduce the need for extensive surgical exploration in cases in which the MCL is clearly intact on MR imaging. In addition, MR imaging may be useful for problem solving in patients who develop recurrent symptoms after surgery for medial or lateral epicondylitis.

In skeletally immature individuals, the flexor muscle-tendon unit may fail at the unfused apophysis of the medial epicondyle. Stress fracture, avulsion, or delayed closure of the medial epicondylar apophysis may occur in young baseball players secondary to overuse (Little Leaguer's elbow).[52] With MR imaging, particularly STIR sequences, it is possi-

ble to identify soft tissue or marrow edema about the medial epicondylar apophysis, useful in detecting these injuries before complete avulsion and displacement.[1]

Lateral Epicondylitis and Lateral Collateral Ligament Injury

Lateral epicondylitis, also known as tennis elbow, is caused by degeneration and tearing of the common extensor tendon.[33,53] This condition often occurs as a result of repetitive sports-related trauma to the tendon, although it is seen far more commonly in nonathletes.[34,38,54] In the typical case, the degenerated extensor carpi radialis brevis tendon is partially avulsed from the lateral epicondyle.[53] Scar tissue, formed in response to this partial avulsion, is susceptible to further tearing with repeated trauma. Recent histologic studies have shown angiofibroblastic tendinosis with a lack of inflammation in the surgical specimens of patients with lateral epicondylitis, suggesting that the abnormal signal seen on MR images is secondary to tendon degeneration and repair rather than to tendinitis.[33,49] Local steroid injections, commonly used to treat lateral epicondylitis, may actually increase the risk of tendon rupture.[55,56] Signal alteration in the region of a local steroid injection should not be confused for primary muscle pathology on MR imaging (Fig. 10-27).

Overall, 4% to 10% of cases of lateral epicondylitis are resistant to conservative therapy,[33,34] and MR imaging is useful in assessing the degree of tendon damage in such cases. Tendon degeneration (tendinosis) is manifested by normal to increased tendon thickness with increased signal intensity on T1-weighted images that does not increase in signal intensity on T2-weighted images. Partial tears are characterized by thinning of the tendon, which is outlined

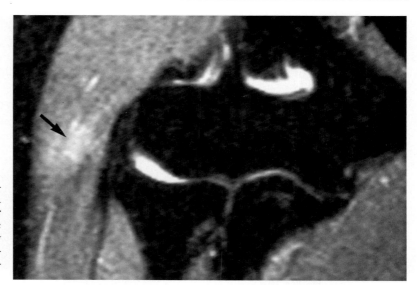

FIGURE 10-27. Clinically suspected tennis elbow in a patient who did not respond to a local steroid injection. A STIR coronal image reveals a normal common extensor tendon adjacent to an area of increased signal within the extensor carpi radialis longus muscle (*arrow*) secondary to the recent steroid injection. Abnormal signal may persist for weeks after an injection and be mistaken for primary muscle pathology on MR imaging.

by adjacent fluid on T2-weighted images. Tendinosis and tearing typically involve the extensor carpi radialis brevis portion of the common extensor tendon anteriorly (Fig. 10-28). Complete tears may be diagnosed on MR imaging by identifying a fluid filled gap separating the tendon from its adjacent bony attachment site (Fig. 10-29).

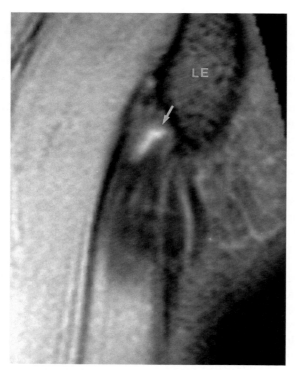

FIGURE 10-28. Partial tear of the extensor carpi radialis brevis. A T2*-weighted gradient-echo sagittal image reveals a small tear (*arrow*) involving the anterior attachment of common extensor tendon to the lateral epicondyle (LE).

At surgery for lateral epicondylitis, 97% of the tendons appear scarred and edematous and 35% are shown to have macroscopic tears[33,53] (Fig. 10-30). MR imaging is useful in identifying high-grade partial tears and complete tears that are unlikely to improve with rest and repeated steroid injections. In addition to determining the degree of tendon damage, MR imaging also allows a more global assessment of the elbow, thereby facilitating detection of additional pathologic conditions that may explain the lack of a therapeutic response. For example, unsuspected ruptures of the lateral collateral ligament complex may occur in association with tears of the common extensor tendon (Fig. 10-31). Morrey[57] recently reported a series of 13 patients who underwent reoperation for failed lateral epicondylitis surgery. Stabilization procedures were required in 4 patients with either iatrogenic or unrecognized lateral ligament insufficiency. Iatrogenic tears of the lateral ulnar collateral ligament (LUCL) may occur secondary to an overaggressive release of the common extensor tendon[58] (Fig. 10-32). Operative release of the extensor tendon may further destabilize the elbow when rupture of the LUCL and subtle associated instability is not recognized clinically (Fig. 10-33). MR imaging can reveal concurrent tears of the LUCL and common extensor tendon in patients with lateral epicondylitis, as well as isolated LUCL tears in patients with posterolateral rotatory instability. Moreover, the lack of a significant abnormality involving the common extensor tendon on MR imaging may prompt consideration of an alternative diagnosis, such as radial nerve entrapment, which may mimic or accompany lateral epicondylitis.[59–61]

The radiohumeral meniscus is a normal variant that has an appearance similar to the meniscal homologue in the wrist or the glenoid labrum in the shoulder on MR imaging.[62] Chronic trauma and fibrosis of this meniscus-like invagi-

text continues on page 788

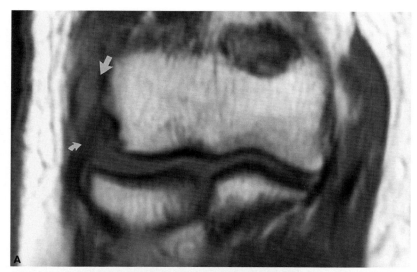

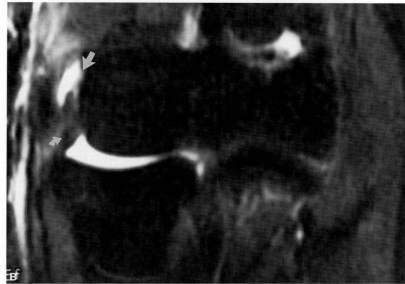

FIGURE 10-29. Tennis elbow secondary to rupture of the common extensor tendon. T1-weighted (**A**) and STIR (**B**) coronal images reveal tearing of the common extensor tendon from the lateral epicondyle (*straight arrow*). The underlying lateral collateral ligament (*curved arrow*) is intact.

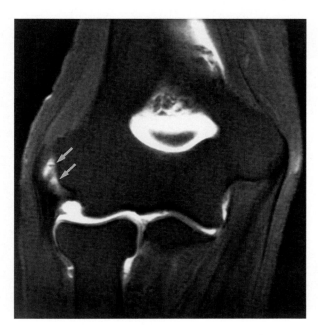

FIGURE 10-30. Partial tearing of the common extensor tendon. MR arthrography with injection of dilute gadolinium into the elbow joint. There is contrast delineating high-grade tearing of the extensor carpi radialis brevis from the lateral epicondyle on this fat-suppressed T1-weighted coronal image (*arrows*).

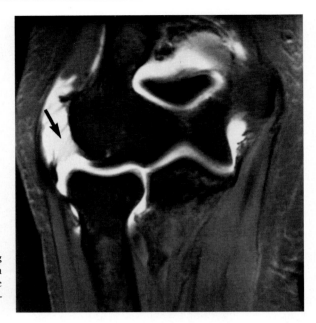

FIGURE 10-31. Massive tear of the common extensor tendon and underlying lateral collateral ligament. MR arthrography with injection of dilute gadolinium into the elbow joint. There is contrast extending through a large defect in the lateral capsule and common extensor tendon on this fat-suppressed T1-weighted coronal image (*arrows*).

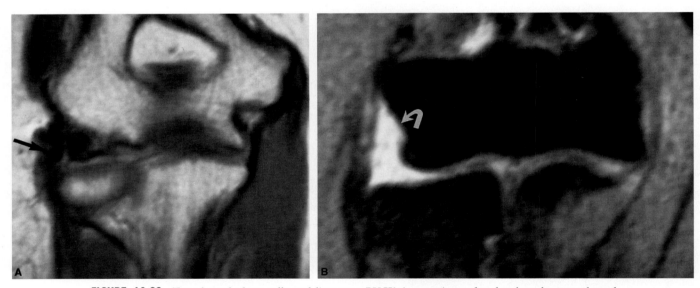

FIGURE 10-32. Torn lateral ulnar collateral ligament (LUCL) in a patient who developed posterolateral rotatory instability after extensor tendon release. T1-weighted (**A**) and STIR (**B**) coronal images reveal complete absence of the common extensor tendon and lateral ulnar collateral ligament adjacent to the lateral epicondyle (*curved white arrow*). Micrometallic artifact is noted from prior surgical release (*black arrow*).

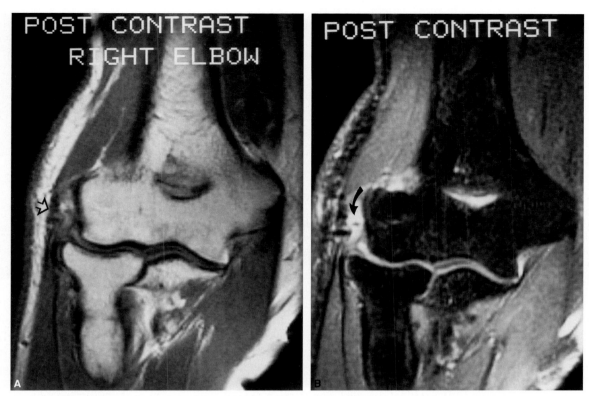

FIGURE 10-33. Torn lateral ulnar collateral ligament (LUCL) in a patient whose symptoms of instability and pain worsened after extensor tendon release. T1-weighted (**A**) and fat-suppressed T1-weighted (**B**) coronal images obtained after intravenous injection of gadolinium reveal complete absence of the common extensor tendon and lateral ulnar collateral ligament adjacent to the lateral epicondyle (*curved arrow*). Micrometallic artifact is noted from prior surgical release (*open arrow*).

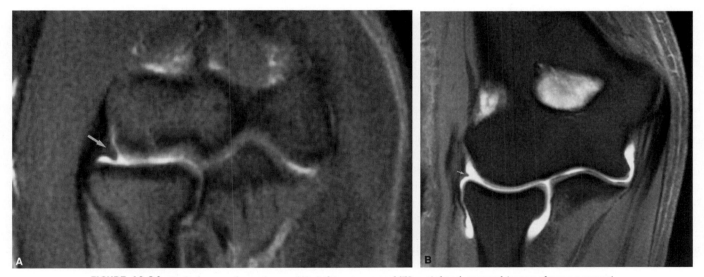

FIGURE 10-34. Radiohumeral meniscus. (**A**) A fat-suppressed T2-weighted coronal image shows a prominent meniscus-like structure (*arrow*) that extends into the lateral margin of the radiohumeral joint. (**B**) A thin lateral synovial fringe is seen in a different patient on a fat-suppressed T1-weighted coronal image obtained after intra-articular injection of gadolinium.

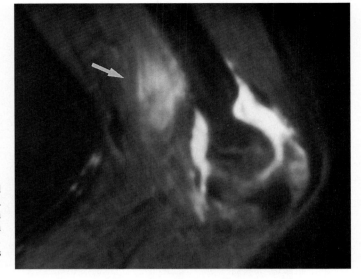

FIGURE 10-35. Transient posterior dislocation in a 7-year-old child with evidence of an effusion and no fracture identified on x-rays. A STIR sagittal image in partial flexion reveals increased signal within the brachialis muscle (*arrows*) compatible with strain or contusion injury. Although there is an effusion, there is no evidence of fracture. Full extension of the elbow is usually not possible in these patients due to pain and muscle spasm.

nation of the lateral capsule has been advanced as a possible cause of lateral elbow pain that may mimic symptoms of a loose body or lateral epicondylitis[62] (Fig. 10-34). The radiohumeral meniscus seen on MR imaging is probably the same structure that has been termed a symptomatic lateral synovial plica[63] of the elbow at arthroscopy. The lateral synovial plica of the elbow, like the more familiar symptomatic medial patella plica in the knee, may be encountered at arthroscopy as a thickened fold or fibrotic fringe of synovial tissue at the lateral margin of the radiocapitellar articulation.[64] Relief of symptoms has been described in several cases after arthroscopic resection of a fibrotic lateral synovial plica of the elbow.[63,65]

Posterior Dislocation Injury and Instability

Although posterior dislocation of the elbow is a relatively unusual event, it is the second most common major joint dislocation (after the shoulder) in adults and it is the most common dislocation in children younger than 10 years of age.[31] Children are predisposed to elbow dislocation due to the relative lack of congruity of the immature cartilaginous articulation compared with the constrained bony articulation of adults. Recurrent complete dislocation of the elbow is unusual, but occurs more frequently in children and adolescents than in adults.[66,67] In children, many dislocations go unrecognized because there is spontaneous reduction and the only finding is a swollen tender elbow.[68] MR imaging in such cases usually shows an effusion as well as a contusion or strain of the brachialis muscle (Fig. 10-35). Bone contusions may be seen at the posterior margin of the capitellum as well as at the radial head and coronoid process.

The usual mechanism of dislocation involves a fall on the outstretched hand.[69] A hyperextension force has been classically proposed to explain posterior dislocation of the

elbow. More recent investigation by O'Driscoll and associates[16,70] has resulted in a clearer understanding of how the flexed elbow may subluxate posterolaterally and may then dislocate. This mechanism involves hypersupination, valgus stress, and axial compressive loading of the elbow, such as may occur during a fall on the outstretched hand.

Elbow instability occurs as a spectrum from subluxation to dislocation that has been divided into three stages.[70] Each of these stages is associated with progressive soft tissue injury that extends from lateral to medial. In stage 1, there is posterolateral subluxation of the ulna and radius relative to the humerus, with disruption of the ulnar part of the lateral collateral ligament that has also been termed the lateral ulnar collateral ligament (LUCL) (Figs. 10-36 and 10-37). Rupture of the LUCL is considered the essential lesion of posterolateral rotatory instability. In stage 2, there is incomplete dislocation, so that the coronoid appears perched on the trochlea (Fig. 10-38). There is further disruption of the lateral ligamentous structures in stage 2 as well as tearing of the anterior and posterior joint capsule. In stage 3, there is complete posterior dislocation with progressive disruption of the MCL complex. There may be disruption of the posterior bundle of the MCL only (stage 3A), in which case the elbow is stable to valgus stress. Stage 3B is characterized by disruption of the anterior bundle of the MCL so that the elbow is unstable in all directions (Fig. 10-39). Complete disruption of the MCL (stage 3B) is the most common finding after complete dislocation. The common flexor and extensor tendons are often disrupted when there is complete posterior dislocation of the elbow[71–73] (Fig. 10-40).

The clinical assessment of elbow instability is difficult, in part because the physical examination is often compromised by guarding and pain. The recently described pivot-shift test of the elbow is a clinical test for posterolateral rotatory instability of the elbow due to insufficiency of the LUCL.[16] The pivot-shift test of the elbow is analogous to

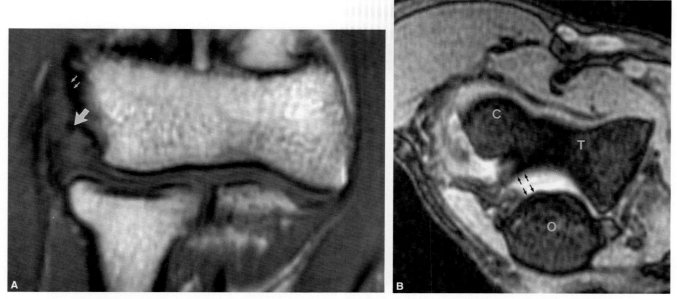

FIGURE 10-36. Stage 1 instability. (**A**) A T1-weighted coronal image reveals tearing of the common extensor tendon (*small arrows*) and the lateral ulnar collateral ligament (*large arrow*). (**B**) A T2*-weighted gradient-echo axial image reveals widening of the posterolateral joint space (*arrows*) due to posterolateral rotatory subluxation of the elbow. C, capitellum; T, trochlea; o, olecranon.

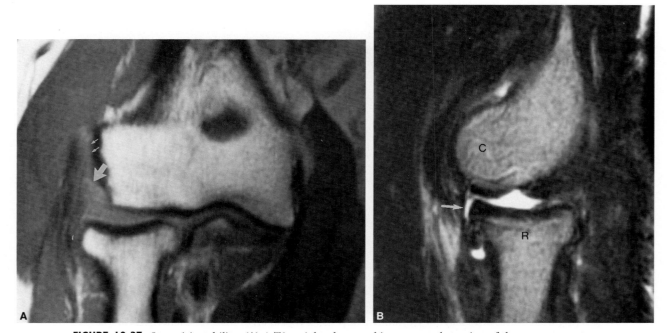

FIGURE 10-37. Stage 1 instability. (**A**) A T1-weighted coronal image reveals tearing of the common extensor tendon (*small arrows*) and the lateral ulnar collateral ligament (*large arrow*) from the lateral epicondyle. (**B**) A T2-weighted sagittal image reveals posterior subluxation (*arrow*) of the radius (R) relative to the capitellum (C).

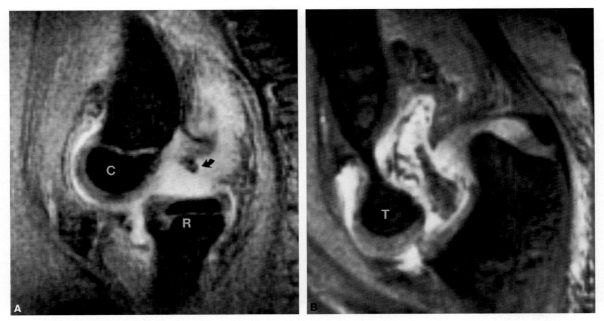

FIGURE 10-38. Stage 2 instability in 13-year-old child with a history of instability and recurrent elbow dislocation. **(A)** A T2*-weighted gradient-echo sagittal image reveals posterior dislocation of the radius (R) relative to the capitellum (C). Rupture of the lateral ulnar collateral ligament (*arrow*) is seen at the posterolateral aspect of the joint capsule. **(B)** The trochlea (T) is perched on the posteriorly subluxed coronoid process.

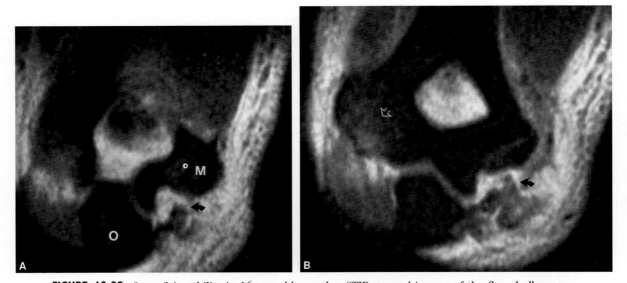

FIGURE 10-39. Stage 3 instability in 16-year-old wrestler. STIR coronal images of the flexed elbow progressing from posterior to anterior (**A** through **C**) reveal a contusion of the capitellum (*open arrows*) as well as a tear of the LUCL (*arrowheads*) and a tear of the MCL (*curved arrows*) due to a recent posterior dislocation. The posterior bundle of the MCL is detached from the medial epicondyle (M), but remains attached to the olecranon (O). The anterior bundle of the MCL is also detached from the medial epicondyle, but remains attached to the coronoid (C). *continued*

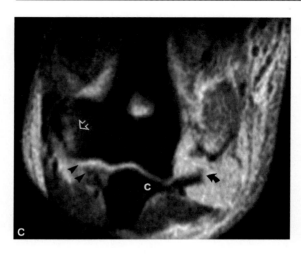

FIGURE 10-39. *Continued*

the widely known pivot-shift test of the knee, used to determine the integrity of the anterior cruciate ligament. A supination/valgus moment is applied during flexion, causing the radius and ulna to subluxate posteriorly. Further flexion produces a palpable and visible clunk as the elbow reduces. This subluxation/reduction maneuver creates apprehension, however, and is usually not possible to perform in the awake patient. Thus, clinical confirmation of recurrent instability of the elbow may require examination under anesthesia to elicit a pivot-shift maneuver.[73]

We have found MR imaging quite reliable for the detection of rupture of the LUCL. This ligament usually tears proximally, at the lateral margin of the capitellum, and is best evaluated on coronal and axial images (Fig. 10-41). LUCL tears may appear as an isolated finding on MR imaging in patients with posterolateral rotatory

instability in stage 1 (see Figs. 10-37 and 10-38), or they may be detected in association with rupture of the MCL in stage 3B (see Fig. 10-39). Disruption of the LUCL is commonly seen in patients with severe tennis elbow who also have tears of the common extensor tendon on MR imaging. Iatrogenic causes of LUCL disruption resulting in posterolateral rotatory instability include overaggressive extensor tendon release for lateral epicondylitis (common extensor tendinosis) and radial head excision for comminuted fractures of the radial head.[57]

Recurrent instability of the elbow involves a common pathway of posterolateral rotatory subluxation due to insufficiency of the LUCL.[73] Surgical correction is performed by reattaching the avulsed LUCL to the humerus or reconstructing it with a tendon graft placed isometrically through tunnels in the ulna and the humerus.[20,74]

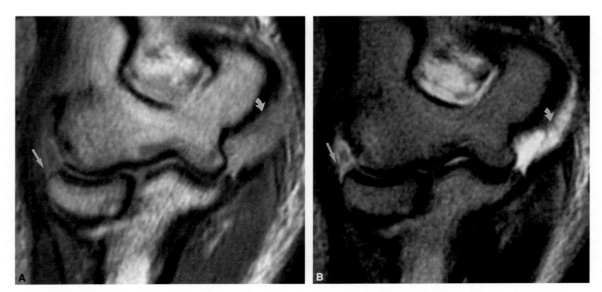

FIGURE 10-40. A 45-year-old woman with a history of recurrent elbow dislocation. Proton density (**A**) and T2-weighted (**B**) coronal images reveal complete avulsion of the medial collateral ligament and the common flexor tendon (*curved arrows*) from the medial epicondyle. Avulsion of the lateral collateral ligament (*straight arrows*) and partial tearing of the common extensor tendon is also seen.

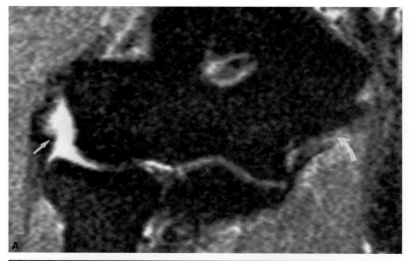

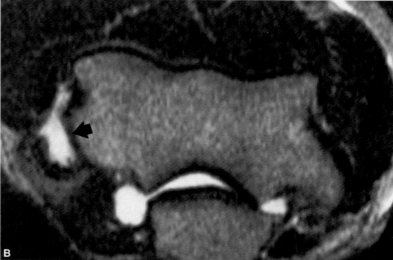

FIGURE 10-41. A 36-year-old man with recurrent instability. (**A**) A STIR coronal image reveals disruption of the LUCL (*arrow*) and partial tearing of the proximal MCL (*curved arrow*). (**B**) A T2-weighted axial image shows fluid at the normal site of the LUCL adjacent to the lateral epicondyle.

Fractures

Radiographically occult or equivocal fractures about the elbow may be assessed with MR imaging. Moreover, MR imaging performed with the patient in a cast does not suffer significant degradation of image quality. If the cast is large, a larger surface coil, such as the head coil, may be needed. In general, the findings of bone injury are somewhat subtle on proton density, T2-weighted, and T2*-weighted sequences and are more conspicuous on T1-weighted, fat-suppressed T2-weighted, and STIR sequences.

The coronoid is an important structure for stability of the elbow. A fracture of the coronoid process (which may be subtle on standard radiographs, especially when small or nondisplaced) is highly characteristic of a previous posterior dislocation or subluxation of the elbow[75] (Fig. 10-42). These fractures may predispose to recurrent posterior instability, depending on the size of the fracture fragment and the presence of associated collateral ligament rupture.[76] Coronoid process fractures occur as a result of direct shear injury by

the trochlea during posterior dislocation or subluxation.[73] They are not hyperextension avulsion injuries, as the tip of the coronoid is an intraarticular structure that does not have a capsular attachment. The anterior capsule and the brachialis muscle insert further distally on the ulna. Anterior capsular injury and contusion or strain of the adjacent brachialis muscle, as well as medial and lateral collateral ligament injury, are commonly seen after posterior elbow dislocation[17,71,72,77] (see Fig. 10-42). Frequently, the common flexor and extensor tendons also rupture with posterior dislocation (see Fig. 10-40). Rarely, if the common flexor tendon is torn or the medial epicondyle is avulsed, the median nerve may become entrapped within the elbow joint during posterior dislocation.[78,79] It is important, therefore, that each of these structures be carefully evaluated when a coronoid process fracture is identified on MR imaging.

Fractures of the coronoid process have been classified into the following three types by Regan and Morrey.[75,76] Type I fractures are small shear fractures that do not destabilize the joint (Fig. 10-43). They should be recognized,

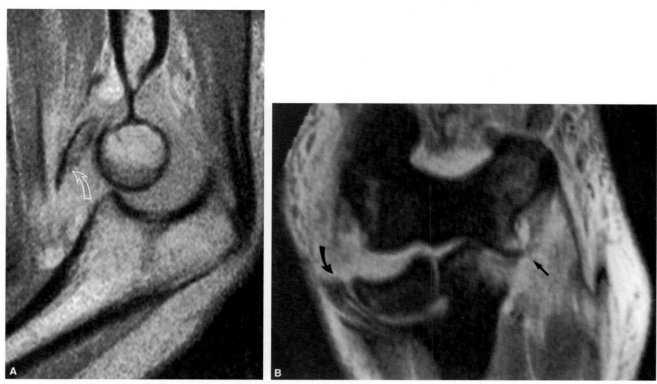

FIGURE 10-42. Type III coronoid fracture. **(A)** A proton density sagittal image reveals posterior subluxation of the ulna and a large fracture of the coronoid process that is superiorly displaced (*open arrow*). Increased signal is also seen within the brachialis muscle and the anterior capsule just anterior to the fracture fragment. **(B)** A STIR coronal image reveals disruption of the lateral collateral ligament proximally (*curved arrow*) and disruption of the anterior bundle of the medial collateral ligament distally (straight arrow).

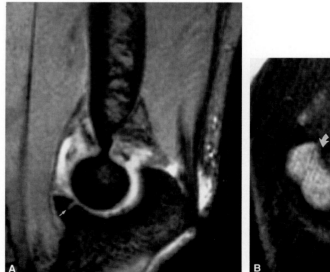

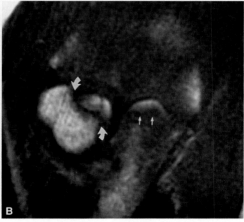

FIGURE 10-43. Posterior dislocation/subluxation injury from a fall on the outstretched hand in a 30-year-old jogger. T2*-weighted gradient-echo sagittal **(A)** and T1-weighted coronal **(B)** images reveal a nondisplaced fracture of the tip of the coronoid process (*small arrows*) and an impacted fracture of the radial head (*curved arrows*). The fracture of the radial head is caused by impaction of the capitellum whereas the coronoid fracture is caused by the adjacent trochlea.

however, as an indicator of posterior elbow dislocation/subluxation injury that may be associated with significant soft tissue disruption. Type II fractures involve less than 50% of the coronoid. Fixation is necessary if the joint remains dislocated or subluxed. Type III fractures involve more than 50% of the coronoid and have a poor prognosis. Type III fractures, as well as malunions and nonunions of the coronoid in patients with instability, also require fixation.[73,76]

Approximately 10% of elbow dislocations result in fractures of the radial head; conversely, about 10% of patients with a radial head fracture have an elbow dislocation[80] (Fig. 10-44). When there is ligamentous disruption and instability, displaced fractures of the radial head are best treated with internal fixation.[73,76] Prosthetic replacement may be necessary to maintain stability when the radial head is comminuted and cannot be repaired. CT is the technique of choice when additional information about the fracture morphology or degree of comminution is needed. MR imaging is useful for detection and character-

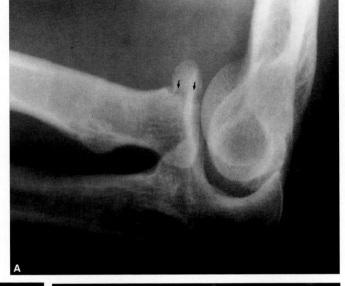

FIGURE 10-44. Signs of posterior elbow dislocation injury on MR imaging. An angled radiographic view of the radial head and (**A**) a T1-weighted sagittal image (**B**) reveal a fracture of the anterior aspect of the radial head (*arrows*). A STIR sagittal image (**C**) shows the radial head fracture (*arrows*) as well as a contusion (black arrowhead) at the posterior margin of the capitellum as a consequence of posterior dislocation/relocation injury. (Courtesy of Mark Anderson, MD.)

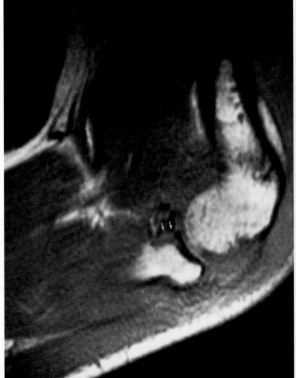

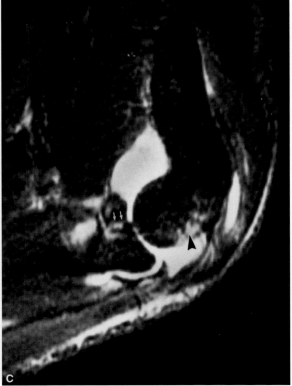

ization of radial head fractures, and is also helpful in the exclusion of associated collateral ligament injury that may contribute to instability (Fig. 10-45). The integrity of the MCL is especially important if excision of the radial head is being considered.

Bone Contusions

Radiographically, occult bone injury produces changes seen in the medullary space that are variously called a bone contusion, bone bruise, trabecular microfracture, or bony trabecular injury.[81-86] The exact nature of the abnormal signal remains speculative, but it is likely secondary to trabecular disruption (microfracture) of the cancellous bone with hemorrhage and edema extending into the medullary space. Typical findings on T1-weighted images include poorly marginated loss of signal intensity relative to fatty marrow that is localized to the site of impaction injury (Fig. 10-46). The area of decreased signal on T1-weighted images increases in signal intensity on T2-weighted images.

Bone contusions are most conspicuous on STIR and other fat-suppressed sequences[86] (Fig. 10-47). Fat-suppressed sequences, which sacrifice signal-to-noise for contrast-to-noise and conspicuity,[86] are often the most diagnostic and important images obtained. These images are not without problems, however, including artifacts related to incomplete fat suppression throughout the image. Heterogeneous fat suppression may be confusing if it is not recognized as a technical pitfall and is instead mistaken for pathologic change (Fig. 10-48). Furthermore, the ability to confidently identify abnormalities is lost in that portion of the image with incomplete fat suppression. In general, it is more difficult to obtain consistent homogeneous fat suppression with spectroscopic chemical-shift methods than with STIR and fast STIR techniques. This is especially true when imaging the elbow with the patient supine and the arm at the side. In this position, the elbow lies in the periphery of the magnet where the magnetic field is less uniform and suboptimal fat suppression may occur.

Bone contusions are well visualized on T1-weighted images if there is predominantly fatty marrow to provide

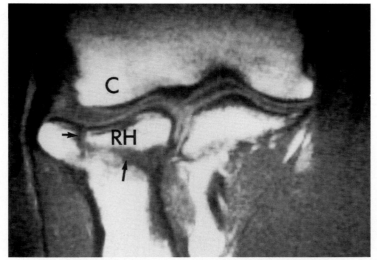

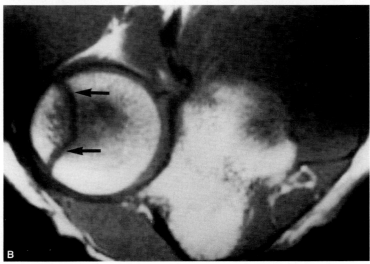

FIGURE 10-45. Radial head fracture. T1-weighted coronal (**A**) and axial (**B**) images reveal a minimally displaced, comminuted fracture of the radial head. The ligaments about the elbow are normal.

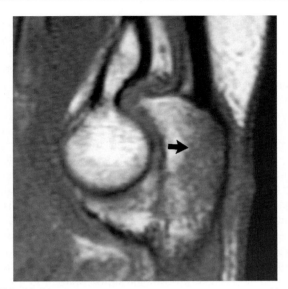

FIGURE 10-46. Olecranon bone contusion in a 32-year-old tennis player who complained of persistent pain while serving. She had suffered a direct blow to the olecranon during a fall 3 weeks previously. A T1-weighted sagittal image reveals abnormal decreased signal (*arrow*) throughout the posterior aspect of the olecranon as well as infiltration of the overlying subcutaneous fat at the site of the olecranon bursa.

background contrast. Bone contusions, as well as other types of marrow pathology, may be inconspicuous on proton density and T2-weighted images, because marrow edema and marrow fat may be of similar signal intensity. Artifactual loss of signal intensity due to magnetic susceptibility differences among trabecular bone, edema, and fat also results in unreliable marrow contrast on gradient-echo T2*-weighted sequences.[87] Gadolinium administration may produce enhancement of bone contusions, and in this setting enhancement is most conspicuous when fat-suppressed T1-weighted images are obtained. Although experience with MR follow-up of patients with bone contusions is relatively limited, it seems that symptoms resolve within 3 months and the MR appearance returns to normal within 6 weeks to 3 months after the injury.[81,82] In one study, bone contusions about the knee were identified on T1- and T2-weighted images in 71% of 98 patients with clinically diagnosed anterior cruciate ligament (ACL) injuries. No contusions, however, were seen on scans performed more than 6 weeks after injury.[84] If not adequately protected during trabecular healing, bone contusions may represent regions of bone theoretically at risk for the subsequent development of insufficiency fractures or osteochondral sequelae.[81,83] For injuries in the lower extremity, some

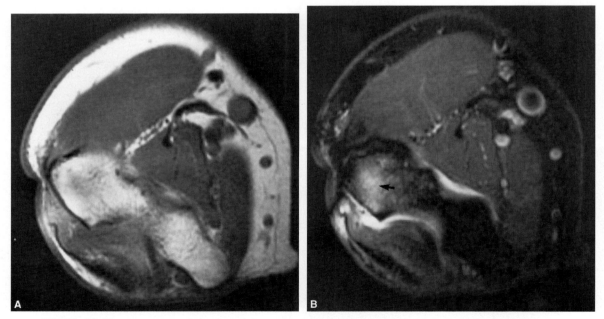

FIGURE 10-47. Contusion of the lateral humeral condyle. T1-weighted (**A**) and STIR (**B**) axial images reveal abnormal signal that is much more conspicuous on the STIR image (*arrow*).

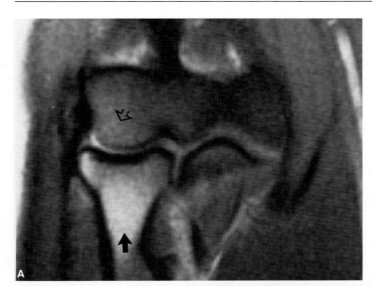

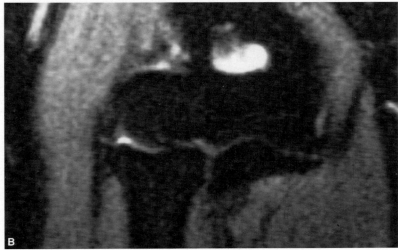

FIGURE 10-48. Technically inadequate fat suppression with the chemical-shift technique resulting in potential misdiagnosis. A fat-suppressed fast spin-echo proton density (4000/40) coronal image (**A**) reveals increased signal throughout the proximal radius (*solid black arrow*). Less prominent signal alteration is seen in the lateral aspect of the capitellum (*open arrow*). The signal within the lateral subcutaneous fat was also not suppressed, providing a clue to the artifactual nature of the increased signal in the radius and capitellum. A fast STIR coronal image (**B**) with uniform fat suppression throughout the image reveals no abnormalities.

authors advocate a delay before resuming full weight bearing and resumption of sports activities, both for the alleviation of pain and to lessen the risk of potential progression of these regions of trabecular disruption into complete fractures.[81,88]

The differential diagnosis of poorly defined marrow edema includes small cortical avulsions that may be radiographically subtle or occult. Avulsion of the joint capsule, ligaments, or tendons may result in marrow edema that is the most conspicuous finding on MR imaging.[89,90] Careful inspection of the cortex, as well as review of the plain films or additional radiographic views, may be necessary to recognize these avulsion fractures.

Other processes also result in nonspecific bone marrow edema on MR imaging. Differential considerations include transient bone marrow edema syndrome, early osteonecrosis, osteomyelitis, edema associated with primary or metastatic tumors, and edema associated with osteochondral defects. Transient bone marrow edema syndrome is more common in the lower extremity, especially the hip, but may occasionally be seen in the bones about the elbow. Marrow edema

may be seen adjacent to osteochondritis dissecans and Panner's disease in the capitellum. Osteomyelitis may also result in the appearance of bone marrow edema on MR imaging.[91] Identification of bony destruction (Fig. 10-49), an abscess, a sequestrum, or a sinus tract may help to recognize this process. Gallium 67 scans or indium 111 labeled white blood cell scans may add specificity if osteomyelitis is suspected.

Bone marrow edema is a conspicuous finding in many neoplasms, especially infiltrative neoplasms and chondroblastoma.[92] It may be the sole MR finding on MR imaging of an osteoid osteoma, resulting in an erroneous diagnosis unless plain films are also reviewed.[93-95] Osteoid osteoma may involve the elbow and present a confusing appearance of marrow edema on MR imaging.[94,96,97] CT may be necessary to detect the nidus of a small osteoid osteoma. Reactive marrow edema is also often seen adjacent to foci of articular cartilage loss associated with various arthropathies about the elbow.

Typically, plain films are performed before MR imaging, and these films should be reviewed for evidence of a fracture,

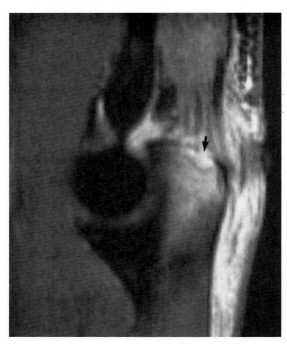

FIGURE 10-49. Osteomyelitis of the olecranon secondary to cellulitis and septic bursitis. A STIR sagittal image reveals increased signal throughout the olecranon with a cortical defect noted superiorly (*arrow*). There is increased signal and thickening of the posterior soft tissues compatible with cellulitis. Bony destruction was subsequently visualized on a lateral plain film (not shown).

bony destruction, sclerosis, osteochondral defects, or other findings that may explain the cause of bone marrow edema on MR imaging. Bone scans are usually abnormal when STIR images reveal marrow edema. However, bone scans may be useful when unexplained marrow edema is identified on MR imaging if a multifocal process, such as metastatic disease, is suspected.

In cases of repetitive trauma and overuse, a stress reaction or stress response can also result in a nonspecific pattern of marrow edema. This process may be followed with limited STIR scans to evaluate various treatment regimens (Fig. 10-50). A stress reaction is differentiated from a stress fracture on MR imaging by the presence of a fracture line. Stress fractures of the middle one third of the olecranon may occur in throwing athletes as a consequence of overload by the triceps mechanism[98–100] (Fig. 10-51). These fractures have the potential to displace and usually are treated surgically. Chronic extension overload in adolescent baseball pitchers leads to nonunion of the olecranon physeal plate that also may require surgery.[101] MR imaging is useful in detecting these lesions, which may be difficult to diagnose clinically and radiographically.

A stress reaction, unlike a bone contusion, is usually associated with a history of overuse rather than acute trauma. As in all of the differential considerations described earlier, the clinical history is extremely important in identifying the cause of marrow edema and in reaching the correct diagnosis on MR imaging.

Pediatric Elbow Fractures

Fractures of the medial epicondyle usually occur in children between the ages of 9 and 15 years and are secondary to a valgus stress, which produces traction and avulsion at the unfused apophyseal growth plate. The epicondyle is displaced inferiorly, due to the pull of the attached flexor muscles (Fig. 10-52). The medial epicondyle may become entrapped within the medial aspect of the joint if there is associated rupture of the MCL and opening of the joint space at the time of valgus stress. Entrapment of the medial epicondyle is typically associated with posterior dislocation of the elbow and rupture of the collateral ligaments.[102–104] This diagnosis can ordinarily be made on plain films, but it is important to remember the sequential appearance of the ossification centers about the elbow so that the entrapped medial epicondyle is not mistaken for a normal trochlear ossification center. MR imaging may be needed to evaluate this complication when the medial epicondyle has not yet

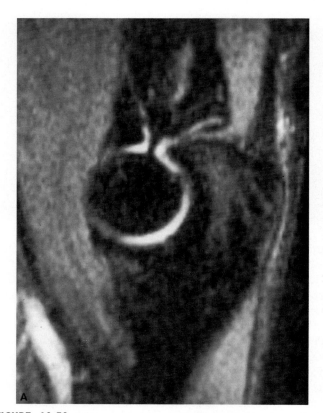

FIGURE 10-50. Olecranon stress reaction secondary to posterior impingement and overuse in a professional baseball pitcher. (**A**) A STIR sagittal image reveals increased signal throughout the olecranon. A bone scan finding was also positive at this time. (**B**) After 6 weeks of rest, the abnormal signal has resolved on this STIR sagittal image. Spurring of the anterior olecranon is evident (*open arrow*). (**C**) Symptoms returned when the patient resumed pitching, and an arthroscopic posterior decompression was performed. A postoperative STIR sagittal image shows the site of bony resection (*arrows*). Although the patient was able to pitch without pain for several months, he ruptured his medial collateral ligament the following season. *continued*

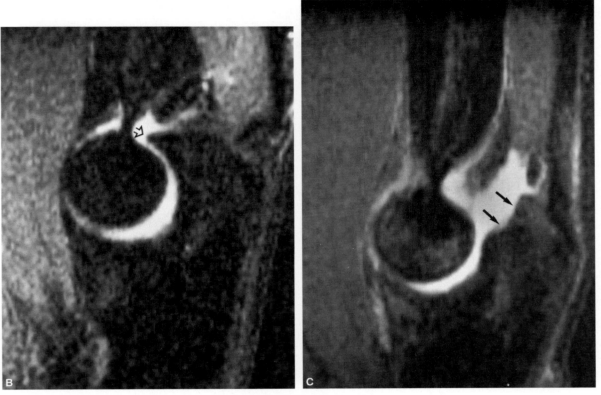

FIGURE 10-50. *Continued*

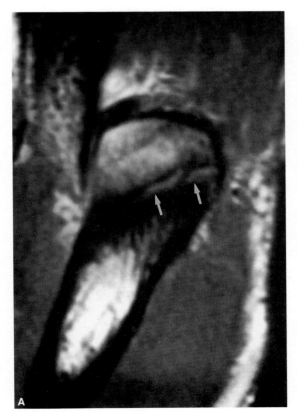

FIGURE 10-51. Chronic stress fracture of the olecranon in a professional baseball pitcher. T1-weighted (**A**) and STIR (**B**) coronal images, as well as a proton density sagittal image (**C**), show fluid within a minimally displaced fracture line (*arrows*) and surrounding sclerosis. The fracture line is perpendicular to the pull of the triceps tendon due to cubitus valgus deformity. Delayed closure or fracture of the olecranon growth plate due to overuse and traction of the triceps in a young pitcher could have a similar appearance.   *continued*

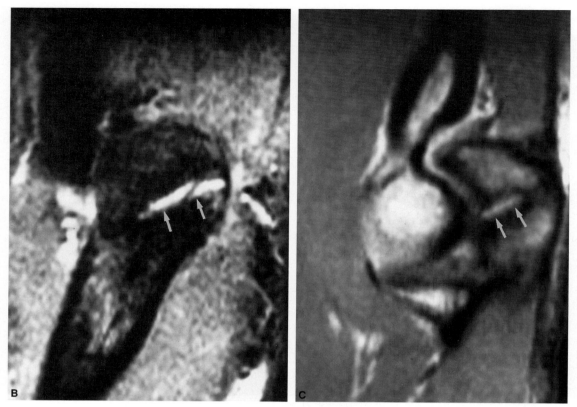

FIGURE 10-51. *Continued*

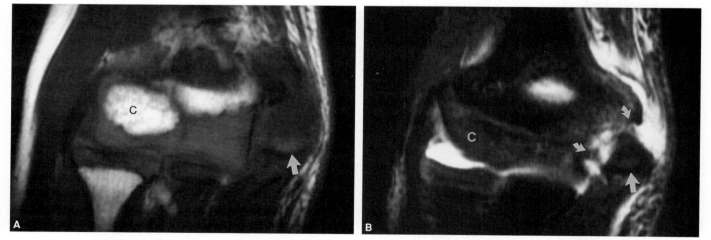

FIGURE 10-52. Avulsion fracture of the medial epicondyle in a 5-year-old boy with medial elbow pain after a fall on his outstretched arm. Radiographs (not shown) revealed partial ossification of the capitellum, radial head, and medial epicondyle with apparent distal displacement of the medial epicondyle compared with the uninjured elbow. T1-weighted (**A**) and STIR (**B**) coronal images reveal distal avulsion of the medial epicondylar apophysis (*arrows*) that is just beginning to ossify. The fracture (*curved arrows*) is well delineated on the STIR sequence. C, capitellum.

ossified. The ulnar nerve is commonly displaced within the joint along with the medial epicondyle, and MR imaging may be used to evaluate the status of the ulnar nerve in such cases. Moreover, chronic tension stress injury and avulsion fractures in young baseball pitchers (Little League elbow) may also be evaluated with MR imaging.[1]

Treatment of medial epicondyle fractures is controversial and depends on the degree of displacement as well as the functional requirements of the patient.[103,105,106] Cases with significant displacement or injuries in young athletes who require a stable elbow for throwing are generally treated surgically. However, both function and range of motion of the elbow was uniformly good in one series of 56 children followed for 21 to 48 years after conservatively treated fractures of the medial epicondyle.[105] Unfortunately, late development of ulnar neuropathy is a common complication of conservatively treated cases[105] (Fig. 10-53).

Extraarticular fracture of the medial epicondyle should be differentiated from the more complicated intraarticular fracture of the medial humeral condyle. Intraarticular frac-

tures of the medial humeral condyle are unusual, but can be confused with avulsion fractures of the medial epicondyle in younger children in whom the trochlea is unossified.[103] The presence of an effusion or significant displacement of the medial epicondyle are plain film clues to the diagnosis of a fracture of the medial humeral condyle.[107] If this diagnosis is not made, and the injury is treated nonsurgically, a poor functional result can be anticipated.[108] MR imaging, rather than arthrography, can be used to exclude involvement of the unossified trochlear cartilage.

MR imaging can also be used to identify or exclude the more common radial head fractures in adults and supracondylar fractures in children, when there is radiographic evidence of a joint effusion and a fracture is not visualized (Fig. 10-54). In children, supracondylar fractures that do not involve the physis are more common than all physeal injuries about the elbow combined.[108,109] However, the elbow is a relatively common site of physeal injury—only distal radial and distal tibial physeal fractures are more common.[3] Fractures of the lateral humeral condyle are the most common

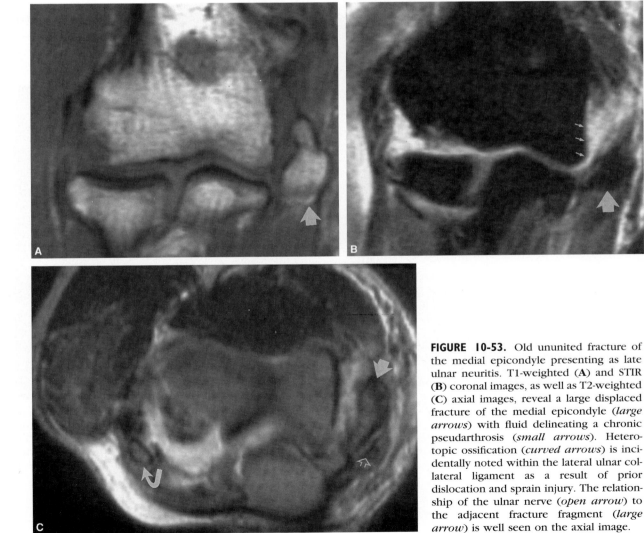

FIGURE 10-53. Old ununited fracture of the medial epicondyle presenting as late ulnar neuritis. T1-weighted (**A**) and STIR (**B**) coronal images, as well as T2-weighted (**C**) axial images, reveal a large displaced fracture of the medial epicondyle (*large arrows*) with fluid delineating a chronic pseudarthrosis (*small arrows*). Heterotopic ossification (*curved arrows*) is incidentally noted within the lateral ulnar collateral ligament as a result of prior dislocation and sprain injury. The relationship of the ulnar nerve (*open arrow*) to the adjacent fracture fragment (*large arrow*) is well seen on the axial image.

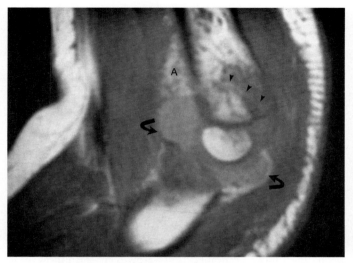

FIGURE 10-54. Radiographically occult elbow fracture in an 8-year-old boy with a positive fat pad sign on x-ray. A T1-weighted sagittal image reveals a supracondylar fracture (*arrowheads*) with adjacent decreased signal. A large effusion is noted (*curved arrows*) elevating the anterior fat pad. A, anterior fat pad.

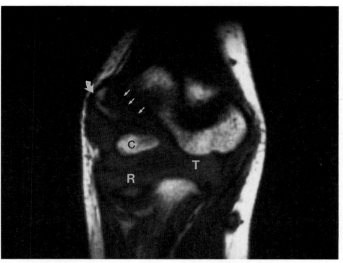

FIGURE 10-55. Radiographically subtle elbow fracture. T1-weighted coronal image reveals a Salter-Harris type II fracture (*arrows*) with mild lateral displacement of the lateral humeral condyle (*curved arrow*). The fracture does not extend into the capitellum (C). T2-weighted images (not shown) excluded extension of the fracture into the unossified trochlear epiphysis. This 5-year-old child did well with closed reduction. R, unossified radial head cartilage; T, unossified trochlear cartilage.

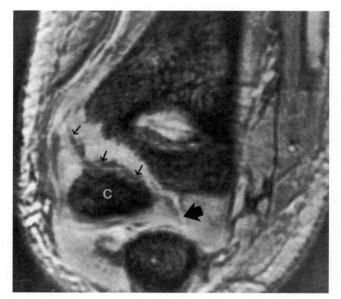

FIGURE 10-56. Salter-Harris type IV fracture of the lateral humeral condyle. T2*-weighted gradient-echo coronal image of a partially flexed elbow reveals the thin metaphyseal fracture fragment (*small arrows*), as well as extension of the fracture through the unossified trochlear epiphysis (*large arrow*). These fractures usually require open reduction and internal fixation. C, capitellum. (Courtesy of Phoebe Kaplan, MD.)

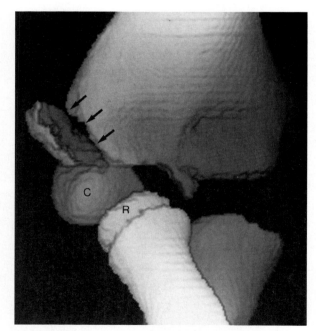

FIGURE 10-57. Fracture of the lateral humeral condyle in a 6-year-old boy. An anterior oblique three-dimensional CT reconstruction reveals the bony extent of the fracture. However, the clinically significant potential extension of the fracture into the cartilaginous epiphysis cannot be assessed on CT scans. C, capitellum; R, radial head.

specific type of physeal injury about the elbow (Fig. 10-55). They occur in children between the ages of 2 and 14 years but are most common between 6 and 10 years of age. A fracture of the lateral humeral condyle is usually a longitudinal Salter-Harris type IV fracture, which is both intraarticular and transphyseal[108] (Fig. 10-56). The intraarticular fracture line is usually entirely through cartilage and is therefore not visible on x-rays or CT (Fig. 10-57). Injury to the physis and the unossified epiphyseal cartilage may be assessed with arthrography or MR imaging in these cases.[3,110,111] This information is important because Salter-Harris type IV fractures of the lateral humeral condyle tend to be unstable and require surgical intervention, whereas Salter-Harris type II fractures can be treated successfully with closed reduction (see Figs. 10-55 through 10-57). Unrecognized Salter-Harris type IV fractures of the lateral humeral condyle are frequently complicated by malunion and nonunion that results in deformity, loss of motion, degenerative arthrosis, and tardy ulnar neuropathy.[108] MR imaging with gradient-echo technique may be useful to depict physeal bars and growth arrest after growth plate injuries[3,110,111] (Fig. 10-58).

Osteochondritis Dissecans

Chronic lateral impaction may lead to osteochondritis dissecans of the capitellum or radial head in adolescent pitchers or gymnasts.[112–114] Repeated valgus stress and a relatively tenuous blood supply within the capitellum has been proposed to explain the frequent occurrence of osteochondritis

dissecans in this location.[115] Stable osteochondral lesions are usually treated with rest and splinting, whereas unstable lesions and loose bodies are usually excised.[116–118] Unless a large acutely displaced defect is encountered, a procedure to stimulate a healing response—such as abrasion chondroplasty or microfracture of the osteochondral defect—is generally performed rather than internal fixation or bone grafting.[64,117] Long-term follow-up has shown that osteochondritis dissecans of the capitellum ultimately leads to osteoarthritis in more than half of patients.[119]

MR imaging can reliably detect and stage osteochondritis dissecans. However, the accuracy of staging is improved by performing MR arthrography using dilute gadolinium.[120] Unstable lesions are characterized by fluid or contrast encircling the osteochondral fragment on T2-weighted images. Loose in situ lesions also may be diagnosed by identifying a cyst-like lesion beneath the osteochondral fragment[121] (Fig. 10-59). At surgery, these cyst-like lesions are typically found to contain loose granulation tissue, explaining why they may enhance after intravenous administration of gadolinium (Fig. 10-60). There is limited published experience with intravenous gadolinium-enhanced scans to evaluate osteonecrosis and osteochondritis dissecans in the elbow.[122] Delayed scans after intravenous gadolinium injection result in predictable enhancement of fluid within the joint.[123] This technique may potentially provide a less invasive method of opacifying the joint fluid and staging osteochondral lesions.

Osteochondritis dissecans should be distinguished from the pseudodefect of the capitellum that represents an MR

text continues on page 806

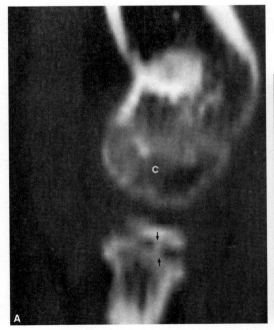
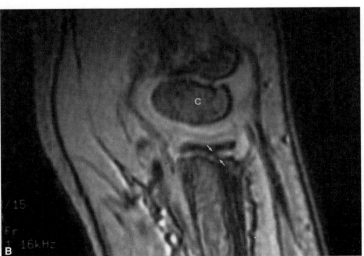

FIGURE 10-58. Focal physeal growth arrest after a fracture of the radial head in a child. A two-dimensional sagittal CT reformation (**A**) and a T2*-weighted gradient-echo sagittal image (**B**) through the medial aspect of the radial head reveal a bony physeal bar (*arrows*). The normal growth plate of the proximal radius is increased in signal on the gradient-echo images. C, capitellum.

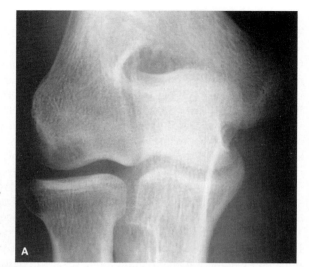

FIGURE 10-59. Osteochondritis dissecans of the capitellum in a 17-year-old boy with completed ossification. (**A**) A radiolucent lesion is seen on this AP radiograph. (**B**) A T1-weighted coronal image reveals a sclerotic rim (*black arrows*) delineating the margins of osteonecrosis as well as slight separation of the cortex overlying the lesion (*white arrows*). (**C**) A T2*-weighted gradient-echo axial image reveals a cyst-like lesion (*white arrows*) that suggests instability of the overlying cortex and articular cartilage (*black arrows*).

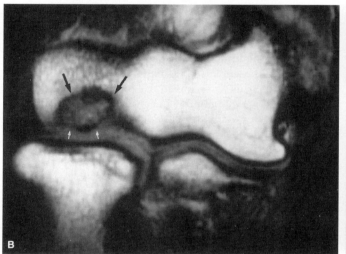

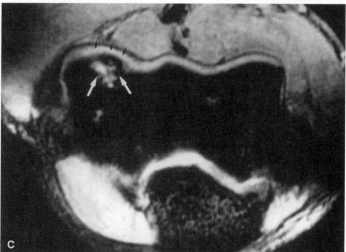

FIGURE 10-60. Osteochondritis dissecans in a 14-year-old boy. (**A**) A T1-weighted axial image reveals an area of osteochondritis dissecans (*open arrow*) in the anterolateral aspect of the capitellum. (**B**) A fat-suppressed T1-weighted axial image after intravenous gadolinium administration reveals an enhancing area of granulation tissue (*open arrow*) beneath a thin osteochondral flap (*curved arrow*). Enhancement of thickened synovium (*small arrows*), compatible with synovitis, is noted. *continued*

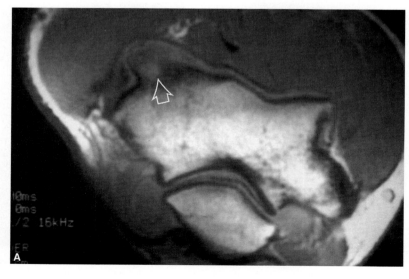

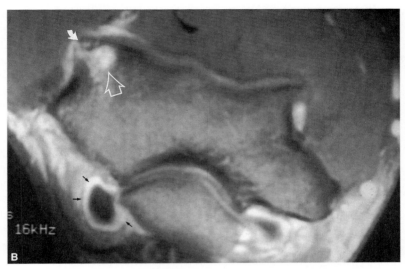

FIGURE 10-60. *Continued*

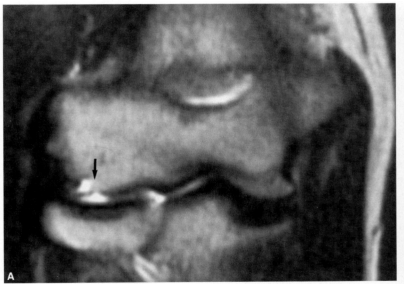

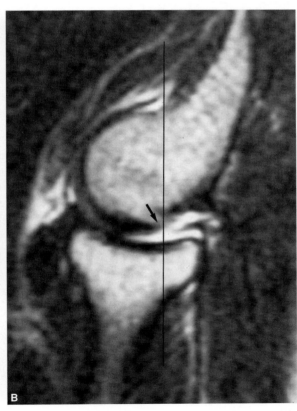

FIGURE 10-61. Pseudodefect of the capitellum. **(A)** A T2-weighted coronal image reveals an apparent discontinuity of the cortex at the inferolateral margin of the capitellum (*arrow*). **(B)** A T2-weighted sagittal image shows the abrupt posterior termination of the cortex and articular cartilage of the capitellum (*arrow*). A vertically orientated black line shows the location of the coronal image illustrated in **A**. R, radius.

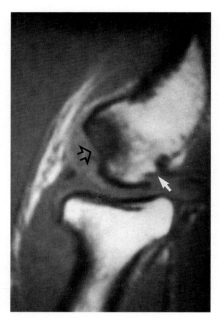

FIGURE 10-62. Osteochondritis dissecans in a 14-year-old boy. A T1-weighted sagittal image reveals a typical defect in the anterior aspect of the capitellum (*open black arrow*). The pseudodefect of the capitellum occurs posteriorly (*white arrow*) on sagittal images through the lateral aspect of the capitellum.

imaging pitfall related to the normal anatomy of the radiocapitellar articulation. Familiarity with the typical appearance and location of the pseudodefect is important to avoid an erroneous diagnosis of an osteochondral defect or an impaction fracture of the capitellum (Fig. 10-61).

The capitellum is an anteriorly directed prominence that arises from the lateral aspect of the distal humerus and resembles one half of a sphere. The articular cartilage of the capitellum extends through an arc of approximately 180° from superior to inferior.[11,124] Osteochondritis dissecans and osteochondral defects typically involve the anterior aspect

of the capitellum,[125,126] whereas the pseudodefect of the capitellum occurs at the abrupt transition between the posterolateral margin of the capitellum and the adjacent nonarticular portion of the lateral humeral condyle (Fig. 10-62). Fluid or contrast in the posterior aspect of the lateral compartment further highlights this abrupt transition between the normal overhanging margins of the capitellum and the rough nonarticular portion of the humerus that simulates an osteochondral defect (Fig. 10-63). This pseudodefect is also conspicuous because of the normal incomplete articulation between the capitellum and the radial head that occurs when the elbow is extended. The absence of contact between the posterolateral aspect of the radial head and the capitellum is a normal feature of the extended elbow joint. However, this further creates the illusion of an osteochondral defect as the cartilage of the radial head opposes the rough nonarticular portion of the humerus.

The capitellum has a tapered appearance from anterior to posterior that accounts for the lack of contact with the posterolateral radius and the appearance of the pseudodefect (see Fig. 10-63D). Sagittal images through the lateral aspect of the capitellum may have the appearance of a posteroinferior defect (see Figs. 10-61B and 10-63B), whereas coronal images through the posterior aspect of the capitellum may have the appearance of a inferolateral defect (see Figs. 10-61A and 10-63A). It is important to note that in a recent study of the capitellar pseudodefect, the variable conspicuity of the pseudodefect was found to depend on the presence of fluid and the angle of the sagittal and coronal images.[127] The pseudodefect is present and more conspicuous when coronal images are truly parallel to the plane of the humeral epicondyles (see Fig. 10-63D) and sagittal images are truly perpendicular to these ''oblique'' coronal images.

Osteochondritis dissecans should be distinguished from osteochondrosis of the capitellum, which is known as Panner's disease. Age is an important factor in making this distinction. Osteochondritis dissecans typically is seen in 13-

FIGURE 10-63. Pseudodefect of the capitellum at MR arthrography. Fat-suppressed T1-weighted coronal (**A**), sagittal (**B**), and axial (**C, D**) images were performed after dilute gadolinium was injected into the elbow joint. Multiple small air bubbles (*small white arrows*) should not be mistaken for loose bodies. The coronal image (**A**) depicts a typical pseudodefect of the capitellum (*open arrow*). The normal posterior tapering of the capitellum (*small black arrows* on **D**) accounts for the pseudodefect at its inferolateral margin. A white line shows the location of the coronal section shown in **A**. *continued*

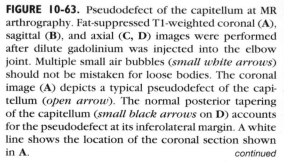

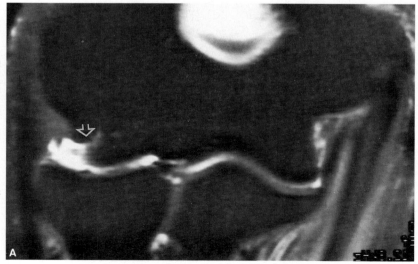

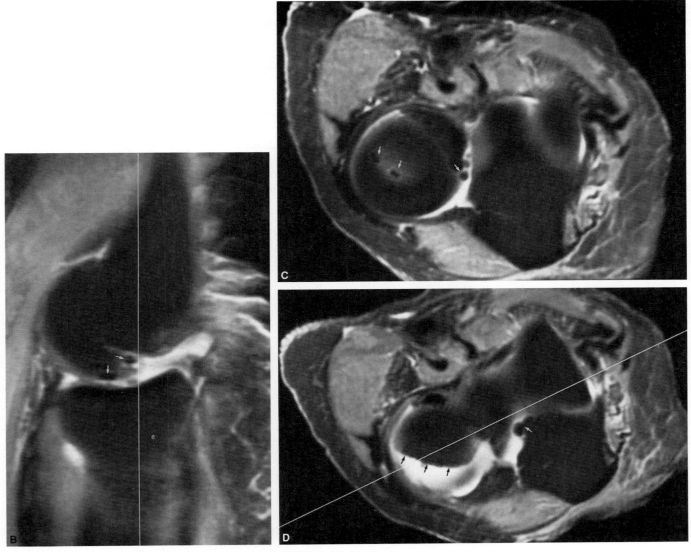

FIGURE. 10-63. *Continued*

to 16-year-old children, whereas Panner's disease typically is seen in 5- to 11-year-old children, before ossification of the capitellum is complete. Loose body formation and significant residual deformity of the capitellum are concerns in osteochondritis dissecans, but are usually not seen in Panner's disease.[128,129] On T1-weighted images, Panner's disease is characterized by fragmentation and abnormally decreased signal intensity within the ossifying capitellar epiphysis, similar in appearance to Legg-Calvé-Perthes disease in the hip (Fig. 10-64). Panner's disease is believed to represent avascular necrosis of the capitellar ossification center that occurs secondary to trauma. Subsequent scans reveal normalization of these changes with little or no residual deformity of the capitellar articular surface. The articular surface typically

remains intact and does not undergo fragmentation or loose body formation (Fig. 10-65).

Loose Bodies

After the knee, the elbow is the second most common site of loose bodies.[130] Loose bodies are thought to arise from a small nidus of bone or cartilage within the joint. The nidus may result from fragmentation of the articular cartilage associated with osteoarthritis or from an osteochondral fracture (Fig. 10-66). The small nidus grows in a laminar fashion, receiving nutrition from the synovial fluid,[131,132] and the

text continues on page 812

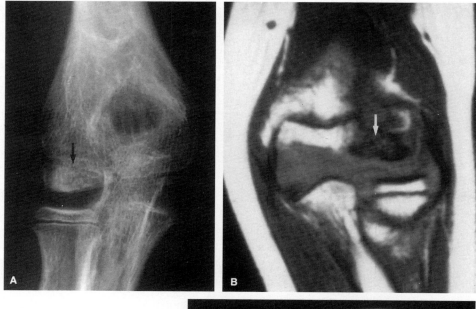

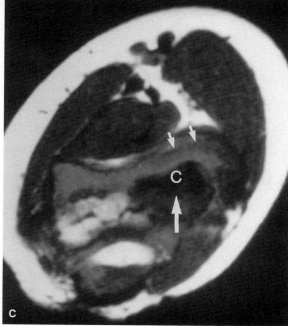

FIGURE 10-64. Panner's disease (osteochondrosis) in a 9-year-old girl. **(A)** Sclerosis within the capitellar ossification center is seen on this AP radiograph. **(B)** A T1-weighted coronal image reveals decreased signal throughout the capitellum (*arrow*). **(C)** A T1-weighted axial image reveals decreased signal throughout the capitellum (*large arrow*). The overlying articular cartilage is intact (*small arrows*). C, capitellum.

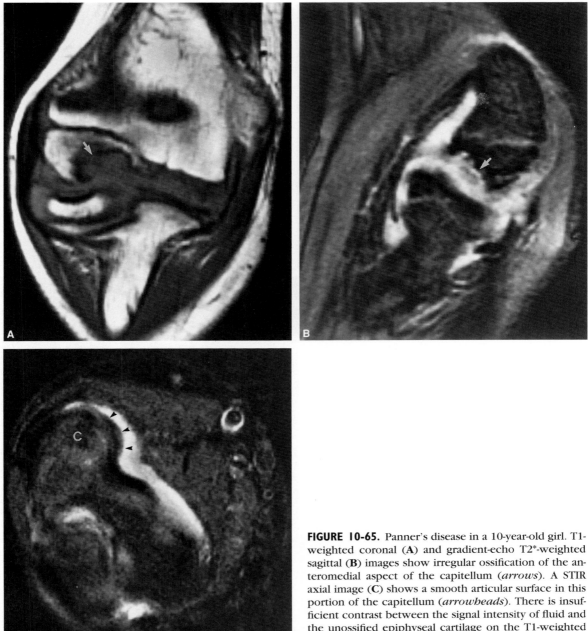

FIGURE 10-65. Panner's disease in a 10-year-old girl. T1-weighted coronal (**A**) and gradient-echo T2*-weighted sagittal (**B**) images show irregular ossification of the anteromedial aspect of the capitellum (*arrows*). A STIR axial image (**C**) shows a smooth articular surface in this portion of the capitellum (*arrowheads*). There is insufficient contrast between the signal intensity of fluid and the unossified epiphyseal cartilage on the T1-weighted (**A**) and the T2* weighted (**B**) scans to determine if the surface of the cartilage is intact. C, capitellum.

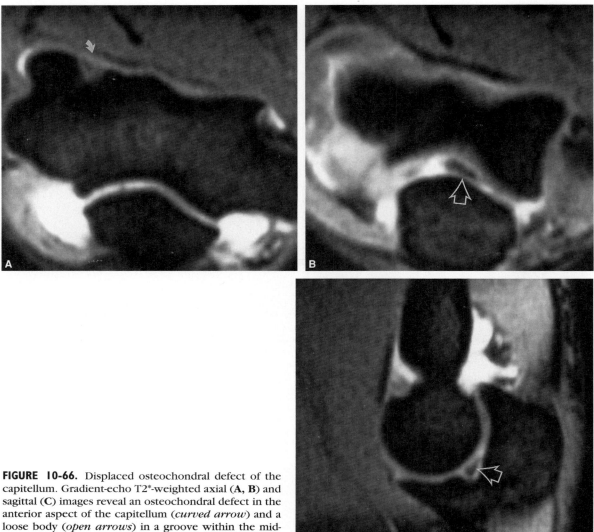

FIGURE 10-66. Displaced osteochondral defect of the capitellum. Gradient-echo T2*-weighted axial (**A, B**) and sagittal (**C**) images reveal an osteochondral defect in the anterior aspect of the capitellum (*curved arrow*) and a loose body (*open arrows*) in a groove within the mid-portion of the trochlear notch of the ulna.

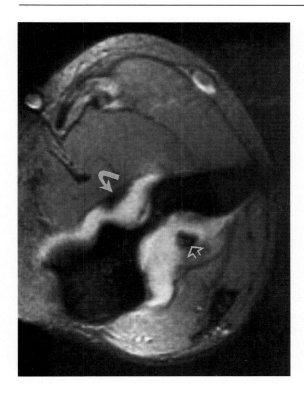

FIGURE 10-67. Loose bodies. The loose body in the anterior compartment (*curved arrow*) is apparently attached to the synovium since it does not appear to respect gravity and sink posteriorly toward the humerus. A posterior compartment loose body (*open arrow*) is also noted on this gradient-echo T2*-weighted axial image.

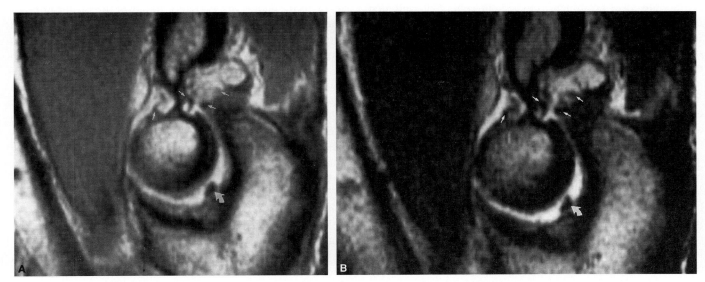

FIGURE 10-68. Loose body and synovitis. Proton density (**A**) and T2-weighted sagittal (**B**) images reveal a small loose body in the central aspect of the trochlear notch of the ulna (*curved white arrows*). Curvilinear foci of synovial thickening (*small white arrows*) should not be mistaken for loose bodies.

growth process may continue as long as the loose body is exposed to synovial fluid. Loose bodies may attach to the synovium or may float freely within the joint space (Fig. 10-67). A change in position of a loose body over sequential imaging studies indicates that it is freely mobile. Similarly, movement of a loose body with changes in position of the elbow joint on a particular imaging study also indicates that the loose body is not firmly attached to the synovium.

Large loose bodies are well seen with MR imaging, especially when an effusion is present.[133] Small loose bodies may be more difficult to detect and differentiate from other foci of signal void, such as thickened synovium (Fig. 10-68). Air bubbles may also mimic loose bodies on MR images.[134] Small air bubbles may arise naturally from vacuum phenomenon or may be introduced iatrogenically during aspiration or injection of fluid (Fig. 10-69; see Fig. 10-63). Vacuum phenomenon is unusual in the elbow joint, but small bubbles are commonly seen with MR arthrography. Even with good arthrographic technique, it is not uncommon to inject several small air bubbles into the joint that may mimic loose bodies on MR images. Air bubbles can be recognized by a characteristic margin of high signal adjacent to the signal void (due to a magnetic susceptibility artifact) which is not found along the margins of a real loose body. Multiple foci of magnetic susceptibility artifact have a similar appearance and may also be seen at the site of micrometallic deposition associated with prior surgery. These foci of magnetic susceptibility artifact are most prominent on gradient-echo T2*-weighted images. Loose bodies may become quite large and result in mechanical symptoms such as locking and limitation of motion. Most patients present with loss of motion, usually extension. Pain is variably present and usually occurs with a sensation of grating or locking.[130] Symptomatic loose bodies are usually arthroscopically removed when detected, because they may lead to premature degenerative arthritis in addition to their effects on joint function.[135]

The group of patients who benefit most from elbow arthroscopy are those with loose bodies.[136,137] Accurate diagnosis of loose bodies is important prior to arthroscopy to avoid the unnecessary expense and potential complications of a surgical procedure. Plain films are routinely obtained prior to arthrography, but may be unreliable. Indeed, in one recent study, there was no radiographic demonstration of loose bodies in 7 of 23 patients treated with arthroscopic removal.[136] Osteophytes and periarticular ossification may be mistaken for intraarticular loose bodies on radiographs. Noncalcified chondral loose bodies cannot be visualized on CT or radiographs, but can be identified with MR imaging. Calcified loose bodies are quite conspicuous on MR imaging, especially with gradient-echo T2*-weighted sequences. They may appear slightly larger than their actual size on gradient-echo T2*-weighted images as a result of magnetic susceptibility effects that are normally dampened by the 180° refocusing pulse on spin-echo images.

Loose bodies may lie anywhere within the elbow joint but are most commonly seen anteriorly.[138] In throwing ath-

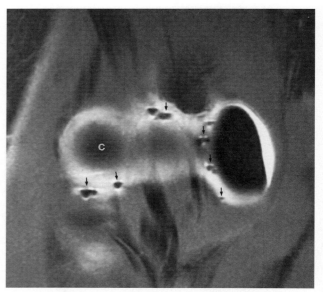

FIGURE 10-69. Air bubbles inadvertently injected at MR arthrography. A fat-suppressed T1-weighted coronal image performed after dilute gadolinium was injected into the elbow joint. Multiple small air bubbles are noted anteriorly that should not be mistaken for loose bodies (*small black arrows*). Fewer air bubbles, as a consequence of a diagnostic aspiration or therapeutic injection, may be more confusing than this case, especially if the radiologist is unaware that such a procedure was done. C, capitellum.

letes, loose bodies are typically found in the posterior compartment as a result of the incongruity of the olecranon and the olecranon fossa that develops from chronic valgus stress.[139,140] Loose bodies may also lodge in the midportion of the trochlear notch of the ulna (see Figs. 10-66 and 10-68). The predilection of loose bodies for this location may be explained by the normal anatomy of the trochlear notch, also referred to as the greater sigmoid notch of the ulna. The midportion of the trochlear notch contains a variably sized bare area that is normally devoid of articular cartilage. A deep groove with a strip of synovium and fat extends transversely across the trochlear notch at the junction of the olecranon and the coronoid portions of the proximal ulna[11] (Fig. 10-70). Loose bodies may lodge in this transverse groove or at the margins of this groove, where the ulna is normally somewhat constricted. This normal waist or constriction in the midportion of the trochlear notch should not be mistaken for an osteochondral defect (see Fig. 10-70). A thin transverse bony ridge may also extend across this portion of the trochlear notch, which lacks articular cartilage and should not be mistaken for an intraarticular osteophyte or a loose body on a single sagittal MR image.[141]

Os Supratrochleare Dorsale

The os supratrochleare dorsale is an accessory ossicle that lies within the olecranon fossa of the humerus.[130,142–144] Although it may be asymptomatic and discovered as an inci-

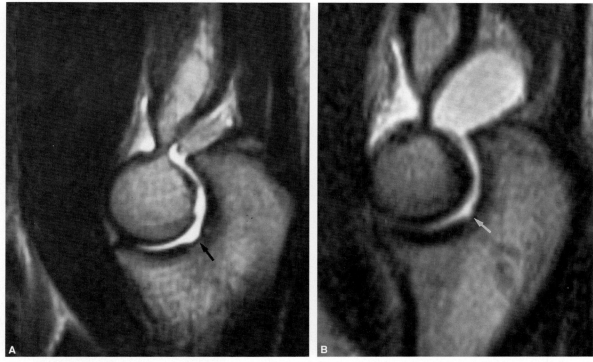

FIGURE 10-70. (A, B) Normal groove within the central aspect of the trochlear notch in two different patients. A variably sized nonarticular groove is seen in the midportion of the trochlear notch (*arrows*) and should not be mistaken for an osteochondral defect of the ulna. Loose bodies may lodge in this groove that is normally devoid of articular cartilage.

dental finding on radiographs or MR imaging, it also may be associated with pain and progressive loss of elbow extension (Fig. 10-71). The os supratrochleare dorsale may be subjected to trauma and impaction during forced elbow extension or hyperextension. Although it almost always involves the dominant arm and is more common in male patients, it is generally considered an accessory bone that is congenital or developmental rather than posttraumatic.

The precise origin of this ossicle is controversial because of its intraarticular location.[144,145] It is thought to arise from a separate ossification center that is partially within the olecranon fossa. In asymptomatic cases, the os supratrochleare dorsale tilts to allow the olecranon to enter the olecranon fossa during full extension.[145] In symptomatic cases, there is progressive enlargement of the ossicle through synovial nutrition, resulting in loss of elbow extension. Deepening and remodeling of the olecranon fossa may occur as the ossicle enlarges (Fig. 10-72; see Fig. 10-71). Fragmentation and sclerosis of the ossicle may occur as a result of forced extension or hyperextension of the elbow. In such cases, the appearance of the olecranon fossa on MR imaging may be useful to differentiate posttraumatic osteochondral loose bodies from a fragmented os supratrochleare dorsale (Fig. 10-73). Differentiation of these entities is not clinically significant, however, since the treatment is the same whether the loose body was caused by trauma or not or was an os supratrochleare

dorsale that was subjected to trauma. If an os supratrochleare dorsale is painful owing to a direct impact, the symptoms should resolve with conservative treatment. If persistent pain, progressive loss of extension, locking, or catching is present, the ossicle can be removed arthroscopically or through a limited arthrotomy.[130]

MR imaging is also used to confirm the intraarticular location of a symptomatic os supratrochleare dorsale prior to arthroscopic removal. Posterior and superior displacement of the posterior intraarticular fat pad of the elbow and joint fluid along the margins of the ossicle on sagittal images confirm its location within the joint (see Figs. 10-71 and 10-72). The relatively large size of these ossicles at the time of presentation allows for accurate characterization with MR imaging. In general, small loose bodies are more difficult to accurately identify with MR imaging, because foci of synovitis, scarring, and small loose bodies also appear as foci of signal void on T2-weighted images (see Fig. 10-72). Routine radiographic correlation may be useful when attempting to identify loose bodies and to differentiate foci of synovitis.[133] CT is occasionally useful as a problem-solving examination when there is uncertainty regarding the presence of a small loose body on MR imaging. CT arthrography or MR arthrography may also help to differentiate periarticular ossification from intraarticular loose bodies by clearly delineating the joint space with contrast. In general, when there is a high clinical suspicion of loose bodies and the

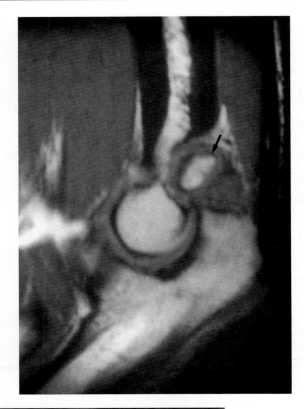

FIGURE 10-71. Symptomatic os supratrochleare dorsale in an 18-year-old man with posterior elbow pain and gradual loss of extension. A T1-weighted sagittal image reveals a large ossicle (*arrow*) within the posterior compartment of the elbow joint.

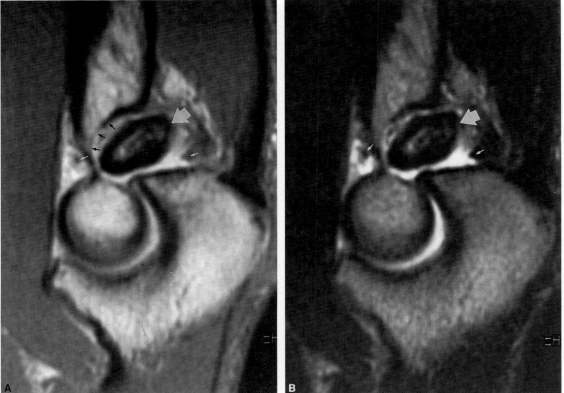

FIGURE 10-72. Symptomatic os supratrochleare dorsale and synovitis. Proton density (**A**) and T2-weighted axial (**B**) images reveal a large intraarticular ossicle (*large white arrows*). There is enlargement and remodeling of the olecranon fossa (*small black arrows*), probably caused by gradual enlargement of the adjacent os supratrochleare dorsale. Foci of synovial thickening (*small white arrows*) should not be mistaken for loose bodies.

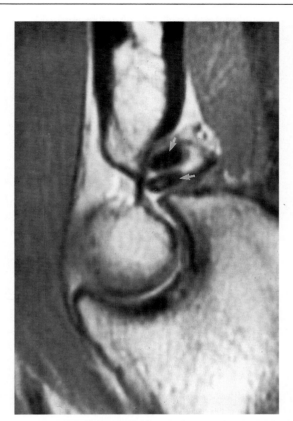

FIGURE 10-73. Posterior compartment loose bodies. A proton density sagittal image reveals two sclerotic loose bodies (*arrows*) that were treated by subsequent arthroscopic removal. There is no deepening and remodeling of the olecranon fossa to suggest fragmentation of a previous os supratrochleare dorsale.

initial radiographs are negative or equivocal, conventional MR imaging is the next best study. MR arthrography is then used if there is little fluid in the elbow on conventional MR imaging and the results are negative or uncertain.

Idiopathic Synovial Osteochondromatosis

Synovial osteochondromatosis is an uncommon disorder characterized by metaplasia of the subsynovial soft tissues that results in cartilage formation within the synovium.[146] This benign proliferative process may involve any joint, but predominates in the knee, hip, and elbow. It is almost invariably a monarticular process that occasionally arises within a bursa or tendon sheath. It may be sharply localized, multifocal, or diffusely present within the synovium of a particular joint (Figs. 10-74 through 10-76).

The average age of patients with synovial osteochondromatosis is about 40 years, and it occurs more commonly in male than in female patients (in a ratio of 2:1).[146] The disease process is typically predictable and self-limiting. In the elbow, there is usually a several year history of pain and swelling with progressive limitation of motion. Gross distension of the joint space may occasionally cause entrapment of

various nerves about the elbow.[147,148] Malignant degeneration has been rarely reported.[146]

This process may be called synovial chondromatosis or synovial osteochondromatosis, depending of the presence of enchondral bone formation within the multiple cartilaginous nodules. Some clinicians use the term synovial osteochondromatosis to encompass each of the progressive stages of this condition. The terms idiopathic synovial osteochondromatosis and primary synovial osteochondromatosis are used to differentiate this condition from the more common secondary causes of loose bodies, such as osteochondral fractures and osteoarthritis with degenerative fragmentation of the articular surface.[112,130,149]

Three progressive phases of idiopathic or primary synovial osteochondromatosis have been identified.[150] In the initial phase, there is active intrasynovial disease without loose body formation. In the transition phase, there is both active intrasynovial proliferation and multiple loose bodies, which may or may not be ossified. In the final phase, the process may apparently become quiescent with multiple osteochondral loose bodies and no active intrasynovial disease. The latter stages of primary synovial osteochondromatosis frequently result in destruction of the articular surfaces and secondary osteoarthritis.[146]

Patients with disease in the initial or transition stages of primary synovial osteochondromatosis are usually treated with complete synovectomy to prevent recurrence. Focal recurrence after surgery is not uncommon, however, as nests of synovium may be left behind.[146] Patients with disease in the final phase may not require synovectomy and may simply be treated with removal of the multiple osteochondral loose bodies.[150] Patients with loose bodies secondary to degeneration or trauma also do not require synovectomy, since the nidus for loose body formation is unrelated to metaplasia within the synovium.

Radiographically, there is usually calcification or ossification of the chondromatosis within the elbow that allows recognition of this condition. Widening of the joint space, bony erosions, and displacement of the intraarticular fat pads may also be seen on plain films. Secondary degenerative changes are frequently visible in the latter stages of the disease. In as many as one third of reported cases, there is no calcification or ossification present, making radiographic diagnosis difficult.[146] In these cases, CT reveals an intraarticular mass of approximately water density, contributing to the diagnostic difficulty and the erroneous impression of a large effusion. Arthrography or MR imaging is useful in identifying the mass of uncalcified chondromatosis in these cases (see Fig. 10-74).

The MR imaging appearance of idiopathic synovial osteochondromatosis reflects the variable gross pathologic appearance of this condition.[151] The most difficult cases to recognize are those that do not have visible calcification or ossification (see Fig. 10-74). The closely packed nodules of cartilage are bright on T2-weighted images and may mimic fluid on MR imaging, especially if the images are not prop-

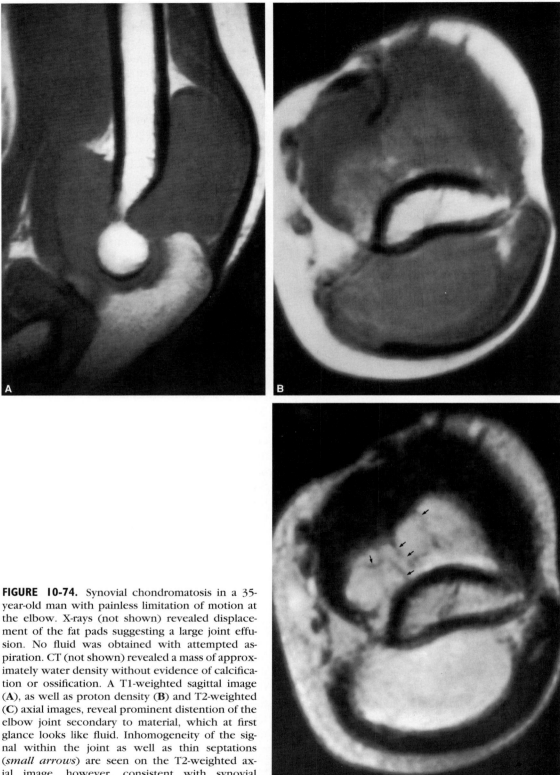

FIGURE 10-74. Synovial chondromatosis in a 35-year-old man with painless limitation of motion at the elbow. X-rays (not shown) revealed displacement of the fat pads suggesting a large joint effusion. No fluid was obtained with attempted aspiration. CT (not shown) revealed a mass of approximately water density without evidence of calcification or ossification. A T1-weighted sagittal image (**A**), as well as proton density (**B**) and T2-weighted (**C**) axial images, reveal prominent distention of the elbow joint secondary to material, which at first glance looks like fluid. Inhomogeneity of the signal within the joint as well as thin septations (*small arrows*) are seen on the T2-weighted axial image, however, consistent with synovial chondromatosis.

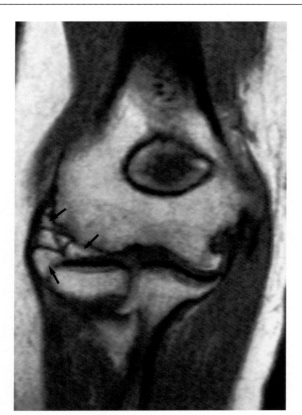

FIGURE 10-75. Localized primary synovial osteochondromatosis. A T1-weighted coronal image reveals multiple faceted bony loose bodies in the lateral compartment of the elbow (*arrows*).

erly windowed. Thin septations of decreased signal and somewhat decreased, heterogeneous signal intensity of the chondromatosis allow for differentiation from a simple effusion. Foci of signal void are present on all pulse sequences when there is calcification within the osteochondromatosis.[151] These foci of signal void are most prominent on gradient-echo T2*-weighted images. Multiple bony loose bodies with a low signal intensity cortical rim and central marrow fat are visible when there is ossification of the synovial chondromatosis in the more advanced stages of this condition (Figs. 10-75 and 10-76). Inhomogeneous enhancement of synovial osteochondromatosis may be seen after intravenous gadolinium administration.[151]

Biceps Tendon Injury

Rupture of the distal biceps tendon was once thought to be an unusual injury. Recently, however, it has become more commonly diagnosed and reported.[152–159] The vast majority of distal biceps ruptures occurs in men, with the injury involving the dominant arm in 80%.[160] The average age at rupture is 55 years, although body builders and weight lifters usually present at a younger age.[153] Anabolic steroid abuse has been implicated in some of these younger patients.[161] Complete rupture of the tendon from its insertion on the radial tuberosity is most commonly observed (Fig. 10-77). Complete tears of the distal biceps are thought to be much more common than partial tears.[154,162] MR imaging is useful in evaluating these injuries because degenerative tendino-

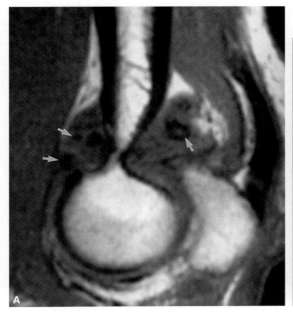

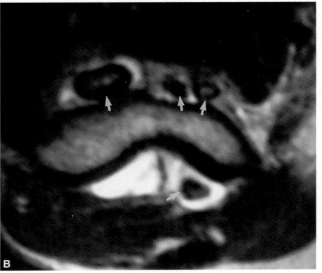

FIGURE 10-76. Diffuse primary synovial osteochondromatosis. T1-weighted sagittal (**A**) and T2-weighted axial (**B**) images reveal multiple osteochondral loose bodies (*arrows*) throughout the elbow joint. Thirty loose bodies were arthroscopically removed.

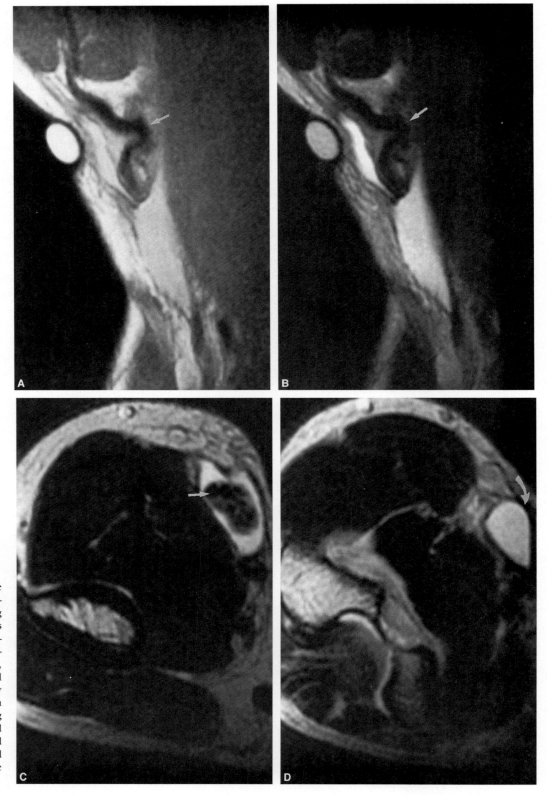

FIGURE 10-77. Rupture of the distal biceps tendon in a 38-year-old man who delayed seeking medical attention until 4 weeks after an acute weight lifting injury. Proton density (**A**) and T2-weighted (**B**) sagittal images, as well as a T2-weighted axial image (**C**), reveal a proximally retracted distal biceps tendon (*arrows*) with surrounding fluid. The tendon is thickened and folded back on itself. Fluid (*curved arrow*) is seen instead of the tendon at the level of the humeral epicondyles (**D**).

sis, partial tears, and complete ruptures may be distinguished.[30,155–158,163]

The biceps brachii is a long fusiform muscle that has two heads proximally and one tendon distally. The long head arises from the supraglenoid tubercle and the superior labrum at the shoulder joint, whereas the short head arises from the coracoid process in a conjoined fashion with the coracobrachialis. The two heads join to form a common muscle belly that ends in a flattened, horizontal distal tendon at the elbow. The distal biceps tendon averages approximately 7 cm in length and rotates laterally about 90° before inserting on the radial tuberosity[161,164] (Fig. 10-78). The tendon is coronally oriented proximally and sagittally oriented distally, at the radial tuberosity. The bicipital radial bursa separates the distal tendon from the anterior aspect of the radial tuberosity just proximal to the tendon insertion.[11] The distal tendon also has a flattened aponeurotic attachment known as the lacertus fibrosus that extends from the myotendinous junction to the medial deep fascia of the forearm. The lacertus fibrosus covers the median nerve and brachial artery that lie medial to the distal biceps tendon. The primary function of the biceps brachii is flexion of the elbow and supination of the forearm. Flexion of the elbow is assisted by the brachialis, which lies just posterior to the biceps. Supination of the forearm is assisted by the supinator muscle.

Rupture of the tendon of the long head of the biceps

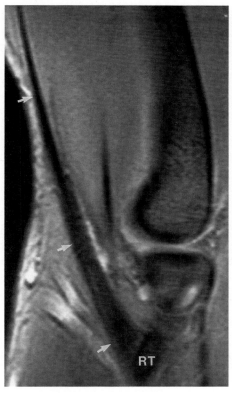

FIGURE 10-78. Normal distal biceps tendon. The biceps tendon (*arrows*) undergoes a 90° rotation as it extends along a 7-cm length from the myotendinous junction to the radial tuberosity (RT) as seen on this gradient-echo T2*-weighted sagittal image.

occurs commonly. It either avulses from the superior labrum or tears within the bicipital groove of the proximal humerus. Rupture of the short head of the biceps is rare. Rupture of the biceps muscle belly or the myotendinous junction, as well as midsubstance rupture of the distal tendon, are considered rare injuries that may occur secondary to direct trauma.[165,166]

The mechanism of distal biceps tendon injury usually involves eccentric contraction of the biceps against resistance, as typically occurs in weight lifters or manual laborers who are attempting to lift a heavy object. The bicipital aponeurosis (lacertus fibrosus) is usually damaged to varying degrees at the time of biceps tendon rupture, but may remain intact (Fig. 10-79). In some cases, the distal biceps tendon may rupture in stages, first with avulsion of the tendon, then followed by secondary tearing of the lacertus fibrosus, which allows proximal retraction of the biceps[154,162] (Fig. 10-80). In cases where the lacertus fibrosus remains intact, there is minimal retraction of the muscle and clinical diagnosis can be difficult.[160] Although flexion power at the elbow may be preserved with an intact lacertus fibrosus, supination of the forearm usually is weakened due to the biceps tendon detachment from the radial tuberosity.

Distal biceps tendinosis is common and has been shown to precede spontaneous tendon rupture.[46] Tendinosis of the distal biceps is probably a multifactorial process that involves repetitive mechanical impingement of a poorly vascularized distal segment of the tendon (Fig. 10-81). Irregularity of the radial tuberosity and chronic inflammation of the adjacent radial bicipital bursa may also contribute.[167,168] There is a zone of relatively poor blood supply within the distal biceps tendon, approximately 10 mm from its insertion on the radial tuberosity.[164] This hypovascular zone may be impinged between the radius and the ulna during pronation. CT and MR studies of pronation in asymptomatic volunteers showed that the space between the radius and ulna progressively narrows (by 50%) during pronation. On average, this space is approximately 8 mm in supination, 6 mm in neutral position, and 4 mm in pronation.[164] Repetitive impingement during pronation, coupled with an intrinsically poor blood supply to the distal biceps tendon, may result in a failed healing response and degenerative tendinosis. Enlargement of the degenerated tendon, as well as irregularity and hypertrophy of the radial tuberosity, may lead to inflammation of the adjacent bursa. Each of these factors may contribute to worsening impingement between the radial tuberosity and the ulna, leading to further degeneration of the distal biceps tendon (Fig. 10-82). This process may ultimately result in complete tendon rupture, or, less commonly, partial tendon rupture or bursitis.

The distal biceps tendon is covered by an extrasynovial paratenon and is separated from the radial tuberosity by the bicipital radial bursa. Inflammation of this cubital bursa may accompany tendinosis and tearing of the distal biceps (Fig. 10-83). Enlargement of the bicipital radial bursa may occasionally present as a nonspecific antecubital fossa mass as

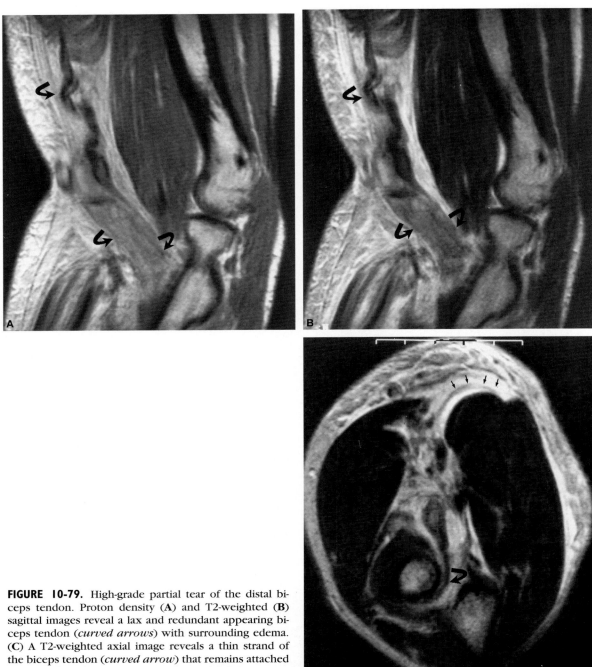

FIGURE 10-79. High-grade partial tear of the distal biceps tendon. Proton density (**A**) and T2-weighted (**B**) sagittal images reveal a lax and redundant appearing biceps tendon (*curved arrows*) with surrounding edema. (**C**) A T2-weighted axial image reveals a thin strand of the biceps tendon (*curved arrow*) that remains attached to the radial tuberosity. Increased signal delineates rupture of the lacertus fibrosus (*small black arrows*).

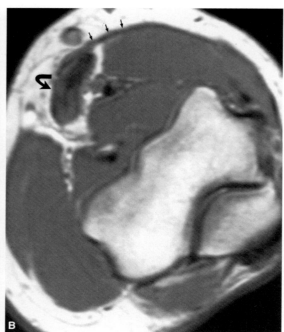

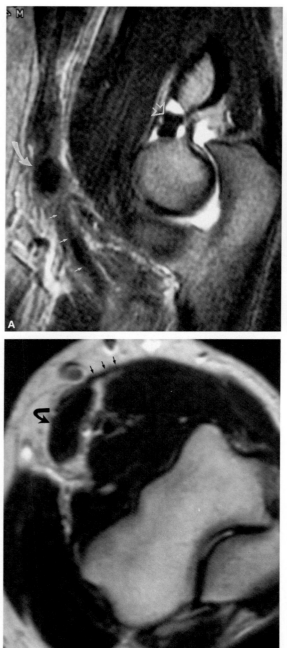

FIGURE 10-80. Old partial biceps tendon tear in a 42-year-old man with painful limitation of elbow flexion. **(A)** A T2-weighted sagittal image displays an unsuspected loose body (*open arrow*) in the anterior aspect of the elbow joint, explaining the loss of full flexion. The proximal biceps tendon is thickened (*curved arrow*), whereas the distal portion of the tendon is abnormally thin (*small white arrows*). Proton density **(B)** and T2-weighted **(C)** axial images reveal increased signal and thickening of the biceps tendon (*curved black arrow*) as well as thickening of the lacertus fibrosus (*small black arrows*), consistent with scarring from a prior partial tear.

large as 5 cm in diameter.[168,169] Intravenous gadolinium is helpful in the recognition of this enlarged bursa on MR imaging, and may allow differentiation of this benign entity from a solid neoplasm.[169] Cubital bursitis, tendinosis, and partial tendon rupture may coexist to differing degrees and may be impossible to distinguish clinically.[154,168] Cubital bursitis and partial tendon rupture may both cause irritation of the adjacent median nerve, further complicating the clinical findings.[168,170]

T2-weighted axial images are most useful for determining the degree of tendon tearing. The axial images should extend from the musculotendinous junction to the insertion of the tendon on the radial tuberosity. Axial images also are useful for evaluating the lacertus fibrosus (see Fig. 10-80). The status of the lacertus on MR imaging is usually not a critical issue because this structure is typically not included in surgical repair of a ruptured biceps tendon. However, surgical repair of a symptomatic lacertus fibrosus rupture has been reported along with repair of a partial tear of the biceps tendon.[162]

MR imaging provides useful information for preoperative planning, including the degree of tearing, the size of the

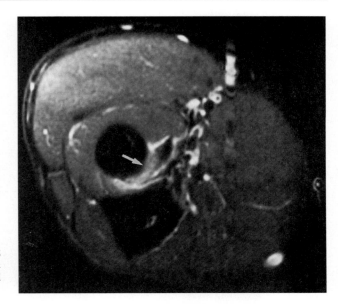

FIGURE 10-81. Distal biceps tendinosis. Axial STIR image demonstrating prominent increased signal within the distal fibers of the biceps tendon (*arrow*), consistent with severe degenerative tendinosis. A discrete partial tear or rupture is not identified.

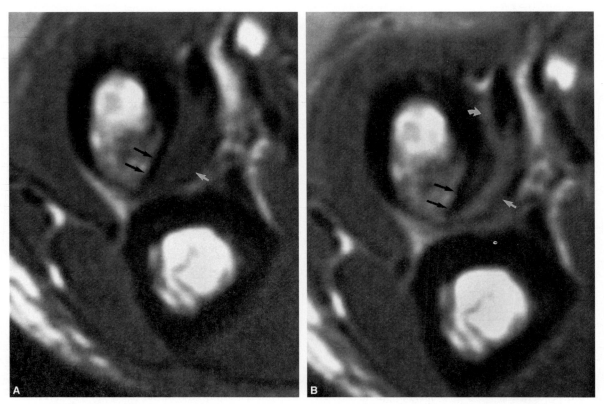

FIGURE 10-82. Distal biceps impingement syndrome. On scans performed with the arm not fully pronated, T1-weighted axial images before (**A**) and after (**B**) intravenous administration of gadolinium reveal prominence of the radial tuberosity (*black arrows*). Further pronation causes impingement of the biceps tendon between the radial tuberosity and the ulna. Abnormal signal is noted in the biceps tendon, which enhances with gadolinium consistent with tendinosis (*straight white arrows*). The synovium within the bicipital radial bursa also enhances with contrast (*curved arrow*).

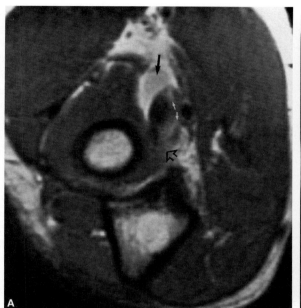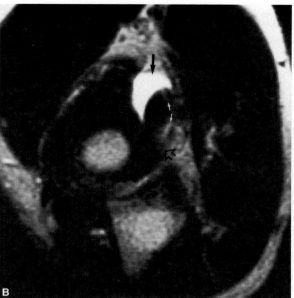

FIGURE 10-83. Bursitis, tendinosis, and mild intrasubstance partial tearing of the distal biceps tendon. Proton density (**A**) and T2-weighted (**B**) axial images reveal prominent distention of the bicipital radial bursa (*black arrows*). The bursa separates the biceps tendon from the radial tuberosity more distally. Moderately increased signal in the biceps tendon (*open arrows*) normalizes in signal on the T2-weighted image, consistent with degenerative tendinosis. A small longitudinal split (*small white arrows*) is seen in the medial aspect of the thickened tendon.

gap, and the location of the tear (see Fig. 10-77). The tendon typically tears from its attachment on the radial tuberosity as a result of attempted elbow flexion against resistance.[38] Other injuries that may occur via the same mechanism include avulsion and strain of the brachialis as well as disruption of the annular ligament with anterior dislocation of the radial head. These rare injuries also may be identified with MR imaging.[155]

Rupture of the distal biceps tendon is generally treated with prompt surgical repair and reattachment to the radial tuberosity to restore flexion and supination strength. Surgical repair may be complicated by radial nerve injury or heterotopic bone formation, resulting in radioulnar synostosis.[171] Early diagnosis of biceps tendon rupture is important because the surgical outcome is improved in patients treated during the first several weeks after injury.[159] After several months, the tendon retracts into the substance of the biceps muscle, making retrieval and reattachment more complicated. In such cases MR imaging may be useful to confirm the clinical diagnosis and to plan reconstructive surgery. Reattachment of a chronically retracted biceps to the radial tuberosity has a significantly higher risk of radial nerve injury.[160] In chronic ruptures, therefore, the retracted distal tendon may be attached to the brachialis muscle or the ulnar tuberosity to avoid injury to the radial nerve. These delayed repairs restore some flexion strength but do not improve supination weakness.

Triceps Tendon Injury

Rupture of the distal triceps tendon is one of the least common tendon injuries, with approximately 60 cases reported in the literature to date. Partial tears of the triceps tendon may occur, but are generally considered to be less common than complete ruptures.[172–174] Triceps tendon injury is being reported with increasing frequency[175–180] and has not been uncommon in our MR imaging practice.

The triceps muscle lies in the posterior compartment of the arm and is composed of three heads. The long head arises from the infraglenoid tubercle of the scapula. The lateral head arises from the lateral and posterior aspect of the humerus, and the medial head arises further distally, from the medial and posterior aspect of the humerus. The triceps is innervated by the radial nerve which passes between the lateral and medial heads in a bony groove along the posterior aspect of the humerus. The distal triceps tendon begins in the middle of the muscle and is initially composed of a small superficial layer and a more substantial deep layer. These layers then combine to form the tendon that inserts on the posterior superior surface of the olecranon. Typically, the triceps tendon tears at or adjacent to its insertion on the olecranon (Fig. 10-84), and usually retracts with a small fleck of bone imbedded in it. This small avulsion fracture may be detected radiographically in approximately 80% of reported cases.[173,174,181] Partial tears usually involve the cen-

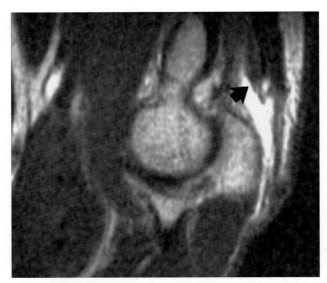

FIGURE 10-84. Acute triceps tendon rupture in a 40-year-old man with a history of surgical excision of the olecranon bursa 4 months before for chronic olecranon bursitis. A T2-weighted sagittal image reveals complete detachment (*arrow*) and retraction of the triceps tendon from the olecranon.

tral third of the tendon, adjacent to the olecranon[182,183] (Fig. 10-85). Rupture of the muscle belly or rupture at the myotendinous junction of the triceps may also occur, but is relatively rare.[184] The mechanism of injury in triceps tendon rupture usually involves forced flexion of the elbow against the resistance of a contracting triceps muscle. Such eccentric contraction of the triceps, which most commonly occurs during a fall on an outstretched arm, results in avulsion of the tendon at its bony attachment to the olecranon. Rupture of the triceps tendon may also occur secondary to a direct blow.[173,174,183,185] The mechanism of injury in sports-related triceps ruptures include a fall on an outstretched arm, a direct blow to the tendon, a decelerating counterforce during active extension, or some combination of these factors. Recent case reports indicate that the triceps tendon may also rupture during sustained extreme concentric contraction while weight lifting.[175,181,186] Both anabolic steroid abuse and local steroid injections have been implicated in rupture of the triceps tendon.[175,179,181,186] The detrimental effects of either systemic anabolic steroids[187] or local corticosteroid injections[56] on the strength of tendons have been documented. Athletes who use anabolic steroids are at risk for tendon ruptures as their excessive muscle strength is exerted on tendons that have become stiffer and absorb less energy prior to failure.[172,187]

The triceps tendon may rupture secondary to minor trauma if there is preexisting degenerative tendinosis.[46] Spontaneous rupture of the triceps has been reported in association with chronic renal failure and secondary hyperparathyroidism, Marfan's syndrome, and osteogenesis imperfecta, as well as in patients treated with oral corticosteroids for systemic lupus erythematosus or rheumatoid arthritis.[160,166]

Olecranon bursitis may mimic or accompany triceps tendon tears. It has also been suggested that olecranon bursitis may predispose to triceps rupture.[188] The presence of underlying triceps tendinosis may explain the association between olecranon bursitis and triceps tendon rupture. An additional factor may be the frequent use of local steroid injections in the treatment of olecranon bursitis. We have seen several cases of triceps rupture in patients who had been treated for olecranon bursitis. Moreover, we have seen both complete and partial tears of the triceps tendon in patients who previously underwent surgery for olecranon bursitis (see Figs. 10-84 and 10-85).

Clinical diagnosis of triceps tendon injury may be difficult due to pain and swelling that limit the physical examination. Clinical assessment focuses on the loss of extension power, which is seen with complete rupture. Unlike the biceps, there are no other muscles that substantially assist in extending the elbow. Indeed, a missed rupture of the triceps may result in severe functional impairment[160] (Fig. 10-86). Immediate surgery is considered the treatment of choice for complete rupture, whereas partial rupture may not necessarily require surgery. However, conservatively treated partial tears must be followed closely to ensure that complete disruption and retraction of the tendon does not develop. Cases that present late with a large gap in the triceps require reconstruction. Reconstruction has less reliable results compared with simple repair at the time of injury.[160,185]

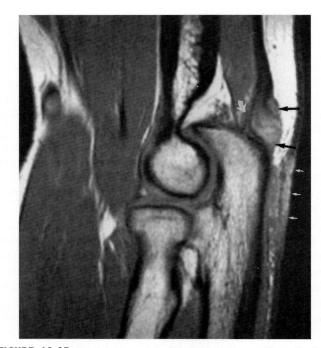

FIGURE 10-85. Partial triceps tendon rupture in a college football player who previously had removal of the olecranon bursa. A T1-weighted sagittal image reveals a gap (*black arrows*) separating the superficial fibers of the triceps tendon from the olecranon. The deep layer of the tendon (*curved arrow*) remains intact. Infiltration of the fat is noted at the site of a prior olecranon bursectomy (*small arrows*).

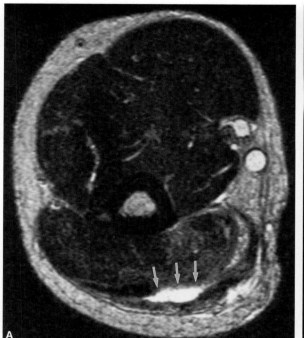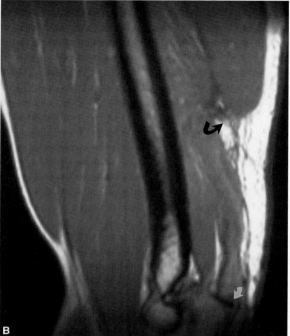

FIGURE 10-86. Chronic, retracted tear of the triceps tendon in a professional football player. **(A)** A T2-weighted axial image through the midportion of the upper arm reveals a fluid-filled defect within the central third of the triceps (*arrows*). This portion of the triceps tendon had retracted even further proximally, resulting in a large gap, atrophy, and functional disability. **(B)** A T1-weighted sagittal image shows prominent superior retraction of the central triceps (*curved black arrow*) from the olecranon (*curved white arrow*).

In patients who have fallen on an outstretched arm, there may be other associated injuries in addition to rupture of the triceps. In one group of 16 patients, concomitant radial head fractures and triceps tendon ruptures were noted.[189] Posterior compartment syndrome may accompany more proximal triceps muscle injury.[190] An interesting association of triceps tendon rupture and ulnar neuritis has been reported in two cases. In both cases, delayed surgery resulted in scar formation about the ulnar nerve.[183,186]

The consequences of overloading the extensor mechanism of the elbow depend largely on the age of the patient and the presence of preexisting tendon degeneration. Most often, the tendon ruptures at a site of degenerative tendinosis. In skeletally immature individuals, separation of the olecranon growth plate may occur and require internal fixation. The growth plate usually fuses at about age 14 in girls and age 16 in boys in an anterior to posterior direction. Closure of the olecranon physis may be delayed in pitchers, secondary to overuse and the repetitive traction of the triceps tendon.[161] This painful persistence of the olecranon growth plate in the throwing elbow usually responds to rest but may require internal fixation.[101] Acute overload of the extensor mechanism in an adolescent with a partially closed olecranon growth plate may result in a Salter-Harris type II fracture. These fractures are often radiographically subtle, and MR imaging may be useful in this setting to evaluate the extensor mechanism and detect occult injury to the growth plate.

Injuries of the triceps tendon and muscle are clearly seen with MR imaging.[30,177,178,191] The normal triceps tendon often appears lax and redundant when the elbow is imaged in full extension or mild hyperextension (Fig. 10-87). This appearance resolves when the elbow is imaged in mild degrees of flexion and should not be mistaken for pathology. Degenerative tendinosis is characterized by thickening and signal alteration of the distal tendon fibers (Fig. 10-88). Acute rupture is clearly seen on T2-weighted or STIR images due to surrounding fluid (Fig. 10-89). Partial tears are much less common than complete rupture and are more difficult to diagnose clinically.[182] MR imaging is useful for differentiation between complete tears that require surgery and partial tears that may heal well with protection and rehabilitation. MR imaging can also help delineate the degree of tendon retraction and muscular atrophy that is present when rupture of the triceps has been missed and a more extensive reconstruction of the defect is required (see Fig. 10-86).

Entrapment Neuropathies

The ulnar nerve is clearly displayed on axial MR images as it passes through the cubital tunnel.[192,193] The roof of the cubital tunnel is formed by the deep fibers of the flexor carpi ulnaris aponeurosis distally and the cubital tunnel retinacu-

text continues on page 828

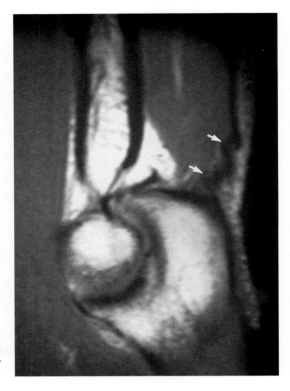

FIGURE 10-87. A T1-weighted sagittal image of the normal triceps tendon imaged in mild hyperextension reveals apparent laxity (*arrows*). This redundant appearance of the tendon is normal and resolves with flexion.

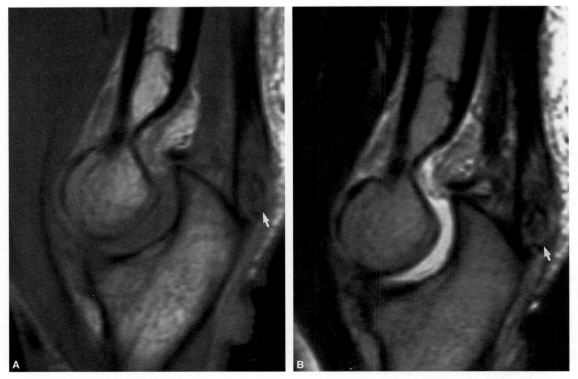

FIGURE 10-88. Degenerative tendinosis in a 57-year-old man. There is prominent thickening and increased signal intensity involving the triceps tendon on these proton density (**A**) and T2-weighted (**B**) sagittal images. A small focus of heterotopic ossification (*arrows*) is seen within the degenerated tendon. An os patella cubiti within the triceps tendon could have a similar appearance.

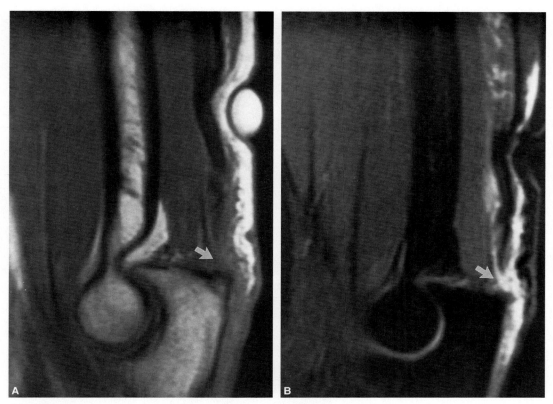

FIGURE 10-89. Acute triceps tendon avulsion in a professional football player. T1-weighted (**A**) and STIR (**B**) sagittal images reveal a small fluid filled gap (*arrows*) that separates the distal triceps tendon from the olecranon. The patient underwent surgical repair 2 days after the injury and recovered well.

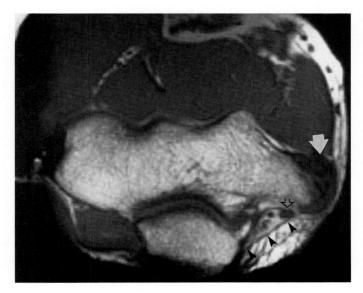

FIGURE 10-90. Anatomy of the cubital tunnel in a 36-year-old golfer with medial epicondylitis. A T1-weighted axial image reveals the normal ulnar nerve (*open arrow*) deep to a thin cubital tunnel retinaculum (*arrowheads*). There is thickening and mild increased signal within the common flexor tendon consistent with degenerative tendinosis.

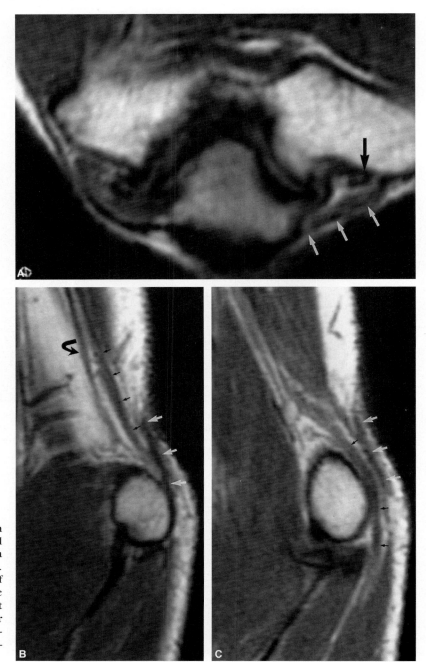

FIGURE 10-91. Thickened cubital tunnel retinaculum in a patient with ulnar neuritis. **(A)** A T1-weighted axial image reveals the ulnar nerve (*black arrow*) deep to a thickened cubital tunnel retinaculum (*white arrows*). **(B, C)** T1-weighted sagittal images show the course of the ulnar nerve (*small arrows*) passing beneath the thickened cubital tunnel retinaculum (*white arrows*) at the level of the medial epicondyle. Proximally, the ulnar nerve is just posterior to the medial intermuscular septum (*curved arrow*). The ulnar nerve then passes between the two heads of the flexor carpi ulnaris.

lum proximally.[194] The flexor carpi ulnaris aponeurosis is a triangular, tendinous arch that extends between the humeral and ulnar heads of the flexor carpi ulnaris muscle and forms the roof of the cubital tunnel just distal to the medial epicondyle and the cubital tunnel retinaculum. The flexor carpi ulnaris aponeurosis is also sometimes referred to as the arcuate ligament, although this term may be confused with the cubital tunnel retinaculum. Normally, during flexion, the flexor carpi ulnaris aponeurosis tenses as the MCL relaxes and bulges superficially.[195] These changes result in decreased volume and increased pressure within the cubital tunnel during.

The cubital tunnel retinaculum (sometimes referred to as the epicondylo-olecranon ligament, or the Osborne ligament or band) is normally a thin fibrous structure that extends from the medial epicondyle to the olecranon[196,197] (Fig. 10-90). Anatomic variations of the cubital tunnel retinaculum may contribute to ulnar neuropathy.[194] These variations in the cubital tunnel retinaculum, and the appearance of the ulnar nerve itself can be identified with MR imaging. A thickened cubital tunnel retinaculum (sometimes called the Osborne lesion; Fig. 10-91) results in dynamic compression of the ulnar nerve during elbow flexion and can be found in 22% of the population.[198] In 11% of the population, the

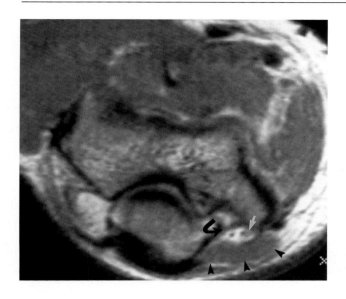

FIGURE 10-92. Anconeus epitrochlearis muscle replacing the cubital tunnel retinaculum. A T2-weighted axial image reveals the ulnar nerve (*white arrow*) deep to an anomalous anconeus epitrochlearis muscle (*black arrowheads*) and superficial to the posterior bundle of the medial collateral ligament (*curved arrow*).

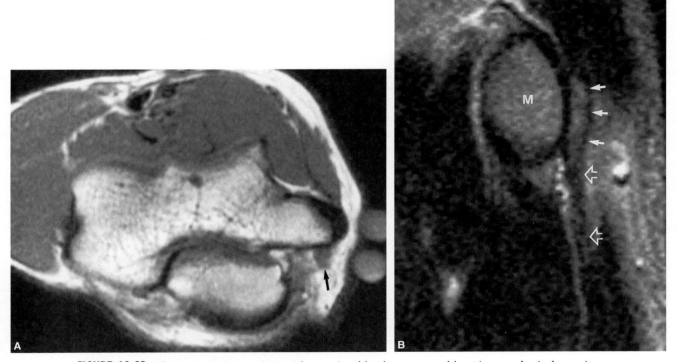

FIGURE 10-93. Ulnar neuritis in a patient with questionable ulnar nerve subluxation on physical examination. **(A)** A T1-weighted axial image reveals prominent enlargement and medial subluxation of the ulnar nerve (*arrow*). The overlying cubital tunnel retinaculum is developmentally absent, allowing anterior dislocation of the ulnar nerve during elbow flexion with subsequent friction neuritis. **(B)** A T2-weighted sagittal image reveals enlargement and increased signal intensity within the ulnar nerve (*solid arrows*) at the level of the medial epicondyle (M). The ulnar nerve appears normal further distally (*open arrows*).

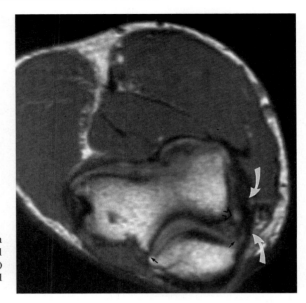

FIGURE 10-94. Ulnar neuritis in a 27-year-old professional pitcher. This proton density axial image shows thickening and medial bowing of the medial collateral ligament (*curved arrows*) as well as a medial loose body (*small open arrow*) and small spurs (*small arrows*) that undermine the floor of the cubital tunnel distal to the medial epicondyle.

cubital tunnel retinaculum may be replaced by an anomalous muscle, the anconeus epitrochlearis, which results in static compression of the ulnar nerve[194] (Fig. 10-92). In 10% of the population, the cubital tunnel retinaculum may be absent, allowing anterior dislocation of the nerve over the medial epicondyle during flexion with subsequent friction neuritis[13] (Fig. 10-93).

The floor of the cubital tunnel is formed by the capsule of the elbow and the posterior and transverse portions of the MCL. Thickening of the MCL and medial bony spurring may undermine the floor of the cubital tunnel and result in ulnar neuropathy[194,199,200] (Fig. 10-94). Heterotopic ossification in the MCL, underlying loose bodies, tumors, scarring, displaced fracture fragments (see Fig. 10-53), or ganglion cysts also may result in ulnar nerve entrapment.

MR imaging signs of ulnar neuritis and entrapment include displacement and flattening of the nerve adjacent to a mass, swelling and enlargement of the nerve proximal or distal to a mass, infiltration of the perineural fat, and increased signal intensity within the nerve on T2-weighted images.[141] Peripheral nerves are normally intermediate in signal intensity on T2-weighted images. The ulnar nerve must be followed carefully to avoid mistaking it for enlargement of the adjacent veins (Fig. 10-95). The posterior ulnar recurrent artery and the deep veins that accompany it are normally small structures that course with the ulnar nerve through the cubital tunnel. Enlargement of a deep vein may appear as a bright tubular structure on T2-weighted, gradient-echo, or STIR sequences, mimicking an edematous ulnar nerve.[141]

Surgical procedures for ulnar nerve entrapment include medial epicondylectomy, decompression of the nerve, and translocation of the nerve[201,202] (Fig. 10-96). Translocation or transfer of the nerve may be subcutane-

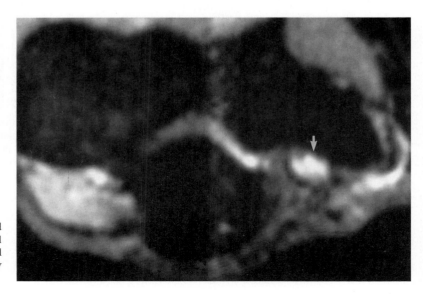

FIGURE 10-95. Ulnar neuritis. There is enlargement and increased signal within the ulnar nerve on this STIR axial image. The nerve was differentiated from adjacent small vessels on other images. Enlargement of these vessels may mimic an edematous nerve.

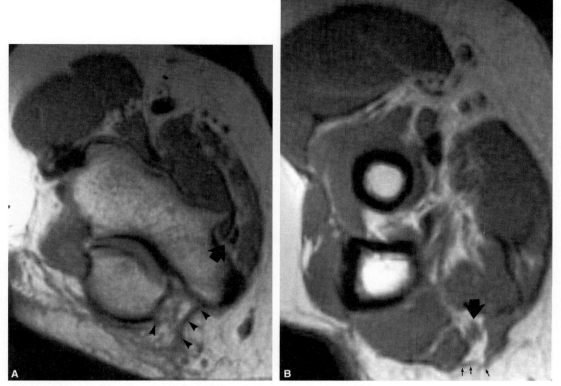

FIGURE 10-96. Appearance of the ulnar nerve after anterior submuscular transfer on proton density axial images. **(A)** The cubital tunnel retinaculum (*arrowheads*) has been divided and the ulnar nerve (*arrow*) has been transferred deep to the pronator teres muscle anteriorly. **(B)** Further distally, the ulnar nerve (*arrow*) has been decompressed by releasing the aponeurosis (*small arrows*) between the humeral and ulnar heads of the flexor carpi ulnaris.

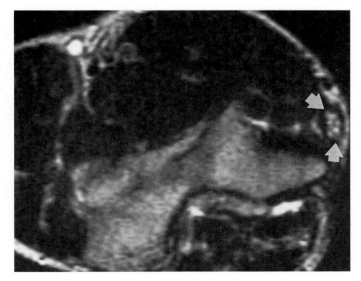

FIGURE 10-97. Appearance of the ulnar nerve after anterior subcutaneous transfer on a T2-weighted axial image. There is increased signal within the enlarged ulnar nerve (*arrows*) consistent with persistent neuritis. A rim of low signal intensity scarring surrounds the nerve.

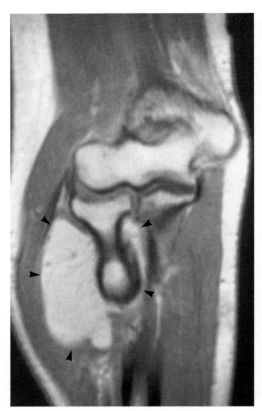

FIGURE 10-98. Radial nerve entrapment secondary to a lipoma. T1-weighted coronal image delineates a mass with fat signal intensity (*arrowheads*) adjacent to the radius, the branches of the radial nerve, and the extensor musculature of the proximal forearm.

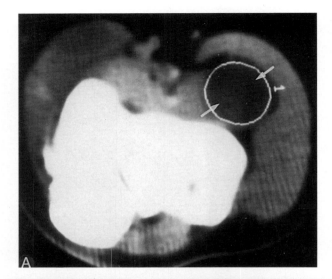

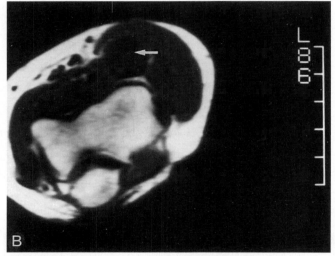

FIGURE 10-99. Entrapment of the radial nerve secondary to a synovial cyst arising from the anterior capsule of the elbow. **(A)** A CT scan shows a fluid density mass lying between the brachialis and brachioradialis muscles at the location of the radial nerve. The mass is isointense with muscle on the corresponding T1-weighted axial image **(B)** and homogeneously increased in signal intensity on the gradient-echo T2*-weighted sagittal **(C)** and axial **(D)** images.

continued

ous, intramuscular, or submuscular.[198] After surgery, low signal intensity scarring may be seen along the margins of the translocated ulnar nerve (Fig. 10-97). This finding also has been observed in patients with ulnar nerve subluxation and friction neuritis.

Entrapment of the median and radial nerves also may be evaluated with MR imaging. Median nerve entrapment may result from a variety of uncommon anatomic variations about the elbow, including the presence of a supracondyloid process with a ligament of Struthers, anomalous muscles, an accessory bicipital aponeurosis, and hypertrophy of the ulnar head of the pronator teres.[201,203] These anatomic variants and pathologic mass lesions (such as an enlarged radial bicipital bursa), which may entrap the median nerve, can be identified with MR imaging. Radial nerve entrapment may be caused by thickening of the arcade of Frohse along the proximal edge of the supinator muscle. In addition, parosteal lipomas may arise from the proximal radius and entrap the radial nerve[204] (Fig. 10-98). Ganglion cysts that arise from the anterior margin of the elbow joint may also compress the radial nerve[205] (Fig. 10-99).

MR imaging may be complementary to electromyography and nerve conduction studies in cases of nerve entrapment about the elbow.[193] In subacute denervation, the affected muscles have prolonged T1 and T2 relaxation times, secondary to muscle fiber shrinkage, and associated increases in extracellular water.[206] Therefore, entrapment of a nerve about the elbow may cause increased signal within the muscles innervated by that nerve on T2-weighted or STIR images (Fig. 10-100). These changes may be followed to resolution or progressive atrophy and fatty infiltration[207,208] (Fig. 10-101). Moreover, the site and cause of entrapment may be discovered with MR imaging by following the nerve implicated from the distribution of the abnormal muscles.[209]

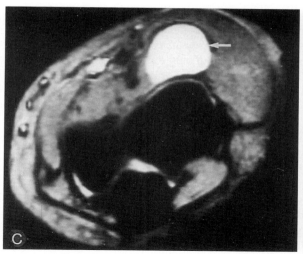
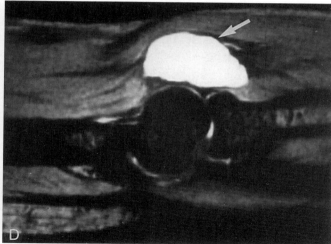

FIGURE 10-99. *Continued*

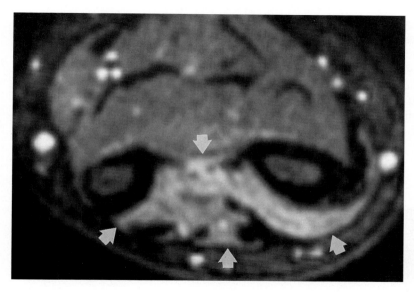

FIGURE 10-100. Subacute denervation of the forearm extensors secondary to entrapment of the posterior interosseous nerve (the deep branch of the radial nerve) at the level of the elbow. There is increased signal within the extensor muscles of the forearm (*arrows*) secondary to subacute denervation on this STIR axial image.

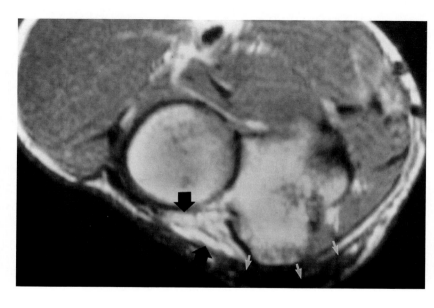

FIGURE 10-101. Fatty infiltration and atrophy of the anconeus muscle secondary to chronic denervation. There is prominent fatty replacement of the anconeus muscle (*large arrows*) on this proton density axial image. Low signal intensity scarring (*small arrows*) is noted at the site of a prior olecranon bursectomy that was complicated by damage to the innervation of the anconeus muscle.

Olecranon Bursitis

The bursae of the human body are generally divided into deep and superficial types. Although most of the deeper bursae are present at birth, superficial bursae, like the olecranon bursa, do not form until childhood in response to movement and function.[210] The subcutaneous olecranon bursa is the most common superficial site of bursitis in the body.[211] Deeper bursae have also been described in the olecranon region, and an intratendinous bursa (in the substance of the distal triceps tendon) may possibly be involved in tears of the triceps tendon and degenerative tendinosis.[211] An association has been also been suggested between subcutaneous olecranon bursitis and triceps tendon rupture.[188] Although a subtendinous bursa (between the triceps tendon and the posterior joint capsule) has also been described, pathology of this deep bursa is rarely identified.

Olecranon bursitis, called miner's elbow or student's elbow, is most commonly due to trauma, either acute or repetitive.[212,213] Traumatic olecranon bursitis is a common football injury, usually associated with artificial turf.[214] Other sports that commonly result in olecranon bursitis include ice hockey and wrestling. Olecranon bursitis may also be secondary to systemic diseases such as rheumatoid arthritis, gout, hydroxyapatite deposition, and calcium pyrophosphate deposition (Fig. 10-102). It is also commonly seen in patients undergoing hemodialysis. In patients with rheumatoid arthritis, the bursa may communicate with the joint, may rupture, or may dissect into the forearm—similar to a popliteal cyst about the knee.[211]

About 20% of patients presenting with acute bursitis have infection, most commonly due to *Staphylococcus aureus*.[215,216] Trauma usually precedes septic olecranon bursitis. In addition, steroid injections have preceded infection in about 10% of cases.[216,217] The source of infection may be hematogenous or it may be from direct spread from abrasions and cellulitis. MR imaging is useful for the identification of osteomyelitis, which sometimes develops in the underlying olecranon (see Fig. 10-49); however, this is thought to be uncommon.[211]

In chronic olecranon bursitis, there is usually chronic synovitis and fibrosis and nodules of granulation tissue are often present.[215] The synovitis and fibrosis may result in a complex appearance on MR imaging, which is difficult to distinguish from a solid mass. Alternatively, a solid neoplasm may occasionally be mistaken for olecranon bursitis (Fig. 10-103). In chronic bursitis, however, there is often spurring of the adjacent olecranon.[212,213] These spurs, as well as the tip of the olecranon, are usually resected in patients in whom conservative treatment has failed and removal of the bursa is necessary.

The MR appearance of olecranon bursitis varies, depending on the conditions that affect the bursa. Acute and chronic hemorrhage, as well as acute and chronic synovitis, result in a complex appearance of the olecranon bursa. In septic bursitis, there may be infiltration of the subcutaneous

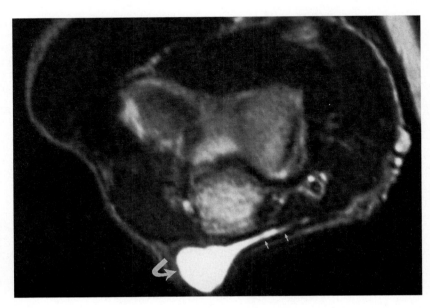

FIGURE 10-102. Olecranon bursitis, secondary to gout. A T2-weighted axial image reveals a well marginated area of homogeneous increased signal (*curved arrow*) as well as a thin pedicle that extends further medially (*small arrows*) consistent with fluid. The fluid lies within the olecranon bursa along the posterior margin of the olecranon and triceps tendon.

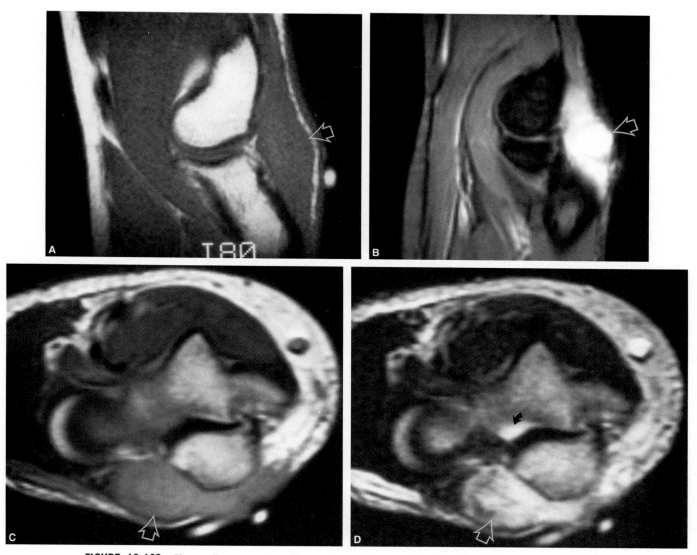

FIGURE 10-103. Clear cell sarcoma initially misdiagnosed as chronic olecranon bursitis on MR imaging. T1-weighted (**A**) and gradient-echo T2*-weighted (**B**) sagittal images reveal a seemingly homogeneous mass (*open arrows*) of increased signal that was mistaken for fluid. Proton density (**C**) and T2-weighted (**D**) axial images reveal a mass (*open arrows*) of heterogeneous increased signal that is less intense than joint fluid (*curved black arrow*).

fat and cellulitis. Osteomyelitis and abnormalities of the adjacent triceps tendon may also be seen on MR imaging.

Osteoarthritis

Osteoarthritis of the elbow is typically seen in patients older than 40 years of age who have a history of work- or sports-related overuse. This condition is more common in manual laborers and occurs much more frequently in men.[218] It involves the dominant extremity in 80% to 90% of cases and is bilateral in 25% to 60% of cases.[219,220] Patients often present with stiffness and loss of motion related to spurring and loose body formation as well as mild to moderate pain.[219] Radiographically, there is usually spurring of the anterior margin of the coronoid and the posterior margin of the olecranon. Both MR imaging and CT may be useful for differentiating bony loose bodies and spurs about the elbow joint.

Articular cartilage loss occurs in predictable locations within the elbow joint. Chondromalacia and chondral defects may be seen in the posterolateral aspect of the trochlear notch in throwing athletes.[221] In elderly individuals, articular cartilage loss is more common in the radiohumeral articulation rather than in the ulnohumeral joint.[10,222] Early chondral degeneration characteristically involves opposing surfaces at the medial margin of the radiohumeral articulation. The medial rim of the radial head and the adjacent crest at the lateral margin of the trochlea are the usual sites of early articular cartilage loss.[10] With progressive degeneration of the articular cartilage, there is usually involvement of the entire radial head and the anteroinferior aspect of the capitellum.

With optimal MR imaging technique, the thin articular cartilage of the elbow is clearly displayed (Fig. 10-104). Fat-suppressed sequences and MR arthrography are especially

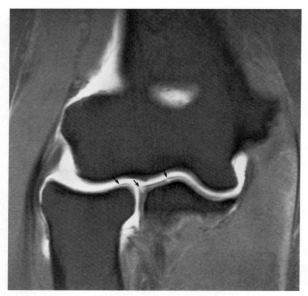

FIGURE 10-105. Mild articular cartilage degeneration. There is thinning of the cartilage overlying the central aspect of the radial head on this fat-suppressed T1-weighted coronal image performed after intraarticular injection of dilute gadolinium. Contrast extends into mild fissuring of the articular cartilage (*arrows*), and is also seen extravasating laterally through a defect in the lateral collateral ligament and common extensor tendon.

useful in demonstrating the chondral surfaces (Fig. 10-105). Deep fissuring or full thickness defects of the articular cartilage often result in abnormalities of the exposed subchondral cancellous bone and greater conspicuity on MR scans (Fig. 10-106). More advanced articular cartilage loss, associated marginal spurring, and loose body formation can all be seen with MR imaging (Figs. 10-107 and 10-108).

Rheumatoid Arthritis

Rheumatoid arthritis usually involves the elbow joint within the first 5 years of diagnosis of this condition.[223] Elbow joint involvement eventually occurs in 20% to 50% of patients. Patients usually present with painful distension of the joint capsule (Fig. 10-109). If synovitis is uncontrolled, there is erosion of the hyaline cartilage on the joint surfaces. Progressive destruction results in joint space narrowing and instability. The synovitis may herniate into the periarticular soft tissues, resulting in compression of the peripheral nerves about the elbow.[223] Rheumatoid synovitis may also produce large intraosseous synovial cysts (Fig. 10-110). These features of rheumatoid synovitis are clearly displayed on MR images. On conventional T1-weighted images, thickened synovium (see Fig. 10-109) is greater in signal intensity than fluid and demonstrates decreased signal intensity on T2-weighted images.[224] Gadolinium-enhancement (actively inflamed synovium enhances after intravenous administration

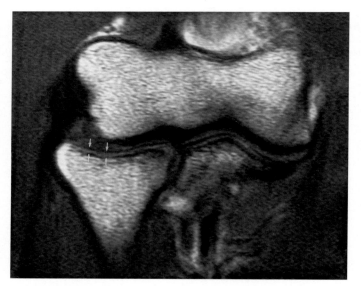

FIGURE 10-104. Normal articular cartilage. A thin layer of articular cartilage is clearly seen on this T1-weighted coronal image acquired with a 12-cm FOV and 512 × 256 matrix.

text continues on page 841

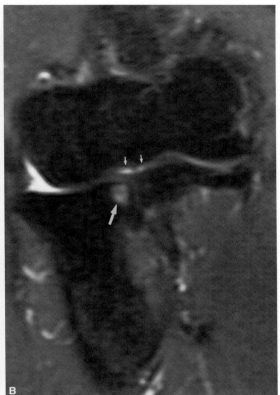

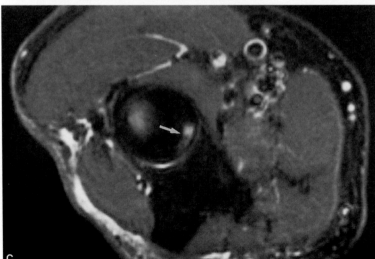

FIGURE 10-106. Mild articular cartilage loss. (**A**) A T1-weighted coronal image reveals small foci of decreased signal (*arrows*) in the medial aspect of the radial head and the adjacent crest at the lateral margin of the trochlea. There is minimal spurring of the capitellum and radius. STIR images in the coronal (**B**) and axial (**C**) planes show increased signal in the medial aspect of the radial head as well as fluid delineating small foci of cartilage loss (*small arrows*) in the crest at the lateral margin of the trochlea.

FIGURE 10-107. Radiohumeral osteoarthritis. There is articular cartilage loss and subchondral sclerosis (*arrows*) involving the radial head (RH) as well as the medial aspect of the capitellum (C) and the adjacent trochleocapitellar groove.

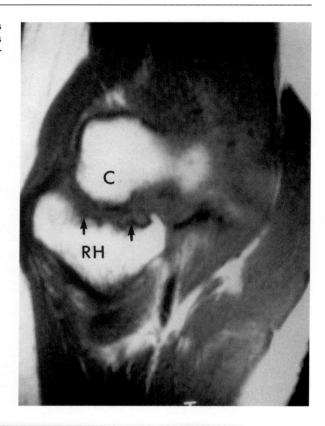

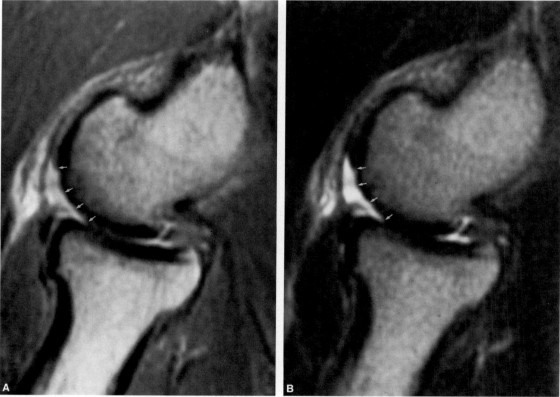

FIGURE 10-108. Osteoarthritis with articular cartilage loss. Fluid can be seen delineating a large chondral defect (*arrows*) in the anteroinferior aspect of the capitellum on proton density (**A**) and T2-weighted (**B**) sagittal images as well as T2-weighted axial images (**C**). There is also loss of articular cartilage covering the radial head as well as minimal marginal spurring throughout the elbow joint. *continued*

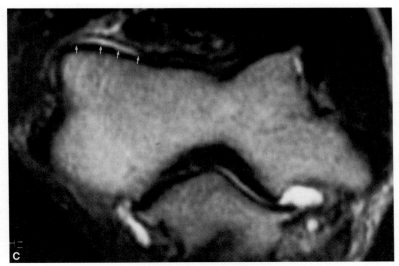

FIGURE 10-108. *Continued*

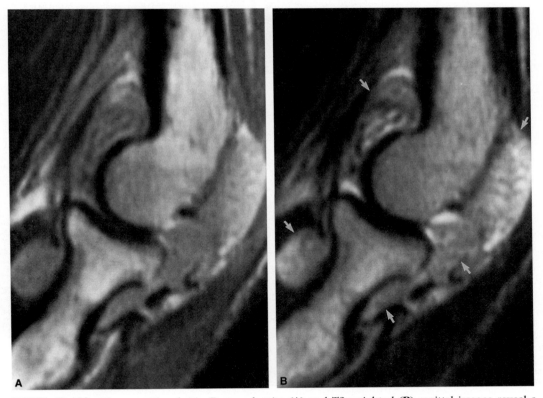

FIGURE 10-109. Rheumatoid arthritis. Proton density (**A**) and T2-weighted (**B**) sagittal images reveal a prominent distention of the elbow joint secondary to thickened synovium and pannus, which display intermediate signal intensity (*arrows*).

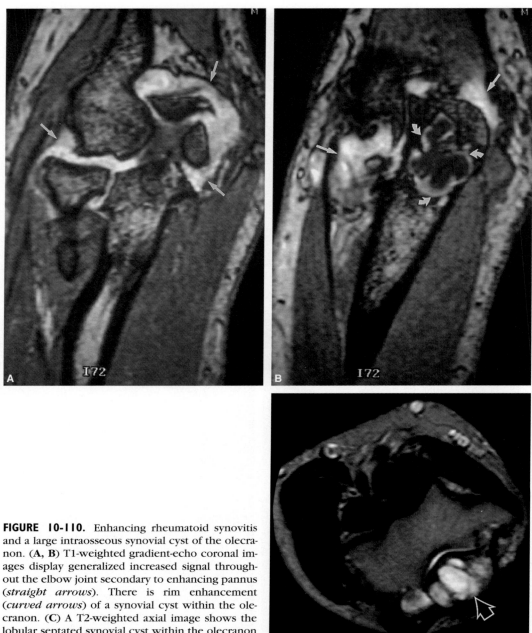

FIGURE 10-110. Enhancing rheumatoid synovitis and a large intraosseous synovial cyst of the olecranon. (**A, B**) T1-weighted gradient-echo coronal images display generalized increased signal throughout the elbow joint secondary to enhancing pannus (*straight arrows*). There is rim enhancement (*curved arrows*) of a synovial cyst within the olecranon. (**C**) A T2-weighted axial image shows the lobular septated synovial cyst within the olecranon (*open arrow*). (Courtesy of Peter Munk, MD.)

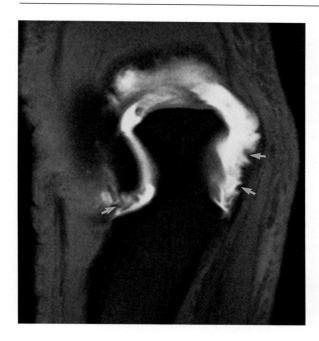

FIGURE 10-111. MR arthrography with intraarticular dilute gadolinium demonstrates mild synovitis. A fat-suppressed T1-weighted coronal image at the level of the olecranon (O) reveals mild corrugation and synovial thickening (*arrows*) in the posterior compartment compatible with synovitis.

of gadolinium [see Fig. 10-110]) may be necessary to differentiate fluid from acute synovitis in some cases.[225–227] MR arthrography, with either saline or dilute gadolinium, is also useful for the identification of synovitis (Fig. 10-111). MR imaging is especially helpful in providing objective evidence of synovitis in the early stages of rheumatoid arthritis, allowing diagnosis institution of treatment in a timely fashion.[228] MR imaging is also useful for characterizing the features of advanced rheumatoid arthritis when clinically indicated (Fig. 10-112).

Chronic pannus and fibrosis in rheumatoid arthritis may occasionally result in low signal intensity synovitis. This MR appearance, however, is more characteristic of the recurrent intraarticular hemorrhage and hemosiderin-laden synovium commonly seen in hemophilia[229–231] and pigmented villonodular synovitis.[232,233] Similar low signal intensity nodular synovial lesions may also be seen in hemodialysis-related amyloid arthropathy,[234] a recently recognized complication of long-term hemodialysis caused by the deposition of a unique form of amyloid derived from circulating beta$_2$-microglobulin.

Cat-Scratch Disease

Cat-scratch disease is a bacterial infection that results in regional adenopathy after inoculation from a scratch or puncture wound[235–238] (Fig. 10-113). The site of inoculation is most commonly in the hands and forearms, resulting in more proximal adenopathy about the elbow, axilla, and neck. Although a cat scratch is not always discovered, 93% of affected patients have a history of exposure to cats. An estimated 22,000 cases are diagnosed each year in the United

States, resulting in more than 2000 hospital admissions. Most cases occur in children and adolescents.[235,236,238]

Cat-scratch disease typically begins with a papule that appears 4 to 6 days after inoculation. The papule progresses to a pustule, which is followed in 3 to 4 weeks by regional adenopathy. The usual clinical picture is a single enlarged node, but multiple nodes are present in 24% of cases.[236] The adenopathy typically resolves within 3 months, but may persist for as long as 1 year.[236,238]

Involvement of multiple nodal sites is suggestive of either multifocal inoculation or dissemination of the disease.[236] Disseminated infection, unusual in immunocompetent patients with cat-scratch disease, may result in splenic or hepatic granulomata, mesenteric adenitis, multifocal osteomyelitis, encephalitis, and meningitis.[235–239] A systemic form of cat-scratch disease may occur in immunocompromised patients following organ transplantation or in patients with HIV infection. In immunocompromised patients with AIDS, the same organism that produces isolated regional adenopathy in immunocompetent patients may produce multiple lytic bony lesions as well as cutaneous proliferative vascular lesions.[240]

Histologic study of the affected lymph nodes in cat-scratch disease shows granulomas, stellate abscesses, and a nonspecific inflammatory cell infiltrate. The presence of each of these findings in the same specimen is highly suggestive of cat-scratch disease.[238] The causative organism, *Bartonella henselae* (formerly known as *Rochalimaea henselae*), is a gram-negative bacillus that may be identified on tissue stains.[241] Isolation of the organism responsible for cat-scratch disease has recently led to the development of an indirect fluorescent antibody test that has become widely available

text continues on page 845

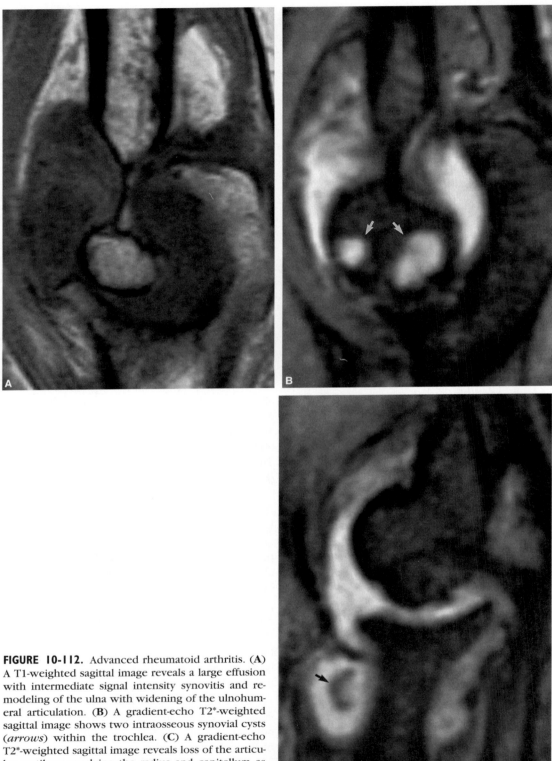

FIGURE 10-112. Advanced rheumatoid arthritis. **(A)** A T1-weighted sagittal image reveals a large effusion with intermediate signal intensity synovitis and remodeling of the ulna with widening of the ulnohumeral articulation. **(B)** A gradient-echo T2*-weighted sagittal image shows two intraosseous synovial cysts (*arrows*) within the trochlea. **(C)** A gradient-echo T2*-weighted sagittal image reveals loss of the articular cartilage overlying the radius and capitellum as well as a loose body (*arrow*).

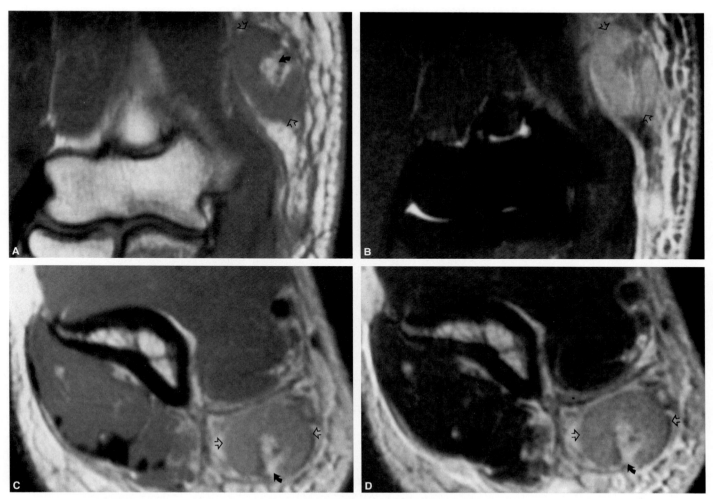

FIGURE 10-113. Cat-scratch disease. T1-weighted (**A**) and STIR (**B**) coronal images as well as proton density (**C**) and T2-weighted (**D**) axial images reveal a 3-cm mass (*open arrows*) in the medial subcutaneous fat just superior to the medial epicondyle. A central area of fat (*curved arrows*) that represents the hilum of an enlarged epitrochlear lymph node is noted. There is lymphatic infiltration and marked swelling of the adjacent tissue compatible with cellulitis.

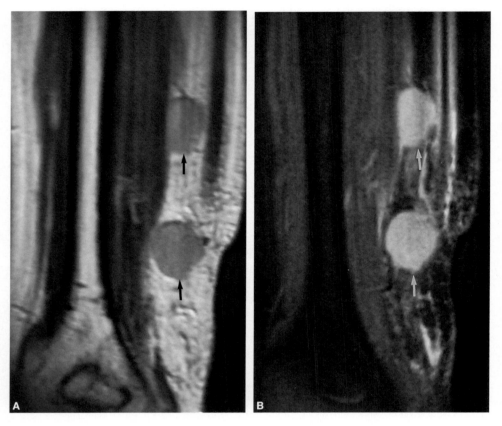

FIGURE 10-114. Biopsy proven cat-scratch disease in a 27-year-old woman believed to have a soft tissue sarcoma. T1-weighted (**A**) and STIR (**B**) coronal images reveal two adjacent masses (*arrows*). Mild swelling and lymphatic infiltration is seen in the adjacent subcutaneous fat, suggesting an inflammatory process.

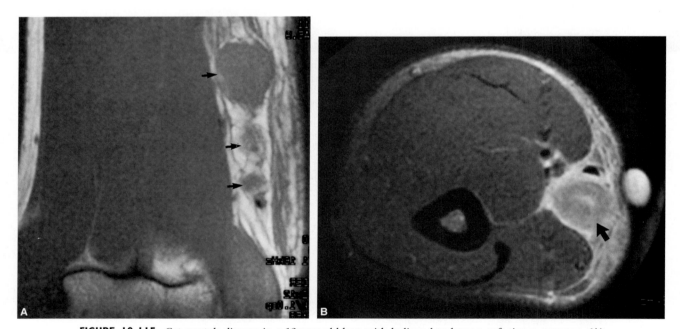

FIGURE 10-115. Cat-scratch disease in a 13-year-old boy with believed to have a soft tissue sarcoma. (**A**) A T1-weighted coronal image reveals a chain of three epitrochlear lymph nodes with swelling (*arrows*) and lymphatic infiltration of the adjacent subcutaneous fat. (**B**) A fat-suppressed T1-weighted axial image obtained after intravenous gadolinium administration shows enhancement of the largest epitrochlear lymph node (*arrow*) and enhancement of the surrounding cellulitis. The adenopathy gradually resolved without treatment over the next 2 weeks.

in the United States for serologic diagnosis.[238] Treatment of uncomplicated cat-scratch disease is controversial: some believe that the disease is self-limited, and antibiotics have not been shown to alter the course of the disease in immunocompetent patients.[230,233,237]

Epitrochlear adenopathy from cat-scratch disease may be mistaken clinically for a hematoma or sarcoma about the elbow, leading to MR imaging for further characterization of the mass[239,242] (Fig. 10-114). MR scans typically reveal a nonspecific mass of low to intermediate signal intensity on T1-weighted images and intermediate to high signal intensity on T2-weighted images. Gadolinium administration produces enhancement of the mass and surrounding lymphedema (Fig. 10-115). Central fluid that does not enhance with gadolinium may be present if there is central necrosis and liquefaction.[242] Suppuration of lymph nodes occurs in about 15% of cases,[238] and nodes typically range in size from 1 to 5 cm.[236] Lymphedema and infiltration of the surrounding fat due to cellulitis are characteristic.[242] The mass is located at the site of epitrochlear lymph nodes, adjacent to the medial neurovascular bundle and just proximal to the elbow. There may be associated axillary adenopathy. Additional clues to diagnosis on MR imaging include a central fatty hilum indicating a lymph node (see Fig. 10-113) or a series of contiguous soft tissue masses indicating a chain of nodes (see Fig. 10-114). Clinical correlation and serologic studies usually lead to the diagnosis of cat-scratch disease presenting as an epitrochlear mass on MR imaging. Recognition of the characteristic appearance of this condition may avoid an unnecessary biopsy (see Fig. 10-115).

References

1. Patten RM. Overuse syndromes and injuries involving the elbow: MR imaging findings. AJR 1995;164:1205.
2. Herzog RJ. Efficacy of magnetic resonance imaging of the elbow. Med Sci Sports Exerc 1994;26:1193.
3. Beltran J, Rosenberg ZS, Kawelblum M, Montes L, Bergman AG, Strongwater A. Pediatric elbow fractures: MRI evaluation. Skeletal Radiol 1994;23:277.
4. Potter HG, Hannafin JA, Morwessel RM, DiCarlo EF, O'Brien SJ, Altchek DW. Lateral epicondylitis: correlation of MR imaging, surgical, and histopathologic findings. Radiology 1995;196:43.
5. Schwartz ML, Al-Zahrani S, Morwessel RM, Andrews JR. Ulnar collateral ligament injury in the throwing athlete: evaluation with saline-enhanced MR arthrography. Radiology 1995;197:297.
6. Kingston S. Diagnostic imaging of the upper extremity. In: Jobe FW, ed. Operative techniques in upper extremity sports injuries. St Louis: Mosby-Year Book, 1996:31.
7. Ho CP. Sports and occupational injuries of the elbow: MR imaging findings. AJR 1995;164:1465.
8. Fritz RC. MR imaging of the elbow. Semin Roentgenol 1995;30:241.
9. Mirowitz SA, London SL. Ulnar collateral ligament injury in baseball pitchers: MR imaging evaluation. Radiology 1992;185:573.
10. Murata H, Ikuta Y, Murakami T. An anatomic investigation of the elbow joint, with special reference to aging of the articular cartilage. J Shoulder Elbow Surg 1993;2:175.
11. Morrey BF. Anatomy of the elbow joint. In: Morrey BF, ed. The elbow and its disorders, 2nd ed. Philadelphia: WB Saunders, 1993:16.
12. Conway JE, Jobe FW, Glousman RE, Pink M. Medial instability of the elbow in throwing athletes: treatment by repair or reconstruction of the ulnar collateral ligament. J Bone Joint Surg [Am] 1992;74:67.
13. Morrey BF. Applied anatomy and biomechanics of the elbow joint. Instr Course Lect 1986;35:59.
14. Morrey BF, An KN. Functional anatomy of the ligaments of the elbow. Clin Orthop 1985;201:84.
15. Jordan SE. Surgical anatomy of the elbow. In: Jobe FW, ed. Operative techniques in upper extremity sports injuries. St Louis: Mosby-Year Book, 1996:402.
16. O'Driscoll SW, Bell DF, Morrey BF. Posterolateral rotatory instability of the elbow. J Bone Joint Surg [Am] 1991;73:440.
17. O'Driscoll SW, Morrey BF, Korinek S, An KN. Elbow subluxation and dislocation: a spectrum of instability. Clin Orthop 1992;280:186.
18. Cohen MS, Hastings H. Rotatory stabilizers of the elbow: the lateral stabilizers. J Shoulder Elbow Surg 1995;4:S10.
19. Olsen BS, Vaesel MT. The lateral collateral ligament of the elbow joint: anatomy and kinematics. J Shoulder Elbow Surg 1995;4:S21.
20. Nestor BJ, O'Driscoll SW, Morrey BF. Ligamentous reconstruction for posterolateral rotatory instability of the elbow. J Bone Joint Surg [Am] 1992;74:1235.
21. Kvitne RS, Jobe FW. Ligamentous and posterior compartment injuries. In: Jobe FW, ed. Operative techniques in upper extremity sports injuries. St Louis: Mosby-Year Book, 1996:411.
22. Fleisig GS, Andrews JR, Dillman C, Escamilla RF. Kinetics of baseball pitching with implications about injury mechanisms. Am J Sports Med 1995;23:233.
23. Joyce ME, Jelsma RD, Andrews JR. Throwing injuries to the elbow. Sports Med Arthosc Rev 1995;3:224.
24. Timmerman LA, Andrews JR. Undersurface tear of the ulnar collateral ligament in baseball players: a newly recognized lesion. Am J Sports Med 1994;22:33.
25. Timmerman LA, Andrews JR. Histology and arthroscopic anatomy of the ulnar collateral ligament of the elbow. Am J Sports Med 1994;22:667.
26. Timmerman LA, Schwartz ML, Andrews JR. Preoperative evaluation of the ulnar collateral ligament by magnetic resonance imaging and computed tomography arthrography: evaluation in 25 baseball players with surgical confirmation. Am J Sports Med 1994;22:26.
27. Bennett JB, Green MS, Tullos HS. Surgical management of chronic medial elbow instability. Clin Orthop 1992;278:62.
28. Sugimoto H, Hyodo K, Shinozaki T, Furuse M. Evaluation of 3D fourier transform imaging for assessing throw injuries of the elbow. Radiology 1994;193P:413.
29. Gore RM, Rogers LF, Bowerman J, Suker J, Compere CL. Osseous manifestations of elbow stress associated with sports activites. AJR 1980;134:971.
30. Murphy BJ. MR imaging of the elbow. Radiology 1992;184:525.
31. Linscheid RL, O'Driscoll SW. Elbow dislocations. In: Morrey BF, ed. The elbow and its disorders, 2nd ed. Philadelphia: WB Saunders, 1993:441.
32. Josefsson PO, Nilsson BE. Incidence of elbow dislocation. Acta Orthop Scand 1986;57:537.
33. Nirschl RP. Elbow tendinosis/tennis elbow. Clin Sports Med 1992;11:851.
34. Coonrad RW, Hooper WR. Tennis elbow, its course, natural history, conservative and surgical management. J Bone Joint Surg [Am] 1973;55:1177.
35. Ollivierre CO, Nirschl RP, Pettrone FA. Resection and repair for medial tennis elbow: a prospective analysis. Am J Sports Med 1995;23:214.
36. Nirschl RP. Muscle and tendon trauma: tennis elbow. In: Morrey BF, ed. The elbow and its disorders, 2nd ed. Philadelphia: WB Saunders, 1993:537.
37. Vangsness CT, Jobe FW. Surgical treatment of medial epicondylitis. J Bone Joint Surg [Br] 1992;73:409.

38. Coonrad RW. Tendinopathies at the elbow. Instr Course Lect 1991;40:25.

39. DeSmet AA, Fisher DR, Heiner JP, Keene JS. Magnetic resonance imaging of muscle tears. Skeletal Radiol 1990;19:283.

40. Fleckenstein JL, Weatherall PT, Parkey RW, Payne JA, Peshock RM. Sports related muscle injuries: evaluation with MR imaging. Radiology 1989;172:793.

41. Fleckenstein JL, Shellock FG. Exertional muscle injuries: magnetic resonance imaging evaluation. Top Magn Reson Imaging 1991;3:50.

42. Fleckenstein JL, Weatherall PT, Bertocci LA, et al. Locomotor system assessment by muscle magnetic resonance imaging. Magn Reson Q 1991;7:79.

43. Speer KP, Lohnes J, Garrett WE. Radiographic imaging of muscle strain injury. Am J Sports Med 1993;21:89.

44. Resendes M, Helms CA, Fritz RC, Genant HK. MR appearance of intramuscular injections. AJR 1992;158:1293.

45. Garrett WEJ. Injuries to the muscle-tendon unit. Instr Course Lect 1988;37:275.

46. Kannus P, Jozsa L. Histopathological changes preceding spontaneous rupture of a tendon: a controlled study of 891 patients. J Bone Joint Surg [Am] 1991;73:1507.

47. Doran A, Gresham GA, Rushton N, Watson C. Tennis elbow: a clinicopathologic study of 22 cases followed for 2 years. Acta Orthop Scand 1990;61:535.

48. Jozsa L, Kvist M, Balint BJ, et al. Alterations in dry mass content of collagen fibers in degenerative tendinopathy and tendon rupture. Matrix 1989;9:140.

49. Regan W, Wold LE, Coonrad R, Morrey BF. Microscopic histopathology of chronic refractory lateral epicondylitis. Am J Sports Med 1992;20:746.

50. Gabel G, Morrey BF. Operative treatment of medial epicondylitis: influence of concomitant ulnar neuropathy at the elbow. J Bone Joint Surg [Am] 1995;77:1065.

51. Kurvers H, Verhaar J. The results of operative treatment of medial epicondylitis. J Bone Joint Surg [Am] 1995;77:1374.

52. Brogdon BG, Crow NE. Little leaguer's elbow. AJR 1960;83:671.

53. Nirschl RP, Pettrone FA. Tennis elbow: The surgical treatment of lateral epicondylitis. J Bone Joint Surg [Am] 1979;61:832.

54. Boyd HB, McLeod AC. Tennis elbow. J Bone Joint Surg [Am] 1973;55:1183.

55. Halpern AA, Horowitz BG, Nagel DA. Tendon ruptures associated with corticosteroid therapy. West J Med 1977;127:378.

56. Unverferth LJ, Olix ML. The effect of local steroid injections on tendon. Am J Sports Med 1973;1:31.

57. Morrey BF. Reoperation for failed surgical treatment of refractory lateral epicondylitis. J Shoulder Elbow Surg 1992;1:47.

58. Morrey BF. Surgical failure of the tennis elbow. In: Morrey BF, ed. The elbow and its disorders, 2nd ed. Philadelphia: WB Saunders, 1993:553.

59. Wittenberg RH, Schaal S, Muhr G. Surgical treatment of persistent elbow epicondylitis. Clin Orthop 1992;278:73.

60. Verhaar J, Spaans F. Radial tunnel syndrome. J Bone Joint Surg [Am] 1991;73:539.

61. Werner CO. Lateral elbow pain and posterior interosseous nerve entrapment. Acta Orthop Scand 1979;174(suppl):1.

62. Rosenberg ZS, Beltran J, Shankman S, Cheung Y. MR imaging of the elbow: potential pitfalls and normal variants. Radiology 1993;189P:310.

63. Clark RP. Symptomatic lateral synovial fringe (plica) of the elbow joint. Arthroscopy 1988;4:112.

64. Martin SD, Baumgarten TE. Elbow arthroscopy in sports medicine. Sports Med Arthosc Rev 1995;3:187.

65. Soffer SR, Andrews JR. Arthroscopic surgical procedures of the elbow: common cases. In: Andrews JR, Soffer SR, eds. Elbow arthroscopy. St Louis: Mosby-Year Book, 1994:74.

66. Osborne G, Cotterill P. Recurrent dislocation of the elbow. J Bone Joint Surg [Br] 1965;48:340.

67. Nevaiser JS, Wickstrom JK. Dislocation of the elbow: a retrospective study of 115 patients. South Med J 1977;70:172.

68. Letts M. Dislocations of the child's elbow. In: Morrey BF, ed. The elbow and its disorders, 2nd ed. Philadelphia: WB Saunders, 1993:288.

69. Timmerman LA, McBride DG. Elbow dislocations in sports. Sports Med Arthosc Rev 1995;3:210.

70. O'Driscoll SW. Classification and spectrum of elbow instability: recurrent instability. In: Morrey BF, ed. The elbow and its disorders, 2nd ed. Philadelphia: WB Saunders, 1993:453.

71. Josefsson PO, Gentz CF, Johnell O, et al. Surgical versus non-surgical treatment of ligamentous injuries following dislocation of the elbow joint. Clin Orthop 1987;214:165.

72. Josefsson PO, Gentz CF, Johnell O, et al. Surgical versus non-surgical treatment of ligamentous injuries following dislocation of the elbow joint: a prospective randomized study. J Bone Joint Surg [Am] 1987;69:605.

73. O'Driscoll SW. Elbow instability. Hand Clin 1994;10:405.

74. O'Driscoll SW, Morrey BF. Surgical reconstruction of the lateral collateral ligament. In: Morrey BF, ed. The elbow. New York: Raven Press, 1994:169.

75. Regan WD, Morrey BF. Fractures of the coronoid process of the ulna. J Bone Joint Surg [Am] 1989;71:1348.

76. Morrey BF. Current concepts in the treatment of fractures of the radial head, the olecranon, and the coronoid. J Bone Joint Surg [Am] 1995;77:316.

77. Josefsson PO, Johnell O, Wendleberg B. Ligamentous injuries in dislocations of the elbow joint. Clin Orthop 1987;221:221.

78. Limb D, Hodkinson SL, Brown RF. Median nerve palsy after posterolateral elbow dislocation. J Bone Joint Surg [Br] 1994;76:987.

79. Hallett J. Entrapment of the median nerve after dislocation of the elbow: a case report. J Bone Joint Surg [Br] 1981;63:408.

80. Morrey BF. Radial head fracture. In: Morrey BF, ed. The elbow and its disorders, 2nd ed. Philadelphia: WB Saunders, 1993:383.

81. Lynch TC, Crues JVI, Morgan FW, Sheehan WE, Harter LP, Ryu R. Bone abnormalities of the knee: prevalence and significance at MR imaging. Radiology 1989;171:761.

82. Mink JH, Deutsch AL. Occult cartilage and bone injuries of the knee: detection, classification, and assessment with MR imaging. Radiology 1989;170:823.

83. Vellet AD, Marks PH, Fowler PJ, Munro TG. Occult posttraumatic osteochondral lesions of the knee: prevalence, classification, and short-term sequelae evaluated with MR imaging. Radiology 1991;178:271.

84. Graf BK, Cook DA, De Smet AA, Keene JS. Bone bruises on magnetic resonance imaging evaluation of anterior cruciate ligament injuries. Am J Sports Med 1993;21:220.

85. Berger PE, Ofstein RA, Jackson DW, Morrison DS, Silvino N, Amador R. MRI demonstration of radiographically occult fractures: what have we been missing? Radiographics 1989;9:407.

86. Kapelov SR, Teresi LM, Bradley WG, et al. Bone contusions of the knee: increased lesion detection with fast spin-echo MR imaging with spectroscopic fat saturation. Radiology 1993;189:901.

87. Sebag G, Moore S. Effect of trabecular bone on the appearance of marrow in gradient-echo imaging of the appendicular skeleton. Radiology 1990;174:855.

88. Anderson IF, Crichton KJ, Grattan-Smith T, Cooper RA, Brazier D. Osteochondral fractures of the dome of the talus. J Bone Joint Surg [Am] 1989;71:1143.

89. Kovalovich AM, Schweitzer ME, Wapner K, Hecht P. Occult calcaneal avulsions: possible cause of pain in recalcitrant plantar fascitis. Radiology 1995;197P:156.

90. Weber WN, Neumann CH, Barakos JA, Petersen SA, Steinbach LS, Genant HK. Lateral tibial rim (Segond) fractures: MR imaging characteristics. Radiology 1991;180:731.

91. Morrison WB, Schweitzer ME, Bock GW, et al. Diagnosis of osteomyelitis: utility of fat-suppressed contrast-enhanced MR imaging. Radiology 1993;189:251.

92. Weatherall PT, Maale GE, Mendelsohn DB, Sherry CS, Erdman WE, Pascoe HR. Chondroblastoma: classic and confusing appearance at MR imaging. Radiology 1994;190:467.

93. Goldman AB, Schneider R, Pavlov H. Osteoid osteomas of the femoral neck: report of four cases evaluated with isotopic bone scanning, CT, and MR imaging (see comments). Radiology 1993;186:227.

94. Woods ER, Martel W, Mandell SH, Crabbe JP. Reactive soft-tissue mass associated with osteoid osteoma: correlation of MR imaging features with pathologic findings. Radiology 1993;186:221.

95. Assoun J, Richardi G, Railhac JJ, et al. Osteoid osteoma: MR imaging versus CT. Radiology 1994;191:217.

96. Moser R Jr, Kransdorf MJ, Brower AC, et al. Osteoid osteoma of the elbow: a review of six cases. Skeletal Radiol 1990;19:181.

97. Otsuka NY, Hastings DE, Fornasier VL. Osteoid osteoma of the elbow: a report of six cases. J Hand Surg [Am] 1992;17:458.

98. Hulkko A, Orava S, Nikula P. Stress fractures of the olecranon in javelin throwers. Int J Sports Med 1988;7:210.

99. Nuber GW, Diment MT. Olecranon stress fractures in throwers. Clin Orthop 1992;278:58.

100. Kviclera DJ, Pedegana LR. Stress fracture of the olecranon: report of two cases and review of the literature. Orthop Rev 1983;12:113.

101. Lowery WD, Kurzweil PR, Forman SK, Morrison DS. Persistence of the olecranon physis: a cause of ''Little League Elbow.'' J Shoulder Elbow Surg 1995;4:143.

102. Inoue G. Neglected intraarticular entrapment of the medial epicondyle after dislocation of the elbow. J Shoulder Elbow Surg 1994;3:320.

103. Wilkins KE. Fractures of the medial epicondyle in children. Instr Course Lect 1991;40:3.

104. Bede WB, Lefebure AR, Rosman Ma. Fractures of the medial humeral epicondyle in children. Can J Surg 1975;18:137.

105. Josefsson PO, Danielsson LG. Epicondylar elbow fracture in children. Acta Orthop Scand 1986;57:313.

106. Hines RF, Herndon WA, Evans JP. Operative treatment of medial epicondyle fractures in children. Clin Orthop 1987;223:170.

107. Harrison RB, Keats TE, Frankel CJ, et al. Radiographic clues to fractures of the unossified medial humeral condyle in young children. Skeletal Radiol 1984;11:209.

108. Peterson HA. Physeal fractures of the elbow. In: Morrey BF, ed. The elbow and its disorders, 2nd ed. Philadelphia: WB Saunders, 1993:248.

109. Klassen RA. Supracondylar fractures of the elbow in children. In: Morrey BF, ed. The elbow and its disorders, 2nd ed. Philadelphia: WB Saunders, 1993:206.

110. Jaramillo D, Hoffer FA. Cartilaginous epiphysis and growth plate: normal and abnormal MR imaging findings. AJR 1992;158:1105.

111. Jaramillo D, Waters PM. Abnormalities of the pediatric elbow: evaluation with MR imaging. Radiology 1992;185P:137.

112. Milgram J, Rogers LF, Miller H. Osteochondral fractures: mechanism of injury and fate of fragments. AJR 1978;130:651.

113. Mitsunaga MM, Adashian DA, Bianco AJJ. Osteochondritis dissecans of the capitellum. J Trauma 1982;22:53.

114. Ruch DS, Poehling GG. Arthroscopic treatment of Panner's disease. Clin Sports Med 1991;10:629.

115. Singer KM, Roy SP. Osteochondrosis of the humeral capitellum. Am J Sports Med 1984;12:351.

116. Morrey BF. Osteochondritis dissecans. In: DeLee JC, Drez D Jr, eds. Orthopaedic sports medicine: principles and practice. Philadelphia: WB Saunders, 1994:908.

117. Baumgarten TE. Osteochondritis dissecans of the capitellum. Sports Med Arthosc Rev 1995;3:219.

118. McManama GB, Micheli LJ, Berry MV, Sohn RS. The surgical treatment of osteochondritis of the capitellum. Am J Sports Med 1985;13:11.

119. Bauer M, Jonsson K, Josefsson PO, Linden B. Osteochondritis dissecans of the elbow: a long-term follow-up study. Clin Orthop 1992;284:156.

120. Kramer J, Stiglbauer R, Engel A, Prayer L, Imhof H. MR contrast arthrography (MRA) in osteochondrosis dissecans. JCAT 1992;16:254.

121. DeSmet AA, Fisher DR, Burnstein MI, Graf B, Lange RH. Value of MR imaging in staging osteochondral lesions of the talus (osteochondritis dissecans). AJR 1990;154:555.

122. Peiss J, Adam G, Casser R, Urhahn R, Gunther RW. Gadopentetate-dimeglumine enhanced MR imaging of osteonecrosis and osteochondritis dissecans of the elbow: initial experience. Skeletal Radiol 1995;24:17.

123. Winalski CS, Aliabadi P, Wright RJ, Shortkroff S, Sledge CB, Weissman BN. Enhancement of joint fluid with intravenously administered gadopentetate dimeglumine: technique, rationale, and implications. Radiology 1993;187:179.

124. Morrey BF. Anatomy and kinematics of the elbow. Instr Course Lect 1991;40:11.

125. Tivnon MC, Anzel SH, Waugh TR. Surgical management of osteochondritis dissecans of the capitellum. Am J Sports Med 1976;4:121.

126. Gryzlo SM. Bony disorders: clinical assessment and treatment. In: Jobe FW, ed. Operative techniques in upper extremity sports injuries. St Louis: Mosby-Year Book, 1996:496.

127. Rosenberg ZS, Beltran J, Cheung YY. Pseudodefect of the capitellum: potential MR imaging pitfall. Radiology 1994;191:821.

128. Vispo-Seara J, Loehr JF, Krauspe R, Gohlke F, Eulert J. Osteochondritis dissecans in children and adolescents. J Shoulder Elbow Surg 1995;4:S21.

129. Shaughnessy WJ, Bianco AJ. Osteochondritis dissecans. In: Morrey BF, ed. The elbow and its disorders, 2nd ed. Philadelphia: WB Saunders, 1993:282.

130. Morrey BF. Loose bodies. In: Morrey BF, ed. The elbow and its disorders, 2nd ed. Philadelphia: WB Saunders, 1993:860.

131. Milgram JW. The classification of loose bodies in human joints. Clin Orthop 1977;124:282.

132. Milgram JW. The development of loose bodies in human joints. Clin Orthop 1977;124:292.

133. Quinn SF, Haberman JJ, Fitzgerald SW, Traughber PD, Belkin RI, Murray WT. Evaluation of loose bodies in the elbow with MR imaging. J Magn Reson Imaging 1994;4:169.

134. Patten RM. Vacuum phenomenon: a potential pitfall in the interpretation of gradient-recalled-echo MR images of the shoulder. AJR 1994;162:1383.

135. Ogilvie-Harris DJ, Schemitsch E. Arthroscopy of the elbow for removal of loose bodies. Arthroscopy 1993;9:5.

136. O'Driscoll SW, Morrey BF. Arthroscopy of the elbow: diagnostic and therapeutic benefits and hazards. J Bone Joint Surg [Am] 1992;74:84.

137. O'Driscoll SW. Elbow arthroscopy for loose bodies. Orthopaedics 1992;15:855.

138. Bell MS. Loose bodies in the elbow. Br J Surg 1975;62:921.

139. Andrews JR, Craven WM. Lesions of the posterior compartment of the elbow. Clin Sports Med 1991;10:632.

140. Andrews JR, Timmerman LA. Outcome of elbow surgery in professional baseball players. Am J Sports Med 1995;23:407.

141. Rosenberg ZS, Beltran J, Cheung Y, Broker M. MR imaging of the elbow: normal variant and potential diagnostic pitfalls of the trochlear groove and cubital tunnel. AJR 1995;164:415.

142. Wood VE, Campbell GS. The supratrochleare dorsale accessory ossicle in the elbow. J Shoulder Elbow Surg 1994;3:395.

143. Gudmundsen TE, ϕstensen H. Accessory ossicles in the elbow. Acta Orthop Scand 1987;58:130.

144. Lawson JP. Clinically significant radiologic anatomic variants of the skeleton. AJR 1994;163:249.

145. Obermann WR, Loose HWC. The os supratrochleare dorsale: a normal variant that may cause symptoms. AJR 1983;141:123.

146. Pritchard DJ, Unni KK. Neoplasms of the elbow. In: Morrey BF, ed. The elbow and its disorders, 2nd ed. Philadelphia: WB Saunders, 1993:843.

147. Field JH. Posterior interosseous nerve palsy secondary to synovial chondromatosis of the elbow joint. J Hand Surg [Am] 1981;6:336.

148. Fahmy NR, Noble J. Ulnar nerve palsy as a complication of synovial osteochondromatosis of the elbow. Hand 1981;13:308.

149. Milgram JW. Secondary synovial osteochondromatosis. Bull Hosp Joint Dis 1979;40:38.

150. Milgram JW. Synovial osteochondromatosis: a histopathological study of 30 cases. J Bone Joint Surg [Am] 1977;59:792.

151. Kramer J, Recht M, Deely DM, et al. MR appearance of idiopathic synovial osteochondromatosis. J Comput Assist Tomogr 1993;17:772.

152. Morrey BF. Distal biceps tendon rupture. In: Morrey BF, ed. The elbow. New York: Raven Press, 1994:115.

153. D'Alessandro DF, Shields CL Jr, Tibone JE, Chandler RW. Repair of distal biceps tendon ruptures in athletes. Am J Sports Med 1993;21:114.

154. Bourne MH, Morrey BF. Partial rupture of the distal biceps tendon. Clin Orthop 1991;271:143.

155. Fitzgerald SW, Curry DR, Erickson SJ, Quinn SF, Friedman H. Distal biceps tendon injury: MR imaging diagnosis. Radiology 1994; 191:203.

156. Strong JA, Melamed JW, Martinez S, Burk DL, Harrelson JM, Spritzer CE. MRI of acute and chronic distal biceps tendon injuries. Presented at 94th Annual Meeting of the American Roentgen Ray Society, New Orleans, 1994:152.

157. Falchook FS, Zlatkin MB, Erbacher GE, Moulton JS, Bisset GS, Murphy BJ. Rupture of the distal biceps tendon: evaluation with MR imaging. Radiology 1994;190:659.

158. Mayer DP, Schmidt RG, Ruiz S. MRI diagnosis of biceps tendon rupture. Comput Med Imaging Graph 1992;16:345.

159. Agins HJ, Chess JL, Goekstra DV, Teitge RA. Rupture of the distal insertion of the biceps brachii tendon. Clin Orthop 1988;234:34.

160. Morrey BF. Tendon injuries about the elbow. In: Morrey BF, ed. The elbow and its disorders, 2nd ed. Philadelphia: WB Saunders, 1993:492.

161. Whiteside JA, Andrews JR. Tendinopathies of the elbow. Sports Med Arthosc Rev 1995;3:195.

162. Nielsen K. Partial rupture of the distal biceps brachii tendon: a case report. Acta Orthop Scand 1987;58:287.

163. Sotje G, Besch L. (Distal rupture of the biceps tendon: a magnetic resonance tomography follow-up). Aktuel Traumatol 1993;23:105.

164. Seiler JG, Parker LM, Chamberland PDC, Sherbourne GM, Carpenter WA. The distal biceps tendon: two potential machanisms involved in its rupture. Arterial supply and mechanical impingement. J Shoulder Elbow Surg 1995;4:149.

165. Heckman JD, Levine MI. Traumatic closed transection of the biceps brachii in the military parachutist. J Bone Joint Surg [Am] 1978;60:369.

166. Kelly JD, Elattrache NS. Muscle ruptures of the shoulder girdle. In: Jobe FW, ed. Operative techniques in upper extremity sports injuries. St Louis: Mosby-Year Book, 1996:360.

167. Davis WM, Yassine Z. An etiological factor in tear of the distal tendon of the biceps brachii. J Bone Joint Surg [Am] 1956;37:1365.

168. Karanjia ND, Stiles PJ. Cubital bursitis. J Bone Joint Surg [Br] 1988;70:832.

169. Kosarek FJ, Hoffman CJ, Martinez S. Distal bicipital bursitis: MR imaging characteristics. Radiology 1995;197P:398.

170. Foxworthy M, Kinninmonth AW. Median nerve compression in the proximal forearm as a complication of partial rupture of the distal biceps brachii tendon. J Hand Surg [Br] 1992;17:515.

171. Failla JM, Amadio PC, Morrey BF, Beckenbaugh RD. Proximal radio-ulnar synostosis after repair of distal biceps brachii rupture by the two-incision technique: report of four cases. Clin Orthop 1990;253:133.

172. D'Alessandro DF, Shields CL. Biceps rupture and triceps avulsion. In: Jobe FW, ed. Operative techniques in upper extremity sports injuries. St Louis: Mosby-Year Book, 1996:506.

173. Tarnsey FF. Rupture and avulsion of the triceps. Clin Orthop 1972;83:177.

174. Farrar ELI, Lippert FGI. Avulsion of the triceps tendon. Clin Orthop 1981;161:242.

175. Klemme WR, Petersen S. Avulsion of the triceps brachii with selective radial neuropathy. Orthopedics 1995;18:285.

176. Kessler KJ, Uribe JW, Vargas L. Triceps rupture: a new mechanism of injury. Contemp Orthop 1994;29:134.

177. Bos CF, Nelissen RG, Bloem JL. Incomplete rupture of the tendon of triceps brachii: a case report. Int Orthop 1994;18:273.

178. Tiger E, Mayer DP, Glazer R. Complete avulsion of the triceps tendon: MRI diagnosis. Comput Med Imaging Graph 1993;17:51.

179. Stannard JP, Bucknell AL. Rupture of the triceps tendon associated with steroid injections. Am J Sports Med 1993;21:482.

180. Viegas SF. Avulsion of the triceps tendon. Orthop Rev 1990;19:533.

181. Bach BRJ, Warren RF, Wickiewicz TL. Triceps rupture: a case report and literature review. Am J Sports Med 1984;15:285.

182. Morrey BF, Regan WD. Tendinopathies about the elbow. In: DeLee JC, Drez D Jr, eds. Orthopaedic sports medicine: principles and practice. Philadelphia: WB Saunders, 1994:860.

183. Anderson KJ, LeCocq JF. Rupture of the triceps tendon. J Bone Joint Surg [Am] 1957;39:444.

184. Aso K, Torisu T. Muscle belly tear of the triceps. Am J Sports Med 1984;12:485.

185. Sherman OH, Snyder SJ, Fox JM. Triceps tendon avulsion in a professional body builder: a case report. Am J Sports Med 1984;12:328.

186. Herrick RT, Herrick S. Ruptured triceps in a powerlifter presenting as cubital tunnel syndrome: a case report. Am J Sports Med 1987;15:514.

187. Miles JW, Grana WA, Egle D, Min KW, Chitwood J. The effect of anabolic steroids on the biomechanical and histological properties of rat tendon. J Bone Joint Surg [Am] 1992;744:411.

188. Clayton ML, Thirupathi RG. Rupture of the triceps tendon with olecranon bursitis. Clin Orthop 1984;184:183.

189. Levy M, Goldberg I, Meir I. Fracture of the head of the radius with a tear or avulsion of the triceps tendon: a new syndrome? J Bone Joint Surg [Br] 1982;64:70.

190. Brumback RJ. Compartment syndrome complicating avulsion of the origin of the triceps muscle: a case report. J Bone Joint Surg [Am] 1987;69:1445.

191. Fritz RC, Brody GA. MR imaging of the wrist and elbow. Clin Sports Med 1995;14:315.

192. Wirth BA. High-resolution MR imaging of the ulnar nerve within the ulnar canal: normal and pathologic appearance of postoperative changes. Radiology 1992;185P:115.

193. Rosenberg ZS, Beltran J, Cheung YY, Ro SY, Green SM, Lenzo SR. The elbow: MR features of nerve disorders. Radiology 1993;188:235.

194. O'Driscoll SW, Horii E, Carmichael SW, Morrey BF. The cubital tunnel and ulnar neuropathy. J Bone Joint Surg [Br] 1991;73:613.

195. Apfelberg DB, Larson SL. Dynamic anatomy of the ulnar nerve at the elbow. Plast Reconstr Surg 1973;51:76.

196. Pecina MM, Krmpotic-Nemanic J, Markiewitz AD. Tunnel syndromes in the upper extremity. In: Pecina MM, Krmpotic-Nemanic J, Markiewitz AD, eds. Tunnel syndromes. Boca Raton, FL: CRC Press, 1991:29.

197. Osborne GV. The surgical treatment of tardy ulnar neuritis. J Bone Joint Surg [Br] 1957;39:782.

198. Jobe FW, Fanton GS, ElAttrache NS. Ulnar nerve injury. In: Morrey BF, ed. The elbow and its disorders, 2nd ed. Philadelphia: WB Saunders, 1993:560.

199. McPherson SA, Meals RA. Cubital tunnel syndrome. Orthop Clin North Am 1992;23:111.

200. Kurosawa H, Nakashita K, Nakashita H, Sasaki S. Pathogenesis and treatment of cubital tunnel syndrome caused by osteoarthosis of the elbow joint. J Shoulder Elbow Surg 1995;4:30.

201. Spinner M, Linscheid RL. Nerve entrapment syndromes. In: Morrey BF, ed. The elbow and its disorders, 2nd ed. Philadelphia: WB Saunders, 1993:813.

202. Spinner M. Nerve decompression. In: Morrey BF, ed. The elbow. New York: Raven Press, 1994:183.

203. Spinner RJ, Carmichael SW, Spinner M. Partial median nerve entrap-

ment in the distal arm because of an accesssory bicipital aponeurosis. J Hand Surg 1991;16A:236.

204. Murphey MD, Johnson DL, Bhatia PS, Neff JR, Rosenthal HG, Walker CW. Parosteal lipoma: MR imaging characteristics. AJR 1994;162:105.

205. Ogino T, Minami A, Kato H. Diagnosis of radial nerve palsy caused by ganglion with use of different imaging techniques. J Hand Surg [Am] 1991;16:230.

206. Polak JF, Jolesz FA, Adams DF. Magnetic resonance imaging examination of skeletal muscle prolongation of T1 and T2 subsequent to denervation. Invest Radiol 1988;23:365.

207. Fleckenstein JL, Watumull D, Conner KE, et al. Denervated human skeletal muscle: MR imaging evaluation. Radiology 1993;187:213.

208. Shabas D, Gerard G, Rossi D. Magnetic resonance imaging of denervated muscle. Comput Radiol 1987;11:9.

209. Uetani M, Hayash K, Matosunaga N, Imamura K, Ito N. Denervated skeletal muscle: MR imaging. Radiology 1993;189:511.

210. Chen J, Alk D, Eventov I, Wientroub S. Development of the olecranon bursa: an anatomic cadaver study. Acta Orthop Scand 1987;58:408.

211. Morrey BF. Bursitis. In: Morrey BF, ed. The elbow and its disorders, 2nd ed. Philadelphia: WB Saunders, 1993:872.

212. Saini M, Canoso JJ. Traumatic olecranon bursitis: radiologic observations. Acta Radiol Diagn 1982;23:255.

213. Canoso JJ. Idiopathic or traumatic olecranon bursitis. Arthritis Rheum 1977;20:1213.

214. Larson RL, Osternig LR. Traumatic bursitis and artificial turf. J Sports Med 1974;2:183.

215. Singer KM, Butters KP. Olecranon bursitis. In: DeLee JC, Drez D Jr, eds. Orthopaedic sports medicine: principles and practice. Philadelphia: WB Saunders, 1994:890.

216. Soderquist B, Hedstrom SA. Predisposing factors, bacteriology, and antibiotic therapy in 35 cases of septic bursitis. Scand J Infect Dis 1986;18:305.

217. Weinstein PS, Canosos JJ, Wohlgethan JR. Long-term follow-up of corticosteroid injection for traumatic olecranon bursitis. Ann Rheum Dis 1984;43:44.

218. Stanley D. Prevalance and etiology of symptomatic elbow osteoarthritis. J Shoulder Elbow Surg 1994;3:386.

219. Morrey BF. Primary degenerative arthritis of the elbow: treatment by ulnohumeral arthroplasty. J Bone Joint Surg [Br] 1992;74:409.

220. Doherty M, Preston B. Primary osteoarthritis of the elbow. Ann Rheum Dis 1989;48:743.

221. Robla J, Hechtman KS, Uribe JW, Phillipon MS. Chondromalacia of the trochlea notch in athletes who throw. J Shoulder Elbow Surg 1996;5:69.

222. Goodfellow JW, Bullough PG. The pattern of aging of the articular cartilage of the elbow joint. J Bone Joint Surg [Br] 1967;49:175.

223. Inglis AE, Figgle MP. Rheumatoid arthritis. In: Morrey BF, ed. The elbow and its disorders, 2nd ed. Philadelphia: WB Saunders, 1993:751.

224. Singson RD, Zalduondo FM. Value of unenhanced spin-echo MR imaging in distinguishing between synovitis and effusion of the knee. AJR 1992;159:569.

225. Adam G, Dammer M, Bohndorf K, Christoph R, Fenke F, Gunther RW. Rheumatoid arthritis of the knee: value of gadopentetate dimeglumine-enhanced MR imaging. AJR 1991;156:125.

226. Bjorkengren AG, Geborek P, Rydholm U, Holtas S, Petterson H. MR imaging of the knee in acute rheumatoid arthritis: synovial uptake of gadolinium-DOTA. AJR 1990;155:329.

227. Kursunoglu-Brahme S, Riccio T, Weisman MH, et al. Rheumatoid knee: role of gadopentetate-enhanced MR imaging. Radiology 1990;176:831.

228. Sugimoto H, Takeda A, Masuyama J, Furuse M. Early-stage rheumatoid arthritis: diagnostic accuracy of MR imaging. Radiology 1996;198:185.

229. Yulish BS, Lieberman JM, Strandjorf SE, Bryan PJ, Mulopulos GP, Modic MT. Hemophilic arthritis: assesment with MR imaging. Radiology 1987;164:759.

230. Idy-Peretti I, Le Balc'h T, Yvart J, Bittoun J. MR imaging of hemophilic arthropathy of the knee: classification and evolution of the subchondral cysts. Magn Reson Imaging 1992;10:67.

231. Baunin C, Railhac JJ, Younes I, et al. MR imaging in hemophilic arthropathy. Eur J Pediatr Surg 1991;1:358.

232. Steinbach LS, Neumann CH, Mills CM, et al. MRI of the knee in diffuse pigmented villonodular synovitis. Clin Imaging 1989;13:305.

233. Goldman AB, DiCarlo EF. Pigmented villonodular synovitis: diagnosis and differential diagnosis. Radiol Clin North Am 1988;26:1327.

234. Cobby MJ, Adler RS, Swartz R, Martel W. Dialysis-related amyloid arthropathy: MR findings in four patients. Am J Roentgenol 1991;157:1023.

235. Shinall EA. Cat-scratch disease: a review of the literature. Pediatr Dermatol 1990;7:11.

236. Margileth AM. Cat-scratch disease. Adv Pediatr Infect Dis 1993;8:1.

237. Spires JR, Smith RJ. Cat-scratch disease. Otolaryngol Head Neck Surg 1986;94:622.

238. Chen SC, Gilbert GL. Cat-scratch disease: past and present. J Paediatr Child Health 1994;30:467.

239. Hopkins KL, Simoneaux SF, Patrick LE, Wyly JB, Dalton MJ, Snitzer JA. Imaging manifestations of cat-scratch disease. AJR 1996;166:435.

240. Baron AL, Steinbach LS, LeBoit PE, Mills CM, Gee JH, Berger TG. Osteolytic lesions and bacillary angiomatosis in HIV infection: radiologic differentiation form AIDS-related Kaposi sarcoma. Radiology 1990;177:77.

241. Bergmans AMC, Groothedde JW, Schellekens JFP, et al. Etiology of cat-scratch disease: comparison of polymerase chain-reaction detection of Bartonella (formerly Rochalimaea) and Afipia felis DNA with serology and skin tests. J Infect Dis 1995;171:916.

242. Dong PR, Seeger LL, Yao L, Panosian CB, Johnson BL, Eckardt JJ. Uncomplicated cat-scratch disease: findings at CT, MR imaging, and radiography. Radiology 1995;165:837.

Magnetic Resonance Imaging in Orthopaedics & Sports Medicine, Second Edition,
edited by David W. Stoller. Lippincott-Raven Publishers, Philadelphia, © 1997.

Chapter 11

The Wrist and Hand

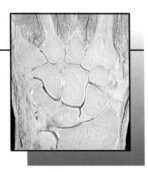

David W. Stoller
Gordon A. Brody

In the evaluation of both normal anatomy and pathology of the wrist and hand, magnetic resonance (MR) imaging has become a subject of increased attention at hand and radiology society meetings. With MR imaging, it is possible for the radiologist to accomplish accurate, noninvasive imaging of specific ligamentous injuries, rendering the vague diagnosis of wrist sprain obsolete. As data on the biomechanics on the carpus are collected, new applications are being developed for kinematic imaging. In addition, as techniques for dynamic MR imaging of the carpus advance, these methods may become the standard for evaluating instability from a physiologic viewpoint. This instability can best be defined as the inability of two bones or groups of bones to maintain a normal physiologic relationship.

STATUS OF IMAGING TECHNIQUES

Standard Radiography

Standard radiographic evaluation of the wrist and hand is restricted primarily to demonstrating the osseous structures. With certain localized pathologic processes, select views, such as a scaphoid and carpal tunnel view, may provide additional information. The scaphoid fat stripe, which can be identified radial to the scaphoid, and the pronator quadratus line, which is frequently obscured by fracture, are shown on posteroanterior (PA) and lateral radiographic views, respectively. However, the usefulness of the scaphoid fat stripe in diagnosing acute scaphoid fracture has been challenged. On a lateral radiograph, the static bony relationships of the radius, lunate, and capitate can be measured in longitudinal axes.

Arthrography

Wrist arthrography has been used to evaluate the integrity of the triangular fibrocartilage (TFC) and the scapholunate (SL) and lunotriquetral (LT) interosseous ligaments.[1-4] Until lately, the three-compartment (ie, triple injection) arthrogram—in which contrast is introduced into the radiocarpal, distal radioulnar, and midcarpal joints—was considered the standard technique.[5,6] More recently, however, single compartment arthrograms of the radiocarpal joint have been shown to have a false-negative rate of only 2% for complete perforations and 10% for complete and partial perforations together. Furthermore, it was found that patient treatment was not affected by the additional information provided by selective second and third injections of the distal radioulnar and midcarpal joints.[7]

Although arthrographic findings correlate quite well with ulnar-sided wrist pain, the technique is far less effective for radial-sided problems. Manaster and colleagues[8] found that although 88% of patients with ulnar pain had LT perforations, only 26% of patients with SL dissociation had SL perforations.[8] Arthrography, therefore, appears to be less useful in assessing the physiologic integrity of the interosseous ligaments on the radial side of the wrist.

Other wrist arthrography studies (using triple-compartment technique) demonstrate poor correlation of the locations of unidirectional or bidirectional communicating defects, as well as noncommunicating defects with the site of wrist pain.[9,10] Another limitation of arthrography is related to the fact that, because of the nature of the arthrography technique, it is impossible to differentiate small, pinhole perforations from those that are large and biomechanically significant. Anatomic studies of aging wrists have shown that degenerative perforations of both the interosseous ligaments and the triangular fibrocartilage complex (TFCC) are quite common in people older than 35 years of age.[11,12] Therefore, arthrography is less diagnostically useful in these patients. Kirschenbaum and colleagues[13] have additionally shown the common arthrographic finding of TFC and intrinsic ligament perforations in young asymptomatic adults.[13] This apparent lack of specificity of arthrography may limit its application, especially in comparison with MR imaging, in which the morphology of the TFC and intrinsic ligaments can be evaluated directly.

Computed Tomography

Computed tomography (CT) has limited but well-defined application in the wrist. It is primarily used to evaluate occult or complex fractures, fracture healing, and lucent defects and to provide improved definition of osseous detail[14] (Fig. 11-1). Although subtle differences in closely related soft-tissue attenuation values cannot be optimally resolved with

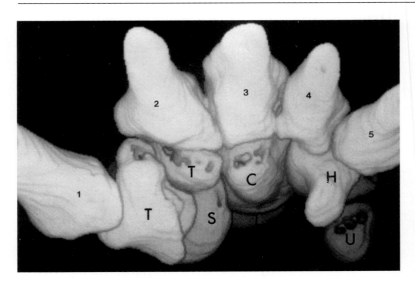

FIGURE 11-1. A 3D CT image of the osseous anatomy of the carpal tunnel shows the metacarpals, labeled 1 through 5. C, capitate; H, hamate; S, scaphoid; T, trapezium proximal to first metacarpal; T, trapezoid proximal to second metacarpal; U, ulna.

CT, it is an excellent modality for defining the location and extent of carpal bone fractures and complex intraarticular fractures of the distal radius.[15,16] Reformatted coronal and sagittal scans, direct coronal scans, and three-dimensional (3D) CT renderings are useful for evaluating fractures and for displaying fracture morphology displacement, nonunion, and alignment through specific anatomic areas (eg, the hook of the hamate).[17,18] Small chip fractures and loose bodies may be identified on thin section (ie, 1.5 mm) CT scans. Axial CT scans of the distal radioulnar joint (DRUJ) can be diagnostic for DRUJ subluxation or dislocation.

Ultrasound and Miscellaneous Techniques

Ultrasound has been used to study the gross motion of the tendons in the carpal tunnel during flexion.[19] Videofluoroscopy and cine CT studies of wrist motion may provide indirect evidence of pathology in tendons, ligaments, and cartilage, without direct imaging or arthroscopy of these structures. Videofluoroscopy is diagnostic of midcarpal instability and may be helpful in evaluating the pathomechanics of other carpal instabilities.

Magnetic Resonance Imaging

Magnetic resonance imaging of the wrist provides the high spatial and contrast resolution of soft-tissue and osseous components needed for evaluation of the small and complex anatomy of the wrist and hand.[20-31] Supporting muscles, ligaments, tendons, tendon sheaths, vessels, nerves and marrow are demonstrated on MR images with excellent spatial resolution using the small fields of view (FOVs) and uniform signal intensity penetration. MR imaging has the potential to replace conventional wrist arthrography in diagnosing tears

involving the intercarpal ligaments and TFCC, by allowing a direct correlation of abnormalities in ligamentous and fibrocartilage morphology with the clinical presentations of pain. Multiplanar images permit direct anatomic and pathologic discrimination in the axial, coronal, sagittal, and oblique planes, without the delayed reconstructions or reformatting required for CT. Sagittal MR images display bone and ligamentous anatomy in a selective "tomography-like" section, without the overlapping of carpal bones seen on lateral radiographs. This facilitates more accurate assessment of carpal instability. Three-dimensional Fourier transform (3DFT) volume imaging allows image acquisition with retrospective reformatting of additional orthogonal or nonorthogonal oblique images. Kinematic imaging in coronal and sagittal orientations provides information regarding carpal bone motion and synchrony with supporting ligamentous structures. This technique, however, which is nonphysiologic, has not been routinely used in clinical imaging. Short TI inversion recovery (STIR) and fat-suppressed T2-weighted fast spin-echo (FSE) techniques have significantly improved visualization of wrist joint fluid, increasing the accuracy of routine wrist MR evaluations relative to MR arthrography.[32] Foo and colleagues[33] have used high resolution spin-echo, two-dimensional, and 3D gradient-recalled acquisitions in the steady state (GRASS), and spoiled GRASS (SPGR) images to optimize trabecular bone detail and anatomy of the wrist[33] (Fig. 11-2). These techniques may need to be used in conjunction with fat-suppression or intraarticular contrast to improve identification of ligament and cartilage pathology. Local gradient coils have been used in 3D gradient-echo imaging and phase contrast angiography of the fingers.[34]

MR imaging is presently used for evaluation of ligamentous pathology, trauma (eg, fracture), avascular necrosis (AVN), and Kienböck's disease (KD), as well as for abnormalities of the TFC and carpal tunnel. In addition, the status of articular cartilage and cortical and subchondral bone response in arthritis can be assessed and categorized.

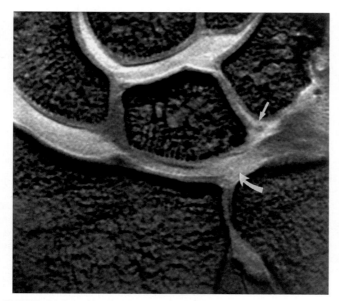

FIGURE 11-2. A 3D fast spoiled GRASS (FSPGR) with intraarticular contrast injected into the radiocarpal compartment. The torn lunotriquetral ligament (*straight arrow*) allows extension of contrast into the midcarpal compartment and the torn radial attachment of the TFC (*curved arrow*) directs contrast into the distal radioulnar joint. Note the superior trabecular bone detail on this image (coronal image; TR, 40.4 msec; TE, 14.5 msec; FOV, 4 cm; slice thickness, 2.0 mm; matrix, 512 × 256; flip angle, 30°).

MAGNETIC RESONANCE IMAGING TECHNIQUES

The wrist and hand are imaged using a dedicated circumferential design quadrature or phased array coil to optimize the signal-to-noise ratio (SNR) (Fig. 11-3) and to obtain high resolution images. With this coil design, the patient's arm may be positioned at the patient's side. Anatomic symmetry of both extremities can be demonstrated in the same FOV

by placing both hands in a large diameter coil. When high spatial resolution images requiring smaller FOVs are necessary for the opposite wrist or hand, separate acquisitions can be performed in the area of suspected pathology and a comparison of normal and abnormal anatomy can be made. Proper positioning requires alignment of the long axis of the distal radius and central metacarpal axis with the wrist in neutral position. Oblique prescriptions are not required to produce orthogonal images with this colinear alignment of the distal radius and carpus. Radial or ulnar deviation and dorsal or volar angulation should be avoided to maintain consistent alignment of the carpus. The wrist is usually positioned in pronation, with the fingers held in extension. The position of the wrist may change relative to the design of the surface coil used. When the wrist is studied in the thumbs-up position, coronal images are obtained by prescribing a sagittal plane acquisition. In this case, oblique imaging may be required to produce orthogonal plane images through the plane of the TFC and intrinsic ligaments of the wrist.

T1-weighted images are obtained in the axial, coronal, and sagittal planes. T1-weighted coronal images are acquired with 3 mm sections, using a 6 cm FOV and a 512 × 256 or 256 × 256 matrix. A repetition time (TR) of 1000 to 1200 msec can be used to increase the number of slices and SNR at 1 excitation (NEX). Pathology of the TFC and intrinsic ligaments is best displayed on STIR (including fast STIR) or fat-suppressed T2-weighted FSE coronal sequences, which create an arthrography-like effect by displaying the high signal intensity of fluid in contrast to the lower signal intensity of ligaments and fibrocartilage. Fat-suppressed T2-weighted FSE sequences use a TR of 3000 msec, an echo time (TE) between 40 and 60 msec, an 8 cm FOV, a 3 mm slice thickness, and a 256 × 256 matrix. 3D FSE techniques will allow the use of even thinner sections (less than 3 mm). Higher matrix and TE values and lower echo train lengths

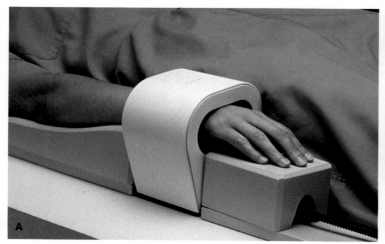

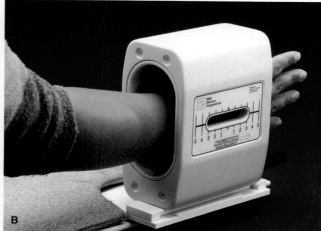

FIGURE 11-3. Dedicated quadrature wrist coils with hand positioned in prone position (**A**) and neutral position (**B**). These coils are usually positioned at a patient's side with the fingers relaxed in extension.

produce images with less blurring. T2*-weighted coronal images also produce excellent contrast between ligaments (the intercarpal ligaments and the TFCC) and fluid. 3DFT volume acquisitions that use gradient-echo protocols are not limited by slice thickness and can be used to reformat anatomy in other planes of section. In 3DFT volume imaging, the imaging time and SNR are proportional to the number of slices, the TR, and the number of excitations. Scan time increases when a higher acquisition matrix (eg, 256 or 512) is used. 3D SPGR techniques are used to display detailed anatomy of the TFCC and intrinsic ligaments. Using these sequences, it is possible to achieve higher resolution MR images with a FOV between 4 and 6 cm and a lower receiver band, ± 8 kHz. Pixel resolution at a 4 cm FOV and 256 × 256 matrix is approximately 100 μm, which allows visualization of trabecular bone detail as well. SPGR techniques may require manipulation of the theta flip angle to less than 30° to achieve a T2-like contrast effect. Fat-suppression is recommended to increase the conspicuity of fluid in abnormal or injured articular cartilage.

An axial STIR or fat-suppressed T2-weighted FSE sequence demonstrates tenosynovitis, ganglia, carpal tunnel syndrome and related changes in the median nerve, and neoplasms. The distinct dorsal, membranous, and volar components of the SL ligament are separated on axial images through the proximal carpal row. The flexor digitorum superficialis and profundus tendons can be differentiated on gradient-echo axial images through the phalanges.

T1-weighted and fat-suppressed T2-weighted FSE sagittal images display the static alignment of the carpal bones, which is important in assessing the capitolunate angle and tilting of the lunate or the degree of scaphoid flexion or extension. The anteroposterior location of TFC tears is determined on fat-suppressed T2-weighted FSE sagittal images. Fluid in dorsal or volar ligaments of the capsule are also shown in this plane.

Administration of intravenous gadolinium DTPA produces enhancement of pannus tissue and subchondral hyperemia in inflammatory arthritides. Scaphoid and lunate vascularity are studied using either a STIR, fat-suppressed T2-weighted FSE coronal, or fat-suppressed T2-weighted intravenous gadolinium-enhanced sequence.

MR arthrography with intraarticular administration of an MR contrast agent or intraarticular saline improves the accuracy of detection of ligamentous disruptions, including flap tears and intercarpal fluid communications. MR identification of small perforations of the TFC and intercarpal ligaments, with characterization of ligament morphology, provides more specific information than simply documenting contrast extension between the radiocarpal and midcarpal joints or radiocarpal and DRUJs, as provided by conventional arthrography.

Coupled 7.5 cm (3 inch) circular surface coils positioned in a kinematic wrist device have been used with gradient-echo protocols to track distal and carpal row motion with

radial and ulnar deviation of the wrist. This information is displayed in a cine loop format, and can be recorded on video or photographed.

Dorsiflexion and plantarflexion motions are best studied in the sagittal plane and require either a greater degree of freedom from the surface coil or pivoting of the coil to accommodate the increased range of motion. It is important to incorporate image quality considerations, however, when designing a surface coil with an increased diameter or anatomic coverage. Separate axial imaging sequences in positions of pronation and supination may be useful in the evaluation of subluxation patterns in the DRUJ. Developments in echo planar imaging technology may facilitate true dynamic joint imaging, which would provide more accurate descriptions of carpal translations and impingements in various instability patterns.

FUNCTIONAL ANATOMY OF THE WRIST

Osseous Structures

The osseous elements of the wrist consist of the distal radius and ulna, the proximal and distal carpal rows, and the bases of the metacarpals. There are three major compartments of the wrist as defined by arthrographic studies: (1) the radiocarpal compartment, (2) the midcarpal compartment, and (3) the DRUJ compartment.

Distal Radioulnar Joint

On its medial side, the distal radius forms a shallow depression for articulation with the ulnar head (Fig. 11-4). The sigmoid notch acts as a seat for the rotating pole of the distal ulna and provides some bony stability to the DRUJ. The DRUJ is inclined 20° distally and ulnarly; this angle of inclination is thought to be important in maintaining forearm rotation. The stabilizing ligaments for the joint include the TFC and the dorsal and volar capsular ligaments (Fig. 11-5). These capsular ligaments are poorly defined and cannot be visualized as distinct anatomic structures. The TFC connects the ulna and radius at their most distal edges and separates the DRUJ from the radiocarpal joint. The TFC runs from the ulnar-most edge of the lunate facet and sigmoid notch to the base of the ulnar styloid, where it inserts into a small depression in the distal ulna known as the fovea. The ulnar insertion consists of two limbs: one distal and one proximal. However, traumatic loss of the soft-tissue stabilizers of the DRUJ, primarily the TFCC, may cause subluxation of the radius on the fixed unit of the ulna.[35] The DRUJ and synovial cavity is identified between the distal radius and ulna and extends across the distal ulna deep to the TFC.[36]

text continues on page 859

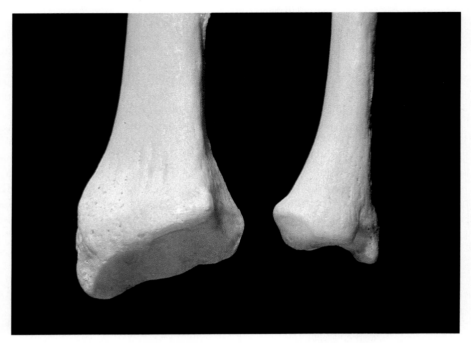

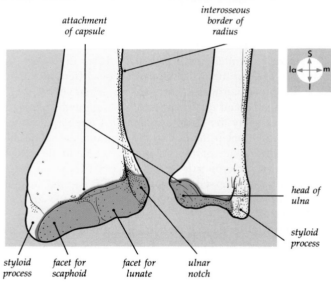

FIGURE 11-4. An anterior view of the distal ends of the radius and ulna. The bones have been separated to reveal the ulnar notch.

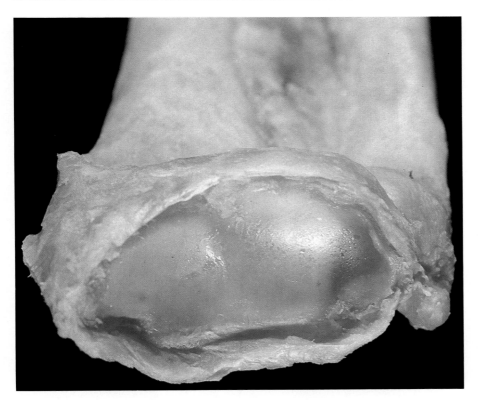

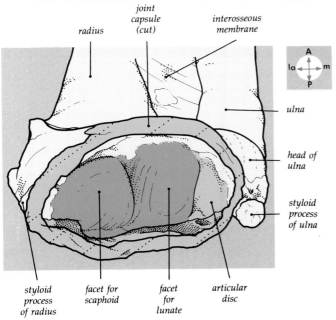

FIGURE 11-5. The articular surface of the distal end of the radius and the adjacent triangular cartilage are exposed by removal of the carpal bones.

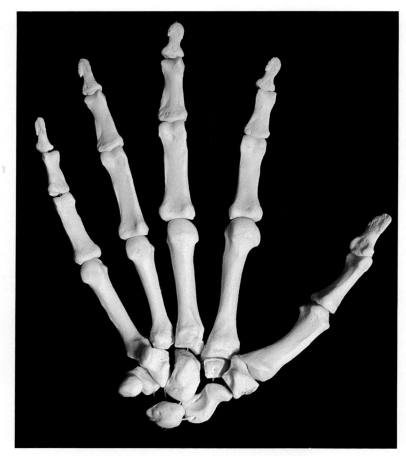

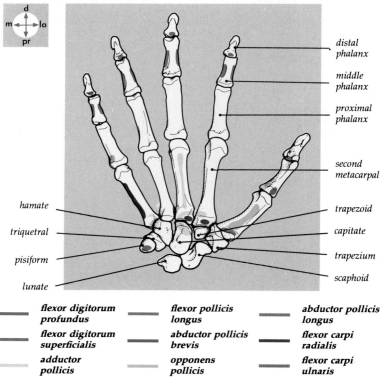

distal
phalanx

middle
phalanx

proximal
phalanx

second
metacarpal

hamate

triquetral

pisiform

lunate

trapezoid

capitate

trapezium

scaphoid

	flexor digitorum profundus		flexor pollicis longus		abductor pollicis longus
	flexor digitorum superficialis		abductor pollicis brevis		flexor carpi radialis
	adductor pollicis		opponens pollicis		flexor carpi ulnaris
	opponens digiti minimi		abductor digiti minimi		

FIGURE 11-6. The bones of the hand. Adjacent bones, particularly in the carpus, have been slightly separated to reveal their articular surfaces.

Radiocarpal Joint

The radiocarpal joint is defined by the TFC and the distal radial surface proximally, and the lunate, triquetrum, and the scaphoid distally. At the site of the radiolunate articulation, the distal articular surfaces of the radius and ulna are usually at the same level (ie, neutral ulnar variance). Alternatively, the ulna may be relatively long (positive ulnar variance), leading to an ulnar abutment syndrome, or relatively short (negative ulnar variance), as is often seen in KD. The distal radius forms two facets that articulate with the scaphoid and lunate of the proximal carpal row. This articulation of the proximal pole of the scaphoid in the scaphoid fossa is quite congruent; even a small degree of malrotation of the scaphoid may cause incongruent loading of the articular cartilage and subsequent degeneration (such as that which accompanies a scapholunate advanced collapse [SLAC] wrist, as described by Watson and Ryu[37]). The lunate facet commonly becomes incongruent following distal radius fractures, especially die punch–type fractures. The interosseous ligaments join the proximal carpal bones at their proximal edges.[36]

Lister's tubercle, the most prominent dorsal radial ridge, separates the extensor pollicis longus tendon (ulnar side) from the extensor carpi radialis and brevis tendons (radial side). This is the site where bone spurs form and attrition ruptures occur in rheumatoid arthritis.

Carpus and Midcarpal Joint

The proximal carpal row consists of the scaphoid, the lunate, and the triquetrum (Figs. 11-6 and 11-7). It is thought that with a congenital bipartite scaphoid, the proximal row should include only the proximal pole of the scaphoid. The distal pole should be thought of as a component of the distal row. The scaphoid, lunate, and triquetrum are linked by strong interosseous ligaments that work together to form a flexible socket or acetabulum that cradles the distal row. Occasionally, anatomic imperfections in this socket lead to arthritic degeneration. The lunate may have a medial facet, which measures 1 to 6 mm in diameter. This facet is present in approximately two thirds of cadaver hands studied, and 44% of these had arthritic degeneration in the proximal pole of the hamate.[38] Hamate arthritis is not seen unless the medial facet was present on the lunate.[38] The distal carpal row consists of the trapezium, the trapezius, the capitate, and the hamate (see Figs. 11-6 and 11-7).

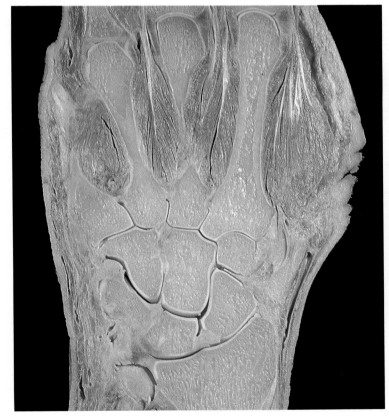

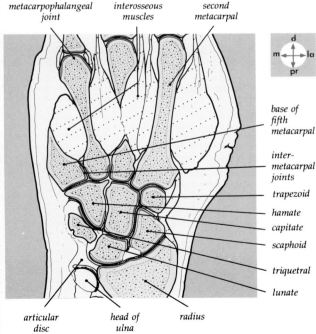

FIGURE 11-7. A coronal section of the hand shows the joints of the carpal region. The thumb and little finger are anterior to the plane of section.

The midcarpal joint is formed between the proximal and distal carpal rows (see Fig. 11-7). The midcarpal joint cavity is located primarily between the distal aspects of the scaphoid, lunate, and triquetrum and the proximal aspect of the distal row. Proximal extension to the midcarpal joint between the scaphoid and lunate and between the lunate and triquetrum are limited by the interosseous ligaments.[36] The three distal extensions of the midcarpal joint are located between the four bones of the distal carpal row. The trapezium-trapezoid or trapezoid and capitate joint spaces may communicate with the second and third carpometacarpal joints. The first carpometacarpal joint does not communicate with the midcarpal joint. The separate joint space between the hamate and the fourth and fifth metacarpals may communicate with the midcarpal joint.

Ligamentous Anatomy

Much of the interest in and appreciation of the ligamentous anatomy of the wrist derives from the advent of wrist arthroscopy. Arthroscopy allows direct examination of the ligaments of the wrist and testing of their physiologic integrity. All arthroscopic portals are, of necessity, dorsally placed, making examination of the volar ligaments especially easy. As a result, the dorsal ligaments initially received less attention, although many investigators are now studying their biomechanics. Definition of pathologic conditions naturally followed elucidation of the ligamentous anatomy, and new treatment procedures have been devised.[39]

The ligaments of the wrist are classified into intrinsic and extrinsic groups[40] (Table 8-1). The extrinsic ligaments extend from the radius, ulna, and metacarpals; and the intrinsic ligaments originate and insert within the carpus. In general, the role of the intrinsic ligaments is to maintain the relationships among the individual carpal bones, whereas the extrinsic ligaments are important in the relationship of the carpus as a whole to the distal radius and ulna, as well as the bases of the metacarpals. Newer anatomic data now show that the extrinsic ligaments, as well as the intrinsic ligaments, are crucial to maintaining the intercarpal relationships. Many investigators object to this classification scheme because it is possible for imbalances of the intrinsic ligaments to cause carpal instability, a condition that was formerly thought to occur only through dysfunction of the intrinsic ligaments. However, this scheme remains useful, if only as an anatomic guide.

Extrinsic Ligaments

RADIOCARPAL LIGAMENTS. The volar extrinsic ligaments are the most constant and the strongest of the extrinsic ligaments. Several mechanically important ligaments originate from the region of the radial styloid and distal radius, including the radial collateral and palmar radiocarpal ligaments. The latter consists of the radioscaphocapitate (RSC) ligament; the radiolunotriquetral (RLT) ligament (also sometimes referred to as the long radiolunate [LRL] ligament); the radioscapholunate (RSL) ligament; and the short radiolunate (SRL) ligament[41] (Fig. 11-8).

TABLE 11-1
Extrinsic and Intrinsic Ligaments of the Wrist

Radiocarpal (Radial Origin)	Ulnocarpal (TFCC ligaments)	Dorsal
Extrinsic Ligaments		
Radial collateral ligament	Dorsal radioulnar ligament	Dorsal radioscapholunotriquetral ligament
Palmar radiocarpal ligament	Volar radioulnar ligament	Scaphotriquetral ligament
Radioscaphocapitate ligament	Ulnolunate ligament	
Long radiolunate ligament or radiolunotriquetral	Ulnotriquetral ligament	
Short radiolunate ligament	Ulnar collateral ligament	
Radioscapholunate ligament	Meniscus homologue	
Radiolunate ligament or ligament of Testut		
Radioscaphoid ligament or ligament of Kuenz		
Intrinsic Ligaments		
Scapholunate ligament		
Lunotriquetral ligament		
Deltoid or arcuate ligaments		
Trapezium-trapezoid ligament		
Trapezoid-capitate ligament		
Capitate-hamate ligament		

TFCC, triangular fibrocartilage complex.

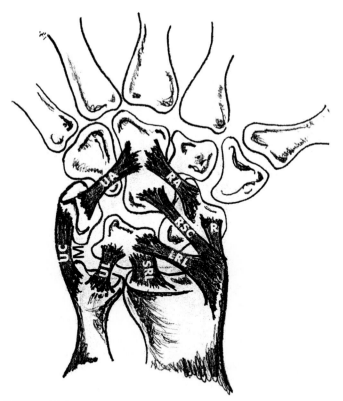

FIGURE 11-8. The volar intrinsic and extrinsic carpal ligaments. **Extrinsic ligaments.** *Radiocarpal (radial origin):* LRL, long radiolunate ligament; R, radial collateral ligament; RSC, radioscaphocapitate ligament; SRL, short radiolunate ligament. *Ulnocarpal:* M, meniscal homologue; UC, ulnar collateral ligament; UL, ulnolunate ligament. The dorsal and volar radioulnar ligaments, the ulnotriquetral ligament, and the radioscapholunate ligament are not shown. **Intrinsic ligaments.** *Arcuate ligaments:* RA, radial arcuate ligament; UA, ulnar arcuate ligament. The scapholunate ligament and lunotriquetral ligament are not shown. The space of Poirier is over the volar aspect of the capitolunate joint.

By virtue of their orientation and mechanical properties, the radiocarpal ligaments maintain the carpus within its radial articulation. Loss of these ligaments allows the carpus to move down the inclined plane of the distal radius and undergo ulnar translation. This condition is not uncommon in rheumatoid arthritis, in which synovitic degeneration of these soft-tissue supporting structures occurs. With ulnar translation, the distance between the radial styloid and the scaphoid increases and the scaphoid and lunate are displaced from their articular fossae. The lunate comes to rest where it articulates with the distal ulna, and the scaphoid becomes perched on the ridge between its own articulation and the lunate fossae. This incongruent loading leads to degeneration of the cartilaginous surfaces and ulnolunate impingement. Overexuberant surgical resection of the radial styloid can destroy the origin of these ligaments and may cause this type of instability. Distal ulna resection (the Darrach procedure) in the rheumatoid wrist may also lead to ulnar translation of the carpus with the loss of the ulnar buttress.

Radial Collateral Ligament.   Although the radial collateral ligament is not a true collateral ligament (because ulnar and radial deviation are normal motion arcs in the wrist, and, by definition, a collateral ligament resists only pathologic or abnormal motion), it has been shown to be mechanically significant and to play a role in the mechanism of midwaist scaphoid fractures by compressing the bone along its longitudinal axis.[42] This ligament originates on the tip of the styloid and inserts into the radial aspect of the scaphoid at its waist. Fibers of the radial collateral ligament also extend from the scaphoid to the trapezium, blending with the transverse carpal ligament and dorsal capsular ligament.[36]

Radioscaphocapitate Ligament.   The RSC ligament is a very stout ligament, readily identified through the arthroscope. It originates from the radial styloid, has a minor insertion into the radial aspect of the waist of the scaphoid, and also inserts on the center of the capitate.[43] The RSC ligament forms a supporting sling at the waist of the scaphoid. As the fibers cross the proximal pole of the scaphoid, there is a fold of synovium that separates them from the bone.[44] In this position, the ligament can be interposed between the fragments of a scaphoid fracture and contribute to nonunion. The RSC ligament, which has a striated appearance on volar coronal MR images, is located distal to the RLT ligament, which has a similar ulnodistal obliquity (Fig. 11-9). Sagittal images demonstrate the volar location of the RSC in cross section ligament relative to the waist of the scaphoid.

Radiolunotriquetral Ligament or Long Radiolunate Ligament.   Progressing ulnarly, the RLT ligament (which is also re-

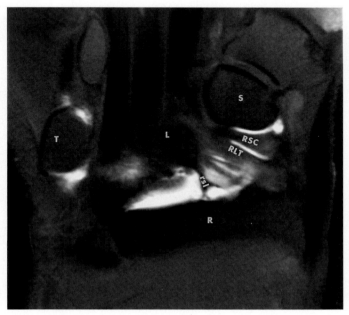

FIGURE 11-9. Anatomy of the radioscaphocapitate (RSC), radiolunotriquetral (RLT), and radioscapholunate (rsl) ligaments at the level of the distal volar radius (R) (fat-suppressed T1-weighted MR arthrogram after radiocarpal injection). T, triquetrum; S, scaphoid.

ferred to as the LRL ligament) is the next ligament seen. It is the largest ligament of the wrist[43] (Fig. 11-10) and originates ulnar to the RSC from the volar lip of the radial styloid process. The RLT has an oblique course attached to the volar aspects of the lunate and triquetrum. On volar coronal MR images, it displays a striated band-like appearance, similar to the RSC ligament. There is an interligamentous sulcus between the RSC and the RLT ligaments on sagittal images (Fig. 11-11). The RLT is a strong ligament that stabilizes

the proximal carpal row on the radius and should be differentiated from the RSL ligament.

Short Radiolunate Ligament. The SRL ligament has been described by Berger and Landsmeer.[44] This ligament originates from the radius in the region of the lunate facet and inserts distally into the volar surface of the lunate (Fig. 11-12). At its insertion, its most radial fibers merge with those of the LRL ligament. The SRL ligament is perhaps

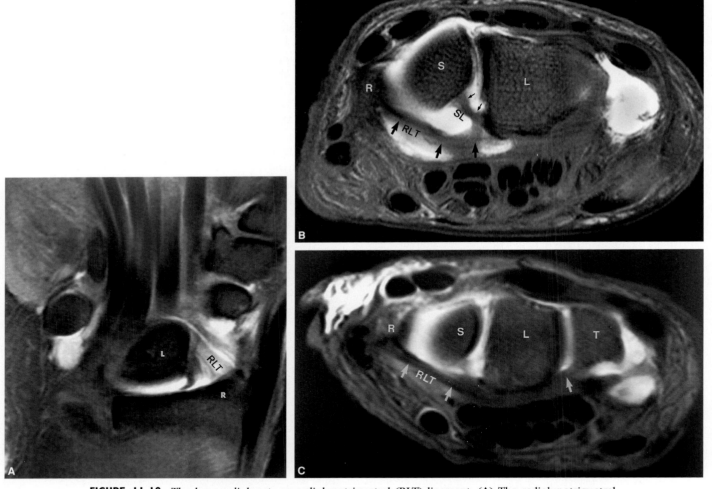

FIGURE 11-10. The long radiolunate or radiolunotriquetral (RLT) ligament. **(A)** The radiolunotriquetral ligament is divided into a radiolunate ligament and lunotriquetral component. The RLT ligament functions as a volar sling for the lunate (volar fat-suppressed T1-weighted coronal MR arthrographic image). L, lunate; R, radius. Fat-suppressed T1-weighted axial MR arthrographic images obtained at the relative level of the proximal **(B)** and distal **(C)** aspects of the radial styloid showing the volar course of the RLT ligament (*large arrows*) from the radial styloid (R) inserting into the lunate (L) and blending with the volar portion of the lunotriquetral interosseous ligament. Note that the lunate attachment of the scapholunate interosseous ligament volar fibers is deep to the lunate attachment of the RLT ligament **(B)**. S, scaphoid; T, triquetrum; SL, scapholunate ligament.

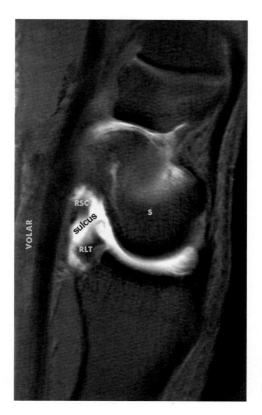

FIGURE 11-11. The interligamentous sulcus between the radioscaphocapitate (RSC) and radiolunotriquetral ligaments is seen on a fat-suppressed T1-weighted sagittal MR arthrogram image at the level of the scaphoid (S). The volar aspect of the wrist is labeled (VOLAR). The RLT ligament is proximal to the RSC ligament.

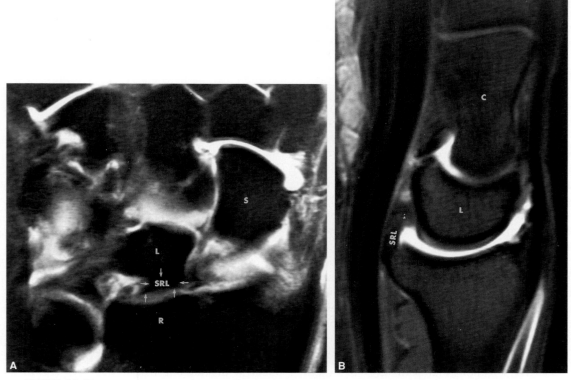

FIGURE 11-12. The short radiolunate ligament. **(A)** The short radiolunate ligament (SRL; *arrows*) can be seen extending volarly to the lunate fossa of the distal radius to its insertion on the radial volar aspect of the lunate (fat-suppressed T1-weighted coronal arthrographic image). S, scaphoid. **(B)** The short radiolunate ligament (SRL) identified on a fat-suppressed T1-weighted sagittal image at the level of the capitate (C) and lunate (L).

the most biomechanically significant volar carpal ligament. It acts as a volar tether to the lunate and plays a major role in preventing the development of dorsal intercalated segment instability (DISI) deformities with lunate extension.

Radioscapholunate Ligament. The RSL ligament is interposed dorsally between the LRL and the SRL ligaments. It arises at the level of the interfacet prominence of the distal radius and inserts into the SL articulation[43] (Fig. 11-13). This structure was first described in detail by Testut, and is often called by his name (ie, the ligament of Testut or the ligament of Testut or Kuenz).[45] The RSL ligament has been studied extensively, and it has been shown to contain the most elastic tissue of any ligament in the wrist. It does not appear to provide any mechanical support to the carpus.

From his work on fetal wrists, Landsmeer described a vascular pedicle that supplies the RSL ligament.[46] It has since been shown that this structure is a neurovascular umbilical cord that may provide a clinically significant blood supply to the proximal pole of the scaphoid via the SL interosseous ligament and a sensory or proprioceptive pathway to the SL joint.[47] The RSL ligament receives its neurovascular supply from the anterior interosseous artery and nerve.

On volar coronal MR arthrographic images, the RSL can be seen as a short ligament with a straight course or minimally convex radial border directed toward the SL interval. The RSL ligament does not have the striations previously described for the RSC and RLT ligaments on coronal images. The proximal attachment of the RSL ligament should never be confused with the normal articular cartilage ridge that separates the scaphoid and lunate fossa of the distal radius (see Fig. 11–13C). This articular cartilage ridge has a broad based attachment to the distal radius.

ULNOCARPAL LIGAMENTS. The ulnar portion of the extrinsic volar ligaments of the wrist is formed by the TFCC (Figs. 11-14 and 11-15). The TFCC consists of the TFC proper (the articular disc), the dorsal and volar radioulnar ligaments, the meniscus homologue, and the ulnolunate and the ulnotriquetral ligaments. The term TFCC was coined to describe all of the ligamentous and cartilaginous structures that were thought to play a role in suspending the distal radius and the ulnar carpus from the distal ulna.[48] The study of the biomechanics of the structures of the TFCC is in its infancy, but there are clinical and laboratory data to support its role in maintaining both the stability of the DRUJ and the stability of the carpus as a whole (preventing pronosupination of the carpus). The TFCC also contributes to stability within the carpus by preventing nondissociative carpal instabilities (CIND) (see ''Carpal Instabilities).

DORSAL LIGAMENTS. Although the palmar or volar radiocarpal ligaments have attracted a great deal of attention in the past, new insights into the biomechanics of the wrist have more recently focused interest on the dorsal ligaments.

The dorsal ligaments do not exist as discrete anatomic entities, and they vary considerably from subject to subject. Two major components can be discerned. The first component is the dorsal radioscapholunotriquetral (RSLT) ligament, a thickening of the dorsal capsule that courses from the dorsal lip of the radius and inserts on the dorsal surfaces of the scaphoid, lunate, and triquetrum. This ligament acts as a checkrein on the proximal carpal row and prevents it from assuming a position of excessive volarflexion. Biomechanical studies have shown that in the final stage of ulnar-sided perilunate instability, it is the RSLT ligament that is injured.[49] Laxity of the RSLT ligament has been implicated in palmar midcarpal instability patterns in which the lunate is allowed to go into volarflexion, leading to instability. The second major component of the dorsal ligamentous structure is the scaphotriquetral (or triquetroscaphoid) ligament. This is a transversely oriented thickening of the dorsal capsular fibers. It runs from the scaphoid to the triquetrum.

Using multiplanar reconstructions with 3DFT MR imaging, Smith[50,51] has demonstrated and described the dorsal carpal ligaments of the wrist. The radiotriquetral ligament can be seen to consist of a single band that arises from the distal radius, adjacent to Lister's tubercle. The dorsal intercarpal ligament is seen either as a broad fused band (a branched structure) with separate triquetroscaphoid and triquetrotrapezoid fascicles, or as completely separate triquetroscaphoid and triquetrotrapezoid fascicles (Figs. 11-16 and 11-17).

Intrinsic Interosseous Ligaments

SCAPHOLUNATE AND LUNOTRIQUETRAL LIGAMENTS. The interosseous ligaments are of paramount importance in maintaining the biomechanical relationship among the carpal bones, especially those of the proximal row (Fig. 11-18). For the proximal carpal row to function properly, the bones must be associated or linked together, and the interosseous ligaments provide this flexible linkage. The SL and LT ligaments are comparable in strength with the anterior cruciate ligament of the knee. They connect the bones at the level of the proximal articular surface and consist of thick dorsal and volar components with thinner membranous portions in between. Most commonly, perforations occur in the thin, membranous portions and may not be mechanically significant.

The SL ligament is triangular on coronal section and is peripherally attached at the SL interval (see Fig. 11-18). The inner apex of the triangular-shaped ligament is not attached to bone and is free within the SL joint.[52] The dorsal fibers of the SL ligament are oriented transversely, or perpendicular to the joint, and form a thick bundle. The dorsal portion of the SL ligament is considered to be the most important component in maintaining carpal stability. The membranous SL ligament fibers course peripherally and obliquely from the scaphoid downward to the lunate. The membranous SL liga-

text continues on page 870

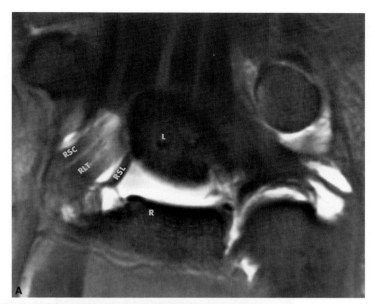

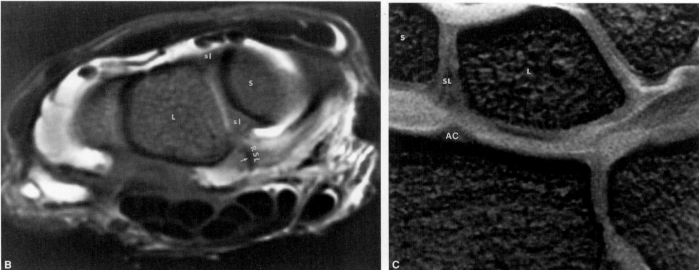

FIGURE 11-13. Anatomy of the radioscapholunate (RSL) and radioscaphocapitate ligaments. (**A**) The RSL ligament represents a neurovascular structure extending from the distal radius into the scapholunate articulation. This ligament, which has also been referred to as the ligament of Testut and Kuenz, is located volar to the intrinsic scapholunate ligament (fat-suppressed T1-weighted coronal MR arthrography image). RSC, radioscaphocapitate ligament; RLT, radiolunotriquetral ligament; L, lunate; R, radius. (**B**) Radioscapholunate ligament (RSL; *arrow*) extending to the scapholunate interval between the scaphoid (S) and lunate (L). Note the relative volar location of the extrinsic RSL to the intrinsic SL ligament (fat-suppressed T1-weighted axial MR arthrographic image). sl, dorsal and volar portions of the intrinsic scapholunate ligament. (**C**) At the level of the distal radius the normal articular cartilage (AC) ridge between the scaphoid fossa and lunate fossa demonstrates a triangular appearance, and is seen in the same plane as the intrinsic scapholunate ligament (spoiled GRASS [SPGR] coronal image at a 4 cm FOV and 1 mm slice thickness). This articular cartilage ridge should not be mistaken for a site of ligamentous attachment.

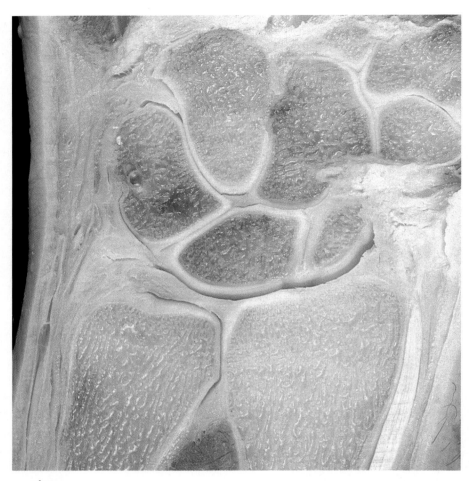

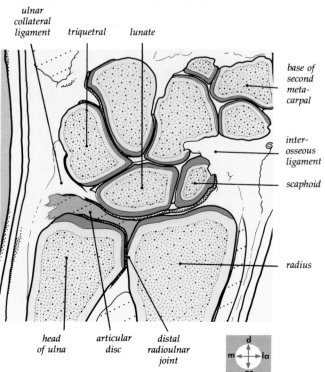

FIGURE 11-14. A coronal section of the wrist joint shows the articular surfaces and triangular cartilage.

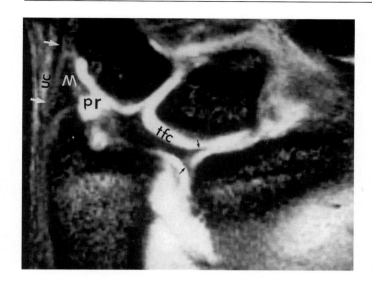

FIGURE 11-15. A T2*-weighted image showing the triangular fibro-cartilage complex. Black arrows, radial attachments of triangular fibrocartilage; white arrows and UC, ulnar collateral ligament; M, meniscus homologue; pr, prestyloid recess; tfc, triangular fibrocartilage.

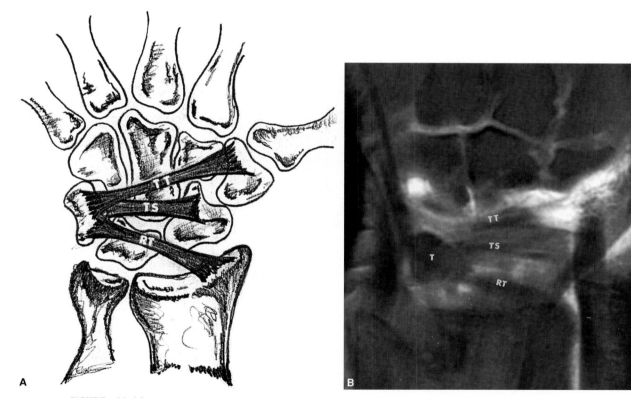

FIGURE 11-16. Patterns of the dorsal carpal ligaments. **(A)** Illustration and **(B)** corresponding fat-suppressed T1-weighted coronal image of a single radiotriquetral ligament (RT) and the triquetroscaphoid (TS) and triquetrotrapezial (TT) fascicles of the dorsal intercarpal ligament. T, triquetrum.   *continued*

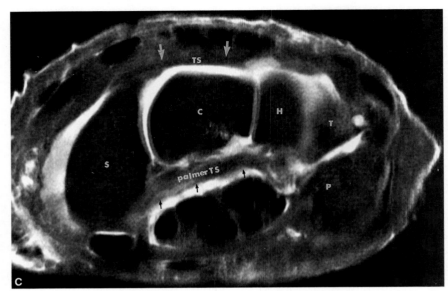

FIGURE 11-16. *Continued.* **(C)** On a fat-suppressed T2-weighted axial image, the triquetroscaphoid fascicle is seen dorsally between the triquetral bone and dorsal pole of the scaphoid (S). The triquetroscaphoid fascicle (TS; *arrows*) extends over the hamate (H) and capitate (C). The palmar triquetroscaphoid ligament is also identified at this level (palmar TS; *arrows*). P, pisiform.

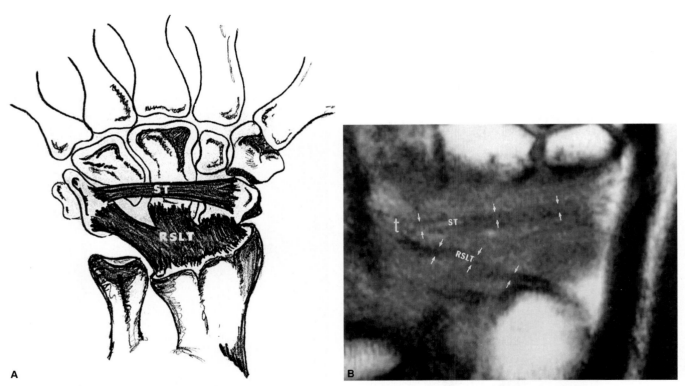

FIGURE 11-17. **(A)** Illustration showing the dorsal intercarpal ligament with a single band (st; *arrows*) without separate triquetroscaphoid and triquetrotrapezial fascicles. The radiotriquetral ligament is labeled from its attachments as the radioscapholunotriquetral ligament (RSLT; *arrows*). **(B)** The dorsal ligaments of the wrist include the dorsal radioscapholunotriquetral ligament (RSLT) or radiotriquetral ligament (RT) (*diagonally oriented white arrows*) and the scaphotriquetral or triquetral scaphoid ligament (ST; *transversely oriented white arrows*). The extensor retinaculum is located proximal to the RT ligament (corresponding T1-weighted coronal image). T, triquetrum.

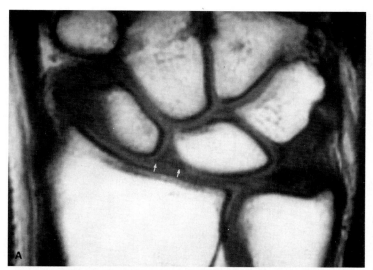

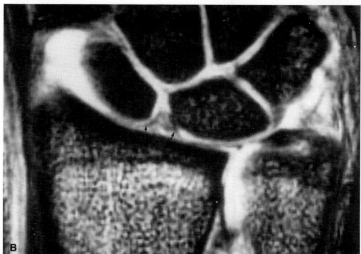

FIGURE 11-18. Anatomy of the scapholunate ligament (*arrows*) on coronal (**A**) T1-weighted and (**B**) T2*-weighted images. There is hyaline cartilage signal intensity at the ligament interfaces with both the scaphoid and lunate. The lunotriquetral ligament, thinner and more linear or horseshoe shaped, is located on the ulnar aspect of the wrist between the lunate and triquetrum. (**C,D**) The volar (v), membranous (m), and dorsal (d) portions of the scapholunate ligament are identified in a separate case. Note the horizontal or transverse orientation of the dorsal fibers which appear tendinous in appearance on **E** (**C**: T1-weighted volar coronal image; **D**: T1-weighted midplane coronal image).

continued

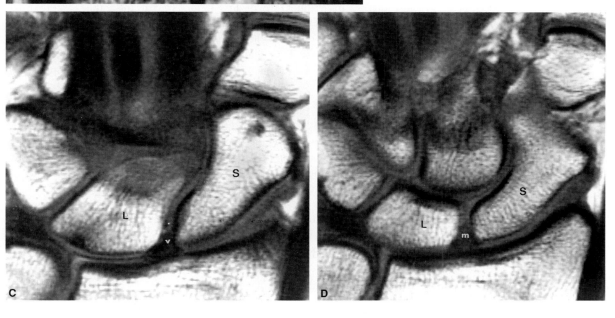

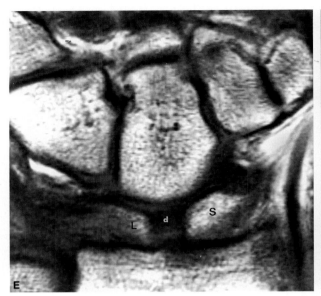

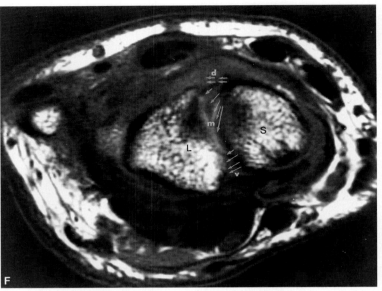

FIGURE 11-18. *Continued.* (E) The volar (v), membranous (m), and dorsal (d) portions of the scapholunate ligament are identified in a separate case. Note the horizontal or transverse orientation of the dorsal fibers which appear tendinous in appearance on E (E: T1-weighted dorsal coronal image). (F) T1-weighted axial image showing the various orientations of the scapholunate interosseous ligament fibers. The dorsal scapholunate ligament (d; *arrows*) is horizontally oriented and is perpendicular to the joint. The fibers of the membranous portion (m; *arrows*) of the scapholunate ligament course peripherally and obliquely from the scaphoid downward toward the lunate in a dorsal-to-volar direction. The volar scapholunate ligament (v; *arrows*) courses obliquely from the scaphoid downward to the lunate. This arrangement of scapholunate fibers biomechanically hinges the joint dorsally at the level of the dorsal transverse fibers. In forced extension, scapholunate ligament failure initiates in its volar aspect. S, scaphoid; L, lunate.

ment fibers attach to both bone and articular cartilage, whereas the dorsal and volar portions of the SL ligament attach directly to bone. The volar SL ligament fibers course obliquely between the volar aspects of the lunate and scaphoid.

The LT ligament is a thin horseshoe-shaped structure that may appear more lax than the SL ligament on MR imaging.[43] The LT ligament does not extend as distally into the LT joint compared with the longer proximal distal dimension of the SL ligament within the SL joint. The volar and dorsal portions of the LT attach directly to bone, whereas its midportion attaches to the hyaline articular cartilage of the LT joint.[43] Smith and Snearly[53] have shown that on coronal MR images the LT ligament is most commonly delta shaped or linear.[53]

ARCUATE LIGAMENTS. More distally, there is a set of ligaments that stabilizes the distal row on the proximal row. These ligaments have been referred to as the deltoid[54] or arcuate ligaments[55] (Fig. 11-19). The ulnar arcuate ligament extends from the volar surface of the lunate and triquetrum to the neck of the capitate, and plays a role in preventing the proximal row from volarflexion (see Fig. 11-19). Progressing radially, the substance of this structure becomes quite thin in the region of the capitolunate articulation. The radial limb (ie, radial arcuate ligament) of this V-shaped ligament runs from the capitate to the distal pole of the scaphoid. The thin tissue between the limbs of the arcuate

or deltoid ligament is known as the space of Poirier. This weak area in the ligamentous floor of the carpus may function as a trap door through which the lunate or capitate may dislocate. The particular functions of these ligaments with respect to midcarpal instabilities are discussed in "Carpal Instabilities." Proximal fibers of the RSC and ulnar arcuate ligament merge volar to the head of the capitate, and are joined by reflected fibers distally from the TFC ligament. This creates a sling-like support for the head of the capitate and hamate.[56] This sling can be appreciated as a thick low signal intensity band extending from the triquetrum to the scaphoid on axial images.

DISTAL CARPAL ROW INTEROSSEOUS LIGAMENTS. Within the distal row, the trapezius and trapezium, trapezoid and capitate, and capitate and hamate are connected by interosseous ligaments. In contradistinction to the interosseous ligaments of the proximal row, these ligaments do not extend from the dorsal to the volar surface; and there is normally communication between the midcarpal space and carpometacarpal joints.

Tendons of the Wrist and Hand

Palm of the Hand

The flexor retinaculum and palmar aponeurosis represent thickened deep fascia of the wrist (Figs. 11-20 through

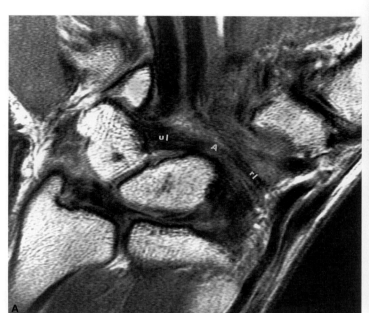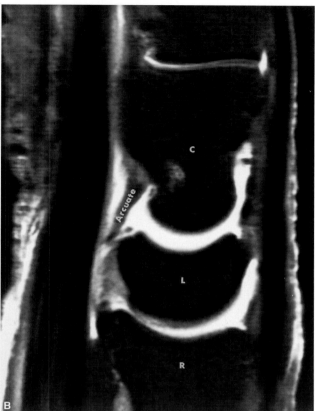

FIGURE 11-19. The arcuate or deltoid ligament. **(A)** The ulnar limb (ul) and radial limb (rl) of the volar intrinsic arcuate ligament are shown in the same volar plane on a T1-weighted coronal image. Both limbs attach centrally to the capitate. **(B)** The arcuate ligament is shown between the capitate (C) and lunate (L) on a midsagittal fat-suppressed MR arthrography image. The ulnar limb of the arcuate or deltoid ligament is the capitoscaphoid arm, and the radial limb of the arcuate ligament is the capitotriquetral arm.

11-22). The superficial palmaris longus tendon is fused to the midline of the flexor retinaculum and expands distally into the palmar aponeurosis. Guyon's canal, a site of potential compression of the ulnar nerve, is formed by an ulnar extension of the flexor retinaculum superficial to the ulnar nerve and artery.

The concave volar surface of the carpus and flexor retinaculum form the anatomic boundaries of the carpal tunnel for passage of the long flexor tendons of the fingers and thumb (Fig. 11-23). The four flexor digitorum superficialis tendons are arranged in two rows, with the tendons to the third (ie, middle) and fourth (ie, ring) digits superficial to the tendons for the second (ie, index) and fifth (ie, little) digits (Fig. 11-24). After entering their respective fibrous flexor sheaths, the tendons of the flexor digitorum superficialis divide into two halves opposite the proximal phalanx and partially decussate around the flexor digitorum profundus tendons. Distal to the site of perforation by the flexor

digitorum profundus, the superficialis tendons pass deep to the flexor digitorum profundus and send slips to attach to the sides of the middle phalanx. The tendons of the flexor digitorum profundus are arranged in the same plane and pass deep to the flexor digitorum superficialis (Fig. 11-25). The tendons of the flexor digitorum profundus attach distally to the base of the terminal phalanx and change from a deep to a superficial location at the partial decussation of the superficialis at the level of the middle phalanx (Fig. 11-26).

Dorsum of the Hand

The extensor digitorum tendons extend across the metacarpophalangeal (MP) joints and contribute to the posterior capsule of this joint, then they broaden out onto the dorsum of the proximal phalanx (Figs. 11-27 and 11-28). The extensor expansion represents the joining of the extensor tendons

text continues on page 879

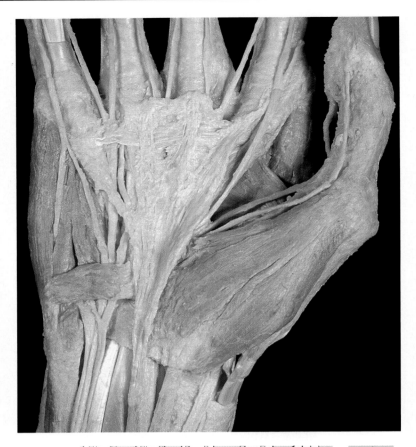

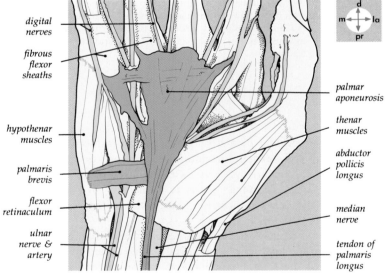

FIGURE 11-20. The palmar aponeurosis is revealed by removing the skin and superficial fascia. The investing fascia has been removed proximal to the flexor retinaculum. R, radius.

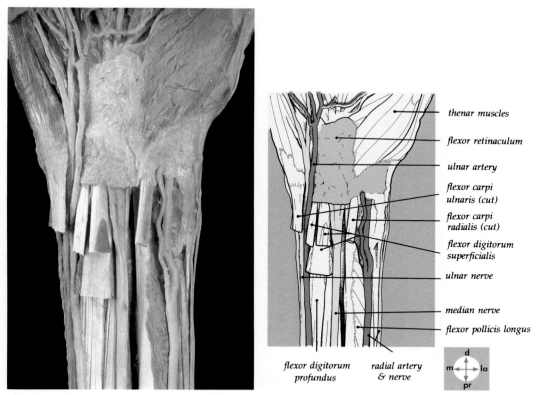

FIGURE 11-21. The flexor retinaculum and its superficial relations and structures are seen entering the carpal tunnel.

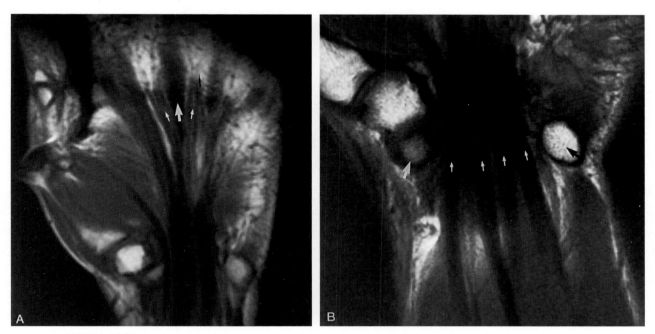

FIGURE 11-22. Volar coronal anatomy. **(A)** A T1-weighted coronal image shows the normal low signal intensity tendon (*large arrow*) and intermediate signal intensity palmar aponeurosis (*small arrows*) distal to the carpal tunnel. **(B)** At a deeper level, a T1-weighted coronal image shows the low signal intensity flexor tendons (*small white arrows*) passing through carpal tunnel. The trapezium (*large white arrow*) and pisiform (*black arrow*) are also seen.

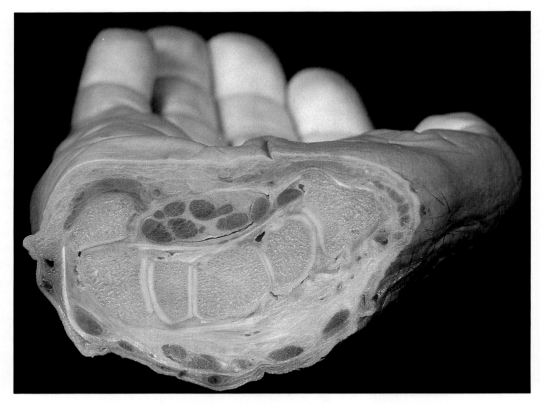

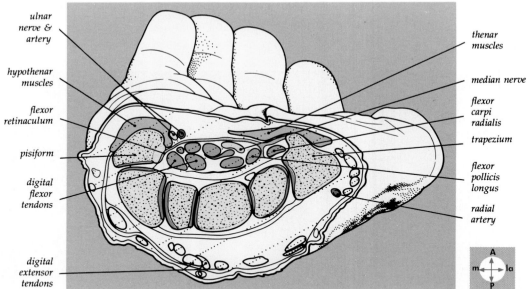

FIGURE 11-23. A transverse section through the carpus shows the carpal tunnel and its contents.

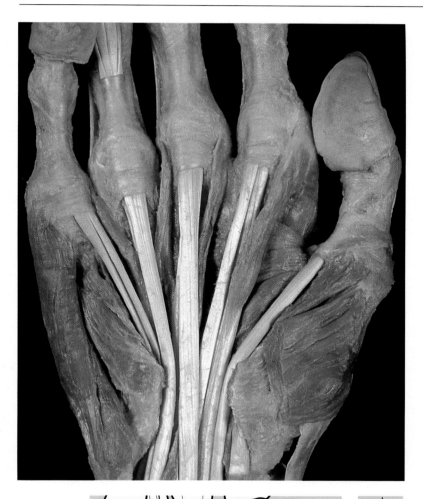

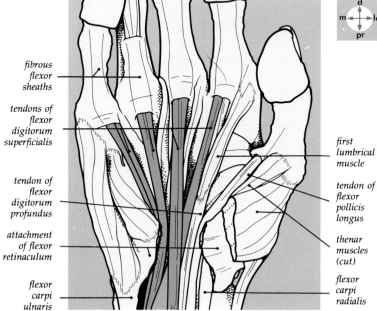

fibrous
flexor
sheaths

tendons of
flexor
digitorum
superficialis

tendon of
flexor
digitorum
profundus

attachment
of flexor
retinaculum

flexor
carpi
ulnaris

first
lumbrical
muscle

tendon of
flexor
pollicis
longus

thenar
muscles
(cut)

flexor
carpi
radialis

FIGURE 11-24. The palmar aponeurosis, flexor retinaculum, investing fascia, and palmar vessels and nerves have been removed to reveal the tendons of the flexor digitorum superficialis in the palm.

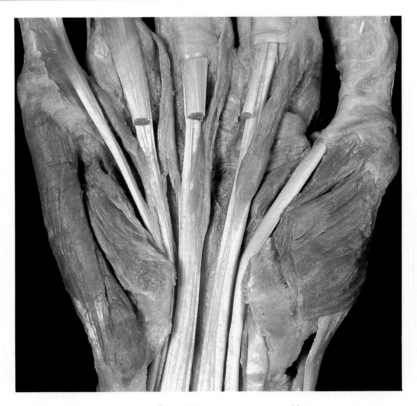

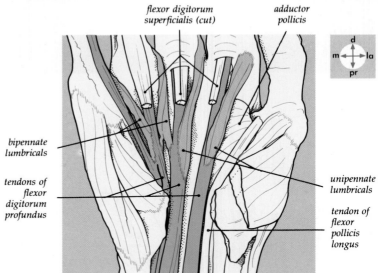

flexor digitorum
superficialis (cut)

adductor
pollicis

bipennate
lumbricals

tendons of
flexor
digitorum
profundus

unipennate
lumbricals

tendon of
flexor
pollicis
longus

FIGURE 11-25. Removal of the tendons of the flexor digitorum superficialis reveals the attachments of the lumbrical muscles to the tendons of the flexor digitorum profundus.

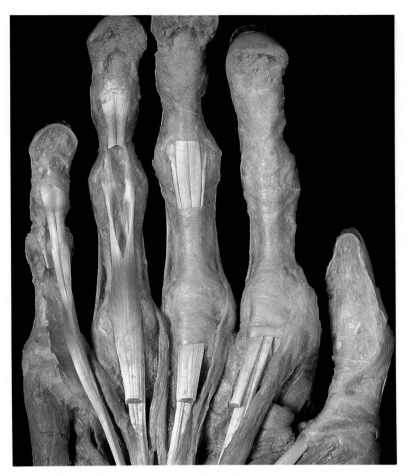

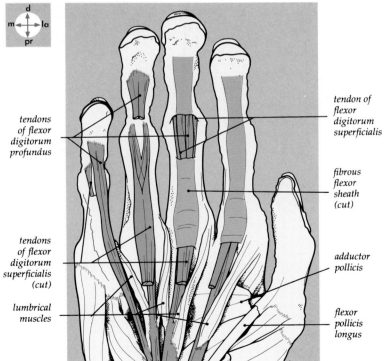

tendons
of flexor
digitorum
profundus

tendon of
flexor
digitorum
superficialis

fibrous
flexor
sheath
(cut)

tendons
of flexor
digitorum
superficialis
(cut)

adductor
pollicis

lumbrical
muscles

flexor
pollicis
longus

FIGURE 11-26. Partial cutting away of the fibrous flexor sheath of the middle finger exposes the tendons of the flexor digitorum superficialis and profundus, revealing the phalangeal attachments in the ring and little fingers.

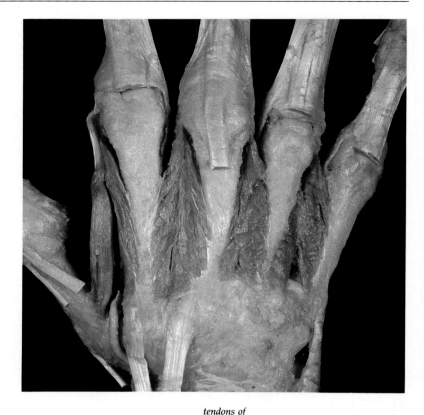

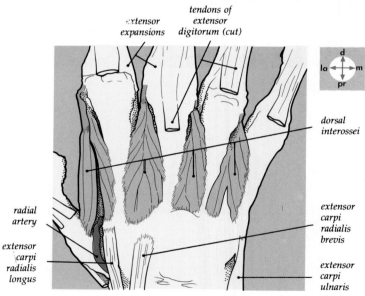

FIGURE 11-27. The dorsal interossei is exposed by removing the deep fascia and the tendons of the extensor digitorum.

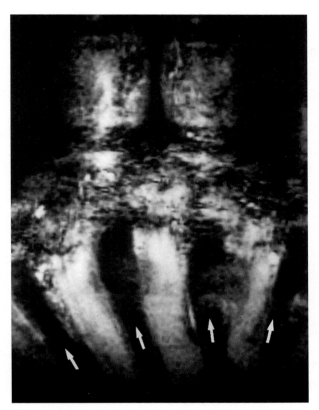

FIGURE 11-28. The low signal intensity tendons of the extensor digitorum (*white arrows*) are seen on a T2*-weighted dorsal coronal image.

and posterior fascia. The extensor tendons and expansion divide into a central slip, which inserts into the base of the middle phalanx, and two lateral or marginal slips, which diverge around the central slip and then converge to insert into the base of the distal phalanx. The interosseous and lumbrical tendons insert onto the dorsal extensor expansion from each of its sides and from its lateral side, respectively.

Ligamentous Support of the Digits

The MP, proximal interphalangeal (PIP), and distal interphalangeal joints are reinforced by palmar and paired collateral ligaments. The palmar ligament, or fibrocartilaginous volar plate, is located between and connected to the collateral ligaments. The palmar ligament blends with the deep transverse metacarpal ligament in the second to fifth MP joints.

NORMAL MAGNETIC RESONANCE ANATOMY OF THE WRIST AND HAND

Axial Images

In the axial plane (Fig. 11-29), the flexor digitorum superficialis and profundus tendons are seen as tubular low signal intensity structures with invested synovial sheaths. In proximal sections, the flexor pollicis longus is seen deep to the median nerve. Distally, it is flanked by the adductor pollicis medially and by the thenar muscles laterally, toward the thumb. At the level of the DRUJ, the volar distal radioulnar

text continues on page 886

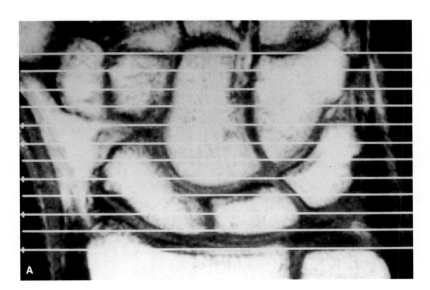

FIGURE 11-29. Normal axial MR anatomy. **(A)** This T1-weighted coronal localizer was used to graphically prescribe axial image locations from **(B)** proximal to **(M)** distal. Images were made at 12 different locations.

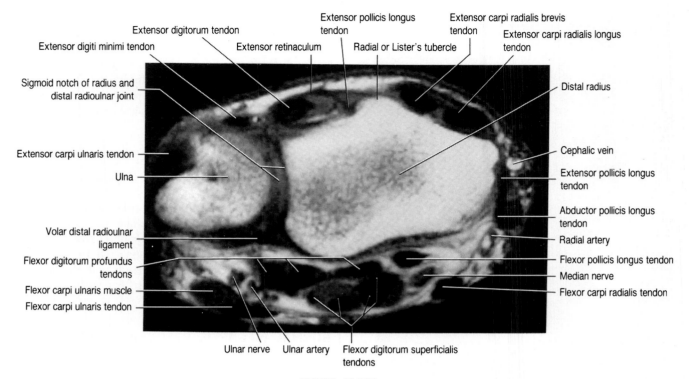

Extensor digiti minimi tendon

Extensor digitorum tendon

Extensor pollicis longus tendon

Extensor retinaculum

Radial or Lister's tubercle

Extensor pollicis longus tendon

Extensor carpi radialis brevis tendon

Extensor carpi radialis longus tendon

Sigmoid notch of radius and distal radioulnar joint

Distal radius

Extensor carpi ulnaris tendon

Ulna

Cephalic vein

Extensor pollicis longus tendon

Volar distal radioulnar ligament

Abductor pollicis longus tendon

Flexor digitorum profundus tendons

Radial artery

Flexor carpi ulnaris muscle

Flexor pollicis longus tendon

Flexor carpi ulnaris tendon

Median nerve

Flexor carpi radialis tendon

Ulnar nerve

Ulnar artery

Flexor digitorum superficialis tendons

FIGURE 11-29B.

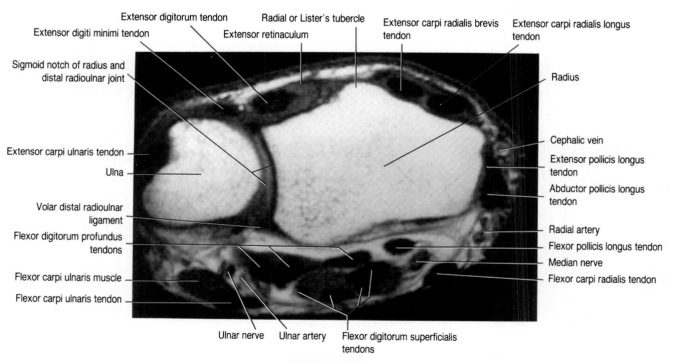

Extensor digiti minimi tendon

Extensor digitorum tendon

Radial or Lister's tubercle

Extensor retinaculum

Extensor carpi radialis brevis tendon

Extensor carpi radialis longus tendon

Sigmoid notch of radius and distal radioulnar joint

Radius

Extensor carpi ulnaris tendon

Ulna

Cephalic vein

Extensor pollicis longus tendon

Volar distal radioulnar ligament

Abductor pollicis longus tendon

Flexor digitorum profundus tendons

Radial artery

Flexor carpi ulnaris muscle

Flexor pollicis longus tendon

Flexor carpi ulnaris tendon

Median nerve

Flexor carpi radialis tendon

Ulnar nerve

Ulnar artery

Flexor digitorum superficialis tendons

FIGURE 11-29C.

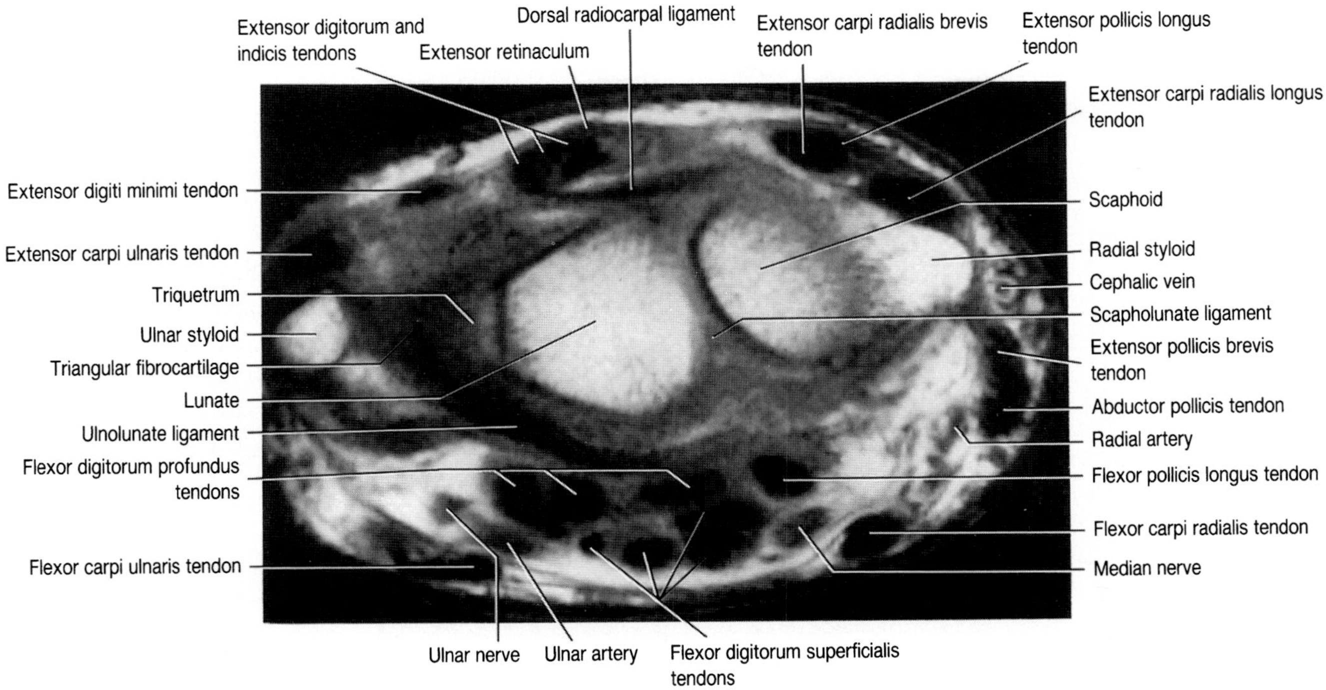

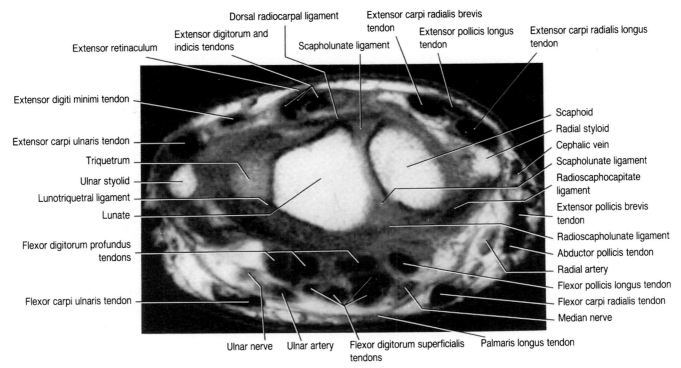

FIGURE 11-29D.

FIGURE 11-29E.

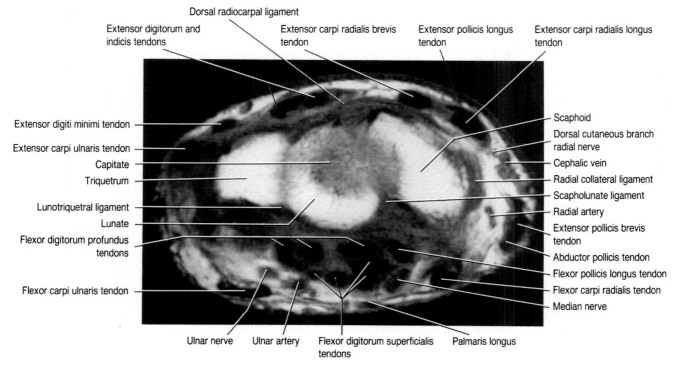

FIGURE 11-29F.

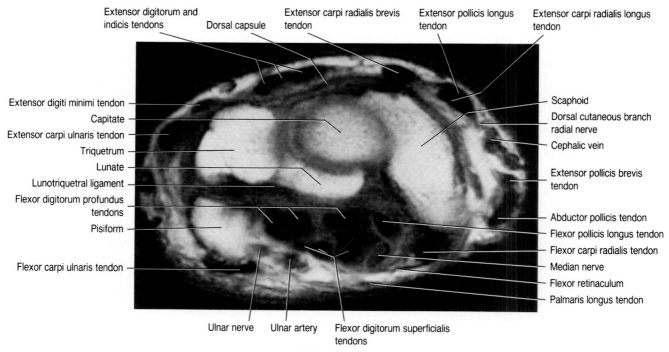

FIGURE 11-29G.

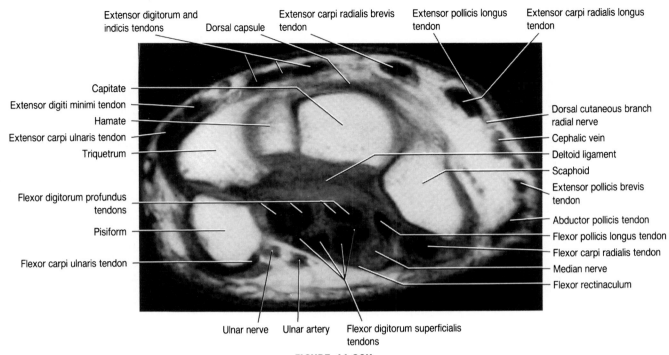

Extensor digitorum and indicis tendons
Dorsal capsule
Extensor carpi radialis brevis tendon
Extensor pollicis longus tendon
Extensor carpi radialis longus tendon

Capitate
Extensor digiti minimi tendon
Hamate
Extensor carpi ulnaris tendon
Triquetrum

Flexor digitorum profundus tendons
Pisiform

Flexor carpi ulnaris tendon

Dorsal cutaneous branch radial nerve
Cephalic vein
Deltoid ligament
Scaphoid
Extensor pollicis brevis tendon
Abductor pollicis tendon
Flexor pollicis longus tendon
Flexor carpi radialis tendon
Median nerve
Flexor rectinaculum

Ulnar nerve   Ulnar artery   Flexor digitorum superficialis tendons

FIGURE 11-29H.

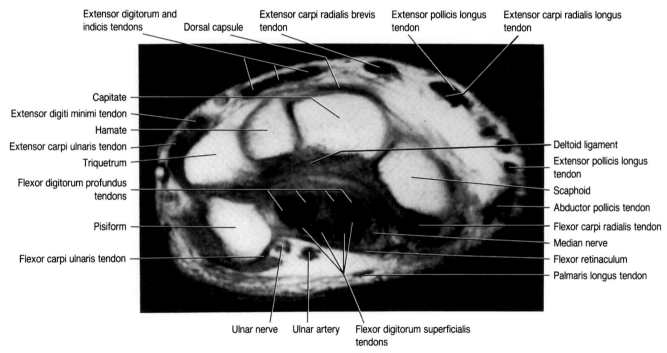

Extensor digitorum and indicis tendons
Dorsal capsule
Extensor carpi radialis brevis tendon
Extensor pollicis longus tendon
Extensor carpi radialis longus tendon

Capitate
Extensor digiti minimi tendon
Hamate
Extensor carpi ulnaris tendon
Triquetrum
Flexor digitorum profundus tendons
Pisiform

Flexor carpi ulnaris tendon

Deltoid ligament
Extensor pollicis longus tendon
Scaphoid
Abductor pollicis tendon
Flexor carpi radialis tendon
Median nerve
Flexor retinaculum
Palmaris longus tendon

Ulnar nerve   Ulnar artery   Flexor digitorum superficialis tendons

FIGURE 11-29I.

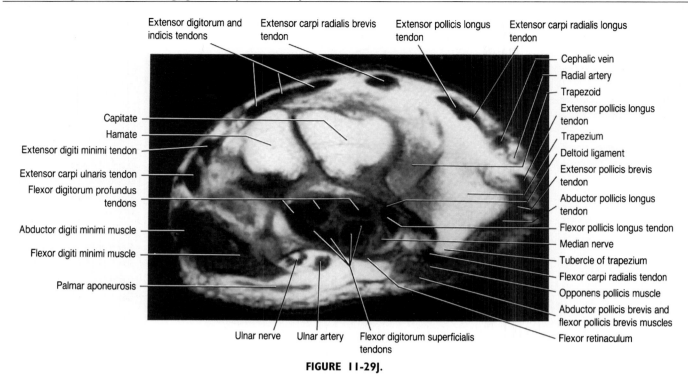

Extensor digitorum and indicis tendons
Extensor carpi radialis brevis tendon
Extensor pollicis longus tendon
Extensor carpi radialis longus tendon

Capitate
Hamate
Extensor digiti minimi tendon
Extensor carpi ulnaris tendon
Flexor digitorum profundus tendons
Abductor digiti minimi muscle
Flexor digiti minimi muscle
Palmar aponeurosis

Cephalic vein
Radial artery
Trapezoid
Extensor pollicis longus tendon
Trapezium
Deltoid ligament
Extensor pollicis brevis tendon
Abductor pollicis longus tendon
Flexor pollicis longus tendon
Median nerve
Tubercle of trapezium
Flexor carpi radialis tendon
Opponens pollicis muscle
Abductor pollicis brevis and flexor pollicis brevis muscles
Flexor retinaculum

Ulnar nerve   Ulnar artery   Flexor digitorum superficialis tendons

FIGURE 11-29J.

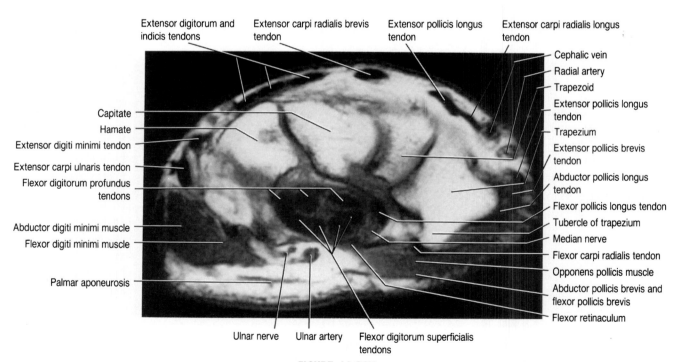

Extensor digitorum and indicis tendons
Extensor carpi radialis brevis tendon
Extensor pollicis longus tendon
Extensor carpi radialis longus tendon

Capitate
Hamate
Extensor digiti minimi tendon
Extensor carpi ulnaris tendon
Flexor digitorum profundus tendons
Abductor digiti minimi muscle
Flexor digiti minimi muscle
Palmar aponeurosis

Cephalic vein
Radial artery
Trapezoid
Extensor pollicis longus tendon
Trapezium
Extensor pollicis brevis tendon
Abductor pollicis longus tendon
Flexor pollicis longus tendon
Tubercle of trapezium
Median nerve
Flexor carpi radialis tendon
Opponens pollicis muscle
Abductor pollicis brevis and flexor pollicis brevis
Flexor retinaculum

Ulnar nerve   Ulnar artery   Flexor digitorum superficialis tendons

FIGURE 11-29K.

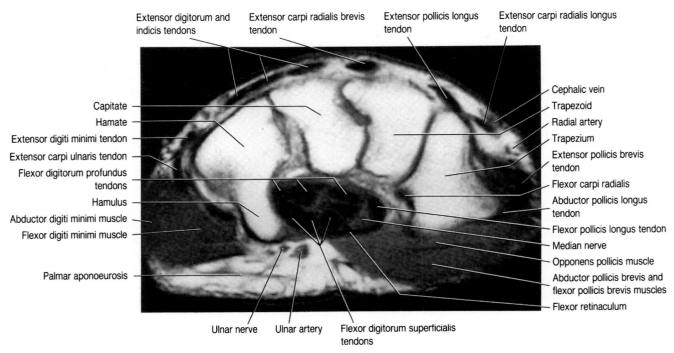

Extensor digitorum and indicis tendons
Extensor carpi radialis brevis tendon
Extensor pollicis longus tendon
Extensor carpi radialis longus tendon

Capitate
Hamate
Extensor digiti minimi tendon
Extensor carpi ulnaris tendon
Flexor digitorum profundus tendons
Hamulus
Abductor digiti minimi muscle
Flexor digiti minimi muscle
Palmar aponoeurosis

Cephalic vein
Trapezoid
Radial artery
Trapezium
Extensor pollicis brevis tendon
Flexor carpi radialis
Abductor pollicis longus tendon
Flexor pollicis longus tendon
Median nerve
Opponens pollicis muscle
Abductor pollicis brevis and flexor pollicis brevis muscles
Flexor retinaculum

Ulnar nerve
Ulnar artery
Flexor digitorum superficialis tendons

FIGURE 11-29L.

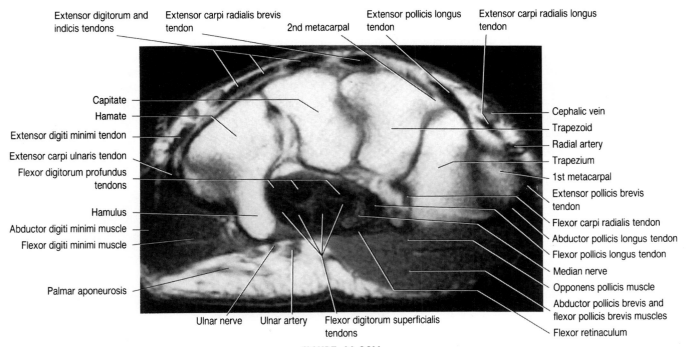

Extensor digitorum and indicis tendons
Extensor carpi radialis brevis tendon
2nd metacarpal
Extensor pollicis longus tendon
Extensor carpi radialis longus tendon

Capitate
Hamate
Extensor digiti minimi tendon
Extensor carpi ulnaris tendon
Flexor digitorum profundus tendons
Hamulus
Abductor digiti minimi muscle
Flexor digiti minimi muscle
Palmar aponeurosis

Cephalic vein
Trapezoid
Radial artery
Trapezium
1st metacarpal
Extensor pollicis brevis tendon
Flexor carpi radialis tendon
Abductor pollicis longus tendon
Flexor pollicis longus tendon
Median nerve
Opponens pollicis muscle
Abductor pollicis brevis and flexor pollicis brevis muscles
Flexor retinaculum

Ulnar nerve
Ulnar artery
Flexor digitorum superficialis tendons

FIGURE 11-29M.

ligament is identified as a thin, low signal intensity band, deep to the flexor digitorum profundus tendons and Parona's space. The position of the distal ulna in relation to the sigmoid notch is determined at this level. The TFCC is displayed on the ulnar aspect of the ulnar styloid. The curve of the ulnolunate ligament is demonstrated at the level of the proximal lunate and distal radius, where it follows the contour of the ulnar and volar aspect of the lunate. The palmaris longus tendon is superficial to the median nerve. The thin low signal intensity flexor retinaculum spans the palmar border of the carpal tunnel. Its distal attachments to the hook of the lunate and tubercle of the trapezium are more reliably defined than the proximal attachments to the tubercles of the pisiform and scaphoid. The separate extensor tendons of the extensor carpi ulnaris, extensor digiti minimi, extensor digitorum and indicis, extensor pollicis longus, and extensor carpi radialis longus are displayed from the ulnar to the radial dorsal aspect of the wrist. The LT and SL and are usually demonstrated at the level of the proximal carpal row. The arcuate ligament is seen volar to the capitate and deep to the flexor tendons. The radial collateral ligament is closely applied to the radial surface of the scaphoid. The palmaris longus tendon is superficial to the median nerve and the flexor retinaculum. The two central tendons of the superficial flexor group are located superiorly within the carpal tunnel before they fan out to their insertions on the middle phalanx. On axial plane images, it is possible to differentiate the four separate tendons of the flexor profundus group. The lumbrical muscle origins are seen deep to the flexor tendons on axial sections through the distal carpal tunnel and demonstrate intermediate signal intensity. The median nerve, also of intermediate signal intensity, can be identified in the superficial radial aspect of the carpal tunnel. On axial images through the midmetacarpals, the flexor tendons are seen anterior to the palmar in-

terossei muscles, whereas the dorsal interossei are seen lying between the metacarpal bones.

Blood vessels display low signal intensity, except in venous structures demonstrated by even-echo rephasing or paradoxical enhancement secondary to slow flow. With gradient-echo techniques, both arterial and venous structures demonstrate high signal intensity.

Sagittal Images

The sagittal imaging plane (Fig. 11-30) is routine in wrist protocols. It is especially useful in the evaluation of static instability patterns and wrist shortening (ie, proximal migration of the capitate) and in viewing the volar-to-dorsal aspect of the TFC. Kienböck's fracture and fracture deformity (ie, humpback scaphoid) are seen on sagittal images, complementary to coronal or axial images. The abductor pollicis longus (APL) and extensor pollicis brevis (EPB) tendons can be seen on radial sagittal images. The scaphoid is identified on sagittal sections through the trapezium and, more dorsally, the trapezoid. The low signal intensity RSC ligament is represented by fibers seen along the volar aspect of the scaphoid between the volar distal radius and the distal pole of the scaphoid. The extensor pollicis longus tendon is dorsal to the radioscaphoid articulation. The pronator quadratus muscle extends along the volar surface of the radial metaphysis and distal diaphysis. The low signal intensity tendon of the flexor carpi radialis is draped volarly over the distal pole of the scaphoid. The long axis (ie, vertical orientation) of the flexor pollicis longus tendon is seen at the ulnar aspect of the scaphoid. The capitate, lunate, and radius are colinearly aligned in sagittal images through the third metacarpal axis.

text continues on page 892

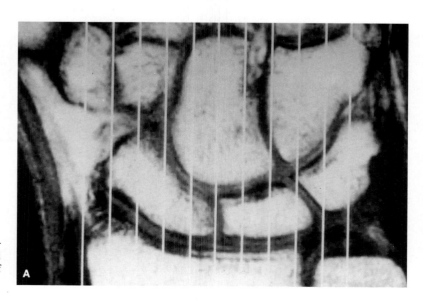

FIGURE 11-30. Normal sagittal MR anatomy. **(A)** This T1-weighted coronal localizer was used to prescribe sagittal image locations from the **(B)** radial to **(L)** ulnar aspect of the wrist.

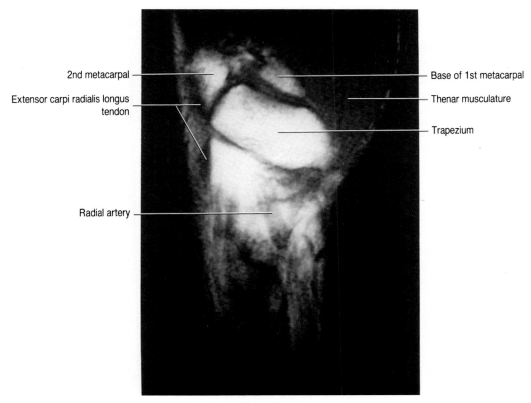

2nd metacarpal

Extensor carpi radialis longus
tendon

Radial artery

Base of 1st metacarpal

Thenar musculature

Trapezium

FIGURE 11-30B.

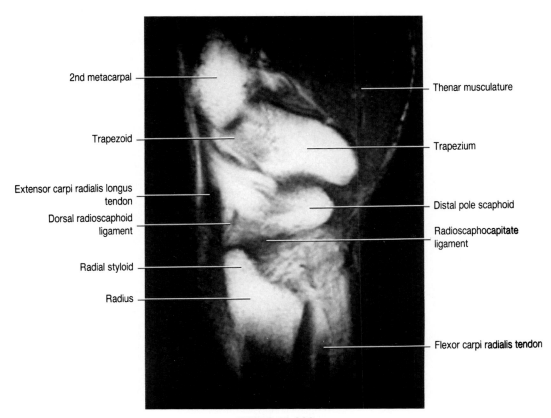

2nd metacarpal

Trapezoid

Extensor carpi radialis longus
tendon

Dorsal radioscaphoid
ligament

Radial styloid

Radius

Thenar musculature

Trapezium

Distal pole scaphoid

Radioscaphocapitate
ligament

Flexor carpi radialis tendon

FIGURE 11-30C.

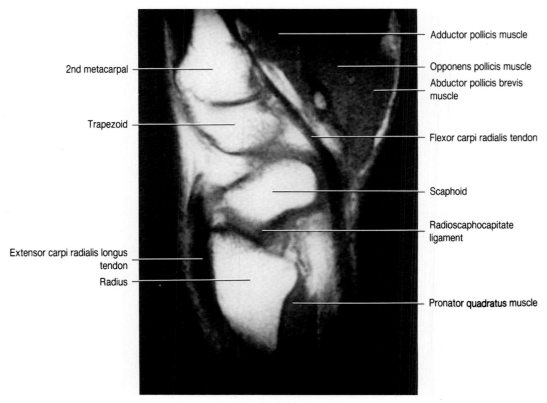

2nd metacarpal

Trapezoid

Extensor carpi radialis longus tendon

Radius

Adductor pollicis muscle

Opponens pollicis muscle

Abductor pollicis brevis muscle

Flexor carpi radialis tendon

Scaphoid

Radioscaphocapitate ligament

Pronator **quadratus** muscle

FIGURE 11-30D.

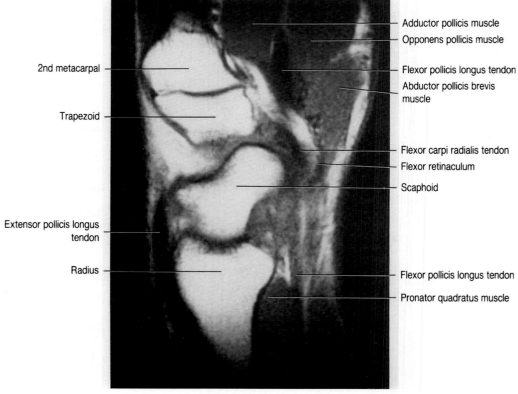

2nd metacarpal

Trapezoid

Extensor pollicis longus tendon

Radius

Adductor pollicis muscle

Opponens pollicis muscle

Flexor pollicis longus tendon

Abductor pollicis brevis muscle

Flexor carpi radialis tendon

Flexor retinaculum

Scaphoid

Flexor pollicis longus tendon

Pronator quadratus muscle

FIGURE 11-30E.

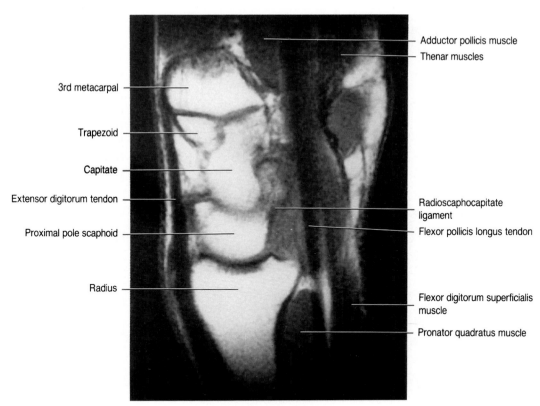

Adductor pollicis muscle

Thenar muscles

3rd metacarpal

Trapezoid

Capitate

Extensor digitorum tendon

Proximal pole scaphoid

Radius

Radioscaphocapitate ligament

Flexor pollicis longus tendon

Flexor digitorum superficialis muscle

Pronator quadratus muscle

FIGURE 11-30F.

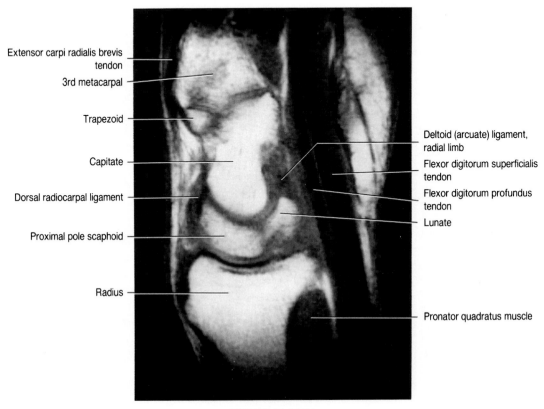

Extensor carpi radialis brevis tendon

3rd metacarpal

Trapezoid

Capitate

Dorsal radiocarpal ligament

Proximal pole scaphoid

Radius

Deltoid (arcuate) ligament, radial limb

Flexor digitorum superficialis tendon

Flexor digitorum profundus tendon

Lunate

Pronator quadratus muscle

FIGURE 11-30G.

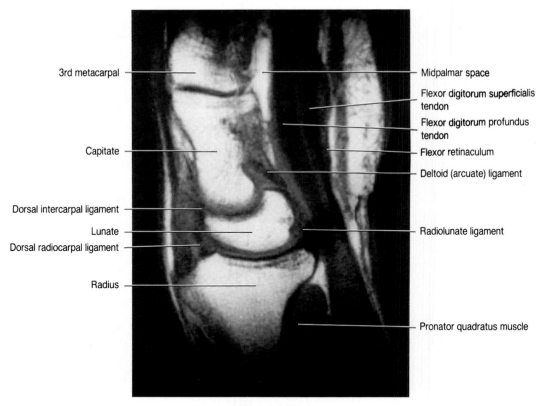

3rd metacarpal — Midpalmar space

Flexor digitorum superficialis tendon

Flexor digitorum profundus tendon

Capitate — Flexor retinaculum

Deltoid (arcuate) ligament

Dorsal intercarpal ligament —

Lunate — Radiolunate ligament

Dorsal radiocarpal ligament —

Radius —

Pronator quadratus muscle

FIGURE 11-30H.

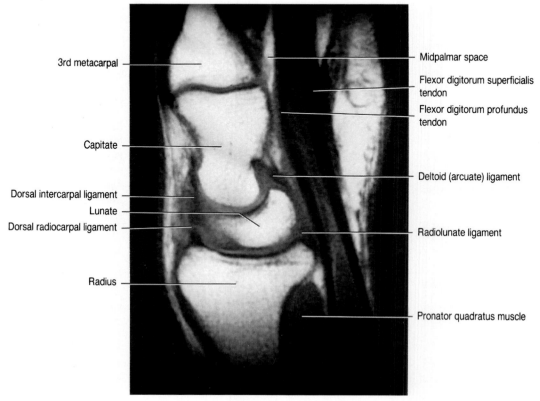

3rd metacarpal — Midpalmar space

Flexor digitorum superficialis tendon

Flexor digitorum profundus tendon

Capitate —

Deltoid (arcuate) ligament

Dorsal intercarpal ligament —

Lunate —

Dorsal radiocarpal ligament —

Radiolunate ligament

Radius —

Pronator quadratus muscle

FIGURE 11-30I.

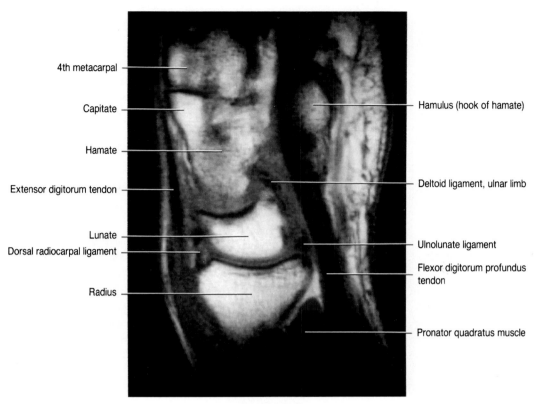

4th metacarpal

Capitate

Hamate

Extensor digitorum tendon

Lunate

Dorsal radiocarpal ligament

Radius

Hamulus (hook of hamate)

Deltoid ligament, ulnar limb

Ulnolunate ligament

Flexor digitorum profundus tendon

Pronator quadratus muscle

FIGURE 11-30J.

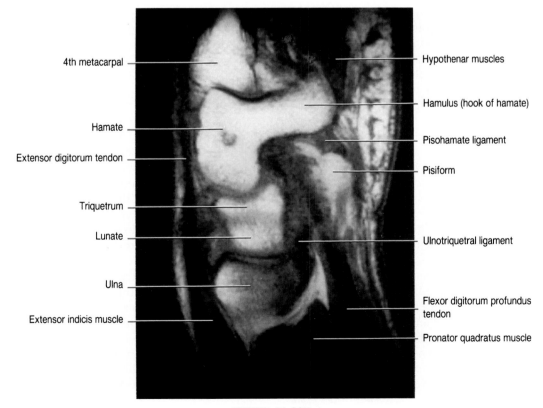

4th metacarpal

Hamate

Extensor digitorum tendon

Triquetrum

Lunate

Ulna

Extensor indicis muscle

Hypothenar muscles

Hamulus (hook of hamate)

Pisohamate ligament

Pisiform

Ulnotriquetral ligament

Flexor digitorum profundus tendon

Pronator quadratus muscle

FIGURE 11-30K.

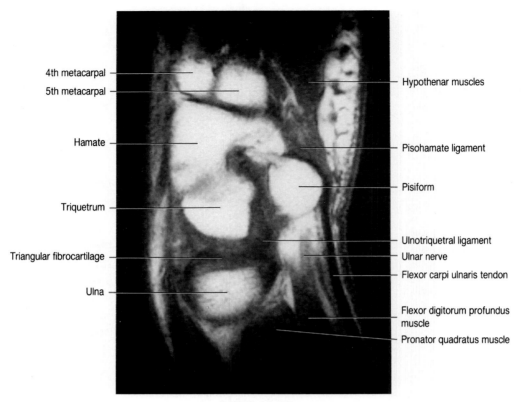

4th metacarpal
5th metacarpal

Hamate

Triquetrum

Triangular fibrocartilage

Ulna

Hypothenar muscles

Pisohamate ligament

Pisiform

Ulnotriquetral ligament
Ulnar nerve
Flexor carpi ulnaris tendon

Flexor digitorum profundus muscle
Pronator quadratus muscle

FIGURE 11-30L.

The radial limb of the deltoid or arcuate ligament extends proximally from the volar aspect of the capitate to the scaphoid. In the sagittal plane, the deltoid ligament may appear to connect to the volar distal surface of the lunate. The radiolunate ligament is located between the volar lunate surface and the distal radius at the radiolunate articulation, deep to the flexor digitorum profundus tendon. The ulnolunate ligament is radial to the TFC. The flexor digitorum superficialis and profundus tendons are best seen volar to the capitate and lunate. The flexor retinaculum is a thin dark line superficial to the flexor digitorum superficialis. The ulnar limb of the arcuate ligament is seen volar to the radial aspect of the triquetrum and the ulnar aspect of the lunate, ulnar to the plane of section through the capitate. The fourth metacarpal, the hook of the hamate, and the triquetrum are seen in the same sagittal section at the most ulnar aspect of the lunate or radial aspect of the ulna. The LT interosseous ligament is also seen at this level. The TFCC is located between the lunate and the ulna and has a concave distal surface. In ulnar sagittal images, the flexor carpi ulnaris extends in a volar direction to insert on the pisiform. The pisohamate and pisometacarpal ligaments attach to the hook of the hamate and the base of the fifth metacarpal, respectively. The intermediate signal intensity ulnar nerve is deep to the flexor carpi ulnaris. The ulnar collateral ligament component of the TFCC extends between the triquetrum and ulna, as can be seen on ulnar sagittal images out of the plane

of the TFC. The thick extensor carpi ulnaris tendon is seen as a groove in the posterior aspect of the distal ulna. In peripheral ulnar sagittal sections, it can be seen to extend dorsal to the triquetrum and insert into the base of the fifth metacarpal.

Coronal Images

Coronal plane images (Fig. 11-31) are important in understanding the relationship between the cartilaginous and ligamentous structures of the wrist. 3DFT volume imaging is more reliable for identification of the volar extrinsic ligaments of the wrist than T2*-weighted techniques with thicker (3 mm or greater) sections. On volar images, the flexor retinaculum is seen superficial to the flexor tendons as a transverse band. En face, the low signal intensity bands of the flexor digitorum tendons are seen passing through the carpal tunnel between the hook of the hamate and the trapezium. The intermediate signal intensity median nerve may also be discerned in this plane of section. The pisohamate and pisometacarpal ligaments are shown in sections at the level of the hook of the hamate and pisiform. The abductor pollicis longus and extensor pollicis brevis tendons border the volar radial aspect of the wrist in sections through the volar

text continues on page 896

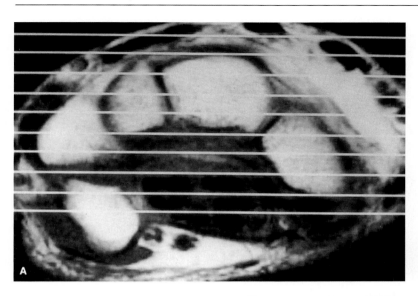

FIGURE 11-31. Normal coronal MR anatomy. **(A)** This T1-weighted axial localizer was used to prescribe coronal image locations from **(B)** dorsal to **(K)** volar.

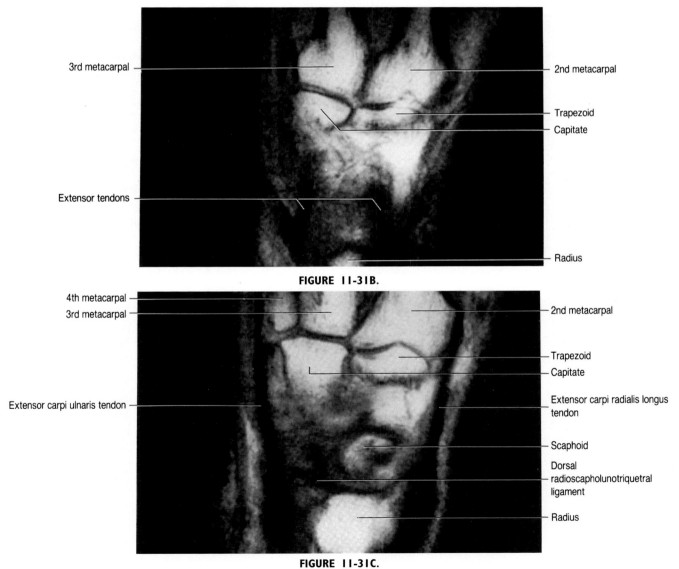

3rd metacarpal

2nd metacarpal

Trapezoid

Capitate

Extensor tendons

Radius

FIGURE 11-31B.

4th metacarpal

3rd metacarpal

2nd metacarpal

Trapezoid

Capitate

Extensor carpi ulnaris tendon

Extensor carpi radialis longus tendon

Scaphoid

Dorsal radioscapholunotriquetral ligament

Radius

FIGURE 11-31C.

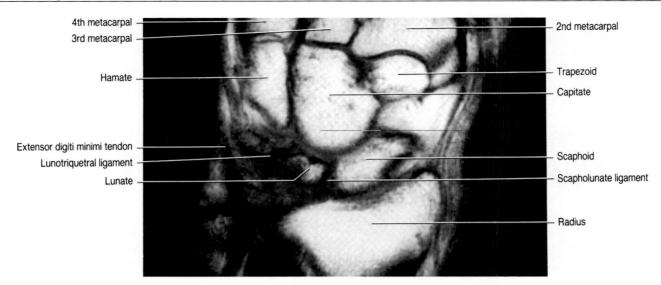

FIGURE 11-31D.

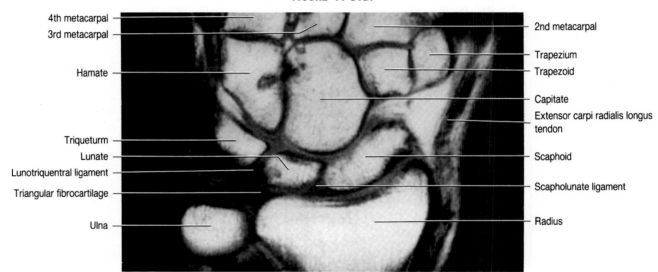

FIGURE 11-31E.

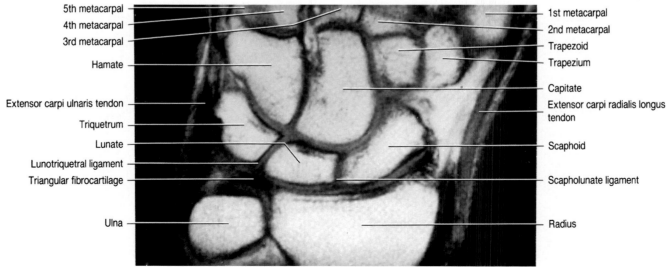

FIGURE 11-31F.

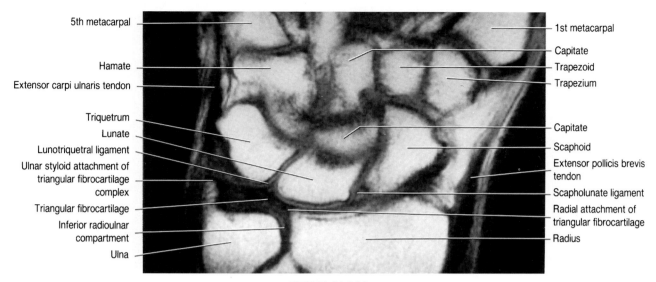

5th metacarpal

Hamate

Extensor carpi ulnaris tendon

Triquetrum

Lunate

Lunotriquetral ligament

Ulnar styloid attachment of
triangular fibrocartilage
complex

Triangular fibrocartilage

Inferior radioulnar
compartment

Ulna

1st metacarpal

Capitate

Trapezoid

Trapezium

Capitate

Scaphoid

Extensor pollicis brevis
tendon

Scapholunate ligament

Radial attachment of
triangular fibrocartilage

Radius

FIGURE 11-31G.

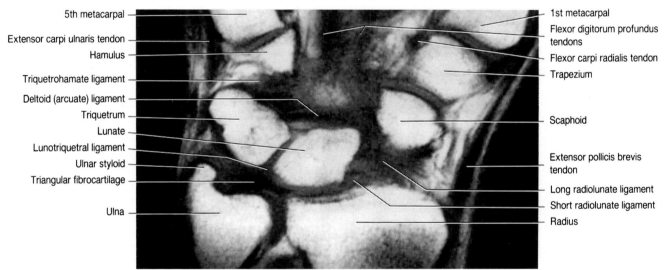

5th metacarpal

Extensor carpi ulnaris tendon

Hamulus

Triquetrohamate ligament

Deltoid (arcuate) ligament

Triquetrum

Lunate

Lunotriquetral ligament

Ulnar styloid

Triangular fibrocartilage

Ulna

1st metacarpal

Flexor digitorum profundus
tendons

Flexor carpi radialis tendon

Trapezium

Scaphoid

Extensor pollicis brevis
tendon

Long radiolunate ligament

Short radiolunate ligament

Radius

FIGURE 11-31H.

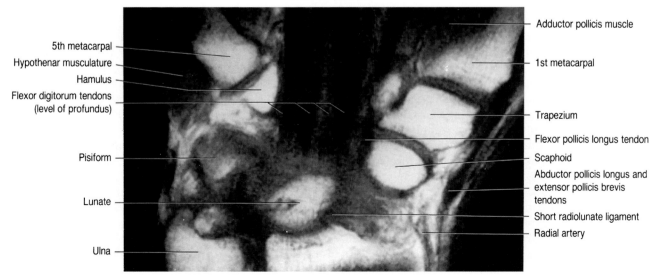

5th metacarpal

Hypothenar musculature

Hamulus

Flexor digitorum tendons
(level of profundus)

Pisiform

Lunate

Ulna

Adductor pollicis muscle

1st metacarpal

Trapezium

Flexor pollicis longus tendon

Scaphoid

Abductor pollicis longus and
extensor pollicis brevis
tendons

Short radiolunate ligament

Radial artery

FIGURE 11-31I.

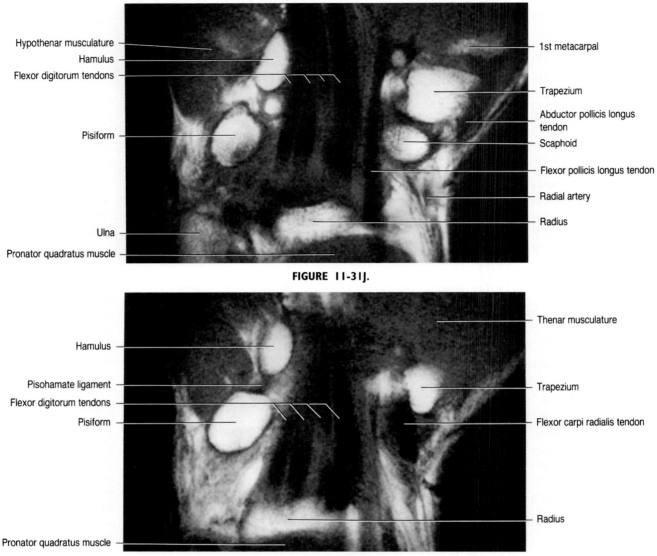

Hypothenar musculature
Hamulus
Flexor digitorum tendons
Pisiform
Ulna
Pronator quadratus muscle

1st metacarpal
Trapezium
Abductor pollicis longus tendon
Scaphoid
Flexor pollicis longus tendon
Radial artery
Radius

FIGURE II-31J.

Hamulus
Pisohamate ligament
Flexor digitorum tendons
Pisiform
Pronator quadratus muscle

Thenar musculature
Trapezium
Flexor carpi radialis tendon
Radius

FIGURE II-31K

surfaces of the scaphoid and lunate. The TFC is seen as a curvilinear bow-tie band of low, homogeneous signal intensity. The band extends horizontally to the base of the ulnar styloid process from the ulnar surface of the distal radius. The meniscal homologue has an intermediate signal intensity on T1- and T2*-weighted images. The RSC and RLT ligaments are visualized volarly and extend from the radial styloid in an ulnar distal direction. These fibers are seen as parallel bands of striations. The more ulnarly located RSL ligament is usually seen in the same plane as the RSC and RLT ligaments, and is a less substantial structure compared with the other volar extrinsic carpal ligaments. The LRL portion of the RLT ligament is represented by obliquely directed fibers extending from the volar radius to the lunate, volar to the proximal pole of the scaphoid. The DRUJ and compartment are separated from the radiocarpal compart-

ment by the TFC. The SL and LT interosseous ligaments are routinely visualized on 3 mm coronal T1- and T2*-weighted images. The extensor carpi ulnaris tendon borders the ulnar aspect of the wrist on the same coronal sections that display the TFC and interosseous ligaments. The radial collateral ligament may be partially visualized between the scaphoid and radial styloid. The articular cartilage surfaces of the carpal bones are of intermediate signal intensity on T1-weighted images and increase in signal intensity on T2*-weighted images. On dorsal images through the carpus, the interosseous ligaments of the distal carpal row can be defined. Dorsally, the obliquely oriented extensor digiti minimi tendon on the ulnar side of the triquetrum and the extensor carpi radialis longus tendon are seen. Lister's tubercle, which contains fatty marrow, is situated between and separates the ulnar aspect of the extensor pollicis longus from the radial aspect of the extensor carpi radialis brevis. The dorsal interossei muscles are demonstrated between the midcarpal shafts.

NORMAL MAGNETIC RESONANCE ANATOMY OF THE FINGERS

Axial Images

Sections through the MP joint (Fig. 11-32) show the flexor digitorum superficialis and profundus tendons as a low signal intensity (ie, dark) structure. Differentiation between the deep profundus and the more volar superficialis is poor. The extensor expansion can be seen dorsolaterally. The four lumbrical muscles that arise from the flexor digitorum profundus attach to the radial aspect to the extensor expansion. The interosseous tendons insert volarly and laterally onto the extensor expansions and the bases of the proximal phalanges. The low to intermediate signal intensity palmar digital artery and the intermediate signal intensity palmar nerve are better visualized than the dorsal neurovascular structures. The intermediate signal intensity palmar ligament (ie, volar plate) is seen between the MP joint and the flexor tendons. The fibrocartilaginous volar plate extends from the base of the proximal phalanx to the metacarpal head. The thin, intermediate signal intensity transverse metacarpal ligaments connect the volar plates of the second through the fifth MP joints. The collateral ligaments are composed of two parts: a weaker fan-like more proximal part, and a stronger cord-like distal part.

At the level of the PIP joints (Figs. 11-33 and 11-34), the flexor digitorum superficialis tendon, having split at the level of the midproximal phalanx, reunites and is deep to (ie, flanks) the flexor digitorum profundus tendon. The proximal and distal interphalangeal joints have palmar ligamentous (ie volar plate) and collateral ligamentous anatomy similar to that of the MP joints.

Sagittal Images

Differentiation between the flexor digitorum superficialis and the profundus is best seen at the mid- and proximal aspects of the proximal phalanx before the superficialis divides (Figs. 11-35 and 11-36). The central band of the extensor tendon and volar plate are identified on the distal and volar aspects of the PIP joints. The volar plate is also easily identified at the level of the MP and distal interphalangeal joints. The dorsal extensor expansion is parallel with and blends with the dorsal, low signal intensity cortex of the proximal phalanx.

Coronal Images

The individual parts of the collateral ligament are seen along the sides of the MP and interphalangeal joints (Fig. 11-37) The lateral bands of the extensor tendon and interosseous tendons are parallel with the proximal phalangeal diaphysis and demonstrate intermediate signal intensity. In the coronal plane, imaging of the collateral ligaments, the flexor digitorum, and the extensor tendons requires thin section (ie, 3 mm or less) imaging (Fig. 11-38).

CARPAL INSTABILITIES

The terms stability and instability, as used in reference to conditions affecting the carpus, must be rigidly defined. Stability refers to the ability of two structures to maintain a normal physiologic spatial relationship under applied physiologic loading. Similarly, two structures are said to be unstable if they cannot maintain this normal relationship under physiologic loading conditions. Carpal instabilities represent deviations from the normal spatial relationships of the carpal bones to each other and their surrounding structures, such

text continues on page 901

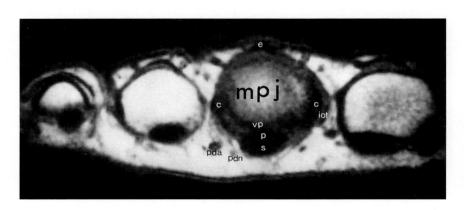

FIGURE 11-32. Axial anatomy as seen through the metacarpophalangeal joint. c, collateral ligament; e, extensor digitorum tendon; iot, interosseous tendon; mpj, metacarpophalangeal joint; p, flexor digitorum profundus tendon; pda, palmar digital artery; pdn, palmar digital nerve; s, flexor digitorum superficialis tendon; vp, volar plate.

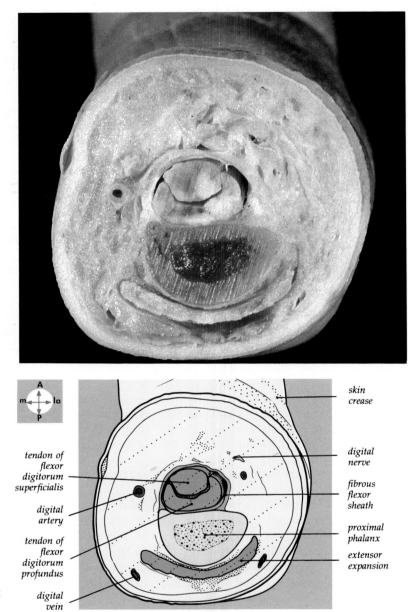

FIGURE 11-33. A transverse section through the index finger at the level of the proximal phalanx.

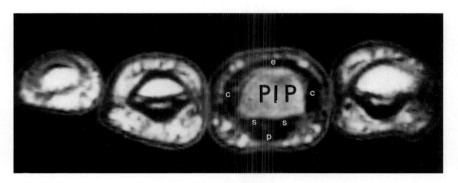

FIGURE 11-34. Axial anatomy as seen through the proximal interphalangeal joint. c, collateral ligament; e, extensor expansion; p, flexor digitorum profundus tendon; pip, proximal interphalangeal joint; s, flexor digitorum superficialis tendon.

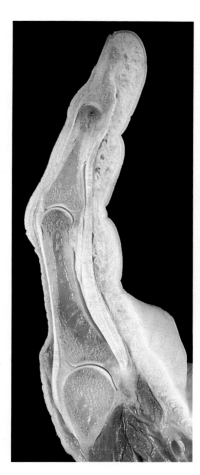

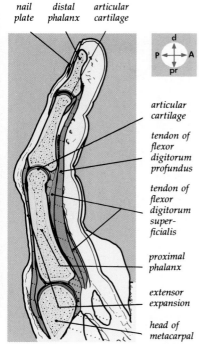

nail
plate
distal
phalanx
articular
cartilage

d
P A
pr

articular
cartilage

tendon of
flexor
digitorum
profundus

tendon of
flexor
digitorum
super-
ficialis

proximal
phalanx

extensor
expansion

head of
metacarpal

FIGURE 11-35. A sagittal section of a finger shows the capsules and the relations of the joints.

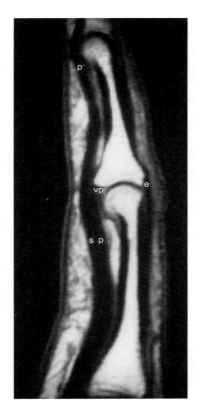

FIGURE 11-36. Sagittal finger anatomy. e, central band of extensor tendon; p, flexor digitorum profundus tendon; s, flexor digitorum superficialis tendon; vp, volar plate.

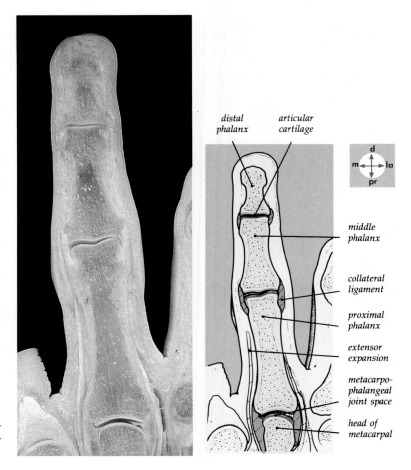

FIGURE 11-37. Coronal section of a finger. The interphalangeal and metacarpophalangeal joint spaces are exaggerated by slight extension of the specimen.

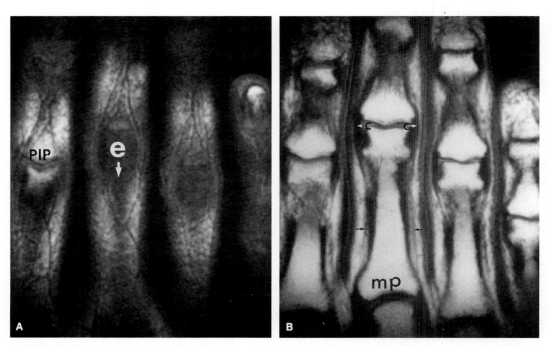

FIGURE 11-38. (**A**) Dorsal and (**B**) midplane coronal views of finger anatomy.

continued

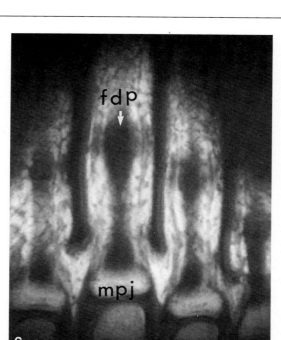

FIGURE 11-38. *Continued.* (**C**) Volar coronal views of finger anatomy. Black arrows, lateral extensor band; c and white arrows, collateral ligament; e, extensor digitorum tendon; fdp, flexor digitorum profundus tendon; mp or mpj, metacarpophalangeal joint; pip, proximal interphalangeal joint.

as the radius, the ulna, and the metacarpals. Since the wrist, like the hip, is virtually always under some load condition, this definition includes instabilities that are seen on routine radiographs as well as those seen on motion studies. Instabilities present on routine radiographs that do not require motion or stress to become evident are referred to as static. Those that require motion or stress to be seen are referred to as dynamic.

MR imaging offers the advantage of revealing associated carpal ligament disruptions when characterizing instabilities in any specified plane of section. Fixed instabilities seen on routine radiographs and coronal or sagittal MR images are often referred to as static, and those that are only revealed by provocative maneuvers in motion studies are referred to as dynamic. Kinematic MR imaging represents a series of static evaluations displayed in a cine loop without true dynamic motion.

In many cases, the difference between dynamic and static instability is a matter of degree of the pathology of the structures that maintain the spatial relationship between the bones. A static instability that is present at all times implies contracture of the soft-tissue constraints. This condition may not be amenable to surgical repair and treatment may require arthrodesis. On the other hand, a dynamic instability that is revealed only by a provocative maneuver may be due to a relatively minor ligament tear or laxity that can be repaired

with a soft-tissue procedure and allows preservation of joint motion.

Stable and Unstable Equilibrium in the Wrist

The normal spatial relationships of the individual components of the wrist (eg, carpal bones, radius, ulna, metacarpals) can be thought of as an example of a stable equilibrium condition. By definition, a stable equilibrium exists when any displacement of a body from its position will result in a restoring force that tends to return the body to its equilibrium position. When all of the supporting constraints of the wrist are normal and intact, any load within physiologic limits may change the spatial relationship of the components, but there will be a simultaneous increase in the tension within these constraining structures that counteracts the deforming force and tends to return the components to their normal spatial relationship. Neutral, dorsiflexion, and palmarflexion motions can be used as an example of the different colinear relationships among the capitate, lunate, and radius (Figs. 11-39 through 11-41).

Conversely, an unstable equilibrium exists when any displacement of a body from its position results in a force that tends to push the body further from the equilibrium position.[57] This condition occurs in the wrist when the constraining structures are incompetent. Constraining or supporting structures about the wrist include not only the ligamentous structures discussed earlier, but also the tendons that cross the joint, as well as the geometry of the carpal bones and their surrounding articular surfaces. The tendency for the wrist to assume a condition of unstable equilibrium when the constraining structures are damaged can be seen as an extension of the normal motions of the carpal bones. To understand these motions, the wrist can be thought of as a flexible spacer interposed between the hand (ie, metacarpals) and the distal radius/ulna. The purpose of this deformable spacer is to maintain a constant distance or space between the base of the third metacarpal and the articular surface of the radius. This theory is supported by the fact that, with radial or ulnar deviation, the carpal height index does not change from its value as measured in the neutral position.[58] This index or ratio is defined as the carpal height measured from the distal capitate surface to the proximal lunate surface, divided by the length of the third metacarpal. In normal individuals, the value is 0.54 ± 0.03. In pathologic conditions such as SLAC wrist or rotatory subluxation of the scaphoid as seen in SL dissociation, this ratio is decreased to values less than 0.49.

In order for this ratio to remain constant with radial and ulnar deviation, there must be a change in the dimensions of the ulnar and radial borders of the flexible spacer between the metacarpals and distal radius and ulna. Since the bones of the distal carpal row are rigidly held in place by their ligamentous restraints and do not move, the normal motions

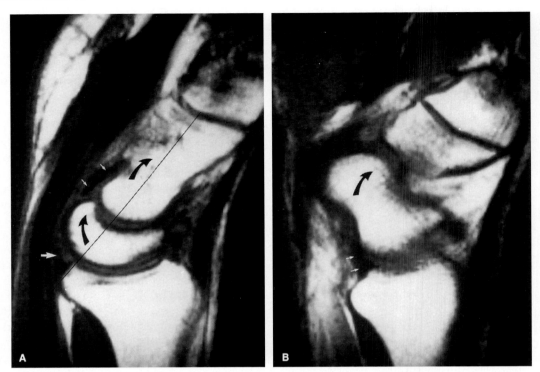

FIGURE 11-39. (A) In wrist dorsiflexion, there is colinear alignment (*long thin black line*) of the dorsiflexed capitate and lunate (*curved arrows*). The deltoid or arcuate ligament (*small white arrows*) and the radiolunate (short radiolunate) ligament (*large white arrow*) are also indicated. Dorsiflexion occurs primarily at the radiocarpal joint. (B) The radioscaphocapitate ligament (*small white arrows*) also tightens during wrist dorsiflexion, locking any motion between the proximal and distal carpal rows and creating a sling across the waist of the scaphoid. Both the scaphoid (*curved arrow*) and capitate are thus dorsiflexed.

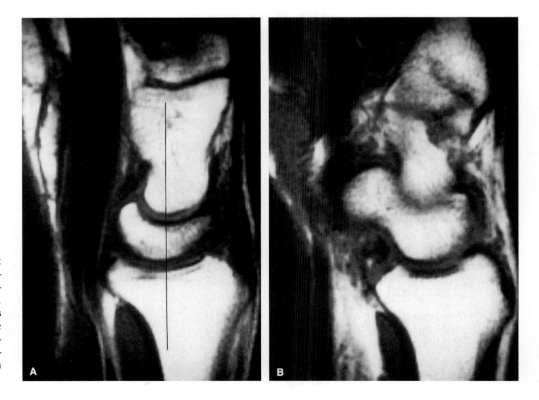

FIGURE 11-40. (A) With the wrist in a neutral position, there is normal colinear alignment of the capitate, lunate, and radius (*black line*). The normal capitolunate angle is between 0° and 30°. (B) When the scaphoid is positioned without dorsiflexion or palmar flexion, the normal scapholunate angle is between 30° and 60°.

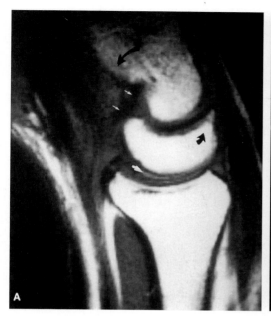
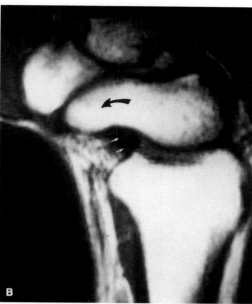

FIGURE 11-41. (A) Palmar flexion occurs primarily at the midcarpal articulation. Palmar flexion of the capitate (*long curved arrow*) and some palmar flexion of the lunate (*short curved arrow*) can be seen. The arcuate or deltoid ligament (*small white arrows*) is more lax. Large white arrow, radiolunate articulation. (B) Flexion of the scaphoid (*curved arrow*) with a lax radioscaphocapitate ligament (*straight arrows*).

of the three bones of the proximal row must account for the changes in the dimensions of the radial and ulnar borders of the wrist.

With radial deviation, the radial border must shorten; this is accomplished by rotation of the scaphoid into a flexed position (Fig. 11-42). The ulnar border is lengthened as the triquetrum slides out from beneath the hamate. On plain radiographs or coronal MR images in this position, the scaphoid is foreshortened and the joint space is evident between the hamate and the triquetrum; no superimposition of these bones occurs. The lunate is linked or associated with the scaphoid and triquetrum through the interosseous ligaments, which are displayed as homogeneous low signal intensity structures on coronal MR images. The SL ligament has a triangular morphology, whereas the LT ligament is more linear in shape. Lunate motion is thus a reflection of this proximal carpal row linkage, as well as the compressive forces placed on it by the capitate. At extreme radial deviation, the summation of these forces produces slight volar-flexion of the lunate. Since the wrist is in a condition of stable equilibrium, the bones of the proximal carpal row return to their neutral position when the force causing radial deviation is removed. Thus, in radial deviation, a flexion torque predominates, and compression of the scaphotrapezial-trapezoid (STT) joint and proximal carpal row flexion produce a physiologic volar intercalated segment instability (VISI) pattern.

With ulnar deviation, the radial side of the flexible spacer must lengthen and the ulnar side must shorten. Therefore, the scaphoid becomes more horizontal or extended to lengthen the radial side, and the triquetrum slides beneath the hamate to shorten the ulnar side. PA radiographs show an elongated scaphoid and superimposi-

tion of the hamate on the triquetrum. Coronal MR images demonstrate the triquetral movement in an ulnar direction on the slope of the hamate (Fig. 11-43). Palmar movement of the triquetrum in relationship to the hamate results in a palmar position of the lunate axis, relative to the capitate. Compression forces transmitted by the capitate produce dorsal rotation or dorsiflexion of the lunate. Associated volar shift of the lunate maintains colinear alignment of the capitate and radius. During lunate dorsiflexion, there is elevation of the distal pole of the scaphoid (ie, scaphoid extension). Thus, in ulnar deviation, an extension torque predominates, and interaction at the triquetrohamate heli-

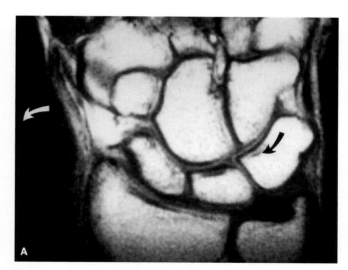

FIGURE 11-42. (A) Radial deviation of the wrist (*curved white arrow*) produces radial and dorsal translation of the triquetrum relative to the slope of the hamate (*curved black arrow*).   *continued*

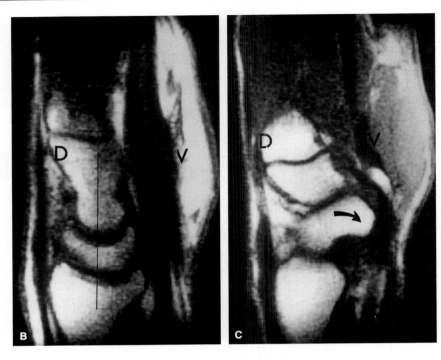

FIGURE 11-42. *Continued.* **(B)** Colinear alignment of the capitate and lunate (*straight line*). There may be mild palmar flexion of the lunate in extreme radial deviation. **(C)** Palmar flexion of the scaphoid (*curved black arrow*). D, dorsal; V, volar.

coid slope and proximal carpal row extension produces a physiologic DISI pattern.

Interosseous Ligament Pathology

Scapholunate Ligament Tear

If an injury to ligamentous constraints occurs, such as a tear of the SL ligament, the linkage between the scaphoid and lunate is removed and these bones become dissociated. An SL ligament tear, however, may exist without a static instability (Fig. 11-44). In this case, the lunate is no longer under the influence of the scaphoid and instead follows the triquetrum, and the loading force of the capitate is not opposed by torque transmitted through the SL ligament from the flexed scaphoid. Similarly, the lunate no longer exerts force on the scaphoid, and there is less opposing force to its flexion.

In this situation, radial deviation produces an exaggeration of the normal motions of the bones of the proximal row. With SL interosseous ligament disruption, the scaphoid becomes more flexed in relation to the lunate, and the SL

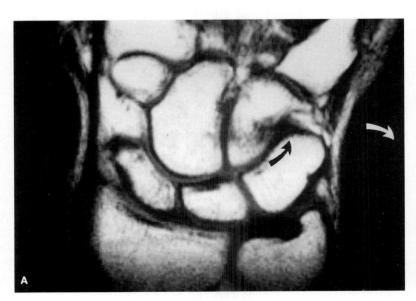

FIGURE 11-43. **(A)** Ulnar deviation of the wrist (*curved white arrow*) produces ulnar translation of the triquetrum relative to the slope of the hamate (*curved black arrow*).

continued

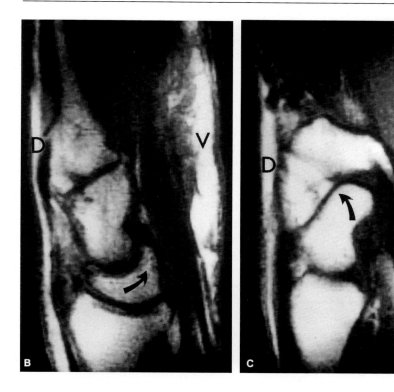

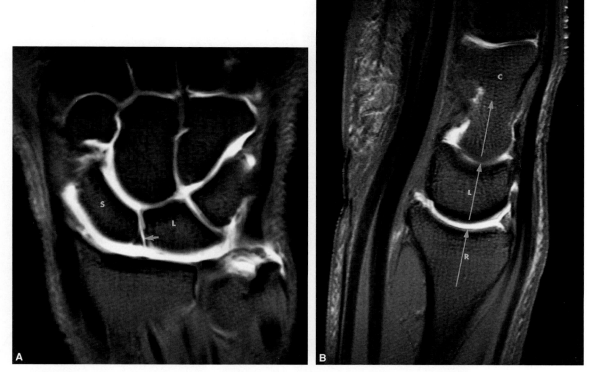

FIGURE 11-43. *Continued.* (**B**) Dorsiflexion of the lunate (ie, dorsal tilt) with associated volar shift (*curved arrow*) allows the capitate to remain colinear with the radius. In contrast, dorsal intercalated segmental instability (DISI) is characterized by dorsal tilting of the lunate without an associated volar shift. Thus, DISI results in dorsal displacement of the capitate relative to the radius and no colinear relationship between the capitate and radius. (**C**) Elevation (ie, extension) of the distal pole of the scaphoid (*curved arrow*). D, dorsal; V, volar.

FIGURE 11-44. Scapholunate ligament tear without carpal instability. (**A**) A fat-suppressed T1-weighted coronal image demonstrates a vertical high signal intensity tear (*arrow*) of the lunate attachment of the scapholunate ligament. The lunotriquetral ligament is absent. (**B**) Corresponding fat-suppressed T1-weighted sagittal image demonstrates colinear (*straight line*) alignment of the capitate (C) and lunate (L) with a normal capitolunate angle. There is no static instability pattern.

angle, normally less than 30° to 60°, increases to more than 70° (Fig. 11-45). The SL angle is determined from two sagittal images to demonstrate the separate lunate and scaphoid axes, which are not shown together in the same sagittal image. The lunate, free of the influence of the scaphoid, tips into a dorsiflexed position in relation to the axis of the capitate. As the scaphoid flexes, a gap appears between the scaphoid and the lunate, and, in time, the capitate will fall into this gap, contributing to a reduction in carpal height.

Rotatory subluxation of the scaphoid, which begins as an SL dissociation, may also occur. In its final stages, as the lunate is dorsiflexed, a DISI pattern is established. On lateral radiographs, there is 10° or more of lunate dorsiflexion relative to the radius. On sagittal MR images, dorsal tilting of the lunate is associated with proximal migration of the capitate and loss of colinear alignment of the capitate, lunate,

and radius. The capitolunate angle, normally 0° to 30°, can be directly measured on sagittal images and may be increased in dorsiflexion ligamentous instability.

Disruption of the SL ligament is shown on T2*-weighted or STIR images as either complete ligamentous disruption or as a discrete area of linear bright signal intensity in a partial or complete tear (Fig. 11-46). In complete tears, synovial fluid communication between the radiocarpal and midcarpal compartments may be identified. Associated stretching (ie, redundancy) or tearing of the radiolunate ligament and the RSC ligament is shown on sagittal images. A flap tear may not be appreciated without the use of MR arthrography. A perforation, identified by communication of fluid across a focal discontinuity, constitutes a communicating defect or tear. Small membranous perforations may exist in the presence of intact dorsal and volar portions of the SL

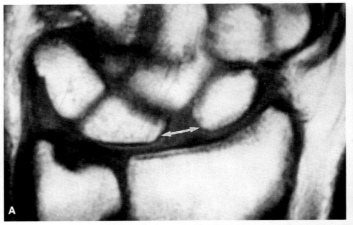

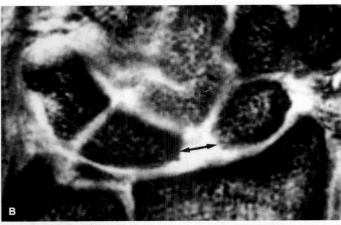

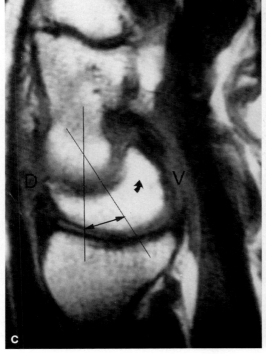

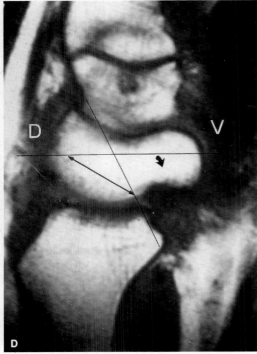

FIGURE 11-45. Coronal **(A)** T1-weighted and **(B)** T2*-weighted images show scapholunate dissociation (*double-headed arrows*) with complete disruption of the scapholunate interosseous ligament in dorsal intercalated segmental instability. **(C)** Dorsal tilting of the lunate (*curved arrow*) without volar shift. Note the dorsal displacement of the capitate relative to the radius. The capitolunate angle (*double-headed arrow*) measures 32°. **(D)** Palmar tilting of the scaphoid (*curved arrow*) causes an abnormally increased scapholunate angle (*double-headed arrow*) of 124°. D, dorsal; V, volar.

ligament (Fig. 11-47). In fact, most degenerative perforations occur in the thin membranous portion of the SL ligament, which is not thought to be biomechanically significant.[59] Partial thickness perforations or noncommunicating defects may be associated with ligamentous tissue degeneration or sprains and may be difficult to appreciate on MR images.[60] A complete SL tear may not be associated with SL interval

diaphysis or static carpal instability as assessed on sagittal images, especially when the volar extrinsic ligaments are intact. Axial MR images are used to distinguish among tears of the dorsal, membranous, and volar portions of the SL ligament (Fig. 11-48). The location of the tear can then be directly correlated with dorsal or volar coronal images. The scaphoid attachment of the SL ligament is more likely to

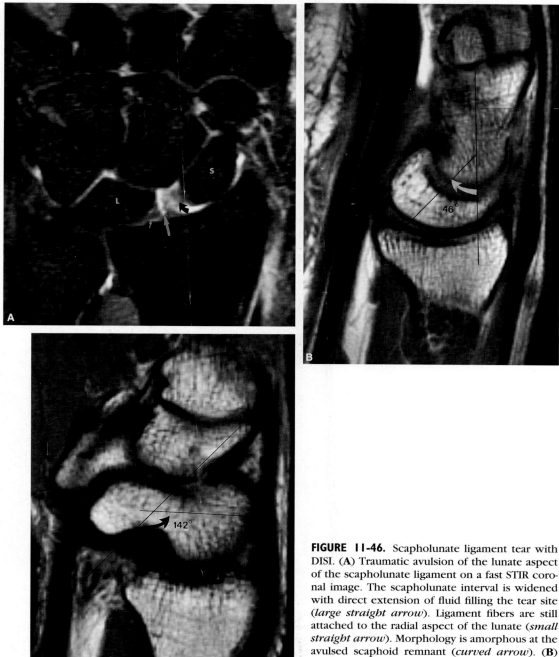

FIGURE 11-46. Scapholunate ligament tear with DISI. **(A)** Traumatic avulsion of the lunate aspect of the scapholunate ligament on a fast STIR coronal image. The scapholunate interval is widened with direct extension of fluid filling the tear site (*large straight arrow*). Ligament fibers are still attached to the radial aspect of the lunate (*small straight arrow*). Morphology is amorphous at the avulsed scaphoid remnant (*curved arrow*). **(B)** The capitolunate angle (*arrow*) is increased to 46°, and there is associated dorsal tilting of the lunate. **(C)** The scaphoid tilts palmarly with an increased scapholunate angle (*arrow*) of 142°.

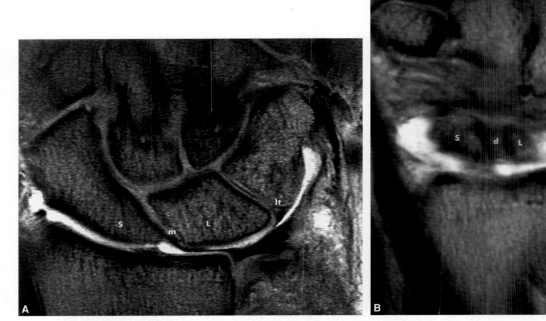

FIGURE 11-47. **(A)** Loss of triangular morphology after debridement of the membranous (m) portion of the scapholunate ligament (*arrow*) on a fat-suppressed T1-weighted coronal MR arthrography image. Note the intact lunotriquetral ligament (lt). **(B)** Normal dorsal (d) fibers of the scapholunate ligament are shown on a more dorsal prescribed fat-suppressed T1-weighted coronal image. This patient was stable without a static or dynamic wrist inability. S, scaphoid; L, lunate.

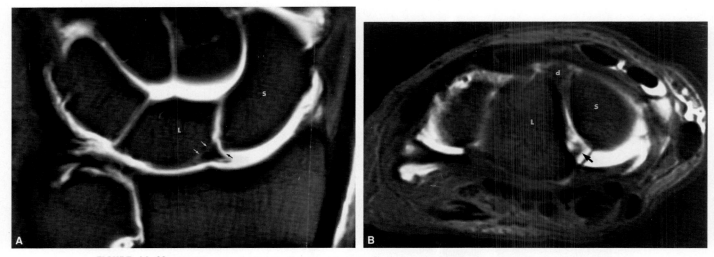

FIGURE 11-48. **(A)** The scapholunate ligament is torn from the weaker hyaline articular cartilage attachment to the scaphoid (*black arrow*). Sharpey's fibers attach the stronger ulnar aspect of the scapholunate ligament directly into cortical and trabecular bone of the lunate (*white arrows*) (fat-suppressed T1-weighted coronal arthrographic image). **(B)** Corresponding fat-suppressed T1-weighted axial image distinguishes torn volar and membranous portions of the SL ligament (*arrow*) with intact dorsal fibers (d). L, lunate; S, scaphoid.

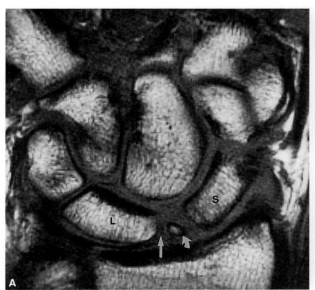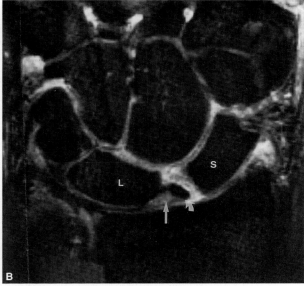

FIGURE 11-49. (**A**) T1-weighted and (**B**) and STIR coronal images of a chronic avulsion fracture of the ulnar aspect of the scaphoid. Note that the scapholunate ligament (*straight arrow*) is still attached to both the lunate and the surface of displaced scaphoid fracture fragment (*curved arrow*). S, scaphoid; L, lunate.

avulse than is the stronger lunate attachment, which has more abundant Sharpey's fibers anchoring the ligament[59] (see Fig. 11-48). The insertion of the SL ligament into hyaline cartilage covering the scaphoid is thus relatively weak. In fact, an SL ligament tear may be associated with a scaphoid avulsion fracture (Fig. 11-49). The SL ligament is uniformly visualized on coronal T2*-weighted images with 3 mm sections. In 90% of coronal plane images, the SL ligament displays a triangular morphology; in 10% of cases, it demonstrates a linear morphology.[51,59] In 63% of cases studied by Smith,[51] the SL ligament was seen as a homogeneous low or low to intermediate signal intensity structure. In 37% of cases, there was intermediate signal intensity areas traversing portions of the SL ligament (part or all of the ligament), which could be potentially mistaken for a tear (Fig. 11-50).

Lunotriquetral Ligament Tear

A loss of linkage (ie, dissociation) between the triquetrum and the lunate—due to a tear of the LT ligament — allows the lunate to follow the scaphoid. Under this influence, volarflexion of the lunate occurs and gives rise to a VISI pattern. VISI may be defined as a carpal instability characterized by proximal and volar migration of the bones of the distal row, associated with flexion of the lunate. The SL angle is decreased to less than 30°, and the capitolunate angle may measure up to 30°. Disruption of the LT ligament is most frequently identified by its absence on T2*-weighted

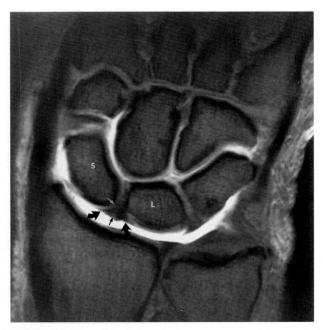

FIGURE 11-50. Normal variations in the appearance of the scapholunate ligament. There is intermediate signal intensity hyaline cartilage at the SL interface with the scaphoid (*white arrow*) and not the lunate bone. Low to intermediate linear signal intensity (*black arrow*) traverses both the proximal and distal surfaces of the SL ligament without tear. The proximal base of the SL ligament extends past the inflection points of both the scaphoid and lunate bones (*curved arrow*) (fat-suppressed T1-weighted coronal MR arthrogram). S, scaphoid; L, lunate.

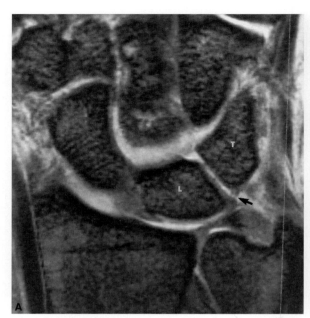 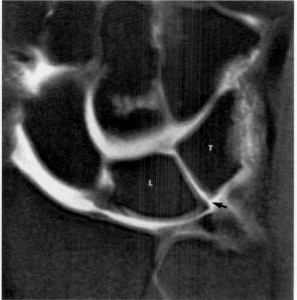

FIGURE 11-51. Tear with absence of the lunotriquetral ligaments (*arrow*) on (**A**) T2*-weighted and (**B**) fat-suppressed T1-weighted MR arthrographic images. The LT ligament tear could be missed using the gradient-echo sequence (**A**) only. L, lunate; T, triquetrum.

or fat-suppressed T2-weighted FSE coronal images (Fig. 11-51). An insertional site tear or perforation is often appreciated on MR arthrography (Fig. 11-52). Fat-suppressed T2-weighted FSE sequences provide sufficient contrast to produce an arthrogram-like effect without injection of contrast (Fig. 11-53). LT ligament tears may be associated with TFC degenerative tears.[43] A VISI pattern usually requires disruption of both the LT intrinsic and dorsal extrinsic ligaments (ie, dorsal radiocarpal ligament). Smith and Snearly[53] described the intact LT ligament as linear in 63% and delta-shaped in 35% of asymptomatic individuals[53] (Fig. 11-54). The intact LT ligament demonstrates homogeneous low signal intensity in 73%, and linear intermediate signal intensity within its substance in 25% of wrists studied.[53] Insertional signal intensity varies with the distribution of hyaline articular cartilage on either side of the LT ligament (see Fig. 11-54). Asymmetric hyaline articular cartilage signal intensity should not be mistaken for an eccentric tear unless fluid signal intensity communication is seen across the ligament cartilage interface. Sagittal MR images are used to assess static VISI instability with palmar tilting of the lunate and scaphoid (Fig. 11-55).

Magnetic Resonance Accuracy

In evaluating SL interosseous ligament pathology, MR imaging has an overall sensitivity rate of 93%, specificity of 83%, and accuracy of 90% when compared with arthrography.[27] In the diagnosis of ligament tears, with arthroscopy as the gold standard, MR imaging is 86% sensitive, 100% specific, and 95% accurate. In the diagnosis of LT interosse-

ous ligament tears, MR imaging is 56% sensitive, 100% specific, and 90% accurate when compared with arthrography, and 50% sensitive, 100% specific, and 80% accurate when compared with arthroscopy.[27] Since the LT ligament is less substantial than the SL ligament, 3DFT coronal images may be needed to improve the sensitivity of diagnosis. In addition, unlike SL ligament dissociations, osseous widening of the LT articulation is uncommon, which may make the detection of LT ligament pathology more difficult, especially in the absence of adjacent fluid (secondary to an effusion or its introduction in MR arthrography).

Thin section axial images may also improve the identification of both SL and LT ligament pathology. MR imaging is superior to conventional arthrography, allowing identification of the size, morphology, and location of an SL or LT ligament tear. This information is important because communication across a pinhole or small perforation or deficiency of the thin membranous portion of the ligament may not be significant in the presence of grossly intact dorsal and volar ligaments. In fact, evaluations of communicating perforations in cadaver wrists have shown that 28% of cadaver wrists have degenerative perforations of the central membranous SL ligament.[59] Degenerative perforations of the membranous LT ligament can be seen in 36% of cadaver wrists. In our experience, degenerative perforations occur twice as often in the LT ligament as in the SL ligament.

MR arthrography has increased the accuracy of evaluation of SL and LT ligament tears, especially in peripheral ligament avulsions where the ligament has not lost its normal morphology. These tears may be difficult to detect on routine

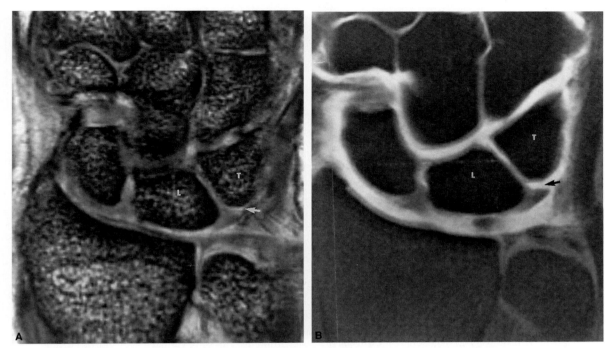

FIGURE 11-52. Avulsed (*arrow*) ulnar aspect of a delta-shaped lunotriquetral ligament on (**A**) T2*-weighted coronal image and (**B**) fat-suppressed T1-weighted coronal MR arthrogram. Note that this flap tear is best visualized in the presence of intraarticular contrast on **B**. The scapholunate ligament is intact. Fluid freely communicates across the lunotriquetral interval between the radiocarpal and midcarpal compartments. L, lunate; T, triquetrum.

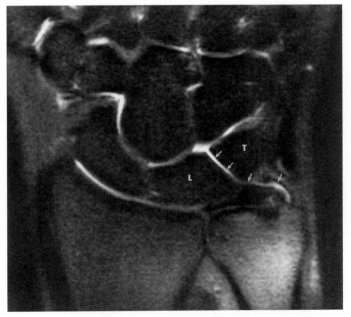

FIGURE 11-53. Direct continuity of fluid (*arrows*) across the lunotriquetral ligament and interval on a fat-suppressed T2-weighted fast spin-echo coronal image without using intraarticular contrast. L, lunate; T, triquetrum.

MR gradient-echo, STIR, or fat-suppressed T2-weighted FSE images unless there is a fluid interface identified between the torn ligament and corresponding osseous attachment.

Classification of Wrist Instabilities

There are numerous classification schemes for instability of the carpus. This is partly due to the fact that the understanding of the biomechanics and treatment of these conditions is rapidly changing. The most useful classification reflects the anatomy and pathophysiology of the condition and indicates treatment.

Amadio has suggested four characteristics to be described in classification of carpal instabilities (Amadio P, personal communication, 1990):

- Severity (which can be categorized as dynamic, static subluxation, or static dislocation)
- Direction of displacement
- Location of injury
- Type of injury.

The direction of displacement may be dorsal (DISI), volar (VISI), or radioulnarproximodistal translation (eg, ulnar,

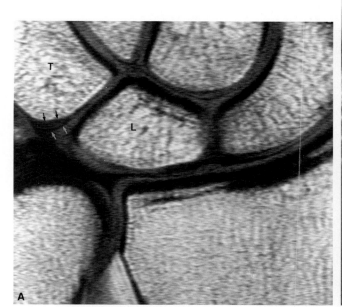
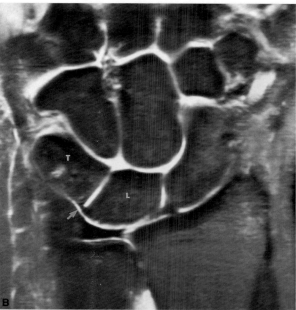

FIGURE 11-54. Normal variants of the lunotriquetral interosseous ligament. (**A**) Eccentric ulnar position of the delta-shaped LT ligament with intermediate signal intensity hyaline cartilage seen on the lunate insertion (*white arrows*) of the ligament. There is direct contact between the LT ligament and the low signal intensity cortex of the triquetrum (*black arrows*). (**B**) Commonly seen linear morphology of the LT ligament (*arrow*). There is no hyaline cartilage signal intensity at the insertion sites of the ligament. T, triquetrum; L, lunate.

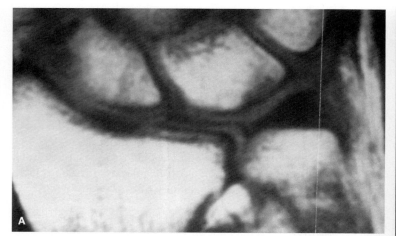
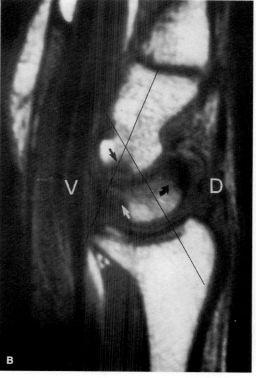

FIGURE 11-55. A volar intercalated segment instability pattern (VISI) is apparent in clinical midcarpal instability. (**A**) A coronal T1-weighted image reveals subchondral sclerosis of the proximal ulnar aspect of the lunate in a patient who presented with clinical midcarpal instability. (**B**) A corresponding sagittal T1-weighted image shows the volar tilt of the lunate (*curved black arrow*), increased capitolunate angle, and subchondral sclerosis of the opposing surfaces of the capitate (*straight black arrow*) and lunate (*white arrow*). The ulnar arm of the arcuate ligament is not visible in this midcarpal instability. MR imaging was the first modality able to document degeneration of the proximal pole of the capitate in subluxation of the capitate on the lunate.

radial, distal, proximal). Proximal or distal displacements are represented by axial carpal dislocations.[61] These are rare traumatic injuries, usually associated with a crush or blast mechanism. There is a longitudinal transarticular derangement of both the carpal and metacarpal transverse arches, with complete loss of the normal relationship between the two columns of the carpus. The radiologic hallmarks are an abnormal widening of any joint between the bones of the distal carpal row, a disruption of Gilula arc III defined by the proximal articular surfaces of the bones of the distal row, and an abnormal gap between the bases of two adjacent metacarpals.[62] The location can be proximal, distal, radial, ulnar, dorsal, volar, radiocarpal, or midcarpal.

Carpal instabilities can be grouped into perilunar (perilunate) instabilities, midcarpal instabilities, and proximal carpal instabilities. Perilunate instabilities may be divided into lesser and greater arc injuries. Lesser arc injuries involve disruptions that follow the contour of the lunate itself, whereas greater arc injuries are transscaphoid, capitate, hamate, or triquetral. Lesser arc injuries involve SL, LT, and complete perilunate instabilities. Greater arc injuries are divided into scaphoid fractures, naviculocapitate syndrome (scaphoid fracture plus perilunate dislocation), and transscaphoid transtriquetral perilunate dislocation. Perilunar instability includes dorsal perilunate dislocation and palmar lunate dislocation.

Mayfield's spectrum of progressive lunate instability is shown in four stages.[63] The stages were defined experimentally in cadaver wrists by in vitro simulation of a fall on an outstretched hand. The wrist was forced into progressive dorsiflexion, ulnar deviation, and intercarpal supination, and progressive injuries were noted. In stage I instability, the SL ligament fails leading to an SL instability. In stage II, there is progression to failure of the midportion of the RSC ligament. Stage III includes failure of the capitolunate and triquetrolunate joints with failure of the radiotriquetral ligaments. In stage IV, there is failure of the dorsal RSLT ligament, resulting in complete palmar dislocation of the lunate.

Midcarpal instabilities are classified as intrinsic (ligamentous laxity) or extrinsic in origin. Intrinsic instabilities include palmar midcarpal instability (a VISI pattern) and dorsal midcarpal instability (a DISI pattern). In patients with palmar midcarpal instability, ulnar deviation with load on the wrist (ie, a clenched fist placing a transcarpal load) produces a painful clunk. This clunk represents relocation of the midcarpal joint as the wrist moves into ulnar deviation. This instability is due to a congenital or acquired laxity of the ulnar arm of the volar arcuate ligament. This is a true transverse laxity, as all of the instability occurs between the proximal and distal rows. This subluxation/relocation can be prevented by a dorsally directed force on the pisiform, which reduces the static VISI of the proximal row. On cine films, the proximal carpal row suddenly snaps from a volar flexed position to a dorsal or neutral position. This movement is in contrast to the smooth, fluid transition seen in the normal

wrist. Dorsal midcarpal instabilities are most commonly seen after malunion of a distal radius fracture that leaves the distal radius articular surface in a dorsiflexed position. Correction with an osteotomy of the distal radius restores the normal volar tilt.

Proximal carpal instabilities are classified as (1) ulnar translocation of the carpus (secondary to rheumatoid disease or trauma, or iatrogenically introduced by excision of the ulnar head or radial styloid), (2) dorsal instability (secondary to a dorsal rim distal radial fracture—a dorsal Barton's fracture), and (3) palmar instability (secondary to a volar rim distal radial fracture—a volar Barton's fracture).

DISI and VISI instabilities can each be further subdivided into CIND and CID. In this context, nondissociative means that the intercarpal ligaments are intact and that the bones of the row are moving together. Dissociative means that one or more of the intercarpal ligaments are incompetent and the bones of the row no longer move together.[64] There are three major types of injuries:

- Carpal instabilities, dissociative (CID)—injuries affecting intracapsular intercarpal ligaments, as described in the earlier examples
- Carpal instabilities, nondissociative (CIND)—injuries involving the capsular ligaments with no dissociation of the carpal bones themselves
- Complex carpal instabilities—injuries that involve both dissociative and nondissociative elements.

The more common pattern of dissociative instabilities includes complete tears of either or both of the intrinsic ligaments of the proximal carpal row (SL and LT), and transscaphoid fractures. A transscaphoid fracture is the equivalent of a tear of the SL ligament, leading to a dissociative instability as the scaphoid and lunate become unlinked through the fracture site.[65] There is usually associated disruption or attenuation of the palmar or dorsal extrinsic ligaments. In nondissociative instabilities, there may be carpal malalignment with intact interosseous ligaments. There may also be attenuation of the palmar or dorsal radiocarpal ligaments. The proximal carpal row is usually palmar (nondissociative VISI). Nondissociative instability may be secondary to distal radius fracture (in which there is loss of normal volar angulation of the distal radius), ulnar plus variance, midcarpal instability, and abnormalities of the STT joint.[66]

CID may be diagnosed if there is radiographic or arthroscopic evidence of dissociation between rows as well as within rows. Disruption affects both the intercarpal and the capsular wrist ligaments. In the dissociated form of DISI (CID-DISI), there is extension of the scaphoid and lunate, whereas in the interosseous ligaments, extension does not occur. The same holds true for VISI. In CID, there is flexion of the scaphoid and triquetrum; in CIND, there is no flexion of these bones.

In SL dissociation, there is dissociative DISI. There is often a history of a dorsiflexion injury, secondary to a fall, and the development of SL interval tenderness. The physical examination is distinctive in these patients. They cannot bear weight on the wrist in dorsiflexion and the Watson-Shuck test, a drawer test for the SL ligament, is positive. Sagittal MR scans, like lateral radiographs, demonstrate an increased SL angle (greater than 60°) with dorsal angulation of the lunate and triquetrum, and an increased capitolunate angle (greater than 15° compared with the normal capitolunate angle of 30°). There is palmar flexion of the scaphoid. On coronal MR images, a SL gap of more than 4 mm may be seen. With nondissociative DISI, a secondary disorder may develop, characterized by proximal row extension in response to dorsal angulation of a malunited distal radius fracture. There may be damage to the ligaments which stabilize the mid-carpal joint.

LT instability represents dissociative VISI. There is a flexed lunate and the SL angle is decreased to less than 30° with lunate and scaphoid volar flexion. Acute LT dissociation is often associated with a history of a rotational injury to the wrist with the development of ulnar-sided pain. In nondissociative VISI, there is a decreased or normal SL angle, lunate flexion, and a decreased capitolunate angle of less than 15°. There is flexion of the proximal carpal row with a normal SL interval. Nondissociative VISI is usually a chronic condition associated with generalized ligamentous laxity.

Midcarpal Instabilities

Midcarpal instabilities are the most frequently recognized wrist injury, and there is greater experience with MR imaging of these injuries. In palmar midcarpal subluxation, first studied by Lichtman and coworkers,[67] patients present with palmar subluxation at the midcarpal joint and a painful clunk with ulnar deviation of the wrist (see Fig. 11-55). This instability is due mainly to laxity of the ulnar arm of the volar arcuate ligament.[67] There is also evidence of increased ligamentous laxity in these patients, and sagittal MR images show palmarflexion of the lunate, as in a VISI pattern. In ulnar deviation, the excessive volar tilt of the lunate allows the head of the capitate to sublux volarly into the space of Poirier. With radial deviation, the lunate dorsiflexes, and there is relocation of the capitate. This type of instability is classified as dynamic CIND, since there is no dissociation of the carpal bones. The intensity of the clunk and the pain increase with loading of the capitolunate joint, as occurs when the fist is clenched. Dorsally directed pressure on the pisiform eliminates this subluxation, and Lichtman and associates have designed dynamic splints that apply this directional force and successfully relieve the symptoms. This dorsally directed pressure on the pisiform can also be used to diagnose palmar midcarpal subluxation. Dynamic midcarpal instability centered on the lunocapitate joints has been de-

scribed as a "CLIP" or capitolunate instability pattern. There is no underlying DISI or VISI pattern of instability.[68]

The pathology in CIND of this type is related to the intrinsic ligaments of the carpus, but there are also extrinsic causes for midcarpal instability of CIND. Taleisnik and Watson[69] have described these extrinsic causes in conjunction with malunited fractures of the distal radius.[69] In these cases, there is dorsal angulation of the distal radial articular surface that results in dorsiflexion of the lunate and dorsal subluxation of the midcarpal row. This instability can be treated with an osteotomy of the distal radius to restore its normal volar tilt.

Another type of CIND, involving the radiocarpal and ulnocarpal joints, occurs more proximally. Ulnar translation of this type is commonly seen in rheumatoid arthritis. Normally, the volar radiocarpal ligaments, which originate from the region of the radial styloid, act as guide to keep the carpal bones (ie, scaphoid and lunate) well-seated in their fossae in the distal radius. In rheumatoid arthritis, however, destructive synovitis weakens the RSC and RL ligaments, and the carpus begins to migrate down the inclined plane of the distal radius in an ulnar direction. The distance between the radial styloid and scaphoid increases, as can be seen in PA radiographs or coronal plane MR images. Resection of the distal ulna (ie, Darrach procedure) also results in loss of the buttressing effect of the ulna and increased ulnar translation.[70] Posttraumatic ulnar translocation of the carpus has also been described.[71]

Proximally occurring cases of CIND may also be seen with dorsal or volar displacements. Patients with malunited dorsal or volar intraarticular fractures lose the stability that the bony contour of the distal radius provides. This allows the proximal row to slip dorsally or volarly, depending on whether the malunited fracture is dorsal or volar.

Other Static Ligamentous Instabilities

In ulnar translocation, the carpal bones are ulnar in position, the SL and CL angles are normal, and the space between the scaphoid and the radial styloid increases. Greater than 50% of the lunate is medial to the radius (as assessed on a neutral PA radiograph). Ulnar translocation may be caused by synovial-based disorders, as well as by severe trauma and the iatrogenic causes mentioned above.

In dorsal subluxation, the carpal bones occupy a dorsal position relative to the midplane of the radius. The SL and CL angles are normal. There is often an associated dorsally impacted distal radius fracture.

In palmar subluxation, the carpal bones are palmar to the midplane of the radius. The SL and CL angles are normal, and there may be associated ulnar translocation.

Treatment of Carpal Instabilities

Treatment for most of the carpal instabilities described earlier remains extremely controversial. This is especially true of CID. In general, the goal of most surgical approaches is to restore the anatomy and biomechanics of the injured part of the carpus.

Carpal Instability: Nondissociative

In the extrinsic forms of CIND caused by malunited fractures of the distal radius, surgical correction of the instability is aimed at restoring the anatomy of the radius. In rheumatoid arthritis, however, the injured soft-tissue constraints seen in CIND with ulnar translation cannot be reconstructed surgically. Reduction of the carpus and radiolunate fusion may be successful in preventing recurrence of ulnar translation. The lunate, when fused to the radius, acts as a doorstop and prevents the carpus from sliding down the inclined plane of the radius.

CIND associated with dorsal midcarpal instability secondary to a malunited distal radius fracture with dorsal tilt of the articular surface can be treated with an osteotomy of the distal radius, which restores normal volar angulation.

CIND with palmar and carpal instability presents a more difficult problem. The pathology is excessive volar tilt of the lunate caused by laxity of the ulnar arm of the volar arcuate ligament. Lichtman and others have devised a soft-tissue reconstruction that consists of tightening the volar arcuate and dorsal radiolunate ligaments to correct the excessive VISI of the lunate. This procedure has been successfully performed in a small number of patients. A more reliable operation is the four corner fusion—an intercarpal fusion of the lunate-triquetrum-capitate-hamate. Although some range of motion is lost with this procedure, it has been quite successful in eliminating the clunk since the subluxing joint is fused.

Carpal Instability: Dissociative

There is little agreement on the treatment of the various forms of CID. In many cases, these conditions remain unsolved problems—SL dissociation is an excellent example. Early cases of ligament rupture without rotatory subluxation can usually be satisfactorily treated by pinning the SL ligament and performing open suture repair of the torn ligament, followed by immobilization.[72] Accurate reduction is necessary to align the ligament fibers for optimal healing. Once rotation of the scaphoid is accomplished, the proximal pole must be reduced in relation to the lunate and a procedure performed to hold it firmly in place. Ligament reconstructions similar in concept to those devised for the anterior cruciate in the knee have met with uniformly poor results.[73] When the scaphoid rotates or flexes, its proximal pole becomes incongruent in the radial fossa. Several methods use intercarpal fusions to ensure that the proximal pole remains congruent in the scaphoid fossa of the radius. Watson and Mempton have reported on the successful use of triscaphe (ie, scaphoid-trapezoid-trapezius) arthrodesis.[74] Others have performed scaphocapitate fusions with similar results. An alterative to intercarpal fusion is dorsal capsulodesis.[75] In this procedure, a strip of the dorsal capsule of the wrist is left attached proximally to the radius on one end, and the other is inserted into the distal pole of the scaphoid. By pulling dorsally on the distal pole, the scaphoid is held in a horizontal, reduced position. If possible, the SL ligament should be repaired.

Lunotriquetral Dissociations

The treatment of LT dissociations can be approached in two ways. If there is no VISI and positive ulnar variance is present, ulnar shortening unloads the LT interval and provides excellent symptomatic relief. The torn LT ligament should be repaired if possible. LT intercarpal fusion is also an option, although meticulous technique is required to avoid pseudoarthrosis. LT fusion is an attractive concept because this is the most common carpal coalition. These coalitions are usually asymptomatic and are often diagnosed in radiographs taken for other reasons. However, achieving a stable LT fusion has proven difficult, and most series show significant rates of nonunion (ie, up to 40%). Newer techniques with larger bone grafts and compression fixation devices have improved the success of this procedure. We have had 100% success in achieving fusion using the Herbert bone screw with precompression of the fusion site.

DISTAL RADIOULNAR JOINT

The ulna articulates with the distal radius through the sigmoid or ulnar notch.[76] The distal or inferior radioulnar compartment extends proximally as far as the synovium-lined recessus sacciformis. The distal ulna is wrapped in the extensor retinaculum but is not directly attached to it. The extensor carpi ulnaris tendon is deep to the extensor retinaculum and has a subsheath attachment to the distal ulna. The articular disc, or TFC, is composed of collagen and elastic fibers, is triangular in shape, and bridges the distal ends of the radius and ulna. The volar aspect of the TFC has strong attachments to the LT and ulnotriquetral ligaments and a weaker attachment to the ulnolunate ligament. There is 150° of forearm rotation at the DRUJ, with rotation of the distal radius around the ulnar head. In pronation and supination, the ulnar head moves dorsally and palmarly, respectively, in the sigmoid notch (Fig. 11-56). Contact between the ulnar head and the sigmoid notch is greatest during forearm midrotation and least in maximum pronation or supination. These are the positions most commonly used in imaging the wrist with a dedicated wrist coil. Relative to the distal radius, the ulnar

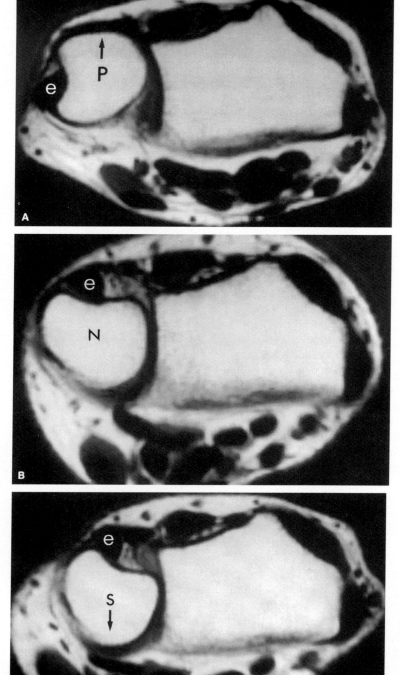

FIGURE 11-56. Normal biomechanics of the distal radioulnar joint. (**A**) Mild dorsal shift (*arrow*) of the ulna relative to the sigmoid notch of the distal radius in full pronation (p) is normal. The extensor carpi ulnaris tendon (e) is located within its groove in the medial distal aspect of the ulna. (**B**) The neutral position (N) of the wrist reveals a symmetric relationship between the position of the distal ulna and sigmoid notch relative to dorsal or volar directions. The extensor carpi ulnaris tendon is seen dorsally, within its ulnar groove. (**C**) Mild volar shift (*arrow*) of the ulna in full wrist supination (s) is normal. The extensor carpi ulnaris tendon (e) may be located within its ulnar groove or subluxed medially in extreme supination.

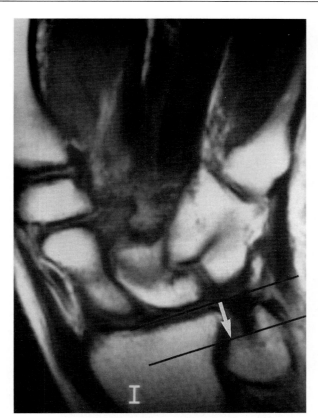

FIGURE 11-57. Negative ulnar variance with the articular surface of the ulna projecting proximal to the articular surface of the radius (*arrow*). Note the secondary deformity of the triangular fibrocartilage. There is an increase in the normal 80% of axial loading forces as supported by the radius, with relative ulnar shortening.

head moves distally in pronation and proximally in supination. The distribution of load across the wrist is 82% through the distal radius and 18% through the distal ulna. The TFCC supports a portion of the ulnar forces that are unloaded in complete excision of the distal ulna.[76] In ulnar deviation, there is increased ulnar load transmission.

Ulnar Variance

The concept of ulnar variance is critical in the management of distal radial fractures, in the pathogenesis of KD, and in TFC pathology. Ulnar variance refers to the relative lengths of the radius and ulna, and can be defined as the relative level of the distal end of the ulna to that of the radius. If the ulna is short, ulnar variance is considered negative (Fig. 11-57). If the ulna is long, the variance is referred to as positive (Fig. 11-58). Neutral ulnar variance occurs when the lengths of the radius and ulna are relatively equal. Radiographically, the relative lengths of the radius and ulna are measured from the centers of their distal articular surfaces. There are three commonly used methods for measuring ulnar variance, and all three are similarly accurate and reliable.[77] It should be noted that wrist position is an important determinant of ulnar variance. Supination causes relative ulnar shortening, and pronation causes lengthening.[78] For this reason, it is critical that ulnar variance be determined with the forearm and wrist in 0° of pronation and supination.

Ulnolunate Abutment Syndrome

The syndrome of ulnolunate abutment (also referred to as the ulnar impaction syndrome, ulnocarpal abutment, and ulnolunate impaction syndrome) occurs when there is exces-

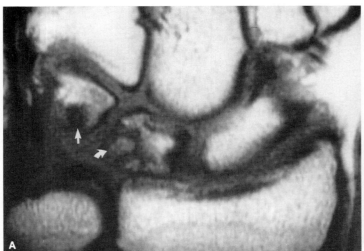

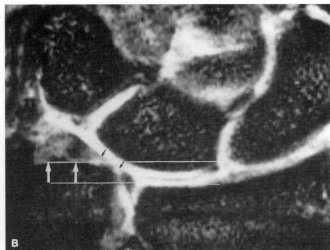

FIGURE 11-58. Ulnolunate abutment syndrome. (**A**) A T1-weighted coronal image shows low signal intensity subchondral degenerative sclerosis involving the ulnar aspect of the lunate (*straight arrow*) and triquetrum (*curved arrow*). (**B**) Positive ulnar variance (*white arrows*), triangular fibrocartilage perforations (*black arrows*), and a torn lunotriquetral ligament are features of ulnolunate (ie, ulnocarpal) abutment syndrome.

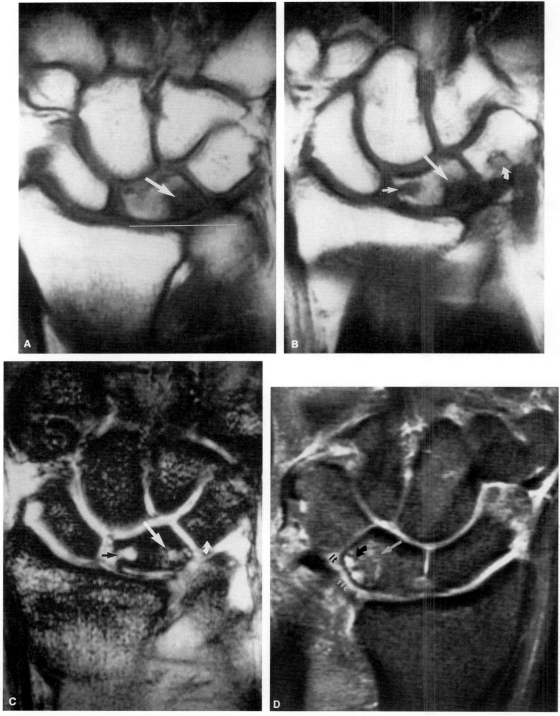

FIGURE 11-59. Ulnolunate abutment syndrome. (**A**) A T1-weighted coronal image shows predominant low signal intensity subchondral sclerosis (*arrow*) affecting the proximal ulnar aspect of the lunate. This sclerosis may be mistaken for Kienböck's disease. Mild positive ulnar variance (*white line*) can also be seen. Coronal (**B**) T1-weighted and (**C**) T2*-weighted images show more extensive subchondral cystic changes (*small straight arrows*), sclerosis (*large straight arrows*), and triquetral involvement (*curved arrows*). There is degeneration of the distal ulnar and proximal lunate articular cartilage surfaces, as well as disruption of the triangular fibrocartilage. (**D**) In a separate case, a fat-suppressed T2-weighted fast spin-echo coronal image displays both ulnar-sided erosions (*curved arrow*) and subchondral marrow edema (*straight arrow*). The triangular fibrocartilage (tfc) and lunotriquetral (lt) ligament are torn.

sive positive ulnar variance.[76] The term ulnar impingement syndrome should be reserved for cases of impingement of the ulna against the shaft of the radius, as may occur after excessive Darrach-type shortening of the ulna. In ulnar abutment syndrome, there is painful compression of the distal ulna on the medial surface of the lunate. It is not unusual to see full-thickness defects of the cartilage of the lunate as well as tears of the TFC. In extreme cases of excessive ulnar length—common in patients with rheumatoid arthritis—there may be dorsal subluxation of the ulna, and supination is blocked. Severe dorsal subluxation with supination of the carpus is common. Attritional ruptures of the extensor tendons of the fourth and fifth compartments often occur due to erosion caused by the prominent ulna.

Magnetic Resonance Findings

With the exception of positive ulnar variance or a prominent ulnar styloid, plain radiographs in patients with early ulnolunate (ie, ulnocarpal) impingement are unremarkable. Later, subchondral sclerosis and cystic degeneration can be seen along the proximal, adjacent borders of the triquetrum and lunate. Bone scintigraphy may show nonspecific uptake in the ulnolunate region. MR imaging may demonstrate central perforations of the TFC in association with neutral or positive ulnar variance (see Figs. 11-58 and 11-59). These tears occur between contact surfaces of the lunate and ulna. MR imaging also allows detection of the earliest development of subchondral sclerosis and cystic changes on the ulnar aspect of the lunate. Sclerotic changes demonstrate low signal intensity on T1-, T2-, and T2*-weighted images. The cystic degeneration demonstrates low or low to intermediate signal intensity on T2-weighted images. Coronal scans reveal the initial degenerative changes in the articular cartilage of the distal ulna, proximal lunate, or proximal triquetral surfaces. These degenerative changes are indicated by either attenuation of articular cartilage or irregularity or denuding of the articular cartilage surface. Another feature of the ulnolunate impingement syndrome that can be documented on coronal and sagittal MR images is LT ligament disruption and resultant instability. Treatment with TFCC debridement and ulnar shortening may be necessary to relieve pain and halt progression of impingement.

Instability of the Distal Radioulnar Joint

Distal radioulnar joint instability may be secondary to a sprain, dislocation or malalignment of a forearm bone fracture, synovitis, or ligamentous laxity.[79,80] The sigmoid notch, the dorsal and volar radioulnar ligament, the interosseous membrane, and the dorsal retinaculum maintain DRUJ static stability. The pronator quadratus, the extensor carpi ulnaris, and the flexor carpi ulnaris contribute to DRUJ dynamic

stability. The carpus, through its dorsal and volar radiocarpal ligament attachments, rotates the wrist radius around the ulna in pronosupination. The distal ulna moves volar to dorsal within the sigmoid notch of the distal radius between supination and pronation. There is associated translation (approximately 1 mm) of the ulna from proximal to distal. In full pronation, the distal ulna is dorsal to the proximal LT surface. A distal ulnar sprain or dislocation usually occurs in the position of pronation. Pronation, extension, and radial deviation place the dorsal radioulnar, the ulnotriquetral, and ulnar collateral ligaments under increased tension, and may force the distal ulna to dislocate dorsally relative to the sigmoid notch. Dorsal instability of the DRUJ is often associated with a supination deformity of the radial carpal complex. Treatment is therefore directed at correction of both the distal ulnar dorsal displacement and the supinated angulation of the carpus relative to the radius.

CT and MR imaging of both wrists in both full pronation and full supination have been shown to be useful in the diagnosis of distal radioulnar subluxation.[81,82] A relatively new technique to evaluate instability at this joint uses a frame that places a calibrated degree of stress on the distal ulna and radius in conjunction with CT scanning.[83] The controlled load placed on the joint is supposed to simulate the physiologic changes in dynamic subluxation, a condition that is difficult to diagnose. Useful quantitation of the degree of subluxation may also be possible with this technique.

The advantage of MR axial imaging in maximum pronation and supination is identification of the relative positions of the distal radius and ulna with soft-tissue contrast information (Fig. 11-60). Axial images display the condition of the dorsal and volar radioulnar ligaments, and volar radioulnar ligament tears may be associated with dorsal instability of the DRUJ. The normal volar distal radioulnar ligament is maximally taut when the wrist is studied in pronation. Ulnar styloid avulsions, TFCC tears, or distal radial fractures may lead to DRUJ instability with subluxation, and the these structures can be assessed during the same examination with MR imaging in the coronal plane. Compared with CT, MR imaging is more accurate in the characterization of associated effusions of the DRUJ, which are a secondary sign of TFC pathology. Axial and sagittal images are useful in demonstrating displacement of the distal ulna in relationship to the TFCC.

TRIANGULAR FIBROCARTILAGE COMPLEX

Gross Anatomy

The TFCC is composed of the dorsal and volar radioulnar ligaments, the ulnar collateral ligament, the meniscus homologue, the articular disc or TFC, the extensor carpi ulnaris sheath, the ulnolunate ligament, and the ulnotriquetral ligament. It is classified as part of the ulnocarpal extrinsic liga-

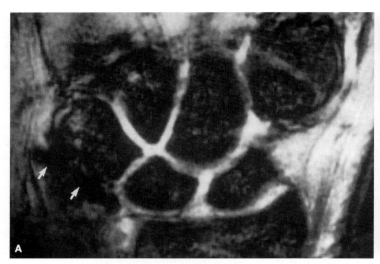 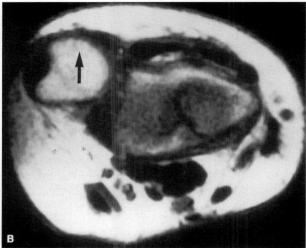

FIGURE 11-60. Postoperative repair of the triangular fibrocartilage. (**A**) A T2*-weighted coronal image shows residual susceptibility artifact (*arrows*) overlying the area of failed TFC repair. (**B**) A T1-weighted axial image shows dorsal displacement of the ulna (*arrow*). The ulnar attachment of the volar radioulnar ligament is not seen.

mentous group, and stabilizes the DRUJ and ulnocarpal articulation. The dorsal and volar radioulnar ligaments reinforce the peripheral margins of the TFC, which is thinned centrally and thickened peripherally. The thickened ulnar collateral fibers that are distal to the TFC comprise the meniscus homologue. These fibers then insert distally into the triquetrum, the hamate, and the base of the fifth metacarpal. The ulnolunate ligament originates on the anterior border of

the TFC and inserts on the lunate. The ulnotriquetral ligament also originates on the anterior aspect of the TFC (the volar aspect of the radioulnar ligament) and extends to the volar-ulnar aspect of the triquetrum. The TFC has a biconcave morphology (Fig. 11-61) and articulates with the distal ulna and triquetrum in the proximal carpal row. With a strong radial attachment of the TFC, the ligaments that have or share TFC attachment function to connect the volar aspect of the carpus to the radius.

TFCC Injuries

Triangular fibrocartilage complex abnormalities can be classified into traumatic injuries (class I) and degenerative injuries (class II).[84] Traumatic injuries are treated by arthroscopic debridement in avascular portions and are repaired in vascularized areas.[79] Degenerative lesions of the TFCC are treated by salvage procedures, including arthroscopic debridement, ulnar shortening, or ulnar head resection. Class I traumatic injuries of the TFCC are further subdivided into (1) class IA injuries (Fig. 11-62), including perforation or traumatic tear of the TFC disc proper; (2) class IB injuries (Fig. 11-63), represented by an ulnar avulsion of the TFCC with or without associated ulnar styloid fracture; (3) class 1C injuries (Fig. 11-64), distal avulsions of the TFCC through its lunate attachment (ulnolunate ligament) or its triquetrum attachment (ulnotriquetral ligament); and (4) class ID injuries (Fig. 11-65), which represent a radial avulsion at the level of the distal sigmoid notch with or without associated sigmoid notch fracture. Class II degenerative lesions demonstrate the spectrum of ulnocarpal abutment syndrome findings. Class IIA injuries represent TFCC wear (Fig. 11-66). Class IIB injuries include TFCC wear with associated lunate and/or ulnar chondro-

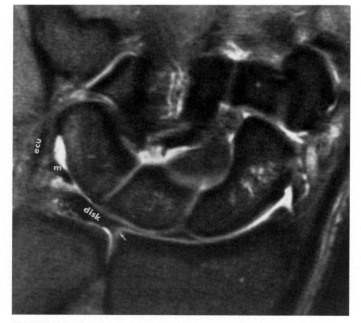

FIGURE 11-61. Fat-suppressed T2-weighted fast spin-echo coronal image of the normal TFCC. The biconcave central disk (disk), extensor carpi ulnaris (ecu), meniscal homologue (m), and cartilage of the radial sigmoid notch (*arrow*) are identified.

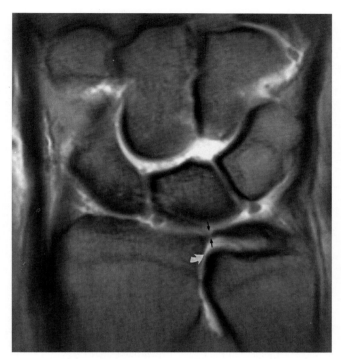

FIGURE 11-62. Class IA lesion with slit-like tear or perforation (*straight arrow*) of the radial aspect of the TFC medial to its radial origin. There is communication of radiocarpal joint contrast (*curved arrow*) with the distal radioulnar joint (fat-suppressed T1-weighted coronal arthrographic image).

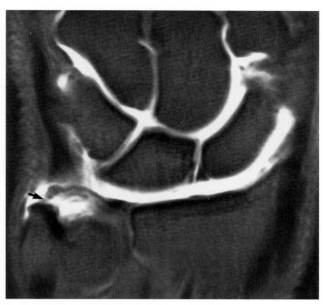

FIGURE 11-63. Class IB lesion with traumatic avulsion of the ulnar attachment of the TFC. There is direct extension of contrast between the ulnar styloid and the avulsed TFC (*arrow*) (fat-suppressed T1-weighted coronal arthrographic image). In addition, this patient has an avulsion of the ulnar aspect of the SL ligament and absent LT ligament.

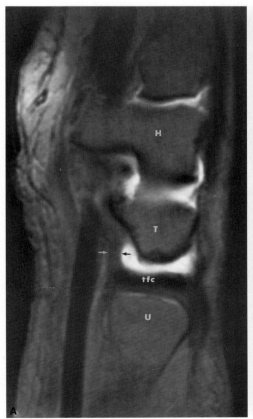

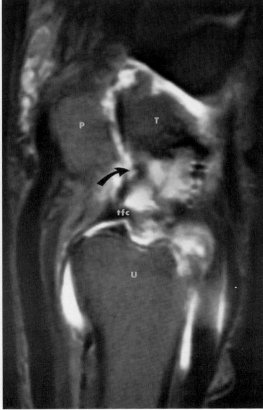

FIGURE 11-64. Fat-suppressed T1-weighted sagittal MR arthrographic images comparing (**A**) intact (*black and white straight arrow*) ulnocarpal (ulnolunate and ulnotriquetral) ligament with (**B**) avulsed osseous insertions (*curved arrow*) of the ulnocarpal ligaments. There is also associated tearing of the dorsal radial aspect of the TFC. Isolated avulsion of the distal ulnolunate or ulnotriquetral ligaments as described in a class IC lesion is not common. H, hamate; T, triquetrum; tfc, triangular fibrocartilage; U, ulna; P, pisiform.

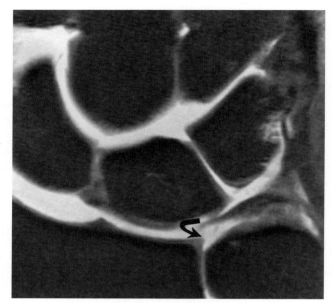

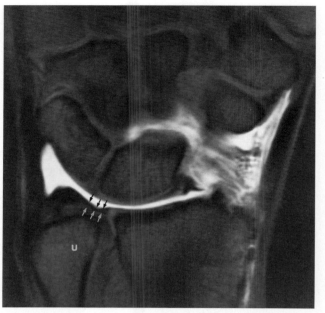

FIGURE 11-65. Traumatic avulsion of the radial attachment of the TFC as described in class ID lesions. Note the exposed articular cartilage at the radial sigmoid notch. Fluid communicates between the radiocarpal and distal radioulnar compartments (*curved arrow*) on this fat-suppressed T1-weighted coronal MR arthrographic image. The LT ligament is absent.

FIGURE 11-66. Class IIA lesion with degenerative thinning (*arrows*) of the TFC without perforation. No lunate chondromalacia is present and the LT ligament is intact. Fat-suppressed T1-weighted coronal MR arthrographic image. U, ulna.

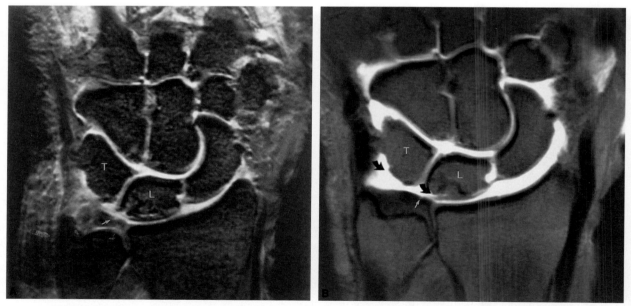

FIGURE 11-67. Class IIB lesion with degenerative fraying of the distal aspect of the TFC (*straight arrow*). There is chondromalacia of the lunate and triquetrum (*curved arrow*) without associated TFC perforation. The LT and SL ligaments are torn (**A**: T2*-weighted coronal image; **B**: fat-suppressed T1-weighted coronal MR arthrographic image).

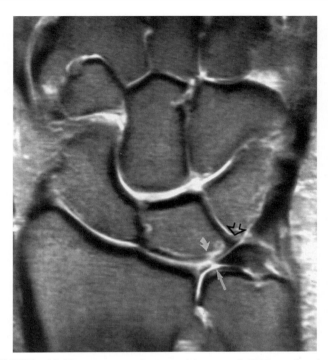

FIGURE 11-68. Class IIC lesion with central TFC perforation (*straight arrow*) and lunate chondromalacia (*curved arrow*) on a fat-suppressed T2-weighted fast spin-echo coronal image. No intraarticular contrast was required to facilitate the diagnosis. The LT ligament is intact (*open arrow*). Tapering of the edges of the TFC is seen in degenerative (class II) lesions whereas traumatic (class I) tears tend to have abrupt or straight margins.

malacia (Fig. 11-67). Class IIC injuries represent a TFCC perforation in association with lunate or ulnar chondromalacia (Fig. 11-68). Class IID lesions (Fig. 11-69) include a TFCC perforation, lunate or ulnar chondromalacia, and an LT ligament perforation. In class IIE injuries (Fig. 11-70) there is the additional finding of ulnocarpal arthritis.

Arthroscopic Evaluation

Anatomy

The TFCC arises from the medial surface of the radius at the level of the articular cartilage. Its origin is flush with the radial articular surface, and the only way to differentiate these structures arthroscopically is by palpation with a probe. As noted earlier, the TFCC courses toward the base of the ulnar styloid to insert into the fovea. The articular disc is continuous with the volar ulnocarpal ligaments as well as the dorsal capsular structures. There is a strong dorsal insertion into the undersurface of the sheath of the extensor carpi ulnaris tendon. More radially, the articular disc of the TFCC is suspended from the dorsal capsular structures of the wrist.

Pathology

When all the suspensory insertions around the periphery of the TFCC are intact, the TFCC is under tension and ballottement under arthroscopy produces a resiliency sometimes called the "trampoline effect." Separation of the peripheral insertions of the TFCC, especially at the fovea or radius, result in a loss of this suspensory trampoline effect.[85]

The central portion, or centrum, of the TFCC is thin and is the most common site of tears. The dorsal and volar portions of the TFCC, which are thicker than the central portion, are sometimes referred to as the dorsal and volar limbi.[35] Whereas the thin central portion can be excised if torn, much like the meniscus of the knee, the limbi should be preserved because they appear to play an important mechanical role in the stability of the DRUJ. On average, the limbi are 4 to 5 mm thick.[86] Tears of the centrum can be associated with a variety of causes. Perforations from excessive loading in patients with positive or neutral ulnar variance and ulnocarpal impingement syndromes are common. As noted earlier,

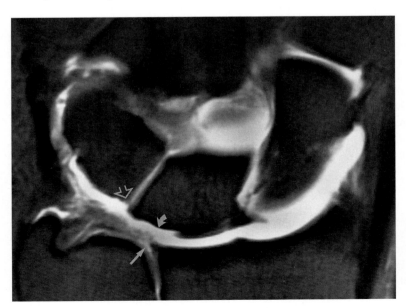

FIGURE 11-69. Fat-suppressed T1-weighted coronal arthrographic image demonstrating class IID injury with perforation of TFC (*straight arrow*), loss of lunate articular cartilage (*curved arrow*), and lunotriquetral ligament disruption (*open arrow*). The intrasubstance enhancement of the TFC is commonly seen in degenerative lesions.

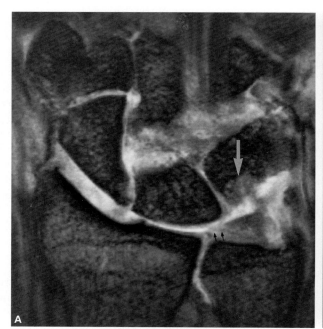 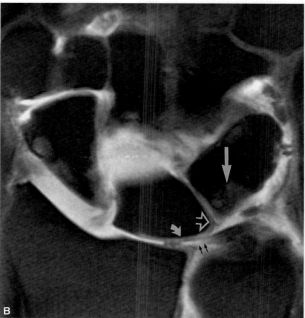

FIGURE 11-70. Class IIE lesion with ulnocarpal arthritis demonstrates a central TFC perforation (*small straight arrows*), lunate (*curved arrow*) and triquetral chondromalacia, lunotriquetral ligament tear (*open arrow*), and triquetral subchondral erosion (*long straight arrow*) (**A**: T2*-weighted coronal image; **B**: fat-suppressed T1-weighted coronal arthrographic image).

these patients may present with findings indicative of cartilage degeneration of the distal ulna and medial lunate. Some patients with ulnocarpal impingement present with a triad of symptoms, including positive or neutral ulnar variance, TFCC perforations, and LT instability. An ulnar unloading procedure, such as ulnar shortening, relieves the pressure on the LT ligament and allows the symptoms to subside. With extreme instability or cartilage degeneration between the lunate and triquetrum, fusion of the LT joint may be necessary in addition to the ulnar shortening.[86]

Studies of the vascular anatomy of the articular disc have shown that, similar to the meniscus of the knee, only the peripheral 15% to 20% of the disc is vascularized. The central portion is avascular.[87] Therefore, although there is a potential for surgical repair of peripheral lesions, central lesions cannot be expected to heal and should be treated by excision. Reinsertion of peripheral ulnar avulsions of the TFCC have resulted in restoration of biomechanical function and symptomatic relief.[85]

The TFC is continuous with the volar ulnolunate and ulnotriquetral ligaments, and these structures provide a strong insertion into the carpus. Tears of these ligaments, implicated in ulnar wrist pain, can be depicted on MR images, and there are reports of successful treatment with arthroscopic debridement.[88]

Magnetic Resonance Evaluation

Anatomy

Both the distal and proximal surfaces of the TFC are depicted on MR images; information not available with wrist arthroscopy or single compartment radiocarpal arthrography. On coronal plane T1-weighted, T2*-weighted, STIR, or fat-suppressed T2-weighted FSE images, the TFC is depicted as a biconcave disc of homogeneous low to intermediate signal intensity. The tendon of the extensor carpi ulnaris is seen on the radial aspect of the ulnar styloid process. Coronal plane images of the TFC disc demonstrate the lateral attachment to the ulnar aspect of the distal radius, with separate superior and inferior bifurcated radial attachments. The inferior radial attachment is not seen on arthroscopic evaluation restricted to the radiocarpal surface of the TFC.

The contours of the TFC (ie, proximal and distal surfaces) and ulnar variance are best assessed on coronal images. The distribution of force across the radial plate is increased by negative ulnar variance and is reduced by positive ulnar variance. The TFC is thus an important contributor to stabilization of the medial aspect of the radiocarpal joint. Disruption of the TFC is associated with various degrees of DRUJ instability. Small volar tears lead to mild dorsal subluxation; small dorsal tears cause volar subluxation; and massive tears can produce subluxation or dislocation in either direction. Volar instability is manifested by supination and dorsal instability by pronation.

On axial images, the TFC is shaped like an equilateral triangle. The apex of the TFCC converges on the ulnar styloid, and the base of the triangle attaches on the superior margin of the distal radial sigmoid notch. Sagittal images show the TFC in sections through the triquetrum. In this plane, the TFC morphology is discoid, as seen from anterior to posterior. The TFC is located immediately distal to the dome of the ulna, and is thinned centrally with broader volar and distal margins (ie, peripheral thickening). This peripheral thickening is composed of lamellar collagen and gives rise to the dorsal and volar radioulnar ligaments. The ulnocarpal ligament arises from the volar distal surface of the TFC and passes distally to the bones of the ulnar carpus.

Totterman and Miller[89] reported on the use of 3D gradient recall echo imaging to routinely visualize the radioulnar and ulnocarpal ligaments.[89] The volar and dorsal radioulnar ligaments are seen as broad striated bands that originate from the volar and dorsal (respectively) radial cortices of the sigmoid notch of the distal radius and extend to the base of the ulnar styloid process. These ligaments course volar and dorsal to the central disc of the TFC. The normal appearance of these ligaments is shown in Figures 11-71 and 11-72.

The ulnolunate and LT ligaments are directly visualized as inhomogeneous intermediate signal intensity structures extending from the volar aspect of the volar radioulnar ligament to the volar ulnar aspect of the lunate and triquetrum.[89] These ligaments appear as thickenings of the capsule originating in the volar radioulnar ligament and are not as well-defined as the previously described volar extrinsic ligaments on the radial side of the radiocarpal joint.

The ulnar styloid attachment of the TFCC is secured with striated fascicles, which are extensions of the radioulnar ligament and central disc.[89] Two types of attachments to the ulna are observed. The more common is composed of two striated fascicles (Fig. 11-73): one inserting at the styloid tip, and the other inserting at the base of the styloid. The low signal intensity striated fascicles are separated by higher signal intensity tissue. The less common type of TFCC attachment is a broad-based striated attachment of fascicles along the entire length of the ulnar styloid (Fig. 11-74).

The meniscus homologue is variably demonstrated on MR images. Its low signal intensity pattern is best observed in its more well-defined dorsal portion (Fig. 11-75). The meniscus homologue has been shown to have an insertion onto the pisiform in cadaver dissections and may provide stability at the level of the pisotriquetral articulation.[90] The prestyloid recess is defined as a high signal intensity area bordered by the meniscus homologue, the styloid attachment of the TFCC, the central disc, the medial carpal capsule, and the extensor carpi ulnaris sheath (see Fig. 11-75).

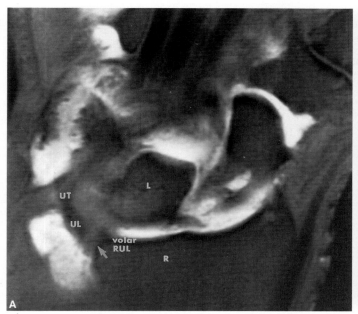

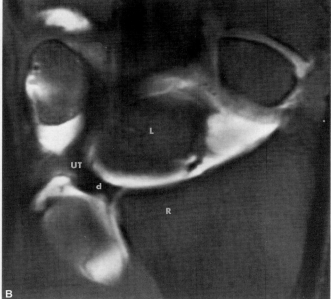

FIGURE 11-71. TFCC—volar aspect. **(A)** Volar fat-suppressed T1-weighted coronal image shows the radial attachment (*arrow*) of the volar radioulnar ligament (volar RUL). The ulnolunate (UL) and ulnotriquetral (UT) ligaments (components of the ulnocarpal ligaments) originate and extend from the volar radioulnar ligament to attach to the volar-ulnar aspect of the lunate and triquetrum. **(B)** The ulnotriquetral ligament (UT) continues in an ulnar distal course toward the triquetrum at the level of the volar aspect of the articular disk (d) (fat-suppressed T1-weighted coronal image).   *continued*

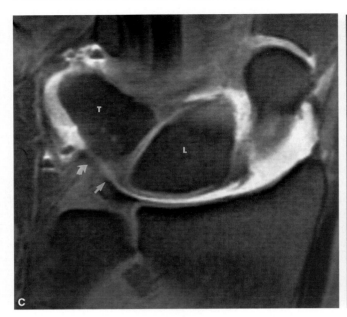

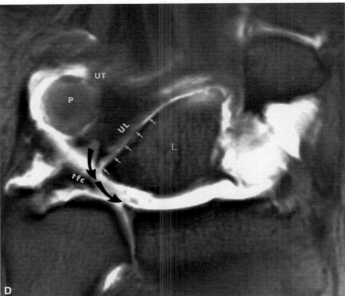

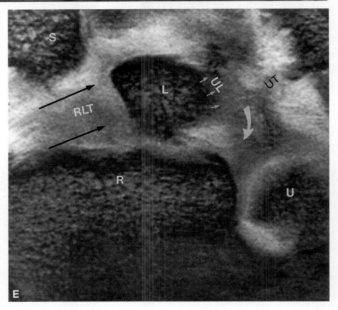

FIGURE 11-71. *Continued.* (**C**) The ulnolunate (*straight arrow*) and ulnotriquetral (*curved arrow*) ligaments are visualized as a merged or confluent extension from the volar aspect of the radioulnar ligament. (**D**) The lunate (L) insertion (*arrows*) and triquetrum insertion of the ulnolunate (UL) and ulnotriquetral (UT) ligaments, respectively, are shown. Note the broad-based common origin of these ligaments from the distal volar aspect of the volar radioulnar ligament (*curved arrow*). The radial aspect of the triangular fibrocartilage (tfc) is torn in this patient (fat-suppressed T1-weighted coronal MR arthrogram). (**E**) A separate case demonstrates the continuity of the hypointense sheet of tissue representing the ulnolunate (UL) and ulnotriquetral (UT) ligaments extending from the volar aspect of the volar radioulnar ligament (*curved arrow*) (coronal spoiled GRASS image). RLT and straight arrow, radiolunotriquetral ligament; R, radius; L, lunate; U, ulna; T, triquetrum; P, pisiform; S, scaphoid.

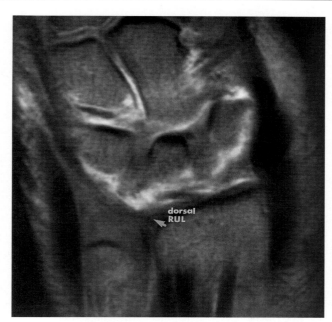

FIGURE 11-72. The dorsal radioulnar ligament (dorsal RUL; *arrow*) attachment to the dorsal distal radius. The dorsal portions of the intrinsic interosseous scapholunate and lunotriquetral ligaments are also seen at this level (fat-suppressed T1-weighted coronal MR arthrographic image).

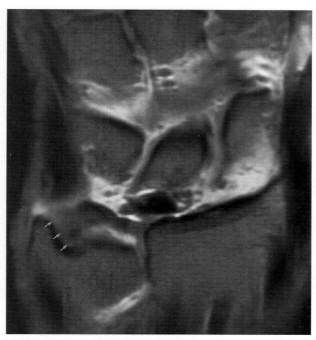

FIGURE 11-74. Single broad base attachment of the TFCC extending from the tip to the base of the ulnar styloid process (*arrows*) (fat-suppressed T1-weighted coronal MR arthrographic image).

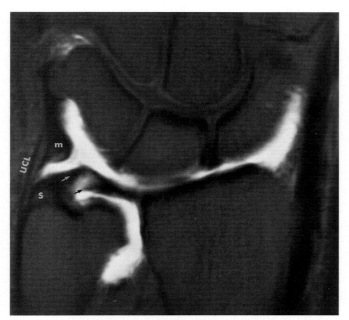

FIGURE 11-73. Insertion of the TFCC into the ulnar styloid (s) process is accomplished by separate groups of fascicles directed to the styloid tip (*white arrow*) and base (*black arrow*). The ulnar collateral ligament (UCL), seen as a distinct structure of the triangular fibrocartilage complex, extends from the outer aspect of the ulnar styloid to the triquetrum, hamate, and fifth metacarpal. The meniscus homologue (m) corresponds to thickening of the longitudinally oriented fibers of the ulnar collateral ligament distal to the triangular fibrocartilage (fat-suppressed T1-weighted coronal MR arthrographic image).

The central disc demonstrates low to intermediate signal intensity on mid-coronal images with a bow-tie morphology.[89] The radial attachment of the disc is thicker than the central portion and is attached to the high signal intensity hyaline articular cartilage of the sigmoid notch (Fig. 11-76). The superficial articular cartilage layer of the lunate fossa is visualized as a thin line of low signal intensity in apparent continuity with the distal surface of the radial aspect of the TFCC disc. The proximal surface of the TFCC central disc is either in direct contact with the high signal intensity articular cartilage of the ulnar head, or is separated from the articular cartilage by the ulnar extension of DRUJ fluid within the distal radioulnar compartment.

Pathology

Magnetic resonance imaging of the TFCC reveals many tears that previously went undetected.[91] These include intrasubstance (ie, horizontal) tears and peripheral lesions of the insertions of the TFCC that do not show contrast leakage.

Central perforations of the TFC are thought to be unusual in the first two decades of life. By the fifth decade of life, however, symptomatic perforations can be identified in 40% of TFC studies, and by the sixth decade, perforations are found in 50% of patients studied.[11,92] This finding may help to explain the poor correlation between clinical findings of wrist pain and communication of contrast across the TFC seen in radiocarpal arthrograms. The fact that radiocarpal compartment communication with the inferior radioulnar

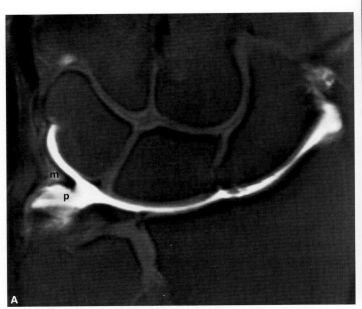

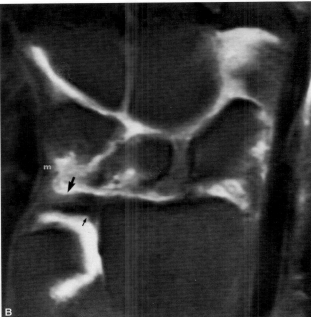

FIGURE 11-75. Meniscus homologue and prestyloid recess. **(A)** The triangular shaped meniscus homologue (m) and prestyloid recess (p) are shown on a fat-suppressed T1-weighted coronal MR arthrographic image. The prestyloid recess is seen proximal to the meniscus homologue and distal to the ulnar styloid attachment of the TFCC. The TFC, or central disk, is located radial to the prestyloid recess whereas the medial capsule defines the ulnar aspect of the recess. The extensor carpi ulnaris tendon sheath courses dorsal to the prestyloid recess. **(B)** A more dorsal coronal image demonstrates the confluence of the meniscus homologue (m) and the radial origin of the dorsal radioulnar ligament (*large arrow*). A fold from the dorsal radioulnar ligament forms the proximal attachment of the TFCC (*small arrow*) (fat-suppressed T1-weighted coronal MR arthrographic image).

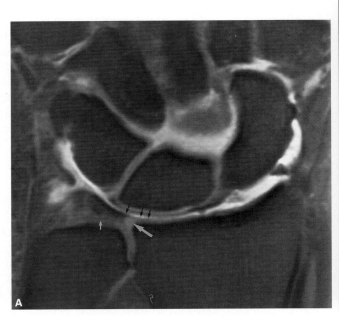

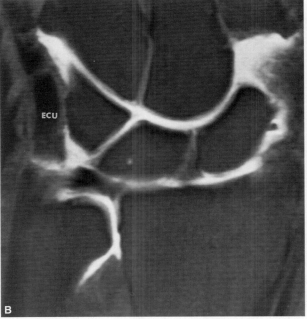

FIGURE 11-76. The TFC. **(A)** The distal aspect of the TFC or central disk is shown to be contiguous with the articular cartilage of the distal surface of the lunate fossa (*small black arrows*). The volar and dorsal radioulnar ligaments contribute to the striated tissue between the ulnar styloid and the central disk. High signal intensity articular cartilage (*large white arrow*) is present at the radial attachment of the central disk to the sigmoid notch of the radius. Note that the central disk is in direct contact with the articular cartilage of the ulnar head in the absence of distal radioulnar joint fluid distention (*small white arrow*). **(B)** The extensor carpi ulnaris tendon and sheath (ECU) are identified on a more dorsal coronal image in the plane of the TFC. The TFC attaches to the sheath of the extensor carpi ulnaris tendon dorsomedially. **(A, B:** fat-suppressed T1-weighted coronal MR arthrographic images.)

compartment is found more frequently in anatomic dissections than with arthroscopic injection can be explained by the existence of partial tears and unidirectional flap tears. In a cadaver study, Tan and colleagues[93] documented congenital perforations of the TFC in the fetus and infants, supporting the frequent finding of perforations in asymptomatic adults. These findings bring into question the significance of identifying fluid communications across the TFC in the presence of grossly normal TFCC morphology.

On T2*-weighted images, the thin layer of hyaline articular cartilage proximal to the radial attachment of the TFC along the ulnar aspect of the distal radius demonstrates bright signal intensity and should not be mistaken for fluid communication with the inferior radioulnar joint or detachment of the radial aspect of the TFC. Intrasubstance degeneration of the TFC is best depicted on T2*-weighted images, and appears as regions of increased signal intensity without extension to the superior or inferior margins of the TFC. The meniscus homologue demonstrates greater signal intensity than the TFC on T2*-weighted images. Partial tears in this area may be more difficult to identify due to the increased signal intensity and inhomogeneity of the meniscal homologue and ulnar attachments. Tears of the TFC may occur either as an isolated injury or in association with subluxations of the DRUJ or perilunate dislocations. Patients with TFC pathology often present with pain, clicking, or both on the ulnar aspect of the wrist. An unstable flap of tissue from a TFC causes catching on the ulnar aspect of the wrist, especially when loaded in extension or ulnar deviation. TFC tears, demonstrated by discontinuity or fragmentation, are most commonly located near or adjacent to the radial attachment.[66] Contour irregularities, especially with associated regions of increased signal intensity, can be identified on T1-, T2-, and T2*-weighted images. Tears on the radial aspect of the TFC frequently have a dorsal-to-volar orientation and extend to both its proximal and distal surfaces (Fig. 11-77).

Associated synovitis, seen as a localized fluid collection or radiocarpal joint effusion on T2- or T2*-weighted images, may be associated with chondromalacia of the lunate, trique-

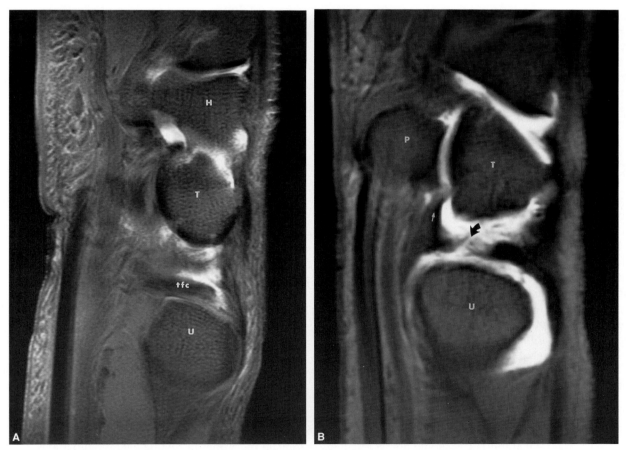

FIGURE 11-77. Comparison of (**A**) an intact TFC with (**B**) a TFC tear on fat-suppressed T1-weighted sagittal MR arthrographic images. The TFC tear (*curved arrow*) involves the radial aspect of the disk without disruption of the volar ulnocarpal ligaments (*straight arrow*). H, hamate; T, triquetrum; tfc, triangular fibrocartilage; P, pisiform; U, ulna.

trum, or ulna. In younger patients, there is a higher incidence of tears on the ulnar aspect of the TFC. Peripheral tears are secondary to traumatic avulsion, whereas central perforations may be associated with findings of TFC degeneration.[94] These degenerative changes, usually histologic mucinous or myxoid degeneration, are seen as increased signal intensity on T1- and T2*-weighted images and thinning or attenuation of the articular disc. Degeneration is common in the thinner central portion of the TFC disc and initially occurs on the ulnar or proximal surface of the TFC.[65] Whereas deformity of the TFC is common in patients with negative ulnar variance, TFC tears are associated with positive ulnar variance.

MR imaging is particularly valuable in assessing postoperative TFC repairs and associated distal joint instability. MR accuracy for detecting TFC tears is reported to be 95% compared with arthrography, and 89% compared with arthroscopy and arthrotomy.[27,91]

Treatment

The significance of TFCC lesions must be evaluated as a part of the whole clinical presentation. As noted earlier, asymptomatic tears become more and more common after 35 years of age.[11] In many cases, a TFCC lesion is not actually responsible for the patient's symptoms, but is rather a clue to the pathologic process. In these cases, treatment modalities are not directed at the TFCC tear itself, but at the underlying pathology. For example, in the patient with positive ulnar variance and a TFCC tear, treatment is aimed at relieving the overloading of the distal ulna rather than merely repairing or debriding the tear. Frequently, there is severe painful chondromalacia of the distal ulna.

TFCC resection and debridement are the treatments of choice for a flap tear of the TFCC—similar to that of the meniscus of the knee—that causes pain. These treatments also are indicated if there is instability of the DRUJ due to the TFCC injury. If repair is not possible, then the structure should be augmented. We use an intraarticular ligament reconstruction to augment tears of the dorsal limbus of the TFCC that lead to DRUJ instability. There are data, however, that indicate that no resection of the TFCC is mechanically benign, even though the avascular, thin centrum of the disc was thought by many to be mechanically insignificant, and the mechanics for stabilizing the DRUJ were thought to be primarily derived from the intact dorsal and volar limbi. Adams[95] has reported that although the dorsal and volar limbi of the TFCC provide the final restraints to DRUJ dislocation, the centrum is an important component for normal motion. Resection of the centrum was found to alter the mechanics of the DRUJ and the remainder of the TFCC.[95] These findings suggest that the TFCC should not be resected with impunity and the methods of reconstruction need to be studied more carefully.

The meniscus homologue consists of a fold of fibrous

tissue interposed between the tip of the ulnar styloid and the triquetrum. This is an evolutionary remnant of the early primate wrist, in which weightbearing was facilitated by an elongated ulnar styloid that articulated, through a free meniscus, with the triquetrum.[96] Occasionally, a free meniscus or an abnormally long ulnar styloid tipped with articular cartilage that impinges against the triquetrum can be seen in humans. Triquetral impingement of the ulnar styloid results in cartilage degeneration of the triquetrum. This impingement can be treated with a limited ulnar styloidectomy. The meniscus homologue forms the entrance to the prestyloid recess seen in arthrographic examination of the wrist.

FRACTURES OF THE DISTAL RADIUS AND CARPUS

Conventional radiography is limited in the detection of nondisplaced or partially displaced fractures of the carpus and distal radius. Trispiral tomography depends on correct planar positioning, or carpal fractures may be underdiagnosed. Results from early bone scintigraphy, performed within 72 hours of an acute fracture, may be negative or equivocal. CT using thin (1.5 mm) sections in either direct coronal or axial planes with reformatting and 3D rendering is the most accurate modality for identifying fractures and for characterizing morphology and associated comminution or displacement. Chip fractures can be detected by CT in patients with negative findings on MR studies. Fracture extent and adjacent marrow hyperemia are clearly demonstrated on MR images. In subacute and chronic fractures, sclerosis demonstrates low signal intensity on T1-weighted images. The temporal stage of a fracture (eg, acute, subacute, chronic) and its location determine the optimal diagnostic imaging plane (eg, coronal, axial, or sagittal). MR imaging shows associated ligamentous injury in isolated or multiple carpal bone trauma. If initial imaging is inadequate, delayed diagnosis and treatment may lead to poor anatomic reduction and loss of function.

Distal Radius Fractures

There are several systems for classifying fractures of the distal radius, but the Frykman classification[97] (Fig. 11-78) has received the most attention. This system differentiates among fractures based on whether they are intraarticular or extraarticular and on the degree to which they involve the DRUJ. Melone's system[98] for classifying articular fractures of the distal radius is based on the degree and direction of displacement of the articular fragments[98] (Figs. 11-79 and 11-80). This system is clinically useful because it indicates when open reduction is necessary to achieve accurate anatomical reduction. In routine lateral radiographs, the normal palmar tilt of the articular surface of the distal radius is 10° to 14°. On PA radiographs, the inclination of the radial

text continues on page 934

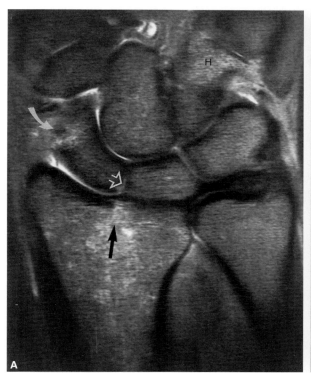

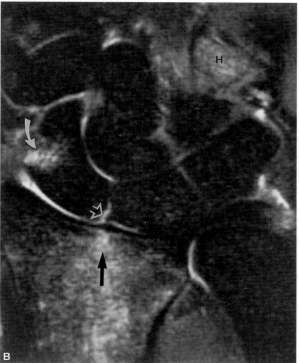

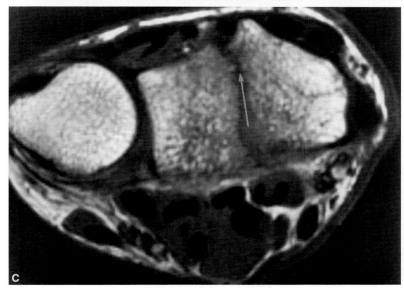

FIGURE 11-78. Nondisplaced intraarticular distal radius fracture (Frykman type III) associated with scapholunate ligament tear, hook of the hamate fracture, and nondisplaced fracture of the distal scaphoid pole. Fracture-related marrow edema is hyperintense on both fat-suppressed T2-weighted fast spin-echo (**A**) and fast STIR (**B**) coronal images. The dorsal-to-volar extension of the fracture is shown on a T1-weighted axial image (**C**). In the Frykman classification of distal radius fractures, intraarticular fractures are classified as class III or higher, based on radiocarpal, distal radioulnar joint, and distal ulnar involvement. Complex intraarticular fractures have a poor prognosis.

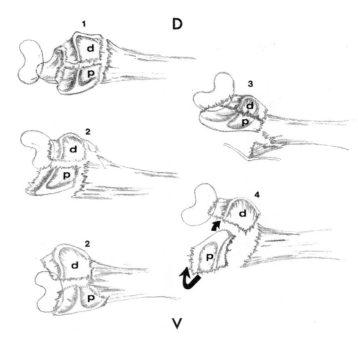

FIGURE 11-79. The Melone classification of distal radius articular fractures. The displacement of the medial complex (which consists of medial fragments and ligamentous attachments to the ulnar styloid and carpus) is the basis for classifying four types of articular fractures. (1) In a type 1 fracture, the medial complex may be displaced or not, with stable reduction and congruity of the joint surface. (2) In a type 2 fracture, there is comminution and the fracture is unstable. The medial complex is posteriorly or anteriorly displaced. (3) In a type 3 fracture, the medial complex is displaced and there is a spike fragment from the comminuted radial shaft. (4) In a type 4 fracture, separation or rotation of the dorsal and palmar medial fragments occurs, with severe disruption of the distal radial articular surface. Small and large curved arrows, rotation of distal and palmar medial fragments; D, dorsal; d, dorsal medial fragment; p, palmar medial fragment; V, volar.

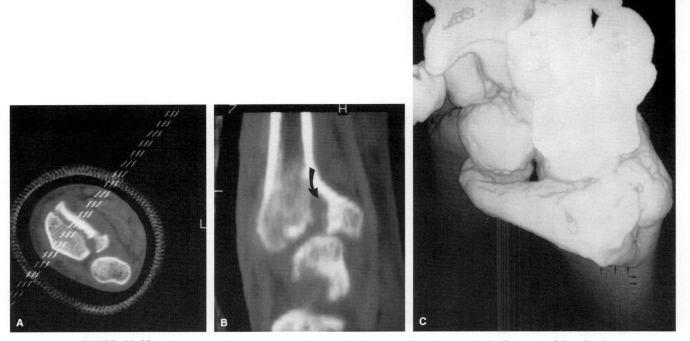

FIGURE 11-80. (A) Axial and (B) sagittal reformatted CT scans show intraarticular fracture of the distal radius with anterior displacement (*curved arrow*) of the palmar articular surface. This is a Melone type 2 fracture, or reverse Barton's fracture, involving the volar and not the dorsal lip of the radius. (C) The corresponding 3D CT shows an intraarticular fracture of the palmar articular surface or volar lip of the radius (*arrows*).

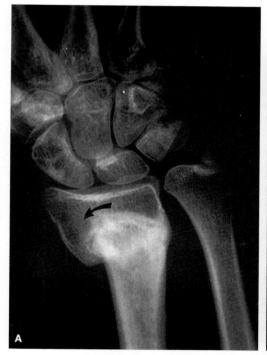

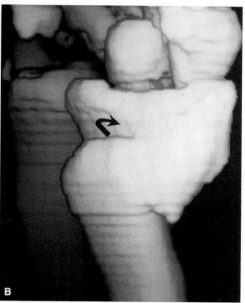

FIGURE 11-81. Colles' fracture. (A) An anteroposterior radiograph shows nonarticular distal radius and ulnar styloid fractures. There is lateral displacement of the distal radius fracture fragment (*arrow*), with associated radial shortening. (B) The corresponding 3D CT image reveals dorsal impaction with apex volar angulation (*arrow*).

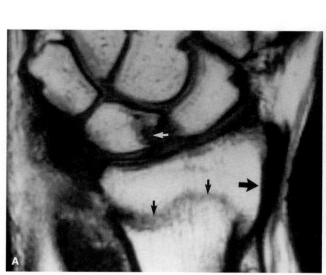

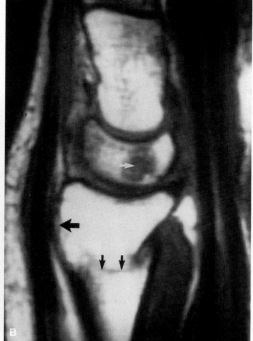

FIGURE 11-82. (A) A T1-weighted coronal image shows a postreduction Colles' fracture (*small black arrows*) with lateral displacement (*large black arrow*). Subchondral cystic erosion is present in the radial aspect of the lunate (*white arrow*). (B) A T1-weighted sagittal image shows dorsal displacement (*large black arrow*) with angulation of the distal fracture fragment. The fracture site (*small black arrows*) and lunate cystic erosion (*white arrow*) are also shown.

articular surface forms an angle of 23° with the long axis of the forearm. These angles must be accurately restored with fracture reduction. If the palmar tilt is not anatomically correct, the range of motion in flexion will be limited and an intercalated instability pattern of the carpus may develop. Loss of the angle of inclination leads to increased loading of the radial articular surface and arthritic degeneration.[99]

Colles' Fractures

Colles' fractures occur secondary to a fall on the outstretched hand, with a pronated forearm in dorsiflexion. The fracture commonly occurs in women older than 50 years of age. The fracture line occurs within 2 to 3 cm of the articular surface of the distal radius (Figs. 11-81 and 11-82). The distal fracture segment may demonstrate dorsal displacement, angula-

tion, or both. There may also be medial or lateral displacement. The transmission of force across the transverse carpal ligament may result in an associated ulnar styloid fracture.

With MR imaging, it is possible to assess the articular surface of the distal radius and to document precise angular deformities in sagittal, axial, and coronal planes. The median and ulnar nerves, which may be involved at the time of injury, are best seen on axial MR images.

Die Punch Fractures

In a die punch fracture, the lunate impacts the distal radius, splitting its fossa in both the coronal and sagittal planes and depressing the articular surface, much like a tibial plateau fracture[100,101] (Fig. 11-83). It is critical to restore the articular surface to anatomic continuity fol-

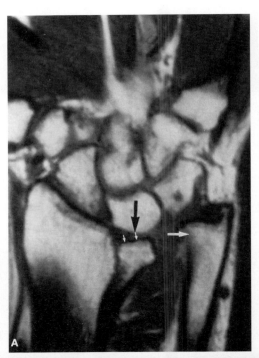

FIGURE 11-83. Die punch fracture. Coronal (**A**) T1-weighted and (**B**) 2D CT reformatted images show splitting and depression of the lunate fossa (*small white arrows*) of the distal radius, with proximal migration of the lunate (*black arrows*). Associated diastasis (*large white arrows*) of the distal radioulnar joint is present, with complete disruption of the triangular fibrocartilage complex. (**C**) The corresponding 3D coronal CT image shows an intraarticular fracture (*vertical arrow*) and distal radioulnar joint diastasis (*horizontal arrow*).

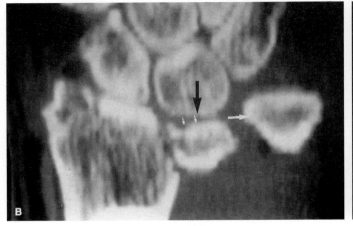

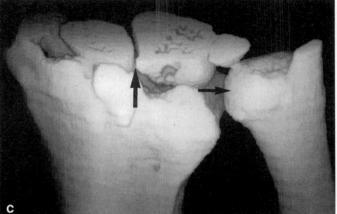

lowing this injury to prevent the development of late traumatic arthritis.

Recent clinical studies have shown that over 90% of young adult patients with incongruity (defined as more than 2 mm of displacement) develop arthritis.[102] Since the die punch lesion is a common cause of incongruity, surgeons have increased their efforts to reestablish normal articular anatomy following these injuries. Newer surgical techniques that show some promise include arthroscopic percutaneous pinning and reduction. Once the depressed articular fragments are reduced, they can be augmented with buttressing bone grafts placed via an extraarticular approach.

Carpal Fractures

Scaphoid Fractures

Scaphoid fractures are the most common fractures of the carpus.[103] Fracture of the scaphoid is frequently associated with dorsiflexion loading and a radial deviation mechanism. A conventional radiographic diagnostic series includes PA, ulnar deviation, oblique, and lateral radiographs. Repeat studies after a 2 to 3 week delay may be necessary if plain film radiograph results are negative. Negative bone scintigraphy findings may require repeat studies 48 hours after the

initial injury. Patients with trauma to the scaphoid often present with pain over the anatomical snuff box.

Fractures with a gap of 1 mm or less of diastasis are considered stable. Although certain types of scaphoid fractures (classified as type B fractures) have an increased rate of complications with nonoperative treatment, in fact all complete scaphoid fractures are potentially unstable, even in the absence of any displacement on initial radiography.[104] Incomplete and tubercle fractures of the scaphoid have a good prognosis with nonoperative treatment. Unstable scaphoid fractures may have a nonunion rate of up to 50% with closed treatment. Seventy percent of scaphoid fractures involve the middle one third, or waist, of the scaphoid, and these fractures have an increased risk for delayed union and AVN[105] (Fig. 11-84). Twenty percent of scaphoid fractures involve the proximal one third of the scaphoid, and 10% involve the distal one third (Fig. 11-85). The blood supply of the scaphoid is primarily through the distal pole, entering via the dorsal ridge from branches of the radial artery. Thus, with fractures through the waist of the scaphoid, blood supply to the proximal pole is poor, accounting for the high rate of AVN and delayed healing. Other complications of scaphoid fractures include deformity, carpal instability, secondary osteoarthritis, carpal tunnel syndrome, and sympathetic dystrophy (Fig. 11-86).

text continues on page 938

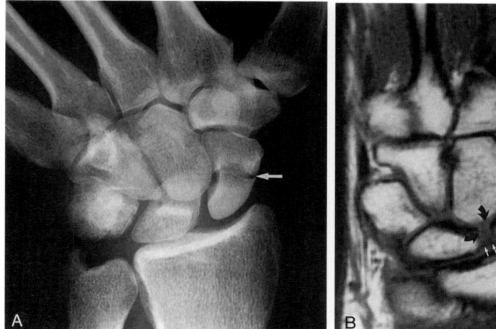
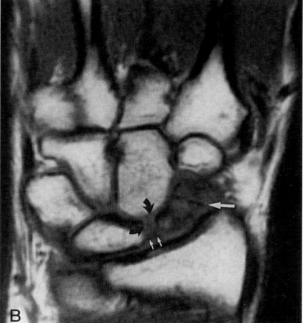

FIGURE 11-84. **(A)** Anteroposterior radiograph showing a scaphoid waist fracture (*arrow*) with avascular necrosis. No sclerosis is demonstrated in the proximal or distal fragments. **(B)** On the corresponding T1-weighted coronal image, the proximal pole necrotic marrow demonstrates lower signal intensity, and the remaining hyperemic marrow demonstrates intermediate to low signal intensity. The low signal intensity scapholunate ligament (*small white arrows*) and fluid in the widened scapholunate space (*curved arrows*) are also seen. The fracture site (*large white arrow*) is also identified.

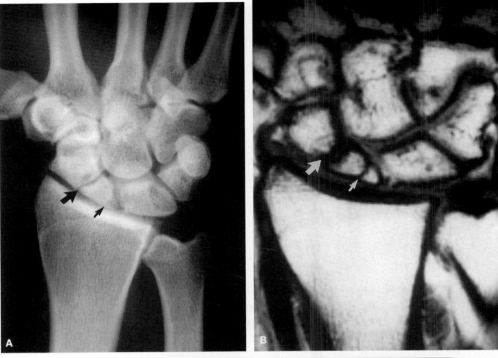

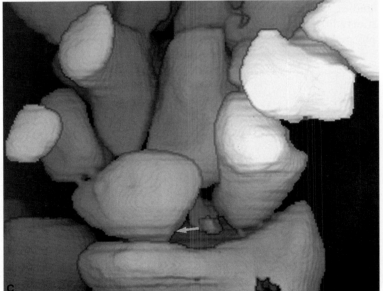

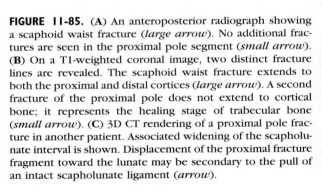

FIGURE 11-85. **(A)** An anteroposterior radiograph showing a scaphoid waist fracture (*large arrow*). No additional fractures are seen in the proximal pole segment (*small arrow*). **(B)** On a T1-weighted coronal image, two distinct fracture lines are revealed. The scaphoid waist fracture extends to both the proximal and distal cortices (*large arrow*). A second fracture of the proximal pole does not extend to cortical bone; it represents the healing stage of trabecular bone (*small arrow*). **(C)** 3D CT rendering of a proximal pole fracture in another patient. Associated widening of the scapholunate interval is shown. Displacement of the proximal fracture fragment toward the lunate may be secondary to the pull of an intact scapholunate ligament (*arrow*).

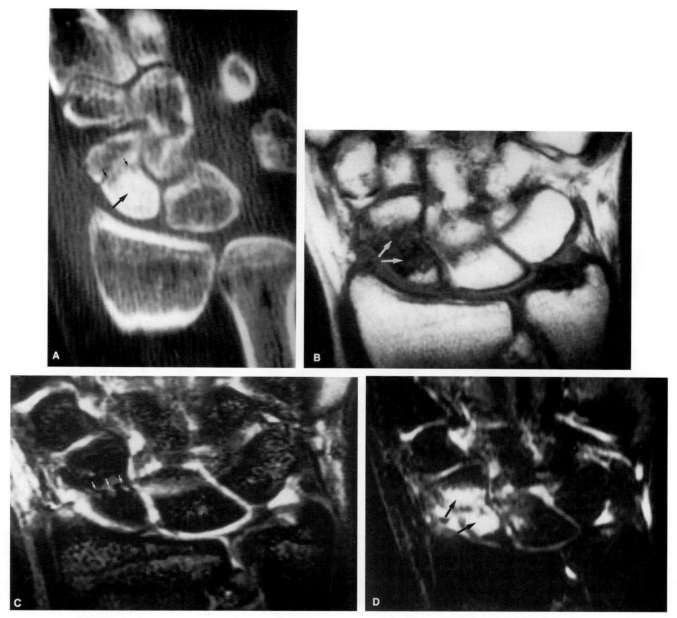

FIGURE 11-86. **(A)** A 2D CT reformatted scan shows a scaphoid waist fracture (*small arrows*) and a sclerotic proximal pole (*large arrow*). **(B)** A T1-weighted coronal image shows low signal intensity marrow on both sides of the fracture site (*arrows*). The scapholunate ligament is intact. **(C)** A T2*-weighted coronal image shows the fracture site morphology (*arrows*) without hyperintense marrow. **(D)** A coronal short TI inversion recovery image shows viable marrow edema in both the sclerotic proximal pole and nonsclerotic bone of the distal pole adjacent to the fracture site.   *continued*

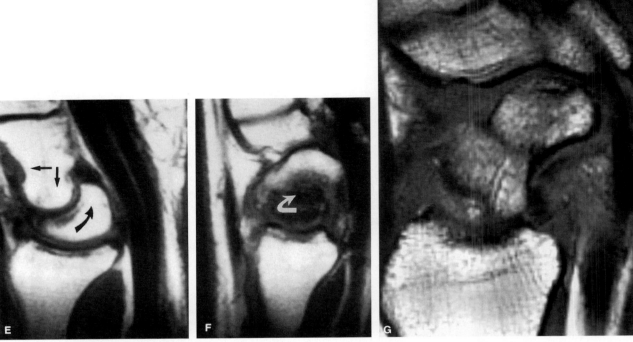

FIGURE 11-86. *Continued.* **(E)** A T1-weighted sagittal image shows a dorsal intercalated segment instability (DISI) pattern with dorsal tilt of the lunate (*curved arrow*), proximal migration, and dorsal displacement of the capitate (*straight arrows*). Disruption of the dorsal capsule is present. **(F)** Humpback flexion deformity of the scaphoid (*curved white arrow*) with distal pole flexion is identified on this T1-weighted sagittal image. **(G)** Healing scaphoid fracture in another patient, without associated humpback flexion deformity.

On MR imaging studies of scaphoid fractures, the low signal intensity fracture line is clearly displayed and may persist, contrasting with the surrounding bright signal intensity of marrow during healing (Fig. 11-87). The identification of extension to cortical bone is necessary to accurately differentiate acute from chronic fractures, and it allows MR imaging to be more sensitive than CT or conventional radiography in evaluating the progress of subacute or chronic fractures.

Sagittal images demonstrate the abnormal morphology of the scaphoid, secondary to fracture fragmentation or suboptimal healing (ie, humpback deformity). This foreshortening of the scaphoid is associated with DISI instability[106] (Fig. 11-88). The presence of Herbert screws produces minimal artifact. The articular cartilage surface of the scaphoid and congruity of adjacent coronal surfaces should be assessed. T2*-weighted images are not as sensitive to the range of contrast as conventional T1-weighted images, and may not identify a nonacute, nondisplaced fracture. Gradient-echo images are, however, useful in demonstrating the integrity of the adjacent SL ligament. The volar capsule (the RSC ligament and RLT ligament) is shown on sagittal images,

and adjacent synovitis or edema of ligamentous structures may be identified on T1- or T2*-weighted images at the level of the scaphoid. Short TI inversion recovery or fat-suppressed T2-weighted FSE sequences are more sensitive to hyperemia (in the proximal pole or in the bone adjacent to the fracture site), which may be misdiagnosed as sclerosis, end-stage necrosis, or both on conventional T1-, T2-, or T2*-weighted images (see Fig. 11-86).

Triquetrum Fractures

Fractures of the triquetrum represent the second most common fracture of the carpus.[103] Correct positioning in lateral and pronated oblique projections is usually required to identify fractures of the triquetrum in standard radiography. CT examination of the triquetrum, however, is not limited by overlapping of the proximal and distal carpal rows, which may obscure identification of a fracture line. Triquetral fractures include chip fractures that involve the dorsal surface and occur secondary to an avulsion injury at the insertional site of the ulnotriquetral ligament or to trauma

text continues on page 942

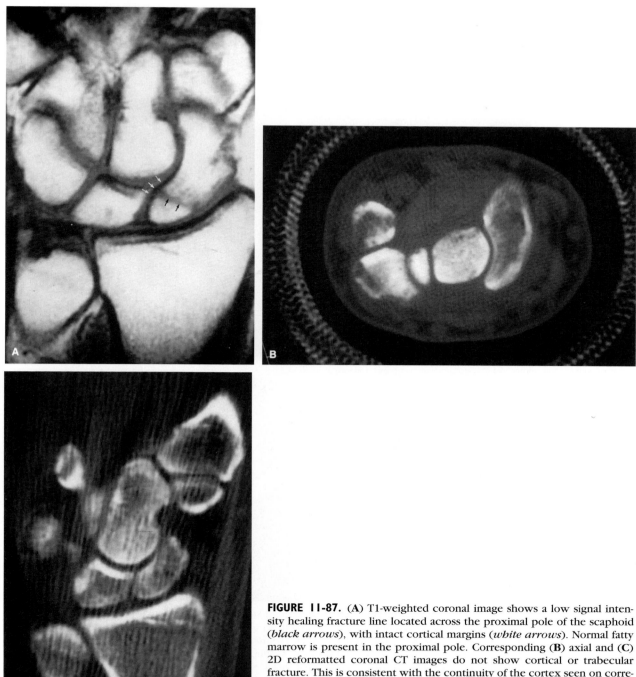

FIGURE 11-87. (**A**) T1-weighted coronal image shows a low signal intensity healing fracture line located across the proximal pole of the scaphoid (*black arrows*), with intact cortical margins (*white arrows*). Normal fatty marrow is present in the proximal pole. Corresponding (**B**) axial and (**C**) 2D reformatted coronal CT images do not show cortical or trabecular fracture. This is consistent with the continuity of the cortex seen on corresponding MR images, which are more sensitive in the initial and healing stages of scaphoid fractures. Small chip fractures of other carpal bones, however, are still best evaluated with thin section CT.

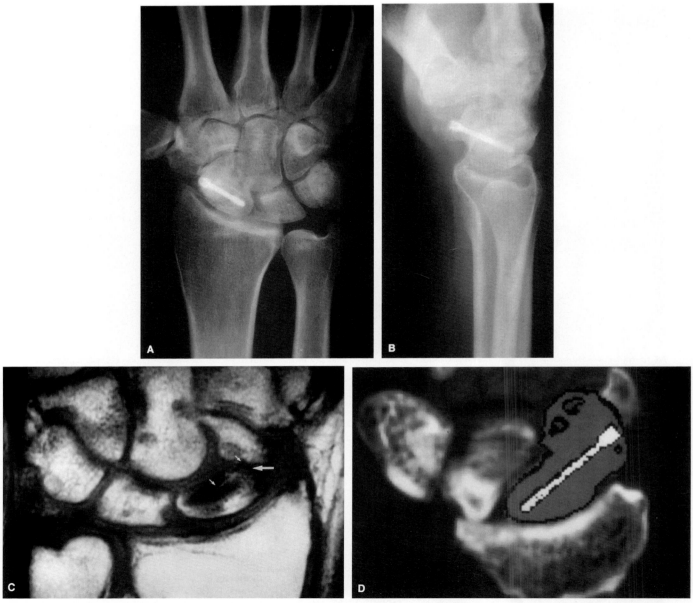

FIGURE 11-88. Scaphoid fracture with dorsal intercalated segment instability (DISI). **(A)** Anteroposterior and **(B)** lateral radiographs show a scaphoid waist fracture fixed with titanium screw. **(C)** A T1-weighted coronal image shows minimal artifact adjacent to the screw (*small arrows*). A low signal intensity fracture line (*large arrow*) is seen in the middle one third of the scaphoid, without development of avascular necrosis of the proximal pole. **(D)** A 2D CT reformatted image shows the morphology of the titanium screw.

continued

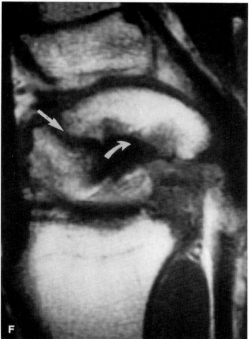

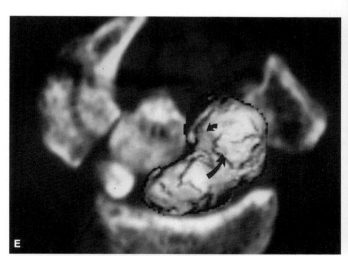

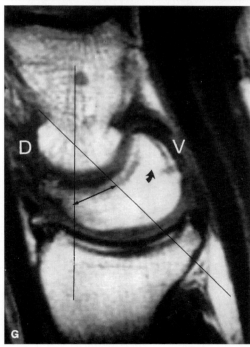

FIGURE 11-88 *Continued.* **(E)** A 3D CT rendering of the fore-shortened scaphoid (*curved arrows*) is displayed on a 2D CT reformatted background. **(F)** A T1-weighted sagittal image illustrates the humpback scaphoid deformity characterized by flexion of the distal pole (*curved arrow*) relative to the fracture line (*straight arrow*) and proximal pole. The radioscapho-capitate ligament is not seen, and there is localized synovitis in its expected location. **(G)** A T1-weighted sagittal image demonstrates DISI secondary to the humpback deformity, and wrist shortening without scapholunate interosseous ligament tear. The dorsal tilt of the lunate (*curved arrow*) and increased capitolunate angle (*double-headed arrow*) are indicated. The capitate is dorsally displaced relative to the radius, as is characteristically seen in DISI instabilities. D, dorsal; V, volar.

to the wrist positioned in hyperextension and ulnar deviation. Fracture through the body of the triquetrum is less common. Triquetral body fractures may be associated with perilunate dislocations or ulnar carpal dissociation.

Multiple fracture lines and acute fracture through the triquetrum may obscure fracture morphology secondary to reactive hyperemia of subchondral bone (Fig. 11-89). T1-weighted images in the axial, coronal, and sagittal imaging planes identify low signal intensity in the area of the fracture. In our experience, CT has been more useful in displaying cortical detail and fracture morphology.

Lunate Fractures

Fracture of the lunate is an uncommon injury that usually occurs secondary to a fall with the wrist in dorsiflexion.[103] In KD, acute fractures of the lunate may be related to single or multiple episodes of compression, but more often they are pathologic fractures through areas of necrotic bone that occur during the advanced stages. Associated perilunate dislocation with ligamentous trauma should be evaluated.

Pisiform Fractures

The pisiform is a sesamoid bone within the flexor carpi ulnaris tendon.[103] Fracture of the pisiform is caused by direct or blunt trauma, such as occurs when the heel of the hand is used as a hammer. It appears as a comminuted or simple fracture. Pisotriquetral arthritis may develop secondary to pisiform fracture. Sagittal and axial T1-weighted images display a larger surface area of the pisiform bone, minimizing the partial volume effect that may complicate coronal images.

Hamate Fractures

Fractures of the hamate, which account for approximately 2% of carpal fractures,[103] may involve either the body or the hook (ie, the hamulus).[107] Fracture of the hook of the hamate may involve an avulsion injury of the transverse carpal ligament. Direct trauma to the volar aspect of the wrist, the most common mechanism of injury, usually occurs in activities that require a grasping movement, such as holding a bat, club, or racket. Ring and little finger flexor tendon attritional rupture may occur with chronic fracture of the hamate (Fig. 11-90). Neuropathy of the deep branch of the ulnar nerve has also been observed in these injuries.[103] Conventional radiographic imaging is often yields negative results in hamate fractures, and diagnosis may require the use of a carpal tunnel projection. T1-weighted axial and sagittal images are best suited for display the anatomy of the hook of the hamate and for identification of hamate fractures (Fig. 11-91). Fat-suppressed T2-weighted FSE or STIR techniques, however, are better for demonstrating associated marrow edema. Thin (1.5 mm) CT scans more accurately identify the extent and location of fractures of the hamate, especially the hook of the hamate. The proximity of the ulnar nerve to the hamate may contribute to the presentation of ulnar wrist pain in patients sustaining hamate trauma.

Capitate Fractures

Fractures of the capitate, which account for 1% to 3% of carpal bone fractures,[103] are similar to scaphoid fractures in that the blood supply of extends through the waist of

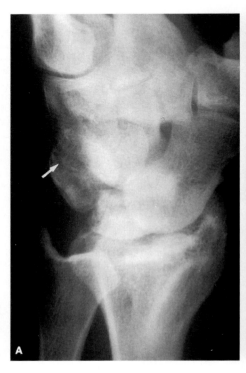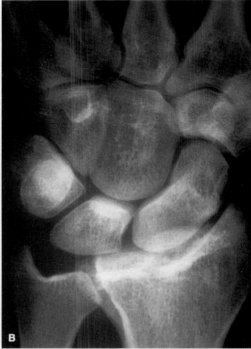

FIGURE 11-89. (A) An oblique radiograph shows a dorsal fracture of the triquetrum (*arrow*). (B) Standard AP projection does not display the fracture. *continued*

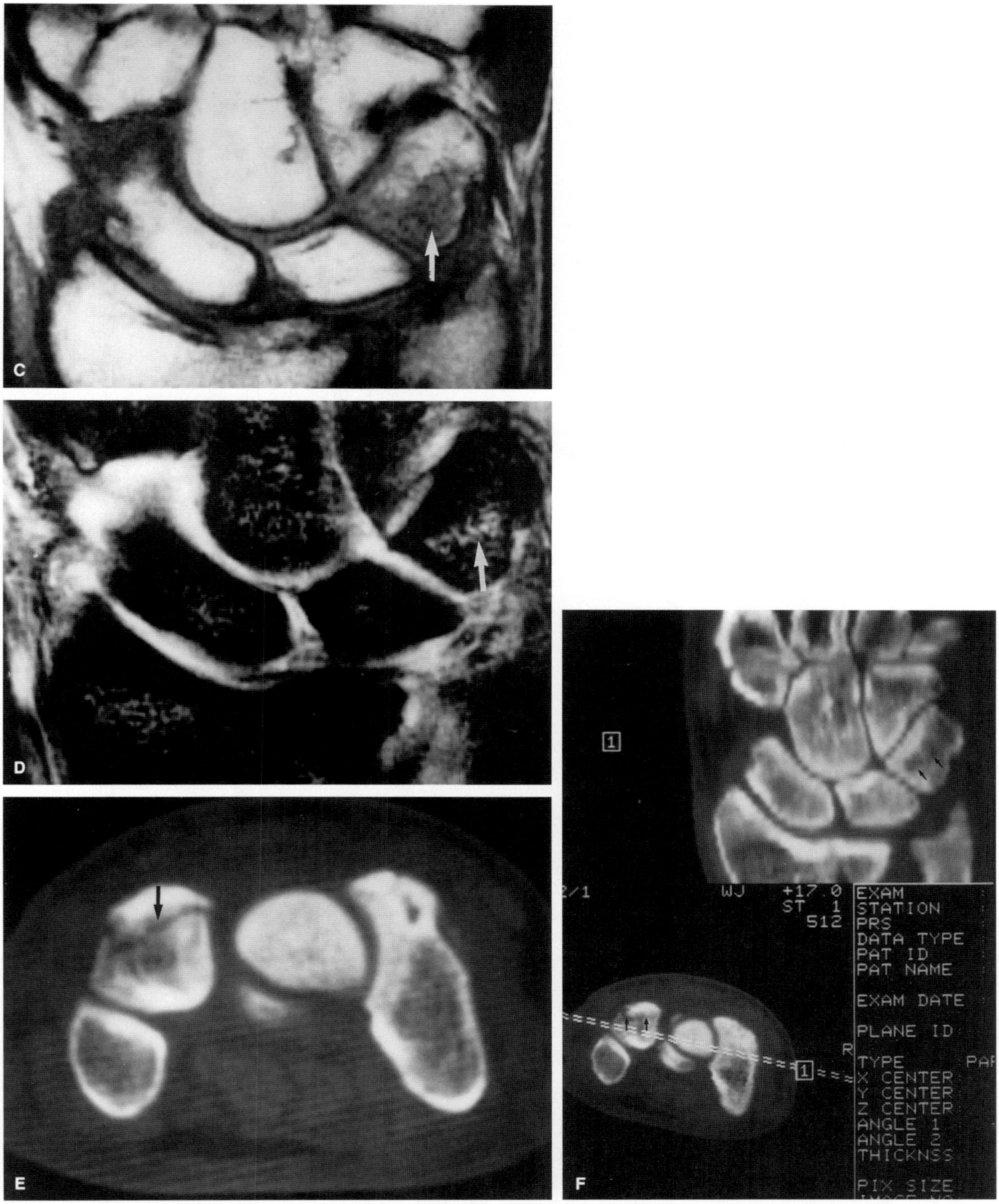

FIGURE 11-89. *Continued.* (**C**) On a T1-weighted coronal image, marrow hyperemia and hemorrhage (*arrow*) demonstrate low signal intensity. (**D**) On a T2*-weighted coronal image, marrow hyperemia and hemorrhage (*arrow*) demonstrate hyperintensity. (**E**) On a direct axial CT image, a complete dorsal fracture is seen (*arrow*). (**F**) A reformatted coronal CT image shows trabecular bone disruption (*arrows*) that corresponds to the area of marrow hemorrhage seen on the T1- and T2*-weighted MR images.

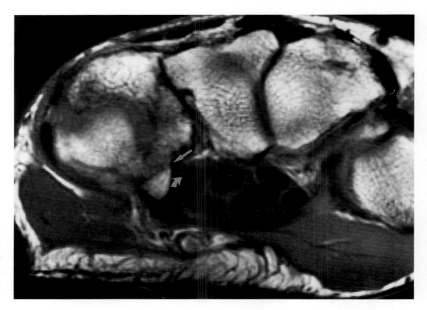

FIGURE 11-90. Hamate fracture associated with a loss of the osseous concavity normally created by the hook of the hamate (*straight arrow*). There is reciprocal flattening with effacement of the carpal tunnel at the level of the ulnar-sided flexor digitorum profundus tendons (*curved arrow*) (T1-weighted axial image).

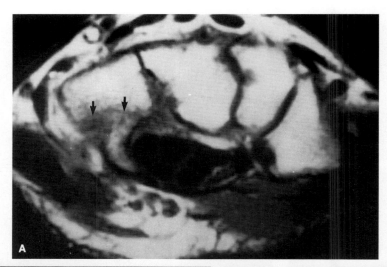

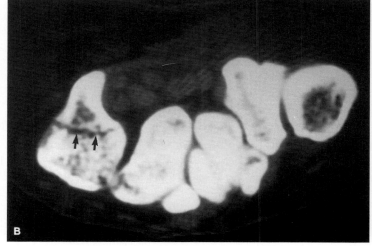

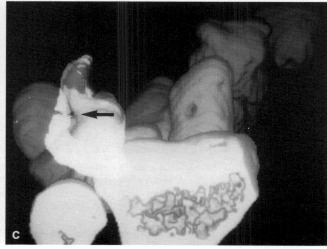

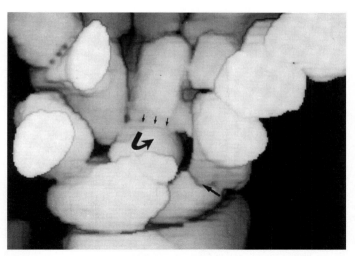

FIGURE 11-92. A 3D CT image demonstrates transscaphoid (*large straight arrow*), transcapitate (*small straight arrows*), and perilunate dislocation with 90° rotation of the proximal capitate fragment (*curved arrow*).

the capitate, making the proximal pole susceptible to AVN. Capitate fractures are caused by either direct trauma or forced dorsiflexion. The most frequent site of fracture involves the waist or neck of the capitate. Sagittal MR images are helpful in assessing rotation at the fracture site. Scaphocapitate syndrome consists of a capitate fracture associated with perilunate dislocation. The mechanism of injury is dorsiflexion in radial deviation (Fig. 11-92). The head of the capitate is fractured and rotated 180°.[103] The proximal end of the capitate demonstrates a squared-off contour.

Trapezium and Trapezoid Fractures

Fractures of the trapezium involve either its body or volar margin.[103] A displaced vertical fracture with lateral subluxation of the first metacarpal is treated with reduction and internal fixation. The trapezoid is the least commonly fractured bone of the carpus.

AVASCULAR NECROSIS OF THE SCAPHOID

Avascular necrosis of the scaphoid is primarily a posttraumatic event that occurs secondary to proximal pole or waist fractures that endanger the dominant blood supply of the scaphoid (Fig. 11-93). There often is sclerosis of the proxi-

mal pole related to osteopenia and hyperemia of adjacent nonnecrotic bone. By the time sclerosis, resorption, and collapse are evident on plain film radiographs, however, the disease is in an advanced state. When AVN of the scaphoid occurs in the absence of fracture, it is called Preiser's disease (Fig. 11-94).

The application of MR imaging to the detection and evaluation of AVN is facilitated by the bright signal intensity contrast generated from the normal fatty marrow content of the carpal bones. MR imaging has been reported to be as sensitive as bone scintigraphy in the detection of AVN, and even more specific.[108-113] On T1-weighted (ie, short TR/TE) sequences, MR sensitivity rates for the detection of decreased marrow signal associated with AVN are 87.5%. With the addition of T2-weighted sequences, specificity is reported to be 100%.

The most common MR appearance of AVN of the scaphoid is low signal intensity in the proximal pole on both T1- and T2-weighted images (Fig. 11-95). In diffuse marrow necrosis, low signal intensity marrow may not be restricted to the proximal pole. T2-weighted images may demonstrate localized fluid accumulation and limited marrow edema of the proximal pole. Reactive marrow hyperemia of the distal pole may be confused with diffuse changes of necrosis (Fig. 11-96). Short TI inversion recovery images can be used to document increased hyperemia of the distal pole marrow as well as proximal pole vascularity, which may not be appreciated on T1-, T2-, or T2*-weighted images. Accurate assessment of vascularity may be limited on gradient-echo sequences. Intravenously administered gadolinium contrast produces enhancement of hyperemic tissue at the fracture site and adjacent subchondral bone marrow.[114] This is assessed on T1-weighted fat-suppressed images. Absence of proximal pole bone marrow enhancement indicates lack of vascular perfusion in the development of AVN. Fracture healing demonstrates hyperemia at the fracture site and adjacent marrow. Nonunion is characterized by persistent low signal intensity on T1, T2, and post-contrast fat-suppressed T1-weighted images. High signal intensity fluid may be seen separating fracture fragments. Callus or fibrous union may also demonstrate low signal intensity on T1- or T2-weighted images. CT is often used to document the extent of bridging bone spatially in a 3D rendering. A vascularized pedicle graft is a treatment option prescribed for scaphoid nonunion with a nonviable proximal fragment.

text continues on page 949

FIGURE 11-91. Hamate fracture. **(A)** A T1-weighted axial image shows a low signal intensity transition (*arrows*) between a fractured hook of the hamate and normal fat marrow signal intensity. Guyon's canal is also seen between the pisiform bone and the hamulus. Corresponding axial **(B)** CT and **(C)** 3D CT images of the carpal tunnel show a transverse nondisplaced fracture (*arrows*) with greater cortical edge detail. MR imaging, however, allows imaging of Guyon's canal and assessment of the ulnar neurovascular structures, which may be secondarily compromised. Fractures of the hook of the hamate are more common than body fractures and may be overlooked on clinical examination or standard radiographs because a carpal tunnel view is required for their identification.

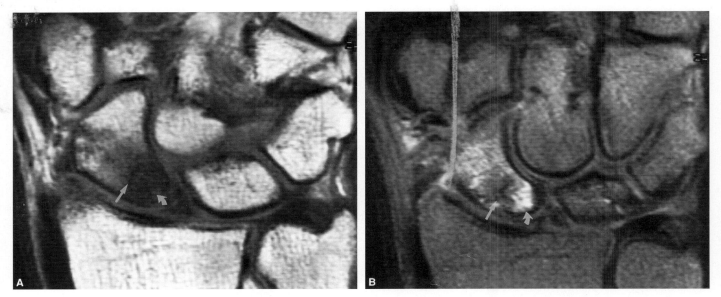

FIGURE 11-93. A scaphoid fracture with avascular necrosis (*curved arrow*) of the proximal pole is hypointense on a T1-weighted coronal image (**A**) and hyperintense in hyperemic viable bone on a fat-suppressed T2-weighted fast spin-echo coronal image (**B**). The fracture line (*straight arrow*) remains hypointense on both pulse sequences. The fat-suppressed T2-weighted fast spin-echo is also more sensitive than the T1-weighted image in detecting distal pole marrow edema.

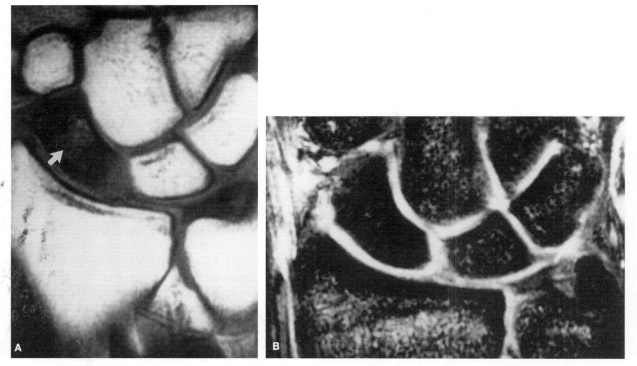

FIGURE 11-94. Preiser's disease. (**A**) A T1-weighted coronal image shows a low signal intensity sclerotic scaphoid (*arrow*) without an identifiable fracture site. (**B**) A T2*-weighted coronal image does not show increased signal intensity.

continued

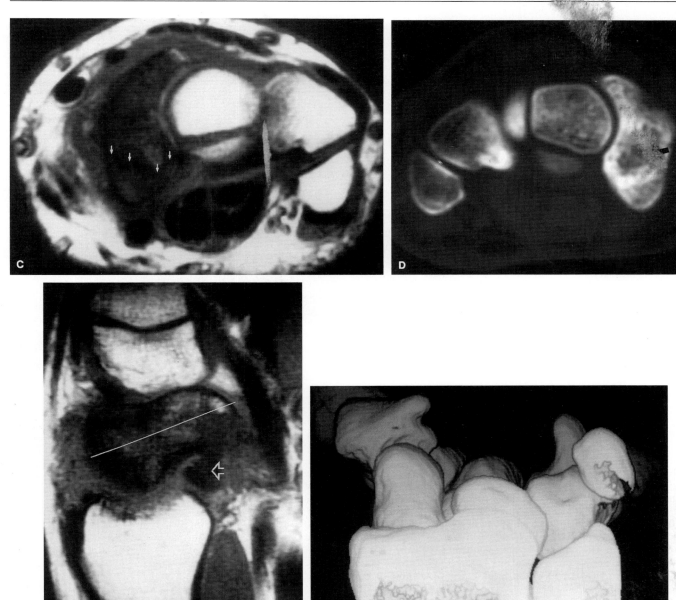

FIGURE 11-94. *Continued.* A T1-weighted axial image (C) and an axial CT scan (D) show stress fracture morphology (*arrows*). (E) A T1-weighted sagittal image shows rotatory subluxation and palmar tilt of the scaphoid (*long white line*) with an edematous, lax radioscaphocapitate ligament (*open arrow*). (F) A 3D CT image shows normal surface morphology of the scaphoid.

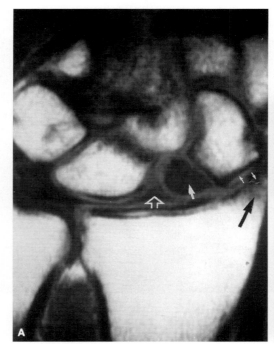

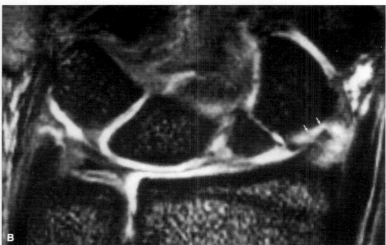

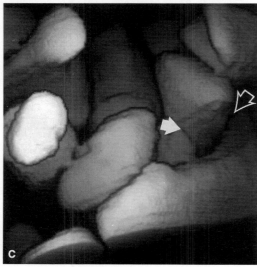

FIGURE 11-95. Avascular necrosis (AVN) of the scaphoid, with early scapholunate advanced collapse (SLAC) wrist. (**A**) A low signal intensity "corner sign" of radial styloid subchondral sclerosis (*black arrow*) is seen in the presence of scaphoid nonunion and AVN of the proximal pole (*large white arrow*) on a T1-weighted coronal image. There is mild narrowing of the radioscaphoid articulation with respect to the distal pole (*small white arrows*). The scapholunate interosseous ligament is intact (*open arrow*). (**B**) Attenuated articular cartilage is seen in the proximal aspect of the distal pole of the scaphoid in early SLAC degeneration (*arrows*) on a T2*-weighted coronal image. The radiolunate joint is characteristically unaffected. (**C**) A 3D CT image shows the fracture site (*solid arrow*) and narrowing of the radioscaphoid articulation at the level of the distal pole of the scaphoid (*open arrow*).

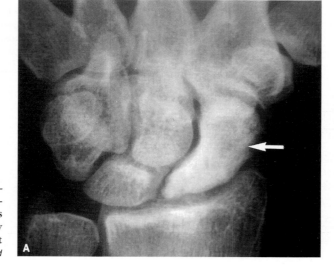

FIGURE 11-96. Scaphoid avascular necrosis. (**A**) An anteroposterior radiograph shows diffuse sclerosis of the scaphoid. The deformity of the proximal aspect of the proximal pole is known as the "nipple sign" and is sometimes seen in association with scaphoid fractures. There is relatively little sclerosis of the distal pole (*arrow*) when compared with that present in the proximal pole.

continued

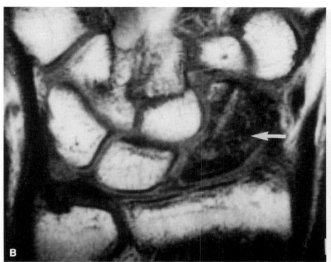 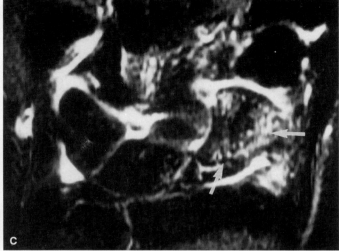

FIGURE 11-96. *Continued.* (**B**) A T1-weighted coronal image shows diffuse low signal intensity sclerosis (*arrow*). (**C**) A short TI inversion recovery coronal image most accurately depicts hyperintense hyperemic marrow in the waist and distal pole of the scaphoid (*arrows*). A discrete scaphoid fracture is not identified.

KIENBÖCK'S DISEASE

Kienböck's disease is a condition marked by AVN of the lunate. The onset of KD, which can be quite insidious, peaks between the ages of 20 and 40 years. There is a 2:1 male-to-female ratio. Although uncommon, bilateral disease does occur. Initially, patients note dorsal tenderness about the lunate and may develop stiffness due to synovitis. The synovitis and inflammation may affect surrounding structures, and one patient presented with acute carpal tunnel syndrome as the first indication of KD. Patients also complain of weakness and decreased grip strength. KD is a great dissembler, and a number of other conditions should be considered. Any history of trauma should be carefully elicited. The differential diagnosis includes dorsal ganglion cysts, rheumatoid arthritis, degenerative or posttraumatic arthritis, synovitis of the wrist from any cause, acute fractures, carpal instabilities, and ulnar impingement syndrome. It is critical that KD be suspected when evaluating dorsally located central wrist pain.

Although the MR appearance of KD is discussed in detail under "Magnetic Resonance Findings," a few comments are in order concerning the early presentation of the disease. In stage I KD, plain film radiograph findings are normal. Before MR imaging became available, the standard test at this stage was the three-phase ^{99m}TC-MDP study.[115] When there is abnormal uptake of technetium, especially in the third or delayed phase, a CT scan should be performed to assess trabecular bone morphology and to identify fractures. The three-phase technetium study is extremely sensitive, but does not provide detail about physiologic changes in the marrow, which can be seen on MR scans. MR imaging is potentially the best first imaging examination after routine

radiographs (Fig. 11-97). MR imaging not only allows assessment of the lunate, but also facilitates ruling out or adding other disorders in the differential diagnosis. MR studies may reveal occult ganglion cysts as well as inflammatory arthritides with synovitis.

Etiology

In 1928, Hulten noted a correlation between negative ulnar variance and the occurrence of KD.[116] He found that 78% of patients with KD had a relatively short ulna, whereas only 23% of patients with normal wrists had negative ulnar variance.[116] Despite his primitive radiographic techniques and measurement methods, this correlation has withstood the test of time. It should be noted that the association between a short ulna and KD is not absolute. Although exceedingly uncommon, KD may also occur in patients with neutral or positive ulnar variance. The significance of negative ulnar variance is that it subjects the lunate to an increased mechanical load compared with that associated with neutral or positive ulnar variance.

As noted earlier, the relative lengths of the ulna and radius vary with the forearm position; it is critical that measurements be made with the forearm in neutral pronosupination. There is no evidence that Hulten was aware of this, and he did not control the forearm position in his studies. When forearm position is carefully controlled, there is virtually no difference in accuracy among the several methods available for measuring variance. Gelberman and colleagues[117] have developed a simple method that requires no special tools. In this technique, a line is extended perpendicularly from the most proximal

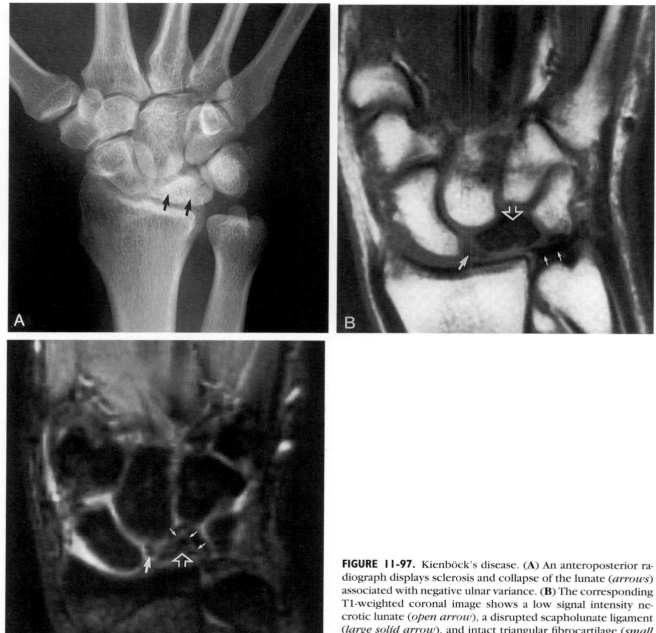

FIGURE 11-97. Kienböck's disease. (**A**) An anteroposterior radiograph displays sclerosis and collapse of the lunate (*arrows*) associated with negative ulnar variance. (**B**) The corresponding T1-weighted coronal image shows a low signal intensity necrotic lunate (*open arrow*), a disrupted scapholunate ligament (*large solid arrow*), and intact triangular fibrocartilage (*small solid arrows*). (**C**) A T2*-weighted coronal image reveals fragmentation (*large solid arrow*) and edema (*small solid arrows*) associated with a necrotic lunate (*open arrow*).

portion of the distal radial articular surface. This point can be found by carefully inspecting PA radiographs for the three sclerotic lines that represent different portions of the articular surface. The most distal line is the dorsal lip of the radius. The middle line, because of the normal volar tilt of the distal radius articular surface, is the volar lip of the radius. The most proximal line is the most proximal portion of the articular surface, and this is where the perpendicular line should originate. The distance between this line and the distal articular surface of the ulna is then measured.

The theory that acute fractures and trauma play a role in the etiology of Kienböck's, an essentially progressive disease, dates as far back as 1843.[118,119] It is the anatomy of the vascular supply of the lunate that places it at risk for the development of AVN. Gelberman and colleagues found that all lunates could be classified into three types based on their intraosseous microvascular anatomy.[120] The extraosseous blood supply was found to be abundant, and AVN could not be ascribed to interruption of these vessels at a single pole of the lunate. However, the subchondral bone adjacent to the radial articular surface was found to be relatively avascular, and this is the area where collapse is most commonly seen. Gelberman and colleagues concluded that AVN is secondary to disruption of the intraosseous blood vessels caused by repeated trauma and compression fractures.

Treatment

The treatment of KD is a subject of great debate among hand surgeons. Because the condition is relatively rare, no single surgeon or center has been able to develop a large enough experience with all stages of the disease to provide truly definitive treatment recommendations. As a result, many types of procedures are recommended in the literature. In general, treatment modalities are tailored to the stage of disease. Early stages—marked by the absence of changes in articular cartilage, minimal collapse of the lunate, and permanent carpal instability patterns—are usually treated with procedures designed to unload and revascularize the lunate. Later stages—with established instability patterns and degenerative arthritis—must be treated with arthrodesis and salvage procedures. As noted later, changes in therapeutic strategy correlate with the transition from stage IIIA to stage IIIB disease.

Staging

The clinical and radiographic characteristics of KD vary according to the stage of the disease.[121] The staging classification devised by Lichtman has the most clinical relevance.[122]

Stage I

In stage I of KD, plain radiographs are normal, with the possible exception of a linear or compression fracture in the lunate. Ulnar variance should be noted. The initial treatment after diagnosis is immobilization and nonsteroidal antiinflammatory drugs (NSAIDs). If there is no improvement with this treatment, then surgical intervention should be considered. A halfway step to an open surgical procedure is the placement of an extended fixation device with distraction to unload the lunate. Although this may help, it is impossible to keep such an appliance in place for more than 3 months, which is insufficient time to allow revascularization. If the patient has negative ulnar variance, then radial shortening is frequently advocated to unload the lunate. Although ulnar lengthening is equally effective, it is technically more demanding. Surgical intervention in stage I is rarely indicated, and all patients should receive a trial of conservative therapy. It is important to remember that until the advent of MR imaging the identification of stage I KD was exceedingly rare, and, therefore, there are very little data on the efficacy of treatment at this stage of the disease. In addition to early detection, MR imaging can be used to document healing during cast immobilization.

Stage II

In stage II, there is a change in the density of the lunate, which, although it has not undergone any changes in its architecture, appears to be quite sclerotic compared with the other bones of the carpus. There is no significant carpal instability, but there may be a slight degree of collapse of the radial side of the lunate. At this stage, conservative therapy is not effective, and unloading, revascularization, or both procedures are necessary. This is probably the optimal time for performing a revascularization procedure. Prior to surgery, CT scans should always be performed to assess bone detail, because a potentially repairable fracture could be identified in this way.

There are two approaches to revascularization. One entails transferring a vascularized bone graft to the lunate, and Braun has successfully used a portion of radial bone for this transfer.[123] Revascularization with transplantation of a vascular pedicle into the lunate was first reported in 1979 and is gaining in popularity.[124] In this procedure, the second intermetacarpal artery with its vena comitantes is passed through a dorsal-to-volar hole in the lunate. Recent studies verify that, as long as the vena comitantes is present, the artery remains patent. Several centers are beginning to report good results with this procedure. Unloading procedures can also be combined with revascularization. Radial shortening or ulnar lengthening are options in the wrist with negative ulnar variance. In the patient with neutral or positive ulnar variance, Almquist and associates[125] have recently introduced the technique of shortening the capitate by osteotomy to unload the lunate.[125] They have shown that shortening the capitate by 2 to 4 mm reduces the load on the lunate significantly and produces a good clinical result.

Intercarpal fusions have also been shown to unload the lunate. Triscaphe (ie, scaphoid-trapezoid-trapezium) and scaphocapitate fusions both appear to be effective.

Stage III

Kienböck's disease is considered to be in a stage III when there is collapse of the entire lunate. Stage III is further subdivided into stages IIIA and IIIB. In stage IIIA, there is lunate collapse but scaphoid rotation is not fixed. There may be dynamic rotatory subluxation, but this can be treated with surgical reconstruction. In stage IIIB, there is lunate collapse with fixed scaphoid rotation and proximal migration of the capitate (ie, CID). There is also a decrease in the carpal height ratio.

Unloading procedures may still be effective in stage IIIA. If a triscaphe (STT) or scaphocapitate fusion is done, the scaphoid fragments can be excised and the space left empty. Formerly, stage IIIA disease was treated by lunate excision and replacement with a silicone prosthesis, but recent reviews have shown a poor functional result and the frequent occurrence of silicone synovitis.[126] This procedure and use of the prosthesis are no longer indicated. In patients with positive ulnar variance, capitate shortening, with or without revascularization with a vascular pedicle, can be used to unload and revascularize the lunate. Radial shortening is substituted for capitate shortening in the patient with negative ulnar variance. During revascularization, every attempt should be made to reconstruct the lunate. When the dorsal cortex is entered, the collapsed articular surface can be elevated and buttressed with a bone graft. The vascular pedicle is then inserted.

In stage IIIB, the fixed rotation of the scaphoid must be corrected. Careful assessment of the scaphoid fossa is important in these patients, and MR imaging can be used for preoperative identification of thinning of the cartilage and arthritic changes in the radial styloid. With fixed rotation of the scaphoid, there is noncongruous loading of the scaphoid fossa. This situation is identical to that in SLAC wrist.

If the cartilage is intact, the procedure of choice fixes the scaphoid in a normal anatomic position with congruous loading of the scaphoid fossa and simultaneously unloads the lunate. A STT or scaphocapitate fusion, with careful attention to reducing the scaphoid, can accomplish this. In most cases, the collapsed lunate should be excised.

Stage IV

Stage IV of KD has all the findings of stage III, with the addition of generalized arthritic changes throughout the carpus. At this point, the disease process is advanced and some type of salvage procedure is necessary. If the articular cartilage in the lunate fossa of the distal radius and the proximal pole of the capitate is in acceptable condition, then a proximal row carpectomy can be performed. Because of the tenuous vascular supply of the lunate, there is usually degeneration in the lunate fossa, although occasionally the distal articular surface of the lunate remains serviceable. In these cases, an RSL fusion may preserve motion at the intercarpal joint. This is not common, however, and arthritic degeneration is usually so advanced throughout the carpus that there is no choice but to perform a panarthrodesis of the wrist. Although there is a total loss of wrist motion, the patient is usually quite happy because of the pain relief.

Magnetic Resonance Findings

Magnetic resonance findings in KD can also be grouped according to the stage of disease.[113]

Stage I

As mentioned earlier, conventional radiographs are usually normal in stage I, although an associated fracture line or compression fracture may be present. At this early stage, bone scintigraphy is both sensitive and nonspecific for the diagnosis of KD. However, bone scintigraphy is poor in differentiating fractures, osteochondral lesions, erosions, and the spectrum of degenerative changes which present as subchondral sclerosis. MR imaging offers comparable or greater sensitivity and improved specificity when compared with scintigraphy or radiographs (Fig. 11-98). With MR imaging, it is possible to characterize the extent of necrosis and the morphology of marrow involvement, as well as the overall morphology of the lunate cortical surfaces, including articular cartilage. Focal or diffuse low signal intensity is seen on T1-weighted images in affected areas of marrow involvement. Coronal plane images best display the largest anterior-to-posterior surface area of involvement. The addition of sagittal or axial images provides more accurate assessment of the volume of marrow involvement. On T2*-weighted images, the lunate demonstrates uniform low signal intensity. Normal lunate marrow or recovering marrow vascularity usually displays a central region of mildly increased signal intensity or inhomogeneity on gradient-echo images. Short TI inversion recovery sequences are more sensitive to hyperemia or vascular dilation and demonstrate increased signal intensity restricted to the lunate.

In early KD, T1-weighted images show unaffected marrow with the high signal intensity of fat, isointense with the other carpal bones of the wrist. The distribution of low signal intensity necrosis may be restricted to a portion of the volar or dorsal coronal plane or may demonstrate an eccentric or central region of involvement. Radiocarpal joint effusions, or more localized synovitis, demonstrate bright signal intensity on T2-weighted, T2*-weighted, and STIR sequences.

Interval MR imaging can be used to show the progression of KD or to document healing with the return of normal

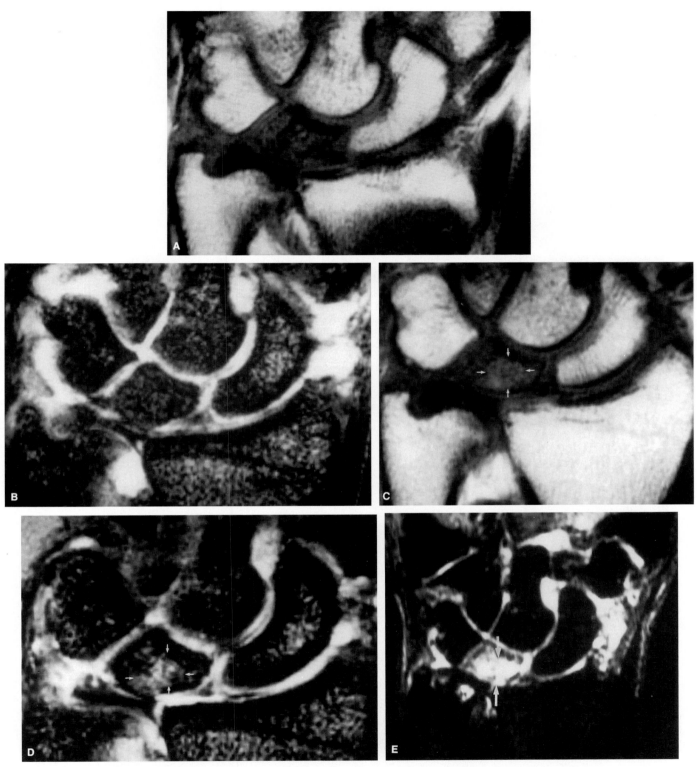

FIGURE 11-98. Stage I Kienböck's disease is treated with cast immobilization. **(A)** Low signal intensity replacement of lunate fatty marrow is seen on a T1-weighted coronal image. **(B)** Uniform low signal intensity lunate marrow is present on the corresponding T2*-weighted coronal image. **(C)** Six months after the initial diagnosis, central fatty marrow signal intensity (*arrows*) is seen on a T1-weighted coronal image. The corresponding T2*-weighted **(D)** and short TI inversion recovery (STIR) **(E)** images show lunate hyperintensity (*arrows*). The STIR image is more sensitive to marrow hyperemia. The increased fatty marrow content of the recovering lunate also contributes to increased signal intensity when using T2*-weighted sequences.

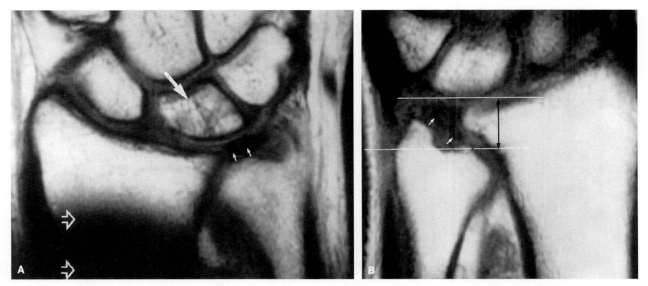

FIGURE 11-99. (A) Recovering fatty marrow signal intensity (*large arrow*) is present after treatment of stage 1 Kienböck's disease of the right wrist. The lunate and triangular fibrocartilage (*small arrows*) is normal. A low signal intensity postoperative artifact secondary to radial shortening is present (*open arrows*). (B) The untreated left wrist shows severe negative ulnar variance (*black double-headed arrow*) and deformed but intact triangular fibrocartilage (*white arrows*). The lunate marrow is unaffected.

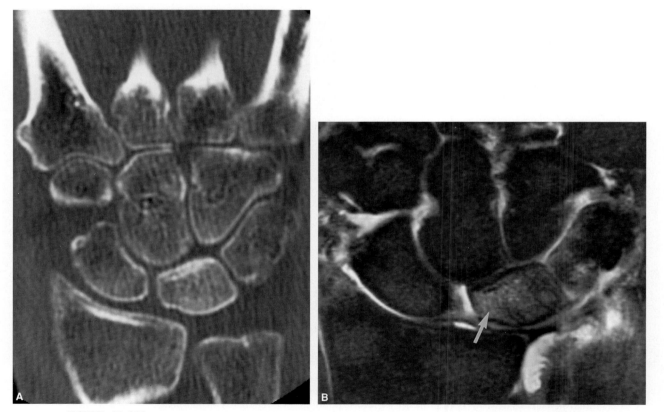

FIGURE 11-100. Stage II Kienböck's disease with (A) increased lunate density (sclerosis) on coronal reformatted CT scan and (B) corresponding marrow hyperintensity on fast STIR coronal image.

marrow signal intensity in stage I disease (see Figs. 11-98 and 11-99). The relative osteopenia of the remaining carpus is not seen using MR techniques. Intravenous gadolinium with fat-suppression displays hyperemic bone with increased signal intensity.

Stage II

In stage II, plain film radiographs show sclerosis of the lunate which corresponds to low signal intensity areas on T1-weighted MR images, areas of viable marrow hyperintensity on short TI inversion recovery images (Fig. 11-100), and low or low to intermediate signal intensity on T2-weighted images. Edema, granulation tissue, and areas of preserved vascularity demonstrate increased or high signal intensity on T2-weighted images. Generally, although morphology and

size are preserved, there is decreased height of the radial aspect of the lunate in late stage II disease (Fig. 11-101).

Stage III

In stage III the lunate undergoes distal-to-proximal collapse in the coronal plane and elongation in the sagittal plane (Fig. 11-102). There is reciprocal proximal migration of the capitate. The absence or presence of SL dissociation with rotatory subluxation of the scaphoid divides patients into stage IIIA and IIIB, respectively. Rotation of the scaphoid may be accompanied by ulnar deviation of the triquetrum. With scaphoid rotation, the inability to see the entire long axis of the scaphoid in a single coronal image is the MR equivalent of the radiographic "ring" sign on conventional

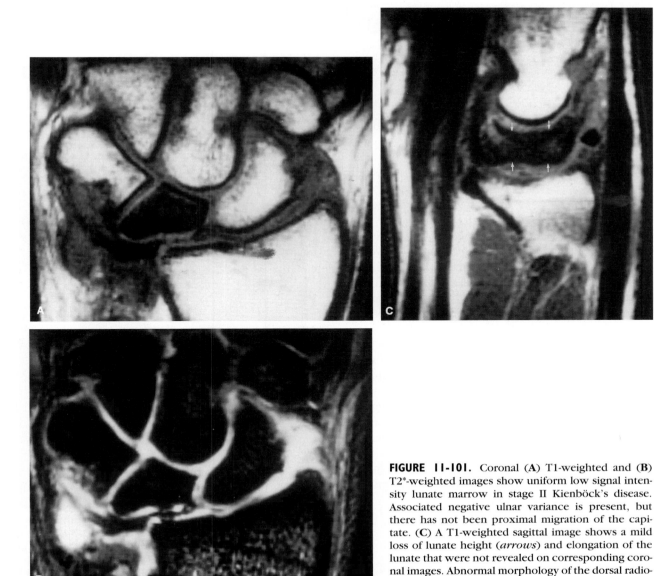

FIGURE 11-101. Coronal **(A)** T1-weighted and **(B)** T2*-weighted images show uniform low signal intensity lunate marrow in stage II Kienböck's disease. Associated negative ulnar variance is present, but there has not been proximal migration of the capitate. **(C)** A T1-weighted sagittal image shows a mild loss of lunate height (*arrows*) and elongation of the lunate that were not revealed on corresponding coronal images. Abnormal morphology of the dorsal radiocarpal ligament is present.

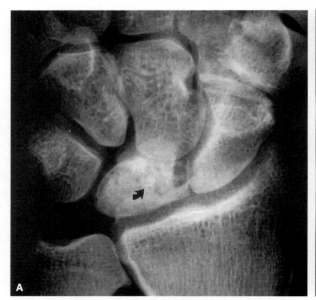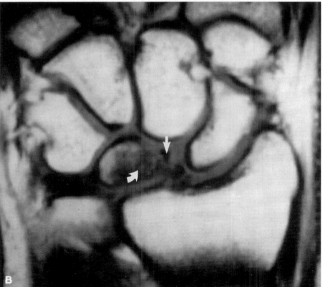

FIGURE 11-102. (A) An anteroposterior radiograph shows lunate collapse (*curved arrow*) and proximal migration of the capitate in stage III Kienböck's disease. (B) A T1-weighted coronal image better depicts necrotic marrow (*curved arrow*) and lunate collapse in the radial border (*straight arrow*).

anteroposterior radiographic projections. Articular cartilage degeneration can be identified in this stage.[127]

Stage IV

Stage IV is characterized by degenerative arthrosis of the lunate and carpus. There are no regions of increased signal intensity on T2*-weighted or STIR images in this advanced stage of the disease, and lunate collapse can be defined in all three orthogonal planes. Splaying of the volar and dorsal poles of the lunate is accompanied by extrinsic effacement and convex bowing of the flexor tendons in the sagittal plane. This may contribute to symptoms of carpal tunnel syndrome, especially if there is associated proximal migration of the flexor retinaculum with wrist shortening. Fragmented portions of the lunate usually demonstrate low signal intensity on T1- and T2*-weighted images. Thin section (1.5 mm) CT scans provide more accurate assessment of cortical fragmentation.

KB may also be associated with Madelung's deformity, a developmental anomaly involving the distal radius and carpus (Fig. 11-103). Synovitis is seen in the advanced stages, characterized by a high signal intensity radiocarpal effusion that often distends synovial recesses. Pannus tissue is low to intermediate in signal intensity on T1- and T2-weighted images and enhances with gadolinium intravenous contrast.

CARPAL TUNNEL SYNDROME

The impairment of motor and/or sensory function of the median nerve as it transgresses the carpal tunnel (ie, carpal

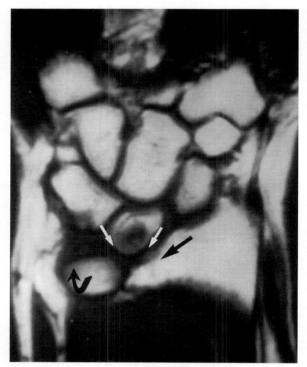

FIGURE 11-103. Madelung's deformity. A T1-weighted coronal image shows the characteristic medial angulation of the distal radial articular surface (*straight black arrow*), dorsal subluxation of the ulna (*curved black arrow*), and triangular configuration of the carpus with the lunate at the apex (*white arrows*). Associated Kienböck's disease is shown as central low signal intensity marrow.

tunnel syndrome) may be caused by fractures and dislocation about the wrist, by intraneural hemorrhage, by infection, by infiltrative disease, and by various soft-tissue injuries. Carpal tunnel syndrome is most often found in patients between 30 and 60 years of age; it has a female-to-male ratio of between 3 to 5:1; and up to 50% of cases are bilateral.[128] The clinical presentation includes pain and numbness with increased nocturnal pain and/or burning. The thumb, index, middle fingers, and radial one half of the ring finger are most commonly affected. Sensory findings range from minimal hypesthesia to complete anesthesia. Muscle atrophy and loss of function are late findings, although the abductor pollicis brevis muscle may show earlier involvement. A positive Tinel's sign (ie, tingling in the digits supplied by the median nerve) indicates nerve entrapment. Phalen's test, tourniquet compression, or direct compression can also be used to elicit signs of medial nerve entrapment. A prolonged sensory conduction or distal motor latency test provide more quantitative information. Electrodiagnostic tests in patients with carpal tunnel syndrome are reported to be 85% to 90% accurate, with a false-negative rate of 10% to 15%.

Related Anatomy

An knowledge of the anatomy of the carpal tunnel is important in understanding the pathophysiology of this syndrome. The carpus has a concave bony contour on its flexor surface and is covered by the flexor retinaculum. The bony carpus thus forms the floor and walls of the carpal tunnel, with the rigid flexor retinaculum as its roof. The flexor retinaculum, or transverse carpal ligament, attaches to the tubercle of the scaphoid, the ridge of the trapezium, and the ulnar aspect of the hook of the hamate and pisiform. The long flexors of the fingers and thumb pass through the carpal tunnel. The separate flexor digitorum superficialis tendons are arranged in two rows, with the tendons to the middle and ring finger volar to the tendons to the index and little finger. The flexor digitorum profundus tendons are arranged in the same coronal plane, and the tendon to the index finger is separated from the adjacent three profundus tendons. All eight flexor tendons are invested in a common synovial sheath. The flexor pollicis longus tendon, invested in its own synovial sheath, is located on the radial aspect of the flexor tendons within the carpal tunnel. The median nerve is deep to the flexor retinaculum and is seen on the lateral side of the flexor digitorum superficialis between the flexor tendon of the middle finger and the flexor carpi radialis. The proximal fibers of the volar carpal ligament contribute to the roof of the carpal tunnel, although this contribution is not as significant as that of the thicker flexor retinaculum.

In dorsiflexion and palmarflexion of the wrist, the median nerve is forced against the transverse carpal ligament. This is compounded by friction forces between the median nerve tendons and the transverse carpal ligament during flexion and extension, with up to 20 mm excursion of the median nerve.

The median nerve is round or oval at the level of the distal radius; it becomes elliptical in shape at the pisiform and hamate. The position and morphology of the median nerve are altered during flexion and extension. With the wrist in a neutral position, the median nerve is seen anterior to the flexor digitorum superficialis tendon of the index finger or posterolaterally between the flexor digitorum tendon of the index finger and flexor pollicis longus tendon. In wrist extension, the median nerve assumes a more anterior position, deep to the flexor retinaculum and superficial to the flexor digitorum superficialis tendon of the index finger. In wrist flexion, the median nerve can be found anterior to the flexor retinaculum or between the flexor digitorum superficialis tendons of the index finger and thumb or middle and ring fingers. In the flexed position, there is flattening of the elliptical shape of the median nerve. Alteration of morphology is less significant in wrist extension.

Etiology

In carpal tunnel syndrome, wick catheter measurements show increased pressures in the carpal canal (ie, 32 mm Hg compared with 2.5 mm Hg in asymptomatic patients).[128] Pressure changes may also be recorded in extremes of dorsiflexion and palmarflexion. CT studies of patients with carpal tunnel syndrome show a decreased cross-sectional area of the carpal canal. Processes that can cause decreased volume or space within the carpal canal include tenosynovitis of the flexor tendons, Colles' fracture, and fracture-dislocation of the carpus and carpometacarpal joints (Fig. 11-104). These processes may also cause posttraumatic scarring, fibrosis, or both, within the carpal tunnel. Inflammatory processes contributing to decreased volume within the carpal tunnel include rheumatoid arthritis, gout, pseudogout, amyloid deposition, and granulomatous infectious processes. All of these can produce a proliferative tenosynovitis with hyperplastic synovium. Tumors of the median nerve (Fig. 11-105) (eg, neurilemomas, fibromas, and hamartomas) as well as tumors extrinsic to the median nerve (eg, ganglia, lipomas, and hemangiomas) produce space-occupying encroachment of the carpal canal.[128,129] Disorders that produce volumetric increase within the carpal tunnel include acromegaly, hypothyroidism, pregnancy, diabetes mellitus, and lupus erythematosus. Volumetric increases are also seen in postmenopausal women. These systemic processes may increase extracapsular fluid retention and produce soft-tissue swelling. Developmental etiologies responsible for carpal tunnel syndrome include a persistent median artery, hypertrophied lumbricals, anomalous muscles, and a distal position of the flexor digitorum superficialis muscle.

The carpal tunnel syndrome can thus be produced by compression or swelling of the median nerve in its synovial

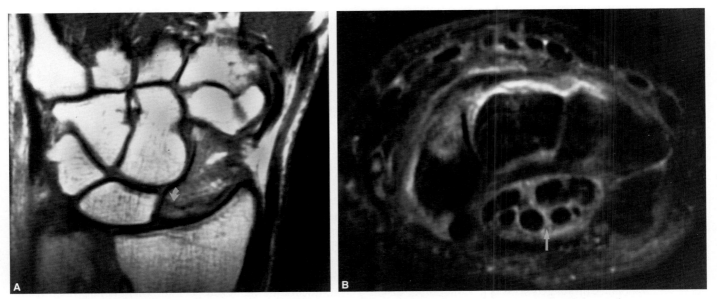

FIGURE 11-104. (A) Scaphoid fracture (*curved arrow*) associated with clinical symptoms of carpal tunnel syndrome (T1-weighted coronal image). (B) Tenosynovitis of the flexor tendons is hyperintense (*straight arrow*) on STIR axial image.

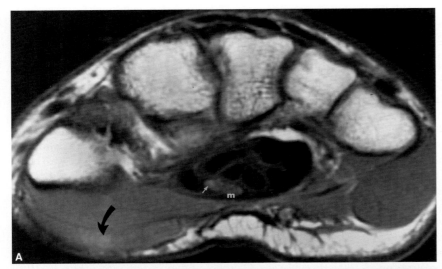

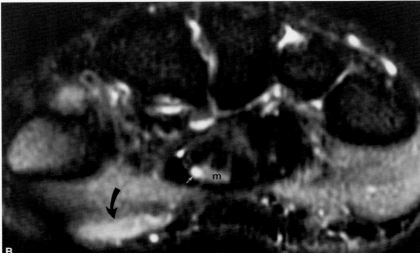

FIGURE 11-105. Neurofibroma (*small straight arrow*) of the motor branch of the median nerve (m) demonstrates intermediate signal intensity on T1-weighted axial image (**A**) and hyperintensity on STIR axial image (**B**). Thenar muscle denervation (*curved arrow*) (corresponding to the affected motor branch of the median nerve) demonstrates increased signal intensity on T1-weighted and STIR axial images. Surgical photograph (**C**) shows the tumor (*arrow*) in situ. D, distal; P, proximal.

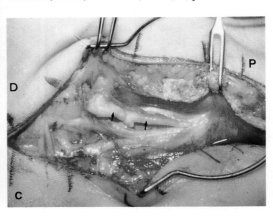

sheath. In the differential diagnosis of carpal tunnel syndrome, it is important to exclude median nerve damage at a more proximal level. In the case of median nerve damage, the palmocutaneous branch of the median nerve may be affected causing weakness of the corresponding flexor muscles of the forearm, including the flexor pollicis longus tendon. This is in contrast to carpal tunnel syndrome, in which the terminal phalanx of the thumb demonstrates normal flexion without motor impairment. Although the median nerve is composed of both sensory and motor nerve fibers, the sensory fibers predominate at the level of the carpal tunnel, explaining the initial findings of sensory deficit with numbness or paresthesias of the thumb, index finger, and middle one half of the ring finger. As the disease progresses, there is wasting and weakness of the thenar muscles, with decreased opposition of the thumb and anesthesia of the three and one half digits on the thumb (radial side) of the hand. There is no anesthesia of the thenar eminence, which is supplied by the cutaneous branch of the median nerve.

Treatment

Initial treatment of carpal tunnel syndrome is conservative and includes splints, NSAIDs, corticosteroids, or a combination of these.[128] Patients who receive the greatest short-term relief with corticosteroid injections have better results with surgical decompression.

Surgical decompression is recommended when there is progressive sensory loss and muscle atrophy plus weakness. The flexor retinaculum, or transverse carpal ligament, is usually divided on its ulnar aspect with complete release. This release may extend proximally into the volar carpal ligament, with an epineurotomy for thickened or scarred epineurium.

Surgical treatment of carpal tunnel syndrome may be complicated by reflex sympathetic dystrophy, scar formation, damage to the branches of the median ulnar nerve, tenosynovitis, flexor tendon adhesions, or bow-stringing of tendons.

Magnetic Resonance Findings

The ability to display the cross-sectional anatomy of the medial nerve and adjacent structures on axial MR images and to trace the flexor tendons on coronal plane images makes MR imaging valuable in characterizing normal anatomy and pathology in the carpal tunnel.[130-134] Early detection of the cause of carpal tunnel syndrome requires soft-tissue discrimination not possible with standard radiographs or CT. Axial and coronal MR imaging of the wrist are useful for evaluating patients with a clinical presentation of median nerve deficits.

In patients with flexor tenosynovitis, axial MR images demonstrate bowing of the flexor retinaculum and the inflamed synovium and tendon sheaths demonstrate low signal intensity on T1-weighted images and increased signal intensity on T2-weighted, T2*-weighted, and STIR sequences (Fig. 11-106).

Regardless of the etiology of carpal tunnel syndrome, the changes in the median nerve are similar[132] (Fig. 11-107). These changes include the following:

- Diffuse swelling or segmental enlargement of the median nerve, best evaluated at the level of the pisiform
- Flattening of the median nerve, best demonstrated at the level of the hamate
- Palmar bowing of the flexor retinaculum, assessed at the level of the hamate[133]
- Increased signal intensity within the median nerve on T2-weighted images (Fig. 11-108).

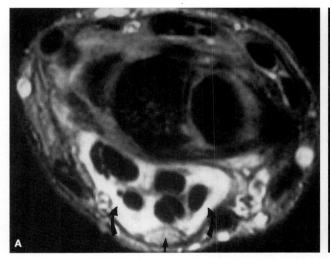 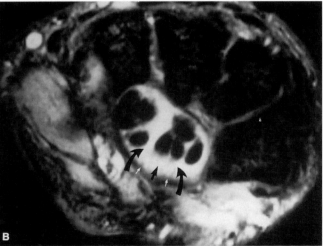

FIGURE 11-106. In carpal tunnel syndrome, T2*-weighted axial images show (**A**) severe, high signal intensity flexor tenosynovitis (*curved arrows*) and swelling of the median nerve proximal to the carpal tunnel (*straight arrow*), and (**B**) hyperintense synovitis (*curved black arrow*) and hyperintense median nerve (*straight black arrow*). The flexor retinaculum is bowed (*white arrows*).

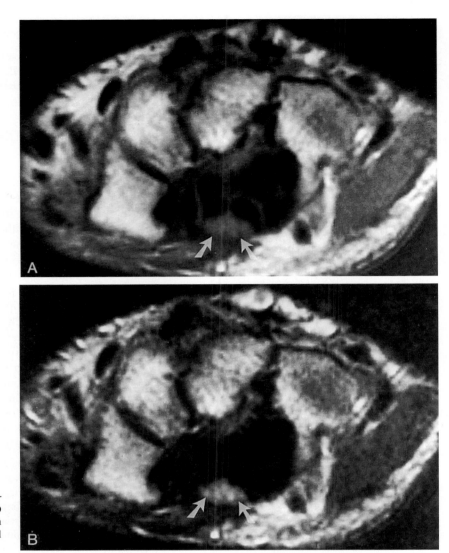

FIGURE 11-107. In carpal tunnel syndrome, an enlarged and edematous median nerve (*arrows*) demonstrates (**A**) intermediate signal intensity on intermediate-weighted images and (**B**) high signal intensity on T2-weighted images.

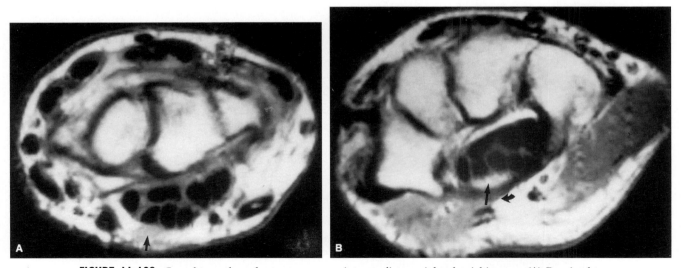

FIGURE 11-108. Carpal tunnel syndrome as seen on intermediate-weighted axial images. (**A**) Proximal to the carpal tunnel, the median nerve demonstrates intermediate signal intensity (*arrow*). (**B**) At the level of the hamate, the median nerve demonstrates high signal intensity (*straight arrow*). Convex bowing of the flexor retinaculum (*curved arrow*) and mild flexor tendon tenosynovitis are also present.

Comparison with the contralateral wrist may be misleading, because involvement is bilateral in one half to two thirds of patients with carpal tunnel syndrome.

Alterations in the median nerve signal intensity are nonspecific, and may represent edema or demyelination within neural fibers. Signal intensity may be decreased when there is fibrosis of the median nerve. Compression and flattening of the median nerve at the level of the hamate may be demonstrated along with bowing of the flexor retinaculum. Ratios of swelling can be calculated by dividing the cross-sectional area of the median nerve at the level of the pisiform and the hamate by the cross-sectional area of the median nerve at the level of the distal radius.[131,132] Significant differences, with doubling of ratios of swelling, have been shown in patients with carpal tunnel syndrome, despite the subjective flattening of the median nerve at the lateral and distal carpus. Ratios of flattening have been used to document statistically significant flattening of the median nerve at the level of the hamate.[132,133] The median nerve may display enlargement or dilation at the level of the pisiform, and compression with flattening at the level of the hook of the hamate.

Increased signal intensity of the median nerve, best demonstrated on axial gradient-echo or STIR images, may be accompanied by an increase in its cross-sectional diameter. Degenerative arthritis and instabilities in advanced arthrosis may cause a decrease in the cross-sectional area of the carpal tunnel and produce symptoms of carpal tunnel disease. Attempts to use MR imaging to measure the diameter of the median nerve, however, require further study. MR imaging is most useful in characterizing space-occupying lesions, whether they be tenosynovitis, ganglia, lipomas, or granulomatous infections (Fig. 11-109).

Enlargement or swelling of the median nerve proximal to the carpal tunnel, referred to as a pseudoneuroma, has also been documented with MR imaging. This condition may actually be associated with constriction of the median nerve within the carpal tunnel, distal to the point of swelling.

Dynamic contrast-enhanced MR imaging can be used to document circulatory disturbance as a cause of carpal tunnel syndrome, separate from deformation or compression of the median nerve.[135] Two abnormal patterns of median nerve enhancement are shown, there is either marked enhancement attributed to nerve edema or lack of enhancement attributed to nerve ischemia. Wrist flexion or extension may alter the pattern from marked enhancement to a lack of enhancement associated with exacerbation of clinical symptoms.

Chronic induration after transverse carpal ligament release is seen on MR scans as an area of neural constriction. Residual hyperintensity of the median nerve within the carpal tunnel may be identified when there is incomplete release of the flexor retinaculum. Release of the transverse carpal ligament from the hook of the hamate may cause the flexor tendons or contents of the carpal canal to demonstrate a volar convexity because of the loss of the normal roof support of the flexor retinaculum. Widening of the fat stripe posterior to the flexor digitorum profundus tendons is a normal postoperative finding. In addition to incomplete release of the flexor retinaculum, MR changes in failed postoperative carpal tunnel surgery include excessive fat within the carpal tunnel, neuromas, and persistent neuritis (Fig. 11-110). Excellent clinical results have been reported for endoscopic carpal tunnel release.[136] However, this procedure may be complicated by ulnar artery and median nerve laceration, partial laceration of the flexor tendons, and fracture of the hook of the hamate.[137] Incomplete release of the transverse carpal ligament may also occur with this technique. MR studies following carpal tunnel release may also demonstrate an increase in carpal canal volume.[138] Carpal tunnel volume increases of up to 24% may be accompanied by a change in shape from a smaller oval to a circular configuration with an increased anteroposterior diameter. A smaller increase in volume was also shown in the mediolateral diameter.

Guyon's Canal

Applications of MR imaging in the evaluation of the ulnar tunnel (or Guyon's canal) are similar to those for the carpal tunnel syndrome.[139] The fibro-osseous ulnar tunnel contains the ulnar nerve and artery and is located in the anteromedial aspect of the wrist (between the pisiform and the hook of the hamate). Anomalous muscles in the canal as well as the diameter of the ulnar nerve (normal mean diameter 3 mm) and the fibromuscular arch at the origin of the flexor digitorum brevis muscle are characterized on axial images. Enlargement of Guyon's canal has been reported following carpal tunnel release.[138] Further study on the usefulness of MR imaging in evaluating patients with ulnar neuropathy is required.

ARTHRITIS

Conventional radiography has been the cornerstone of evaluation and follow-up of arthritides involving the hand, wrist, and elbow. The superior soft-tissue discrimination achieved by MR imaging, however, has proven useful in evaluating patients in both the initial and advanced stages of arthritis. MR imaging achieves noninvasive, accurate delineation of hyaline articular cartilage, ligaments, tendons, and synovium as distinct from cortical bone[140-142] (Fig. 11-111). Alterations in joint morphology or structure can also be identified on MR images before changes can be seen on standard radiographs. Although MR imaging should neither replace radiography nor be used in every patient receiving rheumatologic evaluation, it can, in selected cases, offer specific information that may modify the patient's diagnosis or treatment.

Degenerative Arthritis

Joint space narrowing, loss of articular cartilage, subchondral sclerosis, and cyst formation characterize degenerative

text continues on page 964

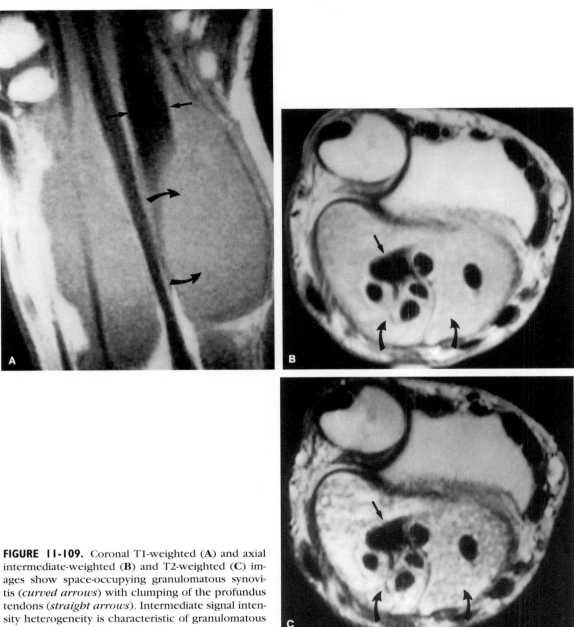

FIGURE 11-109. Coronal T1-weighted (**A**) and axial intermediate-weighted (**B**) and T2-weighted (**C**) images show space-occupying granulomatous synovitis (*curved arrows*) with clumping of the profundus tendons (*straight arrows*). Intermediate signal intensity heterogeneity is characteristic of granulomatous processes in carpal tunnel syndrome.

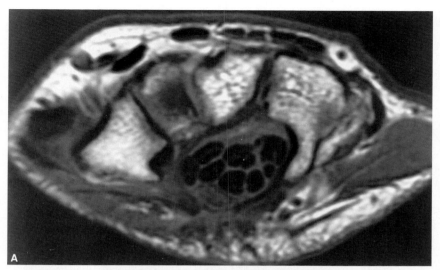

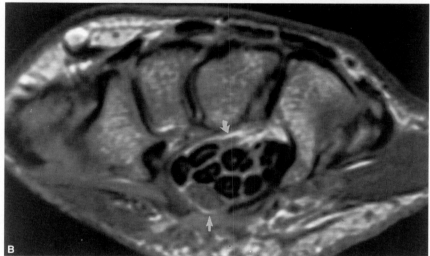

FIGURE 11-110. Persistent symptoms of carpal tunnel syndrome after endoscopic release of the flexor retinaculum. A thin hypointense band (*straight arrow*) is seen overlying the enlarged median nerve on T1-weighted (**A**) and intravenous gadolinium enhanced T1-weighted (**B**) axial images. These findings are consistent with an incomplete release of the flexor retinaculum. Enhancing synovitis is also shown deep to the profundus tendons (*curved arrow*).

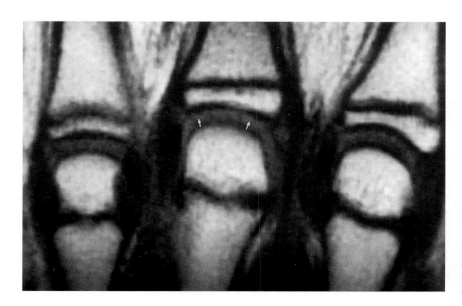

FIGURE 11-111. A T1-weighted coronal image shows the intermediate signal intensity of normal thickness metacarpophalangeal joint hyaline articular cartilage (*arrows*).

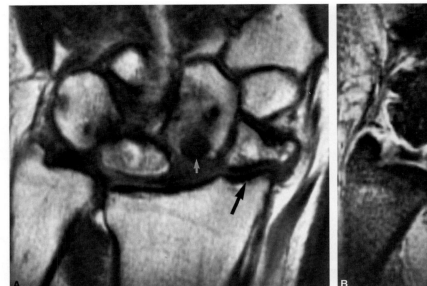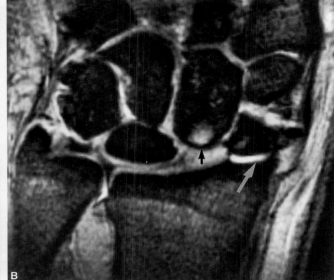

FIGURE 11-112. Scapholunate advanced collapse seen on T1-weighted (**A**) and T2*-weighted (**B**) coronal images. MR findings include rotatory subluxation of the scaphoid, degenerative proximal scaphoradial arthritis (*large arrow*) with loss of articular cartilage, scaphoid collapse, proximal migration of the capitate through the scapholunate interosseous interval, and subchondral cystic change of the proximal capitate (*small arrow*) (a function of an increasing load at the capitolunate joint). Note that the capitate is no longer in contact with the distal radial surface of the lunate and the radiolunate joint is unaffected.

patterns of the carpus (Fig. 11-112). The SLAC wrist develops from incongruent loading and degeneration across the radioscaphoid articulation, related to malalignment of the scaphoid.[143] The SLAC wrist represents the most common form of degenerative arthritis, and is associated with the gradual collapse and loss of ligamentous support. SLAC degeneration may occur with carpal collapse, including that caused by scaphoid nonunion and KD. The earliest changes seen in the SLAC wrist involve spiking at the junction of the articular and nonarticular surfaces on the radial side of the scaphoid, sharpening at the radial styloid tip, and loss of cartilage. Early cartilage loss can be seen clearly on MR scans, and the low signal intensity initial changes in subchondral sclerosis of the radial styloid appear on MR images prior to any visible changes on conventional radiographs (Fig. 11-113). Later in the disease, there is narrowing of the radioscaphoid joint, and the capitolunate joint begins to degenerate. Once the articular space between the capitate and lunate is lost, the hamate impinges against the lunate and degeneration also occurs at this site.

Triscaphe arthritis is the second most frequent form of degenerative arthritis and involves the scaphoid, trapezius and trapezoid articulation.[143] Isolated scaphotrapezial involvement is more common than isolated scaphotrapezoidal involvement. A SLAC wrist may occur in combination with triscaphe degenerative arthritis. Other locations of degenerative arthritis include the area between the distal ulna and the lunate and the LT joints.[143]

Rheumatoid Arthritis

Involvement of the wrist in rheumatoid arthritis characteristically involves the carpus and the MP and PIP joints.[144] Soft-tissue swelling may be caused by joint effusion, edema, and tenosynovitis (Fig. 11-114). Swan-neck and boutonniere deformities are frequent, and, in advanced disease, there are subluxations, dislocations, ulnar deviation in the MP joints, and radial deviation in the radiocarpal articulation. Destructive changes include "main en lorgnette" (ie, telescoping of the fingers), ulnar erosions, SL dissociation, and DRUJ incongruity.

Gadolinium contrast MR imaging can be used to selectively enhance pannus tissue in synovitis involving the DRUJ; the ulnar styloid process; the radiocarpal, intercarpal, and MP joints; and the flexor and extensor tendons.[145] When periarticular enhancement on MR imaging of the wrist or MP and PIP joints of the hand was used as a criterion for the diagnosis of early stage rheumatoid arthritis, sensitivity was 100%, specificity 73%, and accuracy 89%.[146] Coronal fat-suppressed gadolinium-enhanced T1-weighted images of the wrist and hand can be used to evaluate periarticular synovial inflammation as well as subchondral bone marrow edema. Synovial involvement of ligamentous structures frequently affects the ulnolunate and ulnotriquetral ligaments, the TFCC, the DRUJ, the ulnocarpal meniscal homologue, the ulnar collateral ligament, the RSC ligament, the RSL, the LRL, and the SRL.[147] The differential diagnosis of rupture

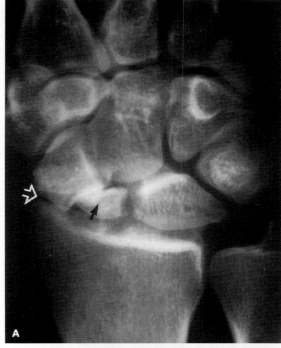

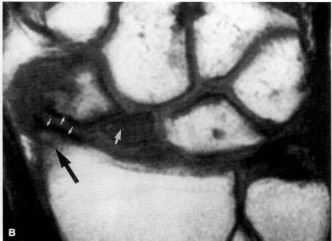

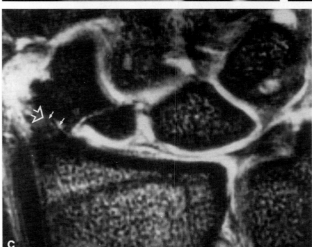

FIGURE 11-113. Scapholunate advanced collapse (SLAC) wrist. (**A**) An anteroposterior radiograph shows nonunion of a scaphoid fracture with degenerative joint-space narrowing between the distal pole of the scaphoid and radius (*open arrow*). There is sclerosis and avascular necrosis (AVN) of the proximal pole (*solid arrow*). Coronal (**B**) T1-weighted and (**C**) T2*-weighted images of SLAC wrist reveal degeneration at the radioscaphoid joint (*open arrow*) and subchondral low signal intensity sclerosis in the radiostyloscaphoid area. Denuded articular cartilage (*small white arrows*) extends proximally only to the level of the nonunion. The proximal pole of the scaphoid functions as a second lunate with preserved articular cartilage. (**B**) Note the low signal intensity "corner sign" of the radial styloid, which is characteristic of early SLAC degeneration (*large black arrow*). AVN of the proximal pole is indicated (*large white arrow*). Increased loading of the capitolunate joint is associated with loss of radioscaphoid cartilage.

of the extensor tendon at the wrist includes MP synovitis, posterior interosseous nerve palsy from rheumatoid disease of the elbow, and extensor tendon pathology overlying the metacarpal heads. With MR imaging, it is possible to identify rupture of the extensor pollicis longus tendon, which may be difficult to assess clinically if the function of the thumb is intact.[147] MR imaging also allows identification of pannus involving the dorsal tendon sheaths and extensor tendons and effusion of the six extensor tendon compartments.[148] TFC tears, dorsal displacement of the ulna, carpal tunnel pathology, and SL dissociation are also assessed on routine coronal, axial, and sagittal studies (Fig. 11-115).

In patients with chronic rheumatoid disease, both plain film radiography and MR studies document the subluxations and erosions affecting the phalanges, carpals, metacarpals, and ulnar styloid. The changes are more pronounced on MR images. Both T1 and T2 tissue relaxation times are prolonged in acute inflammation with edema and in joint effusion; therefore, both conditions demonstrate low signal intensity on T1-weighted images and high signal intensity on T2-weighted images. Inflammatory edema may also extend into the subcutaneous tissues. In contrast, chronically inflamed tissue remains low in signal intensity on both T1- and T2-weighted images. Adjacent areas of fluid collection demonstrate increased signal intensity on T2-weighted acquisitions. Although the signal intensity of localized edematous or inflammatory tissue may be similar to that of synovial fluid,

text continues on page 968

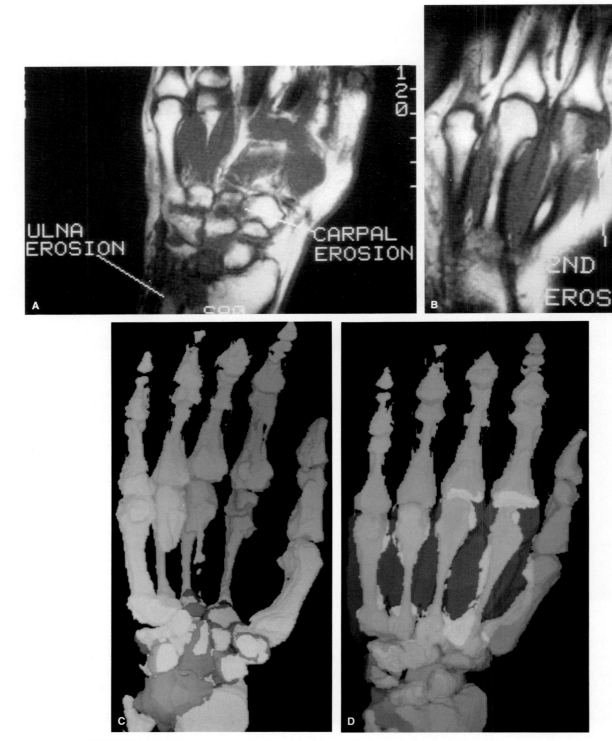

FIGURE 11-114. Rheumatoid arthritis. **(A,B)** T1-weighted coronal images identify rheumatoid erosions of **(A)** the ulnar styloid and carpus and **(B)** the second metacarpal. **(C,D)** The corresponding 3D MR renderings map out pannus formation (*pink*) and inferior distal radioulnar joint effusion (*blue*). The interosseous muscles are shown between the metacarpal bones. **(E)** Unenhanced and **(F)** enhanced T1-weighted coronal images in a different patient demonstrate the application of intravenous gadolinium used to selectively enhance and differentiate pannus from fluid in severe radiocarpal disease. F, low signal intensity fluid; S, enhanced hyperintense synovium. *continued*

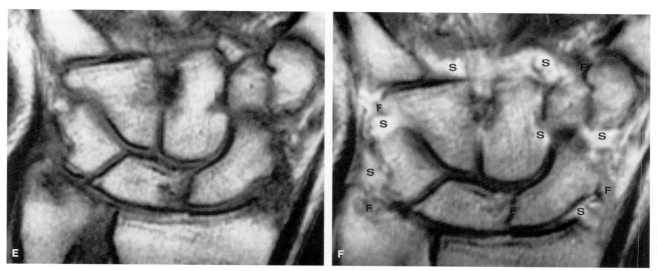

FIGURE 11-114. *Continued.*

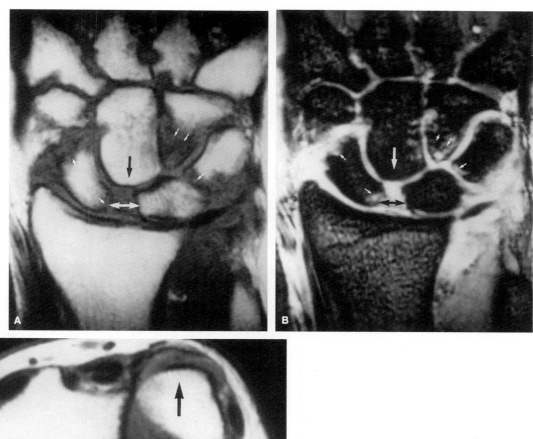

FIGURE 11-115. Rheumatoid arthritis. Coronal **(A)** T1-weighted and **(B)** T2*-weighted images show rheumatoid changes of scapholunate dissociation (*double-headed arrows*), proximal migration of the capitate (*large single arrow*), and multiple erosions involving the scaphoid, triquetrum, and hamate (*small white arrows*). Erosions of the intermetacarpal joints are also present. Note that the carpus has begun to migrate toward the ulna, and the distance between the radial styloid and the scaphoid is increased. **(C)** An axial T1-weighted image shows dorsal subluxation of the ulna (*straight arrow*) and distal radioulnar joint effusion and pannus (*curved arrow*).

noninflammatory effusions in the wrist do not, when imaged on T2-weighted sequences, display an irregular pattern or focal distribution at multiple sites.

Cystic carpal erosions are better delineated on MR images than on corresponding anteroposterior radiographs. Destruction of cartilage and joint arthrosis is seen on T1- and T2-weighted images. Fat-suppressed T2-weighted FSE techniques are more useful in showing changes of articular cartilage involvement. Marrow changes (eg, subchondral sclerosis), present on both sides of the joint or carpal articulation, help to differentiate arthrosis from intramedullary edema.

In patients with juvenile rheumatoid arthritis with wrist involvement, early fluid collections along tendon sheaths, subarticular erosions, and cysts, as well as attenuated intercarpal articular cartilage, can be detected on MR images even when conventional radiographs are normal. Subluxations and areas of bone destruction are equally evident on MR images and on plain film radiographs.

MR imaging has the potential to become an important adjunct in diagnosing and monitoring patients with rheumatoid disease. However, additional studies with large patient populations and comparison with conventional radiographic studies are required before standard indications can be implemented in rheumatoid patients. MR imaging may also prove to be valuable in monitoring a patient's response to drug therapy, including remitative agents such as methotrexate or gold in juvenile and adult rheumatoid disease.

Miscellaneous Arthritides

In evaluating nonrheumatoid arthritic disease, we have had the opportunity to evaluate patients with psoriatic arthritis, Lyme disease, intraosseous sarcoid, hemophilia, calcium pyrophosphate deposition disease (CPPD), and the more commonly found osteoarthritis (Fig. 11-116). Wrist involvement in less common in primary osteoarthritis and secondary degenerative arthritis of the wrist in commonly seen in association with old trauma.

In psoriatic arthritis, MR studies demonstrate destruction of the TFC with pancompartmental joint-space narrowing, erosions, SL ligament disruption, and subchondral low signal intensity sclerosis in the carpus (Fig. 11-117). Synovitis of the flexor carpi radialis tendon, the inferior radioulnar compartment, intermediate signal intensity inflammatory tissue, and dorsal subluxation of the distal ulna can be identified on T1- and T2-weighted axial images. In addition, the integrity of an artificial silastic interphalangeal joint replacement (seen as an area of low signal intensity without artifact) can be assessed on coronal images. The site of fusion of the interphalangeal articulation of the thumb may be degraded by residual metallic artifact, despite prior surgical removal of fixation pins. In diffuse soft-tissue swelling of a single digit secondary to psoriatic arthritis, MR imaging may be successful in excluding the diagnosis of osteomyelitis (Fig. 11-118).

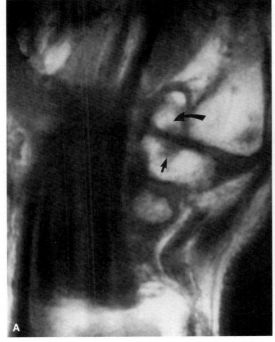
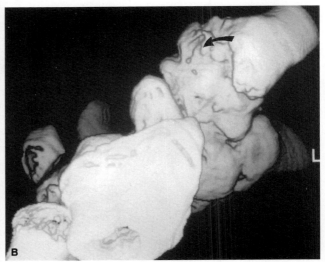

FIGURE 11-116. (A) T1-weighted coronal image and (B) 3D CT image illustrate degenerative osteophytosis of the first carpal metacarpal joint (*curved arrow*) in a patient with osteoarthritis. Low signal intensity subchondral sclerosis of the trapezium is indicated (*straight arrow*).

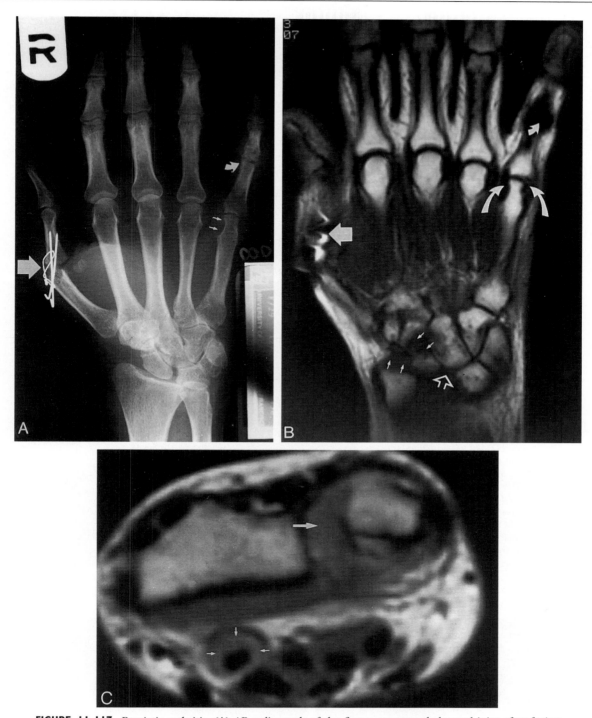

FIGURE 11-117. Psoriatic arthritis. **(A)** AP radiograph of the first metacarpophalangeal joint after fusion for subluxation (*large straight arrow*). Erosion of the fifth metacarpal head (*small straight arrows*) and a proximal interphalangeal joint silastic implant (*curved arrow*) are shown. Diffuse carpal joint-space narrowing is evident. **(B)** The corresponding T1-weighted coronal image shows a first metacarpophalangeal metallic artifact (*large straight solid arrow*), a low signal intensity silastic joint implant (*small curved arrow*), proximal interphalangeal joint erosions and fibrous tissue (*large curved arrow*), scapholunate dissociation (*open arrow*), and subchondral sclerosis of the scaphoid (*small arrows*). **(C)** On axial images, tenosynovitis of a flexor tendon (*small arrows*) and fluid collecting in the radioulnar space (*large arrow*) demonstrate low signal intensity on a T1-weighted image.   *continued*

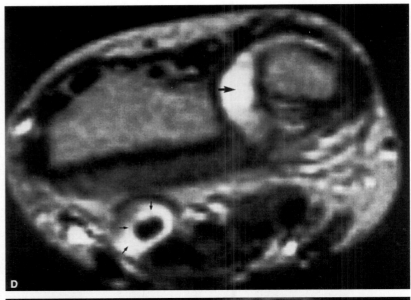

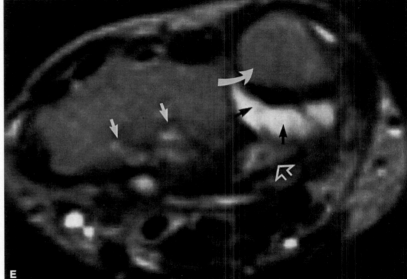

FIGURE 11-117. *Continued.* (D) On axial images, teno-synovitis of a flexor tendon (*small arrows*) and fluid collecting in the radioulnar space (*large arrow*) demonstrate high signal intensity on a T2-weighted image. (E) A distal axial T2-weighted image of the wrist shows dorsal ulnar subluxation (*curved arrow*) with associated joint effusion (*straight solid black arrows*) and intermediate signal intensity synovial hypertrophy (*open arrow*). Erosions of the distal radius are identified (*straight solid white arrows*).

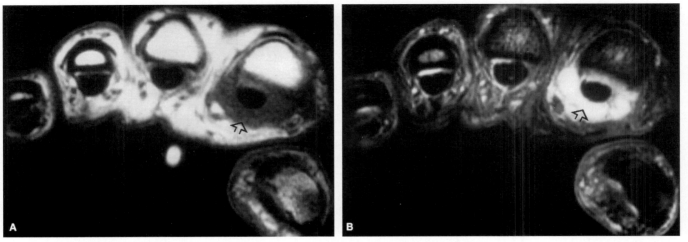

FIGURE 11-118. Psoriatic arthritis. (A) Axial T1-weighted and (B) T2*-weighted images.

continued

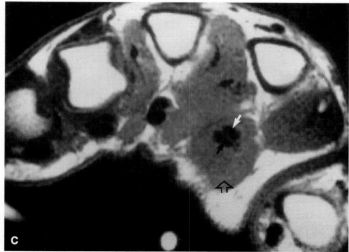

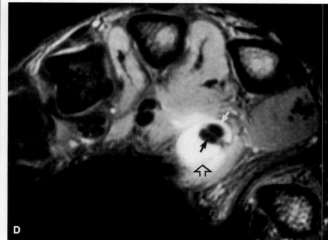

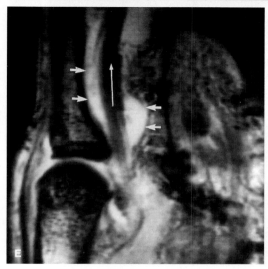

FIGURE 11-118. *Continued.* (**C**) T1-weighted, and (**D**) T2*-weighted images show tenosynovitis (*open arrows*) of the flexor digitorum superficialis (*black arrows*) and profundus (*white arrows*) tendons involving the entire second digit (ie, sausage digit). (**E**) A T2*-weighted sagittal image shows the longitudinal extent of the hyperintense tenosynovitis (*short arrows*) encasing the flexor tendons (*long arrow*) at the level of the distal metacarpal and proximal phalanx.

MR imaging studies in Lyme disease arthritis of the wrist reveal information not available on conventional radiographs. Pockets of fluid collection, characterized by high signal intensity on T2-weighted images, can be detected, as can the scalloped contour of a fluid interface adjacent to inflamed synovium (Fig. 11-119). Joint deformities or cartilaginous erosions are not usually detected.

The hand is a predominant site of involvement in patients who have the relatively rare disorder of skeletal sarcoidosis. In one case we studied, conventional radiographs demonstrated lytic changes characteristic of sarcoid in both the middle and distal phalanges. Although MR images did not provide any additional diagnostic information, the extent of soft-tissue granulomatous proliferation in the cystic defects and areas of cortical destruction were more accurately demonstrated on coronal and axial MR images (Figs. 11-120 and 11-121). The noncaseating, granulomatous tissue typical of sarcoidosis demonstrates low to intermediate signal intensity on T1-weighted sequences and high signal intensity on T2-weighted images.

In hemophilia, acute hemorrhage into soft tissue may produce a fluid-fluid level. Higher signal intensity serum layers above hemorrhagic sediment. More subacute or chronic hemorrhage demonstrates hemosiderin (ie, dark) signal intensity on T1-, T2-, or T2*-weighted images.

Intraosseous cysts (ganglia) of the wrist are hypointense on T1-weighted images and hyperintense on T2- or T2*-weighted or STIR sequences (Fig. 11-122). These cysts, composed of fibrous tissue and mucoid material, are usually asymptomatic and present in a subchondral location.[149]

We have studied several patients with CPPD. The areas of intraarticular calcification are not satisfactorily demonstrated on T1-weighted images, when compared with high-quality magnification radiographs. T2 and T2* weighting and photography at high contrast settings may prove useful in identifying areas of calcified crystalline depositions. The MR changes in CPPD arthropathy include marrow hyperemia, widening of the SL interval, proximal migration of the capitate, and joint space narrowing in the radiocarpal and MP joints (Fig. 11-123). There is trapezioscaphoid

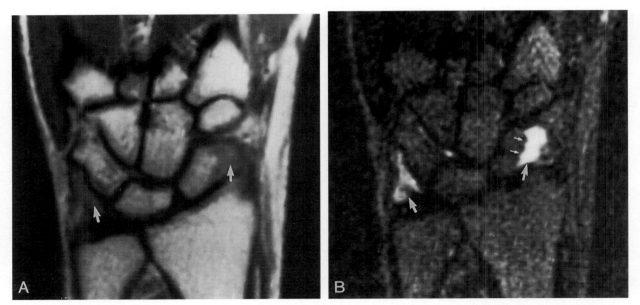

FIGURE 11-119. Synovitis of the wrist with focal fluid pockets (*large arrows*) demonstrates (**A**) low signal intensity on a T1-weighted coronal image and (**B**) high signal intensity on a T2-weighted coronal image. The irregular or corrugated contour of the fluid represents contact with inflamed synovium (*small arrows*).

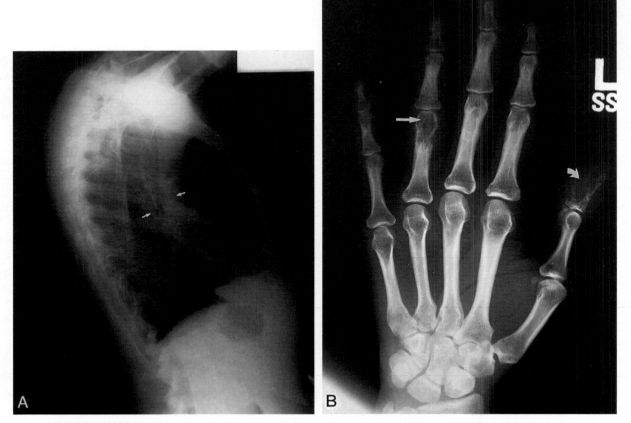

FIGURE 11-120. Skeletal sarcoid. (**A**) A lateral chest radiograph shows hilar lymphadenopathy (*arrows*). (**B**) An anteroposterior radiograph shows lytic lesions of the sarcoid in the proximal phalanx of the fourth digit (*straight arrow*) and the distal phalanx of the thumb (*curved arrow*). continued

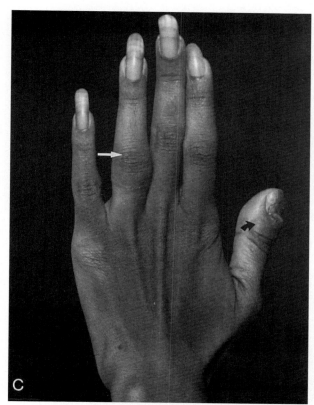

FIGURE 11-120. *Continued.* **(C)** A gross photograph shows soft-tissue swelling of the fourth proximal interphalangeal joint (*straight arrow*). Characteristic nail changes and swelling are seen in the thumb (*curved arrow*).

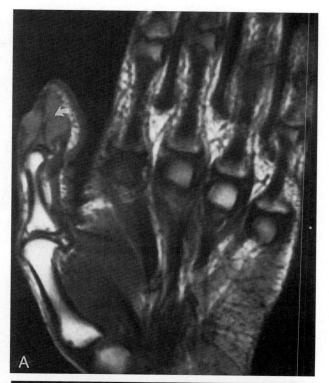

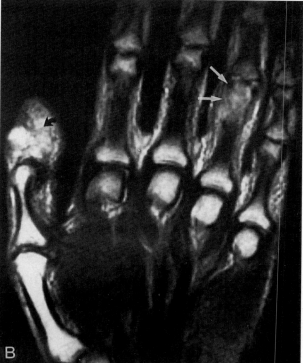

FIGURE 11-121. Skeletal sarcoid. **(A)** A T1-weighted coronal image shows an intermediate signal intensity soft-tissue mass (*curved arrow*) and cortical destruction. **(B)** A T2-weighted coronal image shows high signal intensity granulomatous tissue in the distal phalanx of the thumb (*curved arrow*) and proximal phalanx of the ring finger (*straight arrows*).

involvement, with sparing of the DRUJ.[150] Calcium pyrophosphate deposition may also occur in the TFCC and interosseous ligament. Crystal deposition in ligaments can lead to their rupture. Thus, degenerative changes and SLAC wrist deformity can be seen in CPPD.

The palmar involvement in Dupuytren's contracture has also been defined on MR imaging.[151] Dupuytren's contracture is a fibrosing condition of the hand frequently resulting in progressive flexion contractures of the fingers. Lesions include subcutaneous nodules at the level of the distal palmar crease and cords parallel and superficial to the flexor tendons. These cords demonstrate low to intermediate signal intensity on T1-weighted images and low signal intensity on T2-weighted images. The cords are composed of hypocellular dense collagen. Subcutaneous nodules demonstrate an inhomogeneous intermediate signal intensity on T1- and T2-weighted images. Less common hypocellular nodules demonstrate low signal intensity on both T1- and T2-weighted images.

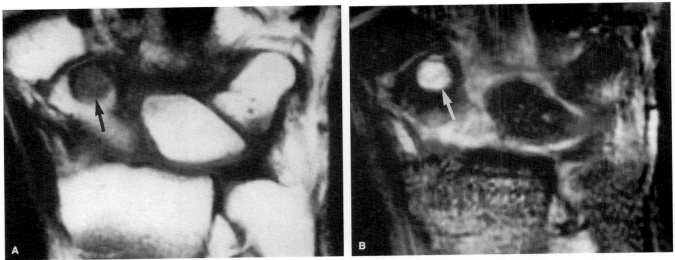

FIGURE 11-122. An intraosseous cyst (*arrows*) of the distal pole of the scaphoid demonstrates (**A**) low signal intensity on a coronal T1-weighted image and (**B**) high signal intensity on a T2*-weighted image.

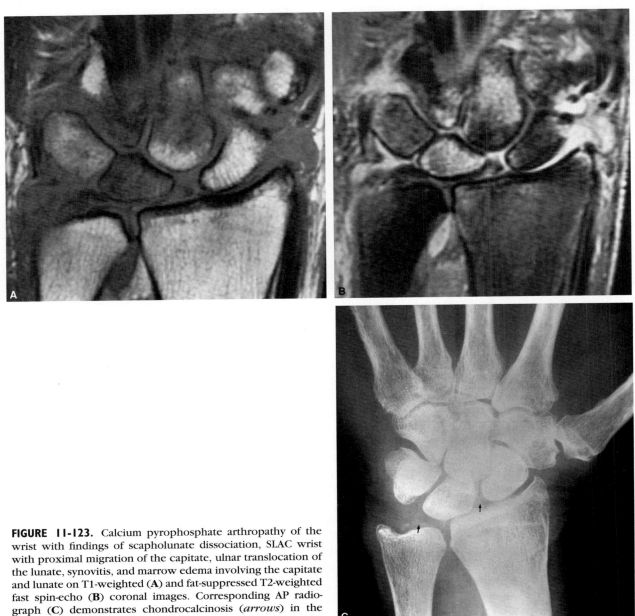

FIGURE 11-123. Calcium pyrophosphate arthropathy of the wrist with findings of scapholunate dissociation, SLAC wrist with proximal migration of the capitate, ulnar translocation of the lunate, synovitis, and marrow edema involving the capitate and lunate on T1-weighted (**A**) and fat-suppressed T2-weighted fast spin-echo (**B**) coronal images. Corresponding AP radiograph (**C**) demonstrates chondrocalcinosis (*arrows*) in the TFCC and scapholunate ligament.

MISCELLANEOUS ABNORMALITIES OF THE WRIST AND HAND

In addition to changes seen in arthritis, other abnormalities including ganglia, tenosynovitis, tendon rupture, and changes of muscle denervation have been characterized on MR images of the hand, wrist, and elbow.

Ganglion Cysts and Giant Cell Tumor of the Tendon Sheath

Cystic swellings overlying a joint or tendon sheath are referred to as ganglia and are thought to be secondary to protrusions of encapsulated synovial tissue[152–154] (Fig. 11-124). On MR images, ganglion cysts generate low signal intensity on T1-weighted images and high signal intensity on T2-weighted images. Fibrous septations may cause loculation of the ganglion. Even with infiltration or edema of adjacent tissues, these lesions are well-demarcated on MR imaging. Intercarpal communication of a ganglion is more frequent than communication with the radiocarpal joint.

MR imaging is used to identify the joint or tendon of origin and to exclude other soft-tissue masses, such as neoplasms, when an accurate preoperative clinical assessment is difficult and wrist arthrography is not satisfactory (Figs. 11-125 through 11-127). Wrist ganglions may be associated with the first carpometacarpal joint, the STT joint, the volar or dorsal wrist capsule, or the flexor carpi radialis tendon (Fig. 11-128). The stalk of the ganglion frequently can be discerned on MR images. Dorsal carpal ganglia including the occult dorsal carpal ganglion are effectively evaluated by MR imaging.[155] MR imaging may show an origin from the dorsal SL ligament.

Pigmented villonodular synovitis of the tendon (ie, giant cell tumor of the tendon sheath) presents as an extraarticular soft-tissue swelling, which may be mistaken for a ganglion.

text continues on page 980

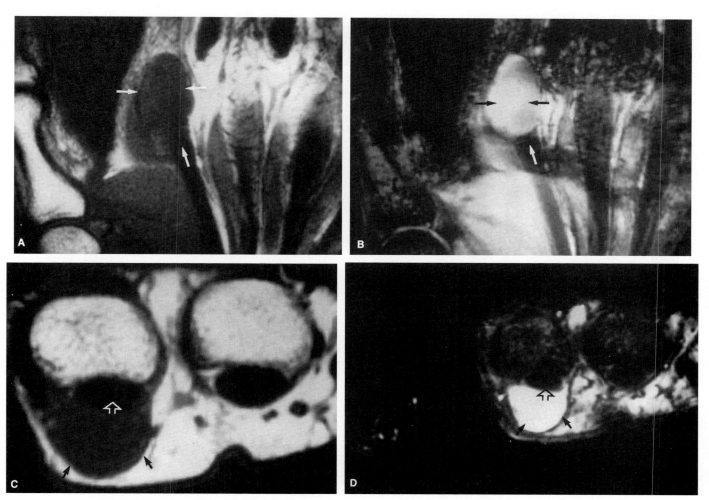

FIGURE 11-124. Coronal (**A**) T1-weighted and (**B**) T2*-weighted images and axial (**C**) T1-weighted and (**D**) T2*-weighted images show a viscous, cystic, synovial fluid-filled volar ganglion (*solid arrows*) of the second digit flexor tendons (*open arrows*).

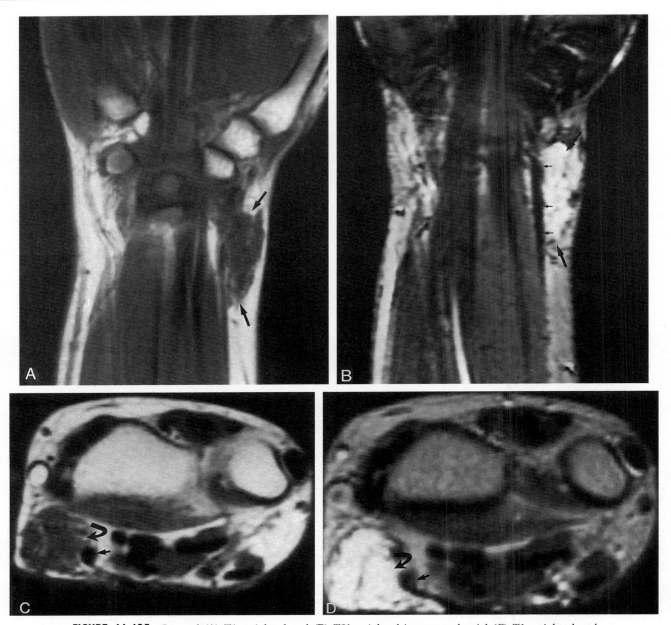

FIGURE 11-125. Coronal (**A**) T1-weighted and (**B**) T2*-weighted images and axial (**C**) T1-weighted and (**D**) T2-weighted images show a synovial ganglion (*large arrows*) associated with the flexor carpi radialis tendon (*small arrows*). The relationship of the cyst (*curved arrows*) to the flexor tendon (*short arrows*) is shown in the axial plane. Mucinous synovial contents demonstrate low signal intensity on T1-weighted images and high signal intensity on T2-weighted images.

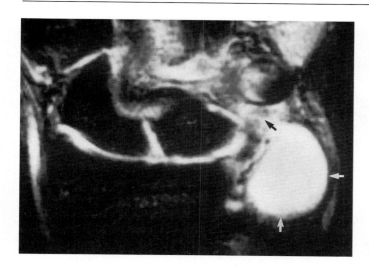

FIGURE 11-126. A large cystic ganglion (*white arrows*) projects from the ulnar aspect of a torn triangular fibrocartilage (*black arrow*).

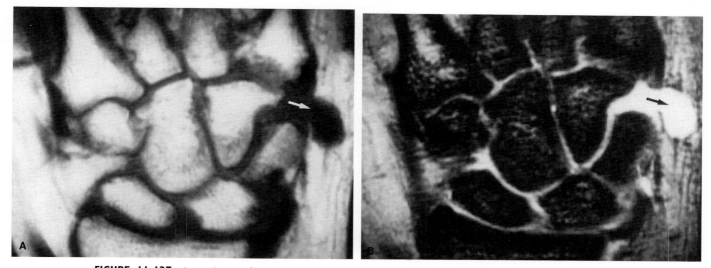

FIGURE 11-127. A cystic ganglion (*arrows*) communicates with the hamate triquetral joint. The lesion demonstrates (**A**) low signal intensity on a T1-weighted coronal image and (**B**) hyperintensity on a T2*-weighted coronal image.

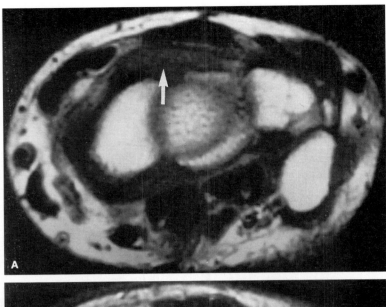

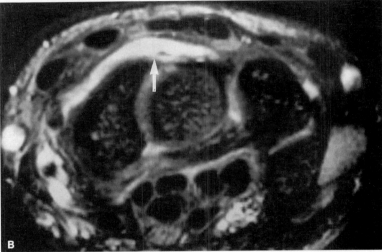

FIGURE 11-128. A dorsal ganglion (*arrows*) projects over the scaphoid and capitate. The lesion demonstrates (**A**) uniform low signal intensity on an axial T1-weighted image and (**B**) high signal intensity on an axial T2*-weighted image.

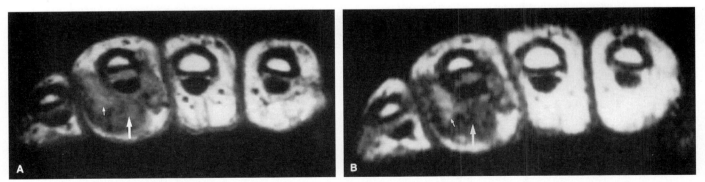

FIGURE 11-129. A giant cell tumor of the tendon sheath (ie, extraarticular pigmented villonodular synovitis; *large arrows*) demonstrates low signal intensity on axial (**A**) intermediate-weighted and (**B**) T2-weighted images. Minimal fluid signal intensity (*short arrows*) is seen.

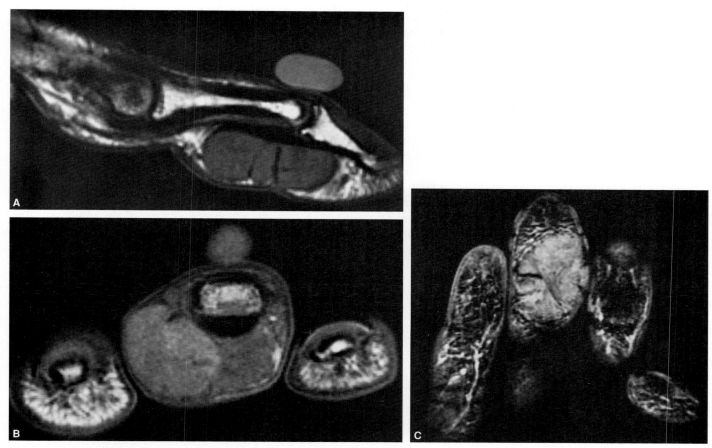

FIGURE 11-130. Giant cell tumor of the flexor tendon sheath is low to intermediate in signal intensity on T1-weighted sagittal (**A**) and axial (**B**) images. On volar T2*-weighted coronal images through the phalanges, however, it demonstrates mild hyperintensity. T2*-weighted sequences are also sensitive to the susceptibility effect of hemosiderin, seen as hypointense foci.

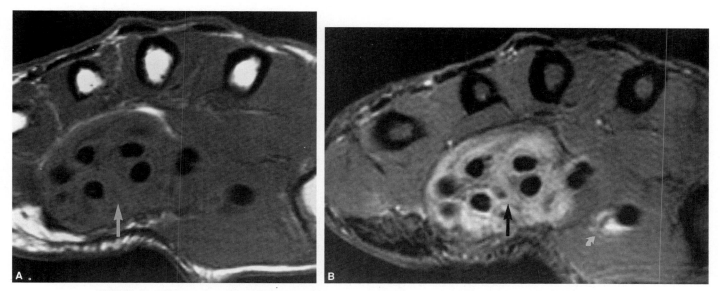

FIGURE 11-131. Tenosynovitis (*straight arrow*) is hypointense on T1-weighted (**A**) and hyperintense on fat-suppressed T2-weighted (**B**) axial images of the profundus and superficialis flexor tendons. Hyperintense inflammation spreads along both the midpalmar and thenar spaces deep to the tendons. Tenosynovitis also targets the flexor pollicis longus tendon in radial bursa (*curved arrow* on image **B**).

Low to intermediate signal intensity on T1- and T2-weighted images is characteristic (Fig. 11-129). Higher signal intensity may be seen on T2*-weighted images (Fig. 11-130).

Tenosynovitis, Tendon Rupture, and Muscle Denervation

Tenosynovitis and capsular synovitis may occur together as part of the spectrum of rheumatoid disease, or they may exist as isolated conditions with a traumatic or infectious etiology (Fig. 11-131). Thickening, swelling, or fluid associated with an irritated synovial tendon sheath may be demonstrated on MR images. An edematous sheath appears as a rim of increased signal intensity on T2-weighted images.

Both flexor and extensor tenosynovitis may occur without a history of infection. Carpal distention may be evident in the small interphalangeal or metacarpal joints when small amounts of synovial fluid accumulate.

The flexor carpi radialis musculotendinous unit can be evaluated on MR imaging. Proximal to the radiocarpal joint, the average length of the flexor carpi radialis musculotendinous unit is 15 cm; proximal to the radial styloid the average tendon length is 8 cm. The flexor carpi radialis tendon occupies a fibro-osseous tunnel at the proximal border of the trapezium[156,157] (Fig. 11-132). A thick septum separates the flexor carpi radialis from the carpal tunnel. The tendon occupies 90% of the space within its tunnel and is in direct contact with the roughened surface of the trapezium. The tendon is in immediate proximity to the distal radius, the

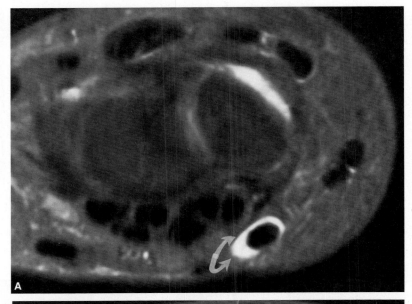

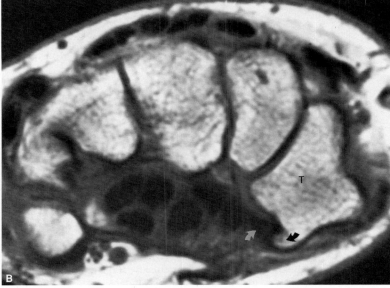

FIGURE 11-132. (**A**) Flexor carpi radialis tenosynovitis (*arrows*) is hyperintense on a fat-suppressed T2-weighted fast spin-echo axial image at the level of the proximal carpal row. (**B**) The vulnerable area of fibro-osseous tunnel narrowing (*white arrow*) occurs beneath the prominent trapezial crest (*black arrow*). Since the tendon sheath forming the rigid fibro-osseous canal narrows and ends at the level of the trapezium (T), MR findings of tendinitis or tenosynovitis are seen proximal to this location.

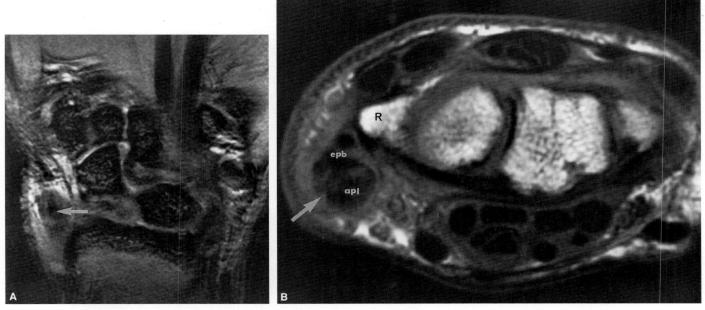

FIGURE 11-133. De Quervain's stenosing tenosynovitis (*arrow*) with inflammation of the abductor pollicis longus (apl) and extensor pollicis brevis (epb) tendons of the first extensor compartment. Inflammation is associated with these enlarged tendons in the fibro-osseous tunnel at the level of the radial styloid (R). Increased signal intensity in the tendon sheath (tenosynovitis) and tendon (tendinitis) coexist in this case. (**A**) T2*-weighted coronal image.(**B**) T1-weighted axial image.

scaphoid tubercle, the STT joint and the carpometacarpal joint of the thumb. This tendon is potentially vulnerable to primary stenosing tenosynovitis and secondary injury with tendinitis associated with distal scaphoid fracture, STT arthritis, and carpometacarpal joint arthritis. Trauma or degeneration of the tendon within the constrained tunnel may be

the predisposing event in the development of flexor carpi radialis tendinitis.

De Quervain's disease is tenosynovitis of the first dorsal compartment affecting the APL and EPB tendons (Fig. 11-133). The APL and EPB tendons are susceptible to tendinitis from repetitive wrist and hand motions.[158] These ten-

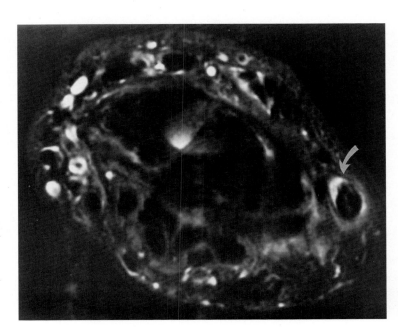

FIGURE 11-134. Tenosynovitis of the extensor carpi ulnaris tendon of the sixth dorsal compartment is shown as fluid hyperintensity of the tendon sheath (*arrow*) on STIR axial image.

dons become inflamed in the fibro-osseous tunnel at the level of the radial styloid. Clinically, there are tenderness and swelling at the radial styloid and a positive Finkelstein's test (radial styloid pain and passive ulnar deviation of the wrist with adduction of the thumb). MR imaging shows enlargement or thickening of the APL tendon sheaths. There is high signal intensity fluid within the tendon sheath, and the involved tendons are thickened. There may be intrasubstance hyperintensity as tendinitis develops.[159] Treatment consists of rest, splinting, and NSAIDs.

Tenosynovitis of the extensor carpi ulnaris tendon presents as dorsal ulnar-sided pain. High signal intensity fluid is visualized surrounding the tendon on T2- or T2*-weighted or STIR images (Fig. 11-134). The tendon sheath is usually thickened, and there is hyperintensity within the tendon. In chronic disease, there is signal void with focal calcifications.[159]

Tenosynovitis of the flexor carpi ulnaris tendon is secondary to chronic injury or repetitive trauma.[159] High signal intensity fluid and tendon sheath thickening are identified on MR images. MR imaging also is used to identify sites of tendon rupture in both the extensor and flexor compartments (Figs. 11-135 and 11-136).

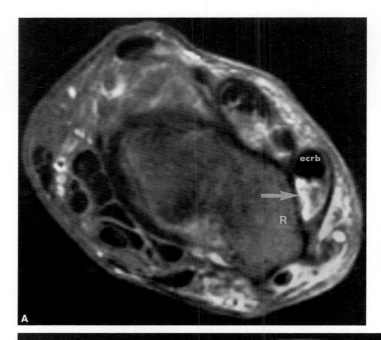

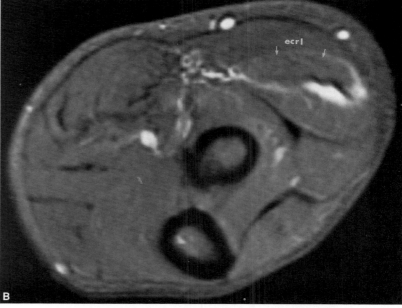

FIGURE 11-135. (A) Rupture (*large arrow*) of the extensor carpi radialis longus tendon at the level of the proximal carpal row after arthroplasty of the thumb. A sling was created by weaving the abductor pollicis longus tenon through the extensor carpi radialis longus tendon. ecrb, extensor carpi radialis brevis; R, radius. (B) Hyperintense edema (*arrows*) of the extensor carpi radialis longus (ecrl) muscle is seen proximal to the carpus in the mid- and proximal forearm. (A, B) Fat-suppressed T2-weighted fast spin-echo axial images.

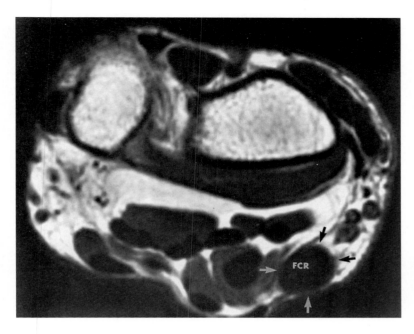

FIGURE 11-136. Enlarged (*arrows*) flexor carpi radialis (FCR) tendon secondary to retraction from a more distal tear. The flexor carpi radialis tendon normally inserts onto the bases of the second and third metacarpals. T1-weighted axial image.

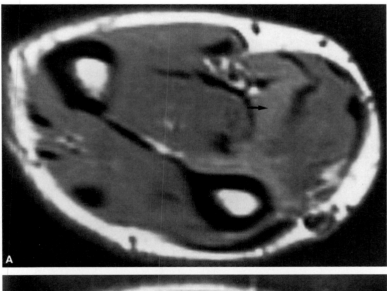

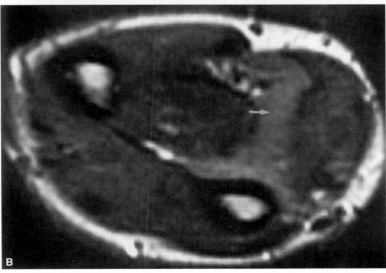

FIGURE 11-137. Proton density (**A**) and T2-weighted fast spin-echo (**B**) axial images demonstrate subacute anterior interosseous nerve paralysis with increased signal intensity (*arrow*) in the distribution of the denervated flexor digitorum profundus and flexor pollicis longus muscles of the forearm. *continued*

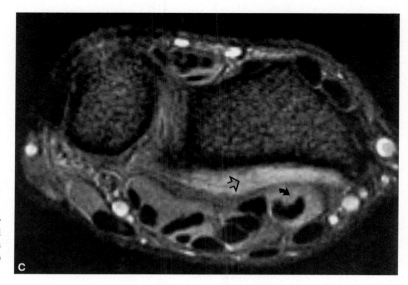

FIGURE 11-137. *Continued.* (**C**) On a T2*-weighted axial image, denervation hyperintensity is shown distally at the level of the distal radius and involves the pronator quadratus (*open arrow*) and flexor pollicis longus (*curved arrow*) muscles.

Changes of subacute muscle denervation demonstrate increased signal intensity on T2 and STIR sequences[160] (Fig. 11-137). Fatty atrophy is associated with chronically denervated muscles. The anterior interosseous branch of the median nerve supplies the flexor digitorum profundus, the flexor pollicis longus, and the pronator quadratus muscles.

PATHOLOGY OF THE FINGER

Ligament Pathology

Ligamentous injuries of the fingers and thumb include disruptions of the collateral ligaments, frequently involving the MP and PIP joints[161] (Figs. 11-138 and 11-139). The PIP joint is a relatively rigid hinge joint and is therefore susceptible to injury through transmission of lateral and torque stress (Fig. 11-140). Masson and coworkers[161] have used MR imaging to identify the separate components of the proper and accessory collateral ligaments of the thumb and finger MP joints (see Fig. 11-138). The more volar accessory component of the collateral ligament inserts onto the lateral margin of the volar plate and is identified deep to the proper collateral ligament on coronal MR images. The volar plate (see Fig. 11-139B) capsular thickening extends from its strong fibrocartilage attachment to the base of the proximal phalanx to a thinner attachment onto the neck of the metacarpal. Volar plate injuries, which are caused by hyperextension,

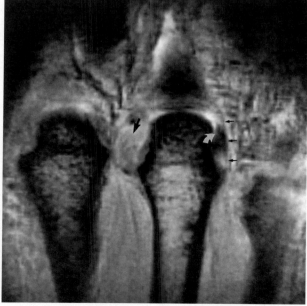

FIGURE 11-138. Distal tear and retraction of the radial collateral ligament (*large straight arrow*) of the third finger metacarpophalangeal (MP) joint on a T2*-weighted coronal image. The radial collateral ligament tears in an ulnar extension mechanism of injury to the MP joint. The intact proper (*small straight arrows*) and accessory collateral (*curved arrow*) ligaments are shown on the ulnar aspect of the MP joint. The accessory collateral ligament originates on the metacarpal head volar to the proper collateral ligament and inserts onto the lateral aspect of the volar plate.

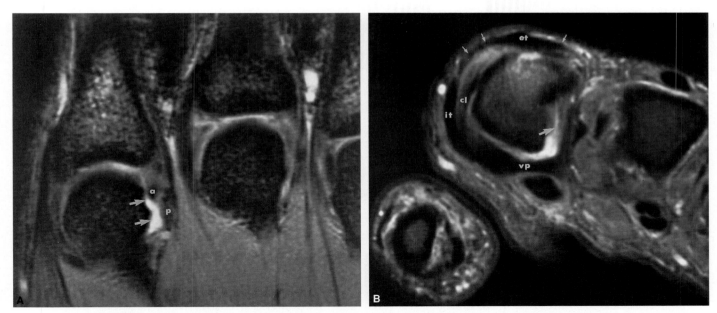

FIGURE 11-139. (**A**) Index metacarpophalangeal joint with direct extension of hyperintense joint fluid across a torn proximal attachment of the ulnar collateral ligament (*arrows*). There is disruption of both the proper (p) and accessory (a) components of the collateral ligament. T2*-weighted coronal image. (**B**) Corresponding T2*-weighted axial image shows the normal insertion of the collateral ligament (cl) into the lateral aspect of the volar plate (vp). The torn and retracted accessory component of the ulnar collateral ligament (*large arrow*) is not seen in continuity with the periphery of the volar plate. The volar plate represents normal capsular thickening forming the floor of the metacarpophalangeal joint. Also shown are the common extensor tendon (et) and sagittal bands (*small arrows*). The sagittal bands of the extensor hood extend from the common extensor tendon to the volar plate and course in the plane between the interosseous tendon (it) and collateral ligament (ct).

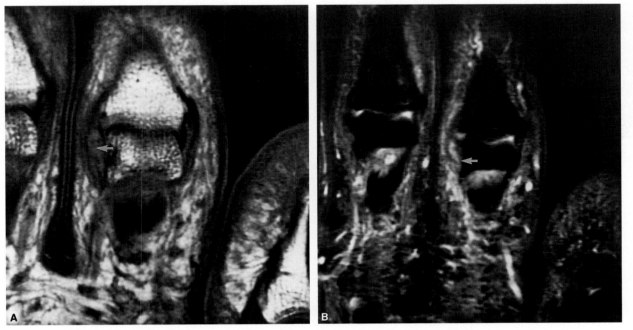

FIGURE 11-140. Proximal attachment ulnar collateral ligament tear (*straight arrow*) of the index finger proximal interphalangeal joint on T1-weighted (**A**) and STIR (**B**) coronal images. The proximal attachment of the ulnar collateral ligament is absent and replaced by hyperintense fluid (*straight arrow*) on the corresponding STIR axial image. *continued*

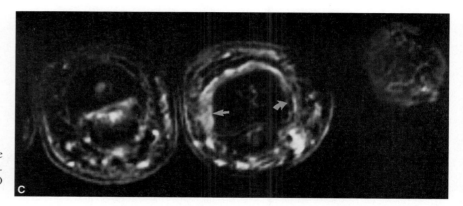

FIGURE 11-140. *Continued.* (**C**), obtained at the level of the distal aspect of the proximal phalanx. Normal radial collateral ligament (*curved arrow*) is shown for comparison.

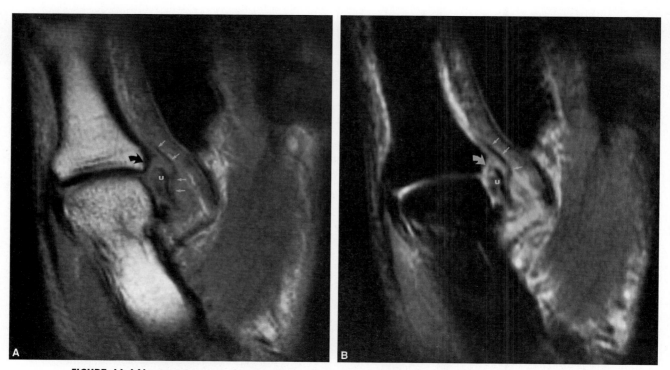

FIGURE 11-141. Gamekeeper's thumb with rupture of the distal attachment (*curved arrow*) of the ulnar collateral ligament (u). The torn ulnar collateral ligament remains deep to the overlying adductor aponeurosis (*small arrows*). In a Stener lesion (not present in this case), the torn ulnar collateral ligament relocates superficial to the adductor pollicis aponeurosis after the abduction injury occurs. (**A**) T1-weighted coronal image. (**B**) STIR coronal image.

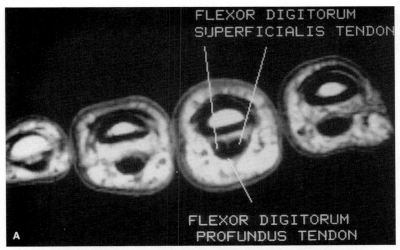

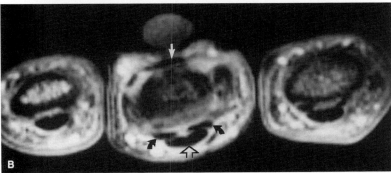

FIGURE 11-142. (**A**) A T1-weighted axial image shows the flexor tendon anatomy at the level of the proximal middle phalanx. (**B**) A T2*-weighted axial image provides superior discrimination of the flexor digitorum superficialis slips (*curved black arrows*) from the flexor digitorum profundus tendon (*open arrow*). The extensor tendon is shown deep to the marker (*white arrow*).

may result in hyperextension or flexion deformities of the joint. Initial treatment for these injuries is short-term splinting in 25° to 30° of flexion.

Ulnar Collateral Ligament Tears of the Thumb

An ulnar collateral ligament tear, sometimes called gamekeeper's thumb, involves disruption of the ulnar collateral ligament of the first MP joint and is frequently associated with a proximal phalanx base fracture[162,163] (Fig. 11-141). This injury may produce instability with abduction stress and is commonly seen in ski-pole, football, hockey, wresting, and baseball injuries. The ulnar collateral ligament may also sustain a partial tear, usually at its distal attachment to the proximal phalanx. Complete ulnar collateral ligament tears result in MP joint instability, with at least 20° greater laxity than the contralateral thumb. T1-, T2-, or T2*-weighted coronal MR images demonstrate edema, thickening, disruption, displacement, or entrapment of the ulnar collateral ligament.[144] The thumb should be positioned so that the radial collateral ligament is included in the imaging plane. Since the adductor pollicis aponeurosis may be interposed between the disrupted

portions of the ulnar collateral ligament, surgical repair is indicated.

Associated displacement of the ulnar collateral ligament proximal and superficial to the adductor pollicis aponeurosis is called the Stener lesion.[162,163] With MR imaging, it is possible to differentiate between ulnar collateral ligament displacement and nondisplaced tears. Spaeth and colleagues[162] reported that MR imaging was 67% specific for identifying all tears.[162] However, it was 100% sensitive and 94% specific for demonstrating ulnar collateral ligament displacement in gamekeeper's thumb. Sonography has also been utilized in the differentiation of displaced and nondisplaced tears of the UCL,[164] although MR imaging has documented better results.[165]

Tendon Injuries

Magnetic resonance imaging has been used to identify the anatomy, site and specific flexor tendon involved in primary tendon tears or postsurgical retears (Figs. 11-142 through 11-145). The differential diagnosis of tendon injury includes motor nerve injuries (which impair active motion but in

text continues on page 990

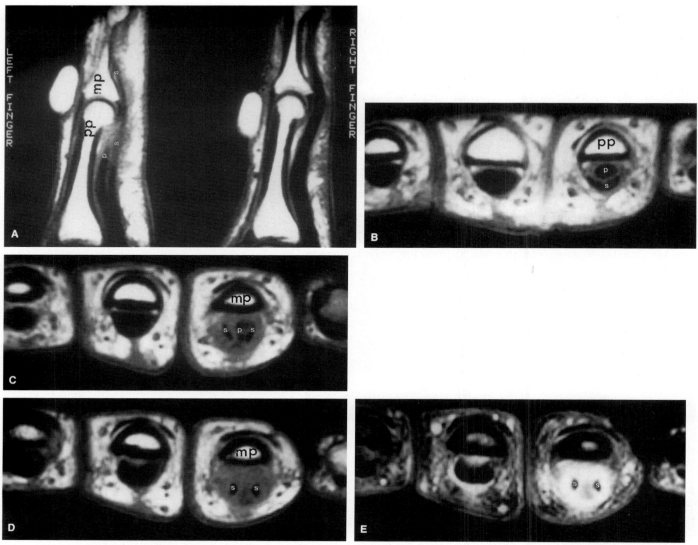

FIGURE 11-143. An isolated flexor digitorum profundus tendon tear. (**A**) T1-weighted sagittal images show the retracted profundus tendon (p) over the left fourth digit at the level of the proximal phalanx (pp). The intact superficialis tendon (s) is shown where it attaches to the borders of the middle phalanx (mp). The normal right finger flexor tendon is shown for comparison. (**B**) A T1-weighted axial image shows the intact flexor digitorum profundus (p) and superficialis (s) tendons at the level of the proximal phalanx (pp). Normally, the superficialis divides into two halves opposite the middle phalanx and passes deep to the profundus tendon, where it decussates and attaches to the middle phalanx. (**C**) A T1-weighted axial image shows the site of flexor digitorum profundus rupture (p) flanked by divided superficialis tendons (s) opposite the middle phalanx (mp). (**D**) A more distal axial T1-weighted image and (**E**) a T2*-weighted image through the middle phalanx (mp) show the absence of the profundus tendon. The flexor digitorum profundus tendon normally inserts onto the anterior aspect of the base of the distal phalanx. The flexor digitorum superficialis (s) divides normally.

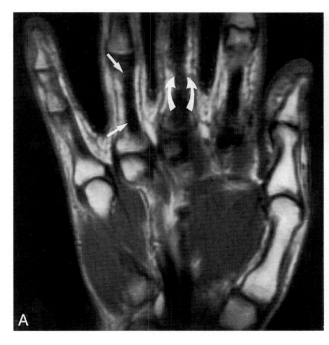

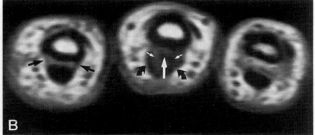

FIGURE 11-144. An intact flexor tendon is shown after repair. (**A**) A T1-weighted coronal image shows the attenuated low signal intensity flexor tendon at the site of primary surgical repair (*curved arrows*). The normal contour of the uninvolved flexor tendon is shown for comparison (*straight arrow*). (**B**) The corresponding axial image demonstrates the central low signal intensity flexor digitorum profundus (*large white arrow*) and the dividing tendons of the flexor digitorum superficialis (*curved black arrows*). Fibrous thickening of the tendon sheaths demonstrates intermediate signal intensity (*small white arrows*). The intact digital fibrous sheaths, which form the fibro-osseous canal, support the flexor tendons (*straight black arrows*).

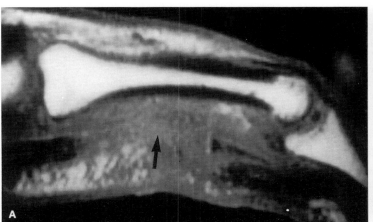

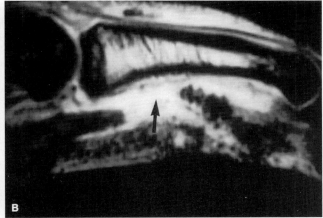

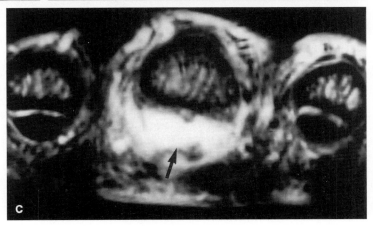

FIGURE 11-145. Complete disruption of the flexor digitorum superficialis and profundus tendons (*arrow*) are seen on (**A**) T1-weighted sagittal, (**B**) T2*-weighted, and (**C**) T2*-weighted axial images after primary tendon repair.

which the viscoelastic muscle tendon unit remains intact), extensor tendon injuries; flexor extensor tenosynovitis, and rupture. These conditions are often difficult to diagnose on clinical examination, and MR studies can be used to evaluate and detect subluxation, synovitis, or tears. Chronic tenosynovitis may lead to tendon attrition and result in tear. MR studies used for follow-up after flexor tendon repair identify specific complications, such as peritendinous adhesions, frank rupture, and rupture with callus. A frank rupture is associated with a larger tendon gap. An elongated callus is characterized by a thin fibrous continuity across the rupture site.[166]

Extensor hood injuries may also be detected on MR images, which display the components of the extensor hood including the sagittal bands.[167]

References

1. Manaster BJ. Digital wrist arthrography: precision in determining the site of radiocarpal-midcarpal communication. AJR 1986;147:563.
2. Braunstein EM, et al. Fluoroscopic and arthroscopic evaluation of carpal instability. AJR 1985;144:1259.
3. Tirman RM, et al. Midcarpal wrist arthrography for detection of tears of the scapholunate and lunatotriquetral ligaments. AJR 1985; 144:107.
4. Hall FM. Wrist arthrography. Radiology 1990;175:585.
5. Palmer A. Arthrography of the wrist. J Hand Surg [Am] 1983;8:15.
6. Zinberg E, et al. The triple injection wrist arthrogram. J Hand Surg [Am] 1988;13:803.
7. Manaster BJ. The clinical efficacy of triple-injection wrist arthrography. Radiology 1991;178:267.
8. Manaster B, Mann R, Rubenstein S. Wrist pain: correlation of clinical and plain film findings with arthrographic results. J Hand Surg [Am] 1989;14:466.
9. Metz VM, Mann FA, Gilula LA. Lack of correlation between site of wrist pain and location of noncommunicating defects shown by three-compartment wrist arthrography. AJR 1993;160:1239.
10. Metz VM, Mann FA, Gilula LA. Three compartment wrist arthrography: correlation of pain site with location of uni- and bidirectional communications. AJR 1993;160:819.
11. Mikic Z. Age changes in triangular fibrocartilage of the wrist joint. J Anat 1978;126:367.
12. Mikic Z. Arthrography of the wrist joint: an experimental study. J Bone Joint Surg [Am] 1984;66:371.
13. Kirschenbaum D, Sieler S, Solonick D, Loeb DM. Arthrography of the wrist: assessment of the integrity of the ligaments in young asymptomatic adults. J Bone Joint Surg [Am] 1995;77A:1207.
14. Stewart NR, Gilula LA. CT of the wrist: a tailored approach. Radiology 1992;183:13.
15. Quinn SF, et al. Advanced imaging of the wrist. Radiographics 1989;9:229.
16. Hindman BW, et al. Occult fractures of the carpals and metacarpals demonstrated by CT. AJR 1989;153:529.
17. Pennes DR, et al. Direct coronal CT of the scaphoid bone. Radiology 1989;171:870.
18. Biondetti PR, et al. Three-dimensional surface reconstruction of the carpal bones from CT scans: transaxial versus coronal technique. Comput Med Imaging Graph 1988;12:67.
19. DeFlaviis L, et al. High resolution ultrasonography of wrist ganglia. JCU 1987;15:17.
20. Weiss KL, et al. High field strength surface coil imaging of the hand and wrist. Part I. Normal anatomy. Radiology 1986;160:143.
21. Baker LL, et al. High resolution magnetic resonance imaging of the wrist: normal anatomy. Skeletal Radiol 1987;16:128.
22. Middleton WD, et al. High resolution surface coil imaging of the joints: anatomic correlation. Radiographics 1987;7:645.
23. Koenig H, et al. Wrist: preliminary report of high resolution MR imaging. Radiology 1986;160:463.
24. Mark S, et al. High resolution MR imaging of peripheral joints using a quadrature coil at 0.35T. ROFO 1987;146:397.
25. Fisher MR, et al. MR imaging using specialized coils. Radiology 1985;157:443.
26. Quinn SF, et al. Advanced imaging of the wrist. Radiographics 1989;9:229.
27. Zlatkin MB, et al. Chronic wrist pain: evaluation with high resolution MR imaging. Radiology 1989;173:723.
28. Greenan T, et al. Magnetic resonance imaging of the wrist. Semin Ultrasound CT MR 1990;11:267.
29. Gundry CR, et al. Is MR better than arthrography for evaluating the ligaments of the wrist? In vitro study. AJR 1990;154:337.
30. Binkovitz LA, et al. Magnetic resonance imaging of the wrist: normal cross sectional imaging and selected abnormal cases. Radiographics 1988;8:1171.
31. Heuck A, et al. Possibilities of MR tomography of diseases of the hand and wrist. Radiologue 1989;29:53.
32. Schweitzer ME, Brahme SK, Hodler J, Hanker GJ. Chronic wrist pain: spin-echo and short TR inversion recovery MR imaging and conventional and MR arthrography. Radiology 1992;182:205.
33. Foo TG, Shellock FG, Hayes CE, Schenck JF. High-resolution MR imaging of the wrist and eye with short TR, short TR and partial-echo acquisition. Radiology 1992;183:277.
34. Blackhand SJ, Chakrabarte I, Gibbs P, Buckley DL. Fingers: three dimensional MR imaging and angiography with local gradient coil. Radiology 1994;190:895.
35. Ekenstam F: The distal radioulnar joint. Uppsala: Acta Universitatis Up Salvensis Uppsala Universitet, 1984.
36. Bogumill GP. Anatomy of the wrist. Philadelphia: WB Saunders, 1988:14.
37. Watson H, Ryu J. Degenerative disorders of the carpus. Orthop Clin North Am 1984;15:337.
38. Viegas S, et al. Medial (hamate) facet of the lunate. J Hand Surg [Am] 1990;15:565.
39. North E, Thomas S. An anatomic guide for arthroscopic visualization of the wrist capsular ligaments. J Hand Surg [Am] 1988;13:815.
40. Cooney W, et al. Anatomy and mechanics of carpal instability. Surg Rounds Orthop 1989;Sept 15.
41. Rominger MB, Bernreuter WK, Kenney PJ, Lee DH. MR imaging of anatomy and tears of wrist ligaments. Radiographics 1993;13:1233.
42. Webster E, Chao E. An experimental approach to mechanism of scaphoid wrist fractures. J Hand Surg [Am] 1978;3:142.
43. Timins ME, Jahnke JP, Krah SF, Erickson SJ. MR imaging of the major carpal stabilizing ligaments: normal anatomy and clinical examples. Radiographics 1995;15:575.
44. Berger R, Landsmeer J. The palmer radiocarpal ligaments: a study of adult and fetal human wrist joints. J Hand Surg [Am] 1990;15:847.
45. Testut L. Traite d'anatomie humaine. Paris: Gaston Doin, 1928:628.
46. Landsmeer J. Atlas of anatomy of the hand. New York: Churchill Livingstone, 1976:11.
47. Berger R, et al. Radioscapholunate ligament: a gross anatomic and histologic study of fetal and adult wrists. J Hand Surg [Am] 1991;16:350.
48. Palmer A, Werner F. The triangular fibrocartilage complex of the wrist/anatomy and function. J Hand Surg [Am] 1981;6:153.
49. Viegas S, et al. Ulnar-sided perilunate instability: an anatomic and biomechanic study. J Hand Surg [Am] 1990;15:268.
50. Smith DK. Volar carpal ligaments of the wrist: normal appearance on

multiplanar reconstructions of three-dimensional fourier transform MR imaging. AJR 1993;161:353.

51. Smith DK. Scapholunate interosseous ligament of the wrist: MR appearances in asymptomatic volunteers and arthrographically normal wrists. Radiology 1994;192:217.

52. Mayfield JK. Pathogenesis of wrist ligament instability. Philadelphia: WB Saunders, 1988:53.

53. Smith DK, Snearly WN. Lunotriquetral interosseous ligament of the wrist: MR appearances in asymptomatic volunteers and arthrographically normal wrists. Radiology 1994;191:199.

54. Taleisnik J. The ligaments of the wrist. In: Taleisnik J, ed. The wrist. New York: Churchill Livingstone, 1985:13.

55. Alexander CE, Lichtman DM. Ulnar carpal instabilities. Orthop Clin North Am 1984;15:2, 307.

56. Totterman SMS, Miller R, Wasserman B, Bleabea JS. Intrinsic and extrinsic carpal ligaments: evaluation by three-dimensional fourier transform MR imaging. AJR 1993;160:117.

57. Resnick R, Halliday D. Physics. New York: Wiley & Sons, 1966.

58. Youm Y, et al. Kinematics of the wrist. Part I. An experimental study of radial-ulnar deviation and flexion-extension. J Bone Joint Surg [Am] 1978;60:423.

59. Smith DK. MR imaging of normal and injured wrist ligaments. MRI Clinics of North America Philadelphia: WB Saunders, May 1995; 3:229.

60. Totterman SMS, Miller RJ. MRI of the wrist and hand. Philadelphia: WB Saunders, 1996:441.

61. Garcia-Elias M, et al. Traumatic axial dislocations of the carpus. J Hand Surg [Am] 1989;14:446.

62. Gilula LA. Carpal injuries: analytic approach and case exercises. AJR 1979;133:503.

63. Szabo RM, Newland CC. Open reduction and ligamentous repair for acute lunate and perilunate dislocation. In: Gelberman RH, ed. New York: Raven Press 1994:167.

64. Ruby LK. Carpal instability. J Bone Joint Surg [Am] 1995;77A:476.

65. Resnick D. Internal derangements of joints, 3rd ed. Philadelphia: WB Saunders, 1995:5:2899.

66. Weber ER. Wrist mechanics and its association with ligamentous instability. In: Lichtman D, ed. The wrist and its disorders. Philadelphia: WB Saunders, 1988:41.

67. Lichtman D, et al. Ulnar midcarpal instability: clinical and laboratory analysis. J Hand Surg [Am] 1981;9:350.

68. Yin Y, Mann FA, Hodge JC, Gilula LA. Roentgenographic interpretation of ligamentous instabilities of the wrist. Static and dynamic instabilities. Philadelphia: WB Saunders, 1996:203.

69. Taleisnik J, Watson H. Midcarpal instability caused by malunited fractures of the distal radius. J Hand Surg [Am] 1984;9:350.

70. Gainer B, Schaberg J. The rheumatoid wrist after resection of the distal ulna. J Hand Surg [Am] 1985;10:837.

71. Rayhack J, et al. Posttraumric uluar translocation of the carpus. J Hand Surg [Am] 1982;12:180.

72. Loeb T, et al. Traumatic carpal instability: putting the pieces together. Orthop Trans 1977;1:163.

73. Glickel S, Millender L. Results of ligamentous reconstruction for chronic intercarpal instability. Orthop Trans 1982;6:167.

74. Watson H, Mempton R. Limited wrist arthrodesis. Part I. J Hand Surg [Am] 1980;5:320.

75. Blatt G. Dorsal capsulodesis for rotatory subluxation of the carpal scaphoid. Presented at the Annual Meeting of the American Society for Surgery of the Hand, New Orleans, 1986.

76. Palmer AC: The distal radioulnar joint. In: Lichtman D, ed. The wrist and its disorders. Philadelphia: WB Saunders, 1988:220.

77. Steyers C, Blair W. Measuring ulnar variance: a comparison of techniques. J Hand Surg [Am] 1989:14:607.

78. Epner R, et al. Ulnar variance: the effect of wrist positioning and roentgen filming technique. J Hand Surg [Am] 1982;7:298.

79. Linscheid RL. Operative treatment for distal radioulnar joint instability. New York: Raven Press, 1994:195.

80. Bruckner JD, Alexander AH, Lichtman DM. Acute dislocations of the distal radio-ulnar joint. J Bone Joint Surg [Am] 1995;77A:958.

81. Olerud C, et al. The congruence of the distal radioulnar joint: a magnetic resonance imaging study. Acta Orthop Scand 1988;59:183.

82. Wechsler R, et al. Computed tomography diagnosis of distal radioulnar subluxation. Skeletal Radiol 1987;16:1.

83. Pirela-Cruz M, et al. Stress computed tomography analysis of the distal radioulnar joint: a diagnostic tool for determining translational motion. J Hand Surg [Am] 1991;16:75.

84. Oneson SR, Scales LM, Timins ME, et al. MR imaging interpretation of the palmar classification of triangular fibrocartilage complex lesions. Radiographics 1996;16:97.

85. Hermandsdorfer J, Kleinman W. Management of chronic peripheral tears of the triangular fibrocartilage complex. J Hand Surg [Am] 1991;16:340.

86. Pin P, et al. Management of chronic lunotriquetral ligament tears J Hand Surg [Am] 1989;14:77.

87. Thiru R, et al. Arterial anatomy of the triangular fibrocartilage of the wrist and its surgical significance. J Hand Surg [Am] 1986,11:258.

88. Mooney J, Poehling G. Disruption of the ulnolunate ligament as a cause for chronic ulnar wrist pain. J Hand Surg [Am] 1991;16:347.

89. Totterman SMA, Miller RJ. Triangular fibrocartilage complex: normal appearance on coronal three-dimensional gradient-recalled-echo MR images. Radiology 1995;195:521.

90. Lubowitz JH, Zunin ID, Lesavoy MA. Ligamentous anatomy of the medial carpal region. Orthop Rev 1993:1129.

91. Golimbu CN, et al. Tears of the triangular fibrocartilage of the wrist: MR imaging. Radiology 1989;173:731.

92. Lewis OJ, et al. The anatomy of the wrist joint. J Anat 1970;106:539.

93. Tan ABH, Yung SW, Wong MK, Kalinga M. Congenital perforations of the triangular fibrocartilage of the wrist. J Hand Surg [Br] 1995;20B:342.

94. Greenan T, et al. Magnetic resonance imaging of the wrist. Semin Ultrasound CT MR 1990;11:267.

95. Adams B. Detrimental effects of resections in the articular disc of the TFCC. Transactions of the 37th Meeting of the ORS 1991;16:212.

96. Lewis O. The development of the human wrist joint during the fetal period. Anat Rec 1970;166:499.

97. Frykman G. Fracture of the distal radius including sequelae: shoulder-hand-finger syndrome. Disturbance in the distal radioulnar joint, and impairment of nerve function: a clinical and experimental study. Acta Orthop Scand 1967;108(suppl):1.

98. Melone C Jr. Open treatment for displaced articular fractures of the distal radius. Clin Orthop 1986;202:103.

99. Werner F, Murphy D, Palmer A. Pressures in the distal radioulnar joint: effect of surgical procedures used for Kienbock's disease. J Orthop Res 1989;7:445.

100. Scheck M. Long-term follow-up of treatment for comminuted fractures of the distal end of the radius by transfixation with Kirschner wires and cast. J Bone Joint Surg [Am] 1962;44:337.

101. Stevens J. Compression fractures of the lower end of the radius. Ann Surg 1920;71:594.

102. Knirk J, Jupiter J. Intraarticular fractures of the distal end of the radius in young adults. J Bone Joint Surg [Am] 1986;68:647.

103. O'Brien ET. Acute. fractures and dislocations of the carpus. In: Lichtman D, ed. The wrist and its disorders. Philadelphia: WB Saunders, 1988:129.

104. Herbert TJ. Open reduction and internal fixation using the Herbert screw. New York: Raven Press, 1994:

105. Fernandez DL, Eggli S. Non-union of the scaphoid. J Bone Joint Surg [Am] 1995;77A:883.

106. Düppe H, Johnell O, Lundborg G, et al. Long-term results of fracture of the scaphoid. J Bone Joint Surg [Am] 1994;76A:249.

107. Gillespy T III, et al. Dorsal fractures of the hamate: radiographic appearance. AJR 1988;151:351.

108. Ruby LK, et al. Natural history of scaphoid nonunion. Radiology 198S;156:856.

109. Reinus WR, et al. Carpal avascular necrosis: MR imaging. Radiology 1986;160:689.

110. Weiss KL, et al. High field MR surface coil imaging of the hand and wrist: normal anatomy. Skeletal Radiol 1987;16:128.

111. Baker LL, et al. High resolution magnetic resonance imaging of the wrist. Normal anatomy. Skeletal Radiol 1987;16:128.

112. Cristiani G, et al. Evaluation of ischaemic necrosis of carpal bones by magnetic resonance imaging. J Hand Surg [Br] 1990;15:249.

113. Desser TS, et al. Scaphoid fractures and Kienböck's disease of the lunate: MR imaging with histopathologic correlation. Magn Reson Imaging 1990;8:357.

114. Golimbu CN, Firooznia H, Rafii M. Avascular necrosis of carpal bones. MRI Clin North Am 1995;3:281.

115. Duong R, et al. Kienböck's disease: scintigraphic demonstration in correlation with clinical, radiographic and pathologic findings. Clin Nucl Med 1982;7:418.

116. Hulten O. Uber anatomische variationen der handgelenkknochen. Acta Radio Scand 1928;9:155.

117. Gelberman R, et al. Ulnar variance in Kienböck's disease. J Bone Joint Surg [Am] 1975;57:674.

118. Peste. Discussion. Bull Soc Anat 1943;18:169.

119. Beckenbaugh R, et al. Kienböck's disease: the natural history of Kienbock's disease and consideration of lunate fractures. Clin Orthop 1980;149:98.

120. Gelberman R, et al. The vascularity of the lunate bone and Kienböck's disease. J Hand Surg [Am] 1980;5:272.

121. Alexander AH, Lichtman D. Kienböck's disease. In: Lichtman D, ed. The wrist and its disorders. Philadelphia: WB Saunders, 1988:329.

122. Lichtman D, et al. Kienböck's disease/update on silicone replacement arthroplasty. J Hand Surg [Am] 1983;7:343.

123. Braun R. Pronator pedicle bone grafting in the forearm and proximal carpal row. Presented at 38th Annual Meeting of the American Society for Surgery of the Hand, March, 1983.

124. Hori Y, et al. Blood vessel transplantation to bone. J Hand Surg [Am] 1979;4:23.

125. Almquist E, et al. Capitate shortening as a treatment for early Kienböck's disease. Presented at the 45th Annual Meeting of the American Society for Surgery of the Hand, March, 1990.

126. Alexander A, et al. Lunate silicone replacement arthroplasty in Kienböck's disease: a long-term follow up. J Hand Surg [Am] 1990; 15:401.

127. Watanabe K, Nakamura R, Imaeda T. Arthroscopic assessment of Kienböck's disease. Arthroscopy 1995;2:257.

128. Coyle MP. Nerve entrapment syndromes in the upper extremity In: Dee R, ed. Principles of orthopaedic practice, vol 1. New York: McGraw-Hill, 1989:672.

129. Cavallaro MC, Taylor JAM, Gorman JD, et al. Imaging findings in a patient with fibrolipomatous hamartoma of the median nerve. AJR 1993;161:837.

130. Middleton WD, et al. MR imaging of the carpal tunnel: normal anatomy and preliminary findings in the carpal tunnel syndrome AJR 1987;148:307.

131. Mesgarzadah M, et al. Carpal tunnel: MR imaging. Part I. Normal anatomy. Radiology 1989;171:743.

132. Mesgarzadah M, et al. Carpal tunnel: MR imaging. Part II. Carpal tunnel syndrome. Radiology 1989;171:749.

133. Healy C, et al. Magnetic resonance imaging of the carpal tunnel. J Hand Surg [Br] 1990;15:243.

134. Zeiss J, et al. Anatomic relations between the median nerve and Hexor tendons in the carpal tunnel: MR evaluation in normal volunteers. AJR 1989;153:533.

135. Sugimoto H, Miyaji N, Ohsawa T. Carpal tunnel syndrome: evaluation of median nerve circulation with dynamic contrast-enhanced MR imaging. Radiology 1994;190:459.

136. Menon J. Endoscopic carpal tunnel release: preliminary report. Arthroscopy 1994;10:31.

137. Rowland EB, Kleinert JM. Endoscopic carpal-tunnel release in cadavera: an investigation of the results of 12 surgeons with this training model. J Bone Joint Surg [Am] 1994;76A:266.

138. Gelberman RH, Eaton R, Urbaniak JR. Peripheral nerve compression. J Bone Joint Surg [Am] 1993;75A:1854.

139. Zeiss J, Jakab E. Khimji T and Imbriglia J. The ulnar tunnel at the wrist (Guyon's canal): normal MR anatomy and variants. AJR 1992;158:1081.

140. Yulish BS, et al. Juvenile rheumatoid arthritis: assessment with MR imaging. Radiology 1987;165:149.

141. Baker LL, et al. High resolution magnetic resonance imaging of the wrist: normal anatomy. Skeletal Radiol 1987;16:128.

142. Meske S, et al. Rheumatoid arthritis lesions of the wrist examined by rapid gradient echo magnetic resonance imaging. Scand J Rheumatol 1990;19:235.

143. Watson KH. Degenerative disorders of the carpus. In: Lichtman D, ed. The wrist and its disorders. Philadelphia: WB Saunders, 1988:286.

144. Renner WR, et al. Early changes of rheumatoid arthritis in the hand and wrist. Radiol Clin North Am 1988;26:1185.

145. Rominger MB, Bernreuter WK, Kenney PJ, et al. MR imaging of the hands in early rheumatoid arthritis: preliminary results. Radiographics 1993;13:37.

146. Sugimoto H, Takeda A, Masuyama J, Furuse M. Early-stage rheumatoid arthritis: diagnostic accuracy of MR imaging. Radiology 1996;198:185.

147. Ellstein JL, et al. Rheumatoid disorders of the hand and wrist. In: Dee R, ed. Principles of orthopaedic practice, vol 1. New York: McGraw-Hill, 1989:646.

148. Rubens D, Blebea J, Totterman SMS, Hooper MM. Rheumatoid arthritis: evaluation of wrist extensor tendons with clinical examination versus MR imaging—a preliminary report. Radiology 1993;187:831.

149. Magee TH, Rowedder AM, Degnan GC. Intraosseous ganglia of the wrist. Radiology 1995;195:517.

150. Yang B, Sartoris DJ, Djukic S, Resnick D. Distribution of calcification in the triangular fibrocartilage region in 181 patients with calcium pyrophosphate dihydrate crystal deposition disease. Radiology 1995;196:547.

151. Yacoe M, Bergman AG, Ladd AL, Hellman BH. Dupuytren's contracture: MR imaging findings and correlation between MR signal intensity and cellularity of lesions. AJR 1993;160:813.

152. Hollister AM, et al. The use of MRI in the diagnosis of an occult wrist ganglion cyst. Orthop Rev 1989;18:1210.

153. Feldman F, et al. Magnetic resonance imaging of para-articular and ectopic ganglia. Skeletal Radiol 1989;18:353.

154. Louis DS, et al. Magnetic resonance imaging of the collateral ligaments of the thumb. J Hand Surg [Am] 1989;14:739.

155. Cardinal E, Buckwalter KA, Braunstein EM, Mih AD. Occult dorsal carpal ganglion: comparison of US and MR imaging. Radiology 1994;193:259.

156. Bishop AT, Gabel G, Carmichael SW. Flexor carpi radialis tendinitis. J Bone Joint Surg [Am] 1994;76A:1009.

157. Gabel G, Bishop AT, Wood MB. Flexor carpi radialis tendinitis. J Bone Joint Surg [Am] 1994;76A:1015.

158. Yates AJ, Wilgis EFS. Wrist pain. In: Nicholas J, ed. The upper extremity in sports medicine, 2nd ed. St Louis: CV Mosby, 1995:471.

159. Klug JD. MR diagnosis of tenosynovitis about the wrist. Philadelphia: WB Saunders, May 1995;3:305.

160. Fleckenstein JL, Watumull D, Conner KE, et al. Denervated human skeletal muscle: MR imaging evaluation. Radiology 1993;187:213.

161. Masson JA, Golimbu CN, Grossman JA. MR imaging of the metacarpophalangeal joints. MRI Clin North Am 1995;3:313.

162. Spaeth HJ, Abrams RA, Bock GW, Trudell D. Gamekeeper thumb:

differentiation of nondisplaced and displaced tears of the ulnar collateral ligament with MR imaging. Radiology 1993;188:553.

163. Hinke DH, Erickson SJ, Chamoy L, Timins ME. Ulnar collateral ligament of the thumb: MR findings in cadavers, volunteers, and patients with ligamentous injury (gamekeeper's thumb). AJR 1994; 163:1431.

164. Noszian IM, Dinkhauser LM, Orthner E, Straub GM. Ulnar collateral ligament: differentiation of displaced and nondisplaced tears with US. Radiology 1995;194:61.

165. Hergan K, Mittler C, Oser W. Ulnar collateral ligament: differentiation of displaced and nondisplaced tears with US and MR imaging. Radiology 1995;194:65.

166. Drape JL, Silbermann-Hoffman O, Houvet P, Dubert T. Complications of flexor tendon repair in the hand: MR imaging assessment. Radiology 1996;198:219.

167. Drape JL, Dubert T, Silbermann O, Thelen P. Acute trauma of the extensor hood of the metacarpophalangeal joint: MR imaging evaluation. Radiology 1994;192:469.

Magnetic Resonance Imaging in Orthopaedics & Sports Medicine, Second Edition,
edited by David W. Stoller. Lippincott-Raven Publishers, Philadelphia, © 1997.

Chapter 12

The Temporomandibular Joint

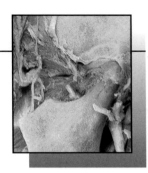

David W. Stoller
Richard L. Jacobson

The primary interest in the temporomandibular joint (TMJ) is in the evaluation of internal disc derangements. Abnormalities in both position and morphology of the TMJ meniscus (disc) have been implicated in myofascial pain syndromes and in biomechanical joint dysfunction. Young and middle-aged women are thought to represent a significant proportion of patients with TMJ abnormalities, mostly caused by bruxism (grinding of the teeth). However, internal disc derangements may also result from direct trauma or indirect trauma (eg, prolonged dental procedures), or they may occur spontaneously. Internal derangements of the TMJ represent one component of craniofacial pain syndromes; other components include myofascial pain dysfunction, abnormalities of the cervical spine, and dental occlusion.

Clinical diagnosis and documentation of TMJ disorders are difficult, and patients may present with symptoms of dysfunction without objective joint disease. However, documentation of internal disc derangements is required by third-party payers before long-term treatment or surgical interven-

tion is approved. Unfortunately, the articular disc cannot be seen by conventional radiography or computed tomography (CT), because these modalities rely on the assessment of osseous structures. Of the available imaging techniques, magnetic resonance (MR) imaging is frequently the procedure of choice to image the TMJ.

CT provides information that enables assessment of maxillofacial trauma; infection, including osteomyelitis; congenital abnormalities; and bony invasion by tumor. However, disc derangements cannot be appreciated by CT. Arthrography indirectly characterizes disc morphology, through either an inferior joint-space injection or dual-space contrast study; however, this is an invasive procedure. Arthrotomography relies on imaging contrast material coating the articular disc relative to the adjacent condyle, the glenoid fossa, and the eminence in closed-, partially open-, and open-mouth positions. With arthrography, the lower compartment of the TMJ is filled with contrast material to assess the position of the disc or, indirectly, the presence of a perforation.[1-7] Arthrog-

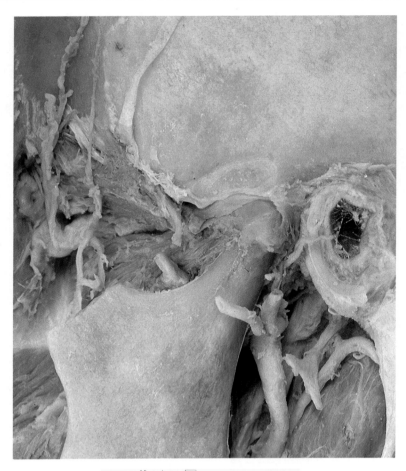

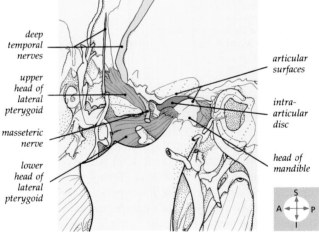

deep
temporal
nerves

upper
head of
lateral
pterygoid

masseteric
nerve

lower
head of
lateral
pterygoid

articular
surfaces

intra-
articular
disc

head of
mandible

FIGURE 12-1. The temporomandibular joint as opened by excision of the lateral part of its capsule.

raphy also is an invasive procedure with associated morbidity, and is limited in accuracy (eg, inability to inject contrast material into the lower joint compartment or injection into both compartments mimics disc perforation). Complications of arthrography include pain, prolonged discomfort, contrast extravasation into retrodiscal and pericapsular tissues, localized hemorrhage, and transient facial paralysis.

CT requires the use of ionizing radiation and only allows imaging of the TMJ disc through the use of reformatted sagittal images obtained from a series of transaxial joint scans.[8-13] The meniscus and bony anatomy are demonstrated in soft-tissue and bone algorithms. CT number highlighting for reformatting sagittal sections may not accurately differentiate the lateral pterygoid tendinous attachment from the articular disc, and is limited in evaluating a thinned or attenuated disc. Direct sagittal scanning has improved resolution over reformatting, and may replace it using the ''identity'' or ''blink'' mode for CT number highlighting. Proper angulation and patient positioning is required to minimize radiation to the orbit and lens.

MR imaging has lately replaced arthrography and CT, and has become the examination of choice in evaluating the TMJ.[13-26] MR studies are noninvasive and provide direct sagittal images that not only display the TMJ meniscus, but also differentiate the cortex, marrow, hyaline cartilage, muscle, fluid, fibrous tissue, and adhesions. This inherent soft-tissue discrimination facilitates thin section acquisitions with specialized surface coils. The development of faster imaging techniques (gradient-echo and fast spin-echo) and dual-coil imaging has facilitated routine bilateral examinations with functional or kinematic positioning of the joint.[27,28] MR imaging has been shown to be 95% accurate in assessing disc position and morphology and 93% accurate in assessing associated osseous changes of the condylar head and glen-

oid fossa.[29] Magnetic resonance can also be used to study other disease processes affecting the TMJ (eg, trauma, arthritis, and neoplasia) as well as to make postsurgical assessments.[30-36]

GROSS ANATOMY OF THE TEMPOROMANDIBULAR JOINT

The TMJ is a synovial diarthroidal joint located between the condyle of the mandible and mandibular fossa of the temporal bone (Fig. 12-1). The joint capsule is composed of loose connective tissue, which allows condylar translation, mandibular protrusion, retraction, and side-to-side excursion.[37,38] The articular disc, or meniscus, partitions the joint into a large superior (ie, upper) joint space and an inferior (ie, lower) joint space. The mandibular condyle divides the inferior joint space into anterior and posterior recesses. The biconcave fibrous fibrocartilaginous disc measures 1 mm centrally, and thickens peripherally into two bands: the anterior and the posterior. The anterior band is 2 mm thick, and the larger posterior band is 2.8 mm thick. Small perforations in the thin, central portion of the disc are normal. However, there is no direct communication between the separate synovium-lined upper and lower compartments. In the closed-mouth position, the bow tie or sigmoid-shaped disc is positioned within the temporal fossa with the posterior band directly superior to the condylar head. The thin, central region of the disc is located between the temporal articular eminence and the anterior condylar head. The anterior band, with the attached superior head of the lateral pterygoid muscle, is located inferior to the articular eminence and anterior to the condylar head.

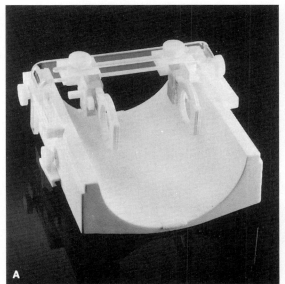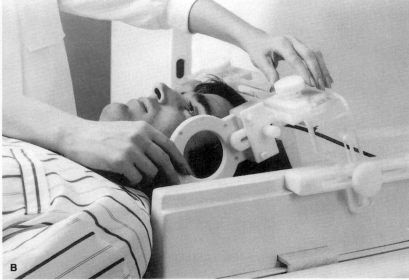

FIGURE 12-2. (**A**) Dual 7.5 cm (3 inch) diameter surface coils and holder. (**B**) Proper patient positioning for use of the imaging coils (GE Medical Systems Design, Milwaukee, WI). (**C**) Similar dual coil set up using a Medical Advances (Milwaukee, WI) design.   *continued*

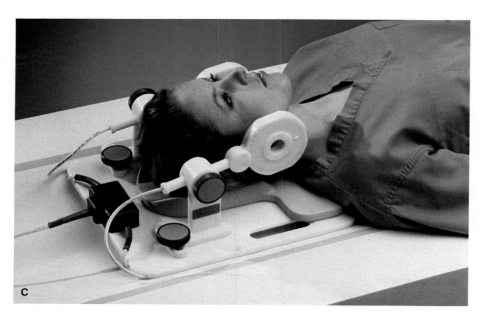

FIGURE 12-2. *Continued*

The posterior attachment of the disc (the bilaminar zone) is a neurovascular area consisting of fat, collagen, and elastic fibers.[39] The posterior-superior ligament of the bilaminar zone is composed of elastin and inserts into the temporal bone of the glenoid fossa. The posterior-inferior ligament of the bilaminar zone has a fibrous, nonelastic insertion into the posterior subcondylar area. Tearing or stretching of this ligament facilitates meniscal displacement.

The lateral pterygoid muscle, which controls mouth opening, consists of superior and inferior heads. The superior head is parallel with the inferior head and inserts onto the anterior joint capsule and condylar neck. The tendinous fibers of the superior head attach directly into the anterior band of the articular disc. The lateral pterygoid muscle produces anterior or forward rotation of the condylar head under the disc, and anterior translation of both the condylar head and the disc below the articular eminence. The medial pterygoid muscle, which is without any disc insertion, attaches onto the medial surface of the angle of the mandible and assists the lateral pterygoid in closing the jaw. The temporalis muscle has a tendinous insertion anteriorly onto the coronoid process of the mandible. The temporomandibular ligament bridges the posterior zygomatic arch and the lateral aspect of the condylar neck, reinforcing the lateral joint capsule. The sphenomandibular and stylomandibular ligaments are located medial and posterior to the TMJ, respectively.

IMAGING PROTOCOLS FOR THE TEMPOROMANDIBULAR JOINT

Direct sagittal images through the TMJ are acquired with the use of a small (7.5 cm [3 inch]) diameter surface coil placed over the region of interest (Fig. 12-2). A high signal-to-noise ratio is achieved by using thin (3 mm) sections, a 12 cm field of view, a 256 × 256 acquisition matrix, and one to two excitations. Axial and coronal images, if obtained, are used as localizers for the sagittal plane acquisition. Oblique prescription lines, oriented in a anteromedial to posterolateral direction, are placed on the axial localizer (Fig. 12-3). A bilateral surface coil setup is used. Oblique images

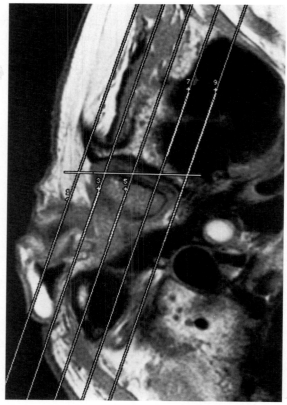

FIGURE 12-3. Oblique sagittal images perpendicular to the long axis of the condylar head as visualized on a T1-weighted axial image. The condylar heads normally angle medially from 15° to 30°.

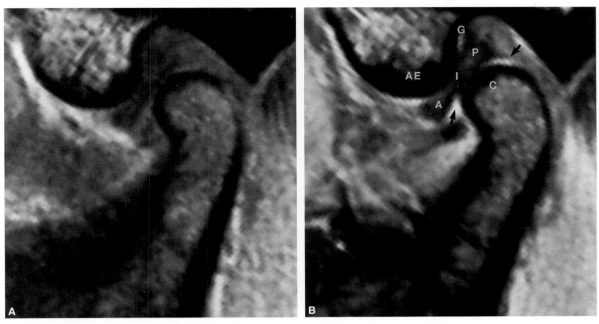

FIGURE 12-4. (A) T1-weighted sagittal image obtained at 3 mm using a 10 cm FOV. (B) Corresponding fat-suppressed T2-weighted fast spin-echo image demonstrating hyperintense joint fluid (*arrows*). G, glenoid fossa; AE, articular eminence of the temporal bone; A, anterior band; I, intermediate zone; P, posterior band; C, condylar head.

can also be prescribed from a coronal localizer, to properly elongate the mandibular condyle. Coronal sequences may be used to improve visualization of medial or lateral disc displacements, especially when there is no component of anterior displacement.[29,40]

A series of sagittal images can provide information about medial and lateral disc position without a separate coronal acquisition. Routine imaging is obtained using a T1-weighted protocol with a repetition time (TR) of 600 msec and echo time (TE) of 17 to 20 msec. A conventional T2-weighted sequence can highlight joint effusions with bright signal intensity, but this doubles imaging time and is not routinely used. With fast spin-echo and fat-suppressed T2-weighted fast spin-echo techniques, delineation of the disc and associated joint effusions is improved and the required imaging time is less than is required by conventional spin-echo imaging[41] (Fig. 12-4). Partial flip-angle fast-scan techniques permit the acquisition of T2*-weighted images of the TMJ in a fraction of the time needed for conventional spin-echo techniques.[28] Using multiplanar gradient-echo software (MPGR; General Electric, Milwaukee, WI), we have used T2* gradient refocused images with a TR of 400 msec, TE of 15 to 20 msec, and a flip angle of 30°.

Gradient-echo three-dimensional Fourier transform volume imaging provides thin section capability in bilateral examinations with the option to reformat images retrospectively in other imaging planes.[42] Gradient-echo techniques are also used in kinematic protocols, which use the Burnett mouth positioning device and display images in the simulated cine mode, to evaluate the TMJ throughout the spectrum of closed- to open-mouth positions. On gradient-echo

imaging, a flow phenomenon within the superficial temporal artery may simulate a loose body.[43] This is seen as a low signal intensity area posterosuperior to the mandibular con-

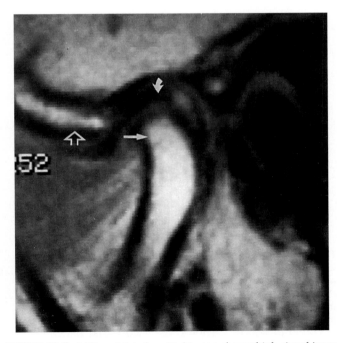

FIGURE 12-5. A T1-weighted sagittal image shows high signal intensity yellow marrow in the articular eminence (*open arrow*) and mandibular condyle (*straight arrow*). The posterior band is located in the expected position, superior to the condylar head (*curved arrow*) (TR, 1000 msec; TE, 40 msec).

dyle. A high signal intensity core mimicking marrow signal may also be seen within the signal void. Contrast enhancement (using dynamic MR imaging) of the posterior disc attachment is associated with joint pain and nonreducing anterior disc displacement.[44]

Simultaneous, bilateral imaging of the TMJ is possible with coil designs that eliminate the need for separate unilateral studies[44,45] (see Fig. 12-2). Although many dentists find studies of only the affected or symptomatic side acceptable, others prefer to routinely evaluate both sides because of the known incidence of bilateral involvement in internal disc derangements. There has been some controversy concerning the position of the mouth (ie, closed, partially open, or open) for optimal MR evaluation of TMJ disc displacements.[46] Advocates of the partially open-mouth position feel that the morphology of the TMJ meniscus is not as distorted in this position as it is in the closed-mouth position. In the closed-mouth position, the articular disc may become compressed between the articular eminence of the temporal bone and the condyle. In studies comparing closed- and partially open-mouth positions, it was found that up to one third of patients inadvertently reduce the meniscus with partial mouth opening.[47,48] Therefore, we routinely evaluate the meniscus in the closed-mouth position. The TMJ is also routinely evaluated in a full open-mouth position to verify meniscal reductions. Although disc reduction is frequently evident on clinical examination, full open– and closed-mouth studies are needed to document meniscus position and degree of reduction in many cases of chronic meniscal derangements. If time permits only one acquisition, then closed-mouth imaging eliminates the possibility of a recaptured disc during forward translation of the condyle.

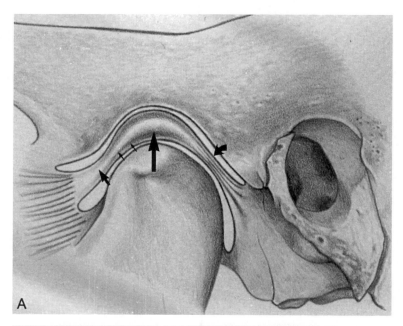

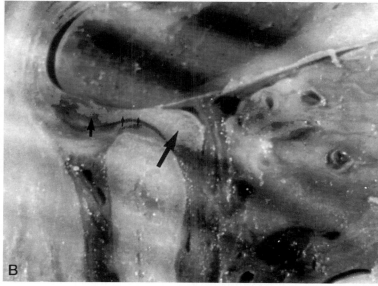

FIGURE 12-6. (**A**) Normal relationships of the temporomandibular joint meniscus to joint landmarks in the closed-mouth position. The posterior band (*large arrow*) is in the 12-o'clock position, superior to the condylar head. The intermediate zone (*small arrows*) is between the articular eminence and the condylar head, and the anterior band (*medium arrow*) is anterior to the condyle and attached to the lateral pterygoid muscle. The bilaminar attachment is seen posteriorly (*curved arrow*). (**B**) A gross anatomic section in the open-mouth position reveals the thick posterior band (*large arrow*), the thin intermediate zone (*small arrows*), and the anterior band (*medium arrow*).

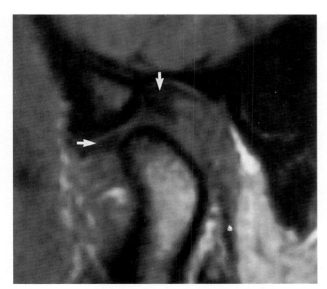

FIGURE 12-7. On a T1-weighted image, the intact TMJ meniscus appears with a central region of intermediate signal intensity in the posterior band (*vertical arrow*). The anterior band demonstrates uniform dark signal intensity (*horizontal arrow*) (TR, 600 msec; TE, 20 msec).

NORMAL MAGNETIC RESONANCE ANATOMY OF THE TEMPOROMANDIBULAR JOINT

Sagittal Images

The articular eminence of the temporal bone and the condyle of the mandible, the bony support of the TMJ, demonstrate the high signal intensity of fatty marrow (Fig. 12-5). Cortical bone, which is of low spin density (ie, dark signal intensity), displays a uniform surface on the condylar head, glenoid fossa, and articular eminence.

The TMJ meniscus is composed of type I collagen, elastic fibers, and glycosaminoglycans.[37,39] It is positioned on the superior surface of the condyle. The disc demonstrates low or dark signal intensity on T1-, T2-, and T2*-weighted images, whereas synovium in the superior or inferior joint spaces demonstrates intermediate signal intensity.

The articular disc is composed of three parts: an anterior band, a thin intermediate zone, and a thicker posterior band[14-22] (Fig. 12-6). Although all three parts of the normal biconcave disc demonstrate low signal intensity, it is not unusual to see a central portion of intermediate signal intensity in the posterior band (Fig. 12-7). The anterior band, positioned in front of the condyle, is anchored to the superior head of the lateral pterygoid muscle, which demonstrates intermediate signal intensity, by tendinous fibers, which demonstrate low signal intensity. The oblique orientation of the lateral pterygoid tends to direct most meniscal displacements in an anteromedial path. The thin intermediate zone is located between the low signal intensity cortical surfaces of the articular eminence and condylar head. The intermediate zone, also referred to as the weight-bearing zone, maintains a consistent relationship to the condyle and temporal eminence during transla-

tion. The thick posterior band is attached to a vascularized bilaminar zone in the retrodiscal tissue complex, which is anchored to the temporal bone (Fig. 12-8). Within the bilaminar zone, a parallel band of low signal intensity may be distinguished, demarcating superior and inferior fibers of the bilaminar zone. The transition between the posterior band and the bilaminar retrodiscal complex may be marked by a vertical line of intermediate signal intensity[49] (Fig. 12-9). In the closed-mouth position, the posterior band occupies a 12-o'clock location in relation to the condylar head. Mild asymmetry between the condylar positions of the articular disc is common (see Fig. 12-9). In the open-mouth position, with forward translation and posterior disc rotation, the posterior band may be seen just dorsal to the 12-o'clock location. The articular disc defines and separates the upper and lower joint compartments. Capsular signal intensity is difficult to differentiate from joint synovial tissue.

Coronal Images

Coronal plane images, which are less frequently used, best demonstrate the articular disc in the plane of section through the posterior band in the closed-mouth position[50] (Fig. 12-10). Although coronal images do not adequately define the anatomy of the intermediate zone, they are preferred for demonstrating the medial and lateral boundaries of the joint capsule, disc displacement, and the lateral supporting tem-

text continues on page 1004

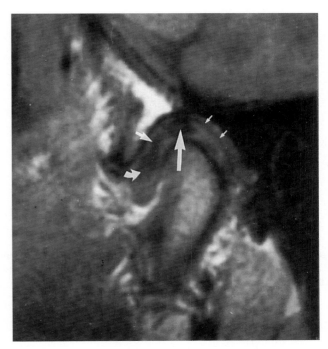

FIGURE 12-8. A T1-weighted image of normal meniscus anatomy shows the anterior band (*curved arrow*), the intermediate zone (*medium straight arrow*), the posterior band (*large straight arrow*), and a low signal intensity band within the bilaminar zone (*small straight arrows*) (TR, 600 msec; TE, 20 msec).

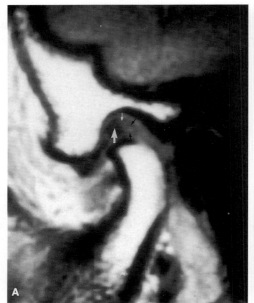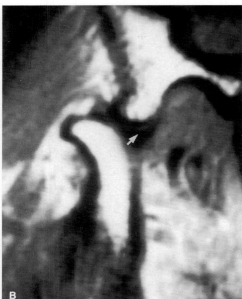

FIGURE 12-9. Disc anatomy. **(A)** In the closed-mouth position, the posterior band (*large white arrow*) is in the 11-o'clock position. A vertical transition between the posterior band and the bilaminar zone can be seen (*small white arrow*). The locations of the superior and inferior bilaminar fibers are also shown (*small black arrows*). **(B)** Normal anterior translation of the condyle relative to the articular eminence occurs in the open-mouth (30-mm) position. The posterior band (*arrow*) can be seen.

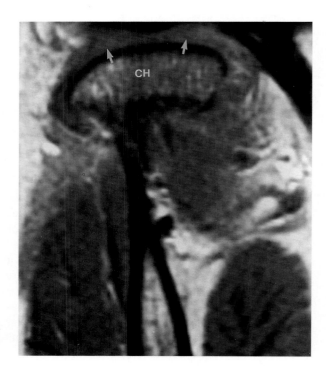

FIGURE 12-10. A T1-weighted coronal image through the condylar head (CH) shows the normal tissue of the posterior disc attachment (*arrows*). There is no lateral or medial disc displacement.

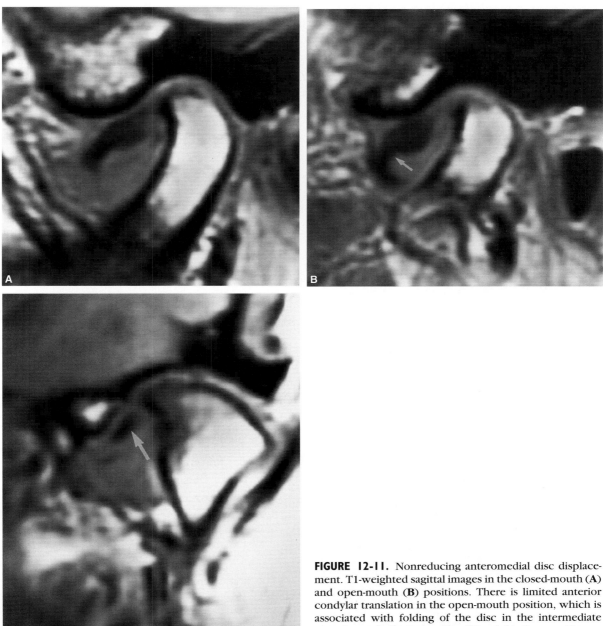

FIGURE 12-11. Nonreducing anteromedial disc displacement. T1-weighted sagittal images in the closed-mouth (**A**) and open-mouth (**B**) positions. There is limited anterior condylar translation in the open-mouth position, which is associated with folding of the disc in the intermediate zone (*arrow*). Corresponding T1-weighted coronal image (**C**) identifies component of medial disc displacement (*arrow*) not appreciated on sagittal images.

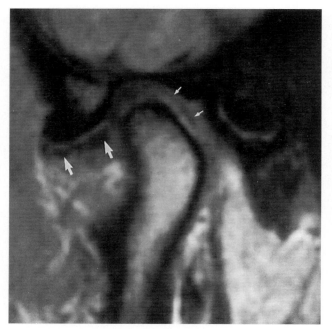

FIGURE 12-12. Complete anterior displacement of the temporomandibular joint meniscus (*large arrows*) on a T1-weighted image. The anterior band, intermediate zone, and posterior band are all anterior to the condylar head. The retrodiscal bilaminar zone (*small arrows*) is seen (TR, 600 msec; TE, 20 msec)

poromandibular ligament (Fig. 12-11). Images through the anterior TMJ display the lateral pterygoid muscle and the more inferior medial pterygoid muscle. The low signal intensity maxillary vessels encased in fat can be seen lateral to the pterygoid muscles and medial to the mandible.

PATHOLOGY OF THE TEMPOROMANDIBULAR JOINT

Internal Derangements

Internal derangements of the TMJ may present with localized pain and tenderness, clicking, joint crepitus, and limited opening of the mouth. The location of the posterior band is used to define the location and degree of disc displacement.

Meniscal Displacement

Internal derangements usually involve anteromedial displacement of the meniscus relative to the condylar head and temporal fossa[14–22,51–53] (Figs. 12-12 and 12-13). Trauma, degeneration, ligamentous laxity, and retrodiscal rents can be contributing factors. Such an anteriorly positioned disc blocks normal forward translation of the condyle, and the patient may present clinically with limited jaw opening and deviation of the mandible toward the affected side.

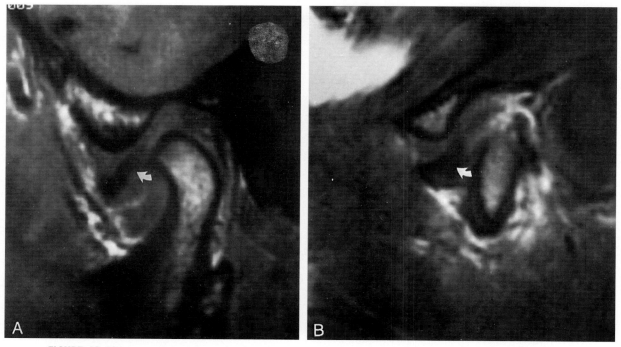

FIGURE 12-13. Anterolateral disc displacement is less common than anterior displacement. The meniscus (*curved arrows*) is located anterior to (**A**) and medial to (**B**) the condylar head.

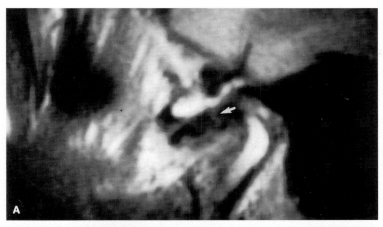

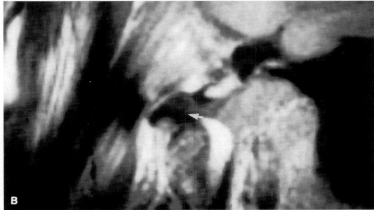

FIGURE 12-14. Anterior disc (ie, meniscus) displacement is seen in the closed-mouth (**A**) and open-mouth (**B**) positions. Secondary changes of disc remodeling with disc flexion, intermediate zone shortening, and enlargement of the posterior band (*arrows*) are present. Intermediate signal intensity in the area of the posterior band represents fibrosis, myxomatous change, and fluid.

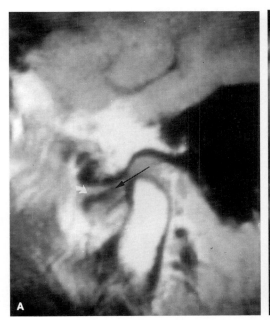

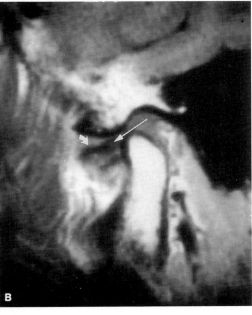

FIGURE 12-15. Remodeling of anterior disc displacement. Irreducible anterior disc displacement (*straight arrows*) is seen in the closed-mouth (**A**) and open-mouth (**B**) positions. Note the limitation of anterior translation relative to the articular eminence. Remodeling, foreshortening, and upward flexion of the intermediate zone (*curved arrows*) are present.

Displacement of the posterior band may be partial or complete, depending on the relative position of the disc between the condyle and articular eminence and on the area of contact between the posterior band and the condyle. The posterior attachment or bilaminar zone also translates anteriorly and is subjected to increased loading between the condyle and articular eminence.

Secondary remodeling may alter the morphology and signal intensity of the abnormally located posterior band, causing enlargement of a portion of the posterior band with associated foreshortening of the intermediate zone[39,54] (Fig. 12-14). Flexion of the disc and remodeling may also be seen in the intermediate zone (Fig. 12-15). More advanced changes include fibrosis of the posterior attachment and loss of the normally distinct anterior and posterior band morphology. Displaced discs display surface irregularities, including fissuring, fibrillation, and fraying, all of which are easily identified on routine MR evaluation. Dystrophic calcification, neovascularization, and perforations may also be associated with internal disc derangements. When remodeling is insufficient to accommodate increased loading of the disc and posterior detachment, the result may be pain, additional disc deformity, and increased susceptibility to injury. The addition of a medial or lateral pull to an anteriorly displaced disc contributes to a more complex rotational displacement.

An opening click is usually associated with reduction of the thick posterior band recaptured by the condylar head in the open-mouth position (Figs. 12-16 and 12-17). This audible or palpable click is often associated with relief of pain as the condyle successfully passes under the posterior band (Fig. 12-18). Less frequently, a reciprocal click occurs during closure, as the posterior band redislocates, anterior to the condyle. The elastic fibers of the bilaminar zone are unable to retract the disc as the condyle moves posteriorly during closing of the mouth. With stretching of the bilaminar zone, the condyle pushes forward to augment the disc during anterior translation and does not pass under the posterior band, therefore, no click is produced (Fig. 12-19).

When the jaw is locked in the closed-mouth position (ie, closed-lock derangement), the meniscus is displaced in both closed- and open-mouth positions, preventing anterior condylar motion (Fig. 12-20). In a closed-lock derangement, early deformations of the disc may be seen during partial mouth opening, which compresses the displaced disc (Fig. 12-21). Eventually, disc deformity is seen in the closed-mouth position, and is characterized by the loss of biconcavity, disc folding, perforation, and a further decrease in disc signal intensity secondary to fibrosis and dystrophic calcification. Thickening of the bilaminar zone directly over the condyle may mimic the appearance of a normal posterior band (Fig. 12-22). With more severe stretching of the bilami-

text continues on page 1011

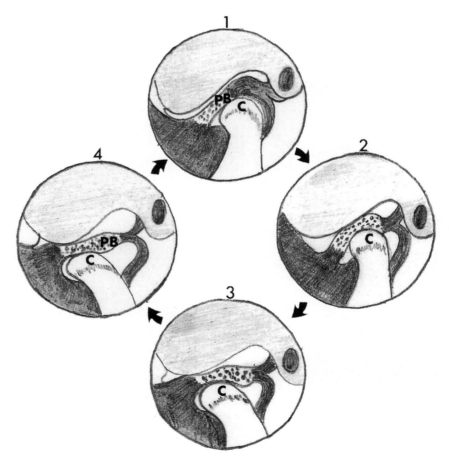

FIGURE 12-16. Progressive stages (1 to 4) of condylar translation, with anterior displaced disc (3) and recapture (4). PB, posterior band; C, condylar head.

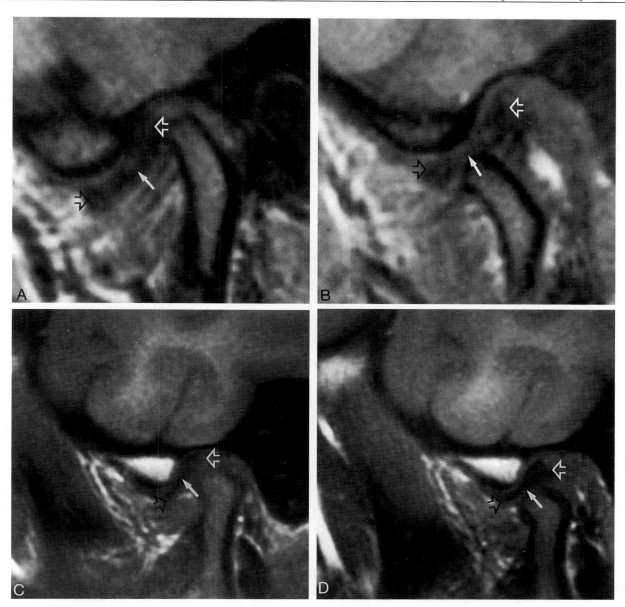

FIGURE 12-17. Disk displacement. (**A, C**) Two examples of an anterior displaced TMJ meniscus as seen in the closed-mouth position. (**B, D**) Recapture of the disc occurs in the open-mouth position. The anterior band (*open black arrows*), intermediate zone (*solid arrows*), and posterior band (*open white arrows*) are seen. In the closed-mouth position, the posterior band is anterior to the condylar head. In the open-mouth position with reduction, the posterior band is directly superior to the condylar head.

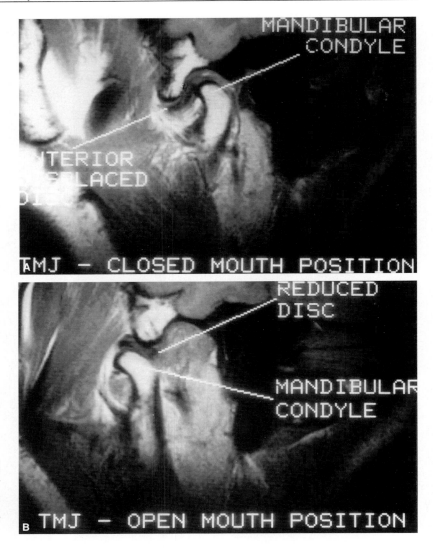

FIGURE 12-18. Reduction of the anterior displaced disc in the closed-mouth (**A**) and open-mouth (**B**) positions. The bilaminar zone is in the 12-o'clock position, the expected normal location of the posterior band. There is adequate anterior translation of the condylar head.

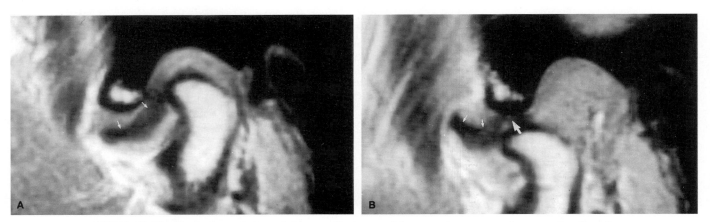

FIGURE 12-19. Blocked translation of the mandibular condyle secondary to complete anterior disc displacement (*small arrows*), as seen in the closed-mouth (**A**) and open-mouth (**B**) positions. A portion of disc tissue (*large arrow*) is identified between the articular eminence and condylar head in the attempted open-mouth position. The bilaminar zone is stretched and no opening click was present during mouth opening.

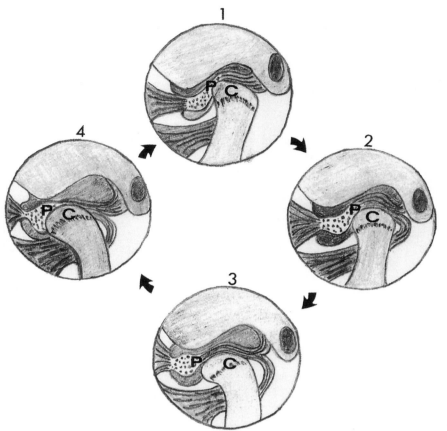

FIGURE 12-20. Deformity of anterior displaced disc occurs with progressive anterior translation (1 to 4). There is no recapture in the closed-mouth (1) and open-mouth (4) positions. P, posterior band; C, condylar head.

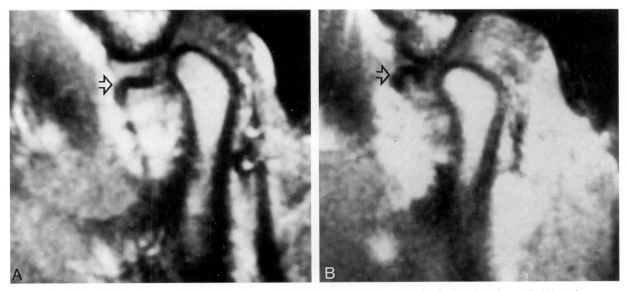

FIGURE 12-21. A nonreducible anteriorly displaced meniscus is seen in both the closed-mouth (**A**) and open-mouth (**B**) positions. Limited condylar translation and deformity of the meniscus is demonstrated in the open-mouth position (**B**). There is loss of normal biconcave disc morphology and irregular folding in the anterior portion (ie, intermediate zone; *arrow*).

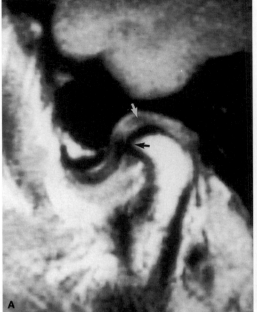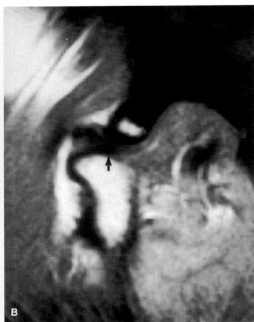

FIGURE 12-22. (A) An anteriorly displaced disc (*black arrow*) is seen in the closed-mouth position with early remodeling and thickening of the bilaminar zone (*white arrow*). (B) The disc is reduced in the open-mouth position (*arrow*).

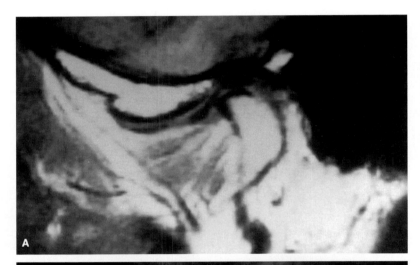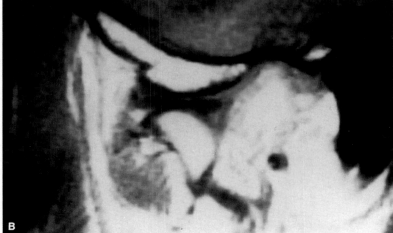

FIGURE 12-23. A grade zero disc shows normal morphology and position of the anterior band, the intermediate zone, and the posterior band in the closed-mouth (A) and open-mouth (B) positions. Grading of disc displacement is independent of disc recapture.

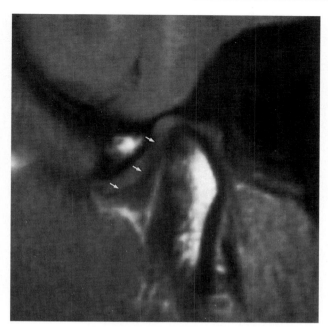

FIGURE 12-24. A T1-weighted image shows grade 1 displacement of the disc with intact morphology (*arrows*) (TR, 600 msec; TE, 20 msec).

nar zone, there may be some degree of anterior condylar translation without contact with the anteriorly displaced disc, giving the clinical appearance of improved mouth opening. In this stage of derangement, however, advanced disc deformity and degeneration are present.

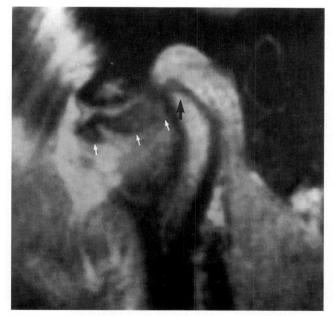

FIGURE 12-25. Grade 1 displacement of the disc (*white arrows*) may show grossly intact morphology, although the intermediate zone is flexed and foreshortened. The condylar head with overlying retrodiscal tissue (*black arrow*) is seen. Normal intermediate signal intensity is present in the posterior band.

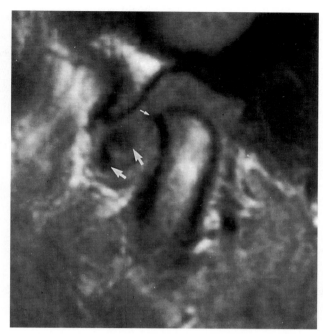

FIGURE 12-26. Grade 2 meniscal derangement with complete loss of normal morphology is seen on a T1-weighted image. The meniscus is redundant compressed anterior to the condylar head (*large arrows*). Associated degenerative change is seen as a low signal intensity anterior osteophyte (*small arrow*) (TR, 600 msec; TE, 20 msec).

A grading system for characterizing disc displacements by morphology has been developed.[48,55,56] The normally positioned meniscus (ie, grade 0; Fig. 12-23) has a drumstick contour and may have a bull's-eye or target region of intermediate signal intensity in the posterior band. In grade 1 meniscal displacement, the meniscus maintains a normal morphology (Figs. 12-24 and 12-25). Abnormal disc morphology (ie, loss of the drumstick shape) represents a grade 2 displacement (Fig. 12-26). A grade 2 meniscus is most likely to be associated with degenerative joint disease, and may not be repairable at surgery. The higher grades of internal disc derangements appear to correlate not only with degenerative joint disease, but also with severity of pain, chronicity, and restriction of joint motion.

A more subjective evaluation of disc displacement includes the observation of decreased posterior band signal intensity relative to the anterior band and intermediate zone. These signal changes are seen in more advanced displacements, especially in association with degenerative joint disease.

With MR imaging, it is possible to both identify a displaced meniscus and to evaluate the severity of the derangement. As a result, it may be used to monitor potential responses to therapy.

In addition to classification by grade, disc displacements may also be classified as acute, subacute, or chronic.[57] Acute displacement is characterized by recapture of the disc in the open-mouth position without alteration in disc size or

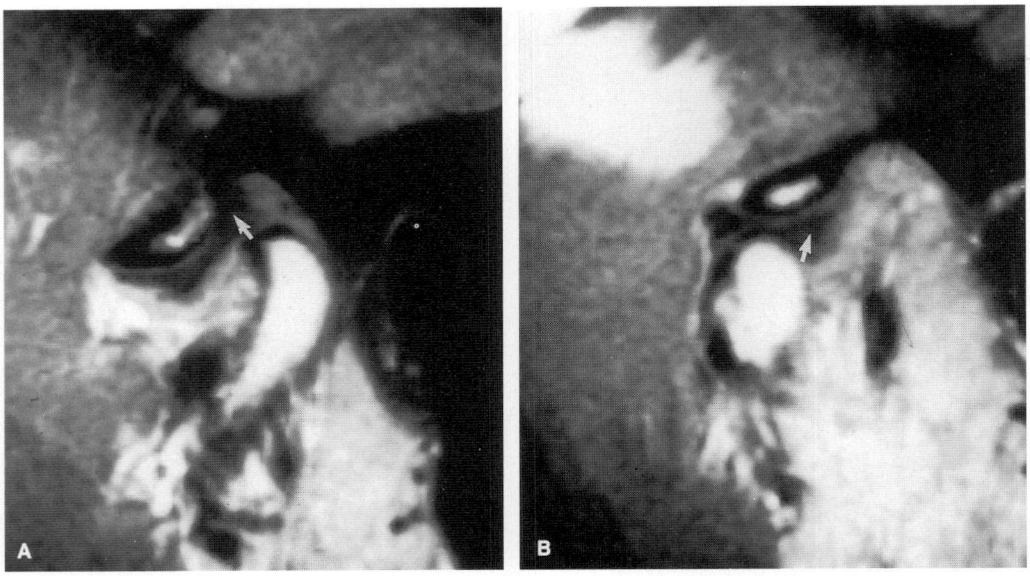

FIGURE 12-27. (A) Acute anterior disc displacement (*arrow*) is seen in closed-mouth centric occlusion, in which there is maximal intercuspation (ie, contact) between opposing occlusal surfaces (*arrows*). (B) The posterior band is in its normal location in the open-mouth position. Normal disc morphology is maintained in closed- and open-mouth positions.

morphology (Fig. 12-27). In subacute displacement, the displaced disc does not reduce with mouth opening and may show signs of deformity, such as folding or flexion atrophy of the anterior band and thickening of the posterior band (Fig. 12-28). In chronic disc displacement, disc perforation, adhesions, fibrosis, and degenerative joint disease may be present.

Scarring or adhesions within the TMJ demonstrate intermediate signal intensity on both T1- and T2-weighted images. In contrast, joint fluid is of high signal intensity on T2-weighted images. Engorged veins in the vascular pterygoid attachments may mimic upper and lower joint compartment fluid and result in a false-positive diagnosis of effusion.

Stuck or Adherent Disc

The stuck or adherent disc does not change position with jaw opening,[58] and remains fixed, relative to the articular eminence and glenoid fossa, in both closed- and open-mouth positions. Adherent discs are caused by pathologic changes in the chemistry of synovial fluid, leading to changes in the TMJ intraarticular pressure. Loss of disc mobility is thought to be associated with the development of intracapsular adhe-

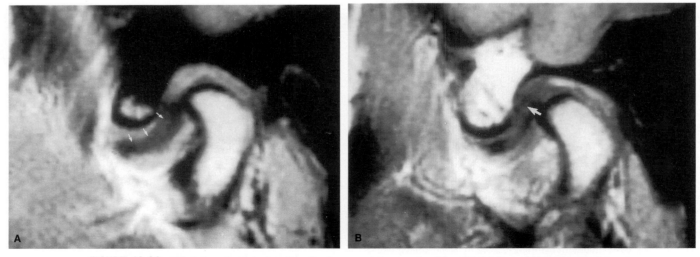

FIGURE 12-28. (A) Subacute anterior disc displacement (*arrows*) with mild folding of the intermediate zone is seen in the closed-mouth position. (B) The disc is not recaptured in the open-mouth position (*arrow*).

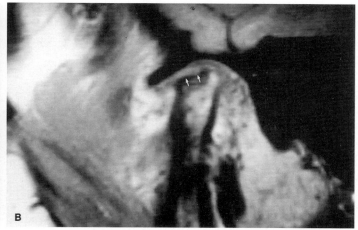

FIGURE 12-29. Degenerative osteoarthritis results in an absent-macerated disc with flattening of the condylar head (*white arrows*) and subchondral low signal intensity sclerosis, as seen in the closed-mouth (**A**) and open-mouth (**B**) positions. Anterior translation is unimpeded (*black arrow*) due to the absent disc.

sions. Abnormal mobility is associated with clinical TMJ dysfunction—limitation of condylar translation results in restricted jaw opening—even when the disc is located in a normal position. Rao and colleagues[58] documented that 20% of joints with the disc in a normal position are actually stuck or adherent.

Synovial adhesions, and the thicker dense fibrous adhesions, can be directly visualized and treated arthroscopically. The majority of stuck discs (71%) demonstrate limited condylar translation as defined by the posterior position of the condyle relative to the articular eminence in the open-mouth position. Since the disc may be stuck in either a normal or displaced position, treatment protocols may need to be modified or changed with respect to attempting to recapture a nonmobile disc. Disc mobility cannot be assessed in the absence of any condylar translation (ie, when the joint is frozen).

Rao and coworkers have proposed a MR classification that incorporates disc mobility and characterizes the normally positioned disc as either mobile, stuck, or associated with a frozen joint.[58] A displaced disc position can be classified as mobile with recapture, mobile without recapture, stuck with recapture, stuck without recapture, or associated with a frozen joint with no condylar translation.

Disc Perforations

Perforations of the meniscus are more difficult to identify on MR images than in arthrograms.[33] With arthrography, a small disc perforation may be demonstrated by communication of contrast material between the superior and inferior joint recesses. However, false-positive rates as high as 20% have been reported with arthrography. In addition, the majority of these perforations are associated with a displaced meniscus that would be detected by MR imaging.

Degenerative Osseous Findings

Degenerative osseous changes associated with disc derangements include sclerosis and an uneven or attenuated cortical surface in the condylar head, articular eminence, and fossa. Flattening of the condylar head and anterior osteophytes are demonstrated on sagittal images (Fig. 12-29). The normally high signal intensity fatty marrow is replaced with low signal intensity subchondral sclerosis on T1-, T2-, and T2*-weighted images (Fig. 12-30). Changes associated with advanced osteoarthritis include bony ankylosis, fibrous an-

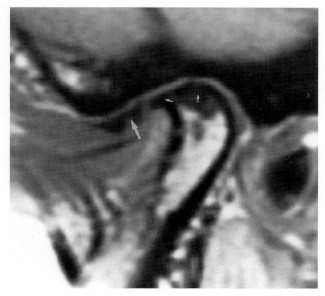

FIGURE 12-30. Low signal intensity subchondral sclerosis is identified in the condylar head and anterior osteophyte (*small arrows*). Anterior displaced disc is shown (*large arrow*).

kylosis, and avascular necrosis of the mandibular condyle. Fibrous tissue decreases the internal signal intensity of normal joint synovium.

Clinical Evaluation and Treatment

The patient presenting with TMJ dysfunction requires comprehensive analysis and careful diagnosis, recognizing the complex multifactorial etiology. If a functional, occlusal, or structural etiology is suspected, the following workup is recommended:

- Submentovertex (base) projection with tomography in the open and closed position (hard tissue evaluation)
- MR imaging in the closed- and open-mouth positions with T1, T2*, or T2-weighted fast spin-echo imaging in the sagittal plane; coronal images are additionally useful in identifying medial and lateral disc displacement
- Lateral cephalometric radiographs and tomograms with two-dimensional analysis; cephalometric techniques take into account the angulations of the condyle with proper head positioning using a head-holder and system of coordinates
- Frontal cephalometric radiographs and tomograms with two-dimensional analysis
- Extraoral and intraoral photographs with a three-dimensional soft-tissue analysis
- Articulated models of the teeth mounted in centric relation.

Conservative treatment often consists of splint therapy that positions the mandible and condyle more anteriorly to recapture the displaced meniscus and to relax the lateral

pterygoid muscle, which may be in spasm. MR studies can be performed both before and after splint application, to assess the location of the TMJ meniscus, and to measure condylar translation (Figs. 12-31 and 12-32). There are numerous types of splints, all designed to fit either on the maxillary upper arch (upper teeth) or the mandibular arch (lower teeth). Most are custom-made to fit the individual, and most splints are temporary. The orthosis most frequently prescribed by dentists is a flat plane stabilizing splint. This type of splint is often constructed on the maxillary arch and worn at night to protect the teeth during possible grinding or clenching of the teeth. Clenching is more detrimental to the TMJ due to the sustained pressure of the condyle directly against the delicate retrodiscal tissue, which is susceptible to injury.

Splints can be made out of various materials. The most commonly used is methylmethacrylate, an acrylic made by mixing a polymer (powder) and a monomer (liquid) together, using either cold or heat curing. The surface of the splint can be modified, by adding or removing acrylic, and is designed to guide the mandible and condyle in three dimensions as the opposing teeth come into contact with the splint surface.

A biotemplate is typically an anatomically constructed splint shaded to match the color of the teeth (Fig. 12-33). It is usually constructed on the mandibular arch for ease of wear and is designed to guide the mandible into a rest position called physiologic centric relation (defined as an un-

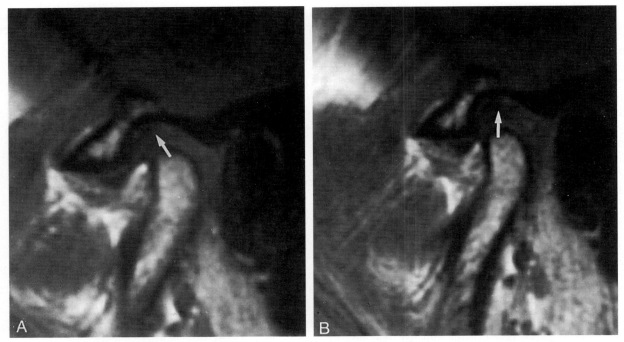

FIGURE 12-31. Splinting of the temporomandibular joint meniscus. **(A)** The posterior band (*arrows*) is seen anterior to the condylar head without the internal splint (ie, mild anterior displacement). **(B)** With insertion of an occlusal splint, the posterior band is positioned directly superior to the condylar head.

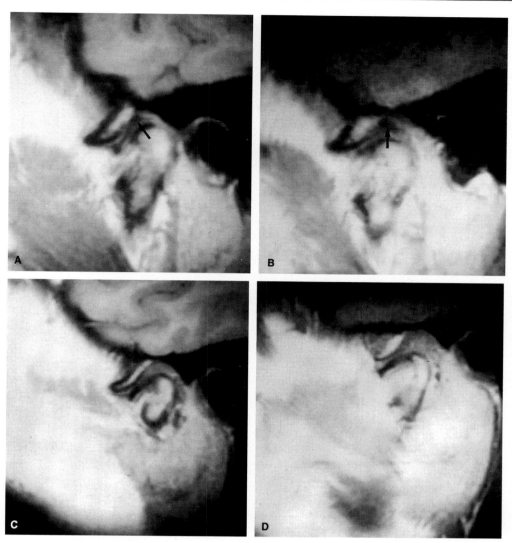

FIGURE 12-32. (A) In the closed-mouth position the posterior band (*arrow*) is in an anterior position in the left temporomandibular joint in a patient without a splint. (B) After placement of an internal splint, the posterior band (*arrow*) is relocated to the 12-o'clock position in the left temporomandibular joint. In the right temporomandibular joint, the disc appears in an anterior position both without (C) and with (D) an internal splint.

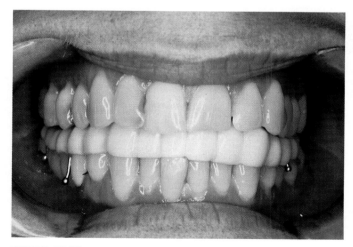

FIGURE 12-33. Biotemplate fitted on the mandibular arch to produce a physiologic centric relation between the glenoid fossa and condylar head.

strained position of the condyle gently seated in the glenoid fossa with the disc in juxtaposition between the condyle and the fossa). Since the surfaces of this type of removable splint can be carefully constructed to function like the surfaces of the teeth, it can be judiciously prescribed for full-time wear for the duration of the therapy.

An important factor in the prescription of any appliance is accurate pretreatment diagnosis as evaluated by corrected tomograms or MR imaging. Complications can develop, for example, in prescribing an appliance such as gnathologic splint without adequate patient evaluation and selection. A gnathologic splint is typically placed on the maxillary arch and is designed with an acrylic surface to guide the mandible into a centric relation. The splint attempts to produce this centric relationship by directing the articular eminence in the most posterior and superior unstrained position of the condyle, symmetrically seated in the glenoid fossa. This type of splint, which functions as the patient bites down, however, should not be used if the disc is anteriorly displaced as documented by MR imaging. If the disc is abnormally posi-

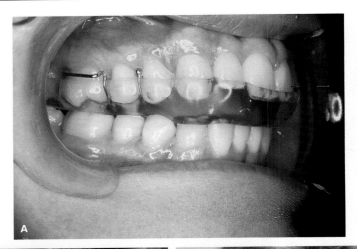

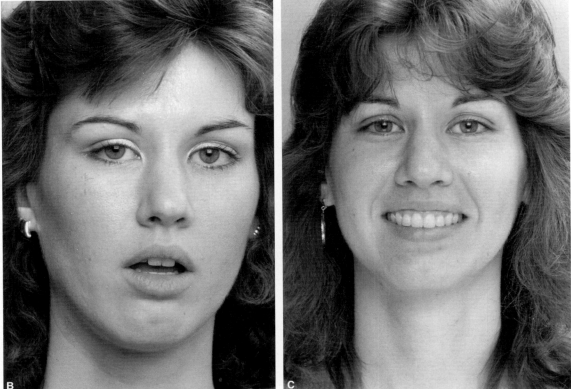

FIGURE 12-34. Complications of splint therapy. Full time use of a gnathologic splint (**A**) for 1 year resulted in the development of a compound bite with resulting mentalis strain (**B**). Orthodontically corrected bite (**C**) was achieved with braces, using a segmental technique—without surgery.

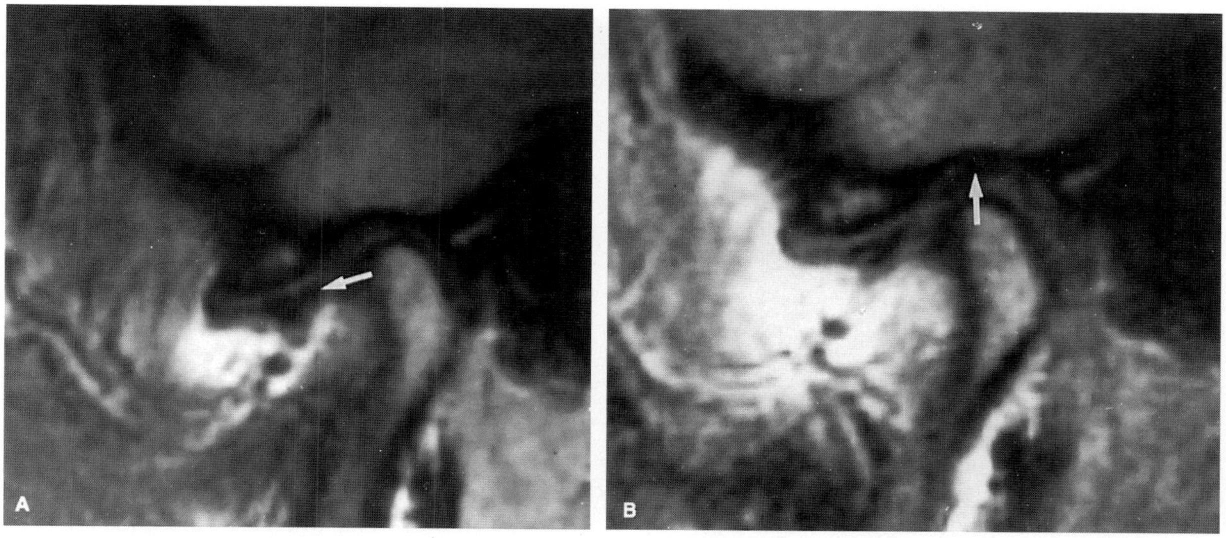

FIGURE 12-35. The temporomandibular joint meniscus (*arrow*) before (**A**) and after (**B**) arthroscopic saline reduction.

tioned, centric positioning of the condyle will not improve TMJ function. Gnathologic splints are indicated in healthy patients without displacement in order to locate a centric relation. In contrast, a biotemplate creates a physiologic rest position. The occlusal surface of this splint can be modified to effectively reposition the condyle and sometimes recapture an acutely displaced disc.

One of the limitations of splint therapy, especially when a gnathologic splint is used full-time for any prolonged period, is the development of malocclusion (Fig. 12-34). For example, a compound open bite can develop, with resulting inability of the teeth to meet together even when the patient is asked to close. Although this can sometimes be corrected orthodontically, using fixed appliances attached to the teeth (braces), orthognathic surgery is often necessary, sometimes in combination with orthodontic treatment. Treatment options are determined by the degree of open bite, and whether it is dental or skeletal.

Sometimes, a displaced disc is treated by an arthroscopic procedure in which saline is injected into the upper compartment to force reduction, and MR imaging has had some limited use for imaging patients undergoing this procedure[59] (Fig. 12-35). However, engorged veins in the vascular pterygoid attachment can mimic upper and lower joint compartment fluid and may result in a false-positive diagnosis of effusion (Fig. 12-36).

Postsurgical plication (Fig. 12-37) and proplast prosthetic replacements for the TMJ meniscus were designed to preserve the normal anatomic relationships of the native disc to the condylar and articular eminences.[60-62] The silastic and proplast/Teflon implants are hypointense on T1-weighted images, but may be associated with a massive surrounding foreign body (giant cell) tissue reaction and

scar formation that is of intermediate signal intensity. In addition, these implants may become fragmented, in which case associated granulation tissue produces condylar head erosions. Because of these complications, which necessitate surgical removal of the disc implant and granulation tissue, TMJ surgery, especially with the use of allo-

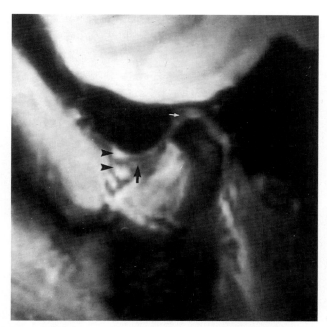

FIGURE 12-36. A T2*-weighted image with high signal intensity in engorged veins (*black arrowheads*) in the lateral pterygoid attachment (*black arrow*) to the temporomandibular joint meniscus. The intact posterior band is seen superior to the condylar head between the 11- and 12-o'clock positions (*white arrow*) (TR, 400 msec; TE, 30 msec; flip angle, 30°).

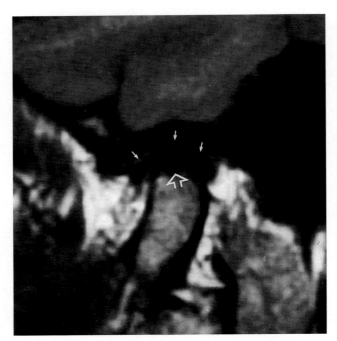

FIGURE 12-37. Postsurgical primary plication of the temporomandibular joint meniscus in the normal position (*small arrows*). A focus of low signal intensity subchondral sclerosis (*open arrow*) can be seen.

plastic disc implants, is generally discouraged.[63] The majority of TMJ dysfunctions should be managed conservatively. Patients may regain relatively normal TMJ function with adequate condylar translation despite the presence of a chronically anteriorly displaced disc.

Loss of the osseous mandibular condyle morphology may be caused by condylar shaving, condylectomy, pyogenic infection, and arthritis (seronegative and seropositive). A metallic prosthetic condylar head and arthroplasties with complete condylar head, neck, and disc replacements (Kent prosthesis) have also been associated with bone resorption and foreign body reactions (Fig. 12-38). The Kent prosthesis has been withdrawn by the FDA, mainly due to the breakdown of the Teflon coating and subsequent giant cell reaction to the breakdown fragments. Teflon could not withstand the pressure generated by the functioning of the TMJ.

Trauma

Mandible fractures include fractures of the condylar head, neck, and process and fractures of the mandibular ramus, angle, body, and symphysis.[63] Fractures of the mandibular condyle are either intracapsular (condylar head) or extracapsular (condyle neck or subcondylar) injuries that present as either nondisplaced or displaced fractures. Malocclusion, TMJ dysfunction, and muscle atrophy are minimized with proper closed or open reduction and internal fixation (for complex fractures). Temporary or short-term interdental fixation followed by early mobilization is often performed in association with closed reduction of the fracture.[63]

In complex fractures about the mandible and TMJ, CT is useful in demonstrating osseous fragments and their degree of displacement.[33,64] In selected cases, MR imaging may provide additional information regarding soft-tissue injury and the integrity of the articular disc (Fig. 12-39). Since forces are transmitted through the condyle, internal derange-

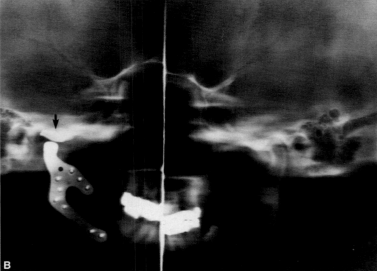

FIGURE 12-38. (**A**) Kent prosthesis with metallic condylar head, neck, and disc replacement. (**B**) The disc component is best visualized on a lateral tomograph (*arrow*). This prosthesis is no longer approved for clinical use.

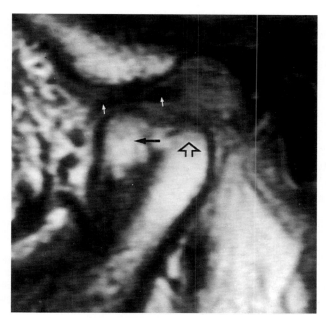

FIGURE 12-39. Pseudo–double-condyle is seen in posttraumatic fracture of the mandibular condyle with displacement of the articular head (*solid black arrow*) anterior to the condylar neck (open black arrow). The associated temporomandibular joint meniscus is seen (*white arrows*).

ment of the TMJ can occur in the absence of fractures. A direct mandibular blow may stretch the meniscus and cause lateral pterygoid spasm and anterior disc displacement. In children, TMJ trauma may result in disruption of the condylar growth center of the jaw.

Arthritis

In the adult, TMJ osteoarthritis may occur as a sequela to trauma and internal disc derangements.[33] The TMJ may also be affected in episodes of gout, rheumatoid arthritis, lupus, or the seronegative arthropathies such as psoriatic arthritis[65] (Fig. 12-40) and ankylosing spondylitis. In the presence of synovitis and articular destruction, the disc is vulnerable to perforation and displacement. MR imaging is more sensitive than conventional radiography (including tomography) for the identification of synovial pannus tissue, which frequently produces condylar erosions. Early detection of synovitis and pannus tissue may correlate with TMJ dysfunction, including limited condylar translation. Administration of intravenous gadolinium causes areas of synovial inflammation to enhance.[66] Changes on radiography—including cartilage loss, bony erosions, joint space narrowing, and subchondral sclerosis—are usually seen in more advanced stages of disease. TMJ pain may be present in the absence of significant appendicular joint involvement.

In osteoarthritis, cortical and articular cartilage thinning, with flattening and deformity of the condylar head,

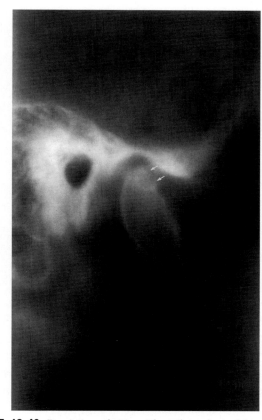

FIGURE 12-40. Psoriatic arthritis with unilateral condylar erosions (*arrows*) shown on lateral tomograph. MR imaging, when clinically appropriate, allows direct visualization of articular cartilage and synovial tissue (pannus).

is seen on MR images. Osteophytes, usually located anteriorly, joint-space narrowing, and erosions of both the temporal eminence and condyle are frequently seen in degenerative joint disease (Figs. 12-41 and 12-42). Extensive subchondral or bony sclerosis in the condylar head, neck, and articular eminence may be seen on both

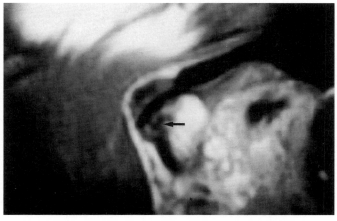

FIGURE 12-41. Mixed sclerosis and fat marrow signal intensity (*arrow*) are seen in a large anterior condylar osteophyte.

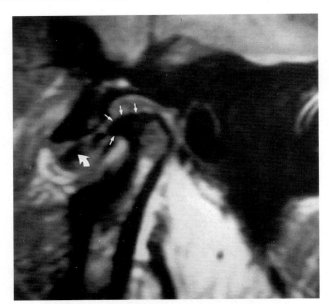

FIGURE 12-42. A low signal intensity large anterior osteophyte (*straight arrows*). Associated anterior meniscal displacement is also present (*curved arrow*).

T1- and T2-weighted images as areas of diffuse low signal intensity (Fig. 12-43). Low signal intensity may also represent the development of avascular necrosis.[61] Joint effusions, articular erosions, and synovial proliferation are all identifiable on T1- and T2-weighted images. On T2-weighted images, hyperplastic synovium and pannus demonstrate intermediate signal intensity, not the high signal intensity seen with associated fluid.

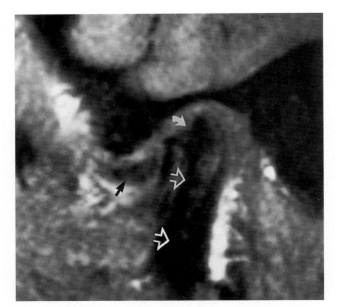

FIGURE 12-43. Low signal intensity degenerative sclerosis (*open arrows*) in the mandibular condyle. The anterior displaced meniscus (*black arrow*) and articular head deformity (*curved arrow*) are shown.

Rarely, the TMJ is a site of cartilaginous metaplasia in synovial chondromatosis[32] and MR images are characterized by small calcifications and an associated soft-tissue mass. Tumors involving the TMJ may present with clinical findings that initially mimic disc pathology (eg, pain, limitation of jaw opening, malocclusion, and facial asymmetry).

References

1. Jacobs JM, Manaster BJ. Digital subtraction arthrography of the temporomandibular joint. AJR 1987;148:344.
2. Kaplan PA, et al. Inferior joint space arthrography of normal temporomandibular joints: reassessment of diagnostic criteria. Radiology 1986;159:585.
3. Kaplan PA, et al. Temporomandibular joint arthrography following surgical treatment of internal derangements. Radiology 1987;163:217.
4. Kaplan PA, et al. Temporomandibular joint arthrography of normal subjects: prevalence of pain with ionic versus nonionic contrast agents. Radiology 1985;156:825.
5. Katzberg RW, et al. Temporomandibular joint arthrography: comparison of morbidity with ionic and low osmolality contrast media. Radiology 1985;155:245.
6. Ross JB. Arthrography compared with MRI for TMJ intracapsular soft tissue diagnosis. TMJ Update 1989;7:31.
7. Duvoisin B, Klaus E, Schnyder P. Coronal radiographs and videofluoroscopy improve the diagnostic quality of temporomandibular joint arthrography. AJR 1990;155:105.
8. Christiansen EL, et al. Correlative thin section temporomandibular joint anatomy and computed tomography. RadioGraphics 1986;6:703.
9. Christiansen EL, et al. CT number characteristics of malpositioned TMJ menisci: diagnosis with CT number highlighting (blinkmode). Invest Radiol 1987;22:315.
10. Larheim TA, Kolbenstvedt A. High resolution computed tomography of the osseous temporomandibular joint. Radiology 1985;157:573.
11. Swartz JD, et al. High-resolution computed tomography. Part V: evaluation of the temporomandibular joint. Radiology 1986;159:823.
12. Manco LG, et al. Internal derangements of the temporomandibular joint evaluated with direct sagittal CT: prospective study. Radiology 1985;157:407.
13. Helms CA, Kaplan P. Diagnostic imaging of the temporomandibular joint: recommendations for use of various techniques. AJR 1990;154:319.
14. Kneeland JB, et al. High-resolution MR imaging using loop-gap resonators. Radiology 1986;158:247.
15. Middleton WD, et al. High resolution surface coil magnetic resonance imaging of the joints: anatomic correlation. RadioGraphics 1987;7:645.
16. Helms CA, et al. Magnetic resonance imaging of internal derangement of the temporomandibular joint. Radiol Clin North Am 1986;24:189.
17. Harms SE, Wilf RM. Magnetic resonance imaging of the temporomandibular joint. RadioGraphics 1987;7:521.
18. Katzberg RW, et al. Normal and abnormal temporomandibular joint: MR imaging with surface coil. Radiology 1986;158:183.
19. Westesson P, et al. Temporomandibular joint: comparison of MR images with cryosectional anatomy. Radiology 1987;164:59.
20. Robers D, et al. Temporomandibular joint: magnetic resonance imaging. Radiology 1985;154:829.
21. Harms SE, et al. Temporomandibular joint: magnetic resonance imaging using surface coils. Radiology 1985;157:133.
22. Laurell KA, et al. Magnetic resonance imaging of the temporomandibular joint. Part 1: literature review. J Prosthet Dent 1987;58:83.
23. Kaplan P, Helms C. Current status of temporomandibular joint imaging for the diagnosis of internal derangements. AJR 1989;152:697.

24. Hansson L, Westesson P, Katzberg RW, et al. MR imaging of the temporomandibular joint: comparison of images of autopsy specimens made at 0.3 T and 1.5 T with anatomic cryosections. AJR 1989;152.

25. Fulmer JM, Harms SE. The temporomandibular joint. Top Magn Reson Imaging 1989;1:75.

26. Rao VM, Farole A, Karasick D. Temporomandibular joint dysfunction: correlation of MR imaging, arthrography, and arthroscopy. Radiology 1990;174:663.

27. Burnett KR, et al. Dynamic display of the temporomandibular joint meniscus by using "fast-scan" MR imaging. AJR 1987;149:959.

28. Stoller DW, et al. Fast MR improves imaging of the musculoskeletal system. Diagnostic Imaging 1988;98.

29. Tasaki MM, Westesson P-L. Temporomandibular joint: diagnostic accuracy with sagittal and coronal MR imaging. Radiology 1993;186:723.

30. Manco LG, DeLuke DM. CT diagnosis of synovial chondromatosis of the temporomandibular joint. AJR 1987;148:574.

31. Kneeland JB, et al. Failed temporomandibular joint prostheses: MR imaging. Radiology 1987;165:179.

32. Nokes ST, et al. Temporomandibular joint chondromatosis with intracranial extension: MR and CT contributions. AJR 1987;148:1173.

33. Murphy WA. The temporomandibular joint. In: Resnick D, Niwayama G, eds. Diagnosis of bone and joint disorders, 2nd ed, vol 3. Philadelphia: WB Saunders, 1988.

34. Schellhas KP. Temporomandibular joint injuries. Radiology 1989;173:211.

35. Larheim TA, Smith HJ, Aspestrand F. Rheumatic disease of the temporomandibular joint: MR imaging and tomographic manifestations. Radiology 1990;175:527.

36. Schellhas KP, Wilkes C. Temporomandibular joint inflammation: comparison of MR fast scanning with T1- and T2-weighted imaging techniques. AJR 1989;153:93.

37. Shannon M, et al. MR of the normal temporomandibular joint. In: Palacios E, et al, eds. Magnetic resonance of the temporomandibular joint. Stuttgart/New York: Thieme, 1990:48.

38. Katzberg RW, Westesson P, Rallents RH, et al. Temporomandibular joint: MR assessment of rotational and sideways disc displacements. Radiology 1988;169:741.

39. Scapino RP. Histopathology of the disc and posterior displacement in disc displacement internal derangements of the TMJ. In: Palacios E, et al, eds. Magnetic resonance of the temporomandibular joint. Stuttgart/New York: Thieme, 1990:63.

40. Brooks SL, Westesson P-L. Temporomandibular joint: value of coronal MR images. Radiology 1993;188:317.

41. Rao VM, Vinitski S, Liem M, Rapoport R. Fast spin-echo imaging of the temporomandibular joint. JRMI 1995;5:293.

42. Wilk RM, Harms SE. Temporomandibular joint: multislab, three-dimensional Fourier transform MR imaging. Radiology 1988;167:861.

43. Crabbe JP, Brooks SL, Lillie JH. Gradient echo MR imaging of the temporomandibular joint: diagnostic pitfall caused by the superficial temporal artery. AJR 1995;164:451.

44. Suenaga S, Hamamoto S, Kawano K, et al. Dynamic MR imaging of the temporomandibular joint in patients with arthrosis: relationship between contrast enhancement of the posterior disk attachment and joint pain. AJR 1996;166:1475

45. Harms SE, et al. Specialized receiver coils for bilateral MR imaging examinations of the temporomandibular joint. Radiology 1987;165:159.

46. Drace JE, Enzmann DR. Defining the normal temporomandibular joint: closed-, partially open-, and open-mouth MR imaging of asymptomatic subjects. Radiology 1990;177:67.

47. Drace J, Enzmann DR. MR imaging of the temporomandibular joint (TMJ): closed-, partially open-, and open-mouth views of the abnormal TMJ. Radiology 1987;165:149.

48. Helms CA, et al. Staging of internal derangements of the temporomandibular joint with MR imaging, and optimal mouth position for diagnosis. Radiology 1987;165:149.

49. Drace JE, Young SW, Enzmann DR. TMJ meniscus and bilaminar zone: MR imaging of the substructure-diagnostic landmarks and pitfalls of interpretation. Radiology 1990;177:73.

50. Schwaighofer BW, Tanaka TT, Klein MV, et al. MR imaging of the temporomandibular joint: a cadaver study of the value of coronal images. AJR 1990;154:1245.

51. Katzberg RW, et al. Magnetic resonance imaging of the temporomandibular joint meniscus. Oral Surg Oral Med Oral Pathol 1985;59:332.

52. Schellhas KP, et al. Temporomandibular joint: diagnosis of internal derangements using magnetic resonance imaging. Minn Med 1986;69:519.

53. Cirbus MT, et al. Magnetic resonance imaging in confirming internal derangement of the temporomandibular joint. J Prosthet Dent 1987;57:487.

54. Palacios E, et al. Internal derangement and other pathology in magnetic resonance imaging of the temporomandibular joint. In: Palacios E, et al, eds. Magnetic resonance of the temporomandibular joint. Stuttgan/New York: Thieme, 1990:75.

55. Helms CA, Doyle GW, Orwig D, et al. Staging of internal derangements of the TMJ with magnetic resonance imaging: preliminary observations. J Craniomandib Disorders 1989;3:93.

56. Helms CA, Kaban LB, McNeil C, et al. Temporomandibular joint: morphology and signal intensity characteristics of the disc at MR imaging. Radiology 1989;172:817.

57. Hasso AN, Christiansen EL, Alder ME. The temporomandibular joint. Radiol Clin North Am 1989;27:301.

58. Rao VM, Liem MD, Farole A, Razek AAKA. Elusive "stuck" disc in the temporomandibular joint: diagnosis with MR imaging. Radiology 1993;189:823.

59. Nitzan DW, Dolwick MF, Martinez GA. Temporomandibular joint arthrocentesis: a simplified treatment for severe, limited mouth opening. J Oral Maxillofac Surg 1991;49:1163.

60. Kneeland JB, et al. MR imaging of a fractured temporomandibular disc prosthesis. J Comput Assist Tomogr 1987;11:199.

61. Schellhas KP, et al. Temporomandibular joint: MR imaging of internal derangements and postoperative changes. AJR 1988;150:381.

62. Schellhas KP, Wilkes CH, el Deeb M, et al. Permanent proplast temporomandibular joint implants: MR imaging of destructive complications. AJR 1988;15:731.

63. Resnick D. Diagnosis of bone and joint disorders, 3rd ed, vol 3. Philadelphia: WB Saunders, 1995.

64. Katzberg RW, et al. Dislocation of jaws. Radiology 1985;1S4:556.

65. Kononen M. Radiographic changes in the condyle of the temporomandibular joint in psoriatic arthritis. Acta Radiol 1987;28:185.

66. Westesson P-L. MRI of the temporomandibular joint. Imaging Decisions 1994;1:2.

Magnetic Resonance Imaging in Orthopaedics & Sports Medicine, Second Edition,
edited by David W. Stoller. Lippincott-Raven Publishers, Philadelphia, © 1997.

Chapter 13

Kinematic Magnetic Resonance Imaging

Frank G. Shellock

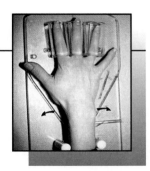

Kinematics, a term borrowed from the science of biomechanics, is used to describe the movement of a body without reference to force or mass.[1] Kinematic magnetic resonance (MR) imaging refers to the assessment of joint function with respect to the various interactions of the soft tissue and bony structures that comprise the joint, as well as the relative alignment of these structures through a specific range of motion.[2] This diagnostic imaging technique was developed to address the fact that many pathologic conditions that affect a joint are position-dependent or are related to the reaction to stress or a "loaded" condition. The functional information obtained using kinematic MR imaging often serves to definitively identify the underlying abnormality or to supplement

the information acquired with standard, static-view MR imaging techniques.

Kinematic MR imaging techniques have been used in evaluation of the temporomandibular joint, the knee, the patellofemoral joint, the wrist, the ankle, the shoulder, and the cervical spine.[2-17] In order to illustrate the usefulness of this technique for diagnosis or elucidation of pathologic conditions, this chapter presents the kinematic MR imaging protocols for the joints most frequently studied using this technique (ie, the temporomandibular joint, the patellofemoral joint, the ankle, and the wrist); describes pertinent normal kinematics and pathokinematics; and reviews the clinical applications for kinematic MR imaging.

GENERAL ASPECTS OF KINEMATIC MR IMAGING

Techniques

Protocols for kinematic MR imaging, which continue to evolve and change, utilize a variety of pulse sequences and joint positioning strategies. In general, kinematic MR imaging methods are divided into four primary types: (1) incremental passive positioning, (2) cine-cyclic, (3) active movement, and (4) active movement against resistance.

The incremental passive positioning technique involves gradual movement and sequential imaging of the joint through a specific range of motion. Typically, images are acquired using either a T1-weighted spin-echo sequence or a gradient-echo pulse sequence.

The cine-cyclic method (also referred to as "motion-triggered" MR imaging) is similar to gated MR imaging, such as that which is used for cardiac studies.[6,18] In this type of kinematic MR imaging, the active, physical motion of the joint is repeated throughout the image acquisition cycle, which may last for 2 to several minutes.[6,18] Scans are performed with a spin-echo pulse sequence.

In the active movement technique, fast gradient-echo pulse sequences or echo planar imaging are used to permit imaging of the joint during dynamic motion. A temporal resolution of one image per second or less is required for good results.

The active movement against resistance method is similar to the active movement technique with respect to the MR imaging requirements. This form of kinematic MR imaging imposes a resistive load that stresses the joint during dynamic motion.

Positioning Devices

Positioning devices are commonly required for kinematic MR imaging examinations. They are used to guide the joint in a specific plane of imaging and through a specific range of motion. These devices must be constructed of components that are compatible with the electromagnetic fields used for MR imaging. In addition, they need to be designed with a thorough understanding of the biomechanical function of the joint. For example, positioning devices for the lower extremity (eg, knee or patellofemoral joint) should permit unrestricted rotational movements in addition to flexion and extension of the joint. Some positioning devices incorporate surface coils that not only facilitate imaging, but may be used to apply resistance to the joint during kinematic MR imaging. Several commercially available positioning devices that address these needs have been developed.

THE TEMPOROMANDIBULAR JOINT

The inability of MR imaging to provide a functional assessment of jaw biomechanics and meniscocondylar coordination was initially seen as a limitation of this diagnostic technique for evaluating temporomandibular joint (TMJ) dysfunction. Therefore, kinematic MR imaging was first applied to the assessment of the TMJ at different increments of mouth opening using an incremental passive positioning technique. This technique has proven to be extremely valuable in the examination and characterization of TMJ abnormalities.[3–5,19]

Kinematic MR Imaging Protocol

Functional abnormalities that affect the TMJ are primarily associated with the position of the meniscus relative to the mandibular condyle. Kinematic MR images obtained with a T1-weighted spin-echo pulse sequence (ie, short echo time [TE] and short repetition time [TR]) best depict the meniscocondylar orientations through the range of motion of this joint.[4,5,19] Partial flip angle or gradient-echo pulse sequences have also been used for kinematic studies,[3] but these techniques have intrinsically poor spatial resolution and are more susceptible to artifacts.[4,5] Furthermore, since the kinematic MR imaging examination is performed using an incremental passive positioning technique, the amount of time saved by using a gradient-echo pulse sequence over a T1-weighted spin-echo sequence is insignificant. Typically, the T1-weighted spin-echo images acquired for kinematic MR study of the TMJ are of sufficiently high quality to both demonstrate the anatomic features of the joint and assess its function.[5]

The high incidence of bilateral abnormalities in patients with internal derangements of the TMJ makes it advisable to perform kinematic MR imaging on both joints simultaneously. Adequate signal-to-noise ratio, to facilitate imaging these small joints, is optimally accomplished with dual 7.5 cm (3 inch) circular surface coils or a quadrature head coil (Fig. 13-1). Simultaneous MR imaging of the right and left joints also permits direct comparison between the joints at the same relative degree of mouth opening. This is especially important in identifying motion-related abnormalities, such as lateral deviation and asymmetrical movements.[4,5]

The mandibular condyle is positioned at oblique angles in both the sagittal and coronal planes.[17] It has been shown that the best orientation for images of the TMJ is with reference to the long axis of the condylar head, because a significant number of both normal individuals and patients have abnormally configured condyles with respect to size, shape, and orientation. Therefore, slice locations for kinematic MR imaging of the TMJ should be determined by the user and selected in planes that are perpendicular (ie, oblique sagittal planes) to the long axis of the condylar head, as viewed in an axial plane localizer scan (Fig. 13-2). This not only provides standardized and consistent information, but also decreases scan time because only slice locations from the anatomic regions of interest are obtained.

A nonferromagnetic positioning device should be used to passively maintain the patient's mouth at predetermined

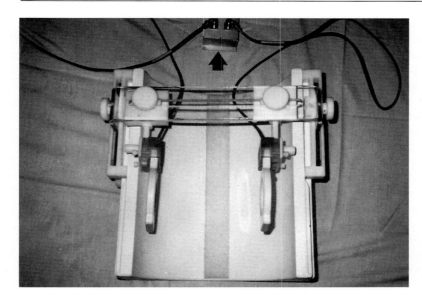

FIGURE 13-1. Dual 6.5 cm receive-only surface coils with a combiner box (*arrow*) are used for simultaneous high-resolution MR imaging of bilateral temporomandibular joints.

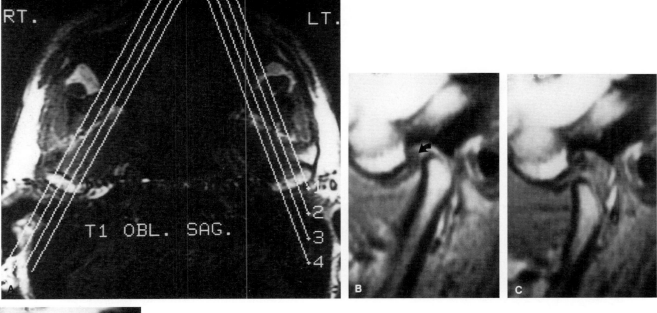

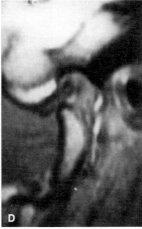

FIGURE 13-2. (**A**) An MR axial plane localizer is used to prescribe the oblique sagittal slice locations for kinematic MR imaging of the temporomandibular joint. The slice locations are selected in an orientation that is perpendicular to the long axis of the right and left condylar heads using graphic prescription software (TR, 400 msec; TE, 20 msec; slice thickness, 5 mm). (**B**) In an example of oblique sagittal plane images obtained for kinematic MR study of the temporomandibular joint, there is anterior displacement of the meniscus in the closed-mouth position (*arrow*). (**C, D**) In the subsequent images, reduction occurs during opening of the mouth as the condylar head moves onto the intermediate zone of the meniscus (TR, 400 msec; TE, 20 msec; slice thickness, 3 mm).

opening-phase increments (Fig. 13-3). MR scans are then performed at each position as the mouth is progressively opened. Prior to kinematic MR imaging study, the range of motion for each patient is determined by having the patient open his or her mouth as wide as possible—without forcing the joint or causing pain—with the positioning device in place. The increments of opening are then based on this information.

Two or three thin slice (≤ 3 mm) images are acquired through the TMJ in the oblique sagittal plane at the following mouth positions: (1) closed-mouth position (ie, maximum intercuspation of the teeth), (2) closed-mouth position with the positioning device in place (note that the distance the patient's mouth is opened at this increment is dependent on the length of the incisors), (3) repeatedly at progressive increments of mouth-opening position using 20% intervals of the range of motion until the full opened-mouth position is attained. In this manner, seven images are obtained for the kinematic MR imaging study of the TMJ.

Total imaging time for a kinematic MR imaging study of the bilateral TMJs takes approximately 15 minutes using the following protocol and obtaining images at seven different increments of opening (TR/TE of 600/20 msec; matrix

size of 128 × 256; a 10 cm field of view; a 3 mm slice thickness; 1 excitation; and six slice locations [three through each condylar head]).

Images may be viewed individually or displayed as a cine-loop using standard software commonly found on most MR systems. For the cine-loop display, the slice locations (obtained through each TMJ at the same location) that best depict the meniscus, condyle, glenoid fossa, and articular eminence should be selected and displayed at a user-controlled speed.

Normal Kinematics

When the mouth is closed, the meniscus is positioned such that the posterior band is in a 12 o'clock position (± 10%) relative to the condylar head.[19] As the mouth opens, the condyle rotates anteriorly and moves onto the intermediate zone of the meniscus. The condyle remains positioned on the intermediate zone as the mouth continues to open, and translates anteriorly until it reaches the base of the articular eminence or slightly anterior to this position. The appearance of this entire movement in kinematic MR imaging is that of rotation and then free gliding or smooth anterior translation of the condylar head (Fig. 13-4).

Pathokinematics

Kinematic MR imaging provides useful diagnostic information for a variety of TMJ abnormalities of varying degrees of severity. The internal derangements best evaluated by kinematic MR imaging are usually anterior displacements of the meniscus. However, abnormal movements of the mandible are also easily identified,[4,5] and there is evidence that adhesions that affect the TMJ may also be identified using kinematic MR imaging.

Anterior Displacement of the Meniscus With Reduction

In evaluating the TMJ with an anteriorly displaced meniscus, many clinicians believe that it is important to determine whether or not the meniscus resumes its normal orientation relative to the mandibular condyle as the mouth opens (ie, reduction of an anteriorly displaced meniscus) as well as the relative position at which this occurs. By using kinematic MR imaging and viewing the joint at different increments between closed and fully opened positions of the mouth, it is possible to ascertain if there is reduction of the meniscus, and the relative position of the mandible at the point at which it occurs (Fig. 13-5). Recapture of an anteriorly displaced meniscus may occur at any point in the range of motion of the TMJ.

Determination of the point at which the meniscus is recaptured is important with respect to the correct application of splint therapy, which is frequently used to treat anterior

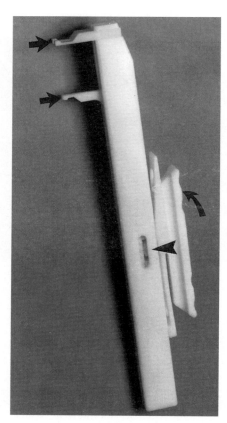

FIGURE 13-3. A special nonferromagnetic positioning device is used to open the patient's mouth at predetermined increments. A gauge (*arrowhead*) is used to determine the degree of mouth opening based on the distance between the disposable mouth pieces (*straight arrows*). Movement of the mouthpieces is controlled by the pressing the patient-activated handle (*curved arrow*).

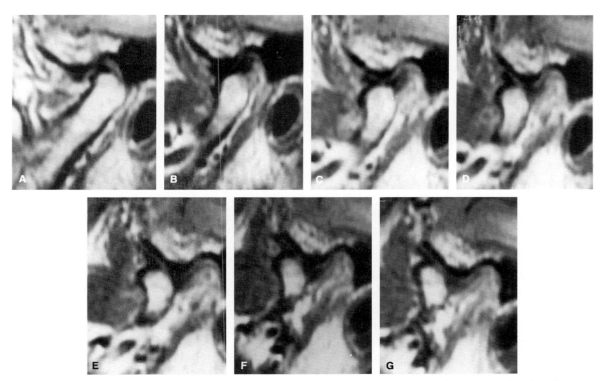

FIGURE 13-4. (**A**) In a kinematic study of the normal temporomandibular joint, the posterior band of the meniscus is in a 12 o'clock position relative to the condylar head in the closed-mouth position. (**B** through **G**) As the mouth progressively opens, the condyle moves onto the intermediate zone of the meniscus. This relative meniscocondylar relationship is maintained throughout the remaining range of motion of the joint, as the condyle translates anteriorly. The range of motion in this subject was 48 mm (oblique sagittal plane images; TR, 600 msec; TE, 20 msec; slice thickness, 3 mm).

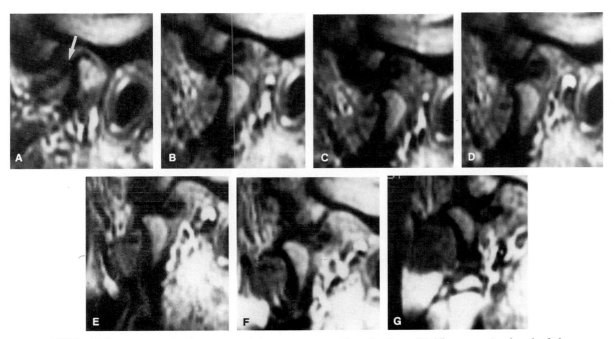

FIGURE 13-5. Anterior displacement of the meniscus with reduction. (**A**) The posterior band of the meniscus (*arrow*) is anteriorly displaced in the closed-mouth position. (**B** through **G**) As the mouth opens, the condylar head moves onto the intermediate zone of the meniscus and recaptures the meniscus (oblique sagittal images; TR, 600 msec; TE, 20 msec; slice thickness, 3 mm).

displacements of the meniscus.[20,21] The size of the splint may be altered accordingly to treat an "early" versus a "late" recapture of the meniscus. If splint therapy is not properly applied, the internal derangement of the TMJ may progress, or, at the very least, may not be corrected. Anteriorly displaced menisci that reduce early are considered less severe than those that reduce late.

Anterior Displacement of the Meniscus Without Reduction

A more severe form of internal derangement of the TMJ is an anterior displacement of the meniscus that is not recaptured (Fig. 13-6). In this case, the kinematic MR imaging examination demonstrates a markedly displaced meniscus on the closed-mouth view that develops a distorted shape during the mouth-opening phases, as it is pushed out in front of the mandibular condyle. This form of abnormal TMJ function is typically associated with a limited range of motion as well as severe laxity of the meniscal attachments or tears of the posterior disk attachment. Other joint abnormalities such as osteophytes, adhesions, and degenerative arthritis may also be found with this more advanced stage of TMJ dysfunction (Fig. 13-7).

Since treatment of anterior displacements of the meniscus that do not reduce typically requires surgical intervention, kinematic differentiation between a meniscus that has a late recapture from one that does not recapture in a fully opened mouth position is especially useful.

Asymmetrical Motion Abnormalities

Since the mandible has a bilateral articulation with the cranium, both TMJs should function synchronously, and any disordered movement is regarded as an abnormality.[4,15,17] Kinematic MR imaging is extremely useful for identifying and characterizing the extent of any asymmetrical motion that may affect the TMJ.[4,5] As mentioned earlier, in normal kinematic MR imaging of the TMJ there is initial rotation of the condylar head, which is followed by smooth anterior translation. Asymmetrical motion may take the form of lateral deviations with opening and closing of the mouth, as well as other more peculiar movements. For example, there may be progressive anterior translation of one condyle while the other moves in a retrograde manner (Fig. 13-8). Asymmetric motion of the TMJ may be caused by muscle spasm, shortened or atrophic muscles, fibrous adhesions, fibrotic contractures, or by other mechanisms. In addition, associated displacements of the meniscus, as well as degenerative alterations in the bony anatomy, may or may not be present.

THE PATELLOFEMORAL JOINT

Disorders of the patellofemoral joint are a primary source of anterior knee pain and occur with a frequency comparable to that of meniscal lesions.[22–26] Patellar malalignment and abnormal tracking, typically produced by incongruency between the patella and the femoral trochlear groove, result in

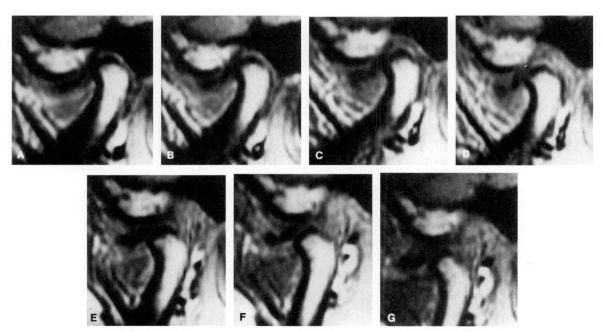

FIGURE 13-6. Anterior displacement of the meniscus without reduction. **(A)** The entire meniscus is anteriorly displaced relative to the condylar head in the closed-mouth position. **(B through G)** As the mouth opens, the condylar head translates anteriorly but does not recapture the meniscus. The meniscus remains in front of the condylar head during progressive mouth opening. In addition, there is a limited range of motion of the joint (oblique sagittal images; TR, 600 msec; TE, 20 msec; slice thickness, 3 mm).

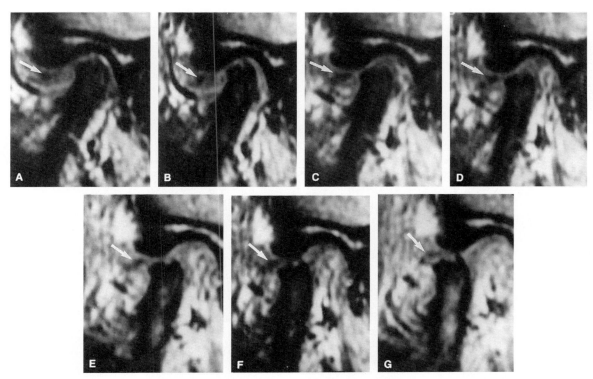

FIGURE 13-7. Anterior displacement of the meniscus without reduction and with advanced degenerative changes. (**A**) The entire meniscus (*arrow*) is anteriorly displaced in the closed mouth position and appears to have lost its posterior attachment. (**B** through **G**) As the mouth opens, the condylar head translates anteriorly and the shape of the meniscus (*arrows*) appears to be distorted, as it remains in front of the condylar head. There is marked degeneration of the joint with substantial sclerosis of the bony anatomy (oblique sagittal images; TR, 600 msec; TE, 20 msec; slice thickness, 3 mm).

instability of the patellofemoral joint.[22–26] Malalignment and maltracking are believed to produce significant shearing forces and excessive contact stresses that lead to lesions and eventual degeneration of the articular cartilage.[27,28] Even in the absence of a detectable cartilage defect, a chronically malaligned patella may also change the load distribution in the patellofemoral joint and cause clinical symptoms.[22,27] Although less common, other possible causes of anterior knee pain that should be considered in the differential diagnosis include reflex sympathetic dystrophy, bursitis, plica syndrome, hyperplasia of the peripatellar fat pad, and synovitis.[22–25]

Detection of patellofemoral joint abnormalities by physical examination alone can be a formidable task. Not only do the clinical signs often mimic other forms of internal derangements of the knee, but coexisting abnormalities are also common.[22–25] In addition, patients with persistent symptoms following patellar realignment surgery present a particular diagnostic challenge.[12,13] Proper classification of abnormal patellar alignment and tracking is crucial for an optimal decision to be made concerning the most appropriate treatment for these conditions.[22–27]

Abnormal conditions of patellar alignment and tracking appear during the earliest portion of the range of motion of this joint, as the patella enters and articulates with the femoral trochlear groove.[22–25,29–33] As flexion of the joint increases, the patella moves deeper into the femoral trochlear groove. At this point, patellar displacement is less likely to occur, because the femoral trochlear groove functions to buttress and stabilize the patella.[23–26]

Since patellofemoral incongruency is most likely to occur during the initial degrees of patellofemoral joint flexion, diagnostic imaging techniques that show the joint during this portion of the range of motion are best suited for the identification of abnormalities.[12,13,25,30–32] Imaging the patellofemoral joint at 25° or more of flexion frequently causes clinically important information to be overlooked.[9,31,32] A number of studies have shown that patellar malalignment and abnormal tracking are not consistently or reliably identified when techniques that image the joint at flexion angles greater than 30° (ie, most plain radiographic methods) are used.[9,31,32–34]

Kinematic MR imaging was first used for the evaluation of the patellofemoral joint in 1988.[11] Since then, several studies have demonstrated that kinematic MR imaging is a useful and sensitive means of evaluating patellar tracking and alignment in patients with patellofemoral joint abnormalities.[6,9,12,18,29,30,34–45] In one recent study, kinematic MR imaging was reported to be more effective than physical examination alone in detecting patellofemoral incongruency.[45]

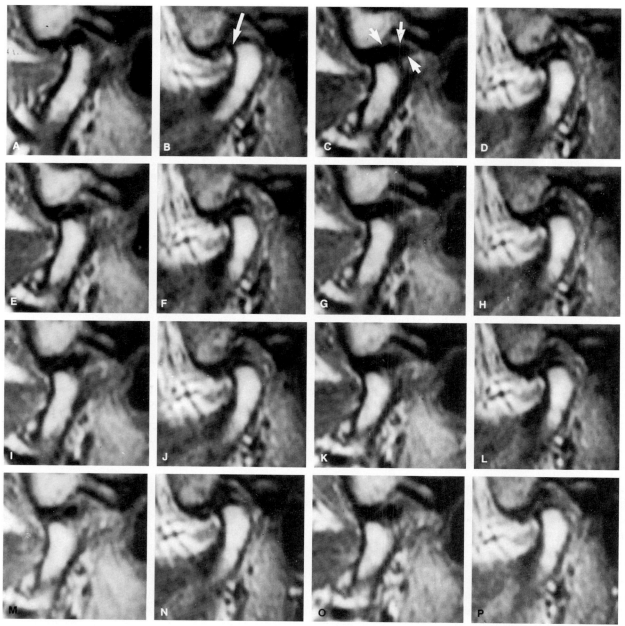

FIGURE 13-8. Asymmetric motion of the temporomandibular joint. (**A**) In the closed-mouth position, the meniscus on the right temporomandibular joint is in a normal position. (**B**) A small spur, however, is seen on the condyle (*arrow*) of the left temporomandibular joint and there is a slight anterior displacement of the meniscus. (**C, E, G, I, K, M, O**) During incremental opening of the mouth, the meniscus becomes slightly deformed during the initial phase of anterior movement of the condyle (*arrows*), and there is progressive anterior translation of the right condyle. (**D**) On the left temporomandibular joint, there is early recapture of the meniscus as the condyle translates anteriorly. (**D, F, H, J, L, N, P**) However, there is retrograde movement of the condyle as it moves back toward the glenoid (**P**). This patient had clinical evidence of lateral deviation of the mandible during opening of the mouth (oblique sagittal images; TR, 600 msec; TE, 20 msec; slice thickness, 3 mm).

Although conventional computed tomography (CT) and cine CT have also been used to perform kinematic studies of the patellofemoral joint,[25,31–33] kinematic MR imaging has the advantage of showing the various soft-tissue components (ie, medial and lateral retinacula, patellar tendon, quadriceps muscles) that are involved in the stability and function of the patellofemoral joint.[9,12,30,35,36,38] This information is frequently useful because irregularities of one or more of these soft-tissue structures is typically responsible for patellar malalignment and tracking abnormalities.[22,34,35,38]

Kinematic MR Imaging Protocols

Each of the previously described techniques for kinematic MR imaging has been applied to the evaluation of the patellofemoral joint.

Incremental Passive Positioning Technique

Early applications of kinematic MR imaging of the patellofemoral joint used the incremental passive positioning technique.[8–13,29,30,32,43,44] This technique involves obtaining multiple axial plane images at different section locations as the patellofemoral joints (since patellofemoral joint abnormalities tend to be bilateral, both joints should be evaluated simultaneously) are passively and incrementally flexed using a patient-activated, nonferromagnetic positioning device[9–12] (Fig. 13-9). The use of this device is essential to avoid displacement of the pa-

tella from direct anterior or lateral pressure that may occur when the patient is placed in a prone position. If it occurs, such displacement may give the erroneous appearance of patellar subluxation (Shellock FG, unpublished observations, 1987).

MR images are obtained using a T1-weighted spin-echo pulse sequence at several different slice locations while the joint is flexed in 5° increments from 5° to 30°. Because the patella and femoral trochlear groove are relatively large structures, comparatively ''low-resolution'' imaging parameters can be used. The body coil may be used to transmit and receive, and the T1-weighted spin-echo images are usually obtained with $\frac{1}{2}$ excitation, a 256 × 128 acquisition matrix, a 34 to 40 cm field of view, and a 5 mm slice thickness.

When the patient is placed prone on the positioning device, special care should be taken to arrange the extremities so that lower extremity alignment (observed while the patient is in an upright position) is maintained. This patient positioning scheme is unique because it allows rotational movements of the lower extremities to occur during flexion of the patellofemoral joints,[9,35,36] which is important because excessive internal or external rotation may be partially responsible for abnormal patellar alignment and tracking.[22–25] It is interesting to note that the kinematics of the patellofemoral joint are the same with prone and supine positioning.[35,38] A variety of studies have shown kinematic MR imaging of the patellofemoral joint using the incremental passive positioning technique to be an acceptable means of evaluating patellar alignment and tracking.[9–12,29,30,35,43,44]

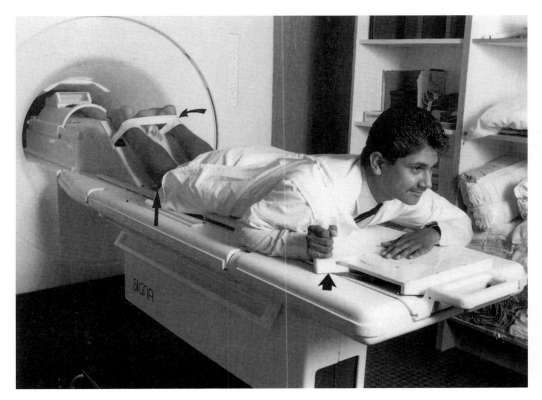

FIGURE 13-9. Nonferromagnetic positioning device used to perform kinematic MR imaging of the patellofemoral joints using the incremental passive positioning technique. This device has a patient-activated handle (*short arrow*) that flexes the knees from extension to 30° of flexion at 5° increments. A gauge indicates the amount of flexion. A cutout area (*long straight arrow*) permits uninhibited movement of the patellofemoral joints with the patient placed on this device in a prone position. A Velcro strap (*curved arrow*) is loosely applied to maintain the relative alignment of the lower extremities without impairing lower extremity rotational movements during joint flexion.

Active Movement Techniques

More recently, MR imaging techniques using fast gradient-echo pulse sequences or echo planar imaging have been developed that provide significant improvements in temporal resolution and allow images to be obtained during active movement of the patellofemoral joint.[37,39,41] The primary advantage of using active movement techniques is they take into account the influence of activated muscles and other related soft-tissue structure on patellar alignment and tracking.[37,39,41] In addition, since a sophisticated positioning device is not needed to incrementally flex the joint passively, the overall examination time is substantially reduced.

For the active movement technique, the patient is placed prone on a nonferromagnetic positioning device and is instructed to move from approximately 45° of flexion to extension while images are obtained at a single section location. The patient should begin to move both patellofemoral joints approximately 1 second after hearing the gradient noise that indicates that imaging has begun, and should continue to move until full extension is reached.[37,41] This maneuver should be practiced two or three times without imaging to ensure that the movement is acceptable (ie, motion was even and constant) to the MR system operator.[37,41]

The following imaging parameters may be used for fast spoiled gradient recalled echo in the steady state (GRASS) active movement kinematic MR imaging (TR/TE of 6.5/2.1 msec; a flip angle of 30°; one signal average; a 256 × 128 matrix; a 36 to 40 cm field of view; and a 7 mm section thickness). With this protocol, six images at a single section location can be acquired in approximately 8 seconds.[37,41] Imaging at the previously described rate of movement and using the imaging parameters just described, the six images at a single section location are evenly spaced through the range of motion achievable within the bore of the magnet. This procedure should be repeated at three different section locations in order to evaluate the entire excursion of the patella as it articulates with the femoral trochlear groove. Compared with the incremental passive positioning technique, active movement kinematic MR imaging studies provide a more physiologic examination, and, in certain instances, abnormal patellar tracking is more apparent with these techniques.[41]

Cine-Cyclic Technique

The cine-cyclic technique of performing kinematic MR imaging of the patellofemoral joint employs a special nonferromagnetic positioning device, incorporating a trigger system that senses the motion of the patella.[6,18] Patellar alignment and tracking may then be assessed during active movement similar to cardiac-gated studies. The patient is placed supine on the positioning device and a single patellofemoral joint is flexed and extended repeatedly while gradient-echo images are obtained using a circular surface coil.[6,18] Motion-triggered cine kinematic MR images show different patellar tracking patterns than those seen on images obtained using the incremental passive positioning technique,[6,18] highlighting the importance of using an active movement technique for evaluation of the patellofemoral joint.[6,18]

Active Movement Against Resistance Technique

In another refinement of kinematic MR imaging of the patellofemoral joint, the examination may be conducted during active movement against an externally applied load.[32,42,45] This particular form of kinematic MR imaging was developed to place stress on the quadriceps muscles and other associated soft tissues in order to show displacement of the patella in the presence of any imbalances in these anatomic structures.[42] When resistance—to stress the patellofemoral joint—is added to the kinematic MR examination, patellar malalignment and tracking abnormalities that may not be observed during unloaded examinations can be elicited, making active movement loaded kinematic MR imaging of the patellofemoral joint an improved diagnostic technique for identifying aberrant positions of the patella in relation to the femoral trochlear groove.[42,45]

A major determinant of the effective function of the patellofemoral joint is the tolerance displayed in reaction to external forces or to the stresses encountered during weight-bearing or movement.[1,46,47] Patients with derangements of the patellofemoral joint usually experience pain or increased symptoms during activity or stress of the joint.[22–25] It is thought that this occurs because of the high magnitude of the quadriceps muscle force that occurs during physical actions that necessitate flexion of the patellofemoral joint.[46,47] As the quadriceps muscle force rises, so does the reaction force imposed upon the patellofemoral joint.[46,47]

The active movement against resistance kinematic MR imaging examination is performed using a nonferromagnetic positioning device (Captain Plastic, Seattle, WA), which incorporates a mechanism that allows adjustable resistance to be applied to the patellofemoral joint in the sagittal plane (Fig. 13-10). With the patient in a prone position, the movement against this resistance primarily requires activation of the extensor mechanism of the knee.[42] The design of this device is such that a bilateral examination is accomplished as the patellofemoral joints move through a range of motion from approximately 45° of flexion to extension.[42] The "loaded" conditions of the active movement kinematic MR imaging technique are imposed during the earliest increments of joint flexion, when the muscle force required and the associated patellofemoral joint reaction forces are greatest.[1,46,47]

A force of 30 foot-pound/second is applied during the active movement kinematic MR imaging examination, a figure selected to apply sufficient resistance to stress the patellofemoral joints of adult patients and to provide a consistent level of work intensity for each individual (Grabiner MD, personal communication, 1992). Such exertion against a constant external load requires isoinertial muscle contraction of the quadriceps.[1] Imaging parameters similar to those

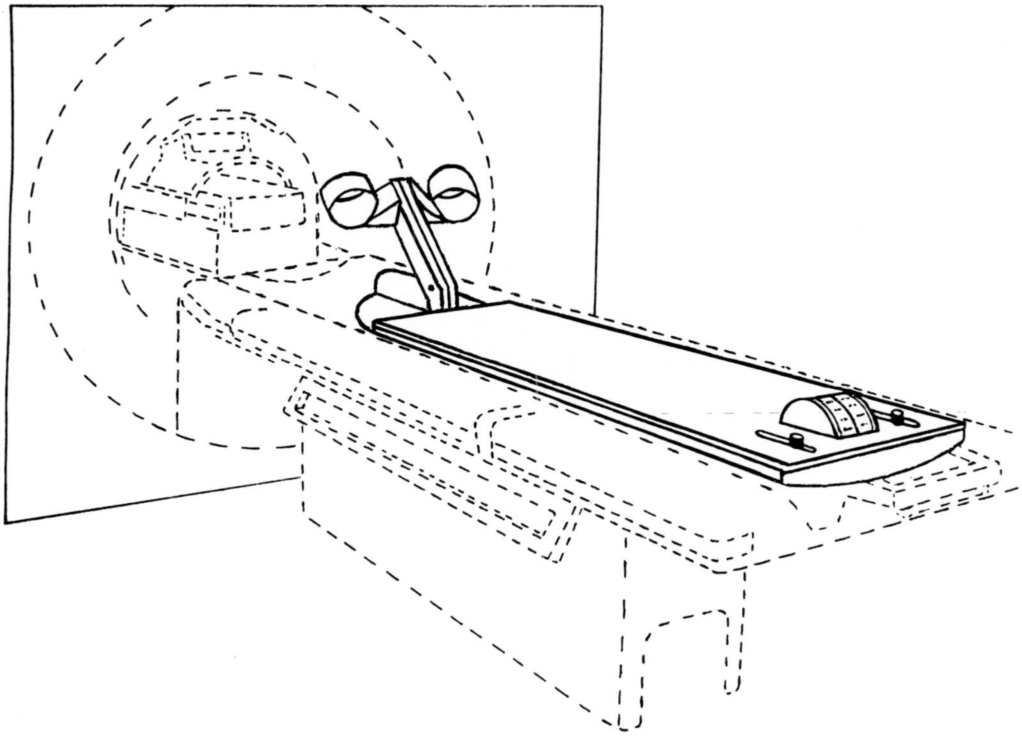

FIGURE 13-10. Nonferromagnetic positioning device used to perform kinematic MR imaging of the patellofemoral joints using the active movement against resistance technique. The patient is placed on this device in a prone position. A gauge indicates the resistance applied. The patellofemoral joints are suspended above the MR system table to allow unrestricted movements. Velcro straps are placed around the lower legs to hold them within small cradles that swivel 360°. There is no impairment of rotational movements of the lower extremities using this positioning device.

used for the active movement technique are used for the active movement loaded kinematic MR imaging study, and the total acquisition time (to obtain six images at three different section locations) is approximately 1 minute and 10 seconds (approximately 10 seconds is required to release and to reapply resistance for the loaded study).[42]

Anatomy of the Patellofemoral Joint

Because the patella articulates with the femoral trochlear groove during knee flexion, congruency of the shapes of the patella and femoral trochlear groove is important for proper function of the patellofemoral joint.[22–25] Dysplastic bony anatomy and/or abnormal soft-tissue structures are commonly observed in conjunction with patellofemoral instability.[22–25,48] Careful inspection of the shapes of the patella and the femoral trochlear groove often provides additional evidence concerning the presence of a patellofemoral joint disorder. However, normal patellar alignment and tracking may exist even in the presence of abnormal morphology.[22–25,27,48]

Evaluation of the anatomic features of the patellofemoral joint is best accomplished by obtaining sequential axial section images with the joint positioned in extension.[9,32,35] In addition, axial plane images obtained with the joint extended are useful for determining the position of the inferior pole of the patella relative to the femoral trochlear groove in order to identify patella alta and patella baja (see later).[9,32,35]

Patellar Anatomy

The patella is a sesamoid bone contained within the quadriceps tendon. It functions both to protect the femoral articular surface as well as to increase the efficiency of the quadriceps mechanism by virtue of the fulcrum effect. The width (51 to 57 mm) and height (57 to 58 mm) of the patella are remarkably constant, although its thickness, measured at the midequatorial plane, is quite variable. The normal anterior patellar surface is convex in all directions and demonstrates a rough cribriform surface that provides attachment for the quadriceps tendon in its upper one third. The inferior third ends in a V-shaped point, which is enveloped by the patellar tendon. The posterior surface can be divided into two parts with the inferior portion, which is usually nonarticular, representing nearly 25% of the total height. The upper three fourths of the posterior surface of the patella is covered by hyaline cartilage, which, in the central portion of the patella, is thicker (5 to 6 mm) than in any other articulation.

The articular surface of the patella is roughly oval in shape and is divided into medial and lateral facets by a vertical ridge that is oriented in the long axis of the patella. The facets may be of equal size, although predominance of the lateral facet is more common. The medial facet demonstrates considerable anatomical variation. It is subdivided by a small vertical ridge (the secondary ridge) into the medial facet proper and a smaller ''odd'' facet along its medial border. The secondary ridge runs in a longitudinal oblique direction and is closer to the midline proximally than distally. The odd facet, which is concave or flat, may be in the same

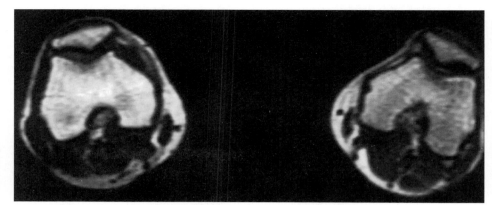

FIGURE 13-11. An axial image showing Wiberg type I patellar shapes. The lateral and medial patellar facets are the symmetrical (TR, 400 msec; TE, 20 msec; slice thickness, 5 mm).

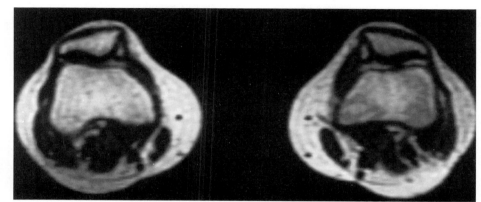

FIGURE 13-12. An axial image showing Wiberg type II patellar shapes. The lateral patellar facets are longer than the medial patellar facets (TR, 400 msec; TE, 20 msec; slice thickness, 5 mm).

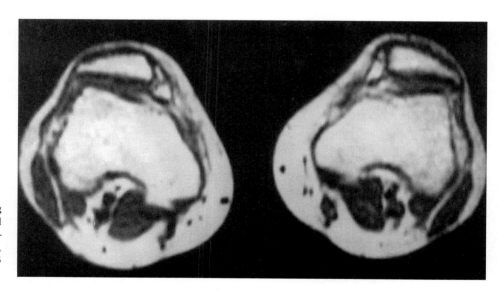

FIGURE 13-13. An axial image showing Wiberg type III patellar shapes. The lateral patellar facets are dominant, with significantly smaller medial patellar facets (TR, 400 msec; TE, 20 msec; slice thickness, 5 mm).

plane as the medial facet or may be oriented at as much as a 60° angle to it. The medial facet is usually flat or convex with articular cartilage of varying thickness. The lateral facet is both longer and wider than the medial facet and is concave in both vertical and transverse planes. Two transverse ridges have been described that divide the patella into upper, middle, and lower thirds. The most constant of these is seen separating the middle and lower thirds of the lateral facet.

In his classic paper, Wiberg[49] proposed a three part classification to describe the majority of patellar facet configurations. The system was based upon the configuration of the subchondral bone of the facets as depicted on tangential conventional radiographs. In the Wiberg type I configuration, both facets are gently concave, symmetrical, and nearly equal in size (Fig. 13-11). In type II the medial facet is smaller than the lateral (Fig. 13-12), which remains concave; the medial facet is flat or convex. Type II is the most common configuration, accounting for up to 65% of patellae. The differences between type I and type II patellae represent a continuum and may be subtle. In the type III configuration (Fig. 13-13), the medial facet is distinctly smaller, and there is marked lateral predominance. This configuration accounts for approximately 25% of patellae. Dysplastic patellar shapes have a variety of unusual configurations (Fig. 13-14) and are commonly observed in conjunction with patellofemoral arthrosis, chondromalacia, recurrent dislocation, and patellofemoral instability.[49] Recent studies using the tomographic capabilities of CT and MR imaging have demonstrated a change in apparent patella configuration from one section location to another, a finding that casts suspicion on the value of this or any similar classification system for patellar shapes.[25,32,34] Use of the Wiberg patellar

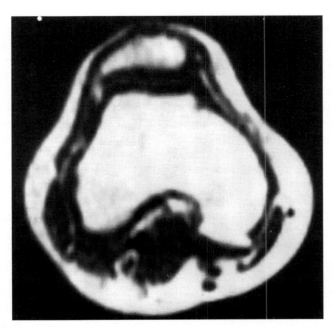

FIGURE 13-14. A dysplastic patella has no well-formed patellar ridge. The femoral trochlear groove is flattened (TR, 400 msec; TE, 20 msec; slice thickness, 5 mm).

shape classification scheme, however, remains common in the orthopaedic literature.

Ficat and Hungerford[23] proposed an alternative classification scheme based upon the angle subtended by the two major facets as depicted on conventional radiographs. The so-called pebble-shaped patella is characterized by an angle greater than 140°. An angle of 90° to 100° most closely corresponds to the Wiberg type III patella. The Alpine hunter's cap deformity is characterized by a patella approaching a single articular facet at a 90° angle. This hemipatella configuration with one articular facet is commonly observed in patients with lateral instability and is associated with hypoplasia of the vastus medialis and decreased depth of the femoral trochlear sulcus. The half-moon patella is characterized by an acute angle with a single articular facet.

Anatomy of the Femoral Trochlear Groove

The femoral trochlear groove provides a mechanical restraint that helps stabilize and serves as a guide for the patella as it articulates with this anatomic site during joint flexion.[22–25,32,34] The normal femoral trochlear shape has a deep sulcus with well-defined medial and lateral facets that are either equal in size or with a slightly larger lateral facet.[22–25] The most important aspect of the shape of the groove is that it conforms to the shape of the patella for proper articulation.[22–25] There is a wide variety of abnormal shapes of the femoral trochlear groove, with hypoplastic or dysplastic medial or lateral aspects (see Fig. 13-14). A shallow or flattened femoral trochlear groove or sulcus may be associated with patellofemoral joint instability.[22–25,32]

Patella Alta and Patella Baja

The height of the patella relative to the femoral trochlear groove is also biomechanically important for proper function of the patellofemoral joint.[30–32] Contact points between the cartilaginous surfaces of the patella and femoral trochlear groove during joint flexion are drastically altered if the patella is positioned too high or too low. Abnormal patellar height may be partially responsible for patellar malalignment and abnormal tracking.[22–24,30–33]

As mentioned earlier, the height of the patella is easily appreciated on kinematic MR imaging studies by inspecting axial plane section locations obtained through the patellofemoral joint while it is in an extended position. This permits visualization of the inferior pole, midplane, and superior aspect of the patella as they are positioned in relation to the femoral trochlear groove. Patellar height is considered to be normal when the inferior pole of the patella is positioned in the superior aspect of the femoral trochlear groove.[31,32,38] Patella alta, an abnormally high position of the patella, is diagnosed when the inferior pole of the patella is positioned above the superior aspect of the femoral trochlear groove with the joint extended[50] (Fig. 13-15). It is associated with various patellofemoral problems, including patellofemoral joint instability, patellar dislocation, and chondromalacia pa-

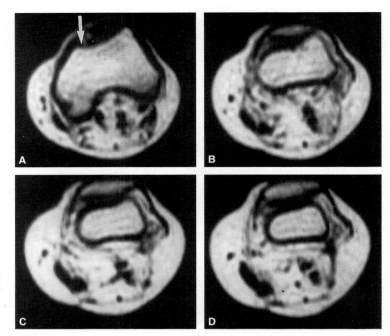

FIGURE 13-15. Sequential axial images demonstrate patella alta. (**A**) The patella is positioned well above the femoral trochlear groove, which has a hypoplastic medial aspect (*arrow*). (**B** through **D**) In addition, the patella is poorly formed (TR, 400 msec; TE, 20 msec; slice thickness, 5 mm).

tella,[50–52] and is found more often in women than men. Patella baja, an abnormally low position of the patella, is diagnosed when the entire patella is positioned in or below the femoral trochlear groove with the joint extended. It is often seen in young adult athletes in conjunction with Osgood-Schlatter disease[51] (a traumatic disturbance in the development of the tibial tuberosity in adolescents). Patella baja may also be found after patellar realignment procedures that involve repositioning or shortening of the patellar tendon or ligament.[51]

Evaluation of Kinematic MR Imaging of the Patellofemoral Joint

In order to determine patellar alignment and tracking and to thoroughly assess the kinematic aspects of the patellofemoral joint, three to four different section locations through the femoral trochlear groove or femoral trochlea (depending on the position of the patella and the positions at which the patella articulates with the femoral trochlear groove or femoral trochlea) should be evaluated during the initial increments of flexion.[32,35,38] The axial plane images obtained during the kinematic MR examination of the patellofemoral joint can be qualitatively analyzed individually or as a cine-loop display (ie, by making a cine-loop of the six or seven axial plane images obtained at a given section location). A cine-loop display of the acquired images facilitates viewing of multiple images obtained at different section locations. Compared with static images of patellar alignment and tracking, the cine-loop display provides considerably better qualitative information about the patellofemoral joint and the various patterns of patellar motion.[32,35,38]

There are significant limitations associated with previously used methods of assessing patellar alignment and tracking. Over the years, a variety of techniques have been suggested for identifying patellofemoral incongruency.[25,31,32,53–55] However, the majority of these were designed for use with plain radiographs obtained at a single increment of joint flexion, usually greater than 30°. These measurements are not practical or helpful for use with kinematic MR imaging, and the multiple images obtained at different increments of joint flexion during kinematic MR imaging, which display the overall pattern of patellar motion, provide more relevant information.

In addition, there is no agreement on the usefulness of quantification techniques for determining patellar malalignment.[23–25,32,33] Abnormal patellofemoral joint function is often associated with anatomic irregularities (eg, dysplastic patellae, dysplastic bony anatomy, patella alta, and patella baja). Unfortunately, these conditions preclude accurate assessment of patellar alignment using quantification schemes because there are no consistent landmarks for reliable measurement of congruent patellofemoral anatomy. Most importantly, quantitative assessment of patellofemoral incongruency has never been used by orthopaedists to guide surgical or rehabilitation procedures designed to treat patellofemoral joint abnormalities.

In view of the limitations associated with measurements of patellofemoral incongruency, qualitative criteria are more useful for the description of the relationship between the patella and the femoral trochlear groove or femoral trochlea during joint flexion.[32,33,35–39,45] The severity of the problem is displayed by the movements of the patella over the range of motion that is examined. It is easy to determine if the abnormal patellar movement patterns are improving, staying the same, or worsening during flexion of the joint. With minor patellar malalignment and abnormal tracking, displacement of the patella is transient, as the patella centralizes or moves into a more normal position during increasing increments of joint flexion. Even minor patellofemoral joint incongruency, however, may cause significant symptoms.[27] With more severe patellar motion abnormalities, the patella is either maintained in its displaced position or is further displaced (ie, progressive subluxation) with increasing increments of joint flexion.

Normal Kinematics

During extension of the patellofemoral joint, there are essentially no forces acting on the patella and, therefore, the patella may be situated medially, laterally, or in a central position relative to the femoral trochlear groove. ''Pseudo-subluxation'' of the patella during extension is considered a normal variant, since it may be found in any of these positions. As previously indicated, images obtained with the patellofemoral joint extended are useful for determining the position of the patella as it enters the femoral trochlear groove—information necessary for the identification of patella alta or baja as well as for assessing the anatomy of the patella and femoral trochlear groove.

During flexion of the patellofemoral joint, forces from various sources act on the patella.[1] Normal alignment and tracking of the patella during flexion is dependent on the interaction of the dynamic stabilizers (primarily the quadriceps muscles), static stabilizers (the patellar tendon, lateral patellofemoral ligament, lateral patellar ligament, medial retinaculum, lateral retinaculum, and fascia lata), bony structures (congruency between the shapes of the patella and femoral trochlear groove), and alignment of the femur and tibia.[1,25,32] Disruption of one or more of these factors is typically responsible for patellofemoral joint dysfunction.[22–25,32]

In normal patellar alignment and tracking, the ridge of the patella is positioned directly in the center of the femoral trochlear groove, and this orientation is maintained throughout the early and later increments of joint flexion, as the patella moves in a vertical plane (Fig. 13-16). Abnormalities of patellar alignment and tracking are apparent on kinematic MR imaging studies when deviation from this normal pattern of patellar movement is exhibited at one or more slice locations at 5° or more of joint flexion.[20,32,35]

Pathokinematics

Lateral Subluxation of the Patella

Lateral subluxation of the patella is a form of patellar malalignment in which the either ridge of the patella is laterally displaced relative to the femoral trochlear groove or the centermost part of the femoral trochlea and the lateral facet

of the patella overlap the lateral aspect of the femoral trochlea (Figs. 13-17 and 13-18). This is the most common form of patellar malalignment and abnormal tracking, and it occurs with varying degrees of severity. Unbalanced forces from lateral soft-tissue structures, possibly combined with insufficient counterbalancing forces from medial soft-tissue structures, are typically the cause of lateral subluxation of the patella. A dysplastic patella, dysplastic femoral trochlear groove, and/or patella alta may also be partially responsible for this patellofemoral joint abnormality.

In some cases of lateral subluxation of the patella, there is a redundant lateral retinaculum (Fig. 13-19). This finding, readily identified by kinematic MR imaging techniques,[9–12] is especially important because it indicates that the subluxated patella is not caused by excessive force from the lateral retinaculum and that surgical release of the lateral retinaculum (a procedure frequently performed in an attempt to realign a laterally subluxated patella) is not the appropriate treatment for this type of patellar malalignment and abnormal tracking.

Lateral Patellar Tilt or Excessive Lateral Pressure Syndrome

Lateral patellar tilt or excessive lateral pressure syndrome (ELPS) was first described by Ficat and Hungerford.[23] This form of patellar malalignment is a clinicoradiologic entity, clinically characterized by anterior knee pain and radiologically illustrated by tilting of the patella with functional patellar lateralization, usually onto a dominant lateral facet.[23,25] A small degree of lateral displacement of the patella may or may not be present during joint flexion, as increasing tension from one or more overly taut soft-tissue structures tilts the patella in a lateral fashion (Fig. 13-20). There are several reasons to believe that the main pathologic component of this abnormality is excessive force from the lateral retinaculum.[25] Because the patellar tilting that occurs with ELPS may be either transient (centralization or correction of the patellar malalignment occurs during joint flexion) or progressive (there is additional tilting with increasing increments of joint flexion), kinematic MR imaging techniques are particularly useful for identifying and characterizing this abnormality.[9,24,32,35] It should be noted that tilting of the patella onto the lateral aspect of the femoral trochlear groove often shifts the patellar ridge medially, and this may be designated as medial subluxation of the patella (see later) rather than ELPS.

The underlying hyperpressure found in ELPS can produce significant destruction of the articular cartilage.[23,25] The excessive lateral pressure may produce lateral joint line narrowing as a result of a decrease in cartilage thickness, or even gross cartilage degeneration along the median ridge and lateral facet of the patella.[23,25] A dysplastic patella and/or femoral trochlear groove is commonly encountered with ELPS. This is particularly likely to occur if ELPS is present during growth and development of the patellofemoral joint, since the final shapes of the patella and femoral trochlea are

text continues on page 1043

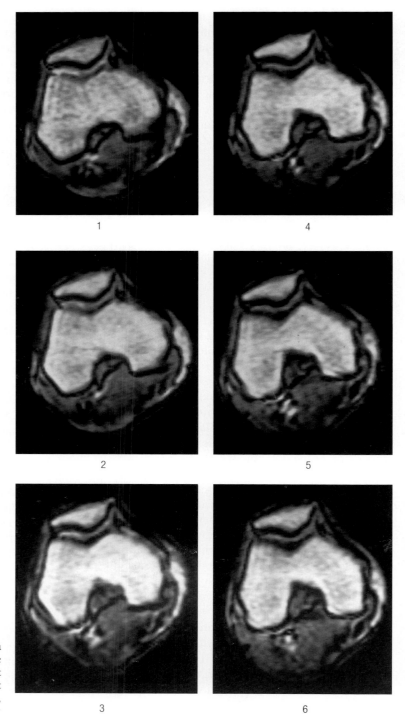

1

4

2

5

3

6

FIGURE 13-16. Normal kinematic study with the patella in a centralized position relative to the femoral trochlear groove throughout the range of motion studied (axial plane fast spoiled GRASS images obtained using the active movement against resistance technique; TR/TE, 6.5/2.1 msec; flip angle, 30°; slice thickness, 7 mm).

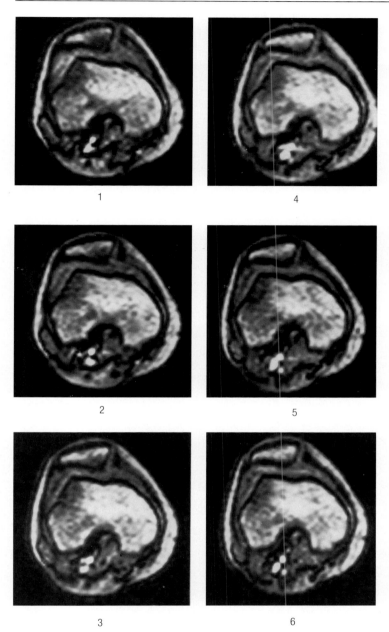

1

2

3

4

5

6

FIGURE 13-17. Lateral subluxation of the patella. Areas of decreased signal intensity in the lateral femoral condyle and median ridge of the patella indicate bone contusions, suggesting that there was a prior traumatic dislocation of the patella (axial plane fast spoiled GRASS kinematic MR images obtained using the active movement against resistance technique; TR/TE, 6.5/2.1 msec; flip angle, 30°; slice thickness, 7 mm).

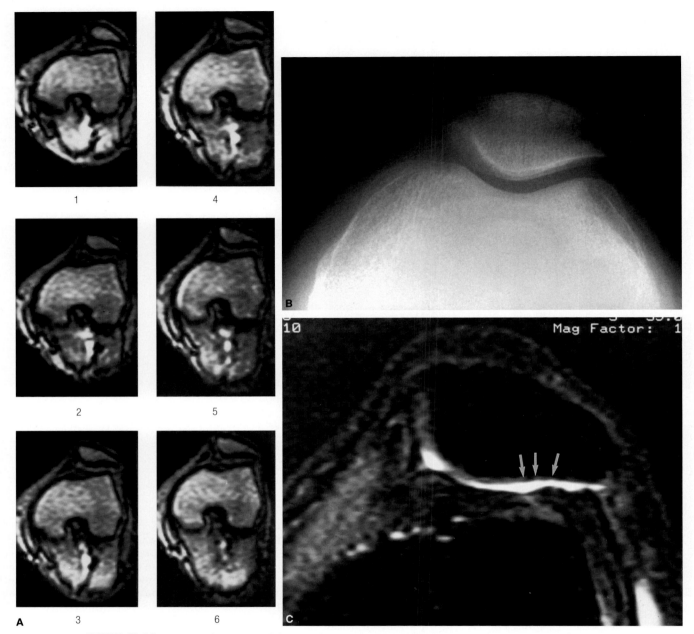

FIGURE 13-18. Lateral subluxation of the patella. **(A)** Kinematic MR imaging examination using the active movement against resistance technique clearly shows lateral subluxation (axial plane fast spoiled GRASS images; TR/TE, 6.5/2.1 msec; flip angle, 30°; slice thickness, 7 mm). **(B)** Plain film of the patellofemoral joint obtained at 45° of flexion showing normal patellar alignment. A comparison of the two images illustrates the relative insensitivity of plain film techniques in the identification of patellofemoral joint abnormalities. **(C)** Axial plane image of the patellofemoral joint obtained using an extremity coil and a fast spin-echo, inversion recovery pulse sequence to visualize the articular cartilage. There is cartilage thinning (*arrows*) that corresponds to the contact points between the patella and femoral condyle seen on the kinematic MR imaging examination (TR/TI/TE, 4000/160/35 msec; slice thickness, 4 mm).

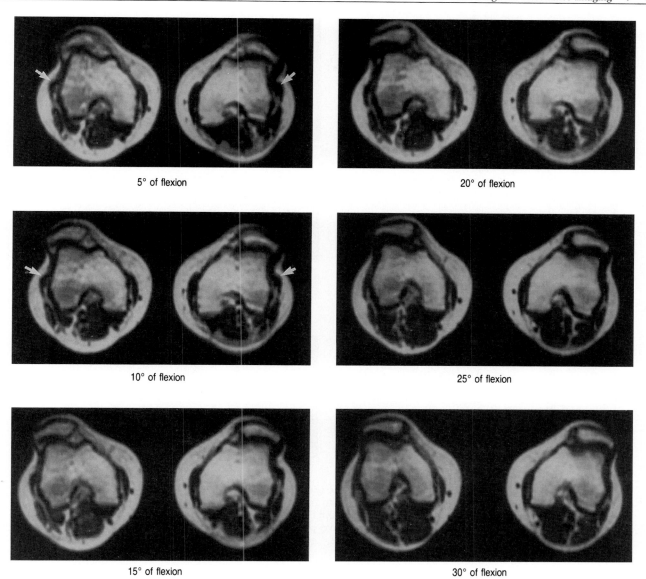

5° of flexion

20° of flexion

10° of flexion

25° of flexion

15° of flexion

30° of flexion

FIGURE 13-19. Bilateral lateral subluxation of the patella with redundant lateral retinacula is noted at initial increments of joint flexion (*arrows*). Each patella is laterally subluxated, especially during the initial increments of joint flexion, and moves toward the center of the femoral trochlear groove by 30° of joint flexion. These laterally subluxated patellae are not considered to be caused by excessive forces from the lateral retinacula (axial plane kinematic MR images obtained using the incremental passive positioning technique; TR, 400 msec; TE, 20 msec; slice thickness, 5 mm).

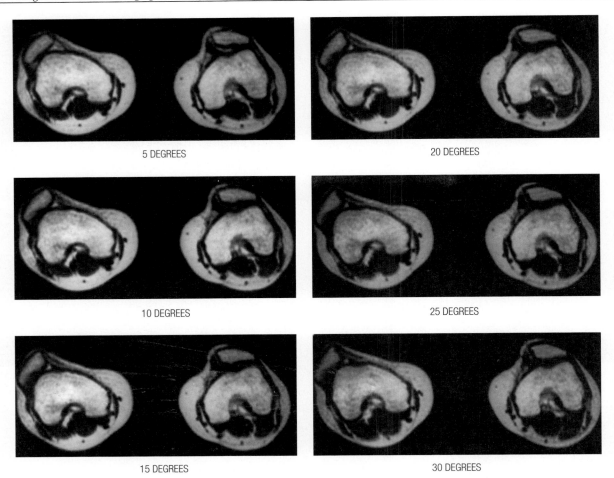

5 DEGREES

20 DEGREES

10 DEGREES

25 DEGREES

15 DEGREES

30 DEGREES

FIGURE 13-20. Excessive lateral pressure syndrome (ELPS) of the left patellofemoral joint and dislocation of the patella in the right patellofemoral joint. Note that the patellofemoral joint with ELPS has a slight lateral tilt, as the patella appears to be separated from the femoral trochlear groove (axial plane kinematic MR images obtained using the incremental passive positioning technique; TR/TE, 400/20 msec; slice thickness, 5 mm).

typically modified by use.[25] Surgical release of the lateral retinaculum is usually effective for treating ELPS.[24,25]

Medial Subluxation of the Patella (Patella Adentro)

Medial subluxation of the patella (patella adentro) involves medial displacement of the patellar ridge relative to the femoral trochlear groove or the centermost part of the femoral trochlea (Figs. 13-21 through 13-23). Recently, medial subluxation of the patella has been characterized and studied extensively by clinical and diagnostic imaging techniques.[8,9,40,56] This type of abnormal patellar alignment and tracking is frequently found in symptomatic patients after surgical patellar realignment procedures in which there has been overcompensation of the lateral tethering or stabilizing mechanisms of the patellofemoral joint[57] (Fig. 13-24). For example, the lateral soft-tissue structures of the patellofemoral joint may be excessively released during a lateral retinacular release procedure, causing a patella that was originally laterally subluxated to become medially displaced.

Medial subluxation of the patella may also be found in patients without previous patellar realignment surgery.[8,9,40,56] Various factors, existing either separately or in combination, may be responsible for producing this type of aberrant patellar alignment and tracking, including an excessively tight medial retinaculum, an insufficient lateral retinaculum, abnormal patellofemoral anatomy, and a quadriceps imbalance. Extreme internal rotation of the lower extremities and atrophy of the vastus lateralis are common clinical findings in patients with medially subluxated patellae.[40,45] Identification of a medially subluxated patella, and distinguishing this particular form of patellar malalignment and abnormal tracking from lateral subluxation, are crucial in order to select and apply appropriate rehabilitative or surgical therapy.

Lateral-to-Medial Subluxation of the Patella

Lateral-to-medial subluxation of the patella is a pattern of abnormal patellar alignment and tracking in which the patella is positioned in a slight lateral subluxation during the initial increments of joint flexion (ie, 5° to 10°), moves into and across the femoral trochlear groove or femoral trochlea as flexion increases, and displaces medially during higher increments of flexion (Fig. 13-25). This relatively uncommon abnormality is typically found in association with patella alta and/or dysplastic bony anatomy, in which there is a lack of stabilization provided by the femoral trochlear groove.[35,38] In addition, lateral-to-medial subluxation of the patella may occur in patellofemoral joints in which surgical attempts at patellar realignment have been unsuccessful.

The actual biomechanical factors responsible for lateral-to-medial subluxation of the patella are obviously quite complicated. Apparently, various disordered or uncoordinated forces that act on the patella during joint flexion cause this pattern of patellofemoral joint instability. As with other types of abnormal patellar alignment and tracking, kinematic MR imaging techniques are particularly well suited to the depiction of the lateral-to-medial subluxation pattern because they show the various positions and motions of the patella at several different increments of joint flexion.[35,38]

Evaluation of Treatment Techniques

In addition to providing diagnostic information pertaining to the patellofemoral joint, kinematic MR imaging is also useful for assessment of conservative methods of treatment, including taping and bracing methods[43,58-60] (Fig. 13-26). For example, kinematic MR imaging of the patellofemoral joint can be used to determine the effects of a brace designed to correct patellar malalignment and abnormal tracking by imaging patients with and without the brace applied (Fig. 13-27). Additionally, rehabilitation methods may be monitored in order to rapidly assess their beneficial effects.

THE WRIST

Kinematic MR imaging is used in a variety of ways to examine the function of the wrist.[2,15,16,61] At present, this modality is primarily employed for detection of subtle abnormalities of carpal motion, instability patterns, transitory subluxation, and instability patterns that are not easily evaluated by routine MR imaging techniques.[2,15,61,62]

Kinematic MR imaging of the wrist offers several advantages over standard wrist fluoroscopy, such as tomographic information and a direct means of viewing the interosseous ligaments.[2,15,16,61] Idiopathic pain syndromes related to motion are often not sufficiently characterized by static-view MR techniques, especially if transitory subluxations are present. Kinematic MR examination provides enhanced imaging of the muscles, tendons, ligaments, and hyaline and fibrocartilaginous structures during controlled motion, which is useful in assessment of impingement or other abnormalities related to movement.[2,15,16] Kinematic MR imaging using a positioning device to hold the wrist in "radial stress" and "ulnar stress" positions while obtaining coronal plane images is useful for detection of interosseous ligament defects, especially those involving the scapholunate and lunotriquetral ligaments.[62] This simple kinematic method appears to improve the diagnostic accuracy of MR imaging for identification of abnormalities that are considered to be particularly challenging using conventional techniques.[62]

Kinematic MR Imaging Protocol

The small size of the wrist makes it necessary to use either single or dual 7.5 or 12.5 cm (3 or 5 inch) receive-only circular surface coils to obtain high-resolution images for kinematic MR imaging studies.[2,35] The same surface coil configuration may also be used to obtain high-resolution static MR views of the wrist. The surface coils are placed

text continues on page 1047

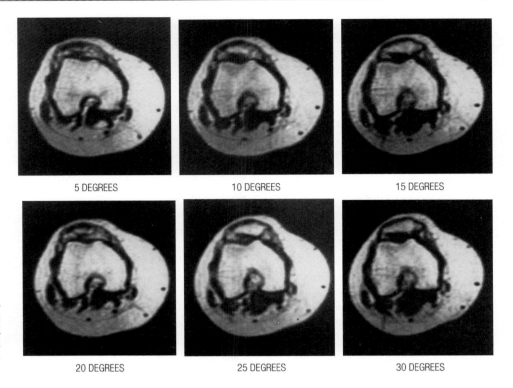

FIGURE 13-21. Severe medial subluxation of the patella in a patient without prior surgery (axial plane kinematic MR images obtained using the incremental passive positioning technique; TR/TE, 400/20 msec; slice thickness, 5 mm).

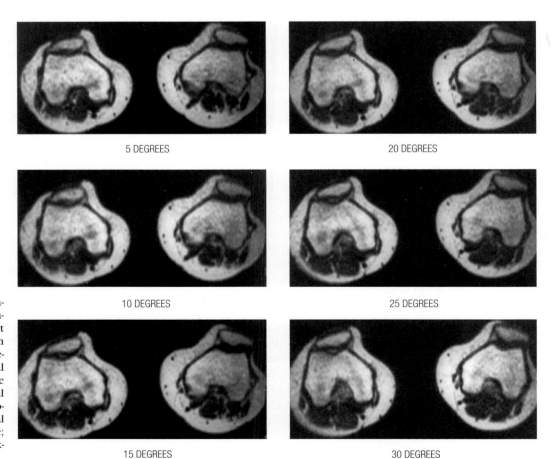

FIGURE 13-22. Lateral subluxation of the patella in the left patellofemoral joint, with slight laxity of the lateral retinaculum seen during the initial increments of joint flexion. Medial subluxation of the patella in the right patellofemoral joint (axial plane kinematic MR images obtained using the incremental passive positioning technique; TR/TE, 400/20 msec; slice thickness, 5 mm).

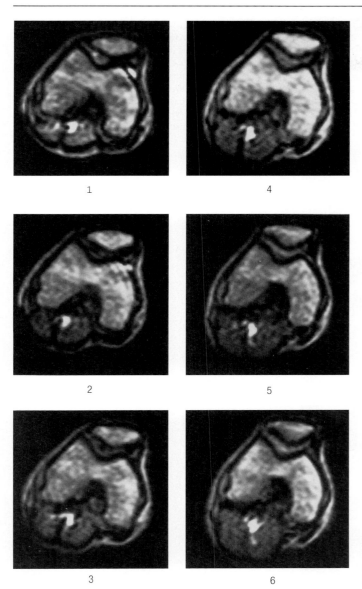

FIGURE 13-23. Medial subluxation of the patella (axial plane fast spoiled GRASS kinematic MR images obtained using the active movement against resistance technique; TR/TE, 6.5/2.1 msec; flip angle, 30°; slice thickness, 7 mm).

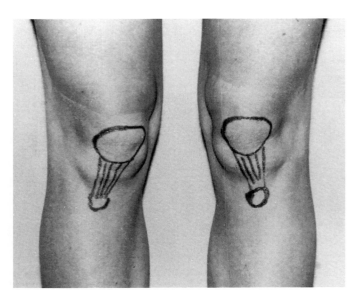

FIGURE 13-24. Bilateral internal rotation of the lower extremities is commonly found in association with medial subluxation of the patella.

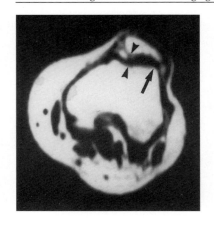
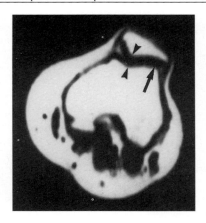
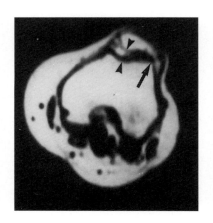
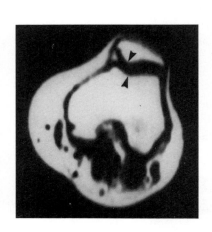
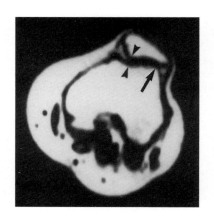
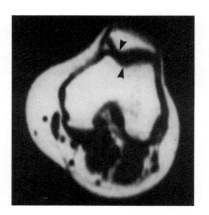

FIGURE 13-25. Slight lateral subluxation of the patella occurs at 5° through 20° of flexion (*long black arrows, alignment of arrowheads*). At 25° of flexion, the patella centralizes (*alignment of arrowheads*). At 30° of flexion, there is slight medial subluxation of the patella (*alignment of arrowheads*). This kinematic pattern is indicative of lateral-to-medial subluxation of the patella (axial plane images; TR, 400 msec; TE, 20 msec; slice thickness, 5 mm).

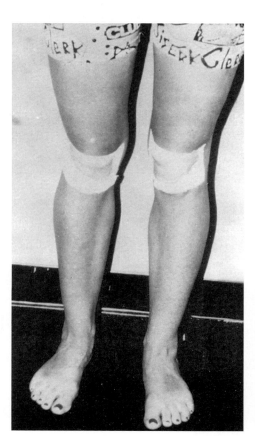

FIGURE 13-26. The McConnel taping technique is used as a conservative method for the treatment of patellofemoral joint abnormalities.

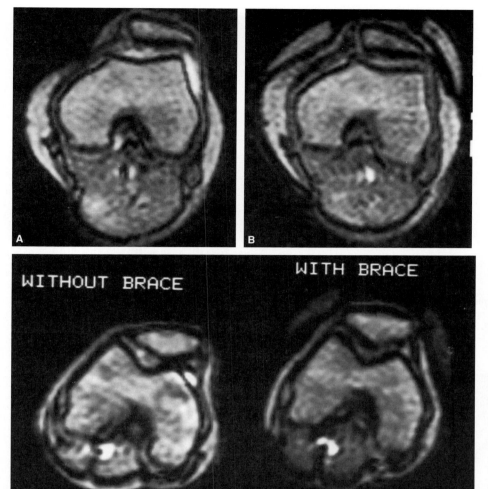

FIGURE 13-27. The kinematic MR imaging examination may be used to assess the effect of conservative treatment techniques, such as the application of braces, to correct abnormal patellar alignment and tracking. Treatment of lateral subluxation before (**A**) and after (**B**) application of a brace. Note that the application of the brace centralized the patella relative to the femoral trochlear groove (axial plane fast spoiled GRASS images; TR/TE, 6.5/2.1 msec; flip angle, 30°; slice thickness, 7 mm; both images were obtained at approximately 40° of flexion). (**C**) Treatment of medial subluxation before and after application of a brace. The application of the brace centralized the patella relative to the femoral trochlear groove (axial plane fast spoiled GRASS images; TR/TE, 6.5/2.1 msec; flip angle, 30°; slice thickness, 7 mm. Both images obtained at approximately 35° of flexion).

above, or, if dual surface coils are used, above and below the wrist. T1- and T2-weighted spin-echo or gradient-echo pulse sequences may be used to obtain images in the coronal plane, using an 8 to 10 cm field of view.

A nonferromagnetic positioning device is used to position the wrist through the range of motion in radial, neutral, and ulnar positions using an incremental passive positioning technique (Fig. 13-28). The patient is placed in a prone position with the elbow extended, and foam padding is placed at various sites under the axilla, arm, and elbow for support and comfort. As with other types of kinematic MR imaging studies, either multiple static images or a cine loop format may be used to view the acquired images. However, the cine loop display is best for demonstrating subtle instability patterns of the carpal bones.

Normal Kinematics

Coronal plane, kinematic MR imaging of normal motion of the wrist in radial, neutral, and ulnar positions show the carpal bones bordered by the radius and ulna, moving in a smooth, symmetrical manner[61,63] (Fig. 13-29). Any deviation from this symmetrical movement of the carpal bones is indicative of instability.

The normal carpal relationships have been described by Gilula[63] as three separate arcs. Arc I follows the main convex curvatures of the proximal surfaces of the scaphoid, lunate, and triquetrum carpal bones. Arc II outlines the distal concave curvatures of these three bones; and arc III traces the main proximal curvatures of the hamate and capitate. Any disruption of these arcs suggests an abnormality at that particular site. The abnormalities may be caused by a torn ligament, laxity of the ligament, or a carpal bone fracture.[1,63,64]

Assessment of intercarpal spacing may also provide evidence of an abnormality.[1,61,63–66] Spacing between the carpal bones should be equal, without any significant or uneven intercarpal widening, proximal or distal movement, or anterior or posterior displacement of the carpal bones.[1,61,63–66] The normal intercarpal space is approximately 1 to 2 mm wide. Increased joint space is suggestive of an abnormal ligament, increased joint fluid, synovial hypertrophy, or other forms of pathokinematics.[1,61–66] Decreased joint space may be caused by an abnormal ligament, loss of carti-

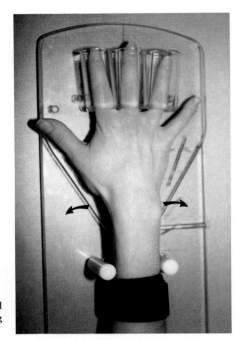

FIGURE 13-28. Nonferromagnetic positioning device used to place the wrist in a neutral position and in ulnar and radial deviation (*curved arrows*) for a kinematic MR imaging examination.

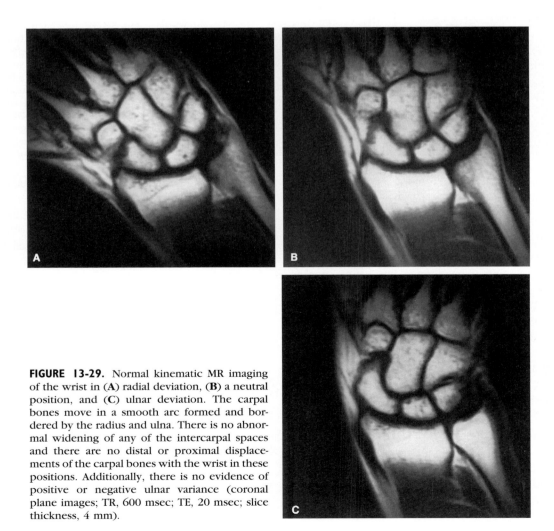

FIGURE 13-29. Normal kinematic MR imaging of the wrist in (**A**) radial deviation, (**B**) a neutral position, and (**C**) ulnar deviation. The carpal bones move in a smooth arc formed and bordered by the radius and ulna. There is no abnormal widening of any of the intercarpal spaces and there are no distal or proximal displacements of the carpal bones with the wrist in these positions. Additionally, there is no evidence of positive or negative ulnar variance (coronal plane images; TR, 600 msec; TE, 20 msec; slice thickness, 4 mm).

lage, carpal coalition, or dislocated or subluxated carpal bones.[1,61-63]

The presence of ulnar variance, whether positive or negative, should also be noted on kinematic MR imaging study of the wrist because it may provide an indication of the mechanism responsible for the abnormality. For example, positive ulnar variance has been associated with tears of the triangular fibrocartilage complex and articular erosions of the lunate and triquetrum.[61] Alternatively, negative ulnar variance is often seen with Kienbock's disease or avascular necrosis of the lunate.[61]

Pathokinematics

Carpal Instability

Carpal bone instability is typically caused by a hyperextension impact injury.[61,63-66] The specific carpal site of the instability depends on the position of the hand (ie, flexed or extended, or in ulnar or radial deviation) at the time of contact.[61,63-66] Early detection and treatment of carpal bone dissociations are crucial for a satisfactory clinical outcome. Conventional plain film x-rays, CT, or static-view MR imaging may be inconclusive in identifying carpal bone instability because the abnormality may be so subtle that it escapes detection unless the wrist is manipulated so that asynchronous motion of the carpals, widening of the joint space, or both may be appreciated. With kinematic MR imaging of the wrist, however, the pathokinematic aspects of carpal instability are depicted[61,63] (Fig. 13-30).

Position-Related Impingement

Kinematic MR imaging of the wrist may also furnish additional useful diagnostic information related to bony and soft-tissue pathologic changes that occur in conjunction with motion-related impingement syndromes.[2] In positive ulnar variance, for example, kinematic MR imaging not only allows identification of the impingement during wrist movement, which is ulnar deviation in this case, but also allows characterization of the abnormality (Fig. 13-31).

THE ANKLE

Clinical applications for kinematic MR imaging of the ankle continue to evolve.[2,14,67] By using a combination of standard high-resolution static MR imaging methods and kinematic

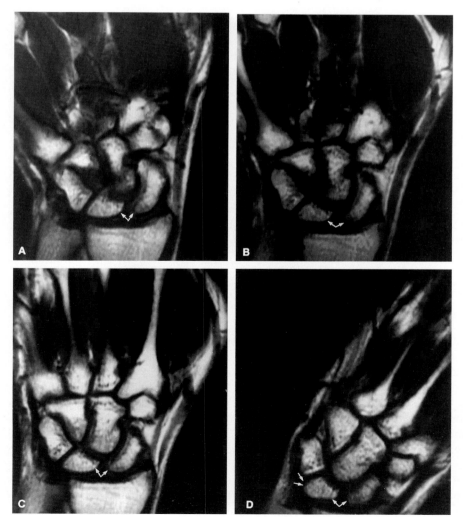

FIGURE 13-30. (**A through C**) Kinematic MR imaging study showing carpal instability with widening of the joint space between the scaphoid and lunate (*joined arrows*). (**D**) This widening is most apparent during radial deviation. In addition, the scaphoid is slightly displaced during radial deviation (*arrows*). There is negative ulnar variance (coronal plane images; TR, 600 msec; TE, 20 msec; slice thickness, 4 mm).

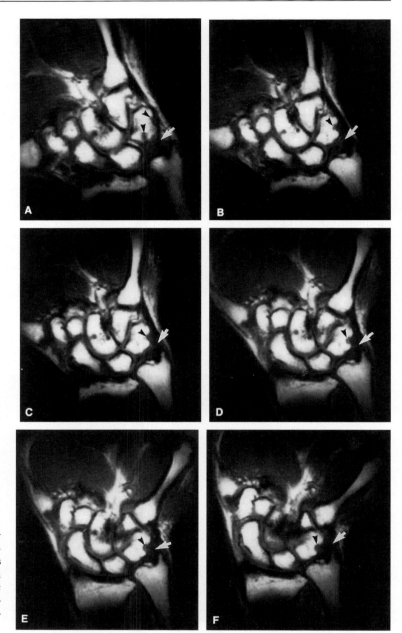

FIGURE 13-31. (**A** through **D**) Kinematic MR imaging study showing cystic degeneration in the triquetrum (*black arrowheads*). There is also positive ulnar variance. Signal changes in the triangular fibrocartilage complex are compatible with a tear (*white arrowheads*). (**E, F**) Impingement between the distal ulna and triquetrum occurs during ulnar deviation (coronal plane images; TR, 600 msec; TE, 20 msec; slice thickness, 4 mm).

MR imaging, a variety of pathologic conditions that affect this joint have been studied.[2,14,67–70] Recent reports indicate that kinematic MR imaging helps to provide a more thorough examination of the ankle, particularly in cases of functional abnormalities associated with bony subluxations or soft-tissue impingement.[2,14,67] Some of the proposed clinical applications include assessment of tibiotalar rotation, evaluation of partial tears of the tendons and ligaments, and determination of loading areas of the talar dome.[2,69] Another important application for kinematic MR imaging of the ankle is assessment of peroneal tendon subluxation.[67]

Kinematic MR Imaging Protocol

The small size and complex anatomy of the ankle make high-resolution kinematic MR views essential for optimal examination of this joint.[2,14,67] Therefore, an apparatus that incorporates dual 12.5 cm (5 inch) receive-only circular surface coils (Captain Plastic, Seattle, WA,) was developed for this procedure (Fig. 13-32). This device permits high-resolution MR imaging for both static and kinematic MR imaging studies.[14]

The patient is placed in a supine position, and the ankle is strapped to a nonferromagnetic positioning device. The kinematic study is performed using an incremental passive position-

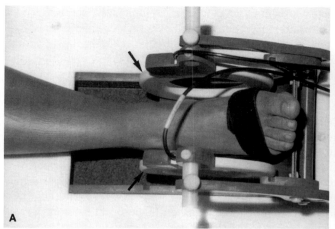
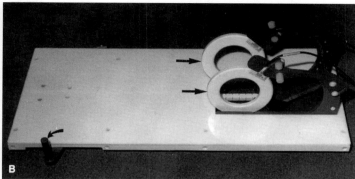

FIGURE 13-32. (**A, B**) Nonferromagnetic positioning device for placing the ankle in dorsiflexed, neutral, and plantarflexed positions for kinematic MR imaging examination using the incremental passive positioning technique. This device has a handle (*curved arrow*) to guide the position of the ankle and incorporates dual 5 inch circular, receive-only surface coils (*straight arrows*).

ing technique with the ankle positioned in dorsiflexion and then progressively moved through a range of motion to plantar flexion. Sagittal or axial T1-weighted spin-echo images are acquired at each increment, using a 10 to 16 cm field of view. Gradient-echo pulse sequences have also been used to examine the ankle without the use of a positioning device.[67] Either static views or the cine-loop format may be used to review the multiple images obtained.

Normal Kinematics

The movement of the ankle joint occurs primarily in the sagittal plane, which permits plantarflexion (extension) and dorsiflexion (flexion) of the foot as the talus rotates beneath the tibia and fibula[1,2,71] (Fig. 13-33). The stability of the ankle is preserved primarily by the configuration of the talus and its conformation to the shapes of the tibia and fibula.[1,2,71] Additional soft-tissue stabilizing structures include the anterior talofibular and calcaneofibular ligaments on the lateral aspect of the joint and the deltoid ligament on the medial side.[1,71-73] The musculotendinous structures that encompass the ankle are involved in stabilization of the joint to a lesser degree.

Abnormalities of the bony anatomy and alterations of the structural soft-tissue restraints markedly affect the stability of the ankle and cause significant malalignment of joint surfaces.[1] These changes are typically manifested as a loss of range of motion, particularly in dorsiflexion.[71-75] Furthermore, slight displacements of the tibiotalar or fibulotalar

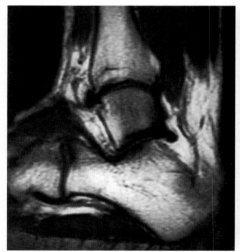
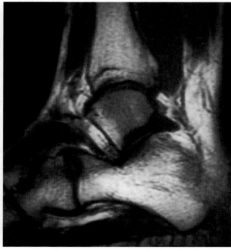
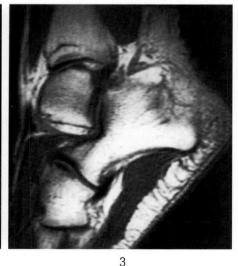

1　　　　　　　　　　　　　　2　　　　　　　　　　　　　　3

FIGURE 13-33. Normal kinematic MR imaging examination of the ankle in (1) dorsiflexed, (2) neutral, and (3) plantarflexed positions using incremental passive positioning technique. There is smooth movement as the talus rotates beneath the tibia (sagittal plane images; TR/TE, 600/20 msec; slice thickness, 4 mm).

articulations can produce substantial changes in loading stress on the ankle causing subsequent pathologic conditions.[1,72,74]

Pathokinematics

Although experience with this technique is limited, sagittal kinematic MR imaging of the ankle is likely to become very useful in evaluating the following pathologic conditions.

Position-Related Impingement

Evaluation of patients with chronic ankle pain is difficult because there are a variety of possible mechanisms potentially responsible for the symptoms, including impingement of soft-tissue structures and/or bony anatomy, osteochondritis dissecans, avascular necrosis, or loose bodies (Figs. 13-34). Kinematic MR imaging combined with high-resolution static-view MR imaging of the ankle provides information that permits differentiation among these various conditions.[2,14,67]

Bony or soft-tissue impingement syndromes that affect the ankle typically cause pain and inhibit motion during dorsiflexion.[71-75] In the past, it was thought that impingement syndromes of the ankle were caused by osseous structures, such as an osteophyte on the anterior aspect of the tibia that impacts with the talus during dorsiflexion. However, soft-tissue impingement syndromes associated with plantarflexion inversion injuries of the ankle have recently been described.[72,73] Following tears of the lateral ankle ligaments (usually the talofibular ligament, the calcaneofibular ligament, or both), the healing process may be accompanied by scarring and capsular hypertrophy in the anterolateral space. This can produce a soft-tissue impingement during dorsiflexion of the ankle.[2,73] In such cases, kinematic MR imaging of the ankle demonstrates impingement of the soft-tissue mass during movement of the ankle.

Subluxation of Peroneal Tendons

Ankle injuries may result in subluxation of the peroneal tendons, which is often unrecognized and frequently misdiagnosed as an ankle sprain, delaying appropriate initial management.[67,75-77] Chronic subluxation of the peroneal tendons can be disabling, particularly if tendon pathology is also present.[75-77] The incidence of peroneal tendon subluxation is on the rise due to an increase in recreational sports activities and an additional awareness of the abnormality.[75-77] Although lateral joint pain and tenderness are characteristic in patients with peroneal tendon abnormalities, other associated lesions may produce identical symptoms.[75-77]

Identification of peroneal tendon subluxation is difficult because the clinical signs may mimic other forms of ankle injuries and because coexisting abnormalities may be present. In the acute injury, clinical evaluation of the peroneal tendons may be hindered by associated swelling and tenderness, which can be partially attributed to disruption of neighboring ligaments or osseous structures.[75-77] Additionally, peroneal tendon subluxation may cause pain over the calcaneofibular ligament,[75-77] confusing the presenting symptomatology. Chronic, recurrent subluxation is also difficult to detect clinically, especially if the displacement is subtle or if the tendons spontaneously move back into position.

Various biomechanic mechanisms of injury have been postulated to explain subluxation of the peroneal tendons, including violent or forced dorsiflexed or plantarflexed positions of the ankle.[75-77] In evaluation of the pathobiomechanics of this abnormality, it is helpful to visualize the peroneal tendons during dorsiflexed and plantarflexed ankle movements using kinematic MR imaging.[72,75-77] This allows direct identification of subluxation of the peroneal tendons, as well as the ability to determine occult displacements, since spontaneous reduction of subluxed tendons is known to occur.[72]

Peroneal tendon subluxation may have serious associated sequellae,[76,77] and the prognosis for subluxation of the peroneal tendons that is not repaired or treated in the early stages following injury is poor.[76,77] Therefore, rapid and accurate diagnosis of this abnormality is critical for appropriate patient management. Kinematic MR imaging of the ankle in the axial plane using the previously mentioned positioning device and incremental passive positioning has recently been described as a useful means of identifying subluxation of the peroneal tendons.[67]

NORMAL KINEMATICS OF THE PERONEAL TENDONS. The normal kinematic function of the peroneal tendons is dependent on the integrity of several elastic structures, especially the superior peroneal retinaculum, and on a morphologically adequate retromalleolar groove.[76,77] The soft-tissue structures and the retromalleolar groove serve to maintain the peroneal tendons in a constant position during movements of the ankle.[76,77]

The peroneal tendon complex is comprised of the peroneus longus and brevis tendons, which are ensheathed by a common synovial membrane. The tendon and sheath bundle course through a fibro-osseous canal, composed primarily of the superior peroneal retinaculum and the undersurface of the distal fibular tip. These structures along with the retromalleolar groove serve to maintain the peroneal tendons in a constant position during movements of the ankle. Therefore, the normal kinematic study of the peroneus longus and brevis tendons shows the tendons in a fixed position relative to the retromalleolar groove of the lateral malleolus during dorsiflexed, neutral, and plantarflexed positions of the ankle (Fig. 13-35). In addition, at the level of the calcaneus, the peroneal tendons should be positioned parallel relative to the lateral aspect of the calcaneus during these movements.

PATHOKINEMATICS OF THE PERONEAL TENDONS. Subluxation of the peroneal tendons occurs when the tendons move laterally over the lateral malleolus. This may occur with varying degrees of severity: from subtle displacements relative to the retromalleolar groove associated with dorsiflexed or plantarflexed movements of the ankle to constant displace-

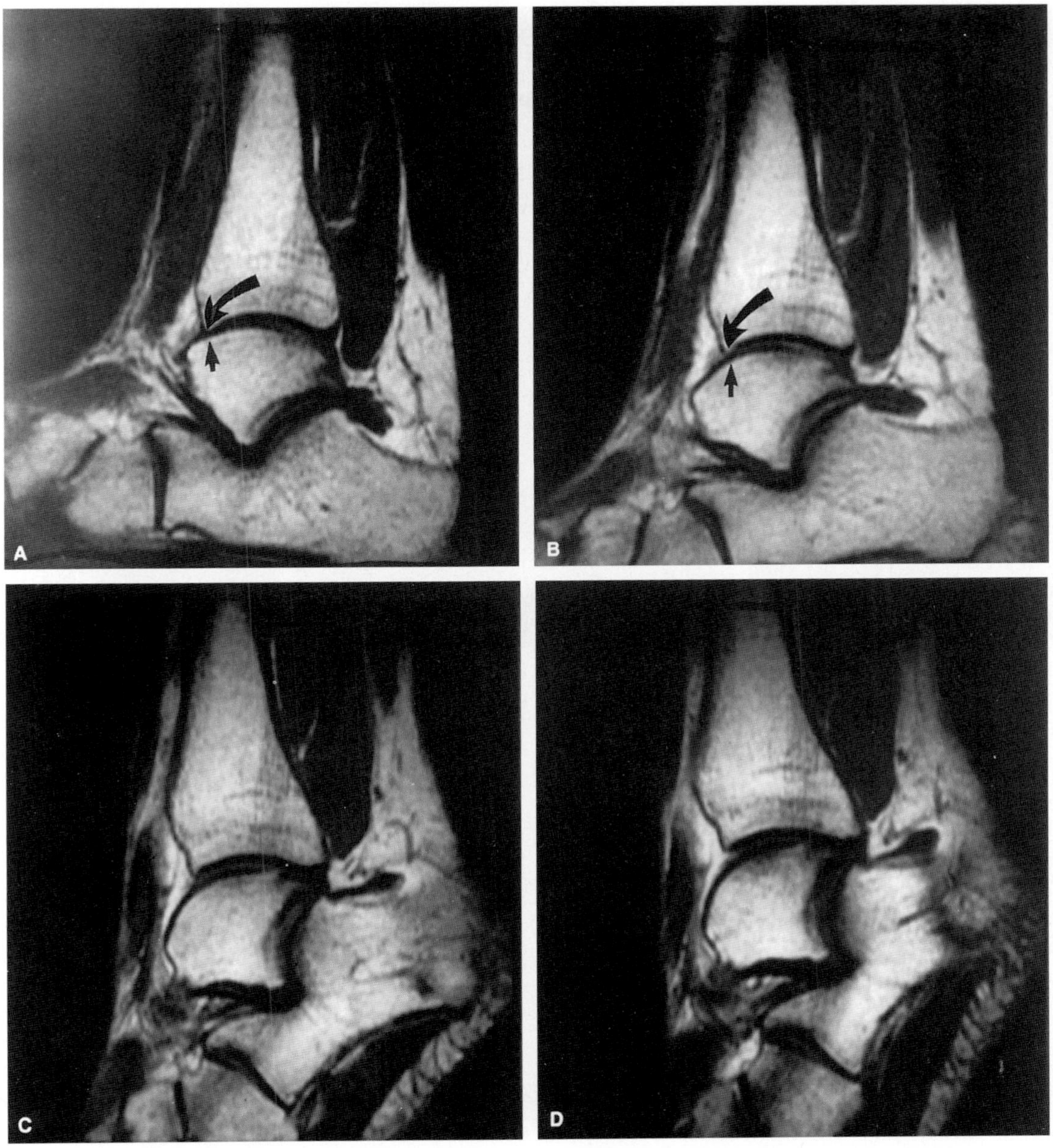

FIGURE 13-34. (**A, B**) Bony impingement (*arrows*) occurs between a small osteophyte on the tibia that impacts with the talus, primarily during dorsiflexion positioning of the ankle. There is also a slight anterior displacement of the talus relative to the tibia. (**C, D**) Bony impingement is not observed during plantar flexion of the ankle (sagittal plane images; TR, 600 msec; TE, 20 msec; slice thickness, 4 mm).

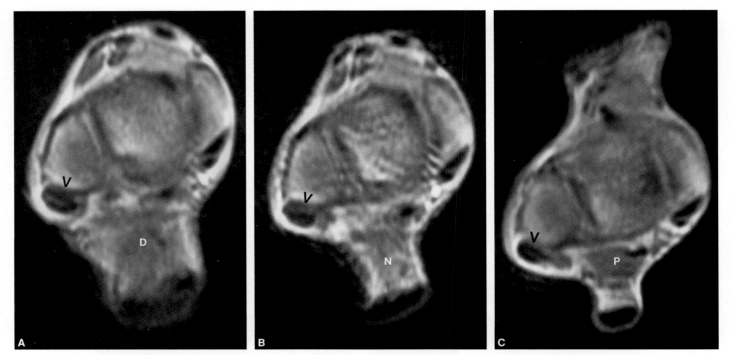

FIGURE 13-35. Kinematic MR imaging examination of the ankle in (**A**) dorsiflexed (D), (**B**) neutral (N), and (**C**) plantarflexed (P) positions using incremental passive positioning technique. The peroneal tendons are maintained in the same position relative to the retromalleolar groove throughout the range of motion of the ankle (*open arrowheads*) (axial plane fast spoiled GRASS images; TR/TE, 6.1/2.5 msec; slice thickness, 5 mm).

ment of the peroneal tendons unrelated to the position of the ankle (ie, the peroneal tendons remain in a displaced position irrespective of the position of the ankle).[67,72,76,77] When an abnormality is demonstrated on axial plane kinematic MR images, the peroneal tendons are either displaced relative to the retromalleolar groove and/or relative to the lateral aspect of the calcaneus, in association with changes in the position of the ankle.[67] In rare cases, medial subluxation of the peroneal tendons may also occur.

The primary causes of peroneal subluxation include those associated with predisposing anatomical disorders—such as a shallow, flat, or convex retromalleolar groove—and/or a weakened peroneal retinaculum. Various forms of retinacular pathology may be responsible for subluxation of the peroneal tendons, including congenital absence of the retinaculum, laxity of the retinaculum in a paralyzed extremity or an extremity in chronic pronation, or retinacular hyperelasticity.[76,77] When retinacular pathology is primarily or solely the cause of peroneal tendon subluxation, the strength of the peroneal retinaculum is usually exceeded during resistance to forced dorsiflexion or plantarflexion ankle movements and the peroneal tendons are displaced.[76,77]

THE SHOULDER

A recent study, conducted to assess the use of kinematic MR imaging of the shoulder during internal and external rotation movements, reported good visualization of the ante-

rior glenoid labrum (AGL) and demonstration of the role of the AGL, in conjunction with the capsular ligaments, in anterior stabilization of the glenohumeral joint.[78] Kinematic MR imaging of the shoulder may be used to demonstrate limitation of the range of motion of the shoulder by entrapment of the AGL at the extremes of motion.[78] Avulsions of the AGL are also well characterized with kinematic MR imaging of the shoulder.[78] Another advantage of kinematic MR imaging of the shoulder is quantification of the degree of subcoracoid impingement, determined by measuring the distance between the lesser tuberosity and the coracoid process.[78] Additional experience with this modality will contribute to further refinement of the role of kinematic MR imaging of the shoulder.

THE CERVICAL SPINE

Functional assessment of the cervical spine may be performed using kinematic MR imaging techniques.[79-81] In many instances, kinematic MR imaging of the cervical spine provides supplemental information to routine, static MR imaging. Since there may be a significant change in spinal canal and cord compression during flexion and extension of the cervical spine, kinematic studies are especially useful for assessment of the cervical spine during these movements. Indications for study include evaluation of spinal stenosis, postoperative status, and suspected spinal instability.[79-81]

Kinematic MR Imaging Protocol

Kinematic MR imaging of the cervical spine may be performed using a specially designed positioning device that incorporates a flexible surface coil to facilitate imaging for an incremental passive positioning technique or active movement kinematic studies.[79–81] Sagittal plane images are obtained with the cervical spine in flexion, a neutral position, and extension (Fig. 13-36). In an alternative method, the cervical spine is placed in just the flexion and extension positions (using foam rubber pads and tape to maintain placement and to restrict motion) while MR images are obtained. T1-weighted, T2-weighted spin-echo, fast spin-echo, and gradient-echo pulse sequences may be used

to obtain images in the mid-sagittal plane, with an 18 to 22 cm field of view.

Evaluation of Kinematic MR Imaging of the Cervical Spine

Sagittal plane images obtained through the cervical spine are typically assessed qualitatively, similar to those acquired using standard MR imaging techniques.[79–81] Attention is directed toward evaluation of position dependent occipitocervical changes, cord narrowing, occult subluxation, or other forms of functional pathology (Fig. 13-37).

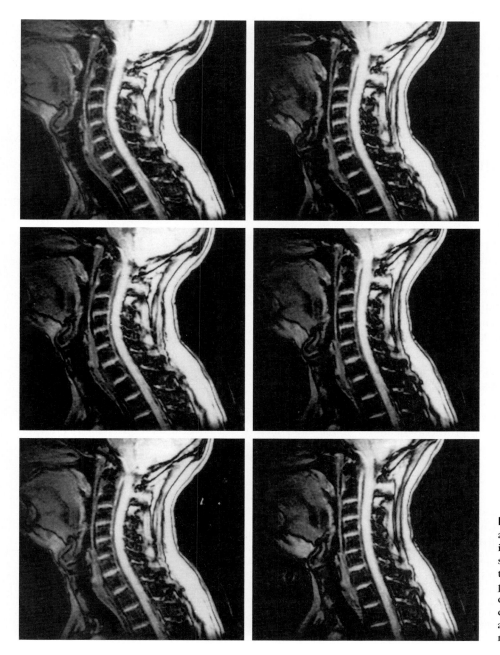

FIGURE 13-36. Kinematic MR imaging examination of the cervical spine using the incremental passive positioning technique shows normal movement and alignment of the cervical vertebrae in flexion, a neutral position, and extension. There is no evidence of subluxation or narrowing of the cord (sagittal plane fast spoiled GRASS images; TR/TE, 8/3 msec; slice thickness, 7 mm).

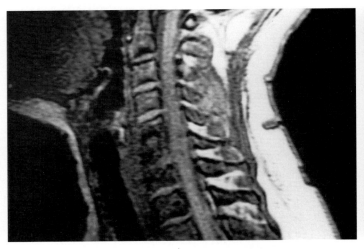
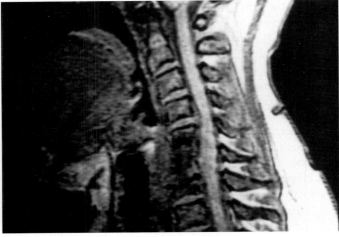

1   2

FIGURE 13-37. Kinematic MR imaging examination of the cervical spine using the incremental passive positioning technique in (1) a neutral position and (2) flexion position shows narrowing of the cord seen during flexion that is not apparent with the cervical spine in a neutral position (sagittal plane fast spoiled GRASS images; TR/TE, 8/3 msec; slice thickness, 7 mm).

FUTURE DIRECTIONS OF KINEMATIC MR IMAGING

The development of fast gradient-echo pulse sequences with increased temporal resolution capabilities has improved rapid imaging of the joints during active motion for kinematic MR imaging examinations. Rapid imaging has allowed a more physiologic and functional assessment, enhancing the usefulness of kinematic MR imaging of joints. The widespread use of fast pulse sequence techniques has allowed further definition and implementation of additional applications of kinematic MR imaging in the clinical setting.

In another technical advancement, echo planar imaging techniques are currently undergoing installation on many MR systems. The imaging speed of these MR systems will likely be used to facilitate performance of kinematic MR imaging of the joints. However, specific protocols need to be developed for appropriate applications. To date, echo planar imaging has shown encouraging results for assessment of the patellofemoral joint with kinematic MR imaging.[39]

MR systems with open-architecture configurations have undergone several technological improvements that make it possible to attain image quality that lends itself to acceptable MR imaging examinations of the joints. Because the patient is more accessible in these MR systems and there is an increased area available for movements of the larger joints (ie, knee, hip, shoulder, and spine), it may be possible to perform MR-guided physical assessments of the joints. This evolution of kinematic MR imaging is presently under development at a number of research centers.

References

1. Nordin M, Frankel VH. Basic biomechanics of the musculoskeletal system, 2nd ed. Philadelphia: Lea & Febiger, 1989.
2. Shellock FG, Mandelbaum B. Kinematic MRI of the joints. In: Mink JH, Deutsch AL, eds. MRI of the musculoskeletal system: a teaching file. New York: Raven Press, 1990.
3. Burnett KR, Davis CL, Read J. Dynamic display of the temporomandibular joint meniscus by using "fast-scan" MR imaging. AJR 1987;149:959.
4. Pressman BD, Shellock FG. Static and kinematic MR imaging of the TMJ. Calif Dental Assoc J 1988;August:32.
5. Pressman BD, Shellock FG. The temporomandibular joint. In: Mink JH, Deutsch AL, eds. MRI of the musculoskeletal system: a teaching file. New York: Raven Press, 1990.
6. Brossman J, Muhle C, Schroder C, Melchert UH, Spielmann RP, Heller M. Motion-triggered cine MR imaging: evaluation of patellar tracking patterns during active and passive knee extension. Radiology 1993; 187:205.
7. Shellock FG, Pressman BD. MR imaging of the temporomandibular joint: improvements in the imaging protocol. AJNR 1989;10:595.
8. Shellock FG, Deutsch AL, Mink JH, Fox JM. Identification of medial subluxation of the patella in a dancer using kinematic MRI of the patellofemoral joint: a case report. Kinesiol Med Dance 1991;13:1.
9. Shellock FG, Mink JH, Deutsch AL, Fox JM. Evaluation of patellar tracking abnormalities using kinematic MR imaging: clinical experience in 130 patients. Radiology 1989;172:799.
10. Shellock FG, Mink JH, Deutsch AL, Fox JM. Kinematic magnetic resonance imaging for evaluation of patellar tracking. Physician Sports Med 1989;17:99.
11. Shellock FG, Mink JH, Fox JM. Patellofemoral joint: kinematic MR imaging to assess tracking abnormalities. Radiology 1988;168:551.

12. Shellock FG, Mink JH, Deutsch AL, Fox JM, Ferkel RD. Evaluation of patients with persistent symptoms after lateral retinacular release by kinematic magnetic resonance imaging of the patellofemoral joint. Arthroscopy 1990;6:226.

13. Shellock FG, Mink JH, Fox JM, Ferkel RD, Friedman M, Molnar T. Kinematic MRI evaluation of symptomatic patients following two or more patellar realignment surgeries. J Magn Reson Imaging 1991; 1:175.

14. Shellock FG, Mink JH, Sullenberger P. High-resolution static and kinematic MRI of the ankle. Society of Magnetic Resonance in Medicine, Berkeley, ninth annual meeting. Book of abstracts, vol 2, 1990:766.

15. Fulmer JM, Harms SE, Flamig DP, Guerdon G, Machek J, Dolinar J. High-resolution cine MR imaging of the wrist. Radiology 1989;173:26.

16. Bergey PD, Zlatkin MB, Dalinka M, Osterman AL, Machek J, Dolinar J. Dynamic MR imaging of the wrist: early results with a specially designed positioning device. Radiology 1989;173:26.

17. Helms CA, Katzberg RW, Dolwick MF. Internal derangements of the temporomandibular joint. San Francisco: University of California Printing Department, 1983.

18. Brossman J, Muhle C, Bull C, et al. Evaluation of patellar tracking in patients with suspected patellar malalignment: cine MR imaging vs. arthroscopy. AJR 1993;162:361.

19. Drace JE, Enzmann DR. Defining the normal temporomandibular joint: closed-, partially open-, and open mouth MR imaging of asymptomatic subjects. Radiology 1990;177:67.

20. Manzione JV, Tallents RF, Katzberg RW, Oster C, Miller TL. Arthrographically guided therapy for recapturing the temporomandibular joint meniscus. Oral Surg Oral Med Oral Pathol 1984;57:235.

21. Tallents RH, Katzberg RW, Miller TL, Manzione JV, Oster C. Arthrographically assisted splint therapy. J Prosthet Dent 1985;53:235.

22. Kummel BM. The diagnosis of patellofemoral derangements. Prim Care 1980;7:199.

23. Ficat RF, Hungerford DS. Disorders of the patello-femoral joint. Baltimore: Williams & Wilkins, 1977.

24. Larson RL. Subluxation-dislocation of the patella. In: Kennedy JC, ed. The injured adolescent knee. Baltimore: Williams and Wilkins, 1979:161.

25. Fulkerson JP, Hungerford DS. Disorders of the patellofemoral joint, 2nd ed. Baltimore: Williams and Wilkins, 1990.

26. Insall J, Falvo KA, Wise DW. Patellar pain and incongruence. II. Clinical application. Clin Orthop 1983;176:225.

27. Moller BN, Krebs B, Jurik AG. Patellofemoral incongruence in chondromalacia and instability of the patella. Acta Orthop Scand 1986;57:232.

28. Moller BN, Moller-Larsen F, Frich LH. Chondromalacia induced by patellar subluxation in rabbit. Acta Orthop Scand 1989;60:188.

29. Kujala UM, Osterman K, Kormano M, Komu M, Schlenzka D. Patellar motion analyzed by magnetic resonance imaging. Acta Orthop Scand 1989;60:13.

30. Kujala UM, Osterman K, Kormano M, Nelimarkka O, Hurme M, Taimela S. Patellofemoral relationships in recurrent patellar dislocation. J Bone Joint Surg [Br] 1989;71B:788.

31. Schutzer SF, Ramsby GR, Fulkerson JP. Computed tomographic classification of patellofemoral joint pain patients. Orthop Clin North Am 1986;17:235.

32. Deutsch AD, Shellock FG, Mink JH. Imaging of the patellofemoral joint: emphasis on advanced techniques. In: Fox J, Del Pizzo W, eds. The patellofemoral joint. New York: McGraw-Hill, 1993.

33. Stanford W, Phelan J, Kathol MH, et al. Patellofemoral joint motion: evaluation by ultrafast computed tomography. Skeletal Radiol 1988; 17:487.

34. Conway WF, Hayes CW, Loughran T, et al. Cross-sectional imaging of the patellofemoral joint and surrounding structures. RadioGraphics 1991;11:195.

35. Shellock FG, Mink JH, Deutsch A, Pressman B. Kinematic MRI of the joints: techniques and clinical applications. Magn Reson Q 1991;7:104.

36. Shellock FG. Patellofemoral joint abnormalities in athletes: evaluation by kinematic MRI. Top Magn Res Imaging 1991;3:1.

37. Shellock FG, Foo TKF, Deutsch A, Mink JH. Patellofemoral joint: evaluation during active flexion with ultrafast spoiled GRASS MR imaging. Radiology 1991;180:581.

38. Shellock FG: Kinematic MRI evaluation of the joints. In: Stoller DW, ed. Magnetic resonance imaging in orthopaedics and rheumatology. Philadelphia: JB Lippincott, 1993.

39. Shellock FG, Cohen MS, Brady T, Mink JH, Pfaff JM. Evaluation of patellar alignment and tracking: comparison between kinematic MRI and ''true'' dynamic imaging by hyperscan MRI. J Magn Reson Imaging 1991;1:148.

40. Shellock FG, Fox JM, Deutsch A, Mink JH. Medial subluxation of the patella: radiologic and physical findings. Radiology 1991;181P:179.

41. Shellock FG, Mink JH, Deutsch AL, Foo TKF. Kinematic MR imaging of the patellofemoral joint: comparison between passive positioning and active movement techniques. Radiology 1992;184:574.

42. Shellock FG, Mink JH, Deutsch AL, Foo TKF, Sullenberger P. Patellofemoral joint: identification of abnormalities using active movement, ''unloaded'' vs ''loaded'' kinematic MR imaging techniques. Radiology 1993;188:575.

43. Koskinen SP, Kujala UM. Effect of patellar brace on patellofemoral relationships. Scand J Med Sci Sports 1991;1:119.

44. Koskinen SK, Hurme M, Kujala UM, Kormano M. Effect of lateral release on patellar motion in chondromalacia: an MRI study of 11 knees. Acta Orthop Scand 1990;61:311.

45. Brown SM, Muroff LR, Bradley WG, Atkinson DJ. Ultrafast kinematic MR imaging of the knee: increased sensitivity with a quadriceps loading device. J Magn Reson Imaging 1993;S29(suppl):(in press).

46. Kaplan E. Some aspects of functional anatomy of the human knee joint. Clin Orthop 1962;23:18.

47. Otis JC, Gould JD. The effect of external load on torque production by knee extensors. J Bone J Surg 1986;68A:65.

48. Insall J. Chondromalacia patellae: patellar malalignment syndrome. Orthop Clin North Am 1979;10:117.

49. Wiberg G. Roentgenographic and anatomic studies on the femoropatellar joint, with special reference to chondromalacia patellae. Acta Orthop Scand 1941;12:319.

50. Shellock FG, Kim S, Mink J, Deutsch A, Fox J. ''Functional'' patella alta determined by axial plane imaging of the patellofemoral joint: association with abnormal patellar alignment and tracking. J Magn Reson Imaging 1992;2P:93.

51. Lancourt JE, Cristini JA. Patella alta and patella infera: their etiological role in patellar dislocation, chondromalacia, and apophysitis of the tibial tubercle. J Bone Joint Surg [Am] 1975;57A:1112.

52. Marks KE, Bentley G. Patella alta and chondromalacia. J Bone Joint Surg [Br] 1978;60B:71.

53. Laurin CA, Dussault R, Levesque HP. The tangential x-ray investigation of the patellofemoral joint: x-ray technique, diagnostic criteria and their interpretation. Clin Orthop 1979;144:16.

54. Merchant AC, Mercer RL, Jacobsen RH, Cool CR. Roentgenographic analysis of patellofemoral congruence. J Bone Joint Surg [Am] 1974;56A:1391.

55. Carson WG, James SL, Larson RL, Singer KM, Winternitz WW. Patellofemoral disorders: physical and radiographic evaluation. II. Radiographic examination. Clin Orthop Rel Res 1984;185:178.

56. Eppley RA. Medial patellar subluxation. In: Fox J, Del Pizzo W, eds. The patellofemoral joint. New York: McGraw-Hill, 1993:149.

57. Hughston JC, Deese M. Medial subluxation of the patella as a complication of lateral release. Am J Sports Med 1988;16:383.

58. Molnar TJ. Patellar rehabilitation. In: Fox J, Del Pizzo W, eds. The patellofemoral joint. New York: McGraw-Hill, 1993:149.

59. Shellock FG, Mink JH, Deutsch AL, Fox J, Molnar T, Kvitne R. Effect of a patellar realignment brace on patellofemoral relationships: evaluation using kinematic MR imaging. J Magn Reson Imaging 1994;4:590.

60. Shellock FG, Mink JH, Deutsch DL, Molnar T. Effect of a newly-

designed patellar realignment brace on patellofemoral relationships: a case report. Med Sci Sports Exerc 1995;27:469.

61. Reicher MA, Kellerhouse LE. Normal wrist anatomy, biomechanics, basic imaging protocol, and normal multiplanar MRI of the wrist. In: Reicher MA, Kellerhouse LE, eds. MRI of the hand and wrist. New York: Raven Press, 1990.

62. Tjin A, Ton ER, Pattynama PMT, Bloem JL, Obermann WR. Interosseous ligaments: device for applying stress in wrist MR imaging. Radiology 1995;196:863.

63. Gilula LA. Carpal injuries: analytic approach and case exercises. AJR 1977;133:503.

64. Culver JE. Instabilities of the wrist. Clin Sports Med 1986;5:725.

65. Lichtman DM, Noble WH, Alexander CE. Dynamic triquetrolunate instability. J Hand Surg [Am] 1984;9:185.

66. Linscheid RL, Dobyns H, Beabout JW, Bryan RS. Traumatic instability of the wrist. J Bone Joint Surg [Am] 1972;54:1612.

67. Shellock FG, Feske W, Frey C, Terk M. Peroneal tendons: use of kinematic MR imaging to determine subluxation. J Magn Reson Imaging 1996.

68. Kneeland B, Macrandar S, Middleton WD, Cates JD, Jesmanowicz A, Hyde JS. MR imaging of the normal ankle: correlation with anatomic sections. AJR 1988;151:117.

69. Hajek PC, Baker LL, Bjorkengren A, Sartoris DJ, Neumann CH, Resnick D. High-resolution magnetic resonance imaging of the ankle: normal anatomy. Skeletal Radiol 1986;15:536.

70. Sierra A, Potchen EJ, Moore J, Smith HG. High-field magnetic resonance imaging of aseptic necrosis of the talus. J Bone Joint Surg [Am] 1986;68:927.

71. Rodgers MM. Dynamic biomechanics of the normal foot and ankle during walking and running. Phys Ther 1988;68:1822.

72. Parlasca R, Shoh H, D'Ambrosia RD. Effects of ligmentous injury on ankle and subtalar joints: a kinematic study. Clin Orthop 1979;140.

73. Perlman M, Leveille D, DeLeonibus J, et al. Inversion lateral ankle trauma: differential diagnosis, review of the literature, and prospective study. J Foot Surg 1987;26:95.

74. Bassett FH, Gates HS, Billys JB, Morris HB, Nikolaou PK. Talar impingement by anteroinferior tibiofibular ligament. J Bone Joint Surg [Am] 1990;72:55.

75. Frey CC, et al. Tendon injuries about the ankle in athletes. Clin Sports Med 1988;7:103.

76. Butler BW, Lanthier J, Wertheimer SJ. Subluxing peroneals: a review of the literature and case report. J Foot Surg 1992;32:134.

77. Geppert MJ, et al. Lateral ankle instability as a cause of superior peroneal retinacular laxity: an anatomic and biomechanical study of cadaveric feet. Foot Ankle 1993;14:330.

78. Bonutti PM, Norfray JF, Friedman RJ, Genez BM. Kinematic MRI of the shoulder. J Comput Assist Tomogr 1993;17:666.

79. Shellock FG, Sullenberger P, Mink JH, et al. MRI of the cervical spine during flexion and extension: development and implementation of a new technique. J Magn Reson Imaging 1994;WIP:S21.

80. Naegele M, Kaden B, Koch FW, Kunze V, Woell B, Bruening R. Dynamic function MR imaging of the cervical spine. Radiology 1992;185P:219.

81. Weidenmaier W, Schnarkowski P, Haeussler MD, Friedrich JM. Dynamics of the cervical spine: functional MR imaging in 50 patients after distention injury. Radiology 1992;185P:219.

Magnetic Resonance Imaging in Orthopaedics & Sports Medicine, Second Edition,
edited by David W. Stoller. Lippincott-Raven Publishers, Philadelphia, © 1997.

Chapter 14

The Spine

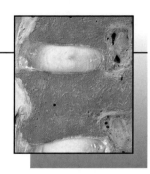

David W. Stoller

Serena S. Hu

Jay A. Kaiser

Accurate diagnosis and evaluation of the cervical, thoracic, and lumbar spines are important in orthopaedics, rheumatology, neurology, and neurosurgery. At best, standard radiographs provide a limited interpretation of nonosseous events occurring in the disks, cord, cerebrospinal fluid (CSF), and ligaments (these structures are not directly seen in plain film radiographs). Myelography, an invasive procedure, provides an indirect evaluation of the disk by displaying the contour of the thecal sac and proximal nerve root sleeves. Computed tomography (CT) is useful in delineating bone detail, and direct axial scans of the spine provide soft tissue discrimination of the disk, nerve roots, and thecal sac.[1-6] Sagittal, coronal, or oblique views, however, cannot be directly acquired and require reformations (Fig. 14-1). Although CT is excellent for assessing postoperative stenosis and pseudoarthrosis, fibrosis and scarring may be difficult to differen-

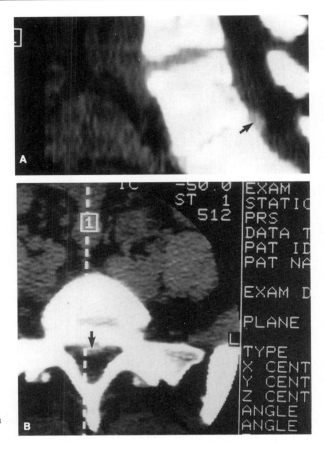

FIGURE 14-1. L5-S1 disk herniation (*arrow*) with soft tissue density seen on (**A**) reformatted CT sagittal images and (**B**) direct axial CT images.

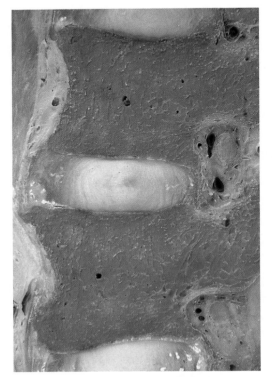

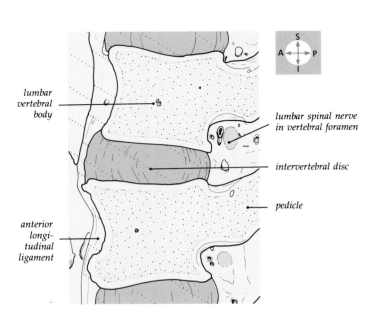

FIGURE 14-2. A sagittal section of the lumbar vertebral column.

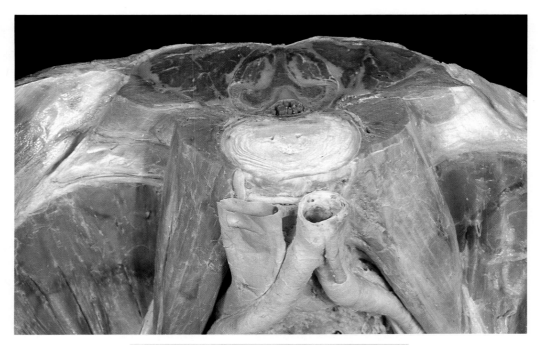

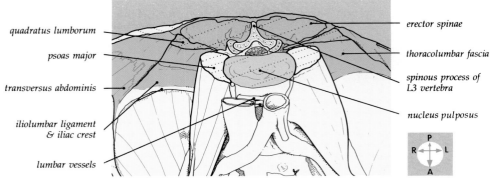

quadratus lumborum

psoas major

transversus abdominis

iliolumbar ligament
& iliac crest

lumbar vessels

erector spinae

thoracolumbar fascia

spinous process of
L3 vertebra

nucleus pulposus

FIGURE 14-3. An oblique view of a transverse section of the lumbar spine and muscles at the level of the disk between the third and fourth lumbar vertebrae.

tiate from disk material, even with the use of contrast enhancement.

Magnetic resonance (MR) imaging supersedes CT and myelography in the routine evaluation of the spine for degenerative disk disease, trauma, infection, neoplasia, and intrinsic cord disease.[7–58] The intervertebral disk consists of the nucleus pulposus, the annulus fibrosus, and the cartilaginous endplate (Figs. 14-2 and 14-3). With MR imaging, the separate components of the disk, including the nucleus pulposus and annulus fibrosus, can be distinguished and assessed in early degenerative disk disease. The disk–thecal sac interface is defined without administration of a contrast agent, the structure of the cord is seen contrasted by surrounding CSF, and the dura and supporting ligaments of the spine are demonstrated in either sagittal or axial images (Figs. 14-4 and 14-5). The conus medullaris is displayed with superior contrast resolution with MR imaging (Figs. 14-6 and 14-7). MR imaging provides the unique advantage of direct marrow imaging in the study of patients with marrow infiltra-

tive diseases, metastasis, infection, or reactive endplate changes.[59–74] The components of the atlantoaxial joint (Fig. 14-8) can be differentiated using MR imaging in any of the three orthogonal planes (Fig. 14-9).

The cervical spine, cord, and paravertebral muscles are enclosed within the paravertebral fascia, and their cross-sectional relationships are best displayed on axial images (Fig. 14-10). The spinal cord is surrounded by the dura, arachnoid, and pia mater (Fig. 14-11). MR imaging of the thoracic spine is obtained with a field of view (FOV) that excludes unwanted information and artifact from mediastinal structures (Figs. 14-12 and 14-13).

MR imaging of the spine has improved as advancements have been made in surface coil design and in software. Oblique imaging, cardiac gating, fast spin-echo techniques, gradient-echo imaging, short TI inversion recovery (STIR) imaging, enhancement with gadolinium contrast (Gd-DTPA; a paramagnetic contrast agent), and most recently, echo pla-

text continues on page 1071

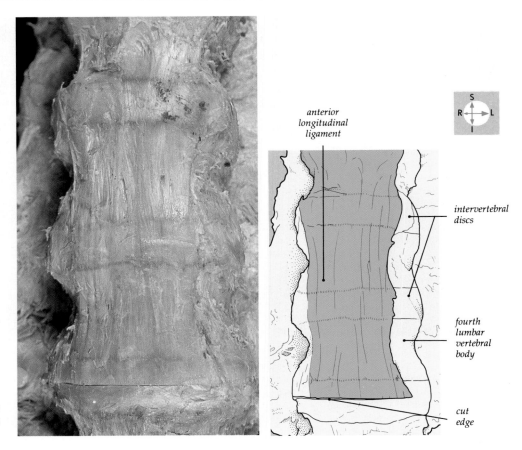

FIGURE 14-4. An oblique view of the anterior longitudinal ligament of the lumbar spine.

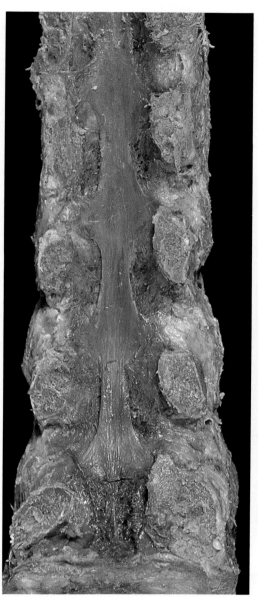

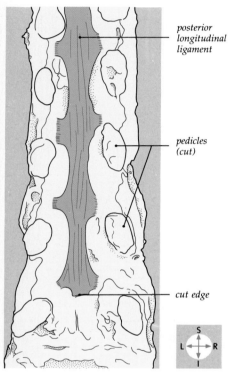

posterior
longitudinal
ligament

pedicles
(cut)

cut edge

FIGURE 14-5. The posterior longitudinal ligament is exposed by removing the vertebral arches, meninges, and spinal cord.

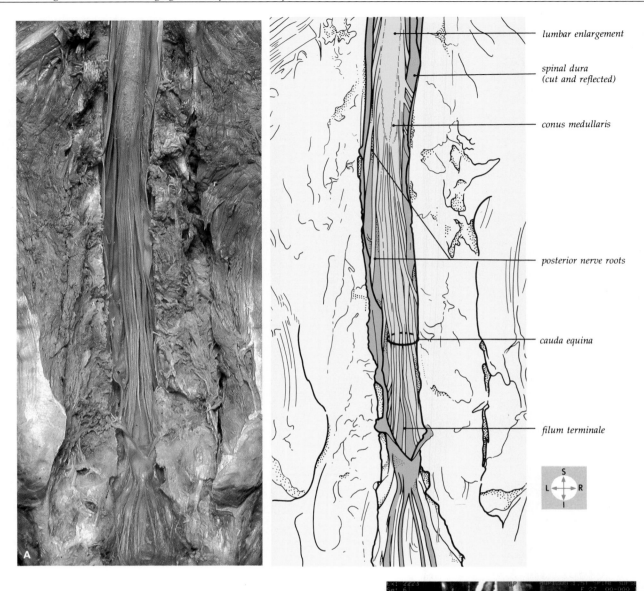

lumbar enlargement

spinal dura
(cut and reflected)

conus medullaris

posterior nerve roots

cauda equina

filum terminale

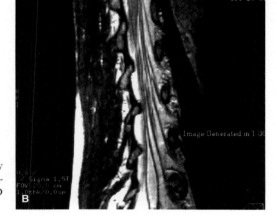

FIGURE 14-6. (**A**) The spinal dura and arachnoid are opened posteriorly and reflected laterally, exposing the lumbar enlargement, conus medullaris, and cauda equina. (**B**) Conus medullaris and cauda equina on 3D fast spin-echo 1 mm thick sagittal oblique image.

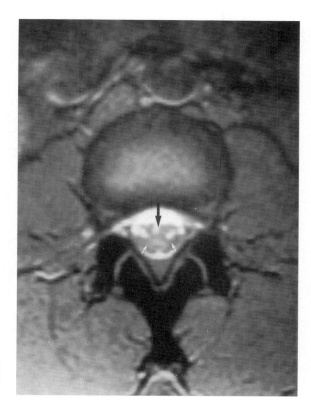

FIGURE 14-7. Normal morphology of the conus medullaris (*black arrow*) at the level of L1-2 is seen on a T2*-weighted axial image. The cauda equina (*white arrows*) are seen posterolaterally.

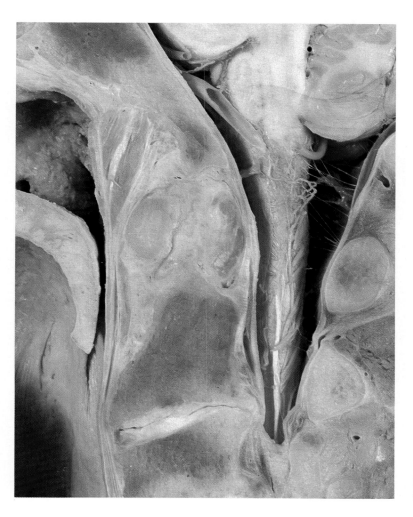

FIGURE 14-8. A near sagittal section through the median atlantoaxial joint.

continued

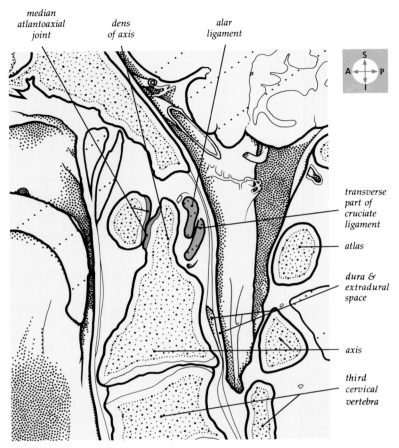

median
atlantoaxial
joint

dens
of axis

alar
ligament

transverse
part of
cruciate
ligament

atlas

dura &
extradural
space

axis

third
cervical
vertebra

FIGURE14-8. *Continued*

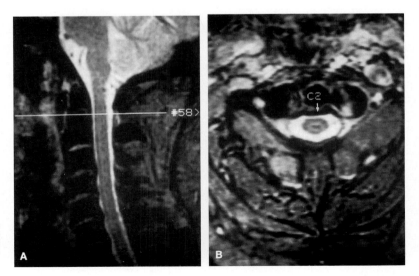

FIGURE 14-9. T2*-weighted (**A**) sagittal and (**B**) axial images at the level of the atlantoaxial joint. The low signal intensity intact transverse ligament is shown on the axial image (*arrow*).

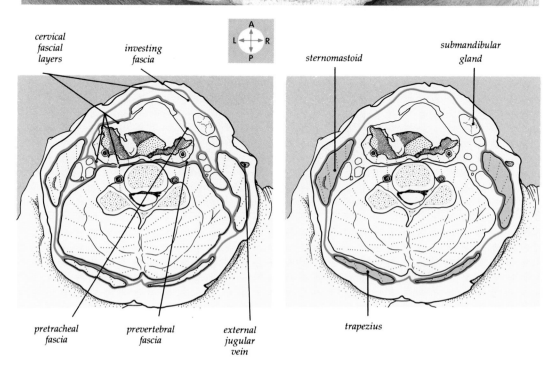

cervical
fascial
layers

investing
fascia

sternomastoid

submandibular
gland

pretracheal
fascia

prevertebral
fascia

external
jugular
vein

trapezius

FIGURE 14-10. A transverse section of the neck at the level of C4 shows the layers of cervical fascia. The layers are shown in separate diagrams.

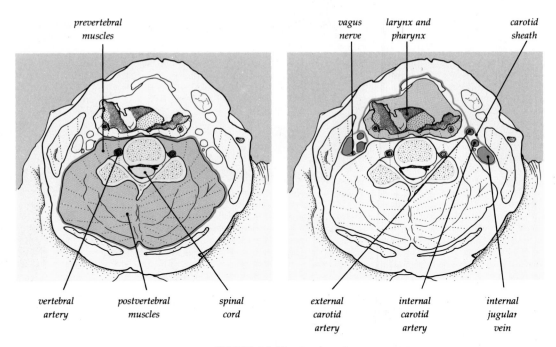

FIGURE 14-10. *Continued*

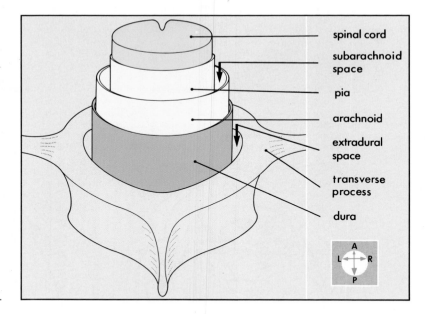

FIGURE 14-11. The spinal meninges.

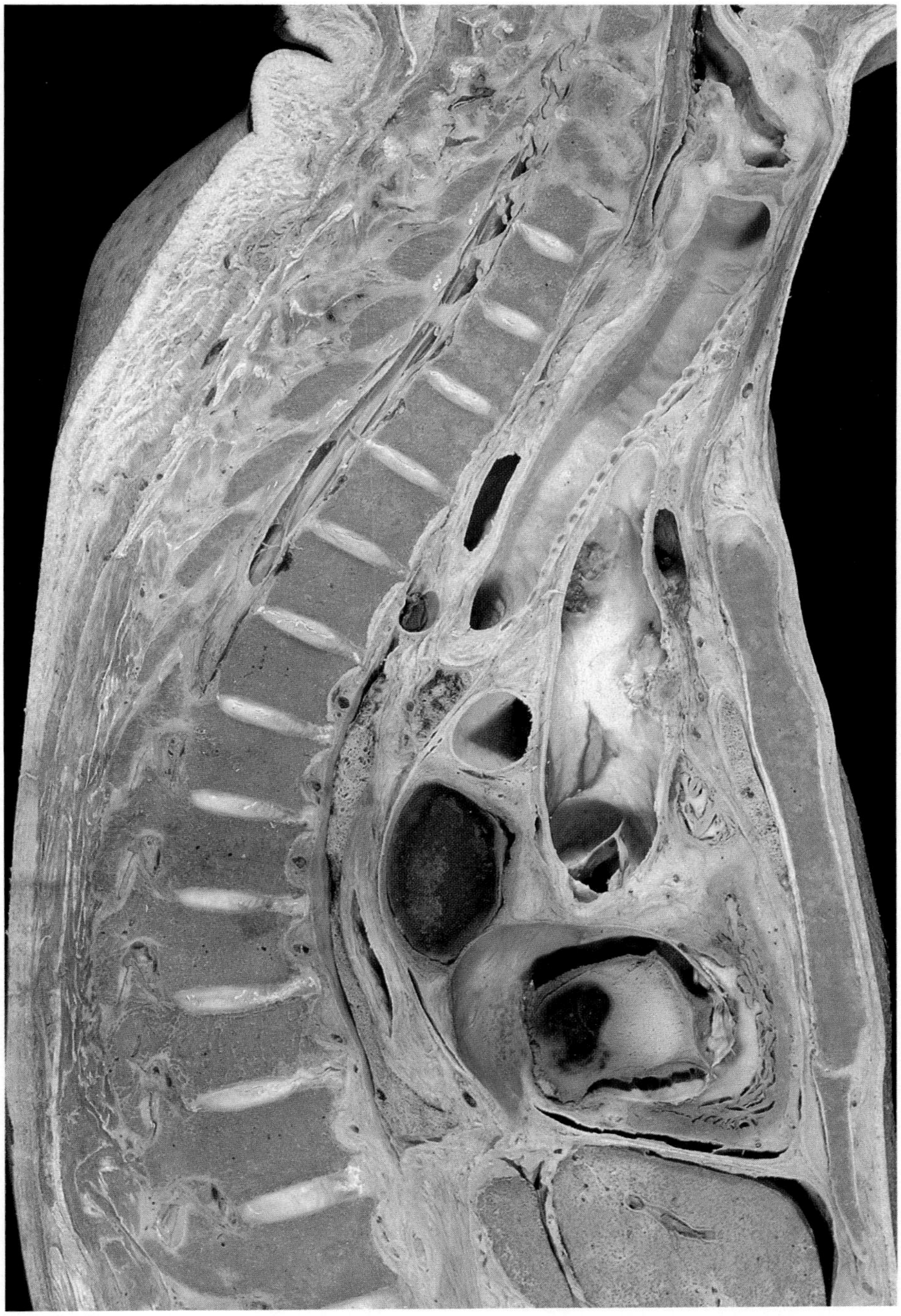

FIGURE 14-12. A near midline sagittal section through the thorax shows some mediastinal structures. *continued*

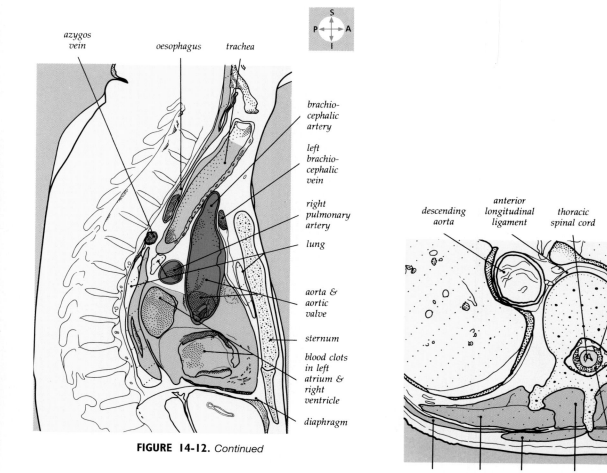

azygos vein

oesophagus

trachea

brachio-cephalic artery

left brachio-cephalic vein

right pulmonary artery

lung

aorta & aortic valve

sternum

blood clots in left atrium & right ventricle

diaphragm

FIGURE 14-12. *Continued*

descending aorta

anterior longitudinal ligament

thoracic spinal cord

extradural space

latissimus dorsi

erector spinae

trapezius

transverso-spinalis

dura

lung

FIGURE 14-13. A transverse section at the level of the seventh thoracic vertebra shows the back muscles and contents of the vertebral foramen.

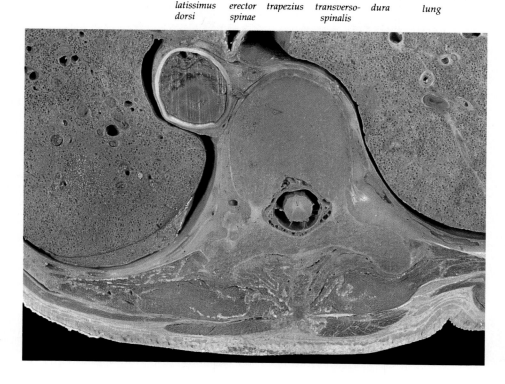

quences permit retrospective reformatting of other orthogonal planes, including oblique imaging through the neural foramen. Kinematic flexion and extension sagittal images, as well as ultrafast scanning dynamic techniques, have been used in selected cases of instability and atlantoaxial subluxations (Fig. 14-17).

IMAGING PROTOCOLS FOR THE THORACIC AND LUMBAR SPINES

The thoracic and lumbar spines are imaged using a planar surface or quadrature coil or a multicoil phased array design. The region of interest can be changed without repositioning the patient if an external spine board housing the surface coil is used or by using phased array multicoil imaging, with selective activation of coils appropriate for the anatomic coverage required. Transitional vertebrae, including sacralization of L5 and lumbarization of S1, can be identified by the morphology of the facets; however, they are more accurately characterized with the addition of a cervicothoracic sagittal scout image to the standard routine lumbosacral sagittal sequences.[77]

Sagittal and axial images of the thoracic and lumbar spines are obtained with conventional T1 and T2 or T2-weighted fast spin-echo sequences. Routine T1-weighted images are acquired at 4 mm slice thicknesses with a 20 to 24 cm FOV, and a 512 × 256, a 256 × 256, or a 256 × 192 acquisition matrix. Conventional T2-weighted images are acquired with a repetition time (TR) of 2000 msec, an echo time (TE) of 20 and 80 msec, a 256 × 192 acquisition matrix, and two signal averages or excitations (NEX). Low signal intensity pulsatile CSF motion artifact, which occurs secondary to spin dephasing, may degrade image quality or obscure pathology in the thoracic space. Cardiac gating of studies in the upper thoracic spine minimizes the effects of flow. Aortic pulsation artifacts may also be problematic in thoracic spine studies that use long TR/TE sequences. Although T2*-

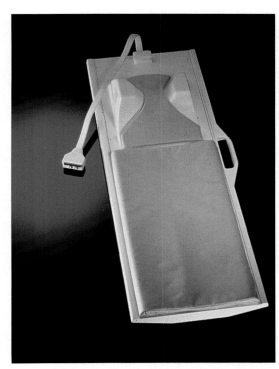

FIGURE 14-14. Phased array coil design (multicoil). During scanning, four coils of this six coil array are activated corresponding to the anatomic area of interest (eg, cervical, thoracic, or lumbar spine).

nar imaging techniques have all been used to maximize the information obtained from MR images. Improved signal-to-noise ratios and excellent spatial and contrast resolution have made it possible to define spinal anatomy in direct sagittal, oblique, and axial planes with MR images obtained from circular and rectangular receive, quadrature, or phased array coils (Figs. 14-14 and 14-15). Three-dimensional Fourier transform (3DFT) volume acquisitions, particularly when used in routine cervical spine studies, allow greater anatomic coverage with thin sections[75,76] (Fig. 14-16). These se-

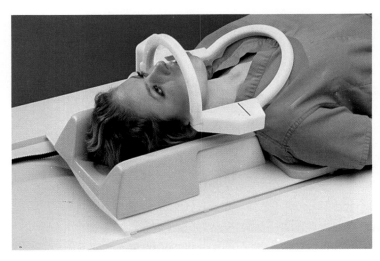

FIGURE 14-15. A cervical quadrature spine coil with demonstration of proper patient positioning.

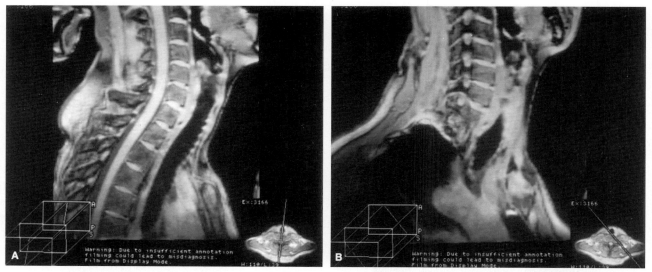

FIGURE 14-16. Three-dimensional Fourier transform volume axial images reformatted in the (**A**) midline and (**B**) sagittal oblique planes provide precise localization of the neural foramen.

weighted contrast has been used to produce relative T2 weighting, contrast properties are not equivalent. For instance, desiccated disks that demonstrate low signal intensity on T2-weighted images may remain isointense with intact intervertebral disks on T2*-weighted refocused images.[78] In general, T2* sequences have been replaced by T2-weighted fast spin-echo sequences. T2-weighted fast spin-echo images can be acquired with a first and second echo using a TR of 3000 to 5000 msec, and a TE of 17 to 30 msec and 90 to

110 msec for the first and second echoes, respectively. Heavily T2-weighted fast spin-echo images, however, cause disks to be blacker, making it difficult to differentiate desiccated nucleus from posterior annulus. A T1-weighted sequence can be used in place of the first echo of a duel echo fast spin-echo sequence. The second echo of the fast spin-echo sequence is then acquired as a single sequence. Infection and metastatic disease are evaluated with STIR or fast spin-echo STIR protocols.

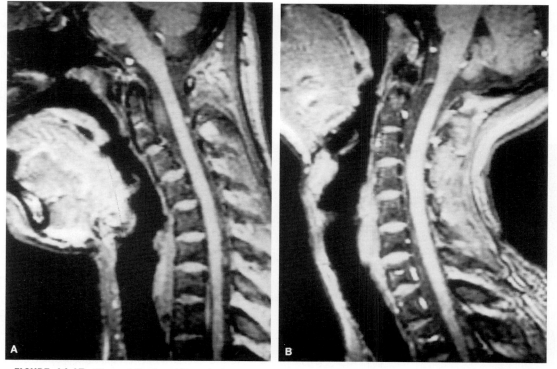

FIGURE 14-17. Normal flexion (**A**) and extension (**B**) of the cervical spine, as seen on sagittal images.

NORMAL MR ANATOMY OF THE THORACIC AND LUMBAR SPINES

Sagittal Images

T1-Weighted Images

In the thoracic spine, the posterior subarachnoid space is larger than the subarachnoid space anterior to the cord (Fig. 14-18). CSF within the subarachnoid space demonstrates low signal intensity, in contrast to the intermediate signal intensity of the cord, and the high signal intensity of the posterior epidural fat. Anterior epidural fat is prominent in the L5-S1 region. Yellow or fatty marrow and mixed elements of cancellous hematopoietic marrow within the vertebral bodies of the thoracic and lumbar spines demonstrate intermediate to high signal intensity, in contrast to the more intermediate signal intensity of intervertebral disks. A focal or diffuse increase in vertebral body marrow signal intensity with aging is attributed to a greater lipid or fatty component in vertebral body marrow stores. Nuclear annular differentiation is not precisely defined on T1-weighted images (Fig. 14-19). The cord demonstrates uniform intermediate signal intensity. The tapered conus medullaris, which is seen in

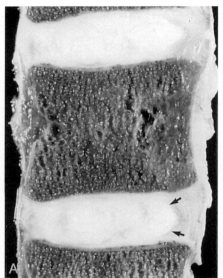

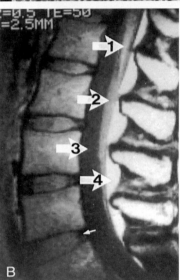

FIGURE 14-19. Lumbar spine. **(A)** A gross sagittal specimen of the lumbar spine demonstrates nuclear-annular separation (*arrows*). **(B)** A T1-weighted midsagittal image of the lumbar spine reveals annular fibers (*small arrow*). 1, conus medullaris; 2, cauda equina, 3, cerebrospinal fluid; 4, epidural fat.

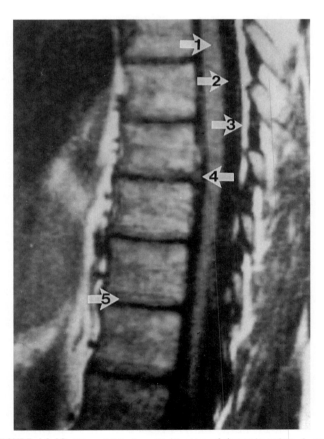

FIGURE 14-18. T1-weighted sagittal image of thoracic spine. 1, spinal cord; 2, cerebrospinal fluid; 3, epidural fat; 4, thoracic disk herniation without cord compression; 5, intervertebral disk.

sagittal images of the lumbar spine with a 24 cm FOV, most commonly terminates posteriorly at the level of L1. The cauda equina is of lower signal intensity than the conus medullaris, secondary to greater surface contrast with surrounding CSF. The fibrous filum terminale may contain fat in up to 5% of normal patients, either focally or along its course as it extends from the conus to the distal thecal sac.[79] On T1-weighted images, anterior and posterior longitudinal ligaments are difficult to distinguish from low signal intensity cortical bone. The exiting nerve roots (spinal nerves) demonstrate intermediate signal intensity within the tear-drop-shaped intervertebral foramina, and are surrounded by

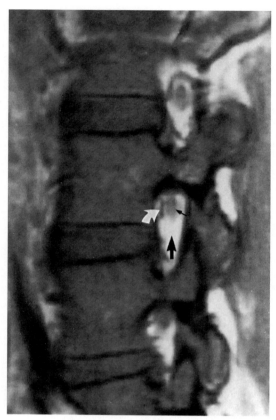

FIGURE 14-20. A parasagittal T1-weighted image of the intervertebral foramina shows high signal intensity epidural fat (*large black arrow*), intermediate signal intensity dorsal root ganglion (*small black arrow*), and low signal intensity radicular vein (*curved white arrow*).

high signal intensity fat (Fig. 14-20). Neural foraminal ligaments appear as low signal intensity linear structures.[80] On parasagittal images, the low signal intensity radicular vein and intermediate signal intensity dorsal root are demarcated by abundant high signal intensity fat within the lumbar neural foramina. Lane and coworkers[81] have proposed that intravascular enhancement of radicular veins, adjacent to or within the endoneurium of nerve roots of the cauda equina, may be mistaken for lumbar nerve root enhancement in the setting of degenerative disk disease.

T2-Weighted Images

On conventional T2 and T2-weighted fast spin-echo images, the low signal intensity cord, conus medullaris, and cauda equina are seen in contrast to high signal intensity CSF (Figs. 14-21 and 14-22). Thoracic and lumbar intervertebral disks demonstrate bright signal intensity on T2, T2-weighted fast spin-echo and T2* weighted images; and epidural fat demonstrates intermediate signal intensity (Fig. 14-23). Vertebral body marrow demonstrates intermediate signal intensity on T2-weighted images and low signal intensity on T2*-weighted images. With T2 techniques, the conus medullaris

demonstrates lower signal intensity than the surrounding bright CSF. The nucleus pulposus and inner annular fibers display increased signal intensity on T2-weighted images, whereas peripheral annular fibers maintain low signal intensity. A low signal intensity band in the midportion of the intervertebral disk is thought to represent an invagination of annular fibers or fibrous tissue commonly seen in the adult spine. The basivertebral vein can be seen as a high signal intensity segment in the midposterior aspect of the vertebral body (Fig. 14-24). The low signal intensity fibrous posterior longitudinal ligament is adherent to the posterior annulus and posterior inferior and superior margins of the vertebral bodies. The anterior and posterior longitudinal ligaments and adjacent cortex and annulus all demonstrate low signal intensity on all imaging sequences.

Axial Images

T1-Weighted Images

In cross-section, the thoracic cord demonstrates intermediate signal intensity, and the surrounding CSF demonstrates low signal intensity. High signal intensity fatty marrow is

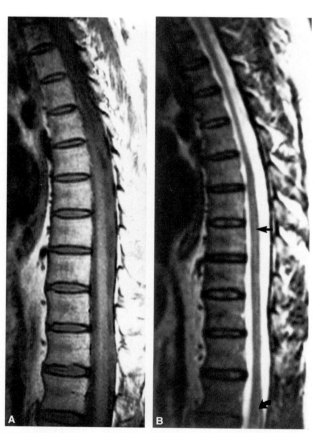

FIGURE 14-21. T1 (**A**) and T2-weighted fast spin-echo (**B**) sagittal images through the thoracic cord (*straight arrow*) and conus medullaris (*curved arrow*). The thoracic cord is hypointense and CSF is hyperintense on the fast spin-echo sequence (**B**).

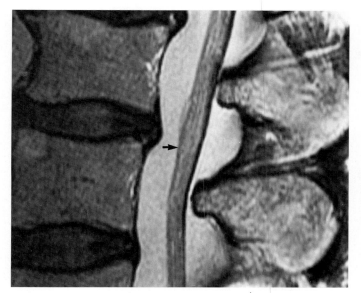

FIGURE 14-22. T2-weighted fast spin-echo sagittal image demonstrates the low signal intensity cauda equina (*arrow*). Degenerative disk disease with protrusions is also present in this patient.

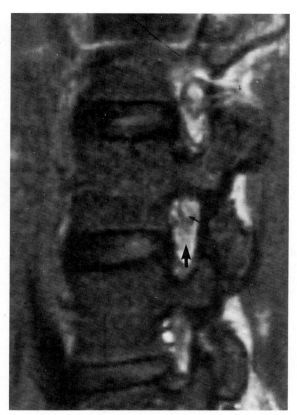

FIGURE 14-23. A conventional T2-weighted parasagittal image of the intervertebral foramina shows poor contrast between intermediate signal intensity neural foraminal fat (*large arrow*) and dorsal root ganglion (*small arrow*).

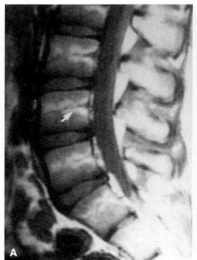
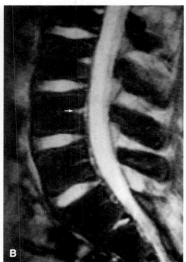

FIGURE 14-24. (**A**) High signal intensity fat (*arrow*) is associated with the basivertebral vein on a T1-weighted sagittal image. (**B**) The basivertebral vein (*arrow*) demonstrates increased signal intensity on a T2*-weighted sagittal image.

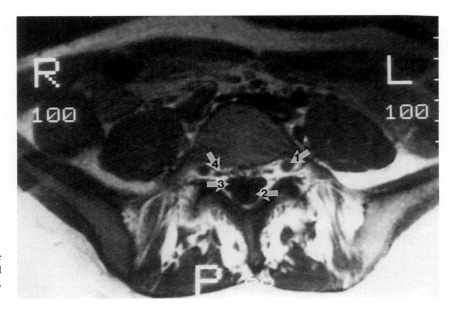

FIGURE 14-25. T1-weighted axial anatomy of the lumbar spine at the level of the superior neural foramina. 1, L5 nerve root sheath; 2, thecal sac; 3, budding S1 nerve root; 4, anterior epidural vein.

seen in the vertebral body, pedicle, lamina, and transverse and spinous processes of the vertebrae. The low signal intensity intraforaminal vein can be seen anterior to the intermediate signal intensity dorsal root ganglion. The dorsal root ganglion and budding and exiting nerve roots are well defined and surrounded by bright signal intensity fat (Fig. 14-25). Exiting nerve roots pass inferior to the pedicle of the corresponding vertebral body. The dorsal root ganglion is located beneath the pedicle and is the most sensitive structure in causing pain from neural impingement (eg, lateral herniations). Nerve roots within the thecal sac occupy a dependent position posteriorly, following the crescentic or curved shape of the thecal sac, with the upper roots positioned more laterally. At lower lumbar vertebral levels, the nerve roots are fewer and become more dispersed within the CSF. A nerve root is conjoined when two nerve roots exit from the same axillary sleeve. Posterior epidural fat can be seen behind the low signal intensity subarachnoid space. The basivertebral vein, retrovertebral plexus, and anterior epidural veins are displayed as low signal intensity structures. The ligamentum flavum demonstrates intermediate signal intensity, parallels the inner surface of the lamina, and blends in with the capsule of the zygapophyseal joint.

T2-Weighted Images

An axial myelographic effect can be generated with T2-weighted fast spin-echo images in less time than that required for conventional spin-echo techniques. On T2-weighted images, the thoracic cord and lumbar cauda equina demonstrate low signal intensity, in contrast to the high signal intensity of the CSF (Fig. 14-26). The cauda equina is seen below the conus, at the L2 level, as a mass of nerve roots in the posterior aspect of the thecal sac (Fig. 14-27). Anterior signal void within the thecal sac is more frequent

with long TR/TE sequences that accentuate CSF pulsation artifacts. Facet hyaline cartilage, 2 to 4 mm thick, demonstrates high signal intensity on gradient-echo images and intermediate signal intensity on conventional T2 and T2-weighted fast spin-echo images. The ligamentum flavum has a high elastin content and therefore displays increased signal intensity on T2*-weighted images.

High signal intensity nuclear material (composed of well-hydrated collagen and proteoglycans) and inner annular fi-

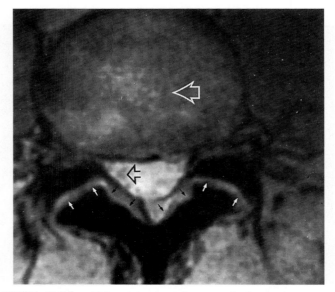

FIGURE 14-26. A T2*-weighted axial image of a lumbar intervertebral disk shows the high signal intensity disk (*open white arrow*), articular cartilage (*solid white arrows*), ligamentum flavum (*solid black arrows*), and low signal intensity cauda equina (*open black arrow*).

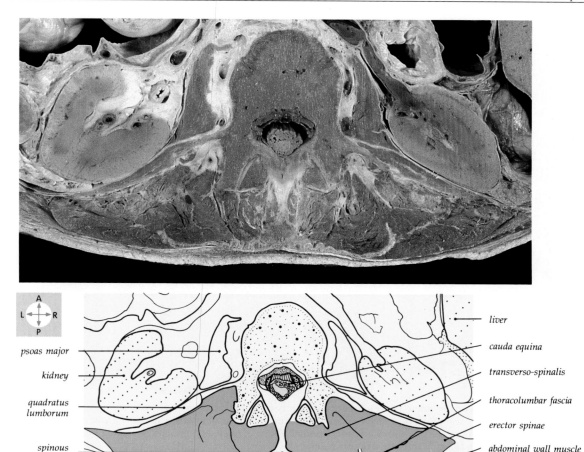

FIGURE 14-27. A transverse section at the level of the second lumbar vertebra shows the back muscles and the contents of the vertebral foramen.

bers can be distinguished from the low signal intensity outer collagen fibers of the annulus (Fig. 14-28). The transition between nucleus pulposus and annulus is not precise, but rather represents a spectrum from a hydrated gelatinous matrix in the nucleus pulposus to a preponderance of type II collagen in the inner annulus and a preponderance of type I collagen in the poorly hydrated outer annulus. Sharpey's fibers and the longitudinal ligaments attach the annulus to the vertebral endplates.

IMAGING PROTOCOLS FOR THE CERVICAL SPINE

The cervical spine is best studied with a custom-designed posterior or anterior quadrature cervical spine coil or phased array coil. Unless properly designed for anterior placement, greater respiratory artifact may be introduced in this position because of closer proximity of the coil to the trachea.

In the sagittal imaging plane, T1-weighted gradient-echo images, which show low signal intensity CSF, are obtained with a TR of 400 to 500 msec, a TE of 9 msec, and a flip angle of 110°. Thin (3 to 4 mm) sections, with or without an interslice gap of 1 mm, are acquired with a 20 cm FOV, a 256 × 192 acquisition matrix, and 4 NEX. Using this protocol, there is some darkening of the vertebral bodies as a result of the T2* effect. Conventional T1-weighted sagittal images, using TRs of less than 600 msec, are acquired before and after Gd-DTPA administration. T2-weighted contrast in the sagittal plane is achieved using either T2 or effective T2 (ie, T2*) weighting, which minimize pulsation artifacts from CSF and cause flow-related enhancement of signal intensity. With long spin-echo acquisition times (long TR/TE), CSF related artifacts are more common, but they can be reduced by gating the acquisition to the cardiac cycle using an electrocardiograph (ECG), pulse trigger, or flow compensation technique.[14,82] For the most part, fast spin-echo

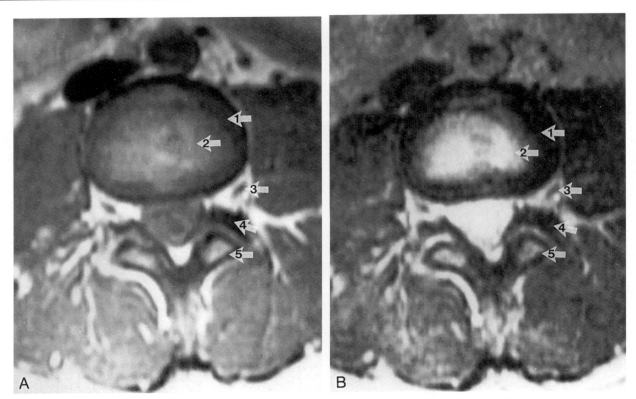

FIGURE 14-28. A conventional T2-weighted axial sequence at an intervertebral disk. (**A**) Intermediate weighted and (**B**) T2-weighted axial images demonstrate increased signal intensity in the nucleus pulposus on T2-weighted contrast. 1, low signal intensity annular fibers; 2, nucleus pulposus; 3, exiting nerve root; 4, superior articular facet; 5, inferior articular facet.

and fat-suppressed fast spin-echo techniques have replaced gradient-echo sequences in the sagittal plane.[83] Fast spin-echo images demonstrate greater CSF cord contrast than do conventional T2 or T2* techniques. Fat-suppressed fast spin-echo images are used to increase the sensitivity to marrow and soft tissue pathology in infection, trauma, and metastatic disease. The ability to differentiate among degenerative disks, osteophytes, and the posterior longitudinal ligament is limited on heavily T2-weighted fast spin-echo sequences. The differentiation between posterior disk and osteophyte is improved with the application of fat-suppression to fast spin-echo sequences. A truncation or "Gibbs" artifact, which produces lines parallel to the CSF–spine interface, may be mistaken for a centrally located syrinx (pseudosyrinx). This artifact is eliminated by increasing the acquisition matrix to 192 or 256 pixels. A phase misregistration from cardiac motion blurs the CSF–cord–extradural interface when the phase encoding direction is anterior to posterior. Reversal of the phase coding from an anterior-to-posterior to superior-to-inferior direction, along with the use of flow compensation, will help to minimize low signal intensity CSF pulsation artifacts.

Axial images are generated with a 3DFT T2*-weighted protocol using a TR of 35 msec, a TE of 15 msec, and a flip angle of 5°. A total of 64 images at 2 mm provides coverage from C1 through T1. Conventional T1-weighted images, if obtained, should be acquired with flow compensation to minimize vascular and CSF flow artifacts. Conventional T2-weighted images in the axial plane have poor signal-to-noise ratios and are degraded by motion artifact unless some form of cardiac gating is employed. Fast spin-echo T2-weighted axial images do, however, provide excellent CSF–cord contrast. A higher acquisition matrix, low echo train values, and longer TE values minimize blurring artifacts. Flow compensation is recommended in the use of fast spin-echo techniques.

Magnetization transfer gradient-echo images have shown improved contrast and delineation of disk herniations, foraminal stenosis, and intrinsic cord lesions compared with nonmagnetization transfer gradient-refocused echo (GRE) and T2-weighted fast spin-echo images.[84]

NORMAL MR ANATOMY OF THE CERVICAL SPINE

Sagittal Images

T1-Weighted Images

On conventional T1-weighted sagittal images of the cervical spine, the yellow or fatty marrow of the vertebral bodies demonstrates bright signal intensity (Fig. 14-29). The

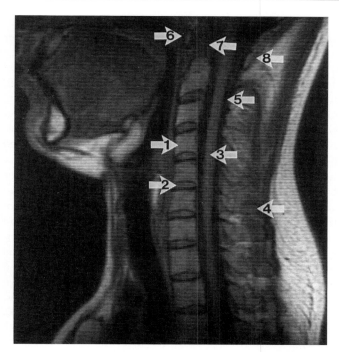

FIGURE 14-29. A T1-weighted image shows the midsagittal anatomy of the cervical spine. 1, bright marrow signal intensity vertebral body; 2, intermediate signal intensity disk; 3, spinal cord; 4, spinous process; 5, low signal intensity cerebrospinal fluid; 6, anterior arch of first cervical vertebra; 7, odontoid; 8, posterior arch of C1.

normal cervical spine should exhibit a cervical lordotic curvature, and C1, which does not have a vertebral body, can be identified by its anterior and posterior arches. The low signal intensity synchondrosis at the base of the odontoid may appear as a dark band, simulating a fracture. The basivertebral veins penetrate the midportion of the posterior cervical vertebral bodies and are connected to the epidural venous system. The short cervical pedicles connect the cervical vertebral body to the articular pillars. From the articular pillars, posteromedially oriented lamina form the spinous process. As in the thoracic and lumbar spines, the superior articular process from the inferior cervical body projects anterior to the inferior articular process, which comes from the cervical vertebral body above. The foramina transversarium of the transverse processes of C2 through C6 contain the vertebral artery and small veins. The anterior-posterior diameter of the cervical canal is tapered from C1 to C3 and is relatively uniform thereafter (ie, from C3 through C7). The low signal intensity anterior and posterior longitudinal ligaments that connect the cervical vertebrae are best seen on sagittal images.

On conventional T1-weighted spin-echo images, the fibrocartilaginous cervical disks display intermediate signal intensity, and CSF, which is of low signal intensity, is seen in contrast to the higher signal intensity of the cord. On T1-weighted gradient-echo images, intervertebral disks demonstrate bright signal intensity, whereas the CSF remains of

low signal intensity. On conventional T1-weighted images, differentiation of posterior cortical bone, longitudinal ligaments, and CSF is difficult because all generate low signal intensity on short TR/TE sequences. The ability to distinguish them is improved by using T1-weighted gradient-echo protocols, which more accurately define endplate and osteophyte anatomy.

The dorsal and ventral roots in the neural foramina are identified on peripheral sagittal images. These structures demonstrate intermediate signal intensity and are surrounded by high signal intensity foraminal fat. A 45° oblique sagittal image is also useful in displaying intervertebral foraminal anatomy in the cervical spine. On gradient-echo images, fat demonstrates intermediate signal intensity in the intervertebral foramina, and these sequences provide less contrast than corresponding T1-weighted images.

Intermediate signal intensity hyaline cartilage can be seen between the obliquely oriented inferior and superior articular facets (Fig. 14-30). The signal void of the anterior vertebral artery can be seen in paramedian sections through the dorsal root ganglion and articular pillars. The subarachnoid space anterior and posterior to the cord are of equal dimensions. The ability to differentiate spinal cord gray and white matter varies, depending on CSF pulsation and truncation artifacts. Truncation artifacts are seen as bands parallel with the cervical cord, and are related to FOV, TR/TE, and pixel size. Bright signal in

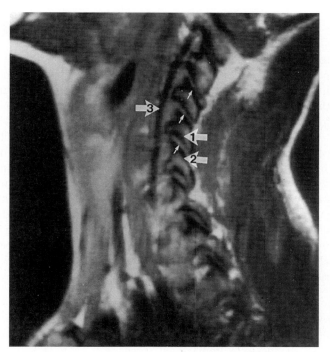

FIGURE 14-30. A T1-weighted image shows the parasagittal anatomy of the cervical spine at the level of the facet joints. The intermediate signal intensity facet cartilage (*small arrows*) is identified. 1, superior articular facet; 2, inferior articular facet; 3, vertebral artery.

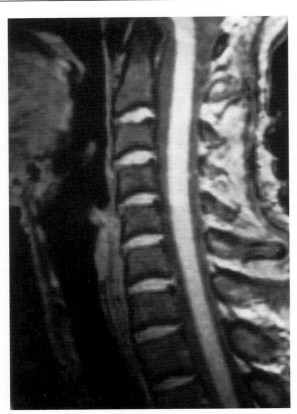

FIGURE 14-31. The disk–thecal sac interface (*arrow*) is clearly defined on a multiplanar gradient-echo MR image with a TE of 9 msec and a flip angle of 110°.

(Fig. 14-32). High signal intensity subarachnoid CSF is seen anteriorly and posteriorly. CSF appears progressively darker with the use of higher flip angles. The marrow and cortex of the cervical vertebrae demonstrate low signal intensity on gradient-echo images, sharply delineating the spinal canal, impinging osteophytes, and the disk–thecal sac interface. On heavily T2*-weighted images, however, disks may not be as easily differentiated from osteophytes, and the posterior disk margin may be overestimated. This can be avoided by comparison with corresponding T1-weighted images, in which the disk is brighter than the adjacent endplates or osteophytes. The basivertebral vein follows a horizontal course through the midvertebral body, and generates bright signal intensity. Facet cartilage, which is intermediate in signal intensity on conventional T1- and T2-weighted images, demonstrates high signal intensity on T2*-weighted images[87] (Fig. 14-33). Flowing arterial and venous blood display high signal intensity. Contrast between the nerve root and fat is diminished on T2- or T2*-weighted images, because fat demonstrates intermediate, not high, signal inten-

tensity from marrow is seen in both the anterior and posterior arches of C1 and in the body of C2. Signal intensity in the body of C2 is higher than that seen in the adjacent odontoid process, and there is a fat pad of high signal intensity directly superior to the odontoid.

T1-weighted gradient-echo images obtained with a TR of 400 to 500 msec, a TE of 9 msec, and a flip angle of 110° demonstrate high signal intensity disks, low signal intensity CSF, and high signal intensity cord (Fig. 14-31). This protocol provides a more accurate characterization of the posterior disk margin from adjacent CSF and vertebral body endplates. Magnetic susceptibility is minimized at a TE of 9 msec. Fat-suppressed T2-weighted fast spin-echo sequences also improve characterization of osteophyte from the posterior annular complex.

T2-Weighted Images

On T2*-weighted images, the intervertebral disks and CSF demonstrate high signal intensity.[41,82,85,86] When flip angles of less than 15° are used, the cord demonstrates low signal intensity. Excellent cord–CSF contrast is also seen on conventional and fast spin-echo T2-weighted protocols

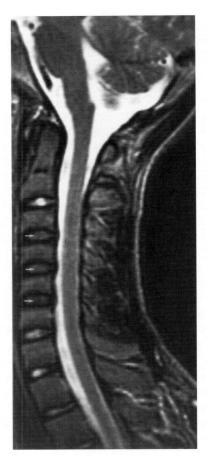

FIGURE 14-32. The low signal intensity cervical cord is clearly differentiated from high signal intensity CSF on a T2-weighted fast spin-echo image. Degenerative disks are hypointense (*small arrows*).

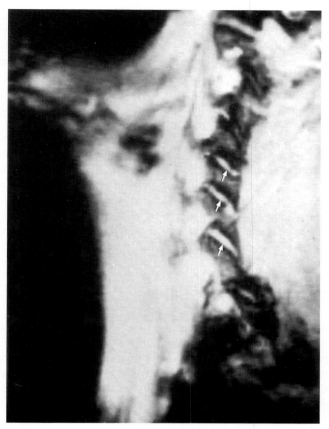

FIGURE 14-33. The facet articular cartilage of the apophyseal joint demonstrates high signal intensity *(arrows)* on a sagittal T2*-weighted image.

Axial Images

T1-Weighted Images

On T1-weighted axial images, either conventional or spoiled gradient refocused acquisition in the steady state, the intermediate signal intensity disk, the black CSF, and the higher signal intensity cord can be differentiated (Figs. 14-34 and 14-35). Differentiation of the nucleus pulposus and annulus, however, is not possible with short TR/TE sequences. The low signal intensity uncinate processes are located lateral to the disk margins, and the facet joints are demonstrated in their oblique orientation, with greater medial-lateral than superior-inferior dimensions. The low signal intensity transverse ligament extends posterior to the odontoid process of C2. The ventral and dorsal nerve roots form a triangle of intermediate signal intensity. The antero-lateral apex of the triangle, including the dorsal root ganglion, is located proximal to the junction of the dorsal and ventral roots in the neural foramen. Anterior to the dorsal root ganglion, the low signal intensity vertebral artery can be seen. At the level of the cervical body, but not the intervertebral disk, high signal intensity neural foraminal fat may outline the intermediate signal intensity nerve roots and sheaths. Vertebrae C1 through C7 have spinal nerve roots that exit the intervertebral nerve root canals (ie, neural foramina) above the corresponding vertebral body level. Low signal intensity epidural veins are located posterior to the

sity. As a result, the anatomy of the neural foramina is not accurately demonstrated on these images. The low signal intensity dura can be identified on T2*-weighted images, but it is not satisfactorily seen on corresponding conventional T1- or T2-weighted images. We have used fat-suppressed T2-weighted fast spin-echo or STIR imaging techniques to evaluate metastatic disease by selectively nulling fat marrow signal intensity. The additive effects of T1 and T2 contrast in STIR techniques produce greater conspicuity than is possible with corresponding conventional T2- or T2*-weighted images.

Fast spin-echo sequences are commonly used in place of conventional T2-weighted protocols. Limitations of fast spin-echo techniques include blurring at lower matrixes, longer echo trains, and lower TE values. The increased signal intensity of fat on T2-weighted fast spin-echo images, compared with conventional spin-echo images, can be compensated for by using relatively higher TR and TE values. The addition of fat-suppression is used to more effectively evaluate marrow and soft tissue pathology and vertebral endplate morphology at the diskovertebral junction.

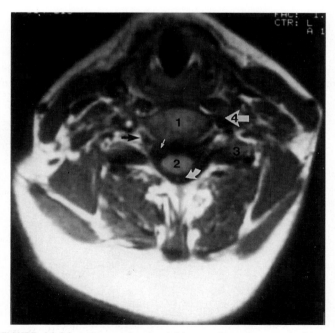

FIGURE 14-34. A T1-weighted axial image through a cervical intervertebral disk shows the root sleeve *(black arrow)*, ventral nerve root *(straight white arrow)*, and cerebrospinal fluid *(curved white arrow)*. 1, intervertebral disk; 2, spinal cord; 3, articular pillar; 4, vertebral artery.

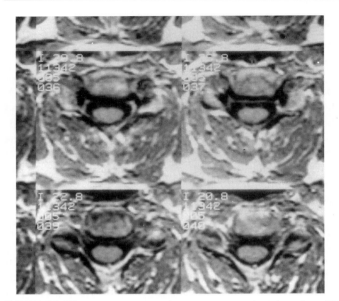

FIGURE 14-35. A volume spoiled GRASS protocol with a short TE (5 msec) and moderate flip angle (45°) produces T1-weighted contrast and eliminates T2 dependence. Cerebrospinal fluid is dark, the spinal cord demonstrates intermediate signal intensity, and fat displays bright signal in this sequence.

vertebral body and surround the vertebral artery in the venous plexus. The epidural venous plexus is enhanced following the administration of Gd-DTPA, especially along the anterolateral aspect of the spinal canal and neural foramen. Gray and white matter can be separately identified on T1-weighted axial images.

T2-Weighted Images

On T2*-weighted images, the intervertebral disk demonstrates high signal intensity, primarily because of the nucleus pulposus[85] (Figs. 14-36 and 14-37). Annular fibers remain

low in signal intensity. The anterior epidural venous plexus generates bright signal intensity, as do the vertebral arteries, allowing the low-to-intermediate signal intensity nerve roots and dorsal root ganglion to be seen. It may be difficult to distinguish the exiting nerve roots, because both the roots and neural foraminal fat are of intermediate signal intensity on these images. The thin line of the dural sac is identified anterior to the subarachnoid CSF. The common carotid artery and jugular vein, both of bright signal intensity, are defined anteromedially and posterolaterally, respectively, on axial planar images. Cortical bone and marrow both demonstrate low signal intensity on gradient-echo refocused images. High signal intensity CSF and low signal intensity cord contrast are improved on fast spin-echo axial images. Fast spin-echo techniques are often preferred when improved contrast is required, as in the assessment of a syrinx.

PATHOLOGY OF THE SPINE

In addition to the assessment of degenerative disk disease in the cervical, thoracic, and lumbar spines, MR imaging is useful in the evaluation of the postoperative spine, infection, trauma, and neoplasia involving osseous structures, soft tissue, and the cord.[7-41,59-62] Malalignment abnormalities, including spondylolisthesis, can be identified and characterized by multiplanar imaging of the pars and facet joints. Direct marrow imaging facilitates early detection in marrow replacement disorders (eg, leukemia, multiple myeloma, metastasis). Functional evaluation of atlantoaxial instability can be achieved by performing separate acquisitions with the patient positioned in flexion and extension.[88] Signal characteristics of cystic lesions (such as syringomyelia and hydromyelia) are similar to those of CSF. Intramedullary lipomas demonstrate high signal intensity on T1-weighted images, intermediate to high signal intensity on T2-weighted images,

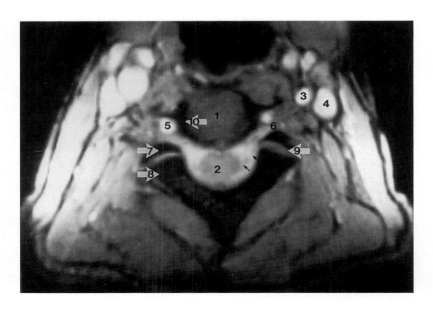

FIGURE 14-36. An axial T2*-weighted image at the midcervical level. 1, intervertebral disk; 2, spinal cord; 3, common carotid artery; 4, jugular vein; 5, vertebral artery; 6, dorsal root ganglion; 7, superior articular process; 8, inferior articular process; 9, facet cartilage; 10, uncinate process.

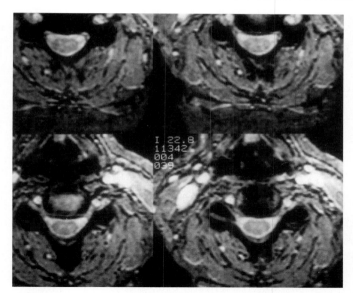

FIGURE 14-37. A protocol of 64 thin section (2 mm), contiguous, T2*-weighted 3D volume images generated with a TR of 35 msec, TE of 15 msec, and a flip angle of 5° produces a myelographic-like image with high signal intensity cerebrospinal fluid and low signal intensity spinal cord, vertebral bodies, and fat.

and are dark on STIR sequences. Lipomas can sometimes be confused with subacute hemorrhage, also bright on T1-weighted images, but hemorrhage shows increased signal intensity on long TR/TE (ie, T2-weighted) sequences. Detection of common intradural extramedullary tumors, such as

neurofibromas[89] and meningiomas, may require the use of intravenous Gd-DTPA. MR imaging is also useful for evaluation of abnormalities of the pediatric spine, including spinal dysraphism.

Degenerative Disk Disease: Disk Herniation

Classification and Terminology

PAINFUL ANNULAR FISSURES (HIZS). The precursor to, and frequently the inciting event in, disk degeneration is felt by many to be tearing of the outer annular fibers, in both concentric and radial orientations. Most of these fissures are not visible on MR imaging, but there is a subset of annular fissures that are bright on T2-weighted sagittal and axial images due to the presence of granulation tissue and edema. They have been termed high intensity zones (HIZs). If heavily T2-weighted sagittal images are performed, they are easily seen with both high field and mid-field MR scanners (Fig. 14-38). Two studies have shown a high correlation between HIZs and concordant pain with diskography.[90,91] Other authors have found this correlation in asymptomatic patients.[92] These painful annular fissures may be the cause of back pain previously unexplained by MR imaging, and may also explain false-negative MR findings as compared with diskography. Further, they may be a marker for internal disk disruption and back pain without radiculopathy. As yet, there are no studies evaluating this marker for use in planning invasive or noninvasive therapy.

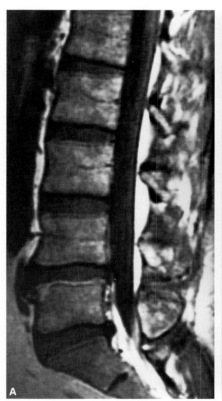
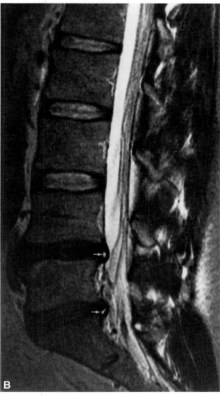

FIGURE 14-38. (**A**) Annular fissures (*arrows*) at levels L4-5 and L5-S1 are not visualized on T1-weighted sagittal image. (**B**) However, they demonstrate focal hyperintensity with the posterior annular complex on T2-weighted fast spin-echo image. Associated hypointense disk degeneration is also shown on T2-weighted fast spin-echo sequence (**B**).

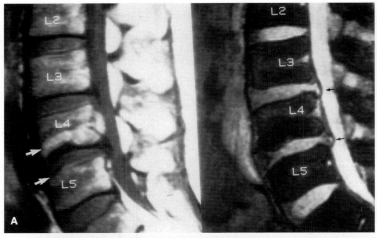

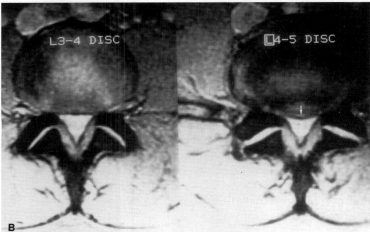

FIGURE 14-39. An L3-4 annular bulge (*arrow*) and mild L4-5 central disk protrusion (*arrow*) is seen on (**A**) T1-weighted (*left*) and T2*-weighted (*right*) sagittal images, and on (**B**) T2*-weighted axial images. Yellow or fatty marrow signal intensity of type II endplate change is shown on the T1-weighted sagittal image (*double white arrows*). There is moderate central canal stenosis at L3-4 and moderate to severe central stenosis at L4-5. The L3-4 annular bulge shows no focal asymmetry of the posterior disk margin in the axial plane. At the L4-5 level, however, there is focal asymmetry of the posterior margin centrally (*arrow*).

TYPES OF DISK HERNIATIONS. The North American Spine Society has agreed to the following nomenclature for disk herniation.

- The nonspecific term *herniation* should be used when a specific diagnosis cannot be made. This situation should only exist when the determination is attempted by CT, CT myelography, myelography, or suboptimal MRI and a definitive diagnosis cannot be made.
- A concentric extension of the disk margins circumferentially beyond the vertebral margins should be termed an annular bulge.
- If there is a focal area of extension of the nucleus beyond the vertebral margin, but it remains beneath the outer annular/posterior longitudinal ligament complex, it should be termed a protrusion.
- The extension of nuclear material completely through the outer annulus into the epidural space is termed an extrusion. Sequestration is a specific type of extrusion in which there is a free fragment of disk.

The practicality of this classification is discussed later with reference to lumbar disk abnormalities.

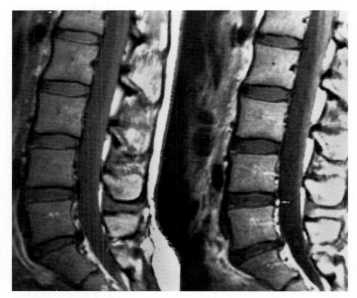

FIGURE 14-40. Enhancing tissue (*arrow*) in an annular bulge is apparent on gadolinium-enhanced T1-weighted sagittal image (*right*). Unenhanced T1-weighted sagittal image (*left*) is shown for comparison.

Disk Herniation in Thoracic and Lumbar Spines

CLASSIFICATION. A recent study reported on the ability of experienced spinal radiologists to be consistent and accurate in the use of the nomenclature described above in assessment of lumbar disk abnormalities.[93] The ability to differentiate among these categories has important implications for treatment.

For instance, an annular disk bulge, a term reserved for a relatively symmetric or generalized extension of the posterior disk margin beyond the posterior borders of the adjacent vertebral body endplates (Fig. 14-39), is a normal finding in the aging spine. This stage of disk degeneration represents stretching or increased laxity of the annulus without focal protrusion.[71] An annular disk bulge may be associated with radial tears of the annulus.

Protrusions are also seen commonly in asymptomatic patients. Disk protrusions are characterized by a focal projection or asymmetry of the posterior disk margin beyond the posterior borders of the adjacent vertebral bodies.[64] A disk protrusion is a contained disk herniation; herniated nuclear material extends through a tear of the inner annulus, but does not extend through outermost annular fibers. Axial images are better than corresponding sagittal images for demonstrating the focal contour changes of the posterior disk margin in a protrusion. In sagittal images, an annular disk bulge and a protrusion may have similar morphology when reviewing a single image. Occasionally, underlying fissuring or tears may be identified on T2-weighted or Gd-DTPA enhanced T1-weighted sagittal images (see Fig. 14-38 and Fig. 14-40). Although, by definition, a disk protrusion is a herniated disk, partial tearing of inner annular fibers cannot

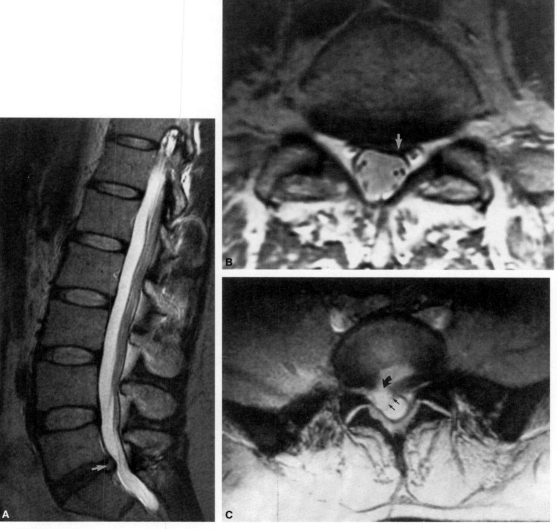

FIGURE 14-41. (**A**) A focal L5-S1 disk protrusion (*arrow*) is shown on a T2-weighted fast spin-echo sagittal image. The annulus remains intact. (**B**) Focal asymmetry of the L5-S1 disk protrusion (*arrow*) is appreciated on intermediate weighted fast spin-echo axial image. (**C**) In a separate case, the path of extruded nuclear disk material is identified (*curved arrow*) in a right paracentral L5-S1 herniation. Indentation of the right ventral lateral aspect of the thecal sac (*small straight arrows*) can also be seen.

be reliably identified with either CT or MR imaging (Fig. 14-41).

Extrusions are not usually seen in asymptomatic patients. In an extruded disk, nuclear disk material extends through all layers of the annulus and produces an extradural mass that often indents the ventral aspect of the thecal sac (see Fig. 14-41). In one study by Jensen and others,[94] no extrusions were found in asymptomatic patients. Differentiation of a prominent disk protrusion from a small disk extrusion may not be possible in the absence of disrupted posterior annular fibers. Extruded disks may extend superior (more common) or inferior to the intervertebral disk either in the midline or more commonly posterolaterally in the lateral recess.

A sequestration, or free fragment, represents disk material that is no longer in continuity with its parent intervertebral disk of origin. It may be adjacent to the disk of origin or it may migrate either cranially or caudally in the spinal canal (Fig. 14-42). Sequestrations are often surrounded by epidural inflammation, which contributes to the epidural mass effect. Intradural extrusion has also been reported.[38,40,95]

The ability to specifically diagnose extrusions and sequestrations has significant implications for planning invasive and minimally invasive therapy. Erkintalo and coworkers[45] reported a positive association between degenerative lumbar disk disease and low back pain in adolescents, al-though the MR findings of degenerative processes were similar in both symptomatic and asymptomatic patients.[45]

MAGNETIC RESONANCE FINDINGS. The accuracy of MR imaging in the assessment of thoracic and lumbar disk herniation has been reported to be equivalent to that for CT myelography[32,34,96–99] (Figs. 14-43 and 14-44). The sagittal plane is sensitive for identification of the posterior disk margin, the outer annular/posterior longitudinal ligament complex, and the interface with the ventral aspect of the thecal sac. It is also valuable in identifying foraminal herniations and foraminal stenosis and associated impingement on the exiting nerve roots. However, sagittal plane findings should be confirmed with corresponding axial images for more accurate assessment of the degree of secondary central canal or lateral recess stenoses and nerve root impingement.

On sagittaiul images, annular disk bulges have a low signal intensity intact posterior annular complex and may be associated with hypointense disk degeneration (Fig. 14-45). Conventional T2 and T2-weighted fast spin-echo weighted images are useful in assessing intervertebral disk degeneration (see Fig. 14-45 and Fig. 14-46). Degenerated disk material, which may be hyperintense on T2*-weighted images, is usually less intense than normally hydrated intervertebral disks at other levels. This greater sensitivity of conventional T2-weighted images to the detection of desic-

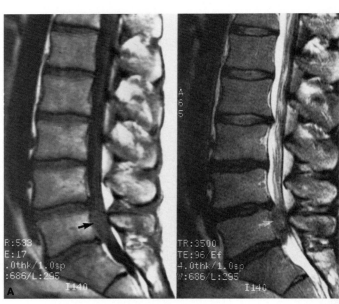
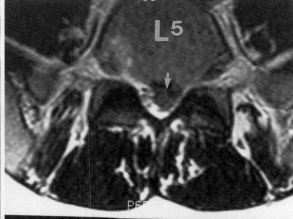
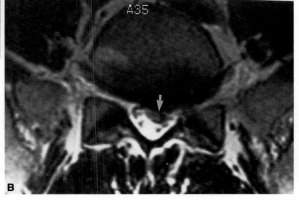

FIGURE 14-42. (A) Large L4-5 sequestered disk fragment (*arrow*) is present posterior to the L5 vertebral body on T1 (*left*) and T2-weighted fast spin-echo (*right*) sagittal images. (B) Corresponding intermediate (*top*) and T2- (*bottom*) weighted axial images demonstrate the relationship of the disk fragment (*arrow*) to the L5 vertebral body (*top*) and inferior extension to the L5-S1 disk level (*bottom*).

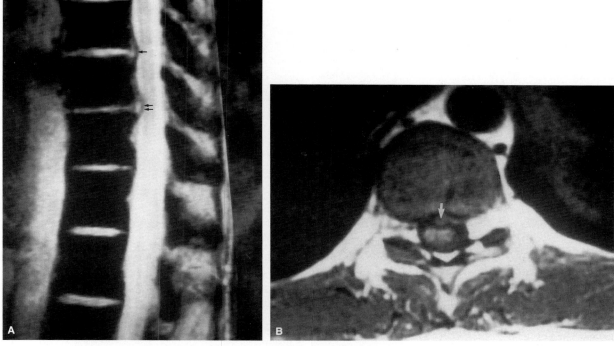

FIGURE 14-43. (A) Two level thoracic disk herniations (*arrows*) demonstrate the high signal intensity of extruded disk material on a T2*-weighted sagittal image. (B) Subligamentous herniation (ie, ruptured annulus fibrosus) produces a central extradural defect (*arrow*) on a T1-weighted axial image.

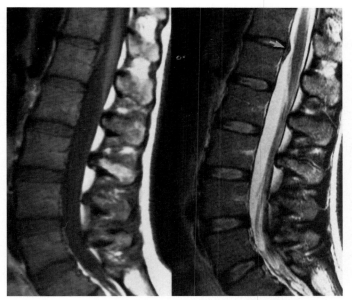

FIGURE 14-44. Lower thoracic disk herniation with an anterior extradural defect at the level of the T12-L1 protrusion (*arrow*). T1 (*left*) and T2-weighted fast spin-echo (*right*) images.

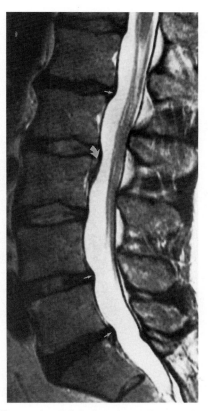

FIGURE 14-45. Annular disk bulges (*straight arrow*) at levels L1-2, L4-5 and L5-S1 on midline T2-weighted fast spin-echo sagittal image. An L2-3 sequestered disk (*curved arrow*) is additionally shown posterior to the L3 vertebral body. Associated disk degeneration is hypointense at the identified levels of annular disk bulges.

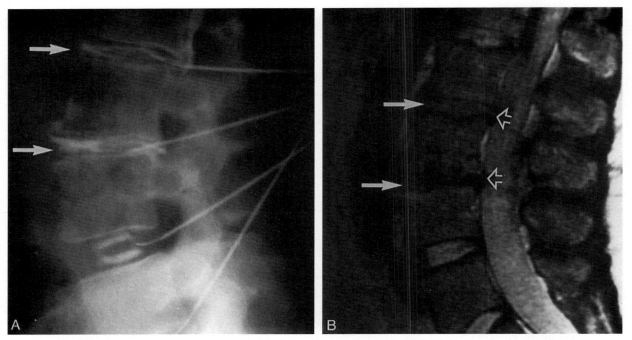

FIGURE 14-46. Degenerative and herniated L2-3 and L3-4 disks demonstrate **(A)** abnormal contrast distribution (*solid arrows*) in a lateral diskogram and **(B)** loss of signal intensity (*solid arrows*) on a T2-weighted sagittal image. Disk bulges that are deforming the ventral aspect of the thecal sac are identified on the sagittal MR image (*open arrows*).

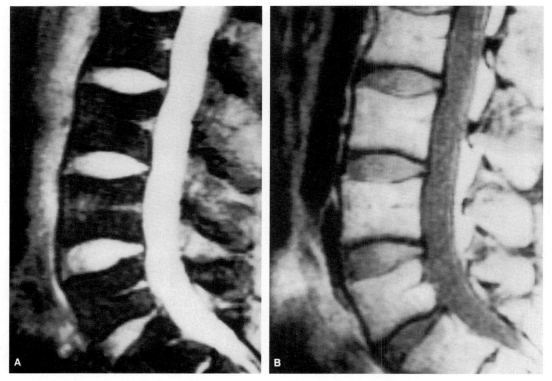

FIGURE 14-47. A comparison of **(A)** T2*-weighted, **(B)** intermediate weighted sagittal, and **(C)** T2-weighted sagittal images in identifying L5-S1 disk desiccation (*arrow*) reveals the greater sensitivity of conventional T2 contrast in detecting low signal intensity disk changes. *continued*

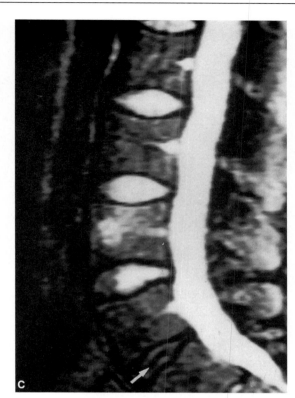

FIGURE 14-47. *Continued.*

cation represents a potential limitation of gradient-echo protocols (Fig. 14-47). T2*-weighted images are particularly sensitive to disk calcifications and nitrogen gas in vacuum phenomena, secondary to magnetic susceptibility (Figs. 14-48 and 14-49).

Most disk protrusions or herniations demonstrate low signal intensity on T1- or T2-weighted images, although the converse is not true (Fig. 14-50). Disks with normal morphology may be desiccated without associated herniation

(Fig. 14-51). Some annular fissures appear as focal areas of bright linear signal intensity within the posterior confines of the annulus on T2- or T2*-weighted sagittal images.[100,101] Disk herniations are subjectively categorized as mild (small), moderate, or severe (large). A mild disk herniation with superimposed spinal stenosis may produce more symptoms than a moderate disk herniation in a capacious canal. Disk–CSF differentiation may be difficult on T1-weighted images, because the posterior disk margin and the thecal sac both demonstrate low signal intensity. Most herniated disks are depicted as degenerative or desiccated on conventional T2 or T2-weighted fast spin-echo images, in contrast to T2*-weighted images. Lateral disk herniations can efface the bright signal intensity neural foraminal fat without compromising the thecal sac (Figs. 14-52 and 14-53). Large posterolateral disk herniations may compromise both the thecal sac and exiting nerve root. The sagittal imaging plane may be more sensitive in defining deformities of the thecal sac at the disk–thecal sac interface, specifically, in demonstrating discontinuity of low signal intensity annular fibers. T2-weighted images increase contrast discrimination between bright signal intensity CSF and low signal intensity annular fibers at the disk–thecal sac boundary. Acute herniations may demonstrate increased signal intensity on both conventional T1- and T2-weighted images[102] (Fig. 15-54). Disk protrusions and extrusions may demonstrate either increased or decreased signal intensity on T2-weighted images (Fig. 14-55). On gradient-echo images, the posterior annular fibers and longitudinal ligament demonstrate low signal intensity, facilitating differentiation of the disk and CSF. On gradient-echo images, the dura of the lumbar spine is depicted as a black line; it may be displaced in posterior disk herniations. Nuclear material extruded from the disk usually demonstrates low signal intensity on conventional T1- and T2-weighted images and high signal intensity on gradient-echo

text continues on page 1093

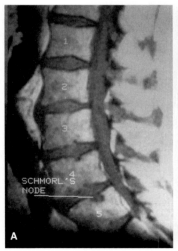

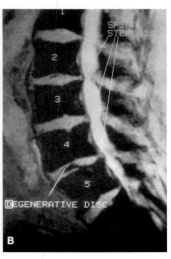

FIGURE 14-48. (A) Schmorl's node superior endplate L5 and (B) low signal intensity degenerative L4-5 vacuum phenomenon. Central stenosis is best displayed with T2*-weighted contrast, which displays the high signal intensity cerebrospinal fluid and the posterior annular complex.

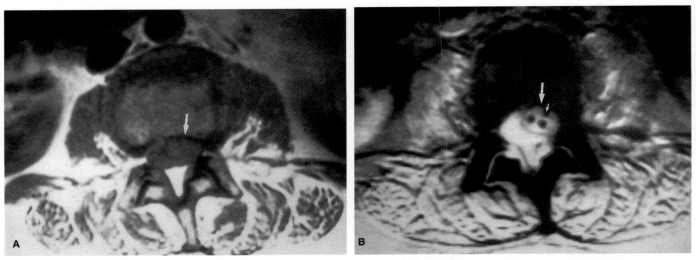

FIGURE 14-49. The low signal intensity susceptibility effects of calcium (*small arrow*) in a sequestered disk (*large arrow*) are seen on (**A**) T1-weighted and (**B**) T2*-weighted axial images.

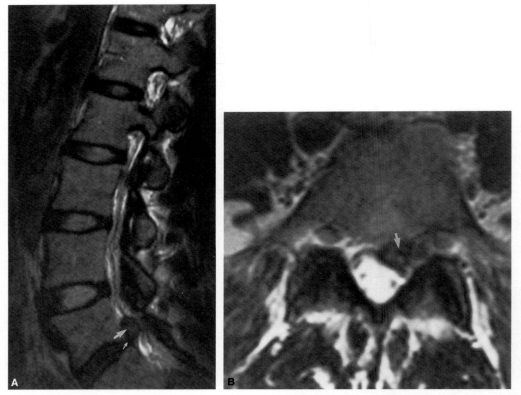

FIGURE 14-50. Left paracentral L5-S1 disk extrusion (*large arrow*), which is connected by a thin pedicle (*small arrow*) to the parent disk. The extruded and parent disk are both hypointense on T2-weighted fast spin-echo sagittal (**A**) and axial (**B**) images.

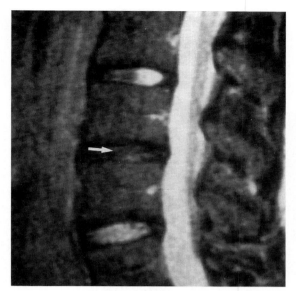

FIGURE 14-51. A desiccated L3-4 disk (*arrow*) without associated herniation shows mild narrowing of the intervertebral disk space on a T2-weighted sagittal image.

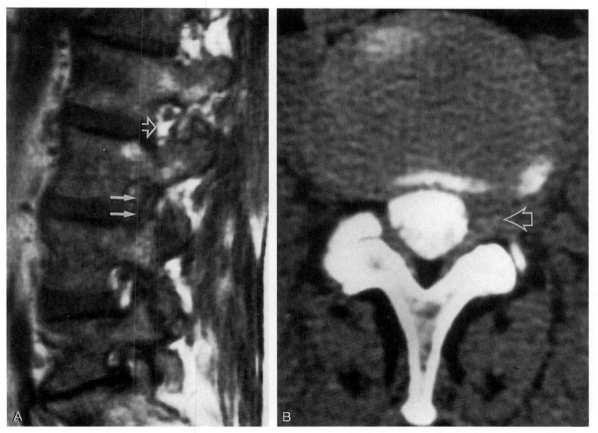

FIGURE 14-52. Lateral disk herniation. (**A**) Foraminal fat in the L3-4 intervertebral foramina (*solid arrows*) is absent, as seen on a T1-weighted parasagittal image. The intact L2-3 disk demonstrates normal high signal intensity foraminal fat for comparison (*open arrow*). (**B**) The corresponding axial CT shows left lateral disk material encroaching on the intervertebral foramina, with resultant stenosis (*open arrow*).

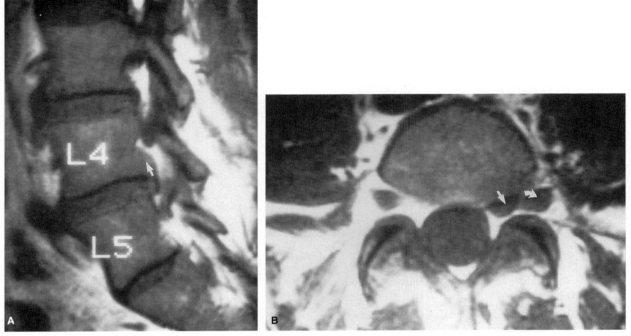

FIGURE 14-53. Left lateral L4-5 disk herniation (*straight arrow*) with superior extension medial to the exiting left L4 nerve root (*curved arrow*) is seen on (**A**) T1-weighted sagittal and (**B**) axial images.

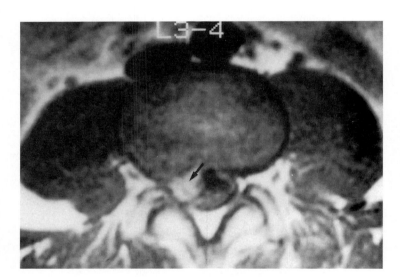

FIGURE 14-54. Extruded nuclear material through the ruptured annulus occurs in acute right paracentral L3-4 disk herniation (*arrow*). Although disk material demonstrates increased signal intensity on this T1-weighted axial image, hyperintensity of nuclear disk material on T1-weighted protocols is uncommon. The right lateral aspect of the thecal sac is compressed.

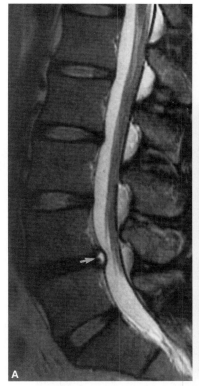
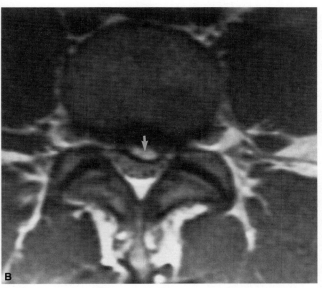

FIGURE 14-55. Hyperintense disk protrusion (*arrow*) of L4-5 level on T2-weighted fast spin-echo sagittal (**A**) and axial (**B**) images.

sequences. Increases in the signal intensity of herniated nuclear material on T2- or T2*-weighted images, however, may be secondary to inflammation or to increased water in the extruded disk.[41,103] Axial images are important in evaluating neural foramina and nerve root effacement in cases of lateral and posterolateral disk herniations (Fig. 14-56). The path of the extruded nuclear material may be outlined on axial T2-weighted images due to a diskogram-like effect. Traversing nerve root enhancement and enlargement (related to nerve root edema) have been reported within the thecal sac above the level of impingement.[104,105] The transient enhancement associated with compression or postoperative inflammation has been attributed to temporary radicular vein stasis.[81]

As mentioned, a free fragment of disk (sequestration) may remain in continuity with the parent disk, and thus be inseparable by MR imaging, especially when surrounded by an associated mass of inflammation. Free fragments may also migrate both cranially and caudally, both in the midline and in the lateral recesses (Fig. 14-57). A low signal intensity (ie, dark) line between a sequestered disk fragment and the parent disk, called the double-fragment sign, may be seen when there has been penetration of the posterior longitudinal ligament[106] (see Fig. 14-57). An intradural disk herniation demonstrates higher signal intensity than CSF on T1-weighted images. Gadolinium may be used to enhance gran-

ulation tissue around the peripheral border of a free fragment (Fig. 14-58). Contrast enhancement is useful in excluding diagnoses such as neurofibroma, epidural fibrosis, and abscesses (although an abscess may also show peripheral enhancement). After Gd-DTPA administration, the central portion of a free fragment or sequestered disk maintains low signal intensity, whereas the periphery is enhanced, producing a bull's-eye appearance (see Fig. 14-58). In the nonoperative spine, enhanced MR images have also been useful in identifying increased signal intensity in annular rents or tears, presumably due to the ingrowth of blood vessels, granulation tissue, or both.[100] It should be noted that calcified cysts of the facet joint may mimic a calcified free fragment (see Fig. 14-40), but usually can be differentiated by their location posterolateral to the thecal sac, as opposed to the anterolateral location of a disk fragment.

Surrounded by high signal intensity epidural fat, a conjoined nerve root (usually two nerve roots that join and exit from the same neural foraminal level) is more clearly depicted on MR images than on CT scans (Fig. 14-59). Conjoined nerve roots appear as asymmetric masses in the anterolateral epidural space and should not be mistaken for disk fragments. This mistake can be avoided by tracking the course of the nerve roots bilaterally at each level. The observation of a conjoined nerve root in conjunction with

text continues on page 1096

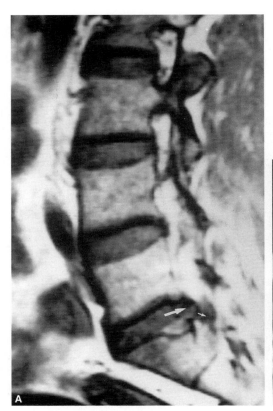
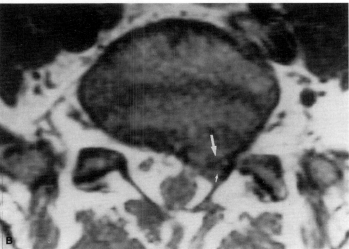

FIGURE 14-56. A large left paracentral L5-S1 herniation (*large arrows*) displaces the left S1 nerve root (*small arrows*) on T1-weighted (**A**) sagittal and (**B**) axial images. The left S1 nerve root is secondarily enlarged.

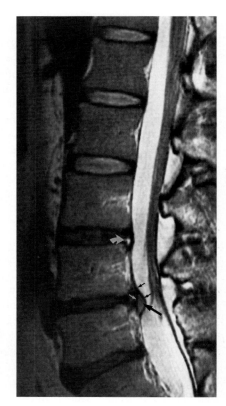

FIGURE 14-57. L4-5 sequestered disk fragment (*large black arrow*) is separated from the L4-5 protrusion, as demarcated by a thin hypointense line (*straight white arrow*). The identification of this line between the parent disk and free fragment indicates a tear in the posterior longitudinal ligament. The low signal intensity posterior longitudinal ligament (*small black arrows*) is posteriorly displaced by the disk fragment. There is mild hyperintensity in the free fragment. An annular fissure is identified at L3-4 (*curved arrow*). T2-weighted fast spin-echo sagittal image.

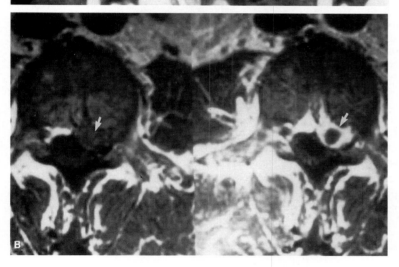

FIGURE 14-58. T1-weighted (**A**) sagittal and (**B**) axial images of an L2-3 free disk fragment (*arrows*) before (*left*) and after (*right*) Gd-DTPA administration. The hyperintense peripheral enhancement reveals an inflammatory reaction in granulation tissue.

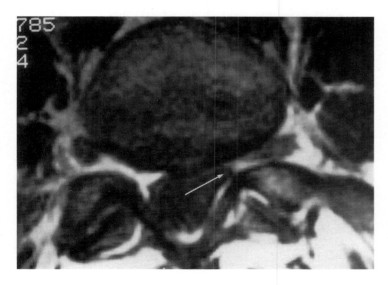

FIGURE 14-59. The L5-S1 left conjoined nerve root (*arrow*) branches off asymmetrically from the thecal sac. The normal right L5 nerve root has exited the intervertebral nerve root canal at this level, as seen on a T1-weighted axial image.

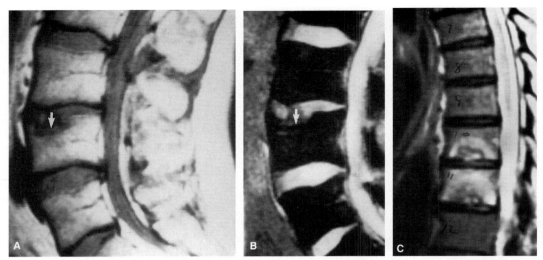

FIGURE 14-60. Schmorl's node (*arrows*) involves the superior endplate of L4 on (**A**) T1-weighted and (**B**) T2-weighted images. Extension of the disk through the superior endplate is best displayed with gradient-echo contrast as an area of high signal intensity. (**C**) Separate case of multiple Schmorl's nodes involving the lower thoracic spine. Immediately adjacent subchondral marrow is hyperintense on T2-weighted image.

an adjacent disk fragment is significant, since the surgeon should be alerted to its presence to prevent unnecessary traction at the time of laminectomy. Schmorl's nodes, which may exhibit enhancement with Gd-DTPA contrast, represent extensions of herniations through vertebral body endplates and demonstrate increased signal intensity relative to vertebral body subchondral bone on T2-weighted images (Fig. 14-60). A limbus vertebra, identified as a defect in the anterior superior vertebral body endplate, is caused by the extension of a herniated disk through the rim apophysis.[101] In a

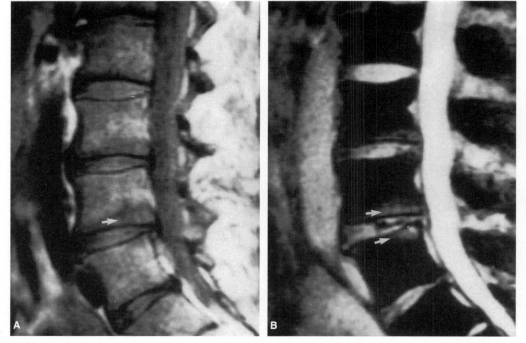

FIGURE 14-61. A type I vertebral body change (*arrows*) demonstrates (**A**) low signal intensity subchondral marrow on a T1-weighted sagittal image, and high signal intensity on (**B**) T2*-weighted and (**C**) gadolinium-enhanced T1-weighted sagittal images.

continued

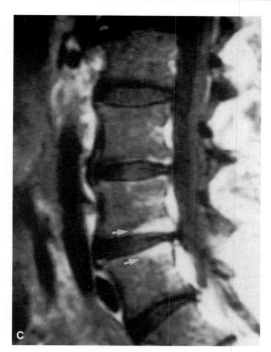

FIGURE 14-61. *Continued.*

comparison of MR imaging, myelography, and postmyelographic CT scan findings with surgical results, Janssen and colleagues[107] reported MR accuracy in predicting operative findings at 96%. Accuracy of myelography (81%), and postmyelographic CT (57%) were significantly less. Myelography and CT together had an accuracy of 84%.

Thoracic disk herniations, which are less frequent than lumbar or cervical herniations, are usually identified in the midthoracic or lower thoracic levels[36,39] (see Figs. 14-43 and 14-44). If no abnormality is found on sagittal images (using a 512 × 256 matrix), oblique axial image prescriptions through all thoracic intervertebral disks are recommended to identify any small extradural defects. In MR studies of asymptomatic individuals, Wood and coworkers[108] reported finding thoracic herniations in 37%, annular bulges in 53%, annular tears in 58%, deformity of the spinal cord in 29%, and Scheuermann's endplate irregularities or kyphosis in 38%.[108]

ENDPLATE CHANGES. Modic and others have characterized changes in vertebral body marrow signal intensity adjacent to the endplates of degenerative intervertebral disks.[64,70,72] In type I endplates, signal intensity is decreased on T1-weighted images and increased on T2- or T2*-weighted images (Figs. 14-61 and 14-62). This pattern is observed on 4% of MR studies for intervertebral disk disease and in 30% of patients after treatment with chymopapain.

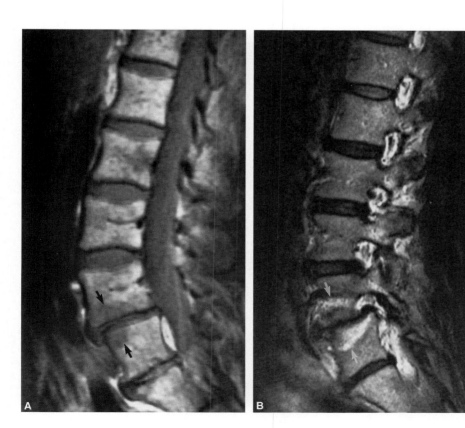

FIGURE 14-62. Type I marrow change (*arrows*) with hypointensity of the L4-5 vertebral body marrow on T1-weighted sagittal image (**A**) and hyperintensity on corresponding T2-weighted fast spin-echo sagittal image (**B**). The L4-5 interspace is narrowed and demonstrates anterior listhesis of L4 on L5.

Type I endplate changes represent subchondral vascularized fibrous tissue associated with endplate fissuring and disruption. Type II endplate changes (Fig. 14-63) include fatty marrow endplate conversion, which demonstrates increased signal intensity on T1-weighted images, isointense to slightly hyperintense signal intensity on T2-weighted images, and isointense signal intensity on T2*-weighted images. Type II changes are seen in approximately 16% of cases and correlate with yellow marrow replacement and associated endplate degeneration or disruption. Type III endplate changes include sclerosis, which demonstrates low signal intensity on T1-, T2-, and T2*-weighted images (Fig. 14-64). It is important not to mistake Gd-DTPA enhancement or increased signal intensity of areas of fibrovascular tissue in STIR images with endplate changes of osteomyelitis that cross the diskovertebral junction. In lumbar spine studies of identical twins, Battie and coworkers[109] have shown a positive genetic influence with respect to endplate changes, desiccation of disk, bulging or herniated disks, and decreased intervertebral disk space height.[109]

OTHER DEGENERATIVE VERTEBRAL BODY AND DISK FINDINGS. The imaging characteristics of an intravertebral body vacuum cleft, a sign of avascular necrosis, can change depending on position. It may be identified in extension, but absent in flexion.[110] An associated fluid-like high signal intensity pattern on T2- and T2*-weighted images has been attributed to the influx of fluid within the intravertebral cleft.

An intervertebral disk vacuum phenomenon may occur adjacent to a collapsed vertebral body, in addition to its more common presentation in association with degenerative disk disease[111] (see Fig. 14-48). Collapse-related vacuum phenomena occur in association with both pathologic and nonpathologic vertebral body collapse due to osteoporosis, multiple myeloma, metastases, acute trauma, and vertebral osteomyelitis.

Disks that are hyperintense on T1-weighted MR images are associated with calcification, thought to correlate with degenerative disk disease.[112] Fat-suppression may decrease the hyperintense signal intensity. Both focal or diffuse hyperintensity patterns have been observed. On T2-weighted images, focal areas of increased signal intensity within a degenerative disk may represent fluid within a cracked and fissured disk (Fig. 14-65).

Jinkins and colleagues[113] have reported normal enhancement characteristics of the lumbar spine after intravenous administration of an expanded dose of gadopentetate dimeglumine including intrathecal linear enhancement, facet joint and intervertebral disk enhancement adjacent to and parallel to the vertebral endplate.[113]

CLINICAL MANAGEMENT

Thoracic Disk Herniation Treatment. Thoracic disk herniation is unusual, accounting for less than 2% of operatively treated disks. It may be incidentally noted on MR imaging and demonstrates an incidence of 7% to 15% in autopsy

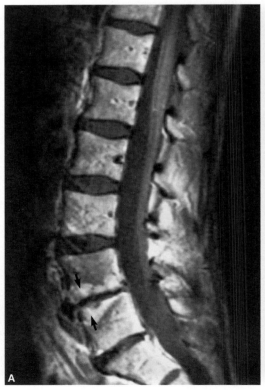
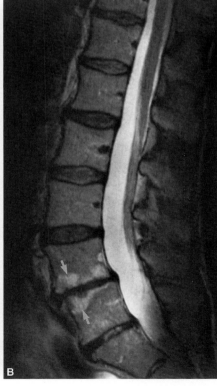

FIGURE 14-63. Type II endplate change (*arrows*) in degenerative disease. (**A**) A T1-weighted sagittal image shows increased signal intensity with yellow marrow replacement in L4-5 subchondral bone. (**B**) T2-weighted fast spin-echo sagittal image demonstrates no further increase in L4-5 marrow fat signal intensity (*arrows*). There is associated disk space narrowing and endplate irregularity.

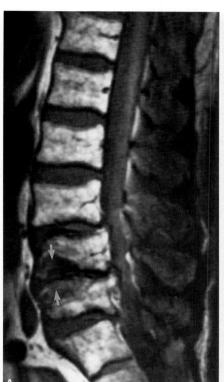
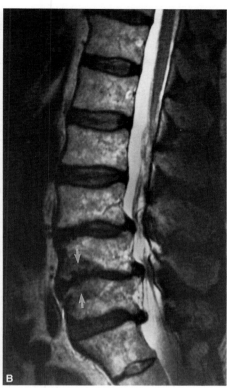

FIGURE 14-64. Type III vertebral body marrow (*arrows*) is hypointense on T1 (**A**) and T2-weighted fast spin-echo (**B**) images at the level of the L4-5 endplates. Type III changes are associated with bony sclerosis on conventional radiographs while type I and II changes do not directly correlate with plain film findings of sclerosis.

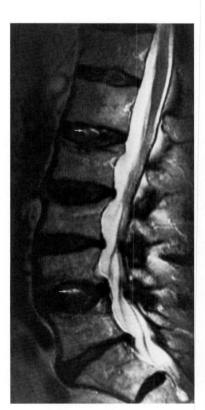

FIGURE 14-65. Focal linear areas of hyperintensity (*arrows*) within degenerative low signal intensity L1-2 and L4-5 disks, as seen on a T2-weighted fast spin-echo sagittal image.

specimens.[114] Most occur in the lower thoracic spine. Patients may present with radicular pain or numbness, extremity weakness, visceral pain, bowel/bladder symptoms, or upper motor neuron signs.[115] If myelopathy is not present, conservative measures such as stretching, extension strengthening, and antiinflammatory agents can be effective.

Surgical intervention is recommended for myelopathy, progressive neurologic deficit, bowel/bladder symptoms, or pain that corresponds to the level of compression and is refractory to conservative care. Anterior diskectomy, which can be accompanied by a local fusion if desired, is performed most safely via a thoracotomy.[116] Recent advancements in endoscopic techniques have resulted in the ability to perform thoracic dissection using thoracoscopy. Although highly technique dependent and not without risk itself, thoracoscopy appears to be a promising technique for removal of herniated thoracic disks with decreased morbidity compared with open thoracotomy.[117]

Lumbar Disk Herniation Treatment. Symptoms of disk herniation generally occur in a younger patient population than do symptoms of spinal stenosis. The classic presentation includes radiculopathy, and pain or numbness in a dermatomal distribution, often associated with weakness of the affected muscle group. The majority of cases occur at the L4-5 and L5-S1 levels. Lateral herniations into the foramen are more common at L3-4, and are frequently seen in an older patient population. This lesion should be suspected in an older patient presenting with anterior thigh pain. A foraminal herniation at this level would comprise the exiting L3 root. At L4-5, a paracentral disk herniation is most likely to compress the L5 nerve root, resulting in weakness of the toe dorsiflexors and pain or numbness over the lateral calf and first dorsal web space. An L5-S1 disk herniation usually compresses the S1 nerve root, resulting in numbness or pain over the lateral aspect and sole of the foot, diminution of the ankle jerk reflex, and weakness of ankle plantar flexion. Approximately half of the patients with lumbar disk herniation recover within 1 month, and over 90% recover by 6 months.[118]

Given the high percentage of patients who recover without surgical intervention, conservative management is the mainstay of treatment. Nonsteroidal antiinflammatory drugs, limited short-term analgesics, and muscle relaxants combined with several days of rest followed by physical therapy can facilitate recovery. Epidural steroids or selective nerve root blocks may decrease the acute sciatic pain.

Surgical intervention is indicated for patients who develop cauda equina syndrome, progressive neurologic deficits, intractable pain, or who do not respond to conservative measures. The standard approach, that of an open diskectomy, supplemented in most cases with loop or microscope magnification, has an 85% success rate if the patient's symptoms correspond to the level of nerve root compression and a radiologic study such as MR imaging or CT confirms a disk herniation. Percutaneous diskectomy, chemonucleolysis, and laser diskectomy have lower success rates, ranging from 57% to 75%.[119,120] Surgical risks for all of these procedures include dural tear, hemorrhage, infection, recurrent or residual disks, nerve deficit, and incorrect level of exploration.

Disk Herniation in Cervical Spine

T1-weighted sagittal images display the subarachnoid disk and cervical cord outlines, allowing direct assessment of cord impingement[7–19,121] (Fig. 14-66). Early degenerative disk disease may be identified on conventional T2-weighted sagittal images and is characterized by loss of signal intensity in a desiccated intervertebral disk. Corresponding gradient-echo images are not as sensitive to changes in intradiskal signal intensity, and only in more advanced stages of degeneration are regions of low signal intensity (from clefting, cavitation, or complete desiccation) demonstrated (Fig. 14-67). T2*-weighted sequences produce a myelographic CSF effect, important in assessing spinal canal stenosis and the disk–thecal sac interface in herniations.[75,76] Gradient-echo techniques use a nonslice selective acquisition without degradation or loss of signal intensity from pulsatile flow columns of CSF. With conventional spin-echo techniques, image quality is degraded by CSF flow artifact, and accuracy in interpreting extradural impressions (eg, disk herniations, osteophytosis) may be compromised. The absence of flow artifact, along with excellent differentiation between the cord and CSF, eliminates the need for cardiac gating in gradient-echo refocused imaging.

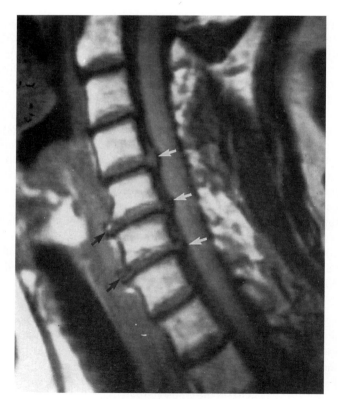

FIGURE 14-66. C3-4, C4-5, and C5-6 disk herniations (*white arrows*) compressing the spinal cord are seen on a T1-weighted sagittal image. Anterior disk bulges (*black arrows*) and loss of disk space height are shown at levels C3-4 and C4-5.

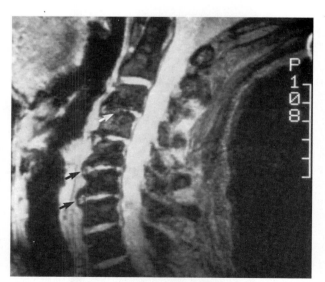

FIGURE 14-67. Cervical osteophytosis is indicated by a degenerative cervical spine with osteophytes (*black arrows*) and an associated C3-4 disk herniation (*white arrow*) on a T2*-weighted sagittal image.

T1, T2-weighted fast spin-echo, fat-suppressed T2-weighted fast spin-echo (which allows for better definition of disk and osteophyte), and gradient-echo sequences define the extent of most cervical disk herniations in the sagittal plane[85,122] (Figs. 14-68 and 14-69). If T2-weighted fast spin-echo images are used alone, however, without a T1 or fat-suppressed sequence, the extent of disk pathology may be overestimated because both osteophyte and disk may appear hypointense (Fig. 14-70). On T2*-weighted sagittal images, magnetic susceptibility artifact also causes overestimation of the degree of cervical disk herniation or stenosis. Parasagittal and axial images are required to evaluate the lateral extension of a herniated disk (Fig. 14-71). Annular disk bulges may also demonstrate a posterior disk convexity on sagittal images. However, the morphology of a contained herniation and the path of extruded disk material is more accurately demonstrated with axial plane images (Fig. 14-72). With 3DFT volume imaging at a slice thickness of 2 mm, cervical intervertebral disks are routinely sectioned at the level of the bright signal intensity nucleus pulposus. Increasing TE or decreasing the flip angle increases the contrast of the low signal intensity cord (Fig. 14-73). Cord compression and edema may be associated with larger disk protrusions. T1-weighted and T2*-weighted gradient-echo images demonstrate small disk herniations that are sometimes missed on conventional T1-weighted spin-echo images because of the paucity of epidural and neural foraminal fat as contrast. A low signal intensity line or boundary between the herniated disk and cord represents the dura and the displaced posterior longitudinal ligament (Fig. 14-74). This dark interface may also be caused by a ridging osteophyte, by calcification, or by flow-related (eg, turbulence) artifact. The most common locations for cervical disk herniations are C5-6 and C6-7. They are usually midline or posterolateral, with the uncinate process offering some protection against lateral cervical herniations[123] (Fig. 14-75). When lateral disk

herniations do occur, they can be seen in peripheral parasagittal and axial images. The superior inferior extension (ie, migration) of disk material is best demonstrated on T1- and T2*-weighted sagittal and axial T2*-weighted images (Figs. 14-76 and 14-77). This may be seen as a dark double line representing a herniated disk fragment crossing the posterior longitudinal ligament. Gd-DTPA administration causes the epidural venous plexus to enhance and aids in the diagnosis of more lateral herniations, although this application is not routine.

We have observed differences in the morphology of a herniated disk in flexion versus extension, which can secondarily change the degree of central canal stenosis. Kinematic flexion and extension MR imaging, however, is better suited to assessing atlantoaxial subluxations.

CLINICAL MANAGEMENT.   Patients with cervical herniated disks generally present with arm or hand pain in a dermatomal pattern, oftentimes with associated numbness or weakness.[124] Neck pain may also accompany a cervical disk herniation. Patients usually respond to conservative measures, such as rest, antiinflammatory drugs, and cervical isometrics. A trial of cervical traction may be indicated if symptoms do not improve.

Surgery is recommended if the extremity symptoms do not improve over time, if weakness progresses, or if long-tract signs such as hyperreflexia develop. Certainly, surgical intervention is recommended only if the level of the herniated disk corresponds to the pain, weakness, or numbness distribution of the nerve root that is being compressed. Anterior cervical diskectomy and fusion is the preferred surgical treatment.[125] Diskectomy alone may result in cervical kyphosis and ultimately in collapse of the disk space and foraminal stenosis. The success rate from combined diskectomy and fusion is high, and adjunctive measures are generally not

text continues on page 1106

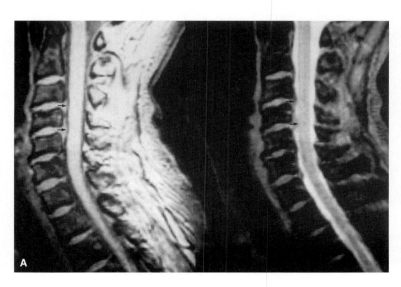

FIGURE 14-68. Mild C3-4 and moderate C4-5 midline cervical disk herniations (*arrows*) are seen on (**A**) gradient-echo sagittal images.   *continued*

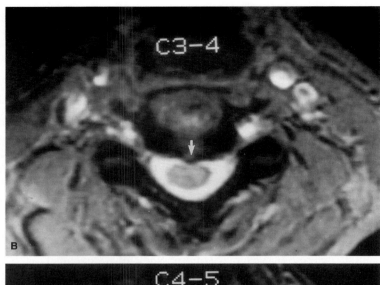

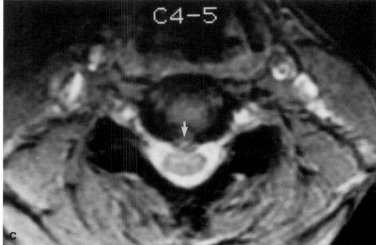

FIGURE 14-68. *Continued.* (**B, C**) Mild C3-4 and moderate C4-5 midline cervical disk herniations (*arrows*) are seen on 3D Fourier transform T2*-weighted axial images.

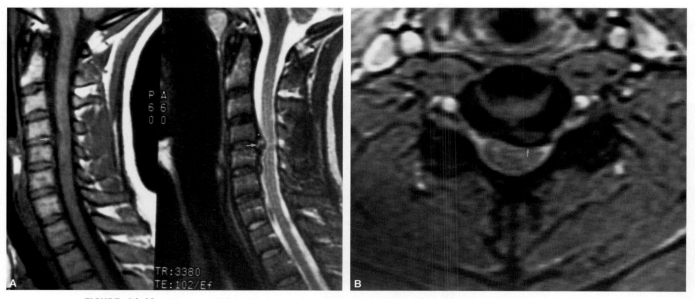

FIGURE 14-69. (**A**) Large C4-5 disk herniation (*arrow*) indenting the anterior aspect of the cord on T1 (left) and T2-weighted fast spin-echo (right) images. There is hyperintensity in the herniated disk material. A smaller herniation is present at C5-6. (**B**) Corresponding 3DFT T2* axial image identifies the indentation on the left ventral aspect of the cord (*arrow*).

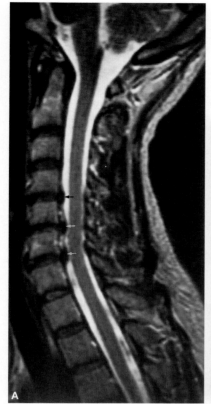

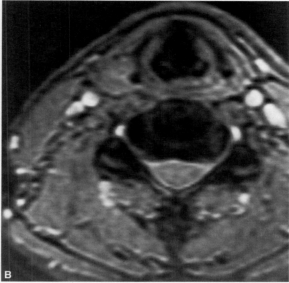

FIGURE 14-70. (A) Cervical spondylosis with hypointense osteophytes (*arrows*) at C4-5, C5-6, and C6-7. The extradural defects may be mistaken for disk protrusions on this T2-weighted fast spin-echo sagittal image. (B) T2* axial image at level C5-6 shows osteophytic ridging and uncinate hypertrophy without associated disk protrusion. There is severe bilateral neural foraminal stenosis.

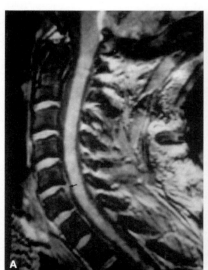

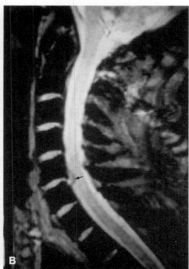

FIGURE 14-71. A C6-7 disk herniation with an anterior extradural defect on (A) a gradient-echo image with 110° flip angle and on (B) a T2*-weighted image. *continued*

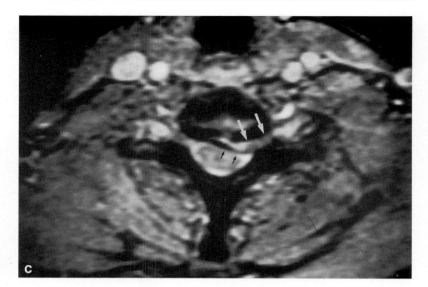

FIGURE 14-71. *Continued.* (**C**) Left paracentral–lateral herniation effaces the left ventrolateral cord (*black arrows*) and causes severe left neural foraminal stenosis (*white arrows*), as seen on a T2*-weighted axial image.

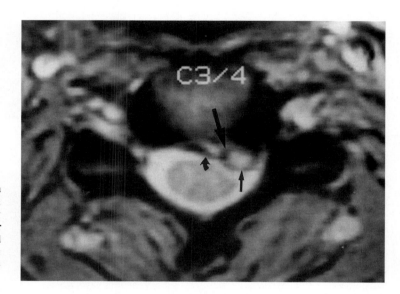

FIGURE 14-72. A severe left paracentral C3-4 disk herniation with "double fragment sign" is seen on a T2*-weighted axial image. The herniated disk demonstrates high signal intensity (*large straight arrow*). A defect in the annulus and posterior longitudinal ligament (*curved arrow*) can be differentiated from the thin dark line between the disk and spinal cord that represents a contribution by the posterior longitudinal ligament and dura (*small straight arrow*).

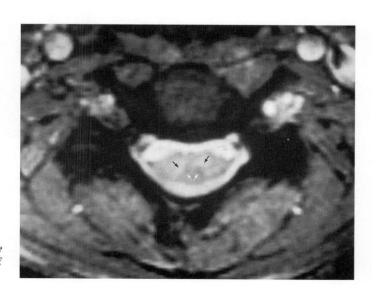

FIGURE 14-73. The white matter of the posterior columns (*white arrows*) demonstrates lower signal intensity than the gray matter of the cord (*black arrows*) on a T2*-weighted axial image.

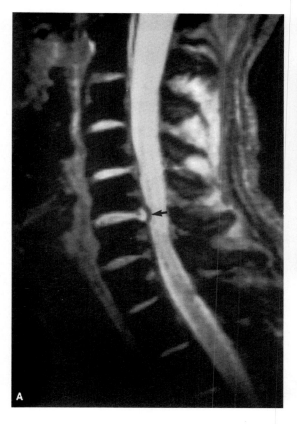

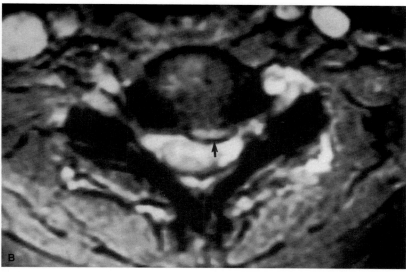

FIGURE 14-74. Moderate C5-6 herniation with a low signal intensity annular—dura interface (*arrow*) is seen on T2*-weighted (**A**) sagittal and (**B**) axial images.

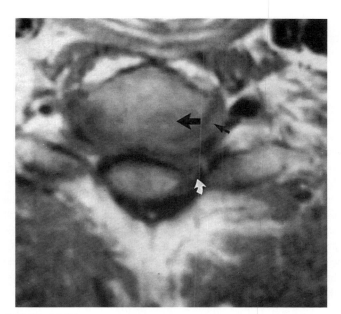

FIGURE 14-75. A T1-weighted axial image shows left lateral disk herniation (*curved white arrow*). The intervertebral disk (*large black arrow*) and uncinate process (*small black arrow*) are seen at this level.

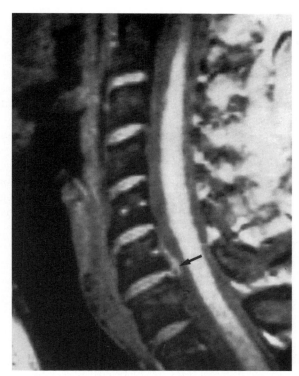

FIGURE 14-76. On a gradient-echo image with a flip angle of 110°, the superior extension of a C6-7 disk herniation demonstrates high signal intensity (*arrow*), in contrast to the low signal intensity of cerebrospinal fluid. The cervical cord is hyperintense.

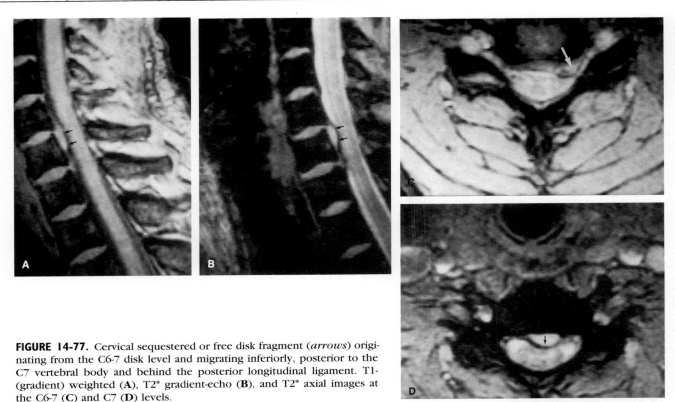

FIGURE 14-77. Cervical sequestered or free disk fragment (*arrows*) originating from the C6-7 disk level and migrating inferiorly, posterior to the C7 vertebral body and behind the posterior longitudinal ligament. T1-(gradient) weighted (**A**), T2* gradient-echo (**B**), and T2* axial images at the C6-7 (**C**) and C7 (**D**) levels.

indicated (Fig. 14-78). However, anterior plating may be indicated in the event of nonunion or if multiple levels (three or more) are being fused. Surgical risks include recurrent laryngeal nerve injury, perforation of local structures, infection, pseudoarthrosis, graft dislodgement, hardware failure or displacement, and neurologic injury.

Lateral disks that impinge on the nerve root (spinal nerve) within the foramen may be addressed posteriorly with a foraminotomy. The nerve root retracts relatively easily compared with the spinal cord, and if the disk herniation is lateral enough, this can be safely performed. A portion of the facet joint must be removed to permit visualization of the foramen and nerve root.

Degenerative Disk Disease: Spinal Stenosis

Stenosis of Thoracic and Lumbar Spines

Spinal stenosis, acquired or congenital, may involve the central canal, the intervertebral foramen, or the lateral recess. In the lumbar spine, stenosis may be bony or secondary to soft tissue (ie, disk) impingement (Figs. 14-79 through 14-81). Indentations of the thecal sac and neural foraminal stenosis are caused by both disk and osteophytic impingement (Fig. 14-82). Facet and ligamentum flavum hypertrophy contribute to neural foraminal

and central canal stenosis (Fig. 14-83). The bright CSF–extradural interface on T2- and T2*-weighted images makes these sequences preferable for the assessment of canal dimensions. The loss or decrease in bright signal intensity epidural fat on T1-weighted images makes these sequences preferable for identifying peripheral or neural foraminal stenosis. Central canal stenosis is common from L2-3 through L4-5, and is frequently characterized by annular disk bulging and facet hypertrophy as components of degenerative disk disease.[106] Loss of bright signal intensity articular cartilage is seen through the facet joints on axial T2*-weighted images. Sclerosis of the facet joint demonstrates low signal intensity on T1-weighted images. Facet effusions, synovial cysts, subchondral cysts, vacuum facets caused by gas formation, osteophyte overgrowth, and joint-space narrowing all contribute to the process of facet arthrosis. Synovial cysts may be unilateral or bilateral and may cause posterior thecal sac compression[126] (Fig. 14-84). Lateral or peripheral stenosis is evaluated both on parasagittal and axial images. The lateral recess and neural foramina are also characterized on T1-weighted images, which show neural stenosis as distinct from bright epidural fat signal intensity.

Thoracic spinal stenosis may result from spinal trauma from a retropulsed vertebral body fragment that compromises the usually spacious thoracic canal.[64]

text continues on page 1111

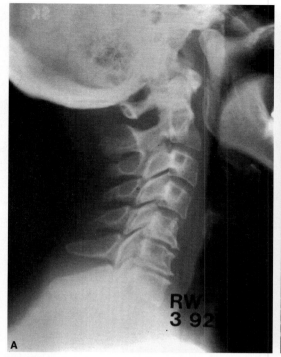

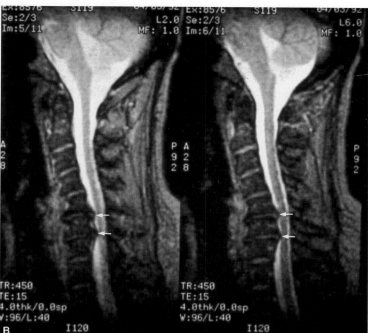

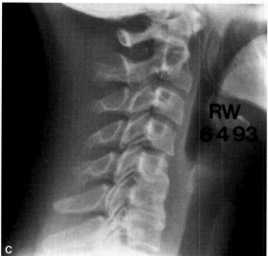

FIGURE 14-78. (**A**) Lateral cervical radiograph of a woman with right arm pain at ulnar aspect of forearm and hand as well as weakness of grip strength and wrist dorsiflexion. Conservative treatment failed to result in sustained relief. (**B**) Sagittal T2*-weighted image demonstrates disk protrusions with osteophyte formation at C5-6 and C6-7 (*arrows*). (**C**) Lateral radiograph after anterior cervical diskectomy and fusion of the two involved levels. Consolidation appears to be complete, and patient denies residual symptoms and has returned to competitive roller skating.

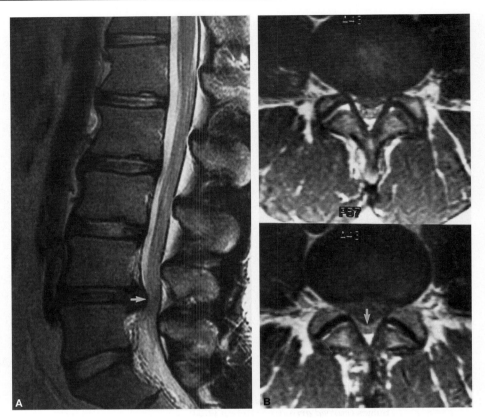

FIGURE 14-79. Central spinal stenosis caused by severe L4-5 disk herniation (*arrow*). T2-weighted fast spin-echo sagittal (**A**) and axial (**B**) images.

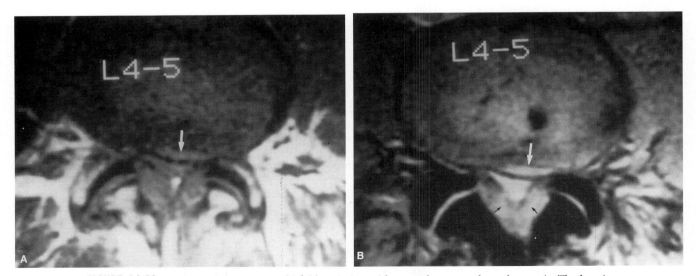

FIGURE 14-80. Moderate left paracentral L4-5 herniation with secondary central canal stenosis. The herniated portion of the disk (*white arrow*) demonstrates intermediate signal intensity on a T1-weighted axial image (**A**) and high signal intensity on a T2*-weighted axial image (**B**). The ligamentum flavum (*black arrows*) is thickened.

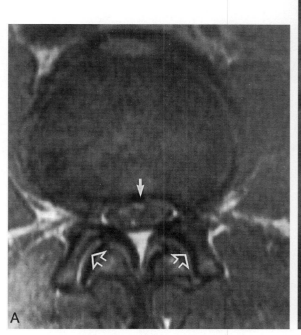

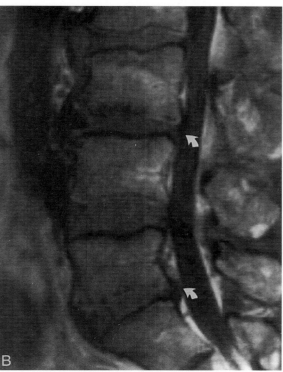

FIGURE 14-81. In congenital lumbar canal stenosis, a narrowed vertebral canal with multiple level disk bulges (*curved arrows*), vertebral bony encroachment, hypertrophied articular facets (*open arrows*), and a small thecal sac (*straight solid arrow*) is shown on T1-weighted (**A**) axial and (**B**) sagittal images.

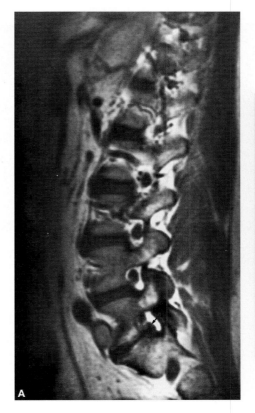

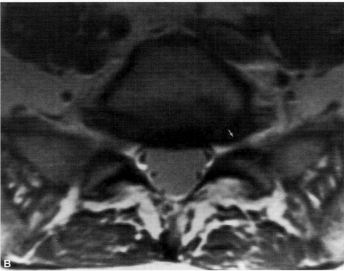

FIGURE 14-82. Left lateral osteophytic ridging (*arrow*) at L5-S1 resulting in left neural foraminal stenosis on T1-weighted sagittal (**A**) and proton density weighted axial (**B**) images.

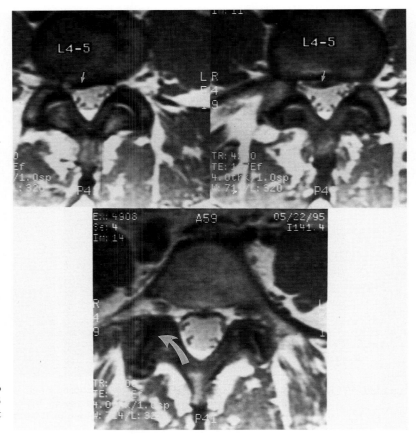

FIGURE 14-83. Mild central canal stenosis secondary to L4-5 disk protrusion (*straight arrow*). There is severe L5 facet hypertrophy (*curved arrow*) contributing to right neural foraminal stenosis.

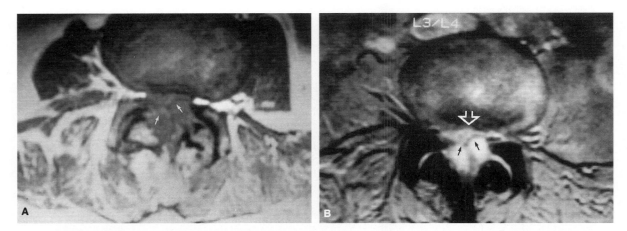

FIGURE 14-84. Bilateral synovial cysts (*solid arrows*) of the L3-4 facet joints result in severe central canal stenosis (*open arrow*). Gelatinous cysts demonstrate low signal intensity on a T1-weighted image (**A**) and high signal intensity on a T2*-weighted image (**B**).

CLINICAL MANAGEMENT OF LUMBAR SPINE STENOSIS. Patients with spinal stenosis generally present with leg pain exacerbated by walking, often with mild to moderate degrees of associated back pain. The leg pain has also been referred to as neurogenic claudication because of its clinical similarities with vascular claudication (ie, leg pain beginning after a relatively fixed distance walking, requiring rest before the patient can proceed). Generally, patients with spinal stenosis must sit or bend forward to relieve their symptoms, because this permits less compression from the infolding of the thickened ligamentum flavum, whereas patients with vascular claudication can stand and rest, permitting blood flow to the extremities to catch up with the muscle demands. Since both conditions affect older patients, examination of distal pulses and workup of the two systems may be appropriate.

The symptoms of spinal stenosis can be improved with a conservative treatment program of physical therapy, including abdominal strengthening, antiinflammatory drugs or use of a lumbar support brace. Although the clinical response is variable, epidural steroids have been used successfully by many patients. Many patients with stenosis are older and have coexisting medical problems, and may be reluctant or even unable to consider surgical intervention.

If conservative treatment fails to adequately improve the patient's mobility and symptoms, surgery may be recommended.[127] Laminectomy, which permits decompression of the stenotic levels, is performed, including removal of the thickened ligamentum flavum and hypertrophic bone of the facet joints. Removal of too much of the facet joints or the need for extensive foraminal decompression, which can weaken the pars interarticularis, may result in destabilization of the lumbar spine and the need to perform a fusion. The presence of degenerative spondylolisthesis or a significant scoliotic deformity is also an indication for concomitant fusion. Pedicle screw instrumentation can be used at the time of fusion to improve the fusion rate and to reduce the likelihood of progressive spondylolisthesis in selected cases. Surgical risks include dural tear, neurologic injury, excessive bleeding, pseudoarthrosis, recurrent stenosis, and hardware failure.

Stenosis of Cervical Spine

A decrease in disk height and bulging of the peripheral annular fibers may contribute to spinal stenosis (Fig. 14-85). Associated osteophytes may project from the anterior and posterior vertebral body margins (Fig. 14-86), and posterior osteophytes may be confused with low signal intensity annular bulges on heavily T2*-weighted images. Low signal intensity osteophytes and endplate sclerosis can be separated from high signal intensity disks on 110° flip angle gradient-echo images (Fig. 14-87). Magnetic-susceptibility artifact on

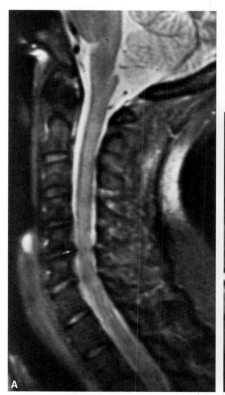
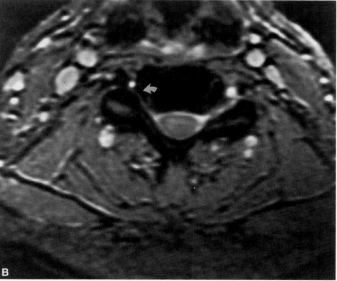

FIGURE 14-85. Posterior osteophytic ridging (*straight arrow*) at the C5-6 level with degenerative loss of intervertebral disc space height associated with mild central canal stenosis and severe right neural foraminal stenosis. Degenerative right uncinate hypertrophy (*curved arrow*) also contributes to the neural foraminal stenosis. (**A**) T2-weighted fast spin-echo sagittal image. (**B**) T2-weighted axial image.

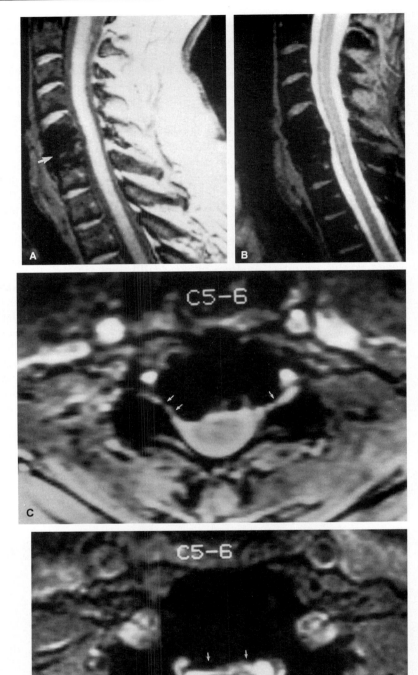

FIGURE 14-86. C5-6 fusion (*arrow*) is seen on (**A**) a gradient-echo sagittal image with a flip angle of 110° and (**B**) a T2*-weighted sagittal image (*right*). (**C**) Severe right (*double arrow*) and moderate left (*single arrow*) neural foraminal stenosis is seen on a T2*-weighted axial image. (**D**) Moderate posterior osteophytic ridging (*arrows*) at the C5-6 fusion level effaces the anterior subarachnoid space on a T2*-weighted axial image.

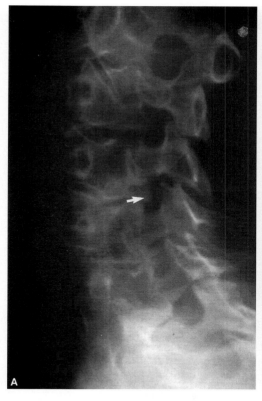

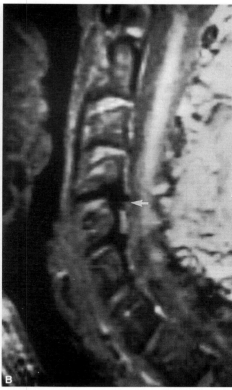

FIGURE 14-87. Stenosis of the left neural foramen on (**A**) an oblique radiograph and (**B**) the corresponding gradient-echo sagittal image. Low signal intensity osteophytic spurring is differentiated from the adjacent vertebral body marrow on the gradient-echo image.

T2*-weighted axial images, may cause overestimation of intervertebral nerve root canal stenosis. Enlarged osteophytes or disk herniation that compromise the subarachnoid space contribute to the development of cord myelopathy[128] (Fig. 14-88). Radiculopathy may result from impingement in the dural sac or root sleeve.[129] Neural foraminal stenosis and associated radiculopathy may also be caused by degenerative changes at the facet and uncinate[130] (eg, uncinate process hypertrophy, uncovertebral spurs) (Fig. 14-89).

Degenerative facet arthrosis may result in vertebral body retrolisthesis, further compromising the anterior-to-posterior sagittal canal diameter.[131] Low signal intensity linear ossification of the posterior longitudinal ligament may also contribute to cord compression, especially when associated with congenital spinal stenosis or hypertrophic changes or spondylosis.[131,132]

CLINICAL MANAGEMENT OF CERVICAL SPINE STENOSIS.

Cord compression secondary to cervical spinal stenosis always requires surgical decompression. Anterior vertebrectomy has been shown to have predictable results if irreversible cord changes have not occurred.[125] The vertebral body or bodies are removed or reconstructed using tricortical iliac crest or fibula, depending upon the length of the defect. Cervical plates have gained in popularity in recent years, to shorten the length of time of immobilization in halo-vest or rigid cervical orthosis.

When cervical stenosis is multiple-level, particularly when secondary to an ossified posterior longitudinal liga-

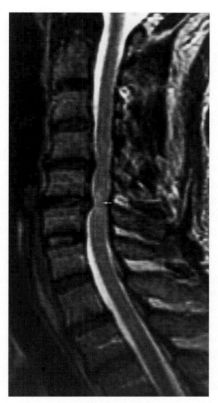

FIGURE 14-88. Cervical myelopathy (*arrow*) with hyperintense changes of myelomalacia at the C5-6 disk level secondary to disk herniation and canal stenosis. T2-weighted fast spin-echo sagittal image.

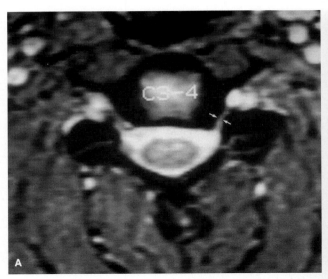

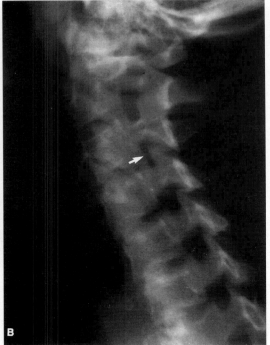

FIGURE 14-89. (A) Left uncinate and facet hypertrophy (*arrows*) produces severe left neural foraminal stenosis. (B) The corresponding oblique radiograph confirms bony left C3-4 neural foraminal stenosis (*arrow*).

ment (OPLL) (Fig. 14-90), posterior laminectomy or laminaplasty can be performed.[133] The latter, popularized in Japan where OPLL is more common than in North America, involves an "open-door" technique, where the lamina are cut on one side of the canal and then hinged on the other, to widen the cervical spinal canal. Local bone can used to prop open the lamina.

Postoperative Spine

Computed tomography plays an important role in assessing bony detail in the postoperative spine, especially in evaluating pseudoarthrosis in lumbar spine fusions.[134] MR imaging, however, is also useful in characterizing endplate and associated marrow changes.[70,72] Stable fusions of the lumbar spine are frequently associated with fatty marrow conversion of the endplates at the corresponding vertebral levels (ie, type II endplate changes).[135] This yellow or fatty marrow conversion demonstrates increased signal intensity on T1-weighted images and becomes isointense with adjacent marrow on T2-weighted images. Focal fatty marrow conversion may also be seen in patients with degenerated disks.[70]

MR imaging has also been used to assess postoperative changes after fusion, laminectomy, chymopapain, and percutaneous nuclectomy.[135-143] The sensitivity and specificity of MR imaging is equal to intravenous contrast CT in distinguishing recurrent disk herniations from scar or fibrosis.

Immediately and for the first few weeks after spine surgery, the MR appearance of immature scar or hematoma is similar to and may be mistaken for the original herniated

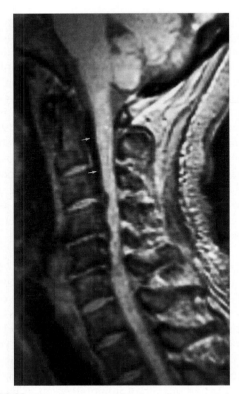

FIGURE 14-90. Hypointense ossification of the posterior longitudinal ligament (*arrow*) easily visualized on T2*-weighted sagittal image secondary to the increased susceptibility effect of heterotopic bone when using gradient-echo sequences.

FIGURE 14-91. L4-5 epidural mass effect (*straight arrow*) with peripheral rim enhancement (*curved arrow*) in the early postoperative period. (**A**) Enhanced T1-weighted sagittal image. (**B**) T1-weighted axial image. (**C**) Enhanced T1-weighted axial image. A recurrent disc and/or scar may produce this appearance.

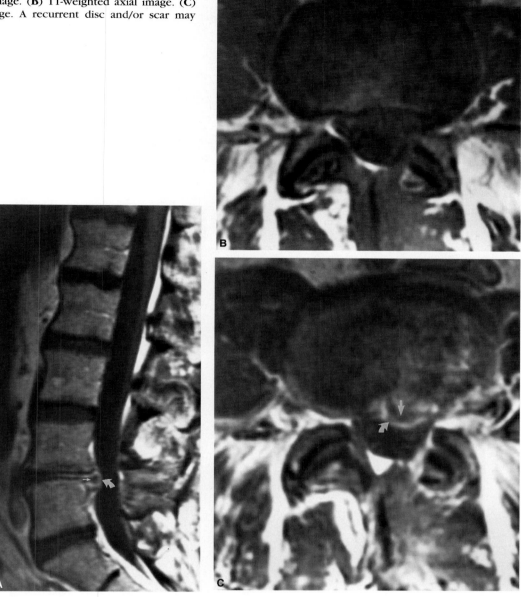

disk. This extradural soft tissue mass effect decreases 2 to 6 months postoperatively[144] (Fig. 14-91) but may be seen as long as a year after surgery. There is progressive enhancement and resorption or contraction of the soft tissue mass on sequential MR studies.[145] Epidural fat inferior to the postsurgical site of herniation has heterogeneous signal intensity. Epidural fibrosis may be in continuity with the parent disk, producing a mass effect. The epidural scar, however, is usually irregularly marginated compared with the smooth configuration of a recurrent herniation (Fig. 14-92).

Recurrent disks may be demarcated by a hypointense rim adjacent to the increased signal intensity herniation. Peripheral enhancement at the site of the original disk herniation decreases from 38% 3 weeks postoperatively to 12% 3

months postoperatively.[146] In addition, the peripheral enhancement pattern at 3 weeks postoperatively changes to a more diffuse enhancement pattern at 3 months (Fig. 14-93). Thus, in the early postoperative period (prior to resorption of the soft tissue mass and associated changes in the enhancement pattern), soft tissue contiguous with the parent disk may be mistaken for residual or recurrent herniation. In addition, the pattern of postoperative enhancement depends on the composition of herniation and granulation tissue and on the maturity of the granulation tissue or scar. Scar tissue enhances earlier and is more intense than adjacent disk material. Organized scar tissue enhances more rapidly than poorly organized scar tissue, and younger scar tissue enhances to a greater extent than that observed in older scar tissue.

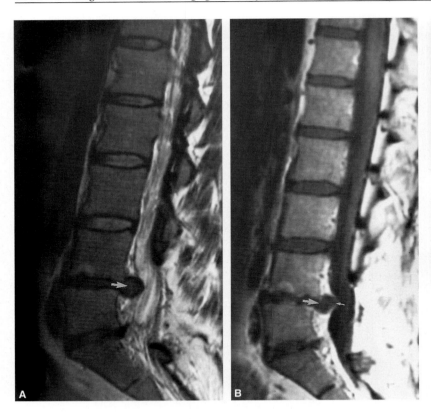

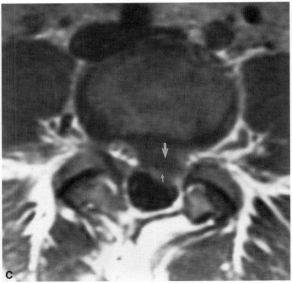

FIGURE 14-92. Large L4-5 recurrent disk herniation (*arrow*) without enhancement. A thin border or rind of enhancing scar tissue (*small arrow*) outlines the herniation. There is associated compression of the left ventral thecal sac. (**A**) T2-weighted fast spin-echo sagittal image. (**B**) Enhanced T1-weighted sagittal image. (**C**) Enhanced T1-weighted axial image.

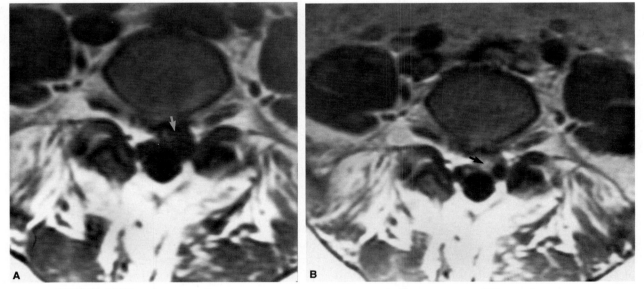

FIGURE 14-93. Three months after surgery, scar tissue (*arrow*) demonstrates a diffuse enhancement pattern adjacent to the enlarged left S1 spinal nerve. No thecal sac deformity is present. (**A**) T1-weighted axial image. (**B**) Enhanced T1-weighted axial image.

Scar tissue location also affects signal intensity properties. On T2-weighted sequences, anterior scar tissue is hyperintense in 82% of cases, lateral scar tissue is hyperintense in 47% of cases, and posterior scar tissue is hyperintense in only 20% of cases.[145] On T1-weighted images, posterior scar demonstrates heterogeneous intermediate signal intensity. Immediately after laminectomy, posterior scar is isointense to hyperintense on T2-weighted images, compared with diskectomy scar, which is hyperintense. With time, the thecal sac deformity resolves by contraction, decreasing the mass effect of the epidural scar (Fig. 14-94).

Both symptomatic and asymptomatic patients may demonstrate nerve root enhancement perioperatively and postoperatively. Boden and colleagues[147] reported enhancement of nerve roots in 62% of patients 3 weeks after surgery, which was absent at 6 months postoperatively. Nerve root enhance-

ment may occur in the absence of arachnoiditis.[147] Symptomatic nerve roots demonstrate enhancement in the preoperative and postoperative period with a strong clinical correlation, whereas enhancement in asymptomatic patients is restricted to the early postoperative period (ie, enhancement is not present 6 months after surgery).

Postoperative diskitis is indicated by decreased signal intensity within the vertebral body marrow on T1-weighted images, hyperintensity on T2-weighted images, and enhancement of vertebral marrow after intravenous contrast administration. Indistinctness or destruction of the cortical endplate is also seen. Similar findings may be present after extensive diskectomies, especially if cortical endplate curettage was performed. A secondary sign of infection is induration of the paravertebral fat. Epidural fluid collections representing abscesses may also be seen. The differentiation of

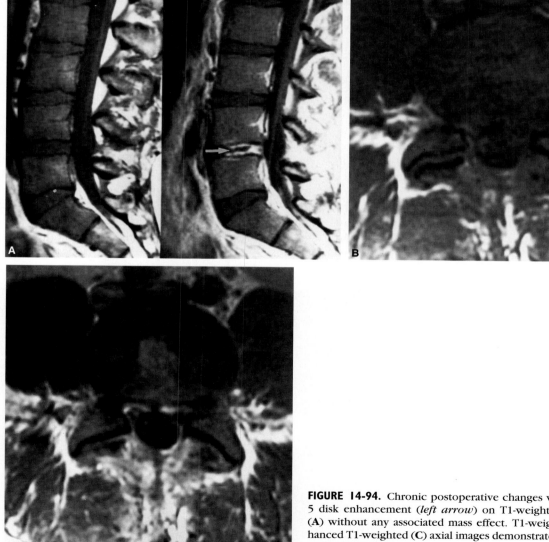

FIGURE 14-94. Chronic postoperative changes with posterior L4-5 disk enhancement (*left arrow*) on T1-weighted sagittal image (**A**) without any associated mass effect. T1-weighted (**B**) and enhanced T1-weighted (**C**) axial images demonstrate epidural fibrosis surrounding the thecal sac and S1 spinal nerves. A posterior laminectomy defect is present.

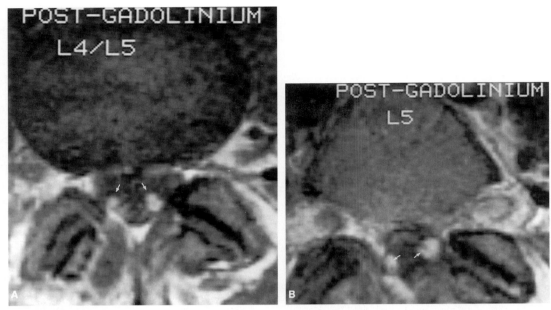

FIGURE 14-95. Arachnoiditis (*arrows*), with asymmetric high signal intensity peripheral clumping of nerve roots within the distal thecal sac, is seen on enhanced T1-weighted axial images at the (**A**) L4-5 and (**B**) L5 levels.

normal postoperative changes from diskitis often requires correlation with the erythrocyte sedimentation rate (ESR) to exclude diskitis. Normally, the ESR returns to baseline within 4 months of surgery. In many instances, percutaneous aspiration or core biopsy may be required to make the diagnosis of diskitis, as well as to obtain an culture sample in order to identify the causative organism for optimally effective antibiotic therapy.

Fat-suppressed gadolinium-enhanced imaging of the postoperative spine may obviate the need for precontrast scanning.[106] In differentiating between recurrent disk herniations and scar tissue, the contrast between bright signal inten-

sity fibrosis and adjacent low signal intensity disk and CSF is superior to that seen with conventional T2-weighted or gradient-echo techniques. On gradient-echo images, herniated disk material may appear isointense or hyperintense relative to adjacent fibrosis or scar. Heavily weighted T2-weighted fast spin-echo sequences have shown potential for the differentiation of hypointense recurrent disk herniations from hyperintense scar tissue without the use of contrast. This observation requires further documentation. When interpreting MR studies of the spine with a metallic artifact, the increased sensitivity to magnetic susceptibility with gradient-echo imaging must be taken into account.

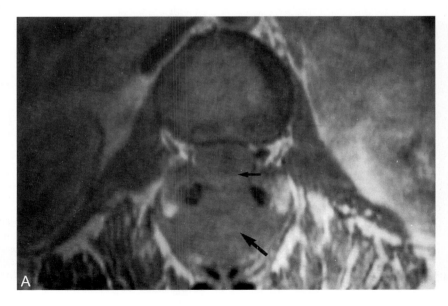

FIGURE 14-96. Postoperative pseudomeningocele (*large black arrows*) demonstrates (**A**) low signal intensity on an intermediate weighted image.

continued

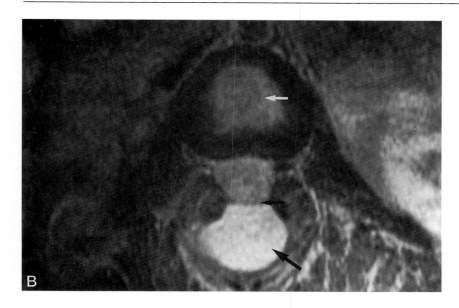

FIGURE 14-96. *Continued.* Postoperative pseudo-meningocele (*large black arrows*) demonstrates (**B**) high signal intensity on a T2-weighted image. Thecal sac–fluid interface (*small black arrows*) and the bright signal intensity nucleus pulposus (*white arrow*) are best seen on the T2-weighted image.

Clumping and irregular separation of the nerve roots are characteristic findings on MR images of arachnoiditis,[148] and T2-weighted axial images are usually necessary to display the distortion of the thecal sac and intrathecal nerve roots (Fig. 14-95). Arachnoiditis is grouped into several MR categories based on the morphology of the separate nerve roots. Group 1 consists of central conglomerations of nerve roots within the thecal sac. In group 2, the nerve roots are clumped peripherally to the meninges, producing an apparent empty thecal sac. In group 3, MR images show an area of increased soft tissue signal intensity occupying the thecal sac with no discrimination of nerve roots.

The signal characteristics of a postoperative fluid collection (ie, pseudomeningocele) are analogous to CSF; they both demonstrate low signal intensity on T1-weighted images and high signal intensity on T2-weighted images (Fig. 14-96).

Focal collections of Pantopaque in the thecal sac have a characteristic appearance on MR imaging; they display high signal intensity on T1-weighted images and low signal intensity on T2-weighted images[149] (Fig. 14-97). Lipomas also show increased signal intensity on T1-weighted images and may be confused with residual Pantopaque. Lipomas, however, may have associated spinal dysraphism.[150]

Laminectomy and laminotomy defects—with loss of continuity of corresponding cortical bone, marrow, and ligamentum flavum—are seen on conventional T1, T2*, and T2-weighted fast spin-echo weighted axial or lateral parasagittal

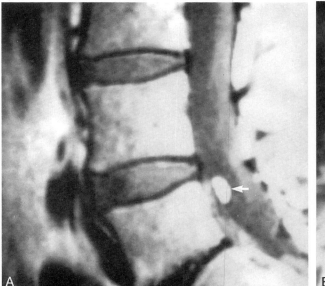

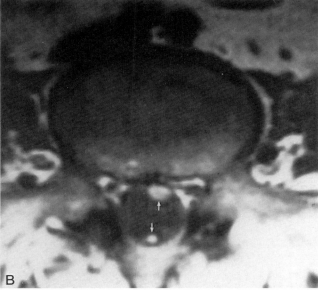

FIGURE 14-97. High signal intensity Pantopaque (*arrows*) is seen on T1-weighted (**A**) sagittal and (**B**) axial images.

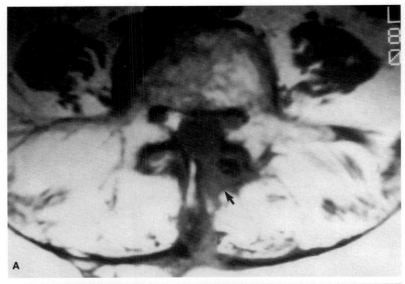

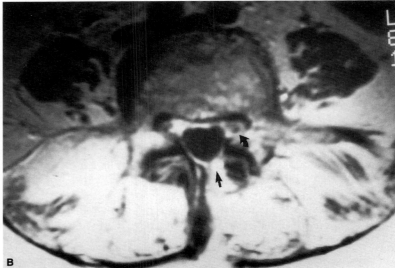

FIGURE 14-98. A left hemilaminectomy defect (*straight arrows*) with enhancing epidural fibrosis surrounding left L5 nerve root (*curved arrow*) is seen on T1-weighted axial images (**A**) before and (**B**) after contrast administration.

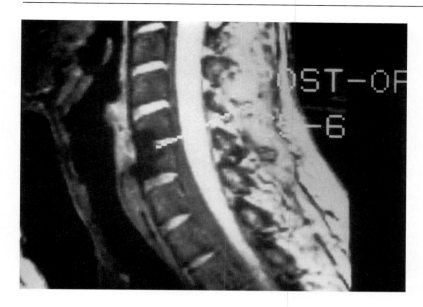

FIGURE 14-99. Uncomplicated anterior interbody fusion of C5-6, without central stenosis or herniation, is seen on a gradient-echo sagittal image.

images (Fig. 14-98). Vertebral body resection demonstrates low signal intensity on T1 and increased signal intensity on T2-weighted images. Soft tissue edema and neovascularity, which demonstrate intermediate signal intensity on T1-weighted images and is hyperintense on T2-weighted images, may persist up to 6 months postoperatively, until it is replaced by scar tissue. In the immediate postoperative period, prior to formation of epidural fibrosis, edema may be enhanced after Gd-DTPA administration. In the postoperative cervical spine, bony stenosis and herniations of adjacent disk levels are also evident (Fig. 14-99).

MR imaging is of limited usefulness for evaluation of percutaneous lumbar diskectomy, and preoperative MR studies may not predict clinical outcomes.[151] Postoperative spinal fusion hardware may limit the usefulness of MR studies because of associated artifacts. When necessary, results are evaluated on a case-by-case basis to assess the fixation technique, type of hardware, and region of interest.[152–154]

Spondylolisthesis

Spondylolisthesis may be either lytic or degenerative.[155,156] In lytic spondylolisthesis, anterior displacement of one vertebra onto another occurs secondary to bilateral fractures or defects in the pars interarticularis (Fig. 14-100). There is forward displacement of the superior vertebral body, and the posterior joints and neural arch are aligned with the posterior elements of the inferior vertebral body.[157] Peripheral parasagittal images, particularly T2*-weighted images or T1-weighted images acquired without an interslice gap, demonstrate the defects in the pars interarticularis. MR imaging is less sensitive than CT (especially if multiplanar reformations are used) in demonstrating completed fractures of the pars interarticularis. Characteristically, the anteroposterior diameter of the spinal canal is increased in the presence of spon-

dylolytic spondylolisthesis, and is narrowed in degenerative spondylolisthesis.[158] Hypertrophic bone and fibrocartilaginous overgrowth at the pars defect often produce lateral recess or central canal stenosis. The vertebral canal is decompressed; therefore, neural foraminal stenosis may occur without central canal stenosis (Fig. 14-101). The posterior aspects or margins of the two involved vertebrae may be seen in the same axial image. Axial images at the level of the spondylolytic defect demonstrate low signal intensity sclerosis, fragmentation, or a discontinuity in the region of the pars defect. An associated disk herniation or spinal nerve entrapment can contribute to impingement of the exiting nerve root.[159] Reactive marrow changes (similar to those described for endplate changes and degenerative disk disease) may be seen in the adjacent pedicles in 40% of patients with spondylolysis and have been described by Ulmer and co-workers.[160] A type 2 pedicle change (hyperintensity on T1-weighted images and isointensity or hyperintensity on T2-weighted images) is the most frequent pattern of pedicle signal intensity observed in spondylolisthesis. Acute spondylolytic spondylolisthesis is usually associated with major trauma, and these injuries are unstable.[161] It may also, however, be seen in younger patients, where it may be associated with sports-related activities involving hyperextension (eg, gymnastics, football, and soccer). Fat-suppressed or STIR images can be used to demonstrate an acute pars fracture.

In degenerative spondylolisthesis, there is forward displacement of the superior vertebral body secondary to medial superior erosion of the inferior facet and is often associated with vertically oriented facet joints. (Fig. 14-102). This facet erosion allows forward movement of the inferior articular facet of the superior vertebral body. In the absence of a pars defect, which would decompress the central canal, narrowing of the anteroposterior diameter of the spinal canal occurs, causing severe central spinal stenosis in addition to lateral

text continues on page 1124

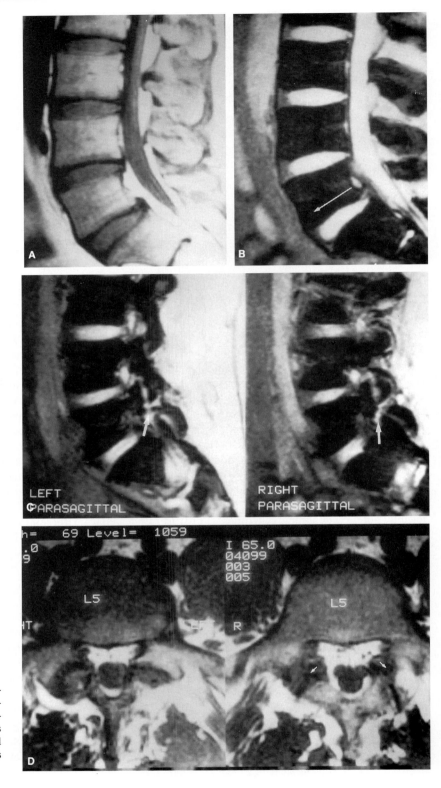

FIGURE 14-100. (A) T1-weighted and (B) T2*-weighted sagittal images show grade I lytic spondylolisthesis of L5 on S1 (*arrows*). (C) T2*-weighted sagittal images show bilateral defects or fractures (*arrows*) of the pars interarticularis. (D) T1-weighted axial images show sclerotic low signal intensity pars defects (*arrows*).

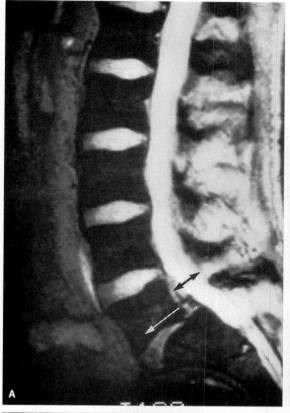

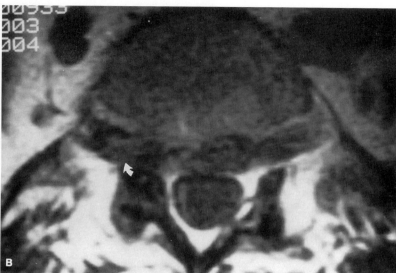

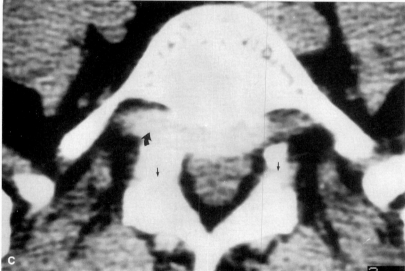

FIGURE 14-101. (A) A T2*-weighted sagittal image shows grade I lytic spondylolisthesis with forward movement of the L5 on S1 vertebral body (*white arrow*). The increase in anterior-to-posterior central canal diameter (*black arrows*) is characteristic. The corresponding (**B**) T1-weighted axial and (**C**) axial CT images show pars defects or fractures (*straight arrows*). There is severe right neural foraminal stenosis (*curved arrows*).

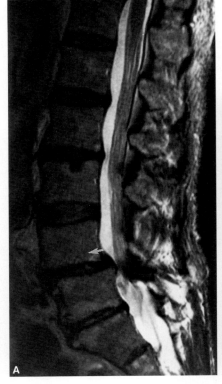
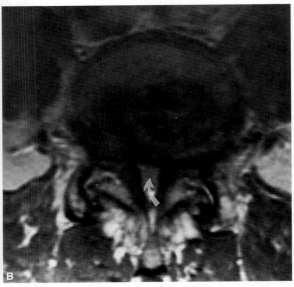

FIGURE 14-102. Degenerative spondylolisthesis of L4 on L5 (*straight arrow*) with intact pars interarticularis and degenerative facet joints as shown on T2-weighted fast spin-echo sagittal image (**A**) and T1-weighted axial image (**B**). There is severe secondary central canal stenosis (*curved arrow*) with narrowing of the anterior-to-posterior diameter of the spinal canal.

recess stenosis, neural foraminal stenosis, or both. The contours of the thecal sac may have an hourglass or constricted outline. Neural foraminal and pars anatomy in lytic or degenerative spondylolisthesis is accurately displayed on CT scans. Posterior displacement or retrolisthesis of an involved vertebral body relative to an inferior level is also a manifestation of degenerative disk disease or facet arthrosis.[162]

Clinical Management

The most common types of spondylolisthesis are isthmic and degenerative. The latter is seen more often in patients with disk space collapse, and usually occurs at L4-5. The former is due to a defect at the pars interarticularis and is generally felt to be developmental in nature. It occurs in the preadolescent, although symptoms may not occur until later in life. It is most commonly seen at L5-S1, secondary to a pars defect at L5.

Patients with isthmic spondylolisthesis present with back pain, often exacerbated by hyperextension activities. The condition is more common in athletes such as gymnasts, divers, and football players.[163,164] Hamstring tightness can be seen in younger patients. Bone or fibrous scar at the pars defect site may result in nerve root impingement and leg pain, numbness, or weakness. In most patients, symptoms can be treated by avoidance of hyperextension activities, bracing, and abdominal strengthening.[165] In a skeletally immature patient, however, slippage greater than 50% relative to the superior aspect of the sacrum indicates a high risk for progression of slippage,

and surgical fusion is indicated. Fusion is also indicated for patients who do not respond to conservative measures. The majority of adolescents have satisfactory results with bilateral lateral fusion in situ.[166] Older patients are more likely to need decompression. Because of the risk of progression of slippage after decompression, fusion is generally performed at the time of decompression. Pedicle screw instrumentation has been used to improve fusion rate and decrease the immobilization period in such patients, although the risk of neurologic injury as well as infection may be increased by their use.

Other surgical options for isthmic spondylolisthesis include (1) pars repair (for levels other than L5, in young patients with minimal slippage); (2) fusion with fibular strut graft (Fig. 14-103; if the patient has a high-grade slip, is too small for instrumentation, and the surgeon desires more immobilization than a cast and bed rest would afford); and (3) fusion with reduction (if the patient's lumbosacral kyphosis results in an inability to stand upright). Although fusion with reduction does have an increased risk for neurologic and other complications, it may be appropriate for a small number of patients.[167–170]

As noted, degenerative spondylolisthesis occurs in older patients. The combination of forward slippage and facet disease results in spinal stenosis, so that these patients generally present with back pain and neurologic claudication. Management is similar to that of spinal stenosis, including antiinflammatory drugs, exercises, and epidural steroids. In patients who are refractory to con-

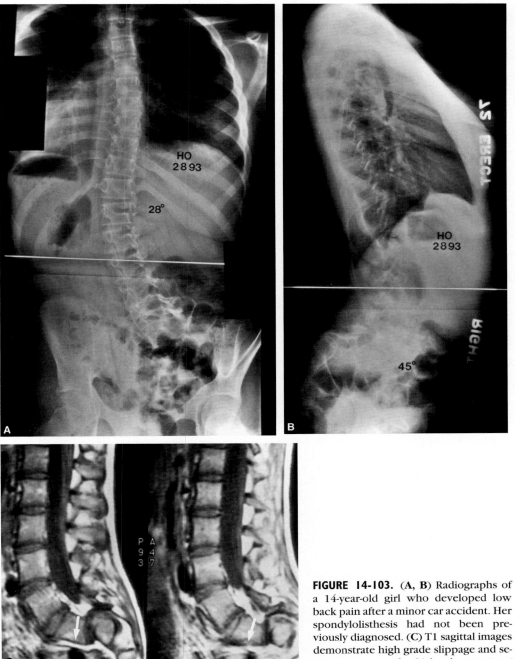

FIGURE 14-103. (A, B) Radiographs of a 14-year-old girl who developed low back pain after a minor car accident. Her spondylolisthesis had not been previously diagnosed. **(C)** T1 sagittal images demonstrate high grade slippage and severe stenosis at the S1 level.   *continued*

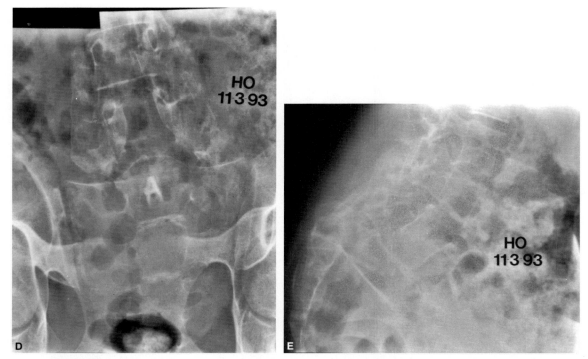

FIGURE 14-103. *Continued.* (**D, E**) Patient underwent a posterior fusion in situ from L3 to the sacrum, augmented by a fibular strut from the sacrum to L5. It can be easily seen as the triangular density at the midsacral level on the AP view.

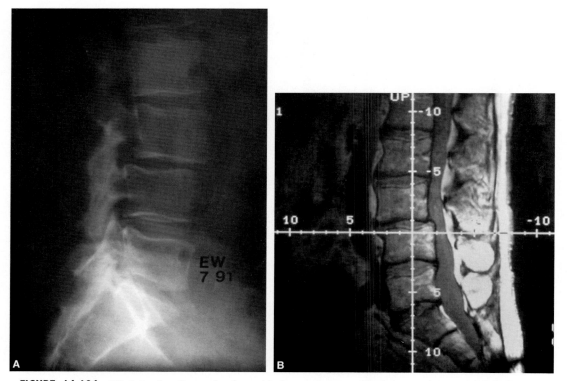

FIGURE 14-104. (**A**) Lateral radiograph of an elderly gentleman with degenerative spondylolisthesis at L3-4, whose chief complaint was low back pain and neurogenic claudication. (**B**) MR image demonstrating disk space narrowing and stenosis at this level. *continued*

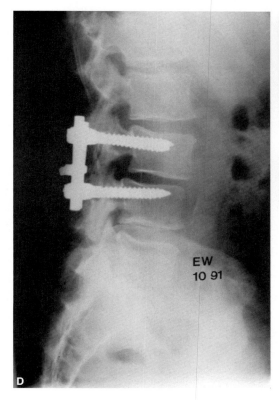

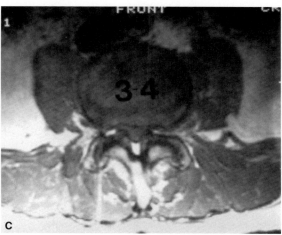

FIGURE 14-104. *Continued.* (**C**) MR image demonstrating disk space narrowing and stenosis at this level. (**D**) The patient underwent a decompression and fusion of L3-4 using pedicle screw instrumentation, with successful relief of symptoms.

servative therapy, or if neurologic compromise occurs, surgical decompression and fusion is indicated. Studies have shown that patients with degenerative spondylolisthesis do better if fusion is performed at the time of decompression[171] (Fig. 14-104). The surgeon may choose to use pedicular instrumentation to improve the fusion rate or to prevent further slippage while the fusion consolidates.

Fractures and Cord Trauma

Magnetic resonance has been used to assess traumatic and nontraumatic vertebral body fractures.[97,162,172–176] In traumatic fractures, retropulsed fracture fragments can be identified relative to the cord, thecal sac, and neural foramina (Figs. 14-105 through 14-107). In 28% of cases, supraspinous ligament disruptions associated with thoracolumbar burst fracture are identified on MR scans[177] (Fig. 14-108). Conventional radiography is not sensitive to posterior ligament disruption (Fig. 14-109). In acute and subacute stages, hemorrhage or edema demonstrate low signal intensity on T1-weighted images and high signal intensity on T2-weighted, T2*-weighted, or STIR images. A chronic fracture does not demonstrate increased signal intensity on long TR/TE sequences. In cases of cord trauma, MR evaluation reveals changes of posttraumatic myelopathy, characterized by low signal intensity on T1-weighted images, isointensity on

text continues on page 1130

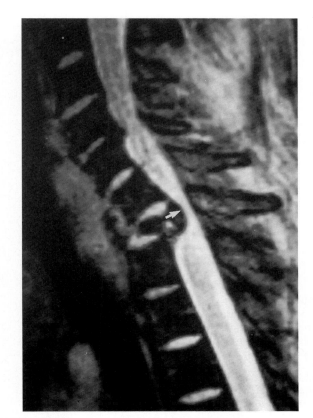

FIGURE 14-105. A C7 burst fracture (*arrow*) with secondary cord compression is seen on a T2*-weighted sagittal image.

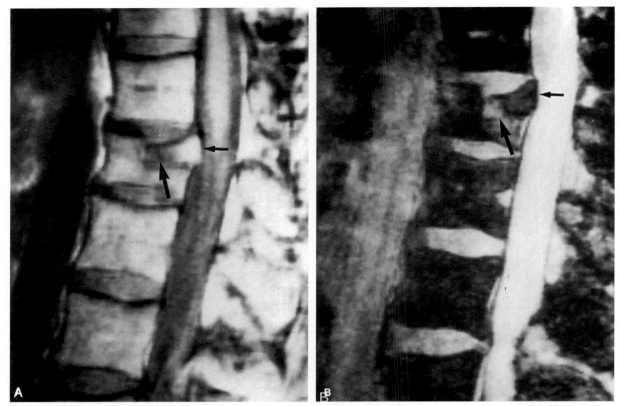

FIGURE 14-106. A posttraumatic L1 vertebral body fracture (*large arrows*) demonstrates (**A**) low signal intensity hemorrhagic marrow on a T1-weighted image and (**B**) increased signal intensity on a T2*-weighted image. A retropulsed fracture segment (*small arrows*) can be seen pressing on the thecal sac.

FIGURE 14-107. Posttraumatic fracture (*straight arrow*) of the posterior inferior corner of L3 secondary to a gunshot injury with disruption of the cauda equina and nerve roots at L2-3 level. Indentation of the ventral aspect of the thecal sac is caused by the fracture fragment. Irregular gadolinium enhancement of the transected traversing nerve roots of the cauda equina is shown (*curved arrow*). (**A**) T2-weighted fast spin-echo sagittal image. (**B**) Enhanced T1-weighted sagittal image.

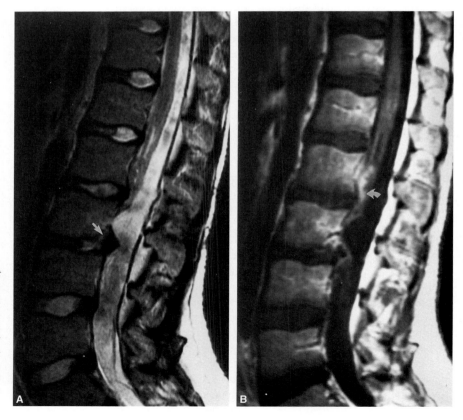

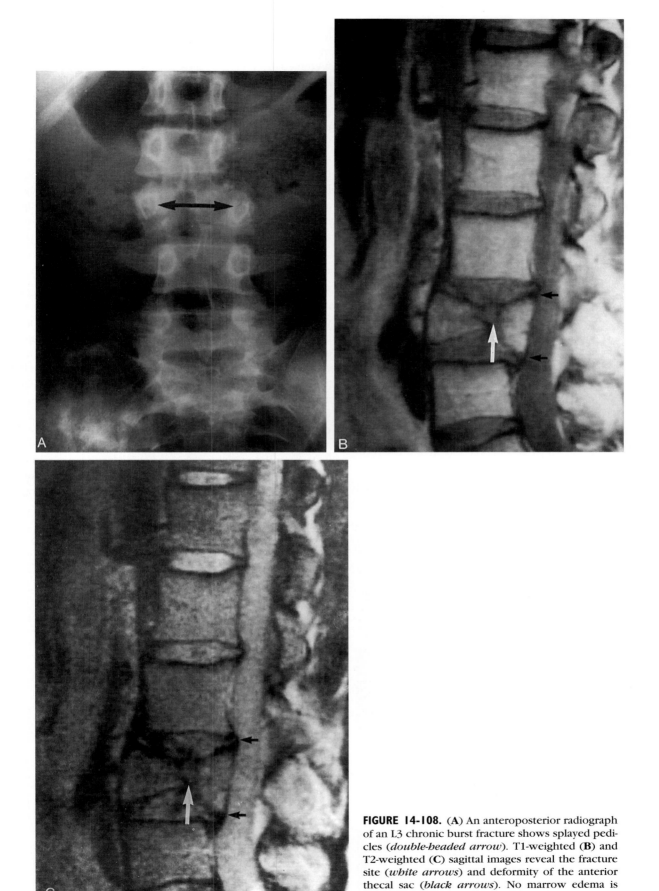

FIGURE 14-108. (**A**) An anteroposterior radiograph of an L3 chronic burst fracture shows splayed pedicles (*double-beaded arrow*). T1-weighted (**B**) and T2-weighted (**C**) sagittal images reveal the fracture site (*white arrows*) and deformity of the anterior thecal sac (*black arrows*). No marrow edema is associated with this chronic fracture.

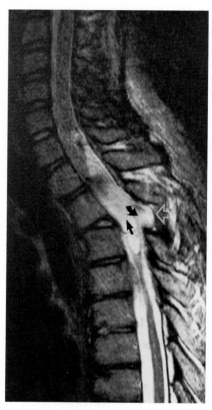

FIGURE 14-109. Posttraumatic injury (*straight arrow*) of the cervical-thoracic cord with disruption of posterior elements (*open arrow*), ligamentum flavum (*curved arrow*), and interspinous ligaments. There is associated atrophy and myelomalacia of the cord parenchyma. (T2-weighted fast spin-echo sagittal image.)

intermediate weighted images, and hyperintensity on T2-weighted or STIR images. Microcystic degeneration may lead to the development of a syrinx cavity. A traumatic syrinx demonstrates hyperintensity on T2-weighted images (Fig. 14-110). Myelomalacia (Fig. 14-111), gliosis-induced microcystic degeneration of the cord parenchyma, is isointense or mildly hyperintense to cord on T1-weighted images (Fig. 14-112). In contrast to a syrinx, myelomalacia is not improved by surgical decompression. A posttraumatic cyst is hypointense on T1-weighted images. Both myelomalacia and posttraumatic cysts are hyperintense on T2-weighted images (Fig. 14-113). Fluid motion and CSF pulsation effects are only visualized in cysts.

Fracture Types

C1 (atlas) injuries include (1) bilateral vertebral fractures through the arch, (2) Jefferson fractures (burst fractures involving anterior and posterior arches, which are unstable if they involve disruption of the transverse ligament), and (3) atlantoaxial rotary displacement (rotary locking of the facets). C2 (axis) injuries include odontoid fractures (type 2 transverse fractures of the base of the odontoid are unstable) and Hangman's fractures (unstable, hyperextension injuries with bilateral neural arch fractures). Flexion injuries are divided into (1) anterior wedge, (2) hyperflexion sprain–anterior subluxation (20% of which show delayed instability), (3) unilateral locked facet injuries (secondary to flexion, distraction, and rotation with common involvement of C4-5 and C5-6), (4) bilateral locked facet injuries (secondary

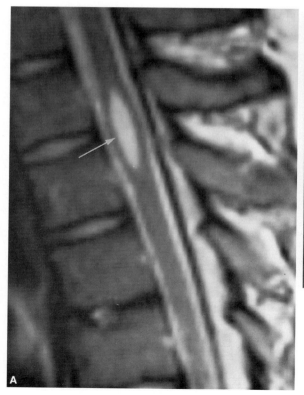

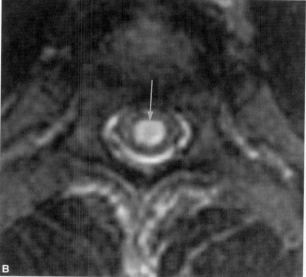

FIGURE 14-110. Post-traumatic syrinx of the lower cervical cord in a high school football player. The syrinx is hyperintense on T2-weighted fast spin-echo sagittal (**A**) and axial (**B**) images. Note the lateralized increased diameter of the cord at the level of the syrinx.

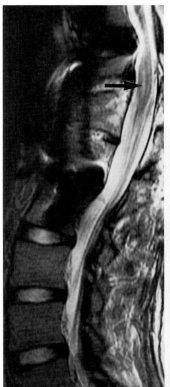

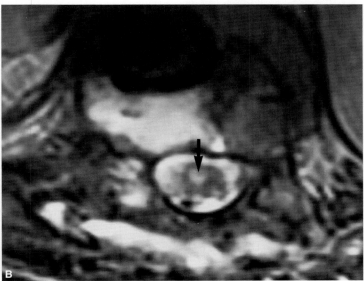

FIGURE 14-111. Posttraumatic T12 burst fracture treated with tibial strut graft. Focal 3 mm hyperintensity (*arrow*) to the right of midline at the T11-12 level represents myelomalacia and corresponds to the patient's presentation with a right lower extremity motor defect. T2-weighted fast spin-echo sagittal (**A**) and axial (**B**) images.

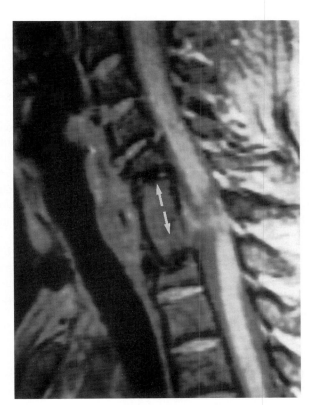

FIGURE 14-112. Cord myelomalacia as a complication of severe cord compression from a fracture flexion dislocation injury. Treatment was by cervical fusion (*white arrows*).

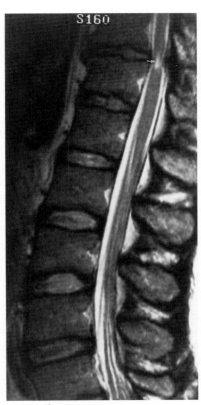

FIGURE 14-113. Focal hyperintense myelomalacia (*arrow*) of the lower thoracic cord associated with mild cord atrophy. T2-weighted fast spin-echo sagittal image.

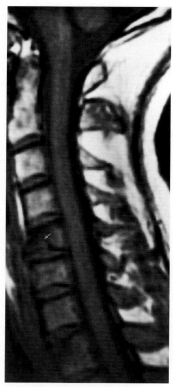

FIGURE 14-114. Extension tear drop fracture (*arrow*) demonstrating a triangular fragment at the anterior inferior corner of C5, without associated involvement of the posterior elements. Unlike the flexion tear drop fracture, this extension injury is stable. T1-weighted sagittal images.

to flexion and distraction with 50% anterior displacement of the vertebral body—these injuries are unstable and are complicated by cord injury), (5) clay shoveler's fractures (spinous process avulsion at C6 or C7), and (6) teardrop burst fractures (unstable fractures with anteroinferior triangular fragment and posterior body displacement into canal).[178] Extension injuries may be associated with prevertebral soft tissue swelling, posterior body displacement or disk vacuum phenomena, or anterior inferior margin avulsion fracture of C2 or C3 (Fig. 14-114). Lumbar spine injuries include compression fracture, fracture-dislocation or burst fracture, and chance fracture (transverse fracture through posterior elements with or without vertebral body involvement).

Cord Injury

A complete functional transection of the cord or transverse myelopathy (complete sensory and motor loss below the lesion), represents the most common cord syndrome associated with cervical spine trauma (see Fig. 14-109). Other cord syndromes include (1) anterior cord syndrome (complete loss of voluntary motor function below the lesion and loss of pain and temperature sensation), (2) acute central cord syndrome (greater motor loss in upper extremities with varying sensory loss), (3) Brown-Séquard syndrome (trans-

verse hemisection of cord—eg, burst fracture—with ipsilateral motor paralysis, loss of position and vibratory sense below the lesion, and contralateral loss of pain and temperature sensation one to two segments below the transverse hemisection), and (4) posterior column syndrome (bilateral loss of vibratory sense and proprioception below the lesion).

Compression Fractures

On T1-weighted images, osteoporotic or nontraumatic compression fractures may be characterized by low signal intensity bands that are parallel with the endplate and demonstrate an increase in signal intensity on T2-weighted images (Fig. 14-115). Osteoporotic fractures frequently are wedge shaped, with relative preservation of posterior vertebral body height (Fig. 14-116). In some cases, compression fractures cannot be differentiated from metastatic disease, although associated convexity or bulging of the posterior vertebral body margin suggests neoplastic disease and a pathologic fracture (Fig. 14-117). On T2-weighted images, the branching pattern of the high signal intensity basivertebral plexus may simulate fracture. If the etiology of the fracture is unclear, Gd-DTPA administration frequently causes enhancement of neoplastic or metastatic disease within a pathologic fracture (Fig. 14-118). However, enhanced areas of metastatic disease may be isointense with adjacent normal, uninvolved vertebral body marrow. Acute and subacute compression fractures may also demonstrate varying degrees of enhancement.

Sacral Stress Fractures

Sacral insufficiency fractures may mimic metastatic disease, demonstrating low signal intensity on T1-weighted images and hyperintensity on STIR or fat-suppressed T2-weighted fast spin-echo sequences (Fig. 14-119). These fractures are commonly symmetric, but may demonstrate asymmetry, and the signal intensity changes may be diffuse without identification of specific fracture morphology. Corresponding CT images with bone windows demonstrate sclerotic linear areas, usually horizontally oriented, representing trabecular fracture. Sacral insufficiency fractures should not be confused with the hyperintensity seen in sacroiliitis in patients with spondyloarthropathy. In sacroiliitis, sacral hyperintensity is parallel to and within the SI joint and may be associated with erosions and irregular cortical margins (Fig. 14-120). Sacroiliitis may be detected in the early stages of development on contrast-enhanced MR studies.[179]

Clinical Management of Fractures

There are two major concerns when a patient sustains a fracture of the spine. First, is there a neurologic deficit secondary to bone or soft tissue compression, and second, is the fracture stable?

text continues on page 1137

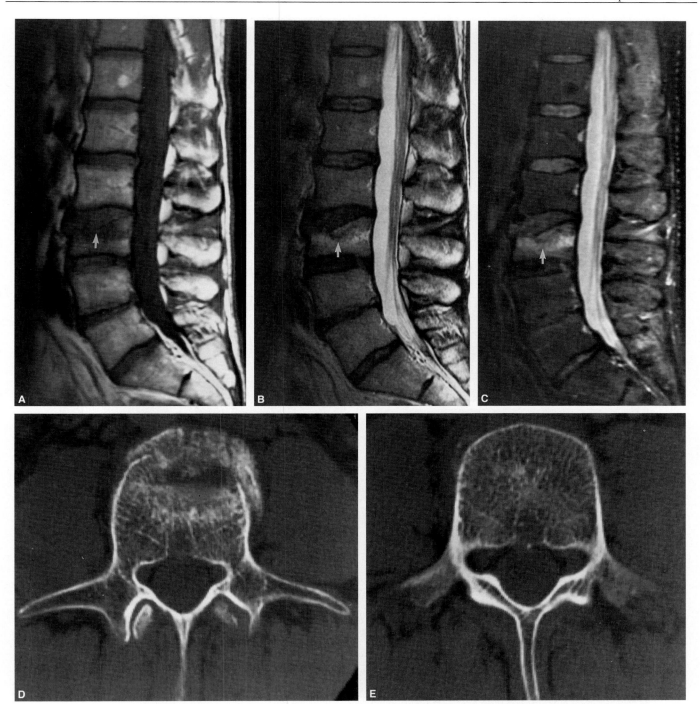

FIGURE 14-115. Nonpathologic compression fracture (*arrow*) of L3 with band of hypointense subchondral marrow on T1-weighted sagittal image (**A**), and hyperintense signal on T2-weighted fast spin-echo (**B**) and fast spin-echo STIR (**C**) sagittal images. Corresponding CT scans demonstrate compression of the superior endplate of L3 (**D**) with normal trabecular morphology within the remaining L3 vertebral body (**E**).

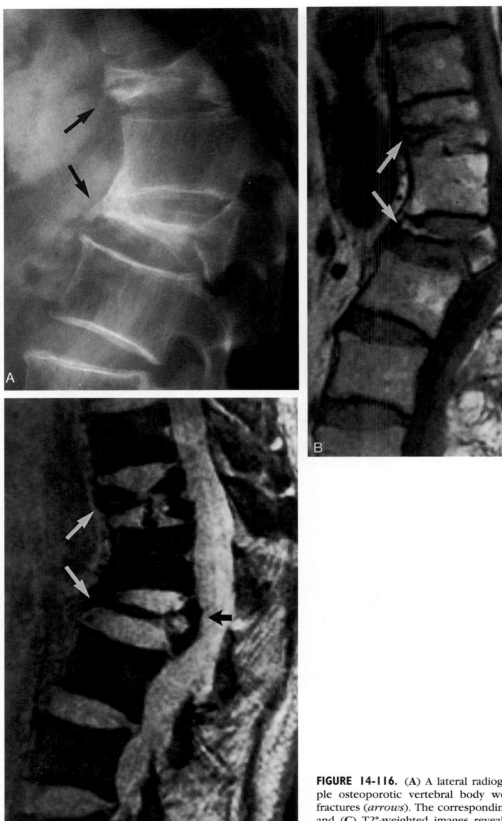

FIGURE 14-116. (A) A lateral radiograph shows multiple osteoporotic vertebral body wedge compression fractures (*arrows*). The corresponding (**B**) T1-weighted and (**C**) T2*-weighted images reveal the compression fractures (*white arrows*) and deformity of the thecal sac (*black arrows*).

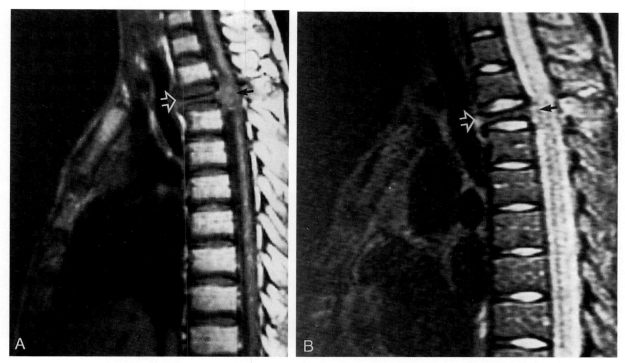

FIGURE 14-117. Pathologic fracture. (**A**) T1-weighted and (**B**) T2-weighted sagittal images show thoracic vertebral body collapse (*open arrow*) with posterior convexity (*solid arrow*) and soft tissue mass in a patient with non-Hodgkin's lymphoma. The soft tissue component demonstrates increased signal intensity, isointense with cerebrospinal fluid, on the T2-weighted image.

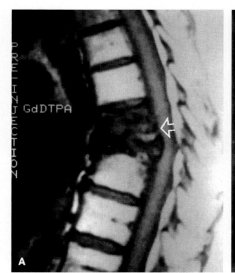
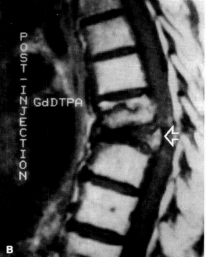

FIGURE 14-118. Pathologic fracture secondary to metastatic lung cancer is seen (**A**) before and (**B**) after Gd-DTPA administration on T1-weighted sagittal images. Note the posterior convexity of the involved vertebral cortex and its hyperintensity postinjection (*arrow*).

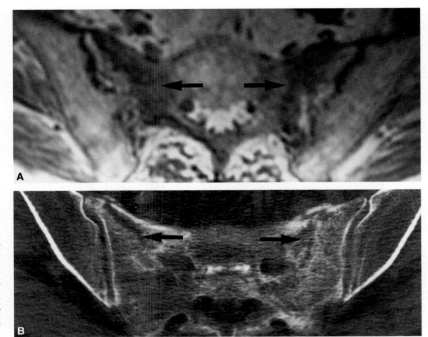

FIGURE 14-119. Bilateral symmetric insufficiency fractures (*arrows*) in a 77-year old woman with a history of breast cancer who complained of bilateral sacral pain. The stress reaction is hypointense on the T1-weighted axial image (**A**) and there is sclerosis of both sacral alae on the CT image (**B**). These fractures demonstrate hyperintensity on fat-suppressed T2-weighted fast spin-echo and STIR sequences.

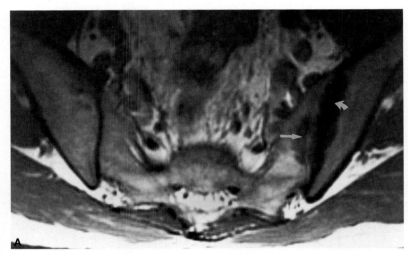

FIGURE 14-120. (**A**) Sacroiliitis with low signal intensity subchondral marrow changes (*straight arrow*) on T1-weighted axial image in association with irregular and sclerotic left sacroiliac joint (*curved arrow*). (**B**) Fast spin-echo STIR coronal sequence identifies hyperintensity in affected subchondral marrow (*arrow*). continued

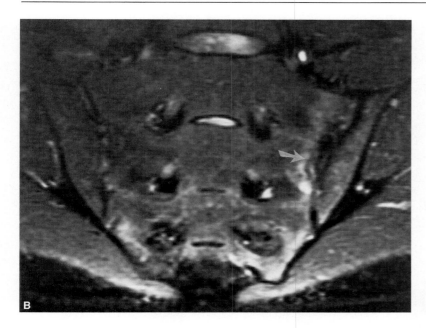

FIGURE 14-120. *Continued*

Examination of the patient requires a detailed neurologic examination including sensory, motor, reflex, and rectal examinations (the last to help determine whether sacral sparing is present). Patients with incomplete neurologic injuries who have evidence of compression of the neural elements should be considered for surgical decompression. Burst-type fractures may result in retropulsion of the fracture fragments. Although posterolateral decompression can be performed for such fractures, an anterior approach is more direct, does not require retraction of neural elements, and can more readily restore bone stock to the anterior spine.[180–182] Some burst fractures result in laminar fractures, which can expand at the time of injury and then close down to entrap nerve roots. Patients with deficits with this fracture pattern may be better approached posteriorly, since a large dural tear and exposed nerve roots may be encountered and the dural sac may need to be repaired.

The question of spinal stability is one of ongoing debate. The spine must be able to withstand physiologic loads without causing neurologic compromise or resulting in progressive deformity. CT scans and MR imaging can be useful in determining the extent of bony and soft tissue injury, the latter of which, especially, can be difficult to determine on plain radiographs. Cervical facet dislocations in particular may be associated with disk disruption, which can result in canal impingement at the time of fracture reduction.[183] Ligamentous injuries are more likely to result in incomplete healing and, therefore, may permit progressive deformity. If early immobilization with a brace, cast, or halo device is not possible, or if long-term instability is anticipated, surgical stabilization with instrumentation and fusion may be indicated. There are numerous options for instrumentation, both anterior and posterior. The goal should be a stable, pain-free spine with maintenance of as much mobility as possible. The sagittal contour in particular should be restored, since excess kyphosis, particularly in the lumbar spine where lordosis is the normal configuration, can result in severe disability.

Infection

Magnetic resonance imaging is more sensitive than either conventional radiography or CT for the detection of vertebral osteomyelitis.[184–186] MR specificity is also superior to corresponding nuclear scintigraphic studies. On T1-weighted images, infection of vertebral bodies and adjacent intervertebral disk spaces is seen as areas of low signal intensity (Fig. 14-121). On T2-weighted images, high signal intensity is observed crossing the involved bone and disk space, with irregularity of cortical margins (Fig. 14-122). In advanced stages of infection, such as tuberculous spondylitis, a soft tissue mass that demonstrates low signal intensity on T1-weighted images and high signal intensity on T2-weighted images is frequently observed[187] (Fig. 14-123). Tuberculous spondylitis is characterized by intraosseous and paraspinal abscess formation, subligamentous extension of infection, destruction and collapse of the vertebral body, and epidural space extension.[188] Spinal instability and deformity may necessitate treatment to avoid neurologic complication. Atypical MR presentations of spinal TB may require biopsy to differentiate tuberculosis from other spinal infections or from neoplasm.[189] Unlike neoplastic disease, infection is associated with loss of disk space height and a low signal intensity intranuclear cleft normally seen on T2-weighted images.

Diskitis, now recognized to be a form of infectious spondylitis in a child, involves the vertebra-disk-vertebra unit by pyogenic infection and requires antibiotic treatment.[190] MR findings are similar to those seen in adult vertebral osteomyelitis, including anterior and posterior soft tissue involvement.

text continues on page 1142

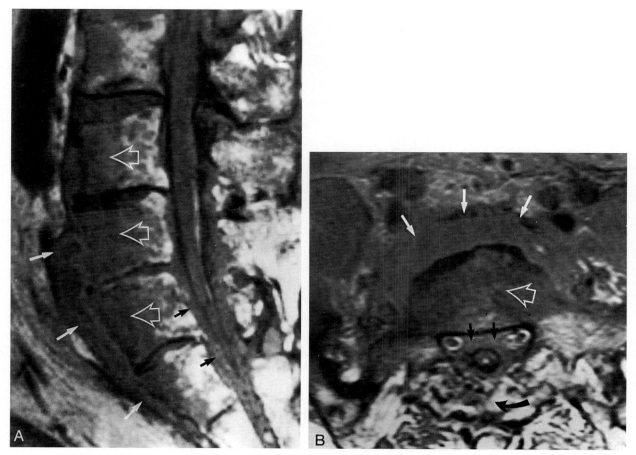

FIGURE 14-121. *Escherichia coli* osteomyelitis. T1-weighted (**A**) sagittal and (**B**) axial images show a low signal intensity *E coli* abscess anterior to the L4 through S2 vertebral bodies (*solid white arrows*). There is adjacent cortical and cancellous destruction. Low signal intensity marrow involvement (*open white arrows*) and epidural spread (*straight black arrows*) are shown. Old posterior fusion mass (*curved black arrow*) is seen on the axial image.

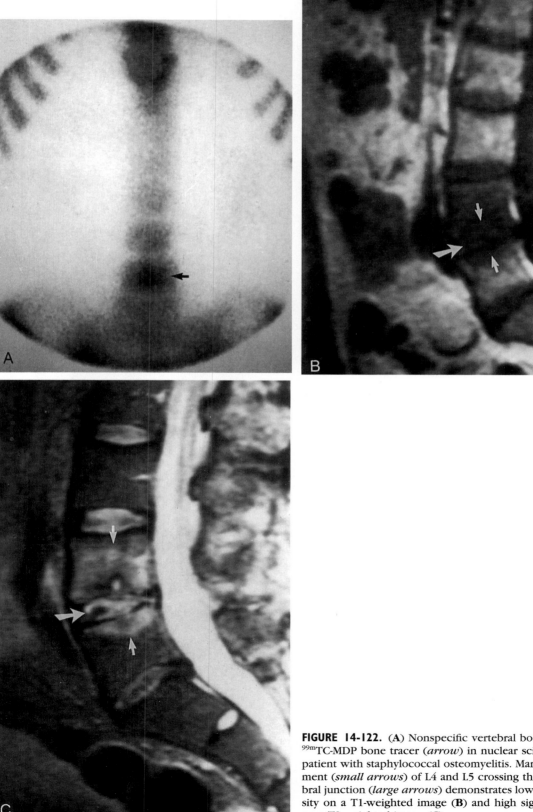

FIGURE 14-122. (**A**) Nonspecific vertebral body uptake of ⁹⁹ᵐTC-MDP bone tracer (*arrow*) in nuclear scintigraphy in patient with staphylococcal osteomyelitis. Marrow involvement (*small arrows*) of L4 and L5 crossing the diskovertebral junction (*large arrows*) demonstrates low signal intensity on a T1-weighted image (**B**) and high signal intensity on a T2-weighted image (**C**).

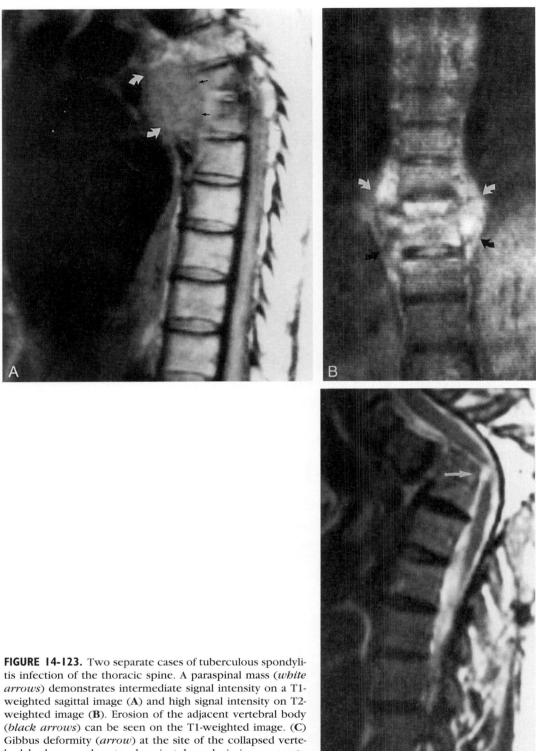

FIGURE 14-123. Two separate cases of tuberculous spondylitis infection of the thoracic spine. A paraspinal mass (*white arrows*) demonstrates intermediate signal intensity on a T1-weighted sagittal image (**A**) and high signal intensity on T2-weighted image (**B**). Erosion of the adjacent vertebral body (*black arrows*) can be seen on the T1-weighted image. (**C**) Gibbus deformity (*arrow*) at the site of the collapsed vertebral body secondary to chronic tuberculosis in a separate patient.

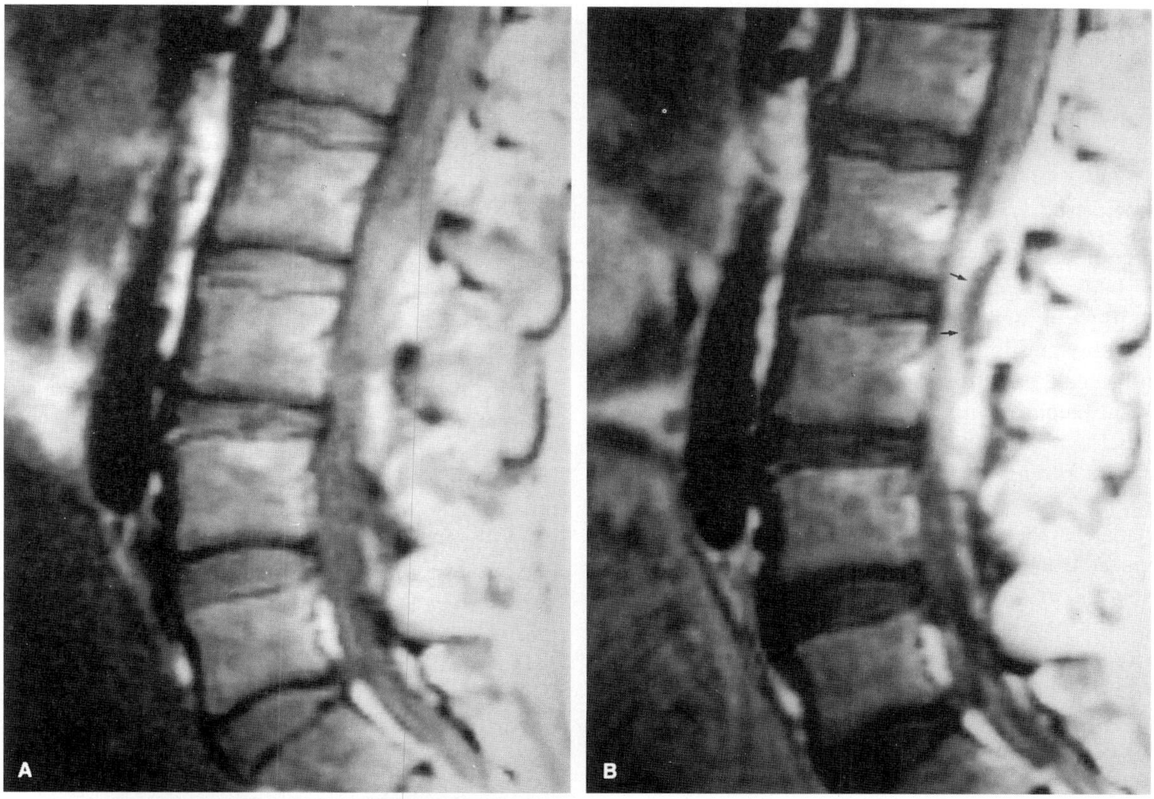

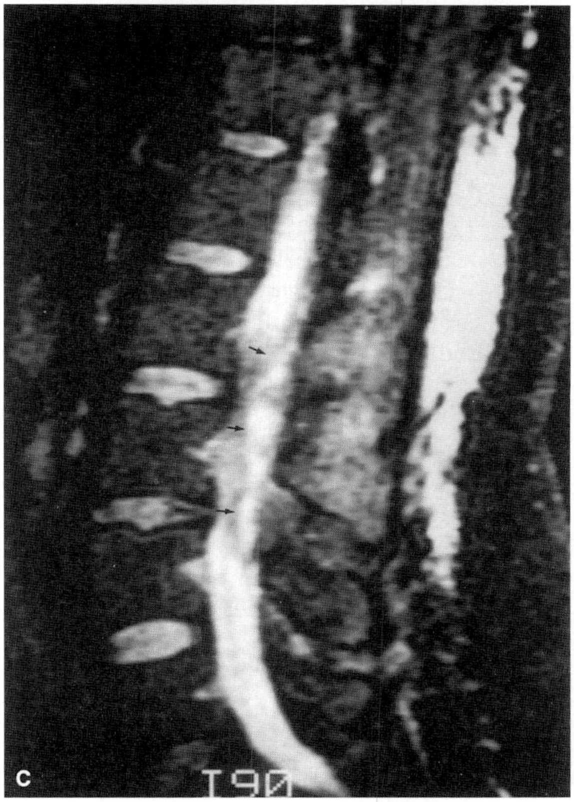

FIGURE 14-124. An epidural staphylococcal abscess (*arrows*) is seen on T1-weighted (**A**), enhanced T1-weighted (**B**), and short TI inversion recovery (**C**) sagittal images. A confluent posterior epidural mass extends from the L2 to the L4 level, deforming the thecal sac.

Epidural abscesses containing pus or granulation tissue, most commonly caused by *Staphylococcus aureus*, are best demonstrated on T2*-weighted or STIR images (Fig. 14-124). Gadolinium enhancement defines the peripheral outline of infected fluid.[191]

Clinical Management

Patients with infections of the spinal column generally complain of back pain and may also have fever, positive laboratory studies, or signs of nerve compression. Because the symptoms may be subtle, there is often a delay in diagnosis. Tubercular osteomyelitis may have a more insidious onset. Bacterial osteomyelitis is most commonly caused by *Staphylococcus aureus*, but infection with *Pseudomonas aeruginosa* is becoming increasingly common.

MR imaging appears to be useful for early diagnosis, since changes are evident days to weeks before radiographic changes appear. Bone scans allow early detection but are much less specific.

Osteomyelitis can be treated successfully with intravenous antibiotics.[192] Appropriate antibiotics may be selected after positive results on blood cultures or with the assistance of needle biopsies. CT-guided needle biopsies are particularly useful in the spine to permit safe sampling of tissue despite the proximity of vascular, pulmonary, and neurologic structures.

If neurologic compromise develops, if the patient develops progressive deformity, or if the patient fails to respond to intravenous antibiotics, surgery is indicated. Most osteomyelitis begins in the anterior spinal structures, so that an anterior approach is generally preferred for nerve decompression. After debridement of the infected and compressive material, bone grafting of the site is used to reconstruct the vertebral body. If accurate debridement has been performed, there is usually no problem with subsequent infection of the bone graft.[193]

Epidural Hematomas

Magnetic resonance imaging is useful for the diagnosis of a spontaneous collection of blood in the epidural space, which can simulate a disk herniation both clinically and on imaging with CT and myelography. These epidural collections of blood produce symptoms of acute onset of back and leg pain (identical to disk herniations) and are not associated with bleeding dyscrasias or anticoagulation. MR scans demonstrate a smoothly marginated mass that is of intermediate to high in signal intensity on both T1- and T2-weighted images. Depending on the age of the hematoma, the signal intensity may vary, be inhomogeneous, and exhibit areas of signal dropout related to hemosiderin. The blood is thought to be contained by the peridural membrane limiting its cranial or caudal extension, although it is not uncommon to see the clot dissect cranially to almost the next disk level or into

the foramen. A prominent epidural venous plexus is often visualized, and there is invariably an underlying small disk protrusion. The differentiation of an extruded disk fragment from epidural hematoma is best made on T2-weighted images. On these scans, the extrusion shows low signal intensity (similar to the parent disk) as opposed to the intermediate-to-high signal intensity seen with a hematoma. Gadolinium administration produces surrounding enhancement, secondary to the extensive epidural inflammation caused by the blood. When the diagnosis of epidural hematoma is suspected, watchful waiting, even in the presence of neurologic deficit is suggested, since epidural hematomas usually resolve in 4 to 6 weeks with consequent resolution of symptoms. If there is significant epidural inflammation, epidural steroid injection at the level of the hematoma is often quite useful. Although extruded disk fragments do often degenerate and shrink, complete resolution in this short time frame is not possible, and it is likely that many of the disappearing disks described in the past were in fact epidural hematomas. Rarely, these collections of blood may encapsulate and become chronic. In this case, the MR appearance is that of a cystic mass with a well-defined capsule that may have a very low signal intensity as a result of hemosiderin deposition. Mass effect persists, and many of these patients have continuing radiculopathy, making them candidates for decompression.[56]

Multiple Sclerosis

Mixed intracranial and spinal cord involvement with multiple sclerosis is more common than isolated spinal disease.[194] In the cervical spine, dual echo (ie, TE of 15 msec and 30 msec) T2*-weighted, T2-weighted fast spin-echo, or STIR images can be used to identify areas of demyelination (Fig. 14-125). Gadolinium-enhanced images are sensitive in identifying more active areas of plaque development in the cervical and thoracic cords (Fig. 14-126). Multiple sclerosis plaques have a linear or elongated morphology and affect single or multiple levels. There is preferential involvement of the dorsal and lateral segments of the cord.[195] Localized swelling of the cord may be seen in more acute inflammatory stages of the disease.

Spinal Tumors

Soft tissue tumors are extradural, intradural, extramedullary, or intramedullary. Extradural tumors consist of primary and metastatic tumors with osseous, soft tissue, and neural elements represented by both benign and malignant processes.[196–198] Intradural extramedullary lesions include meningiomas (Fig. 14-127), nerve sheath tumors (neurofibromas) (Fig. 14-128), embryonal lesions (epidermoids and dermoids [Fig. 14-129] and lipomas), and metastases. Intramedullary neoplasms include gliomas (ependymomas, astro-

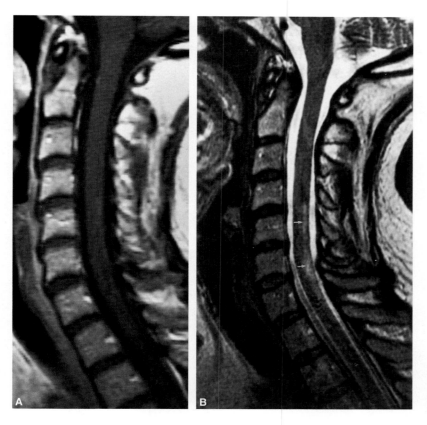

FIGURE 14-125. Detection of extensive hyperintense lesions of multiple sclerosis (*arrows*) on a T2-weighted fast spin-echo sequence. (**A**) T1-weighted sagittal image for comparison. (**B**) T2-weighted fast spin-echo image.

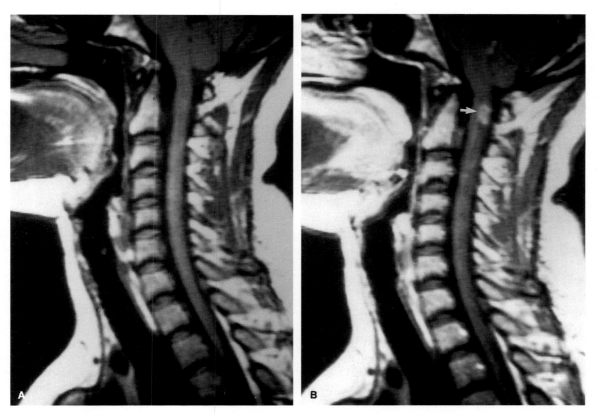

FIGURE 14-126. A multiple sclerosis plaque (*arrows*) demonstrates (**A**) low signal intensity or is isointense on a T1-weighted sagittal image and (**B**) is hyperintense on a Gd-DTPA–enhanced T1-weighted sagittal image.

continued

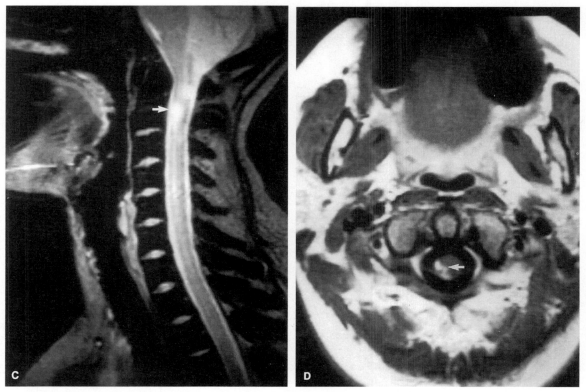

FIGURE 14-126. *Continued.* **(C)** The high signal intensity plaque is poorly differentiated from the cord on a T2*-weighted sagittal image. **(D)** The corresponding enhanced T1-weighted axial image shows the left lateral localization of the demyelinating plaque.

cytomas, oligodendrogliomas, and medulloblastomas), hemangioblastomas (which are uncommon), lipomas, dermoids, epidermoids, and rarely, metastatic disease.

Vertebral bone tumors include hemangioma (Fig. 14-130), osteoid osteoma (requires the use of fat-suppressed T2-weighted fast spin-echo or STIR sequences to detect areas of hyperemia), bone islands (demonstrating low signal intensity on all pulse sequences), expansile osteoblastoma (Fig. 14-131), expansile aneurysmal bone cysts, giant cell tumors (destructive and expansile lesions that favor the sacrum), chordomas (Fig. 14-132), myeloma (destructive lesion of the vertebral body with expansile characteristics), osteogenic sarcoma (hyperintense on T2-weighted images except for the osteoblastic presentation, which is hypointense), chondrosarcoma (calcified matrix), and metastases.[195]

Hemangiomas, aneurysmal bone cysts, and chordomas have characteristic MR findings. Hemangiomas (see Fig. 14-130) demonstrate increased signal intensity on T1- and T2-weighted images, in part related to adipose elements. Vertebral hemangiomas with a content that is predominantly fat represent a more inactive form, whereas more vascular hemangiomas, which demonstrate lower signal intensity on T1-weighted images, are frequently more aggressive and are associated with compression fractures.[199] Focal fatty marrow deposition does not display increased signal intensity on T2-weighted images, and is dark on fat-suppression or STIR

protocols. Aneurysmal bone cysts (see Fig. 14-131) are blood filled and expansile, and demonstrate inhomogeneous signal intensity on T1- and T2-weighted images due to paramagnetic influence. Chordomas (see Fig. 14-132) are aggressive lesions related to notochord remnants located in the sacrococcygeal and basisphenoid regions. On T1-weighted images, they range from hypointense to isointense, and are hyperintense on T2-weighted images.

Drop metastases (Fig. 14-133) represent metastatic implants within the subarachnoid space carried from a primary tumor through the CSF.[200] Medulloblastoma, ependymoma, pineal teratoma, and glioblastoma multiforme can metastasize in this pattern along CSF pathways. With drop metastases, MR imaging may demonstrate hyperintensity on T2-weighted images (T2-weighted fast spin-echo) or enhancement with gadolinium along the outer aspect of the spinal cord, nerve roots, or nerve root axillary pouch.

Lipoma of the Filum Terminale

The fibrous filum terminale extends from the conus to the distal thecal sac and contains fat elements in 4% to 6% of normal individuals[87] (Figs. 14-134 and 14-135). In evaluating the filum terminale, associated cord tethering must be excluded.[201] Intradural lipomas have a relatively

text continues on page 1150

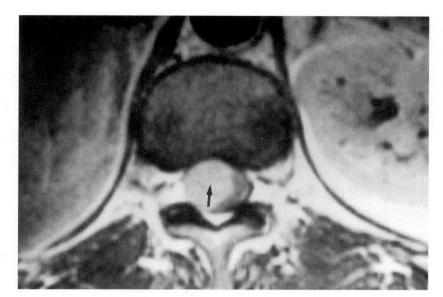

FIGURE 14-127. An extramedullary intradural meningioma (*arrow*) demonstrates increased signal intensity on an enhanced T1-weighted axial image.

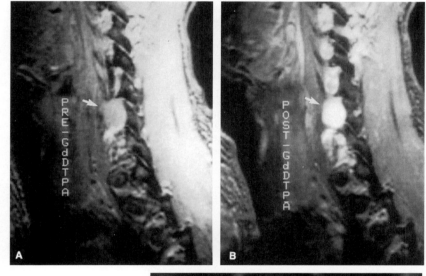

FIGURE 14-128. Right parasagittal C5-6 neurofibroma (*arrows*) is seen before (**A**) and after (**B**) intravenous Gd-DTPA administration. (**C**) Hyperintense dumbbell-shaped neurofibroma (*arrow*) extends through the right intervertebral nerve root canal, as seen on an enhanced T1-weighted axial image. (**D**) In a separate case, a neurilemmoma (schwannoma) is also shown to enhance with Gd-DTPA on a T1-weighted axial image. Neurilemmomas arise from Schwann cells of the nerve sheath (*arrow*).

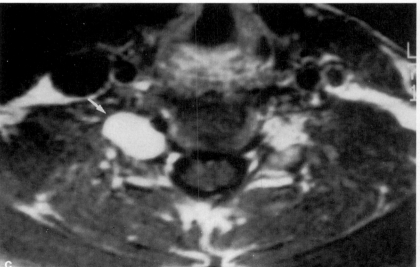

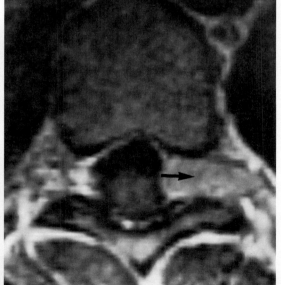

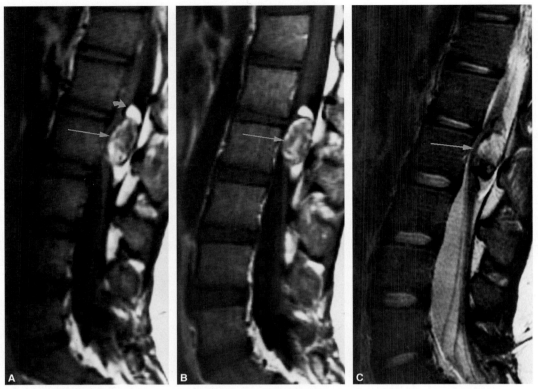

FIGURE 14-129. Intradural-extramedullary dermoid (*straight arrow*) displacing the conus medullaris. The tumor has hyperintense lipid signal (*curved arrow*) on T1-weighted sagittal image (**A**) and displays enhancement on Gd-DTPA enhanced image (**B**). Heterogeneity with low and high signal intensity areas are seen on T2-weighted fast spin-echo image (**C**). This heterogeneity may be secondary to both hemorrhage and fat components.

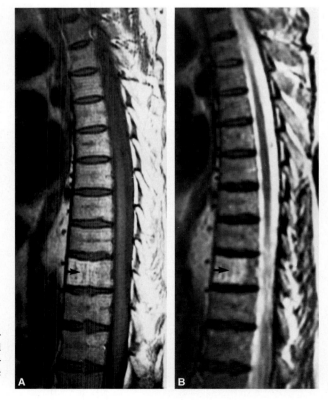

FIGURE 14-130. Vertebral hemangioma (*arrow*) with increased signal intensity shown on both T1 (**A**) and T2-weighted fast spin-echo (**B**) sagittal images. Adipose, or fat tissue, contributes to the hyperintensity on T1-weighted sequences whereas more cellular components are responsible for hyperintensity on T2-weighted sequences.

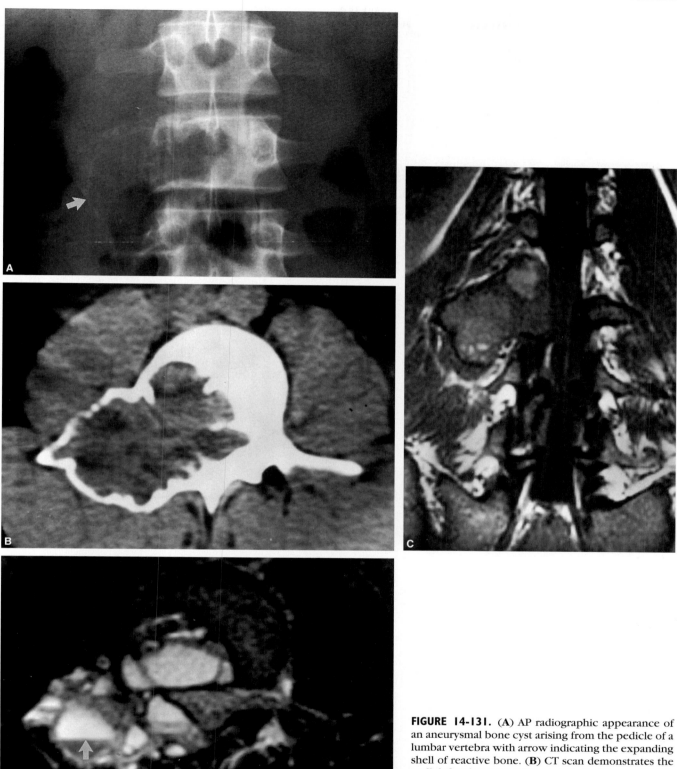

FIGURE 14-131. (A) AP radiographic appearance of an aneurysmal bone cyst arising from the pedicle of a lumbar vertebra with arrow indicating the expanding shell of reactive bone. (B) CT scan demonstrates the well-defined aneurysmal outer shell of bone. (C) T1-weighted coronal image. (D) T2-weighted axial image with arrow pointing to fluid-fluid level of hemorrhagic cyst.

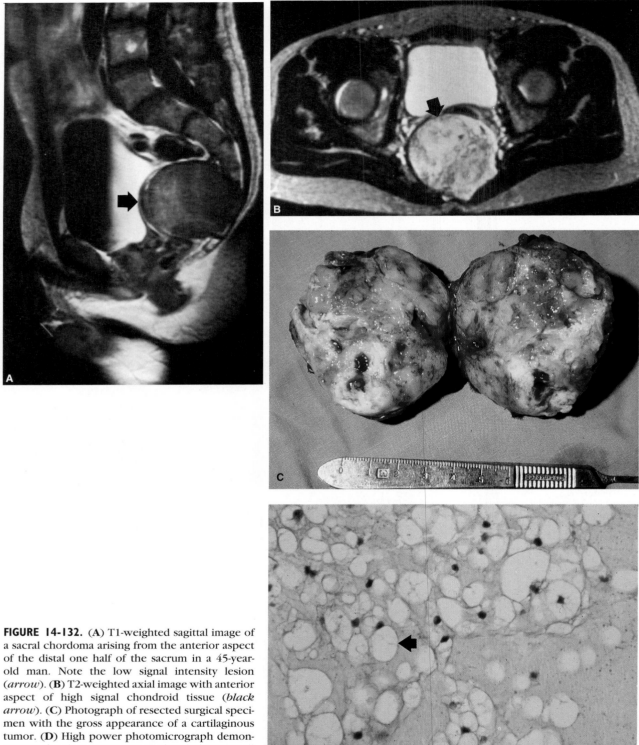

FIGURE 14-132. (**A**) T1-weighted sagittal image of a sacral chordoma arising from the anterior aspect of the distal one half of the sacrum in a 45-year-old man. Note the low signal intensity lesion (*arrow*). (**B**) T2-weighted axial image with anterior aspect of high signal chondroid tissue (*black arrow*). (**C**) Photograph of resected surgical specimen with the gross appearance of a cartilaginous tumor. (**D**) High power photomicrograph demonstrating the clear signet ring or physaliphorous cell (*arrow*) typical of the chordoma.

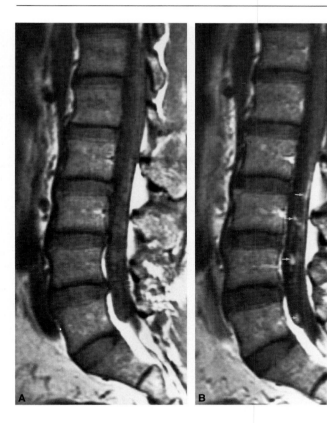

FIGURE 14-133. Intradural drop metastases (*arrows*) demonstrating enhancement of multiple nodules along the course of the cauda equina. T1 (**A**) and Gd-DTPA enhanced T1- (**B**) weighted sagittal images.

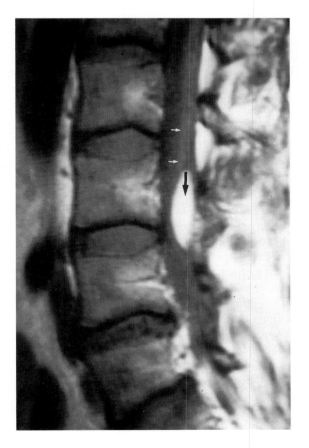

FIGURE 14-134. A T1-weighted sagittal image shows an intradural fusiform high signal intensity lipoma (*black arrow*) of the distal conus (*white arrows*). The lipoma tapers superiorly and inferiorly.

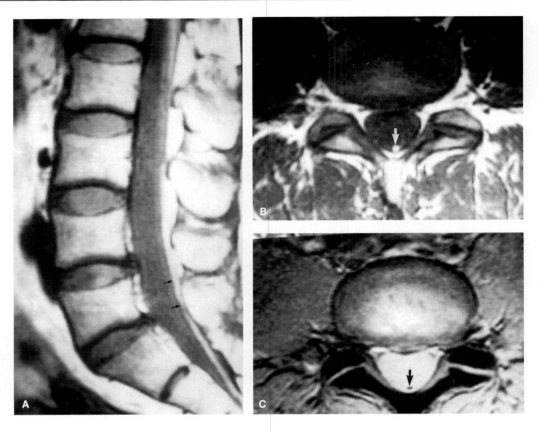

FIGURE 14-135. (A) On a T1-weighted sagittal image, fat (*arrow*) in the filum terminale demonstrates high signal intensity. (B) On a T1-weighted axial image, fat demonstrates high signal intensity. (C) On a T2*-weighted axial image, fat demonstrates low signal intensity.

fusiform morphology and may cause expansion of the filum. Extradural filum lipomas, however, are more diffuse. Lipomas of the conus medullaris may coexist with lipoma of the filum.

Metastatic and Marrow Disease

On MR images, fatty or yellow marrow demonstrates high signal intensity and hematopoietic or red marrow demonstrates low signal intensity in both normal and pathologic states.[202-208] T1- and T2-weighted spin-echo imaging, fat-suppressed T2-weighted fast spin-echo, and STIR sequences have complementary roles in showing the replacement of normal marrow in primary, metastatic, and infiltrative disease processes.[54,63-69,209] MR imaging is also useful in identifying benign processes that may mimic malignancy on conventional radiography.

Most metastatic tumors are characterized by long T1 and T2 values; therefore, there is good contrast discrimination between normal adult marrow and marrow infiltrated by metastatic processes.[210] On STIR images, signal from normal yellow marrow is suppressed, and T1 and T2 prolongation effects are additive. Metastatic lesions from carcinoma of the breast, prostate, lung, colon, and testes, from Ewing's sarcoma, and from multiple myeloma demonstrate increased signal intensity on conventional T2-weighted images, T2*-weighted images, and STIR images, even in cases where nuclear scintigraphy was equivocal (Fig. 14-136). Blastic lesions generally demonstrate low signal intensity, regard-

less of the pulsing parameters. On STIR images, however, increased signal intensity metastatic foci within a blastic reaction have been observed.[211] Epidural involvement with posterior cortical disruption is best seen on T2, T2*, STIR, or Gd-DTPA–enhanced studies[212-214] (Fig. 14-137). After Gd-DTPA administration, neoplastic tissue demonstrates increased signal intensity on short TR/TE sequences as a result of T1 and T2 shortening, and adjacent CSF remains dark.[196] This precisely defines the boundary between the tumor and thecal sac, which is not possible with conventional T2 weighting or even with STIR images, in which the CSF and tumor both demonstrate bright signal intensity.

MR imaging is also sensitive in detecting replacement of marrow-fat with tumor cell populations that have T1 values significantly longer than those of normal yellow marrow.[207,211] Marrow infiltrates from leukemia and lymphoma can be successfully identified on STIR sequences as areas of bright signal intensity within a black or gray background of nulled fat signal from uninvolved marrow. In the spine and pelvis, lymphomatous involvement of marrow may be patchy or nodular, and MR localization prior to biopsy can reduce the number of false negatives from sampling error.

Fatty replacement of affected marrow in patients undergoing radiation and chemotherapy can be demonstrated on T1, T2, and STIR sequences.[215] Normal red or hematopoietic elements in the spine demonstrate gray contrast on STIR sequences, whereas fatty or yellow marrow replacement is seen as areas of dark nulled signal.

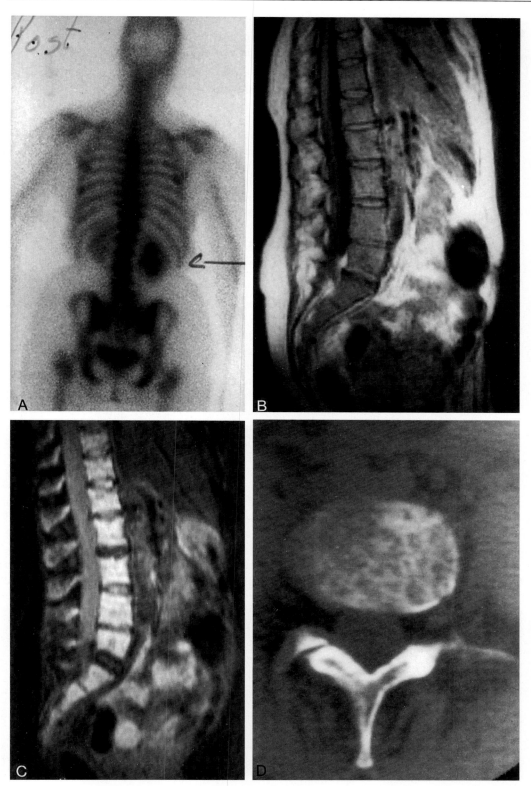

FIGURE 14-136. (A) An unremarkable bone scan result in a patient with aggressive metastatic breast carcinoma. (B) T1-weighted and (C) short TI inversion recovery images show low and high signal intensity, respectively, from diffuse marrow involvement of the entire thoracic and lumbar spines. (D) A corresponding axial CT scan confirms the lytic destruction of cancellous cortical bone.

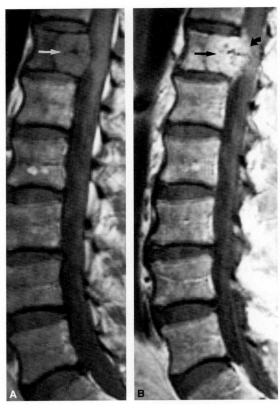

FIGURE 14-137. Metastasis (*straight arrow*) from renal cell carcinoma (*arrow*) on T1 (**A**) and enhanced T1 (**B**) sagittal images. There is anterior epidural extension (*curved arrow*) with compression of the ventral aspect of the thecal sac. Metastasis is hypervascular, demonstrating multiple hypointense vascular foci. The lesion demonstrates marked enhancement with Gd-DTPA (**B**).

Extramedullary cysts of the meninges may present with adjacent bone erosion secondary to chronic local CSF pressure and without the more aggressive bone destruction of metastatic disease. Meningeal cysts may present with or without nerve root involvement (Figs. 14-138 and 14-139).

The sacral plexus may be involved (plexopathy) secondary to metastatic disease as well as from involvement of primary bone and soft tissue lesions[216] (Fig. 14-140).

CLINICAL MANAGEMENT. Most patients with metastatic or infiltrative involvement of the spine present with pain. Bony destruction can be seen on plain radiographs; however, CT scans are better at delineating the extent of bone loss. MR imaging is useful for determining the extent of soft tissue canal encroachment in cases of metastatic tumor involvement. Skeletal metastases are most likely with primary cancer of the prostate, breast, kidney, thyroid, and lung. Metastases to the spinal column occur more frequently than any other bones.

Patients become symptomatic when skeletal metastases cause either microfractures or impending fractures, or when tumor involvement compromises the spinal canal sufficiently to cause pain or neurologic deficit. If the primary tumor has not been diagnosed, it should be sought and treated. Tissue biopsy from the bony lesion may be useful and can be performed via CT guidance.[217] Many metastatic lesions can be successfully treated palliatively with radiation therapy or chemotherapy, and these modalities may be useful particularly when lesions are noted during metastatic workup. However, because the tumor destroys bone, the likelihood of fracture increases. In the spine, bracing, in conjunction with radiation or chemotherapy, may be appropriate. Once neurologic compromise occurs, however, consideration should be given to surgical decompression and stabilization.[218,219] Radiation may be useful in patients with limited life expectancy and incomplete neurologic compromise. Progressive paraplegia or quadriplegia, unless the patient is immediately terminal, should be treated with a surgical decompression and stabilization. Many tumor surgeons use methylmethycrylate (bone cement) for immediate fixation and pain relief. However, even when reinforced by metal instrumentation, such a construct has limited durability.[220] For patients who are

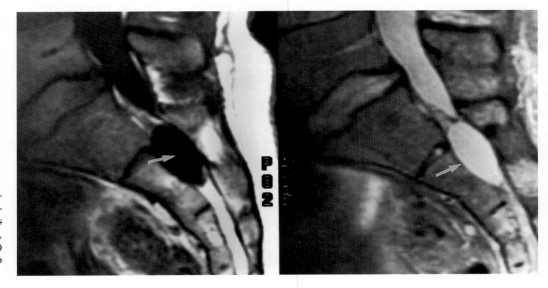

FIGURE 14-138. A Tarlov cerebrospinal fluid cyst (ie, meningeal cyst with nerve roots) is present at the S2 level (*arrow*), as seen on T1-weighted (*left*) and T2-weighted fast spin-echo (*right*) sagittal images.

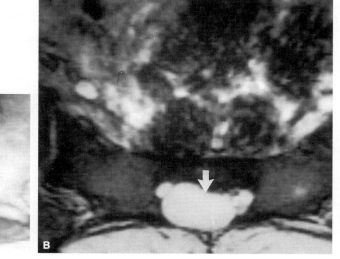

FIGURE 14-139. An extradural meningeal cyst (*arrows*) at the sacral level demonstrates (**A**) low signal intensity on a T1-weighted axial image and (**B**) high signal intensity on a T2*-weighted axial image. There is pressure erosion of the adjacent sacral cortex. This cyst does not involve nerve roots and represents a dural diverticula in continuity with the thecal sac.

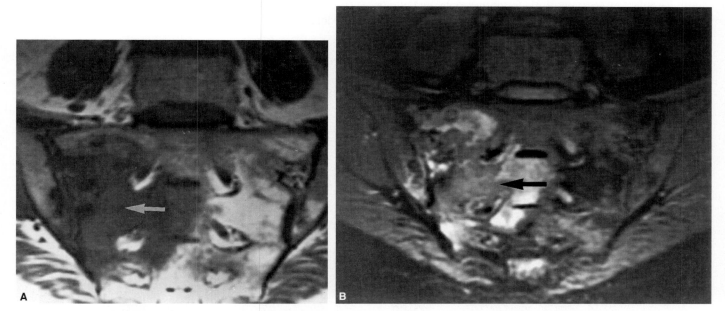

FIGURE 14-140. Metastatic breast carcinoma (*arrow*) with destruction of right sacral segments S1, S2, and S3 on T1-weighted coronal image (**A**) and fast spin-echo STIR image (**B**). Tumor is inhomogeneous with areas of hyperintensity on the STIR image (**B**).

expected to live longer than 6 months and who have significant spinal column involvement, spinal fusion is preferable.[218,219] This, of course, can be difficult to achieve in the face of chemotherapeutic agents and radiation, and so treatment planning for patients with metastatic tumors requires a team approach with oncologists, radiation therapists, and surgeons all closely involved.

Pediatric Pathology

Spinal Dysraphism

CHIARI MALFORMATIONS. In Chiari I malformation, there is tonsillar herniation without an associated spinal dysraphism.[221] Chiari II malformation (Fig. 14-141), which is the most common Chiari type, demonstrates spinal dysraphism usually as a lumbosacral myelomeningocele. Hydromyelia is seen in 20% to 70% of patients. There is caudal elongation of the cerebellum and brain stem. A vermial peg, medullary kink, hypoplastic falx and tentorium, gyral interdigitation, beaking of the quadrigeminal plate–collicular complex, an enlarged massa intermedia, small crowded gyri, a small diverticulum of the anterior third ventricle, low position of the fourth ventricle, and corpus callosal dysgenesis are features seen in Chiari II.[195] In Chiari III malformations there is a craniocervical encephalocele, and these deformities may be associated with cord dysraphism.

MENINGOCELE AND MYELOMENINGOCELE. Meningoceles, which are relatively uncommon, are enlargements of the thecal sac without inclusion of neural elements.[195] Myelomeningoceles and lipomyelomeningoceles (Fig. 14-142) are associated with myelodysplasia (spreading of the lumbosacral lamina). The neural placode is a merging of a clefted spinal cord with dorsal cutaneous tissue. Myelomeningocele is typically associated with the Chiari II malformation. The conus is usually low lying (tethered) and extends posteriorly toward the bifida and placode. Scoliosis, kyphosis, hydromyelia, and diastematomyelia are frequently associated findings. MR imaging is used to document a tethered cord in a dysraphic spine, especially when there is progression of a neurologic deficit or scoliosis is present. The presence of a tethered cord is often not appreciated at the time of closure of the bifida defect in the newborn. In lipomyelomeningocele, there is invagination of subcutaneous fat between the lamina defect and into the spinal canal fused to the placode.

ISOLATED TETHERED CORD SYNDROME. In isolated tethered cord syndrome (tight filum terminale syndrome), the conus medullaris either extends below the L1-2 level with or without

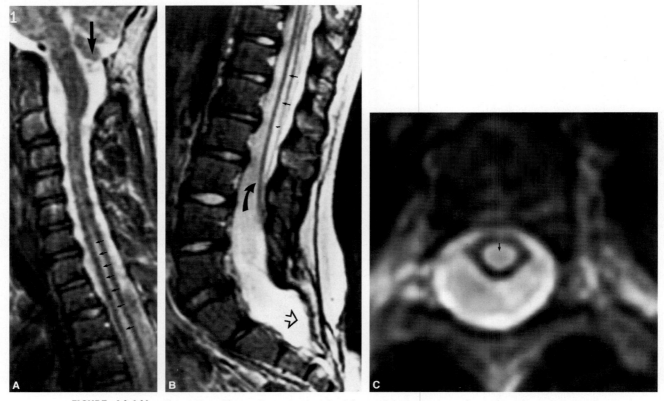

FIGURE 14-141. Chiari II malformation associated with caudal elongation of a tethered cord (*curved arrow*), hydromyelia (*small straight arrows*), and postrepair myelomeningocele (*open arrow*). T2-weighted fast spin-echo sagittal images of the cervical (**A**) and thoracolumbar (**B**) spines. Corresponding T2-weighted fast spin-echo axial image (**C**) is shown through the thoracic cord hydromyelia.

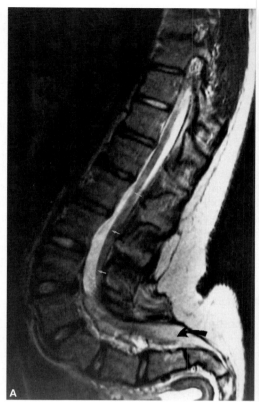

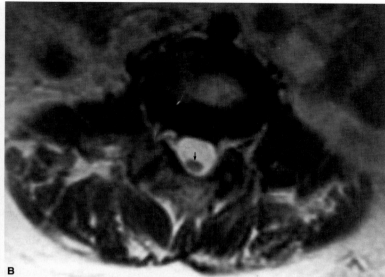

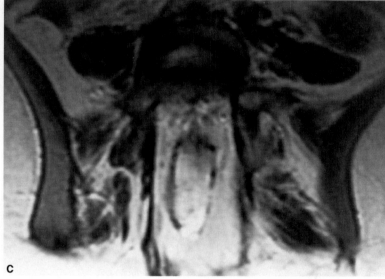

FIGURE 14-142. Lipomyelomeningocele. (**A**) Tethered cord (*small arrows*) in a postoperative lipomyelomeningocele (*curved arrow*). (**B**) Tethered cord (*small arrow*) is identified at the L4-5 level. (**C**) Dysraphic spina bifida (*open arrow*) is present from L5 through the sacrum. T2-weighted fast spin-echo sagittal (**A**) and axial (**B, C**) images.

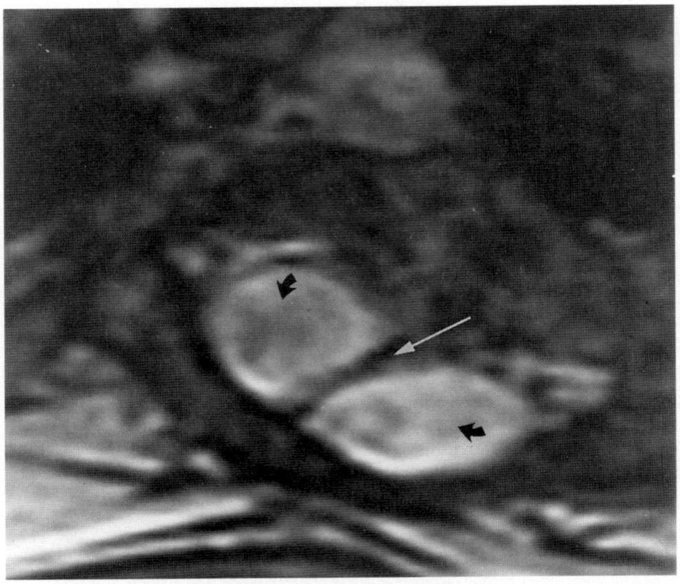

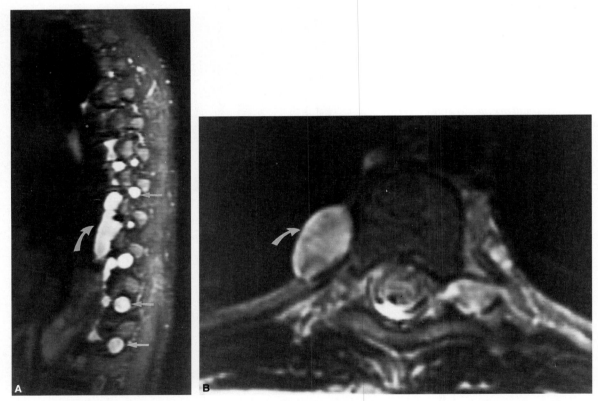

FIGURE 14-143. Diastematomyelia of the thoracic cord with an osseous space (*straight arrow*) separating the cord into two hemicords (*curved arrows*).

a thick filum, or presents with a thick filum and the conus at a normal level.[221] Patients have scoliosis, muscle weakness, foot deformity, abnormal reflexes, and bladder dysfunction.[195]

DIASTEMATOMYELIA. Diastematomyelia is a spinal dysraphism with a partial or complete sagittal spinal cord cleft producing asymmetric hemicords in the lower thoracic and upper spinal spines[195] (Fig. 14-143). This dysraphism may also extend into the cervical region. The hemicords may fuse proximal to the conus or remain separate. The dural sac may also split to accommodate each hemicord.[221] Sometimes there is an osseous or cartilaginous spur that separates the cord into two parts. More commonly, the split cord has no associated spur and occupies a single dural sac. Associated findings include tethered conus, lipoma, hydromyelia, myelomeningocele, lipomyelomeningocele, scoliosis, and hypertrichosis. The bony spur and split cord can be identified on both axial and coronal planar images. The level of the cord separation and fusion can be precisely determined.

Neurofibromatosis

Spine abnormalities seen in neurofibromatosis include scoliosis, kyphosis of the cervical or lumbar spine, posterior vertebral body scalloping, spinal canal enlargement with du-

FIGURE 14-144. Multiple intradural and extradural neurofibroma (*straight arrows*) in association with cystic-appearing thoracic meningoceles (*curved arrow*). Both the dumbbell neurofibromas and lateral meningoceles are hyperintense on fat-suppressed T2-weighted fast spin-echo sagittal image (**A**) and T2-weighted fast spin-echo axial image (**B**).

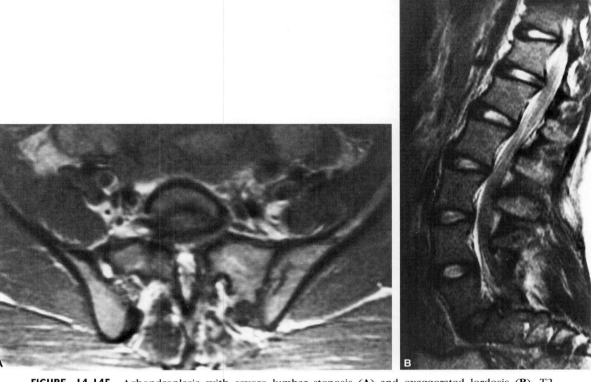

FIGURE 14-145. Achondroplasia with severe lumbar stenosis (**A**) and exaggerated lordosis (**B**). T2-weighted fast spin-echo axial (**A**) and sagittal (**B**) images.

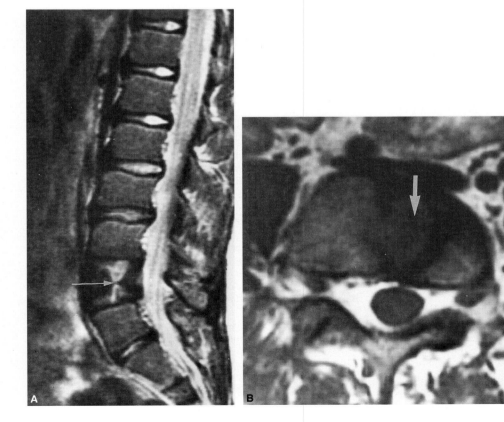

FIGURE 14-146. Butterfly vertebra with central cleft (*arrow*) of L4 seen on T2 sagittal (**A**) and T1 axial (**B**) images. A butterfly vertebra represents a segmentation abnormality. Hemivertebrae and block vertebrae may also be seen in congenital scoliosis.

ral ectasia, cystic dilatation of the nerve root sleeve, lateral thoracic meningoceles, schwannomas, and neurofibromas (dumbbell type with intradural and extradural components) (Fig. 14-144).

Neurofibromatosis type 1 (NF-1), or peripheral neurofibromatosis, is characterized by café-au-lait spots, iris hamartomas, plexiform neurofibromas, bone dysplasia, optic gliomas, astrocytoma, and also occult spinal tumors.[222] Neurofibromatosis type 2 (NF-2), or central neurofibromatosis, is more common than NF-1. Associated abnormalities include schwannomas (bilateral acoustic), multiple meningiomas, ependymomas, and gliomas. Spinal tumors in NF-2— including ependymomas, meningiomas, schwannomas, and neurofibromas—have been reported in 89% of patients studied by Mautner and colleagues.[223]

Achondroplasia

This common form of dwarfism is associated with a narrow spinal canal (Fig. 14-145) and small foramen magnum.[195] In the lumbosacral spine there is characteristic anteroposterior diameter stenosis of the central canal, attributed to premature fusion of the neurocentral synchondrosis and periosteal bone overgrowth. Thoracolumbar kyphosis and atlantoaxial subluxation may contribute to neurologic symptoms associated with spinal stenosis.

Atypical Scoliosis

Atypical idiopathic scoliosis (convex left thoracic or thoracolumbar) has been shown to be associated with MR findings of hydrosyringomyelia (syringomyelia is a cystic process lined by glial cells and hydromyelia is considered to be present if ependyma cells line the cyst). It is usually congenital in origin and is seen in association with dysraphic abnormalities.[224] Atypical features of scoliosis include early onset, rapid development, pain, neurologic symptoms, associated syndromes, a convex left thoracic or thoracolumbar curve, kyphosis, and pedicle thinning. In addition to hydrosyringomyelia, less common MR findings include dural ectasia, Chiari I malformation, and cord astrocytoma. Schwend and colleagues[225] used MR imaging to document a syrinx in 12 of 14 patients with an intraspinal abnormality from a retrospective review of 95 patients with idiopathic scoliosis. Vertebral body abnormalities are often identified in cases of congenital scoliosis (Fig. 14-146). Congenital scoliosis is associated with Chiari I and II malformations, a tethered cord, a syrinx or hydromyelia, and myelomeningocele.

References

1. Dixon AK, Bannon RP. Computed tomography of the postoperative lumbar spine: the need for, and optimal dose of, intravenous contrast media. Br J Radiol 1987;60:215.
2. Braun IF, et al. Contrast enhancement in CT differentiation between recurrent disc herniation and postoperative scar: prospective study. AJNR 1985;6:607.
3. Zinreich SJ, et al. CT myelography for outpatients: an inpatient/outpatient pilot study to assess methodology. Radiology 1985;157:387.
4. Helms CA, et al. CT of the lumbar spine: normal variants and pitfalls. RadioGraphics 1987;7:447.
5. Weiss T, et al. CT of the postoperative lumbar spine: value of intravenous contrast. Neuroradiology 1986;28:241.
6. Zinreich SJ, et al. Three-dimensional CT imaging in post-surgical "failed back" syndrome. J Comput Assist Tomogr 1990;14:574.
7. Mills DG. Imaging of the cervical spine. Proceedings of the MR Clinical Symposium, vol 3, no. 5. Milwaukee: GE Medical Systems, 1987.
8. Berger PE, et al. High resolution surface coil magnetic resonance imaging of the spine: normal and pathologic anatomy. RadioGraphics 1986;6:573.
9. Smoker WRK, et al. MRI versus conventional radiologic examination in the evaluation of the craniovertebral and cervicomedullary junction. RadioGraphics 1986;6:953.
10. Maravilla KR, et al. Magnetic resonance demonstration of multiple sclerosis plaques in the cervical cord. AJNR 1984;5:685.
11. Kulkarni MV, et al. Acute spinal cord injury: MR imaging at 1.5T. Radiology 1987;164:837.
12. Modic MT, et al. Cervical radiculopathy: value of oblique MR imaging. Radiology 1987;163:227.
13. Rubin JB, Enzmann DR. Optimizing conventional MR imaging of the spine. Radiology 1987;163:777.
14. Enzmann DR, et al. Cervical spine MR imaging: generating high signal CSF in sagittal and axial images. Radiology 1987;163:233.
15. Modic MT, et al. Magnetic resonance imaging of the cervical spine: technical and clinical observations. AJNR 1984;5:15.
16. Flannigan BD, et al. MR imaging of the cervical spine; neurovascular anatomy. AJR 1987;148:785.
17. Burnett KR, et al. MRI evaluation of the cervical spine at high field strength. Appl Radiol 1985.
18. Yu S, et al. Facet joint menisci of the cervical spine: correlative MR imaging and cryomicrotomy study. Radiology 1987;164:79.
19. Teresi LM, et al. Asymptomatic degenerative disc disease and spondylosis of the cervical spine: MR imaging. Radiology 1987;164:83.
20. Ross JS, et al. Thoracic disc herniation: MR imaging. Radiology 1987;165:511.
21. Modic MR, et al. Magnetic resonance imaging of intervertebral disc disease: clinical and pulse sequence considerations. Radiology 1984;152:103.
22. Grenier N, et al. Degenerative lumbar disc disease: pitfalls and usefulness of MR imaging in detection of vacuum phenomenon. Radiology 1987;164:861.
23. Ramsey RG. MRI's reputation grows in herniated disc evaluation. Diagn Imaging 1987;120.
24. Pech L, Haughton VM. Lumbar intervertebral disc: correlative MR and anatomic study. Radiology 1985;156:699.
25. Chafetz Nl, et al. Recognition of lumbar disc herniation with NMR. AJR 1983;141:1153.
26. Schellinger D, et al. Facet joint disorders and their role in the production of back pain and sciatica. RadioGraphics 1987;7:923.
27. Grenier N, et al. Normal and degenerative posterior spinal structures: MR imaging. Radiology 1987;165:517.
28. Ross JS, et al. Lumbar spine: postoperative assessment with surface-coil MR imaging. Radiology 1987;164:851.
29. Nokes SR, et al. Childhood scoliosis: MR imaging. Radiology 1987;164:791.
30. Heithoff KBN. Spontaneous lumbar epidural hematoma. Proceedings of the MR Clinical Symposium, vol 3, no.3. Milwaukee: GE Medical Systems, 1987.
31. Glenn WV, et al. Magnetic resonance imaging of the lumbar spine: nerve root canals, disc abnormalities, anatomic correlations and case examples. Milwaukee: GE Medical Systems, 1986.

32. Haughton VM. MR imaging of the spine. Radiology 1988;166:297.

33. Krause D, et al. Lumbar disc herniation: value of oblique magnetic resonance imaging sections. Neuroradiology 1988;15:305.

34. Winter DDB, et al. CT and MR lateral disc herniation: typical appearance and pitfalls of interpretation. Can Assoc Radiol J 1989;40:256.

35. Osborn AG, et al. CT/MR spectrum of far lateral and anterior lumbosacral disc herniations. AJNR 1988;9:775.

36. Williams MP, et al. Thoracic disc herniation: MR imaging. Radiology 1988;167:874.

37. Yu S, et al. Anulus fibrosus in bulging intervertebral discs. Radiology 1988;169:761.

38. Masaryk TJ, et al. High-resolution MR imaging of sequestered lumbar intervertebral discs. AJNR 1988;9:351.

39. Williams MP, et al. Significance of thoracic disc herniation demonstrated by MR imaging. J Comput Assist Tomogr 1989;13:211.

40. Schellinger D, et al. Disc fragment migration. Radiology 1990;175:831.

41. Murayama S, et al. Diagnosis of herniated intervertebral discs with MR imaging: a comparison of gradient-refocused-echo and spin-echo pulse sequences. AJNR 1990;11:17.

42. Boden SD. The use of radiographic imaging studies in the evaluation of the patients who have degenerative disorders of the lumbar spine. J Bone Joint Surg [Am] 1996;78A:114.

43. Modic MT, Ross JS, Obuchowski NA, et al. Contrast-enhanced MR imaging in acute lumbar radiculopathy: pilot study of the natural history. Radiology 1995;195:429.

44. Smoker WRK. Craniovertebral junction: normal anatomy, craniometry, and congenital anomalies. RadioGraphics 1994;14:255.

45. Erkintalo MO, Salminen JJ, Alanen AM, et al. Development of degenerative changes in the lumbar intervertebral disk: results of a prospective MR imaging study in adolescents with and without low-back pain. Radiology 1995;196:529.

46. Thornbury JR, Fryback DG, Turski PA, et al. Disk-caused nerve compression in patients with acute low-back pain: diagnosis with MR, CT myelography, and plain CT. Radiology 1993;186:731.

47. Thornbury JR, Fryback DG, Turski PA, et al. Disk-caused nerve compression in patients with acute low-back pain: diagnosis with MR, CT myelography, and plain CT [errata]. Radiology 1993;187:880.

48. Markus JB, Franchetto AA, Fairbrother J. Magnetic resonance imaging and computed tomography of hyperacute spinal epidural hematoma. Can Assoc Radiol J 1994;45.

49. Orrison WW Jr, Benzel EC, et al. Magnetic resonance imaging evaluation of acute spine trauma. Emerg Radiol 1995;2:120.

50. Georgy BA, Hesselink Jr. MR imaging of the spine: recent advances in pulse sequences and special techniques. AJR 1994;162:923.

51. Seidenwurm DJ, Litt AW. Natural history of lumbar spine disease. Radiology 1995;195:323.

52. Ahmadi J, Bajaj A, Destian S, et al. Spinal tuberculosis: atypical observations at MR imaging. Radiology 1993;189:489.

53. Silverman CS, Lenchik L, Shimkin PM, et al. Value of MR in differentiating subligamentous from supraligamentous lumbar disk herniations. AJNR 1995;16:571.

54. Mehta RC, Marks MP, Hinks RS, et al. MR evaluation of vertebral metastases: T1-weighted, short-inversion-time inversion recovery, fast spin-echo, and inversion-recovery fast spin-echo sequences. AJNR 1994;16:281.

55. Petersilge CA, Pathria MN, Emery SE, Masaryk TJ. Thoracolumbar burst fractures: evaluation with MR imaging. Radiology 1995;194:49.

56. Gundry CR, Heithoff KB. Epidural hematoma of the lumbar spine: 18 surgically confirmed cases. Radiology 1993;187:427.

57. Haddad MC, Sharif HS, Aideyan OA, et al. Infection versus neoplasm in the spine: differentiation by MRI and diagnostic pitfalls. Radiol 1993;3-5:439.

58. Jones KM, Schwartz RB, Mantello MT, et al. Fast spin-echo MR in the detection of vertebral metastases: comparison of three sequences. AJNR 1994;15:401.

59. Porter BA. MR may become routine for imaging bone marrow. Diagn Imaging 1987.

60. Porter BA, et al. Magnetic resonance imaging of bone marrow disorders. Radiol Clin North Am 1986;24:269.

61. Kaplan PA, et al. Bone marrow patterns in aplastic anemia: observations with 1.5T MR imaging. Radiology 1987;164:441.

62. McKinstry CS, et al. Bone marrow in leukemia and aplastic anemia: MR imaging before, during and after treatment. Radiology 1987;162:701.

63. Vogler JB III, et al. Bone marrow imaging. Radiology 1988;168:679.

64. Modic MT, et al. Degenerative disorders of the spine. In: Modic M, Masaryk T, Ross J, eds. Magnetic resonance imaging of the spine. Chicago: Year Book Medical Publishers, 1989:75.

65. Pennes DR, et al. Bone marrow imaging. Radiology 1989;170:894.

66. Stevens SK, et al. Early and late bone marrow changes after irradiation. AJR 1990;154:745.

67. Rosenthal DI, et al. Fatty replacement of spinal bone marrow due to radiation: demonstration by dual energy quantitative CT and MR imaging. J Comput Assist Tomogr 1989;13:463.

68. Carmody RF, et al. Spinal cord compression due to metastatic disease: diagnosis with MR imaging versus myelography. Radiology 1989;173:225.

69. Avrahami E, et al. Early MR demonstration of spinal metastases in patients with normal radiographs and CT and radionuclide bone scans. J Comput Assist Tomogr 1989;13:598.

70. Modic TJ, et al. Degenerative disc disease: assessment of changes in vertebral body marrow with MR imaging. Radiology 1988;166:193.

71. Modic MT, et al. Imaging of degenerative disc disease. Radiology 1988;168:177.

72. Saywell WR, et al. Demonstration of vertebral body end plate veins by magnetic resonance imaging. Br J Radiol 1989;62:290.

73. Modic MT. Intervertebral disc: normal age-related changes in MR signal intensity. Radiology 1990;177:332.

74. Sether LA, et al. Intervertebral disc: normal age related changes in MR signal intensity. Radiology 1990;177:385.

75. Russell EJ. Cervical disc disease. Radiology 1990;177:313.

76. Tsuruda JS, et al. Three-dimensional gradient-recalled MR imaging as a screening tool for the diagnosis of cervical radiculopathy. AJNR 1989;10:1263.

77. Hahn PY, Strobel JJ, Hahn FJ. Verification of lumbosacral segments on MR images: identification of transitional vertebrae. Radiology 1992:182:580.

78. Wasenko JJ, Rosenbaum AE, Yu SF, et al. Gradient echo imaging of the lumbar spine. Comput Med Imaging Graph 1994;18:357.

79. Okumura R, et al. Fatty filum terminate: assessment with MR imaging. J Comput Assist Tomogr 1990;14:571.

80. Nowicki BH, Haughton VM. Neural foraminal ligaments of the lumbar spine: appearance at CT and MR imaging. Radiology 1992;183:257.

81. Lane JI, Koeller KK, Atkinson JDL. MR imaging of the lumbar spine: enhancement of the radicular veins. AJR 1996;166:181.

82. Stoller DW, Genant HK. MRI helps characterize disorders of the spine. Diagn Imaging 1987;9:128.

83. Sze G, Kawamura Y, Negishi C, et al. Fast spin-echo MR imaging of the cervical spine: influence of echo train length and echo spacing on image contrast and quality. AJNR 1993;14:1203.

84. Finelli DA, Hurst GC, Karaman BA, et al. Use of magnetization transfer for improved contrast on gradient-echo MR images of the cervical spine. Radiology 1994;193:165.

85. Enzmann DR, Rubin JB. Cervical spine: MR imaging with a partial flip angle, gradient refocused pulse sequence. Part I. General considerations and disc disease. Radiology 1988;166:467.

86. Stoller DW, Genant HK. Fast imaging of the spine. In: Genant HK, ed. Spine update. San Francisco: Radiology Research and Education Foundation, 1987:47.

87. Xu GL, et al. Lumbar facet joint capsule: appearance at MR imaging and CT. Radiology 1990;177:415.

88. Reynolds H, et al. Cervical rheumatoid arthritis: value of flexion and extension views in imaging. Radiology 1987;164:215.

89. Burk DL, et al. Spinal and paraspinal neurofibromatosis: surface coil MR imaging at 1.5T. Radiology 1987;162:797.

90. April C, Bogduk N. High intensity zone: a diagnostic sign of painful lumbar disc on magnetic resonance imaging. Br J Radiol 1992;65:361.

91. Schellhas K, et al. Lumbar disc high intensity zone: correlation of MR and discography. Spine (in press).

92. Kent DL, Haynor DR, et al. The clinical efficacy of magnetic resonance imaging in neuroimaging. Ann Intern Med 1994;120:856.

93. Brant-Zawadski MN, Jensen MC, et al. Interobserver and intraobserver variability in interpretation of lumbar disc abnormalities: a compassion of two nomenclatures. Spine 1995;20:1257.

94. Jensen MC, Brant-Zawadski MN, et al. Magnetic resonance imaging of the lumbar spine in people without back pain. N Engl J Med 1994;331:69.

95. Holtras S, et al. MR imaging of intradural disc herniation. J Comput Assist Tomogr 1989;11:353.

96. Reicher MA, et al. MR imaging of the lumbar spine: anatomic correlations and the effects of technical variations. AJR 1986;147:891.

97. Modic MR, et al. Magnetic resonance imaging of the spine. Radiol Clin North Am 1986;24:229.

98. Edelman RR, et al. High resolution MRI: imaging anatomy of the lumbosacral spine. Magn Reson Imaging 1986;4:515.

99. Berger PE, et al. High resolution surface coil magnetic resonance imaging of the spine: normal and pathologic anatomy. RadioGraphics 1986;6:573.

100. Ross JS, et al. Tears of the anulus fibrosus: assessment with Gd-DTPA-enhanced MR imaging. AJR 1990;154:159.

101. Yu S, et al. Tears of the anulus fibrosus: correlation between MR and pathologic findings in cadavers. AJNR 1988;9:367.

102. Yussen PS, Swartz JD, Semin US. Acute lumbar disc herniation: imaging diagnosis. CT MR 1993;14:389.

103. Glickstein MF, et al. Magnetic resonance demonstration of hyperintense herniated discs and extruded disc fragments. Skeletal Radiol 1989;18:527.

104. Crisi G, Carpeggiani P, Trevisan C. Gadolinium-enhanced nerve roots in lumbar disk herniation. AJNR 1993;14:1379.

105. Georgy BA, Snow RD, Hesselink JR. MR imaging of spinal nerve roots: techniques, enhancement patterns, and imaging findings. AJR 1996;166:173.

106. Czervionke LF, et al. Degenerative disease of the spine. In: Atlas SW, ed. Magnetic resonance imaging of the brain and spine. New York: Raven Press, 1991:795.

107. Janssen ME, Bertrand SL, Joe C, Levine MI. Lumbar herniated disk disease: comparison of MRI, muelography, and post-myelographic CT scan with surgical findings. Orthopedics 1994;17:121.

108. Wood KB, Garvey TA, Gundry C, Heithoff KB. Magnetic resonance imaging of the thoracic spine: evaluation of asymptomatic individuals. J Bone Joint Surg [Am] 1995;77A:1631.

109. Battie MC, Haynor DR, Fisher LD, et al. Similarities in degenerative findings on magnetic resonance images of the lumbar spines of identical twins. J Bone Joint Surg [Am] 1995;77A:1662.

110. Malghem J, Maldague B, Labaisse MA, et al. Intravertebral vacuum cleft: changes in content after supine positioning. Radiology 1993;187:483.

111. Lafforgue PF, Chagnaud CJ, Daver, LMH, Daumen-Legre VMS. Intervertebral disk vacuum phenomenon secondary to vertebral collapse: prevalence and significance. Radiology 1994;193:853.

112. Bangert BA, Modic MT, Ross JS, Obuchowski NA. Hyperintense disks on T1-weighted MR images: correlation with calcification. Radiology 1995;195:437.

113. Jinkins JR, Rauch RA, Gee GT, et al. Lumbosacral spine: early and delayed MR imaging after administration of an expanded dose of gadopentetate dimeglumine in healthy asymptomatic subjects. Radiology 1995;197:247.

114. Arce CA, Dohrmann GJ. Herniated thoracic discs. Neurol Clin 1985;3:383.

115. Brown CW, et al. The natural history of thoracic disc herniation. Spine 1992;17:97.

116. Bohlman H, Zdeblick T. Anterior excision of herniated thoracic discs. J Bone Joint Surg [Am] 1988;70:1038.

117. Regan JJ, Mack MJ. Endoscopic anterior thoracic discectomy: a prospective evaluation of the first 36 cases. Presented at the 10th Annual Meeting, North Am Spine Society, Washington, DC, October 18–21, 1995.

118. Weber H. Lumbar disc herniation: a controlled prospective study with 10 years observation. Spine 1983;8:131.

119. Delamarter RB, Howard MW, Goldstein T, et al. Percutaneous lumbar discectomy: preoperative and postoperative magnetic resonance imaging. J Bone Joint Surg [Am] 1995;77:578.

120. Kahanovitz N, Viola K, Goldstein T. A multicenter analysis of percutaneous discectomy. Spine 1990;15:713.

121. Flannigan BD, et al. MR imaging of the lumbar spine: anatomic correlations and the effects of technical variations. AJNR 1987;8:27.

122. Enzmann DR, et al. Cervical spine: MR imaging with a partial flip angle, gradient-refocused pulse sequence. Part II. Spinal cord disease. Radiology 1988;166:473.

123. Nakstad PH, et al. MRI in cervical disc herniation. Neuroradiology 1989;31:382.

124. Lestini SF, Wiesel SW. The pathogenesis of cervical spondylosis. Clin Orthop 1989;239:69.

125. Herkowitz HN. The surgical management of cervical spondylotic radiculopathy and myelopathy. Clin Orthop 1989;239:94.

126. Liu SS, et al. Synovial cysts of the lumbosacral spine: diagnosis by MR imaging. AJNR 1989;10:1239.

127. Johnsson KE, Rosen I, Uden A. The natural course of lumbar spinal stenosis. Acta Orthop Scand Suppl 1993;251:67.

128. Law MD, Bernhardt M, White AA III. Evaluation and management of cervical spondylotic myelopathy. J Bone Joint Surg [Am] 1994;76A:1420.

129. Czervionke LF, et al. Cervical neural foramina: correlative anatomic and MR imaging study. Radiology 1988;169:753.

130. Fletcher G, et al. Age-related changes in the cervical facet joints: studies with cryomicrotomy, MR and CT. AJR 1990;154:817.

131. Yamashita Y, et al. Spinal cord compression due to ossification of ligaments: MR imaging. Radiology 1990;175:843.

132. Harsh GR III, et al. Cervical spine stenosis secondary to ossification of the posterior longitudinal ligament. J Neurosurg 1987;67:349.

133. Hirabayashi K, Satomi K. Operative procedures and results of expansive open-door laminoplasty. Spine 1988;13:870.

134. Stoller DW, et al. Applications of computed tomography in the musculoskeletal system. Curr Orthopaed 1987;1:219.

135. Lang P, et al. Magnetic resonance imaging in the assessment of functional lumbar spinal stability [abstract]. Sixth Annual Meeting and Exhibition of the Society of Magnetic Resonance in Medicine, New York, August 17–21, 1987:149.

136. Huckman MS, et al. Chemonucleation and changes observed on lumbar MR scan: preliminary report. AJNR 1987;8:1.

137. Onik G, et al. Percutaneous lumbar discectomy using a new aspiration probe. AJNR 1985;6:290.

138. Ross JS, et al. Postoperative lumbar spine. Semin Roentgenol 1988;23:125.

139. Hueftle MG, et al. Lumbar spine: postoperative MR imaging with Gd-DTPA. Radiology 1988;167:817.

140. Sotiropoulous S, et al. Differentiation between postoperative scar and recurrent disc herniation: prospective comparison of MR, CT and contrast-enhanced CT. AJNR 1989;10:639.

141. Ross JS, et al. Gadolinium-DTPA–enhanced MR imaging of the postoperative lumbar spine: time course and mechanism of enhancement. AJNR 1989;10:37.

142. Ross JS, et al. MR imaging of the postoperative lumbar spine: assessment with gadopentetate dimeglumine. AJNR 1990;11:771.

143. Djukic S, et al. Magnetic resonance imaging of the postoperative lumbar spine. Radiol Clin North Am 1990;28:341.

144. Ross JS, et al. MR enhancement of epidural fibrosis by Gd-DTPA: biodistribution and mechanism. Radiology 1987;165:142

145. Dina TS, Boden SD, Davis DO. Lumbar spine after surgery for herniated disk: imaging findings in the early postoperative period. AJR 1995;164:665.

146. Boden SD, Davis DO, Dina TS, Parker CP, et al. Contrast-enhanced MR imaging performed after successful lumbar disk surgery: prospective study. Radiology 1992;182:59.

147. Boden SD, Davis DO, Dina TS, et al. Contrast-enhanced MR imaging performed after successful lumbar disc surgery: prospective study. Radiology 1992;182:59.

148. Ross JS, et al. MR imaging of lumbar arachnoiditis. AJR 1987;149:1025.

149. Hackney DB, et al. MR characteristics of iophendylate (Pantopaque). J Comput Assist Tomogr 1986;10:401.

150. Altman NR, Altman DH. MR imaging of spinal dysraphism. AJNR 1987;8:533.

151. Delamarter RB, Howard MW, Goldstein T, et al. Percutaneous lumbar discectomy: preoperative and postoperative magnetic resonance imaging. J Bone Joint Surg [Am] 1995;77A:578.

152. Slone RM, MacMillan M, Montgomery WJ. Spinal fixation: Part I. Principles, basic hardware, and fixation techniques for the cervical spine. Radiographics 1993;13:341.

153. Slone RM, MaCmillan M, Montgomery WJ, Heare M. Spinal fixation. Part II. Fixation techniques and hardware for the thoracic and lumbosacral spine. Radiographics 1993;13:521.

154. Slone RM, MacMillan M, Montgomery WJ. Spinal fixation. Part III. Complications of spinal instrumentation. Radiographics 1993;13:797.

155. Johnson DW, et al. MR imaging of the pars interarticularis. AJR 1989;152:327.

156. Grenier N, et al. Isthmic spondylolysis of the lumbar spine: MR imaging at 1.5 T. Radiology 1989;170:489.

157. Gado MB. The spine. In: Lee JK, et al, eds. Computed body tomography with MRI correlation, 2nd ed. New York: Raven Press, 1989:991.

158. Ulmer JL, Elster AD, Mathews VP, King JC. Distinction between degenerative and isthmic spondylolisthesis on sagittal MR images: importance of increased anteroposterior diameter of the spinal canal ("wide canal sign"). AJR 1994;163:411.

159. Jinkins JR, Rauch A. Magnetic resonance imaging of entrapment of lumbar nerve roots in spondylolytic spondylolisthesis. J Bone Joint Surg [Am] 1994;76A:1643.

160. Ulmer JL, Elster AD, Mathews UP, Allen AM. Lumbar spondylolysis: reactive marrow changes seen in adjacent pedicles on MR images. AJR 1995;164:429.

161. Hilibrand AS, Urquhart AG, Graziano GP, Hensinger RN. Acute spondylolytic spondylolisthesis: risk of progression and neurological complications. J Bone Joint Surg [Am] 1995;77A:190.

162. Sartoris DJ, et al. Vertebral-body collapse in focal diffuse disease: patterns of pathologic processes. Radiology 1986;160:479.

163. Ciullo J, Jackson DW. Pars interarticularis stress reaction, spondylolysis and spondylolisthesis in gymnasts. Clin Sports Med 1984;4:95.

164. Commandre FA, et al. Spondylolysis and spondylolisthesis in young athletes: twenty-eight cases. J Sports Med 1988;28:104.

165. Frennered AK, et al. Natural history of symptomatic isthmic low-grade spondylolisthesis in children and adolescents: a seven year follow-up study. J Pediatr Orthop 1991;11:209.

166. Frennered AK, et al. Midterm follow-up of young patients fused in situ for spondylolisthesis. Spine 1991;16:409.

167. Balderston RA, Bradford DS. Technique for achievement and maintenance of reduction for severe spondylolisthesis using spinous process wiring and external fixation of the pelvis. Spine 1985;10:376.

168. Bohlman H, Cook SS. One-stage decompression and posterolateral and interbody fusion for lumbosacral spondylolysis through the posterior approach. J Bone Joint Surg [Am] 1990;64:415.

169. Bradford DA, Iza J. Repair of the defect in spondylolysis of minimal

170. HU SS, Bradford DS. Reduction of high grade spondylolisthesis using Edwards instrumentation. Spine 1996;21 (in press).

171. Herkowitz HN, Kurz LT. Degenerative lumbar spondylolisthesis with spinal stenosis: a prospective study comparing decompression with decompression and intertransverse process arthrodesis. J Bone Joint Surg [Am] 1991;73:802.

172. Kaplan PA, et al. Osteoporosis with vertebral compression fractures, retropulsed fragments, and neurologic compromise. Radiology 1987;165:533.

173. Yuh WTC, et al. Vertebral compression fractures: distinction between benign and malignant causes with MR imaging. Radiology 1989;172:215.

174. Wiener SN, et al. Comparison of magnetic resonance imaging and radionuclide bone imaging of vertebral fractures. Clin Nucl Med 1990;14:666.

175. Baker LL, et al. Benign versus pathologic compression fractures of vertebral bodies: assessment with conventional spin-echo, chemical shift, and STIR MR imaging. Radiology 1990;174:495.

176. El-Khoury GY, Whitten CG. Trauma to the upper thoracic spine: anatomy, biomechanics and unique imaging features. AJR 1993;160:95.

177. Pertersilge CA, Pathria MN, Emery SE, Masaryk TJ. Thoracolumbar burst fractures: evaluation with MR imaging. Radiology 1995;194:49.

178. Manaster BJ. Skeletal radiology. In: Osborn AG, Bragg DG, eds. Handbooks in radiology series. Chicago: Year Book Medical Publishers, 1989.

179. Bollow M, Braun J, Hamm B, Eggens U. Early sarcoiliitis in patients with spondyloarthropathy: evaluation with dynamic gadolinium-enhanced MR imaging. Radiology 1995;194:529.

180. Bohlmann HH. Treatment of fracture and dislocations of the thoracic and lumbar spine. J Bone Joint Surg [Am] 1985;67:165.

181. Hu SS. The effect of surgical decompression on neurologic outcome of lumbar fractures. Clin Orthop 1993;288:166.

182. McAfee PC, Yuan HA, Lasda NA. The unstable burst fracture. Spine 1982;7:365.

183. Arena MJ, Green BA. Extrusion of an intervertebral disc associated with traumatic subluxation or dislocation of cervical facets. J Bone Joint Surg [Am] 1991;73A:155.

184. Modic MT, et al. Vertebral osteomyelitis: assessment using MR. Radiology 1985;157:157.

185. Appel B, et al. MRI of the spine and spinal cord: infectious and inflammatory pathology. Neuroradiology 1988;15:325.

186. Smith AS, et al. MR imaging characteristics of tuberculous spondylitis vs. vertebral osteomyelitis. AJR 1989;153:399.

187. deRoss A, et al. MRI of tuberculous spondylitis. AJR 1986;146:79.

188. Shanley DJ. Tuberculosis of the spine: imaging features. AJR 1995;164:659.

189. Ahmadi J, Bajaj A, Destian S, Segall HD, et al. Spinal tuberculosis: atypical obervations at MR imaging. Radiology 1993;189:489.

190. Ring D, Wenger DR. Magnetic resonance imaging scans in discitis: sequential studies in a child who needed operative drainage. A case report. J Bone Joint Surg [Am] 1994;76A:596.

191. Numaguchi Y, Rigamonti D, Rothman MI, Sato S. Spinal epidural abscess: evaluation with gadolinium-enhanced MR imaging. RadioGraphics 1993;13:545.

192. Malpalam TJ, et al. Nonoperative treatment of spinal infections. J Neurosurg 1989;71:208.

193. Emery SD, Chan DP, Woodward HR. Treatment of hematogenous pyogenic vertebral osteomyelitis with anterior debridement and primary bone grafting. Spine 1989;14:284.

194. Edwards M. White matter disease. In: Atlas SW, ed. Magnetic resonance imaging of the brain and spine. New York: Raven Press, 1991:467.

195. Grossman CB. The Spine. In: Magnetic resonance imaging and com-

puted tomography of the head and spine. Baltimore: Wiliams & Wilkins, 1990:380.

196. Parizel PM, et al. Gd-DTPA–enhanced MR imaging of the spine tumors. AJNR 1989;10:249.

197. Valk J. Gd-DTPA in MR of spinal lesions. AJNR 1988;9:345.

198. Takemoto K, et al. MR imaging of intraspinal tumors: capability in histologic differentiation and compartmentalization of extramedullary tumors. Neuroradiololgy 1988;30:303.

199. Laredo, DJ, et al. Venebral hemangiomas: fat content as a sign of aggressiveness. Radiology 1990;177:467.

200. Jungreis CA, Rothfus WE, Latchaw RE. Tumors and infections of the spine and spinal cord. In: Latchaw RE ed. MR and CT imaging of the head, neck and spine. St Louis: CV Mosby, 1991:1183.

201. Raghaven N, et al. MR imaging in the tethered spinal cord syndrome. AJNR 1989;10:27.

202. Sugimura K, et al. Bone marrow disease of the spine: differentiation with T1 and T2 relaxation times in MR imaging. Radiology 1987;165:541.

203. Daffner RH, et al. MRI in the detection of malignant infiltration of bone marrow. AJR 1986;146:353.

204. Kricun ME. Red-yellow marrow conversion: its effect on the location of some solitary bone lesions. Skeletal Radiol 1985;14:10.

205. Hajek PC, et al. Focal fat deposition in axial bone marrow: MR characteristics. Radiology 1987;162:245.

206. Weaver GR, Sandler MP. Increased sensitivity of magnetic resonance imaging compared to radionuclide bone scintigraphy in the detection of lymphoma of the spine. Clin Nucl Med 1987;12:333.

207. Olson D, et al. Magnetic resonance imaging of the bone marrow in patients with leukemia, aplastic anemia and lymphoma. Invest Radiol 1986.

208. Beltran J, et al. Tumors of the osseous spine: staging with MR imaging versus CT. Radiology 1987;162:565.

209. Ross JS, et al. Vertebral hemangiomas: MR imaging. Radiology 1988;165:165.

210. Sarpel S, et al. Early diagnosis of spinal-epidural metastasis by magnetic resonance imaging. Radiology 1987;164:887.

211. Porter BA, et al. Low field STIR imaging of marrow malignancies. Radiology 1987;165:275.

212. Emory TH, et al. Comparison of Gd-DTPA MR imaging and radionuclide bone scans (WIP). Radiology 1987;165:342.

213. Berry I, et al. Gd-DTPA enhancement of cerebral and spinal tumors on MR imaging. Radiology 1987;165P:38.

214. Fulbright R, Ross JS, Sze G. Application of contrast agents in MR imaging of the spine. JMRI 1993;3:219.

215. Ramsey RG, Zacharias CE. MR imaging of the spine after radiation therapy: easily recognizable effects. JNR 1985;6:247.

216. Gierada DS, Erickson SJ. MR imaging of the sacral plexus: abnormal findings. AJR 1993;160:1067.

217. Mink J. Percutaneous bone biopsy in the patient with known or suspected osseous metastases. Radiology 1986;161:191.

218. O'Neill J, Gardner V, Armstrong G. Treatment of tumors of the thoracic and lumbar spinal column. Clin Orthop 1988;277:103.

219. Weinstein JN, McLain RF. Tumors of the spine. In: Rothman RH, Simeone FA, eds. The spine, 3rd ed. Philadelphia: WB Saunders, 1992.

220. Harrington KD. Anterior decompression and stabilization of the spine as a treatment for vertebral collapse and spinal cord compression for metastatic malignancy. Clin Orthop 1988;233:177.

221. Armstrong DC, Harwood-Nash DC. Pediatric spine. In: Stark DD, Bradley WG, eds. Magnetic resonance imaging. St Louis: CV Mosby, 1992:1370.

222. Elster AD. Occult spinal tumors in neurofibromatosis: implications for screening. AJR 1995;165:956.

223. Mautner VF, Tatagiba M, Lindenau M, Fünsterer C. Spinal tumors in patients with neurofibromatosis type 2: MR imaging study of frequency, multiplicity, and variety. AJR 1995;165:951.

224. Haughton VM, Daniels DL, Czervionke LF, Williams AL. Cervical spine. In: Stark DD, Bradley WG, eds. Magnetic resonance imaging. St Louis: Mosby–Year Book. 1992:1271.

225. Schwend RM, Hennrikus W, Hall Ke, Emans JB. Childhood scoliosis: clinical indications for magnetic resonance imaging. J Bone Joint Surg [Am] 1995;77A:46.

Magnetic Resonance Imaging in Orthopaedics & Sports Medicine, Second Edition,
edited by David W. Stoller. Lippincott-Raven Publishers, Philadelphia, © 1997.

Chapter 15

Marrow Imaging

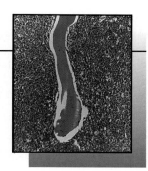

David W. Stoller
Terri M. Steinkirchner
Bruce A. Porter

Conventional radiographic techniques, insensitive to many marrow infiltrations and tumors, are limited in providing accurate bone marrow characterization. Frequently, there is significant trabecular or cancellous destruction before disease progression is detected on standard radiographs. Computed tomography (CT), although accurate for detecting gross metastatic disease of the spine, is of limited use in imaging primary and metastatic marrow neoplasms in the rest of the skeleton. Changes in the CT attenuation value of medullary bone can be nonspecific and do not occur until pathology is well established. Radionuclide bone scanning, the standard method for screening the skeleton for metastatic disease, is relatively insensitive to certain marrow neoplasms, such as leukemia, lymphoma, and myeloma. Very aggressive metastatic tumors may yield false-negative findings on radionuclide scans. Marrow studies with radiolabeled colloids, which have shown promise in research studies, have not become routine in clinical oncology.

Unlike these modalities, magnetic resonance (MR) imaging has the major benefit of imaging bone marrow directly. Multiplanar MR imaging provides the excellent spatial and contrast resolution necessary to differentiate the signal intensities of fatty (yellow) marrow elements from hematopoietic (red) marrow elements. MR imaging may thus become the diagnostic gold standard for diseases that involve or target the bone marrow.

NORMAL BONE MARROW

The normal distribution and MR appearance of bone marrow changes with age.[1–4] An understanding of these variations is important in examining MR patterns in appendicular skeletal locations and determining whether they are potential disease processes or normal variations of marrow. The general status of marrow in adults is best assessed on MR images in the coronal plane of the pelvis, unless symptoms indicate disease elsewhere.

Structure, Function, and Development

The bone marrow is the site of production of circulating blood elements (ie, granulocytes, erythrocytes, monocytes, platelets, and uncommitted lymphocytes). Sustained cellular production is dependent on stem cells, which exhibit properties of both continuous self-replication and differentiation into specific cell lines. The tremendous flexibility of stem cells in the production of blood cellular elements is related to their proliferative activity, which is dependent on the microenvironment (ie, cell-to-cell interaction) and on humoral feedback.[5,6] The earliest stem cells give rise to more restricted stem cells, which exhibit less multipotentiality and decreased ability for self-replication. With further differentiation, committed progenitors are formed that mature along a single hematopoietic pathway. In the presence of colony stimulating factors (CSFs), these progenitor cells can be grown in vitro to form cell colonies known as *colony forming units.*[7]

The marrow cavity is divided into compartments by plates of bony trabeculae. Red, or hematopoietic, marrow is hematopoietically active bone marrow located within the spaces defined by the trabeculae. It is semifluid in consistency and is composed of the various hematopoietic stem cells and their progeny in assorted stages of granulocytic, erythrocytic, and megakaryocytic development. Uncommitted lymphocytes, as well as lymphoid nodules, are also present in the red marrow. The hematopoietic cellular elements are supported by reticulum cells and fat cells. Red marrow contains approximately 40% water, 40% fat, and 20% protein.[8] The vascular system consists of centrally located nutrient arteries that send out branches that terminate in capillary beds within the bone. Postcapillary venules reenter the marrow cavity and coalesce to form venous sinuses. Hematopoietic cell production follows the vascular arrangement, forming active hematopoietic islands between the sinusoids. Bone marrow lacks lymphatic channels.[9,10]

Hematopoietically inactive marrow, or marrow not involved in blood cell production, is referred to as yellow marrow. Because yellow marrow is predominantly composed of fat, it is sometimes called fatty marrow. It contains approximately 15% water, 80% fat, and 5% protein.

Red to Yellow Marrow Conversion

Hematopoiesis begins in utero, at approximately 19 gestational days, within the yolk sac. By week 16 of gestation, the main sites of fetal hematopoiesis are the liver and spleen. After week 24 of gestation, marrow becomes the main organ of hematopoiesis. At birth, active hematopoiesis (ie, red marrow) is present throughout the entire skeleton. Normal physiologic conversion of red to yellow marrow occurs during growth in a predictable and orderly fashion,[11] and is complete by 25 years of age, when the adult pattern is established.

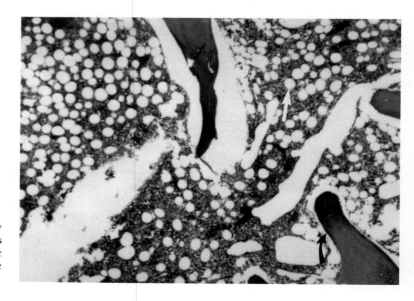

FIGURE 15-1. In a 51-year-old man, normal bone marrow consists of a 50:50 cell-to-fat ratio. Fat (*straight arrow*) is seen as white, round spaces surrounded by hematopoietic cells. The marrow is compartmentalized by trabecular bone (*curved arrow*) (H & E; original magnification ×100).

The cellularity of red marrow varies with age and site. In the newborn, red marrow cellularity approaches 100%. In the adult, fat cells generally occupy approximately 50% of active red marrow (Fig. 15-1). However, the cellularity of marrow also varies with site. For example, at 50 years of age, the average cellularity is 75% in the vertebrae, 60% in the sternum, and 50% in the iliac crests.[10,11] In the adult, red marrow is primarily concentrated in the appendicular and axial (ie, spinal) skeletons. The prevalence of fatty marrow within the spine increases with advancing age. In osteoporosis, fat replacement is associated with loss of cancellous (ie, trabecular) bone. Early in the normal ossification process, yellow marrow replaces the hyaline cartilage template in the epiphysis and apophysis.

Reconversion of Yellow to Red Marrow

Reconversion of yellow to red marrow occurs in the reverse order from that seen in the normal, physiologically maturing skeleton. In other words, it starts in the axial skeleton and proceeds in a proximal-to-distal direction in the appendicular skeleton. For example, hematopoiesis occurs in the proximal metaphysis in the premature skeleton; therefore, reconversion of long bones occurs first in the proximal metaphysis and then in the distal metaphysis. The process of reconversion of yellow to red is triggered by the body's demand for increased blood cell production, which may be caused by stress, anemia, or marrow replacement. The extent of reconversion depends on the duration and severity of the initiating cause. Relatively extensive reconversion is seen in long-standing chronic anemias such as sickle cell anemia or thalassemia major.[12] This process favors sites of residual red marrow stores.

Magnetic Resonance Appearance of Normal Marrow

In yellow marrow, hydrogen protons exist in hydrophobic side groups with short T1 relaxation times.[13,14] The bright signal intensity of yellow marrow reflects the shortened T1

relaxation time of fat. The differences in signal intensities of yellow and red marrow result primarily from differences in their proportional amounts of water and fat; the proportions are approximately equal in red marrow, but there is significantly more fat (80%) in yellow marrow.[3] The role of protein, which constitutes 20% of red marrow and 5% of yellow marrow, in modifying signal intensity is less clear, because protein may exist in either a bound state, with a long T1 relaxation time, or in solution, with a short T1 relaxation time.[13,15]

On T1-weighted and conventional T2-weighted images, yellow marrow demonstrates the bright signal intensity of fat. On heavily T2*-weighted contrast images, yellow marrow appears dark or is of decreased signal intensity. This effect is unrelated to the low signal intensity of yellow marrow on short TI inversion recovery (STIR) images, in which signal from fat is nulled. The signal intensity of fat marrow is also reduced on fat-suppressed T2-weighted spin-echo (SE) or fat-suppressed T2-weighted fast spin-echo (FSE) sequences,[16] and appears darker when using fat suppression techniques with sequences having longer repetition times (TR) and echo times (TE). Red marrow demonstrates low signal intensity on T1-weighted images, reflecting its increased water content, and intermediate signal intensity with progressive T2 weighting. Red and yellow marrow contrast differences become less distinct on heavily T2-weighted protocols with TR greater than 2500 msec.

With suppression of the signal from fat on STIR images, areas of red marrow demonstrate higher signal intensity than areas of yellow marrow. Separation of red and yellow marrow is most difficult on T2*-weighted images, where red marrow stores may actually demonstrate decreased signal intensity relative to adjacent yellow or fatty marrow.

In the newborn, there are no yellow marrow stores, and red marrow signal intensity is equal to or less than that of muscle (Fig. 15-2). On T1-weighted sequences, articular cartilage in epiphyseal centers demonstrates low signal intensity, similar to red marrow. On conventional

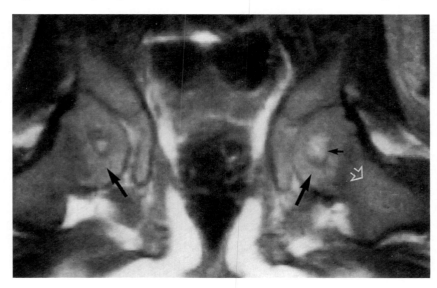

FIGURE 15-2. Intermediate signal intensity epiphyseal cartilage (*large arrows*) with a high signal intensity ossific nucleus (*small arrow*) is seen on a T1-weighted coronal image. Red marrow demonstrates low signal intensity (*open arrow*) (TR, 600 msec; TE, 20 msec).

T2-weighted sequences, articular cartilage is intermediate in signal intensity, and it demonstrates an increase in signal intensity on T2*-weighted sequences (Fig. 15-3). T2*-weighted sequences, however, are not as sensitive as fat-suppressed T2-weighted FSE or STIR techniques for imaging articular cartilage.

As discussed earlier, the maturing skeleton undergoes a process of red to yellow marrow conversion beginning in the hands and feet and progressing to the peripheral and then central skeleton.[1,3] In the long bones of the appendicular skeleton, red marrow conversion occurs first in the diaphysis and progresses to the distal and then proximal metaphysis[17] (Figs. 15-4 through 15-6). In the femoral diaphysis, high signal intensity fatty marrow is observed as early as 3 months of age, with marrow heterogeneity at 12 months, and homogeneous high signal intensity after 5 years of age.[18] In the adult, the proximal two thirds of the femur and humerus contain a higher concentration of red marrow stores, accounting for the appearance on T1-weighted images of low signal intensity inhomogeneity against a background matrix of fatty marrow of bright signal intensity.[19] Uniform fatty marrow within the long bones of the humerus or femur, with-

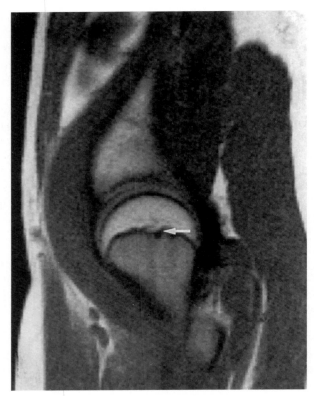

FIGURE 15-4. The low signal intensity physeal plate separates the bright signal intensity metaphyseal red marrow (*arrow*), as seen on a T1-weighted sagittal image (TR, 600 msec; TE, 20 msec).

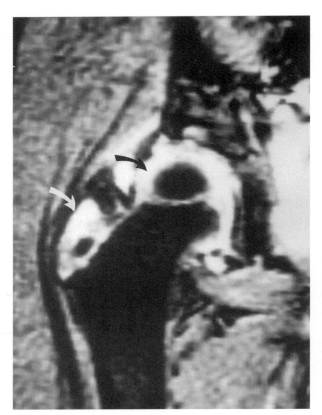

FIGURE 15-3. High signal intensity cartilage in the greater trochanter (*white arrow*) and femoral epiphyses (*black arrow*) can be seen on a T2*-weighted coronal image (TR, 400 msec; TE, 20 msec; flip angle, 25°).

out any red marrow inhomogeneity, is within the spectrum of normal findings. Marrow heterogeneity in the pelvis tends to be most prominent in the acetabulum from birth to 24 years of age. In other locations, marrow signal intensity increases with age.[20] In the sacrum, the lateral masses have a higher fat content and a more heterogeneous signal intensity than the vertebral bodies.[21] In addition, the sacral lateral masses demonstrate brighter signal intensity in male than in female patients.

Mirowitz[22] described finding extension of hematopoietic marrow (residual or reconverted) within the humeral epiphysis. This site, proximal to the humeral metaphysis does not usually contain hematopoietic marrow,[22] although its presence has also been noted in the proximal femoral epiphysis.[23] Although hematopoietic bone marrow is not usually visualized within the epiphysis of long bones in adults, these findings are considered normal. Female patients are more likely to demonstrate epiphyseal hematopoietic marrow, a finding which correlates with a more prominent pattern of hematopoietic marrow within the proximal humeral metaphysis. A curvilinear distribution of marrow usually involves the medial humeral head, and central epiphyseal hematopoietic marrow, in a patchy or globular pattern, is less common.

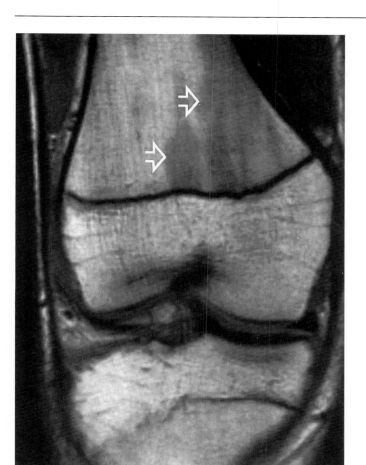

FIGURE 15-5. Residual metaphyseal red marrow in a child is seen as patchy regions of low signal intensity (*open arrows*) on a T1-weighted coronal image (TR, 600 msec; TE, 20 msec).

MARROW IMAGING TECHNIQUES

Spin-Echo and Fast Spin-Echo Imaging

Since both benign and malignant disorders that target the marrow have long T1 and T2 values and high proton density, imaging protocols for marrow characterization use T1-weighted SE sequences. T2-weighted SE sequences have less contrast in the range of commonly used TRs (ie, approximately 2000 msec), and long TR and TE times (ie, TR values between 2000 and 3000 msec and TE values greater than 80 msec) would be necessary to optimize contrast. However, since many lesions become isointense with marrow on intermediate weighted sequences, T1-weighted images with TR values between 400 and 700 msec and short TEs, less than 30 msec, are required.

Lower contrast, as well as artifacts caused by moving high signal intensity fat, may degrade the diagnostic quality of conventional T1- and T2-weighted SE images. Conventional MR imaging may also be of limited value when contrast is intrinsically low due to small differences in signal between tumors and adjacent fat, especially on long TR/TE sequences. The clinical usefulness of marrow MR imaging can be substantially expanded by combining T1-weighted SE and STIR sequences. Fat-suppressed T2-weighted or fat-suppressed T2-weighted FSE techniques, however, have primarily replaced conventional non−fat-suppressed T2-weighted sequences in evaluating marrow pathology.[16] FSE imaging acquires multiple lines of k-space during a single TR. This makes it possible to keep imaging time relatively short when acquiring high-resolution T2-weighted images with ultralong TRs.[24] With FSE pulse sequences, the initial

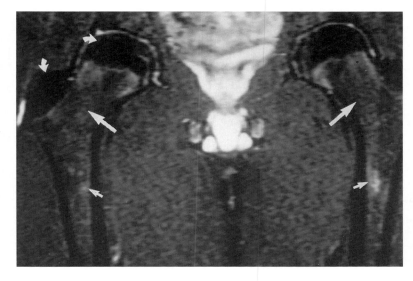

FIGURE 15-6. A coronal STIR image shows normal hematopoietic intermediate signal intensity in the femurs (*large straight arrows*) and dark fatty marrow in the epiphyseal centers and greater trochanter in a 15-year-old boy. Note the early replacement of hematopoietic marrow by fatty marrow in the diaphyses (*small straight arrows*).

90° pulse is followed by the acquisition of 2 to 16 echoes. The echo-train length represents the number of echoes selected. Echo space is the time between each echo. Acquisition time is decreased by increasing the echo train. Because of the high fat signal intensity intrinsic to this sequence, fat-suppression must be added to increase the sensitivity of this technique for routine use in bone marrow imaging. The blurring effect of FSE sequences is decreased with shorter echo-train lengths, longer TEs, and increased matrix resolution (eg, 256 × 256).

Short TI Inversion Recovery Imaging

The STIR technique is highly T1 weighted. The initial 180° radiofrequency (RF) excitation pulse is followed by a standard SE pulse sequence at a given inversion time (TI) (Fig. 15-7). The manner in which this pulse sequence becomes a T1-weighted sequence is shown in Figure 15-8. The strength of the signal that is returned from the SE sequence is proportional to the absolute magnitude of the Z component of the bulk magnetization vector at the instant of the 90° pulse; therefore, a TI can be determined for which fat, which has a short T1, will not emit a signal.

This type of inversion recovery technique (with a short TI) was initially used to eliminate the subcutaneous fat signal responsible for motion and breathing artifacts. It also suppresses the signal from normal medullary fat, which allows the signal emanating from abnormal tissues to be more easily detected, and has, therefore, proven to be highly sensitive for diseases within the medullary space of bone. The following STIR characteristics give rise to the clinical advantages:

- Additive T1 and T2 contrast
- Marked suppression of the high signal from fat
- Twice the magnetization range of SE sequences.

These characteristics produce extraordinarily high contrast that makes the lesion more conspicuous, but preserve the low signal-to-noise ratio. By selecting TI times that occur at the null point during the recovery of signal after an inverting 180° RF pulse, the signal from structures of known TI relaxation times can be selectively suppressed.

The STIR sequence described above suppresses the signal from fat, which is the predominant component of marrow in normal adults. T1 is prolonged in most pathologic conditions affecting the marrow, and the T1 of fatty marrow is short; therefore, there is extreme contrast on STIR images, a considerable advantage over routine SE imaging. On STIR images, fat is black, combinations of red and yellow marrow are light gray (ie, intermediate), and most marrow tumors are bright white. Although red marrow demonstrates increased signal intensity on STIR images, most pathologic conditions involving marrow replacement or infiltration generate greater signal intensities. Fibrous tissue, calcification, and hemosiderin deposits are low in signal intensity, whereas fluid, edema, or recent hemorrhage are all bright. Muscle remains intermediate in signal intensity. STIR sequences reflect the age dependent differences in the percentage of hematopoietic marrow. The FSE STIR technique decreases imaging time significantly and produces diagnostic accuracy comparable with conventional STIR sequences.[24] Either the fat-suppressed T2-weighted FSE or FSE STIR sequences used in conjunction with T1-weighted images represent the key imaging protocols for optimizing marrow tissue contrast.

Gradient-Echo Recall Imaging

Gradient-echo recall techniques (ie, T2*-weighted images) have become increasingly popular, primarily because of their ability to increase the rate of data acquisition and decrease

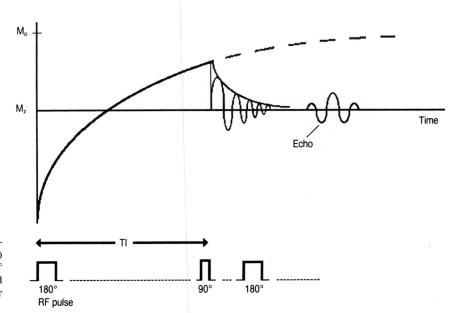

FIGURE 15-7. The inversion recovery pulse sequence is initiated by a 180° radiofrequency (RF) excitation pulse. After a time interval (TI), a 90° pulse followed by a 180° refocusing pulse is used to create a standard spin echo that is sampled for image acquisition.

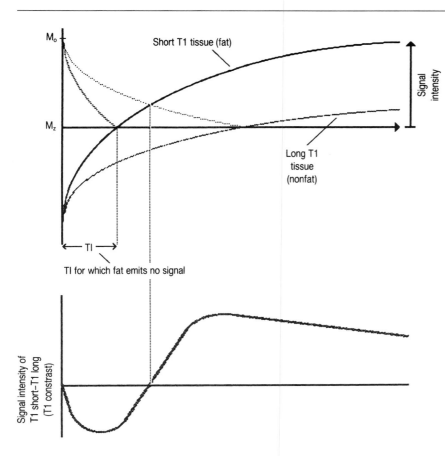

FIGURE 15-8. On T1 contrast using inversion recovery pulse sequences, the strength of the signal intensity with standard inversion recovery pulse sequences is proportional to the absolute value of the Z component of the bulk magnetization vector at the time of signal sampling, which is an imaging time (TI), a variable amount of milliseconds after the initial 180° excitation pulse. A short TI can be chosen so that tissues such as fat, with short repetition time (TR) values, will have a Z component of the bulk magnetization vector near zero at the time of tissue sampling. At this value, fat emits no signal, whereas surrounding tissues with longer TR do emit a signal. This technique can be used to suppress unwanted fat signal when it overwhelms signal from abnormal surrounding tissue in bone marrow disease, or when it is responsible for unwanted motion artifacts.

scan times. A standard gradient recall sequence is shown in Figure 15-9. The initial excitation pulse is an RF pulse that typically possesses a flip angle of less than 90°. If a 90° flip angle is used, the Z component of the bulk magnetization vector is zero after the excitation pulse (Fig. 15-10), and a period of time on the order of T1 is needed for the Z component of the bulk magnetization vector to recover and to allow a second pulse sequence to generate significant signal. If the excitation pulse is less than 90°, however, the Z component of the bulk magnetization vector is not decreased to zero, and the subsequent excitation pulse can be separated from the first by a TR significantly less than T1 (see Fig. 15-10). In addition, the resultant signal is maximized by using free induction decay for data acquisition, instead of a standard SE with its associated long TE and signal drop-off. To balance phase shifts from the readout frequency gradient, so that all phase shifts are only those specifically introduced by the phase and encoding gradients, the initial readout gradient is negative and cancels phase shifts introduced by the positive component of the frequency-encoded gradient during acquisition of the signal. A reversal occurs between the negative and positive gradient; thus, the term *gradient reversal techniques* is used. By using partial flip angles, TR values can be markedly shortened. Because image acquisition time is directly proportional to the value of TR, marked time savings over SE techniques can be attained. However, because the contrast parameters sampled by the gradient-echo

technique are predominantly T2*, the high contrast between soft tissues normally obtained by SE techniques is not routinely seen on gradient-echo images. It is possible to select parameters to provide contrast that is somewhat similar to standard SE imaging (Table 15-1).

Gradient-echo techniques are sensitive to magnetic field inhomogeneities, chemical-shift frequencies, and magnetic susceptibility; therefore, they are prone to motion and distortion artifacts of tissue interfaces with different magnetic susceptibilities. Advantages of gradient-echo techniques, including effective T2 weighting, high resolution, and adequate signal-to-noise ratio without need for interslice spacing, however, make this a useful complement to T1 SE imaging. In addition, three dimensional Fourier transform volume acquisitions, which allow up to 120 images to a slice thickness of 0.7 mm, can be retrospectively reformatted. Susceptibility effects can be used to identify calcium or areas of hemorrhage.

The low signal intensity contrast of T2*-weighted images is not secondary to fat suppression, as with STIR images; therefore, many marrow neoplasms or infiltrative disease processes do not demonstrate increased signal intensity when compared with corresponding STIR images. Red marrow stores do not demonstrate increased signal intensity on T2* gradient-echo images and may be difficult to differentiate from fatty marrow. A high proportion of trabecular bone in areas such as the epiphysis may further modify gradient-echo

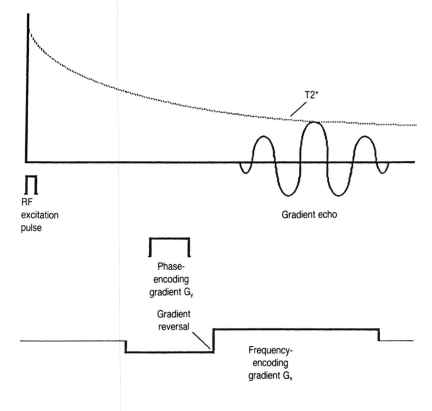

FIGURE 15-9. A highly schematic pulse sequence diagram of a theoretic gradient-echo pulse sequence known as the gradient recall sequence. The sequence is initiated by a radiofrequency (RF) pulse that is typically less than 90°. The initial pulse is followed by a dephasing gradient that is inverted, which rephases the nuclei during data acquisition. This technique allows a phase-encoded gradient as well as a frequency-encoded gradient to be applied during sampling, so that all necessary information to calculate a two-dimensional (2D) image using the 2D Fourier transform method can be obtained during the course of a free induction decay.

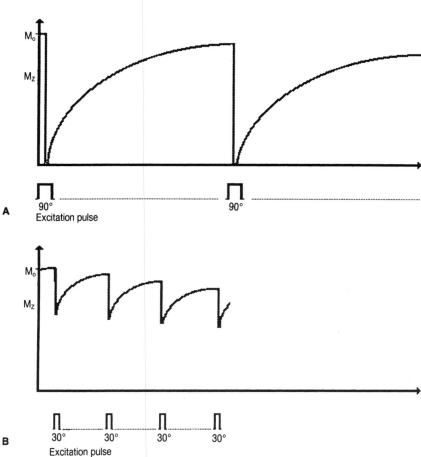

FIGURE 15-10. Small flip angle excitation pulses. After a standard 90° excitation pulse, the Z component of the bulk magnetization vector is zero. (**A**) Time on the order of T1 is required for the Z component of bulk magnetization to recover, so that a second excitation pulse can generate sufficient signal. (**B**) Smaller excitation pulses, such as a 30° pulse, do not decrease the Z component of bulk magnetization vector to zero, and additional excitation pulses can be used with TR values substantially less than T1.

TABLE 15-1
Repetition and Echo Time Pulse Parameters for Variously Weighted Images

	T1-Weighted	Mixed	T2*-Weighted	Proton Density Weighted
TR (msec)	200–400	20–50	200–400	200–400
TE (msec)	12–15	12–15	30–60	12–15
θ (degrees)	45–90	30–60	5–20	5–20

TE, echo time; TR, repetition time; θ, flip angle.
Wehrli FW, Shaw D, Kneeland B. Signal-to-noise, resolution, and contrast. In: Principles, methodology and applications of biomedical magnetic resonance imaging. New York: VCH Publishers, 1987.

contrast (decreasing effective transverse relaxation times), resulting in decreased signal intensity in these areas.[25]

Chemical-Shift Imaging

Chemical-shift imaging is used to produce images that emphasize either the water or fat component of marrow by temporal separation of their respective returning MR signals.[26] Red and yellow marrow differentiation is thus possible on T1-weighted images. Differences in resonant frequencies of fat and water protons (3.5 ppm or 75 to 150 Hz) allow for temporal dephasing after RF pulse excitation. This property is used to develop water and fat images by emphasizing in-phase or out-of-phase tissue properties, thus suppressing fat or water signal.

Magnetic Resonance Survey Evaluation

The protocol for an MR survey examination for marrow evaluation uses T1-weighted coronal images of the pelvis and proximal femurs, which are adult sites of red marrow concentration. These images are acquired with large (40 cm) fields of view to include assessment of lumbosacral spine marrow. Transcoronal STIR images are obtained to null fat signal and identify abnormal T1 or T2 prolongation. Fat-suppressed T2-weighted FSE may be used when thin slice or multiplanar imaging is required in a limited period of time.

Axial T1-weighted, fat-suppressed T2-weighted FSE, or STIR images may be obtained at specific sites of suspected pathologic processes and are important in determining cross sectional marrow involvement. T1-weighted images are particularly valuable in evaluating blastic processes, which are low in signal on STIR and T2*-weighted images. Gadolinium-enhanced axial images may improve the visibility of lesions, especially in cases with soft-tissue or cord involvement. Sagittal T1-weighted and STIR images are routinely acquired to evaluate suspected spinal malignancies.

BONE MARROW PATHOLOGY

Malignant Disorders

Leukemia

ACUTE LEUKEMIAS. Acute leukemias are the 20th most common cause of cancer deaths at all ages, and, as a group, represent the most common malignant disease in childhood. This aggressive group of disorders arises at the primitive stem cell level and is usually classified as either lymphocytic or myelogenous in type, based on the cytologic features of the blast cell. Further classification of the leukemic blasts—based on immunologic markers, cytogenetics, and electron microscopy—provides useful prognostic and therapeutic information. Eighty percent of patients with acute lymphocytic (lymphoblastic) leukemia are children, and 90% of patients with acute myelogenous leukemia are adults.[27,28]

The majority of acute leukemias arise de novo, although they may represent the final stage of a progression from a preleukemic state (eg, myelodysplasia) or the end stage of a chronic myeloproliferative disorder such as chronic myelogenous leukemia. The distinguishing feature of the acute phase is the uncontrolled growth of poorly differentiated blast cells. These cells rapidly accumulate in the marrow, suppressing the normal marrow elements and resulting in the commonly observed clinical symptoms of fatigue, weakness, infections, and hemorrhage.

Marrow involvement in acute leukemia is typically diffuse and is characterized by monotonous infiltration of immature cells in a hypercellular marrow (Fig. 15-11). In occasional cases of myeloblastic leukemia, particularly in very old patients, the marrow is normocellular or even hypocellular.[11] Leukemic expansion in the marrow may elicit symptoms of skeletal tenderness or swelling of the larger joints.[8]

Clinical Assessment. Clinical assessment of leukemia involves posterior iliac crest aspiration for bone marrow biopsy and peripheral blood smear analysis. Peripheral disturbances in hematopoiesis are often nonspecific and frequently occur prior to significant increases in marrow blast cells. At present, the use of MR imaging in childhood leukemias is limited, but this may change as MR imaging becomes more

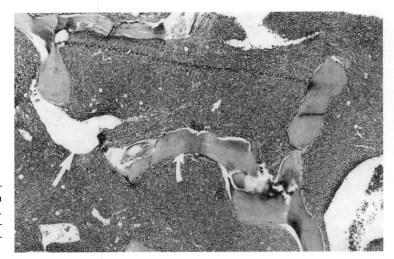

FIGURE 15-11. Acute lymphocytic leukemia. Bone marrow exhibits 100% cellularity consisting of a monotonous population of blast cells (*small arrow*). Fat cells are essentially absent. The vascular sinuses are dilated (*large arrow*), and the trabecular bone is indicated (*curved arrow*) (H & E; original magnification ×100).

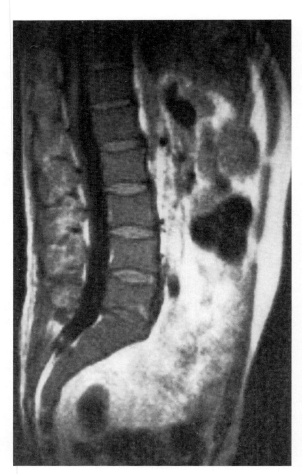

FIGURE 15-12. Diffuse low signal intensity leukemic infiltration of marrow occurs in acute lymphocytic leukemia, as seen on this T1-weighted sagittal image (TR, 600 msec; TE, 20 msec).

commonly used for monitoring the course of relapse and the complications of treatment in these patients.

Acute leukemia in relapse may present with focal or irregular areas of infiltration, which may represent surviving rests of treated tumor cells. This appearance is more patchy and irregularly marginated than that usually seen with focal metastatic disease.

Magnetic Resonance Appearance. In both children and adults, leukemic marrow involvement is homogeneous, diffuse, and symmetric (Fig. 15-12). Focal infiltration is more commonly seen in myelogenous leukemia (Fig. 15-13). On T1-weighted images, leukemic hypercellularity is seen as low signal intensity replacement of higher signal intensity marrow fat (Fig. 15-14). Due to the greater proportion of hematopoietic marrow in children, there is an overlap in the appearance of normal low signal intensity cellular hematopoietic marrow and low to intermediate intensity hypercellular leukemic marrow. Quantitative measurements of T1 relaxation times, still under investigation, have shown prolongation in patients with leukemia and leukemia in relapse.[29–32] These assessments, however, are not specific for the diagnosis of leukemia. Prolongation of T1 relaxation time is also seen in metastatic rhabdomyosarcoma and neuroblastoma. Normal bone marrow has a T1 relaxation time of 350 to 650 msec. At initial diagnosis of leukemia or in leukemia in relapse, T1 relaxation times of 750 msec have been identified. Further studies are needed to confirm the clinical significance of differences in T1 values among initial diagnosis, remission, and relapse.[33]

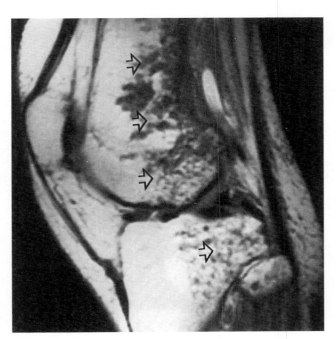

FIGURE 15-13. Low signal intensity leukemic infiltrates (*open arrows*) extending into the epiphysis are seen on a T1-weighted sagittal image. Extension of marrow inhomogeneity crossing the physis is an abnormal finding and is seen with acute myelogenous leukemia (TR, 600 msec, TE 20 msec).

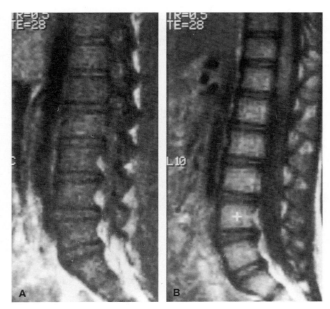

FIGURE 15-14. (A) In a patient with acute lymphocytic leukemia marrow infiltration demonstrates low signal intensity on a T1-weighted sagittal image. **(B)** The spine of a normal age-matched control demonstrates high signal intensity from fatty marrow on a T1-weighted sagittal image (TR, 500 msec; TE, 28 msec).

Conventional T2-weighted images may show increases in signal intensity in acute leukemia. Unlike the situation with metastatic disease, however, T2-weighted images may not be sensitive to leukemic hypercellularity. Quantitative measurement of T2 relaxation times in leukemia has not shown any significant difference from control marrow.

T2*-weighted images, in which T1 and T2 contrast are not additive, are more limited in the evaluation of infiltrative processes of bone marrow. Larger areas or deposits of leukemic involvement may demonstrate hyperintensity on T2*-weighted images, but similarly affected smaller regions may be less conspicuous (Fig. 15-15).

Chemical-shift imaging has also been used to identify pathologic marrow. Relative changes in the fat fraction show the greatest potential for understanding changes in bone marrow signal intensity and changes occurring with relapse.[30,34] Chemical-shift imaging may be more useful in adult patients, because of the greater difference in the fat and water fraction of bone marrow.

Short TI inversion recovery imaging techniques offer superior contrast for demonstrating increased signal intensity in leukemic marrow, exceeding that displayed by normal hematopoietic cells. Nulling of fat signal intensity facilitates the detection of both focal and diffuse leukemic infiltrates.

Postchemotherapy Appearance of Marrow. Patients with acute leukemia or chronic myelogenous leukemia in blast crisis are treated aggressively with myelotoxic drugs. This treatment results in cellular depletion (ie, hypoplasia) of the marrow, accompanied by edema and fibrin deposition. Total depletion of the marrow may occur in a month or less, de-

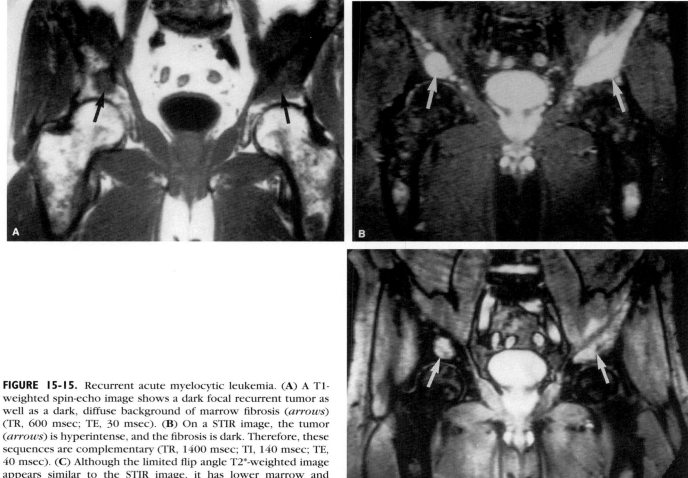

FIGURE 15-15. Recurrent acute myelocytic leukemia. (**A**) A T1-weighted spin-echo image shows a dark focal recurrent tumor as well as a dark, diffuse background of marrow fibrosis (*arrows*) (TR, 600 msec; TE, 30 msec). (**B**) On a STIR image, the tumor (*arrows*) is hyperintense, and the fibrosis is dark. Therefore, these sequences are complementary (TR, 1400 msec; TI, 140 msec; TE, 40 msec). (**C**) Although the limited flip angle T2*-weighted image appears similar to the STIR image, it has lower marrow and soft-tissue contrast (*arrows*) (TR, 400 msec; TE, 20 msec; flip angle, 25°).

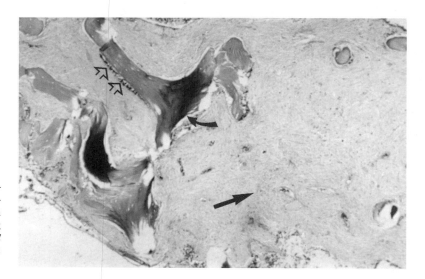

FIGURE 15-16. Extensive myelofibrosis after chemotherapy for acute leukemia. The bone marrow exhibits extensive marrow fibrosis, which appears as spindled cells with an abundant collagen matrix (*solid straight arrow*) filling the marrow space between the trabecular bone (*curved arrow*). Osteoblastic activity can also be seen (*open arrows*) (H & E; original magnification ×100).

pending on the schedule of chemotherapy treatments and the sensitivity of the leukemic cells. As leukemic depletion progresses, fat cells (ie, yellow marrow) regenerate. Normally, this phase of hypoplasia is followed by regeneration of hematopoietic elements (ie, red marrow). Occasionally, however, extensive postchemotherapy fibrosis develops (Figs. 15-16 and 15-17). The fibrosis can be focal or widespread, and may be accompanied by bone formation.[35,36]

Chemotherapy produces a spectrum of MR changes in normal and leukemia marrow, including metastatic disease. Marrow hypoplasia is characterized by the appearance of fatty marrow, which demonstrates high signal intensity on T1-weighted images and intermediate signal intensity on T2-weighted images. With chemical-shift imaging, it is possible to demonstrate sequential increases in bone marrow fat fractions in patients in clinical remission during chemotherapy treatment for acute leukemia.[37] Marrow fibrosis demonstrates low signal intensity on T1- and T2-weighted images. Reconversion of normal fatty marrow to hematopoietic marrow is seen as areas of decreased signal intensity on T1-weighted images and intermediate to mildly increased signal intensity on STIR images. When reconversion takes place adjacent to an area of signal intensity from fat in treated marrow, there is a reversal of the initial imaging signal intensity characteristics from pretreatment bone marrow to postchemotherapy marrow (Fig. 15-18). Immediately after chemotherapy, marrow edema may falsely exaggerate the extent of disease progression. Follow-up examination can be performed to document a more accurate baseline.

In acute myeloid leukemia, MR imaging can demonstrate changes in bulk T1 during treatment which correlate with changes in bone marrow cellularity. However, these findings do not predict a favorable response to treatment.[38]

CHRONIC LEUKEMIAS.   In contrast to the acute leukemias, the malignant cell line in the chronic leukemias has a limited capacity for differentiation and function in the initial stages of the disease process. As the disease progresses, thrombocytopenia and granulocytopenia develop, as they do in patients with acute leukemia. Compared with acute leukemias, the chronic leukemias are characterized by a long course with prolonged survival. Chemotherapy, which is used aggressively in acute myelogenous leukemia and produces significant bone marrow hypoplasia or aplasia, has a secondary role in the management of chronic leukemias, which tend to have a more indolent course.

Chronic Lymphocytic Leukemia.   Chronic lymphocytic leukemia represents the most common form of leukemia in the United States; it is twice as common as chronic myelogenous leukemia. Ninety percent of patients with chronic lymphocytic leukemia are older than 50 years of age, and the disease shows a male predilection.[39] Lymph node involvement is present in the majority of patients. Chronic lymphocytic leukemia is characterized by abnormal clones of immunologically incompetent lymphocytes (Fig. 15-19). Patients may be asymptomatic or the disease may be stable at the time of diagnosis; in this case, treatment with alkylating agents is withheld. Although bone marrow analysis is not required to establish the diagnosis, examination reveals a hypercellular marrow with morphologically mature lymphocytes.

Myeloproliferative Disorders.   The myeloproliferative disorders, a form of chronic leukemia, are a group of syndromes characterized by abnormal proliferation of bone marrow cell lines, which all arise from a common pluripotential stem cell. These stem cells produce the progenitor erythroid, granulocytic, monocytic, and megakaryocytic cell lines. The myeloproliferative syndromes include polycythemia vera, primary myelofibrosis with myeloid metaplasia, essential thrombocythemia, and chronic myelogenous leukemia. All of these disorders result in new clones that have a proliferative advantage over the normal marrow cells, which they gradually replace, and all have genetic instability, which

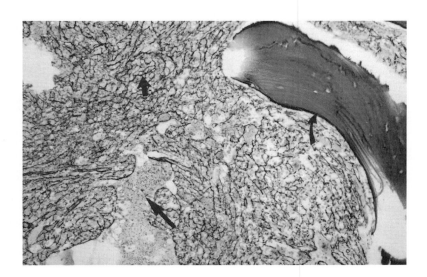

FIGURE 15-17. In myelofibrosis, bone marrow displays abundant reticulin fibers (*short arrow*). Vascular sinusoids (*long arrow*) and trabecular bone (*curved arrow*) can also be seen (silver reticulin; original magnification ×150).

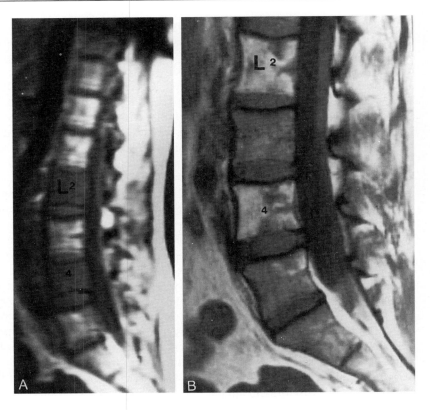

FIGURE 15-18. Marrow response to chemotherapy. T1-weighted images of the lumbar spine (**A**) prechemotherapy and (**B**) postchemotherapy for metastatic colonic carcinoma. Metastatic disease demonstrates low signal intensity at L2 and L4 prior to chemotherapy, and high signal intensity fatty replacement after chemotherapy. Adjacent uninvolved vertebral bodies also show a flip-flop in signal intensity as the red marrow is activated.

predisposes to the development of an acute leukemia. The probability of progression to acute leukemia is greatest in chronic myelogenous leukemia leading to chronic myelogenous leukemia in blast crisis.[40]

The diagnostic features of chronic myelogenous leukemia are the Philadelphia chromosome marker (a translocation between chromosomes 9 and 22) and decreased leukocyte alkaline phosphatase activity in circulating granulocytes. Chronic myelogenous leukemia in blast crisis represents 20% of acute leukemias and usually occurs in the fourth decade of life. Histopathologically, the bone marrow shows granulocytic hyperplasia with marked hypercellular-

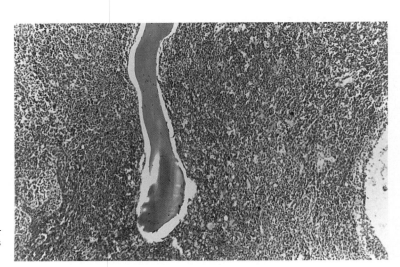

FIGURE 15-19. Chronic myelogenous leukemia. Hypercellular marrow consisting largely of myeloid precursors (H & E; original magnification ×100).

ity, an increased myeloid to erythroid cell ratio, and variable fibrosis.[39,41] Splenomegaly, which is sometimes massive, is found in nearly all cases. Chemotherapy does not increase survival time in chronic myelogenous leukemia, and induction of remission is not possible without bone marrow transplantation.

Splenomegaly, a leukoerythroblastic peripheral smear, and fibrotic marrow with occasional osteosclerosis characterize agnogenic myeloid metaplasia with primary myelofibrosis.[42] The marrow fibrosis commonly results in a dry aspirate. Bone marrow biopsy demonstrates hypercellularity with an increased number of megakaryocytes, increased fibrosis, and decreased fat content (Fig. 15-20). The cause of the myelofibrosis appears to be related to growth factor and factor IV produced by abnormal megakaryocytes.[43] Vascular clumps of hematopoietic cells are found in distended marrow sinusoids. Increased hemosiderin may be present, secondary to repeated blood transfusions to correct associated anemia or to loss of iron uptake due to lack of effective erythropoiesis.

Secondary causes of myelofibrosis are numerous and include metastatic carcinoma, leukemia, lymphomas, tuberculosis, Gaucher's disease, Paget's disease, irradiation, and toxin exposure.[40]

Magnetic Resonance Appearance. Most chronic leukemias tend not to involve yellow marrow areas, and, in adults, are characterized by a moderate to marked decrease in red marrow signal on T1-weighted images (Figs. 15-21 through 15-23). Since red to yellow marrow conversion is complete in adults, leukemic involvement is more likely to be identified in the axial skeleton, pelvis, and proximal femurs. In children, leukemic involvement is more likely to be identified in the more peripheral sites of red marrow stores, such as the metaphysis, with diaphysial or epiphysial extension. Marrow cellularity can also be noninvasively assessed with MR imaging.

In the acute phase of chronic leukemia, particularly in chronic myelogenous leukemia patients in blast crisis, there is almost complete replacement of both red and yellow marrow areas. The decreased signal on T1-weighted sequences represents replacement of marrow fat by tumor cells, which have a significantly longer T1 relaxation time. On STIR images, tumor cells appear as areas of white on a black or gray background.

Severe anemias or other marrow invasive processes may have a similar MR appearance. Myeloma is rather variable, but is generally less symmetrical, more patchy, and irregular in distribution.

In primary myelofibrosis, T1-weighted images show patchy marrow involvement with low signal intensity on T1- and T2-weighted images (Fig. 15-24). T2*-weighted images have been used to evaluate areas of susceptibility where fibrous tissue and hemosiderin have been identified. With STIR techniques, the imaging characteristics of areas of involvement are identical to those of normal hematopoietic marrow (ie, intermediate to mild increased signal intensity). T2*-weighted images, however, do not display typical red marrow imaging characteristics (ie, isointensity with surrounding fat marrow).

Hairy Cell Leukemia. Hairy cell leukemia, representing 2% of all leukemias, is a form of chronic leukemia that evolves from B lymphocytes.[39] It typically occurs in men and classically presents as pancytopenia with splenomegaly. In hairy cell leukemia, the distribution of marrow involvement is irregular and patchy, with a propensity for focal marrow involvement. Focal or extensive involvement with reticulin limits productive marrow aspirations. Bone core biopsy is the definitive diagnostic procedure, and reveals mononuclear cells in clusters or sheets within a fine reticulin mesh in a patchy or diffuse pattern. The marrow may be

text continues on page 1181

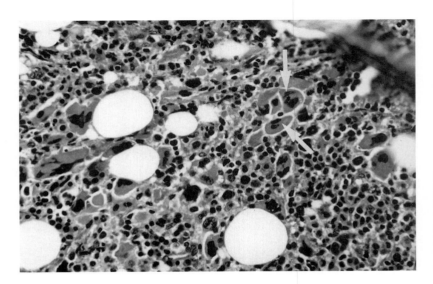

FIGURE 15-20. In myeloproliferative disorders (the cellular phase of agnogenic myeloid metaplasia with primary myelofibrosis), the bone marrow is hypercellular, with an 85:15 cell-to-fat ratio. Abnormal megakaryocytes are increased in number and tend to cluster (*arrows*). Megakaryocytes secrete factors responsible for the extensive marrow fibrosis seen in late stages of the disease (H & E; original magnification ×400).

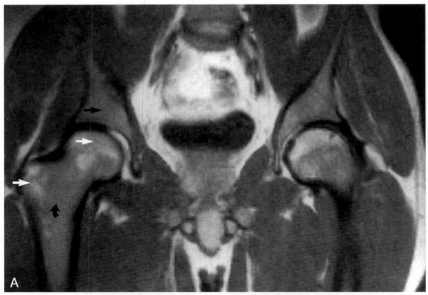

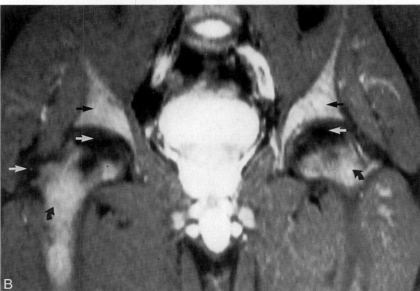

FIGURE 15-21. In chronic myelogenous leukemia, diffuse marrow involvement infiltrates regions of previous red marrow stores in the femurs (*curved arrows*) and acetabulum (*straight black arrows*), and demonstrates (**A**) low signal intensity on a T1-weighted image and (**B**) high signal intensity on a corresponding STIR image. The sites where yellow marrow is spared (the greater trochanter and femoral epiphysis) demonstrate high signal intensity on the T1-weighted image and low signal intensity (from the nulled fat signal) on the STIR sequence (*white arrows*) (**A:** TR, 600 msec; TE, 20 msec; **B:** TR, 1400 msec; TI, 125 msec; TE, 40 msec).

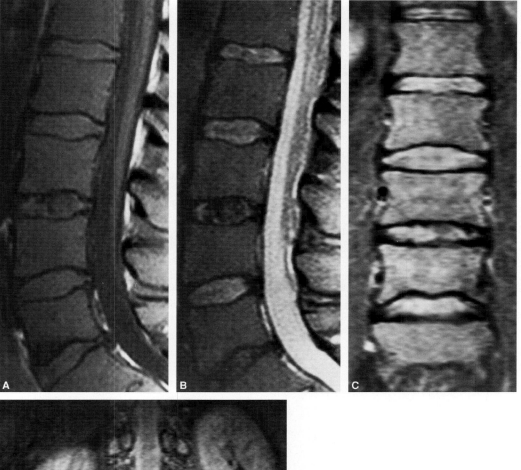

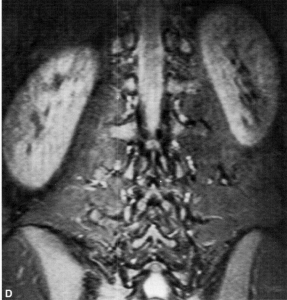

FIGURE 15-22. (A) Chronic myelogenous leukemia with hypointense marrow signal (isointense to the intervertebral disks) on T1-weighted sagittal image. (B) An unremarkable conventional T2-weighted sagittal image. (C) A coronal STIR sequence clearly demonstrates diffuse hyperintensity of the lumbar vertebral bodies. Most leukemias, except those in relapse or hairy cell, present with this diffuse pattern. (D) Abnormal high signal intensity marrow on a coronal STIR imaging approaches that of the kidney and cerebrospinal fluid. The marrow obtained from a posterior iliac crest biopsy is representative of marrow elsewhere.

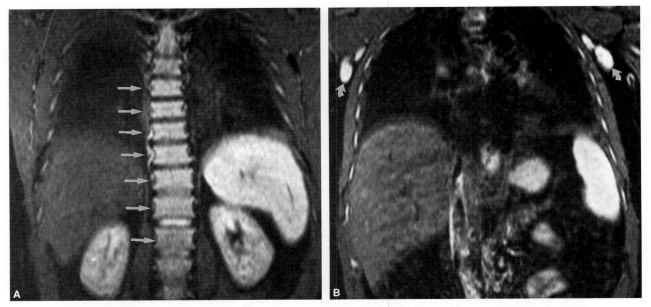

FIGURE 15-23. Chronic lymphocytic leukemia (CLL) in a 52-year-old man. This case is typical of CLL, showing the homogeneous hyperintensity of marrow (*straight arrows*) **(A)** as well as associated axillary adenopathy (*curved arrows*) **(B)** (STIR coronal images).

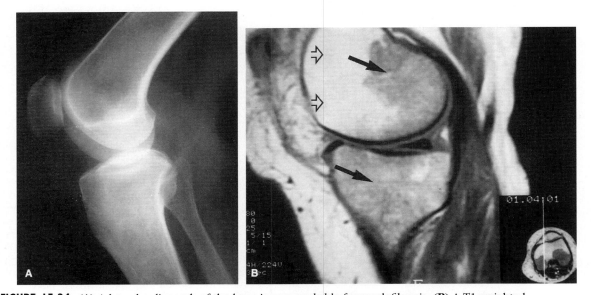

FIGURE 15-24. **(A)** A lateral radiograph of the knee is unremarkable for myelofibrosis. **(B)** A T1-weighted sagittal image shows bright signal intensity normal fatty marrow (*open arrows*) and low signal intensity areas of myelofibrotic marrow (*solid arrows*) (TR, 980 msec; TE, 25 msec). *continued*

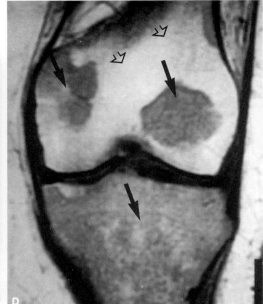

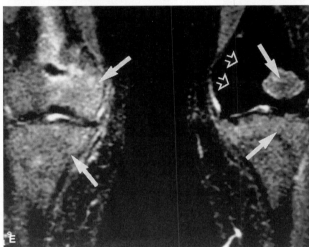

FIGURE 15-24. *Continued.* (**C**) The corresponding T2*-weighted sagittal image shows intermediate signal intensity normal fatty marrow (*open arrows*) and dark signal intensity myelofibrosis (*solid arrows*). The susceptibility of fibrous tissue and hemosiderin contributes to the extreme dark marrow signal intensity (TR, 850 msec; TE, 20 msec; flip angle, 30°). Coronal (**D**) T1-weighted and (**E**) STIR images characterize the patchy involvement of myelofibrosis (*solid arrows*) in contrast to normal fatty marrow (*open arrows*). Fatty marrow is black on the STIR image, whereas myelofibrosis displays intermediate signal intensity resembling red marrow. This may be secondary to compensatory hematopoiesis (**D**: TR, 980 msec; TE, 25 msec; **E**: TR, 1500 msec; TI, 100 msec; TE, 40 msec).

hypercellular or hypocellular[44] (Fig. 15-25). Hairy cells are reactive to tartrate resistant acid phosphatase, which distinguishes hairy cell leukemia from other lymphoproliferative malignancies.[45] MR imaging demonstrates both a patchy lymphoma-like marrow pattern and a second pattern with a diffuse marrow infiltrate that resembles the distribution of chronic myelogenous leukemia[46] (Fig. 15-26).

Hematopoietic Growth Factors

Recent advances in biomolecular research have contributed to the isolation and molecular cloning of the CSFs, which are capable of stimulating bone marrow hematopoietic progenitor cells. Recombinant granulocyte macrophage–colony stimulating factor (sargromostim, GM-CSF) and

granulocyte–colony stimulating factor (filgrastim, G-CSF) have been used to stimulate neutrophil white cell production in many clinical situations including aplastic anemia, myelodysplasia, idiopathic neutropenia (Fig. 15-27), and cyclic neutropenia. These drugs have also been used following myelotoxic chemotherapy for disorders such as pediatric musculoskeletal tumors and breast carcinomas.[47,48] The hematopoietic growth factors predominately induce granulocytosis. Changes in bone marrow treated with GM-CSF and G-CSF include increased marrow cellularity with a significant prominence of myeloid precursors, an appearance which may histologically mimic a myeloproliferative disorder.[49,50]

Reconversion from fatty to hematopoietic marrow may simulate diffuse bone marrow disease by showing hypointensity on T1-weighted images and diffuse hyperintensity on

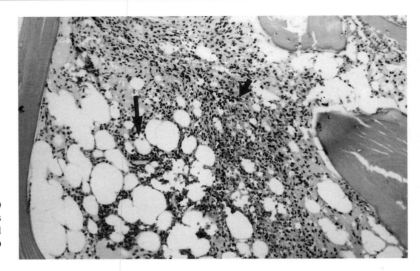

FIGURE 15-25. Bone marrow cellularity is low (ie, 40:60 cell-to-fat ratio) in hairy cell leukemia. Mononuclear cells (*short arrow*) enveloped in reticulin form solid areas and infiltrate between the remaining fat cells (*large arrow*) (H & E; original magnification ×100).

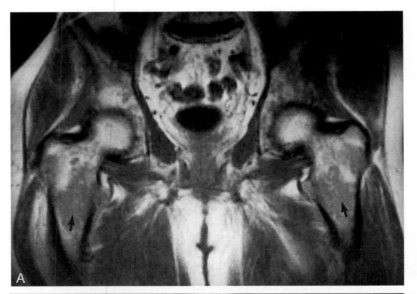

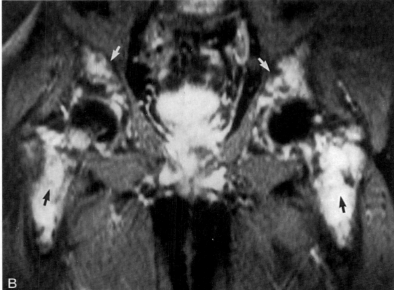

FIGURE 15-26. The patchy pattern of marrow involvement in hairy cell leukemia mimics the appearance of lymphoma. Leukemic infiltration demonstrates low signal intensity (*black arrows*) on a T1-weighted image (**A**) and high signal intensity (*all arrows*) on a STIR sequence (**B**) (**A**: TR, 600 msec; TE, 20 msec; **B**: TR, 1400 msec; TI, 125 msec; TE, 40 msec).

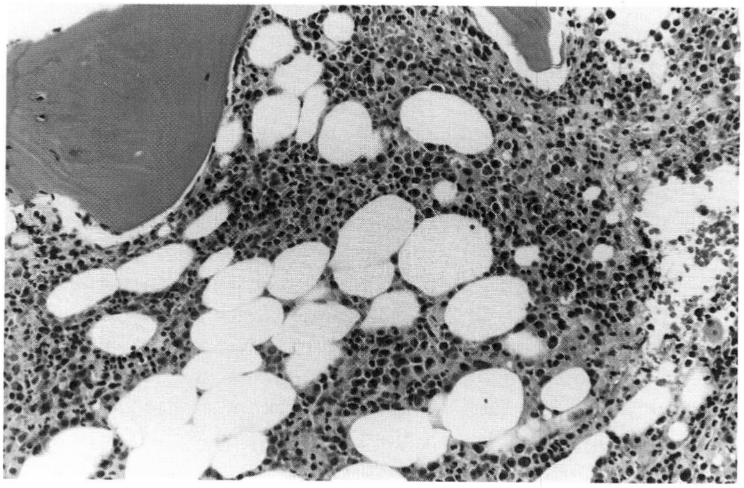

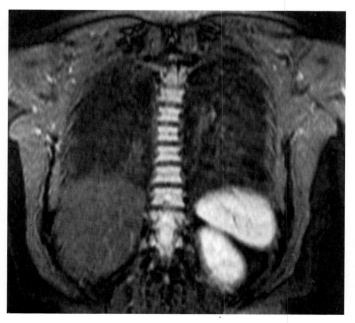

FIGURE 15-27. Idiopathic neutropenia after colony stimulating factor therapy. Immature myeloid precursors can be seen in the interstitial space (H & E; original magnification ×400).

STIR sequences (Fig. 15-28). MR marrow changes usually follow increases in peripheral blood neutrophil levels. The proximal femoral metaphysis and spine are common sites of marrow reconversion.

Bone Marrow Transplantation

Over the last decade, treatment of hematologic malignancies, including the use of maximum dosage multiagent chemotherapy or radiation therapy, has become progressively more intensive. However, maximally intensive multiagent chemotherapeutic regimens result in significant side effects, notably lethal bone marrow cytotoxicity. Bone marrow transplantation is an attempt to circumvent this side effect by providing stem cells to repopulate normal marrow elements. Marrow available for transplantation is of three types: syngeneic (ie, from an identical twin), allogeneic (ie, from an HLA matched donor), and autologous (ie, from the patient).[51] In addition to leukemia treatment, autologous bone marrow transplantation can be used in the management of solid neoplasms such as ovarian tumors, testicular tumors, breast cancers, small cell carcinoma of the lung, Hodgkin's disease, and non-Hodgkin's lymphoma. Preliminary results are encouraging, and increased use of bone marrow transplantation, in conjunction with aggressive chemotherapy, is anticipated.[52]

FIGURE 15-28. Chemotherapy with G-CSF in a 52-year-old woman with inflammatory carcinoma of the breast. This pattern of hyperintensity on STIR may also be seen in patients who are treated with G-CSF after bone marrow transplantation and chemotherapy (when blood counts have "bottomed out"). G-CSF produces hyperintensity which simulates diffuse marrow malignancies or leukemia. Bone marrow biopsy may be recommended in this situation.

PROCEDURE. Prior to bone marrow transplantation, the patient is treated with standard chemotherapy, which ideally induces a state of remission. To eradicate any residual neoplastic cells, the patient then undergoes intensive high-dose chemotherapy, either alone or in combination with total-body irradiation. This also eradicates the patient's immune system, preventing graft resistance in the case of an allogeneic transplantation. After ablation therapy, patients receive donor marrow by intravenous therapy. Histopathologic evidence of stem cell engraftment in the bone marrow is first seen as small clusters of erythroid cells, appearing 1 or 2 weeks after transplantation. Engraftment comprised of erythroid and granulocytic cells is usually seen by 3 weeks. Blood counts start to rise 4 to 8 weeks after transplantation, and normocellular marrow is usually achieved 8 to 12 weeks after transplantation. In the case of autologous bone marrow transplantation, the patient's own marrow is harvested after the induction of a remission state and cryopreserved for later infusion. Various ex vitro techniques (such as centrifugation, monoclonal antibodies, and pharmacologic manipulation) are available, and the ability to purge autologous marrow of contaminating neoplastic cells prior to reinfusion is continuously being improved.[51,53]

GRAFT-VERSUS-HOST DISEASE. Graft-versus-host disease, one of the major complications of marrow transplantation, may occur with allogeneic HLA-matched marrow. It occurs when there is an immunologic reaction by the engrafted T cells against the tissues of the host, particularly the skin, gastrointestinal tract, and liver.[54] The likelihood of graft-versus-host disease increases with patient age, which usually limits this form of marrow transplant to patients younger than 40 years of age. Recent research is exploring the possibility of ex vivo T-lymphocyte depletion from the donor marrow before transplantation to prevent graft-versus-host disease.[55]

MAGNETIC RESONANCE APPEARANCE. Bone marrow transplantation produces characteristic changes on MR studies of vertebral bone marrow.[56] MR changes in the spine can be identified as early as 3 weeks posttransplantation. On T1-weighted images, there is a peripheral zone of intermediate signal intensity, representing repopulated hematopoietic cells, and a central zone of high signal intensity fatty marrow. Short TI inversion recovery images show a reciprocal change, with increased signal intensity in the peripheral zone of hematopoietic cells, and decreased signal intensity in the central zone, because signal from fat is nulled. The alternating zones form a characteristic band pattern. Loss of this band may signify relapse, as a homogeneous area of decreased signal intensity replaces the vertebral body. Repopulation of hematopoietic marrow follows vascular sinusoid pathways, which enter the periphery of the vertebral body, producing the peripheral region of intermediate signal intensity. These sinusoids drain into the basivertebral vein located in the central portion of the vertebral body. On STIR images

used to evaluate repopulated marrow in the spine and pelvis after ablation therapy and bone marrow transplant, it is possible to differentiate red marrow from recurrent tumor (Figs. 15-29 and 15-30).

In patients with chronic myelogenous leukemia, post-transplant increases in marrow signal intensity have been observed in the pelvis and proximal femur, as compared with pretreatment T1-weighted images.[17] The intensity of signal, however, is less than that seen in disease-free marrow. Hypoplastic fatty marrow may be seen prior to hematopoietic repopulation (Fig. 15-31). Bone abnormalities related to total-body irradiation in long term survivors of bone marrow transplantation for childhood leukemia have also been described.[57] Skeletal abnormalities include osteochondroma, metaphyseal abnormalities (sclerosis and vertical striations), and slipped femoral capital epiphysis.

Malignant Lymphoma

Lymphomas represent neoplastic proliferation of the lymphoid cells that normally reside in primary lymphoid tissue such as lymph nodes. The two major types of lymphomas are Hodgkin's disease and non-Hodgkin's lymphoma. Bone marrow examination is an important component of the staging process for patients with malignant lymphoma. Bone marrow involvement is higher in non-Hodgkin's lymphoma (ranging from 25% to 90%) than in Hodgkin's disease (5% to 15%).[58] Demonstration of marrow involvement may advance the stage of disease and contraindicate the use of nodal radiotherapy. After treatment, marrow study is crucial in following the patient for evidence of therapeutic response or lymphomatous relapse.

HODGKIN'S DISEASE. In its most common presentation, Hodgkin's disease is distinguished by its localization to a single group of lymph nodes (ie, cervical, cervicoclavicular, mediastinal, or paraaortic); bimodal age distribution; and infrequent extranodal (eg, bone marrow, CNS, gastrointestinal tract, or skin) involvement. Only when malignant cells enter the blood via a major lymphatic duct does the disease invade the bone marrow—an occurrence that portends a potentially fatal outcome. The disease is usually not generalized in the marrow, but presents focally in nodules (Fig. 15-32). On a microscopic level, Hodgkin's lesions in the bone marrow vary from primarily cellular to primarily fibrotic. The unifying histopathologic feature of Hodgkin's disease is the presence of Reed-Sternberg cells, which are large cells with a bilobed nucleus exhibiting prominent nucleoli set in a polycellular background of inflammatory cells and often fibrosis (Fig. 15-33). The exact cell of origin in Hodgkin's disease is still under debate.

Although four distinct histologic subtypes of Hodgkin's disease have been identified (lymphocyte predominant, nodular sclerosis, mixed cellularity, and lymphocyte depleted), the prognosis of Hodgkin's disease rests primarily in the clinical and pathologic stage of disease rather than its histologic subtype.[59]

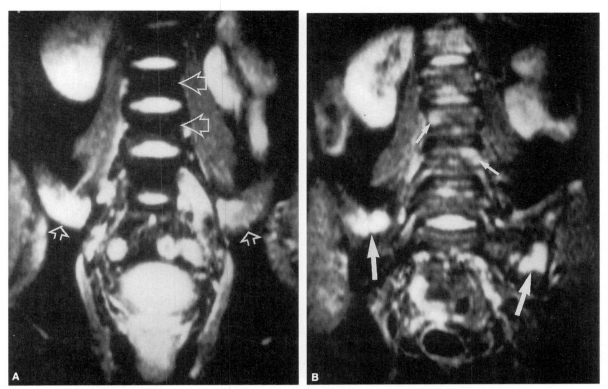

FIGURE 15-29. Recurrent tumor after bone marrow transplantation is seen on coronal STIR images. (**A**) After total body irradiation and bone marrow transplant, there is severe marrow hypoplasia (ie, dark fatty marrow; *large open arrows*) and biopsy edema (*small open arrows*). (**B**) Nine months later, the marrow has been repopulated with hematopoietic cells, which demonstrate intermediate signal intensity, and is spotted with hyperintense recurrent tumor (*arrows*) (TR, 1400 msec; TI, 125 msec; TE, 40 msec).

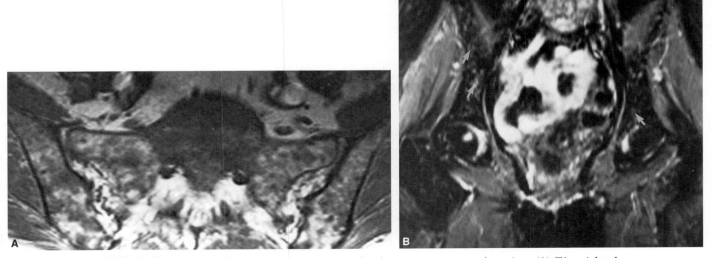

FIGURE 15-30. Recurrent breast carcinoma 1 year after bone marrow transplantation. (**A**) T1-weighted (hypointense) axial image and (**B**) coronal STIR image (hyperintense) demonstrate a miliary pattern of marrow relapse (*arrows*). STIR images are useful since marrow fibrosis or focal sclerotic residual from treated disease may be indistinguishable from recurrent tumor on T1-weighted spin-echo images.

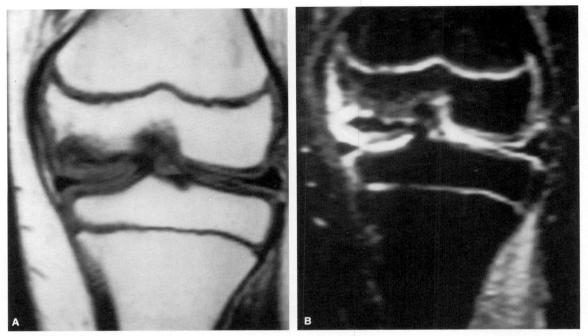

FIGURE 15-31. Knee pain in a 13-year-old girl after a bone marrow transplant for chronic myelogenous leukemia. Hypoplastic marrow demonstrates bright fat marrow signal intensity on coronal T1-weighted images (**A**) and dark fat marrow signal intensity on STIR images (**B**) in the metaphyseal regions of the femur and tibia. A focus of symptomatic osteonecrosis can be identified in the medial femoral condyle (*arrows*) (**A**: TR, 600 msec; TE, 30 msec; **B**: TR, 1400 msec; TI, 125 msec; TE, 40 msec).

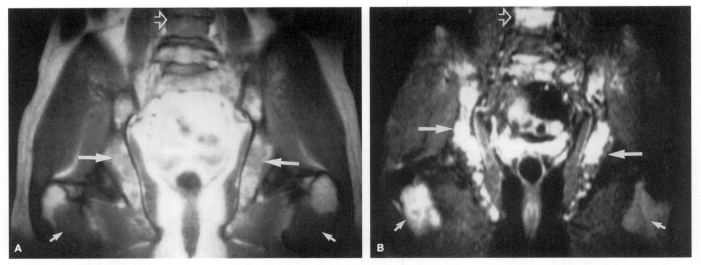

FIGURE 15-32. In the nodular presentation of Hodgkin's disease, there is severe patchy marrow involvement which resembles hairy cell leukemia. Coronal (**A**) T1-weighted and (**B**) STIR images show vertebral body involvement (*open arrow*), iliac crest tumor (*large solid arrows*), and proximal femur tumor (*small solid arrows*) (**A**: TR, 600 msec; TE, 30 msec; **B**: TR, 1400 msec; TI, 140 msec; TE, 40 msec).

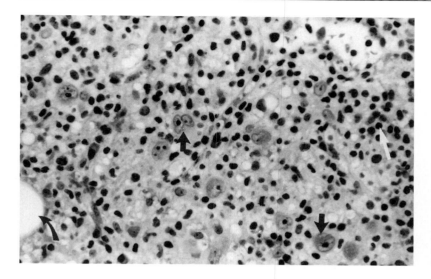

FIGURE 15-33. High magnification photomicrograph of bone marrow displays Hodgkin's cells (*straight black arrows*) scattered among a fibrocellular background. The smaller cells consist of a polymorphous population of lymphocytes, plasma cells, and histiocytes (*white arrows*). Fat cells (*curved black arrow*) are decreased in the areas of Hodgkin's involvement (H & E; original magnification ×400).

NON-HODGKIN'S LYMPHOMA. Malignant lymphomas other than Hodgkin's disease are referred to as non-Hodgkin's lymphoma. Within this classification is a diverse group of diseases that span various morphologic and immunologic types. They range from low-grade indolent processes to highly aggressive lesions which, if left untreated, are rapidly fatal. The various types of non-Hodgkin's lymphoma differ in their response to therapy. In contrast to Hodgkin's disease, the prognosis of non-Hodgkin's lymphoma is more directly related to histologic subtype than to the clinical and pathologic stage.

Low-grade non-Hodgkin's lymphoma, notably small cleaved cell lymphoma (Fig. 15-34) and well-differentiated small lymphocytic cell lymphoma (Fig. 15-35), has a high incidence of marrow involvement. When initially diagnosed, low-grade non-Hodgkin's lymphoma almost always involves widespread lymph nodes at multiple sites in an asymmetrical distribution above and below the diaphragm. In 50% of cases, the bone marrow is affected at the time of diagnosis. On a microscopic level, small cleaved cell lymphomas tend to be focal, patchy, and form nodules in a peritrabecular location. Splenic involvement is usually in the form of small miliary nodules centered in the white pulp zones.[60] Marrow involvement in well-differentiated small lymphocytic lymphoma is most commonly diffuse or interstitial.

High-grade non-Hodgkin's lymphoma (including large cell lymphoma) may be designated as histiocytic or reticulum cell (large cell), immunoblastic, lymphoblastic, Burkitt's, or non-Burkitt's lymphoma. Morphologically and immunologically, high-grade non-Hodgkin's lymphoma is the most heterogeneous type of lymphoma. It is the most common primary lymphoma arising in bone, and the type that occurs most often in acquired immunodeficiency syndrome (AIDS) (Figs. 15-36 and 15-37). In contrast to the low-grade (ie, small cleaved cell) lymphoma, microscopic marrow involvement in high-grade lymphoma can be focal or widespread, but there is no peritrabecular bony preference.

A rapidly growing mass at a single nodal or extranodal site is the typical clinical presentation in large cell lymphoma

text continues on page 1190

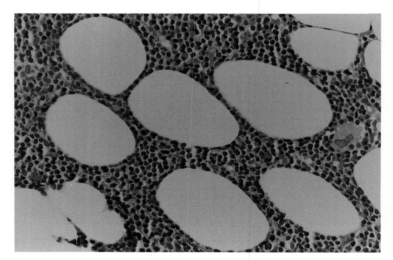

FIGURE 15-34. Malignant lymphoma, predominantly small cleaved cell type. Small cleaved lymphocytes can be seen in the interstitium (H & E; original magnification ×400).

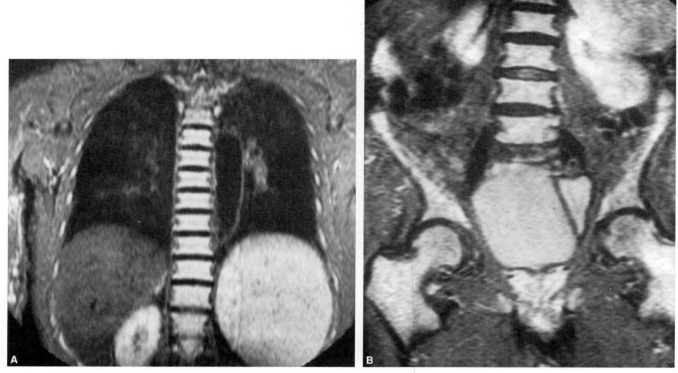

FIGURE 15-35. Low-grade lymphoma in an anemic patient with diffuse marrow involvement. Initial attempts at marrow biopsy produced dry taps. The marrow hyperintensity on these STIR coronal images through the spine (**A**) and pelvis (**B**) were subsequently confirmed as marrow tumor.

FIGURE 15-36. High-grade non-Hodgkin's lymphoma in AIDS. A histologically confirmed large cell lymphoma can be seen on sagittal T1-weighted (**A**) and STIR (**B**) images. Soft-tissue extension (*curved white arrows*), vertebral body infiltration (*large black arrow*), and pedicle infiltration (*small black arrow*) are best seen on the STIR image (**A**: TR, 500 msec; TE, 20 msec; **B**: TR, 2000 msec; TI, 180 msec; TE, 40 msec). T1-weighted axial images before (**C**) and after (**D**) Gd-DTPA administration demonstrate the extent of retroperitoneal soft-tissue (*curved arrow*) and epidural (*straight arrow*) extension (**C, D**: TR, 500 msec; TE, 20 msec).   *continued*

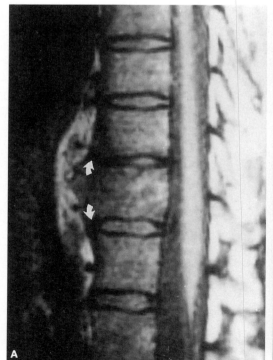

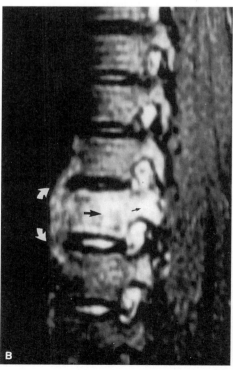

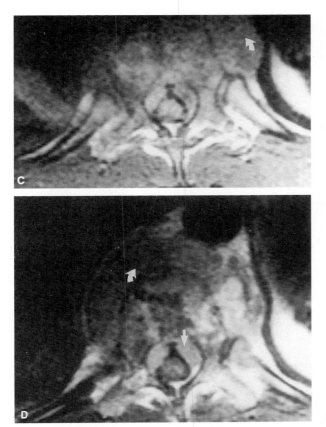

FIGURE 15-36. *Continued*

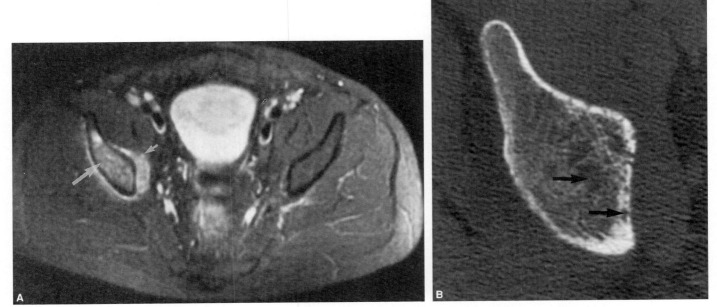

FIGURE 15-37. Large cell non-Hodgkin's lymphoma as presented in AIDS. **(A)** Right iliac bone marrow infiltration (*large arrow*) is hyperintense on first spin-echo STIR image. Perilesional edema and soft extension are associated (*small arrow*). **(B)** Corresponding CT demonstrates aggressive features of trabecular and cortical destruction (*arrows*).

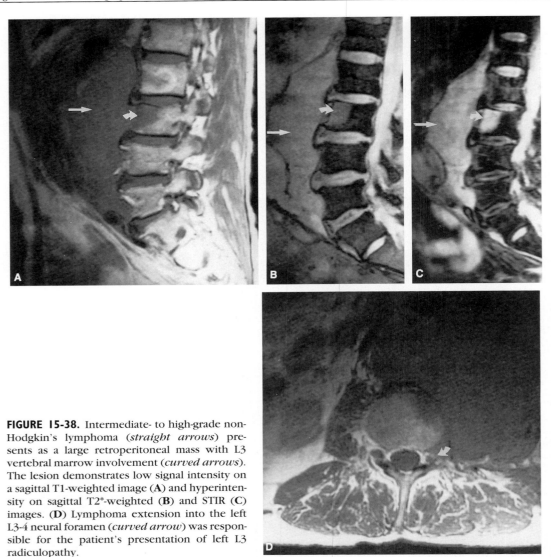

FIGURE 15-38. Intermediate- to high-grade non-Hodgkin's lymphoma (*straight arrows*) presents as a large retroperitoneal mass with L3 vertebral marrow involvement (*curved arrows*). The lesion demonstrates low signal intensity on a sagittal T1-weighted image (**A**) and hyperintensity on sagittal T2*-weighted (**B**) and STIR (**C**) images. (**D**) Lymphoma extension into the left L3-4 neural foramen (*curved arrow*) was responsible for the patient's presentation of left L3 radiculopathy.

(Fig. 15-38). Liver and spleen involvement, not common at the time of diagnosis, consists of large masses, as opposed to the small miliary nodules typical of low-grade lymphomas. Large cell lymphomas are rapidly fatal if not treated. However, with aggressive multiagent chemotherapy, complete remission can be achieved in 60% to 80% of patients. In contrast, low-grade lymphoma is relatively resistant to chemotherapy, although it exhibits an indolent clinical course.[60]

LYMPHOBLASTIC LYMPHOMA. Lymphoblastic lymphoma, also a high-grade lymphoma, is usually diffuse in the bone marrow. It commonly occurs in adolescence, and represents approximately one third of childhood non-Hodgkin's lymphoma. It often progresses to extensive, diffuse bone marrow involvement and frank leukemia. The presentation is usually mediastinal.

BURKITT'S LYMPHOMA. Burkitt's lymphoma is another diffuse, high-grade lymphoma (Fig. 15-39). In nonendemic areas such as the United States, it usually occurs in older children and presents as a rapidly growing abdominal mass with marrow involvement, malignant pleural effusions, and ascites.

MAGNETIC RESONANCE FINDINGS. Unlike leukemia, lymphoma tends to form nodules or marrow tumors[61,62] (Fig. 15-40), although it may at times be diffuse and simulate leukemia on MR images[63] (Fig. 15-41). When diffuse, it can usually be detected by posterior crest marrow biopsy. Frequently, however, sampling error produces a negative marrow biopsy finding, especially when lymphomatous involvement is asymmetric (Fig. 15-42). Bone scanning re-

text continues on page 1194

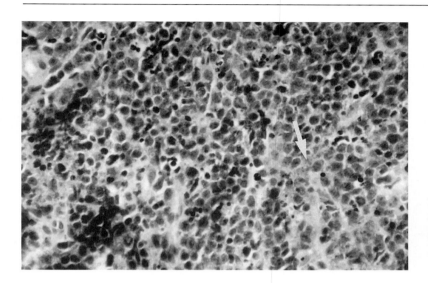

FIGURE 15-39. High magnification photomicrograph of bone marrow that has been extensively replaced by a monotonous population of round immature cells displaying the cytologic features of Burkitt's high-grade lymphoma. There is granular individual cell necrosis (*arrows*) between the cells (H & E; original magnification ×400).

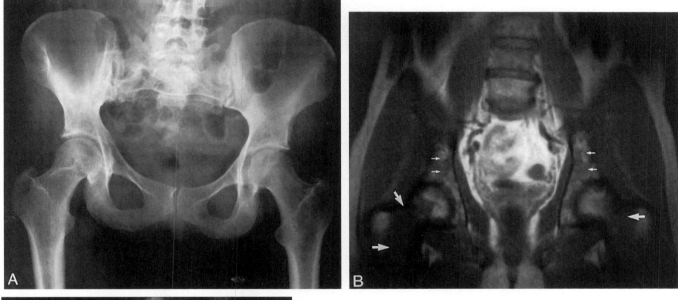

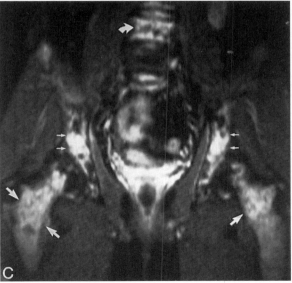

FIGURE 15-40. (A) An anteroposterior radiograph of the pelvis is negative for nodular pattern lymphoma. (B) On a T1-weighted coronal image the proximal femurs (*large arrows*) and acetabula (*small arrows*) display nonspecific low signal intensity. The fatty marrow of the epiphysis and greater trochanter is spared (TR, 600 msec; TE, 20 msec). (C) On a STIR image, there is high signal intensity patchy nodularity of lymphomatous marrow involvement in the proximal femurs (*large arrows*), acetabulum (*small arrows*), and L4 vertebral body (*curved arrow*). The spared yellow marrow of the greater trochanter and femoral epiphysis appears black (TR, 1400 msec; TI, 125 msec; TE, 40 msec).

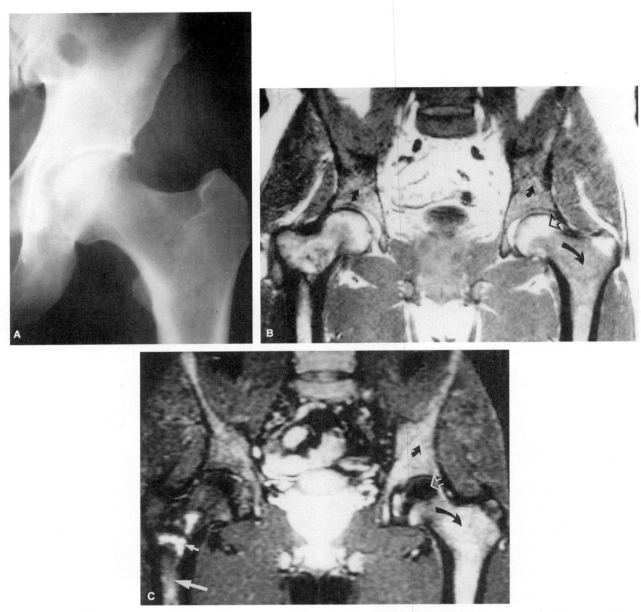

FIGURE 15-41. (A) An anteroposterior radiograph of the left femur and hip is negative for low-grade non-Hodgkin's lymphoma. (B) On a T1-weighted coronal image, diffuse distribution of low signal intensity infiltration, or replacement of normal marrow with histologically proven well-differentiated small lymphocytic cell lymphoma, can be seen. Acetabular (*small curved arrow*) and femoral (*large curved arrow*) sites are shown. Distribution of the tumor corresponds to adult sites of anatomic red marrow. Yellow marrow locations in the femoral head (*open arrow*) and greater trochanter are not involved. The status of the right femur is difficult to assess postradiation. (C) On a coronal STIR image, dark signal intensity postradiation fatty marrow is seen with recurrent tumor (*large solid white arrow*) and postbiopsy fluid (*small solid white arrow*) in the right femur. Hyperintense left acetabular (*small curved arrow*) and femoral (*large curved arrow*) infiltrations are shown on either side of normal femoral head fatty marrow (*open arrow*).

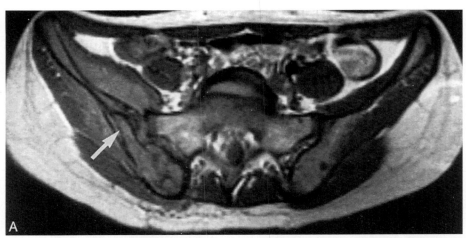

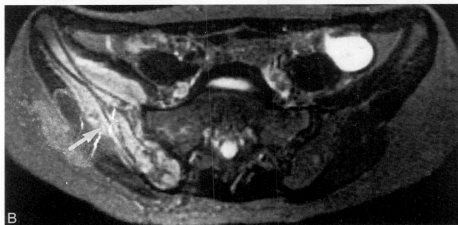

FIGURE 15-42. (A) An asymmetric pattern of low signal intensity lymphoma involving the right ilium (*arrow*) is seen on an intermediate weighted image (TR, 2000 msec; TE, 20 msec). (B) On a T2-weighted image, the lesion demonstrates high signal intensity (*arrow*) (TR, 2000 msec; TE, 60 msec).

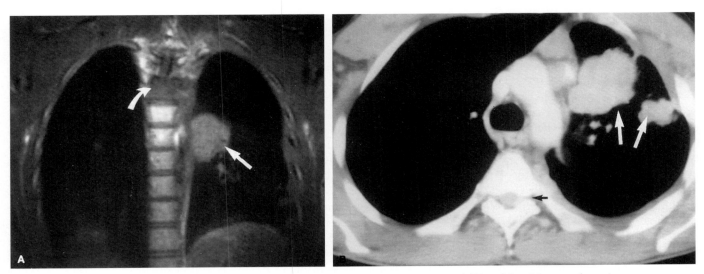

FIGURE 15-43. Recurrent Hodgkin's disease. (A) In a screening coronal T1-weighted image, thoracic vertebral marrow disease is identified in an area of previous irradiation (*curved arrow*). Left hilar adenopathy is also seen (*straight arrow*) (TR, 500 msec; TE, 30 msec). (B) The corresponding CT scan shows hilar involvement (*white arrows*) with equivocal epidural tumor (*black arrow*). T1-weighted sagittal (C) and axial (D) images depict marrow (*arrow* in C) and extensive epidural tumor (*arrow* in D) more accurately than the corresponding CT scans (TR, 600 msec; TE, 30 msec). *continued*

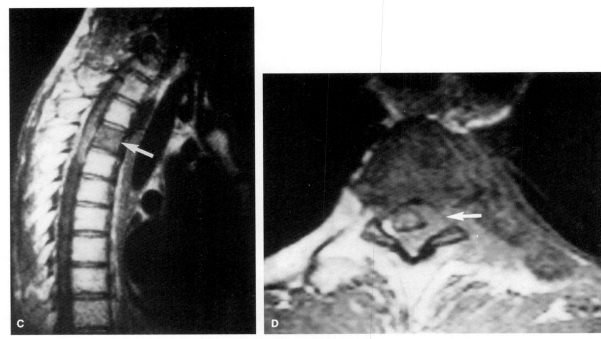

FIGURE 15-43. *Continued*

sults are also frequently negative, even in lymphoma patients with known marrow involvement.

MR imaging, however, has the advantage of being able to sample a large volume of marrow, thus making it possible to detect marrow involvement. Since identification of marrow tumor in patients with lymphoma affects both staging and treatment, this is potentially one of the more important clinical applications for MR imaging of the body. Staging is of particular importance in Hodgkin's disease, because bone marrow involvement portends a potentially fatal outcome and is therefore treated with more aggressive multiagent chemotherapy. Mediastinal tumor is common in the supradiaphragmatic presentation of Hodgkin's disease (Fig. 15-43), and MR imaging can also identify bone marrow involvement not appreciated at the time of diagnosis. An additional benefit of MR imaging, particularly when STIR protocols are used, is the depiction of lymph node invasion (Fig. 15-44). In contrast, CT, although highly accurate for lymph node detection, is insensitive to marrow involvement in the absence of bone destruction. Focal marrow lymphoma may simulate metastatic disease (Fig. 15-45). In contrast to Hodgkin's disease, non-Hodgkin's lymphoma demonstrates early bone marrow involvement.

The AIDS-related lymphomas, which are high grade and of B-cell origin, frequently demonstrate both marrow dissemination and soft-tissue involvement. Short TI inversion recovery contrast is most effective in characterizing these sites of tumor involvement (see Fig. 15-36). MR imaging provides better detail than CT in imaging soft-tissue pathology (Fig. 15-46).

Changes in lumbar vertebral bone marrow have also been characterized on MR scans of patients receiving radi-

ation therapy for Hodgkin's disease.[64,65] In response to treatment with 1500 to 5000 rads, increased signal intensity can be detected on STIR images within 2 weeks. MR changes are thought to reflect marrow edema and necrosis. On T1-weighted images, increased heterogeneity of signal intensity, caused by the predominance of high signal intensity fat, can be identified 3 to 6 weeks postradiation. Late marrow changes, including fatty marrow replacement, occur 6 weeks to 14 months after radiation therapy. On MR scans, these changes are seen as either homogeneous fatty marrow replacement of the vertebral body or as peripheral hematopoietic intermediate signal intensity marrow adjacent to a central zone of fatty marrow. The delineation between irradiated and nonirradiated areas can be sharply defined on STIR images, on which fat displays dark or black signal intensity and adjacent hematopoietic marrow demonstrates intermediate signal intensity. On T1-weighted images, the postradiation identification of low signal intensity vertebral body marrow, especially in the presence of fat marrow signal intensity seen at other levels, is consistent with recurrent disease. T1-weighted and STIR images are most sensitive in identifying recurrent disease in or adjacent to the field of radiation (Fig. 15-47). Coronal T1-weighted and STIR images are also useful in evaluating internal changes in tumor size and recurrent disease in Hodgkin's disease and non-Hodgkin's lymphoma after whole-body irradiation and bone marrow transplantation (Fig. 15-48). Monoclonal antibodies tagged to a radioisotope or chemotherapeutic agent have also been used in lymphoma treatment (Fig. 15-49). On STIR images, red marrow stores can be differentiated from

text continues on page 1198

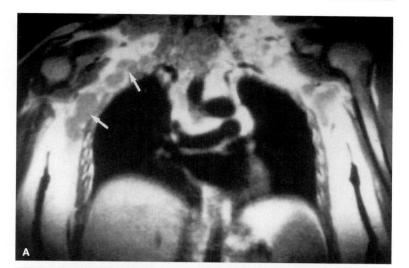

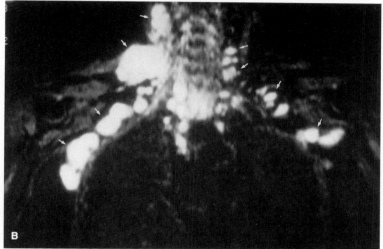

FIGURE 15-44. A 51-year-old woman with aggressive non-Hodgkin's lymphoma (*arrows*). Coronal T1-weighted images (**A**) are not as sensitive as coronal STIR images (**B**) for detection. Nodes and marrow lesions as small as 4 mm can be detected due to their high signal intensity. The marrow is not involved in this patient (**A**: TR, 600 msec; TE, 30 msec; **B**: TR, 1400 msec; TI, 140 msec; TE, 40 msec).

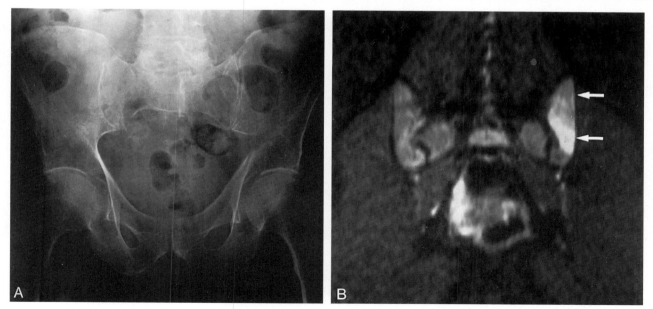

FIGURE 15-45. (**A**) An anteroposterior radiograph is negative for focal pattern lymphoma. (**B**) A STIR sequence shows high signal intensity lymphoma with an asymmetric pattern of marrow involvement (*arrows*) in the posterior ilium (TR 1400 msec; TI 125 msec; TE 40 msec).

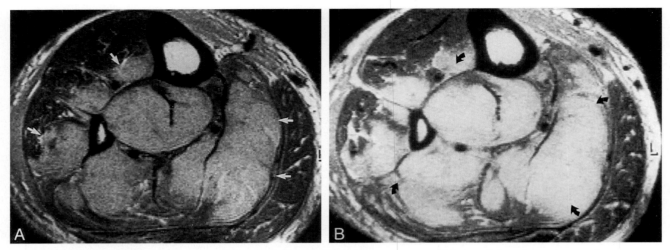

FIGURE 15-46. (**A**) On a T1-weighted axial image, the soft-tissue masses of histiocytic lymphoma (*arrows*) demonstrate intermediate signal intensity (TR, 1000 msec; TE, 40 msec). (**B**) On a T2-weighted sequence, the lesions demonstrate high signal intensity (TR, 2000 msec; TE, 80 msec).

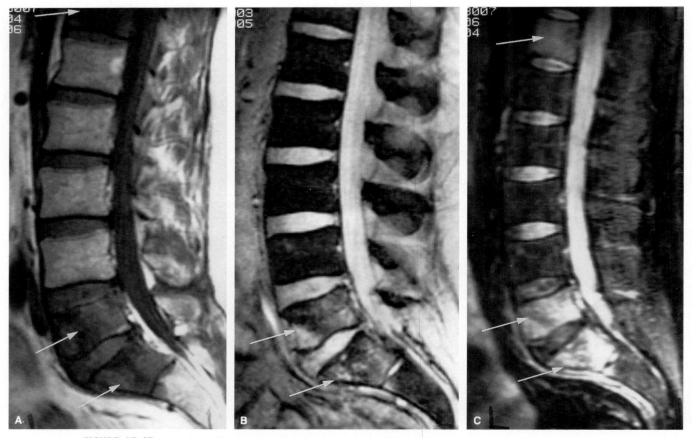

FIGURE 15-47. Hodgkin's disease. Vertebral body marrow infiltration (*arrows*) can be seen in the lumbar and lower thoracic spine on (**A**) T1-weighted, (**B**) T2*-weighted, and (**C**) STIR images. Marrow involvement was clinically unsuspected in this patient, whose status was postsubtotal nodal radiation. Normally, the risk for marrow involvement is higher in patients with advanced disease than it is at the time of diagnosis (**A**: TR, 600 msec; TE, 20 msec; **B**: TR, 400 msec; TE, 15 msec; flip angle, 20°; **C**: TR, 200 msec; TI, 160 msec; TE, 40 msec).

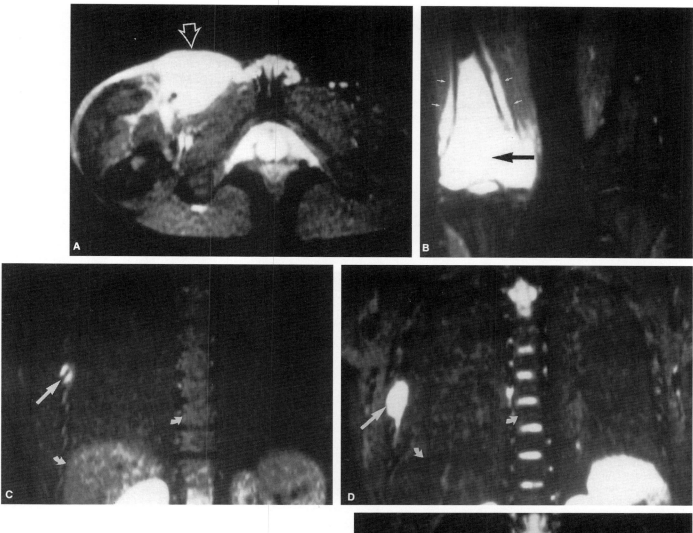

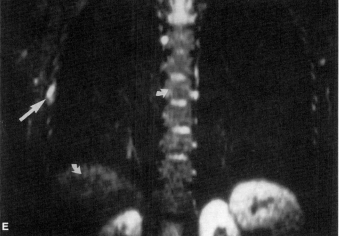

FIGURE 15-48. (**A**) Hyperintense right inguinal adenopathy (*open arrow*) is seen on axial STIR images in a boy with diffuse histiocytic lymphoma. (**B**) STIR sequence also displays a distal femoral tumor (*large arrow*) with adjacent periosteal hyperintensity, either reactive or secondary to tumor infiltration (*small arrows*). (**C**) Rib involvement (*straight arrow*) is revealed on a coronal STIR image. Note the normal STIR signal intensity of the liver and vertebral marrow (*curved arrows*). (**D**) After whole body radiation and bone marrow transplant, the recently treated rib tumor appears larger and more intense (*straight arrow*) on another coronal STIR image. Note the lower signal intensity in the liver and thoracic marrow (*curved arrows*), which indicates increased fat content. (**E**) Nine months after radiation and bone marrow transplant, residual rib signal intensity (*straight arrow*) is still seen on a coronal STIR image. Such lesions may take 12 months to resolve. Liver and marrow signal intensity have normalized (*curved arrows*).

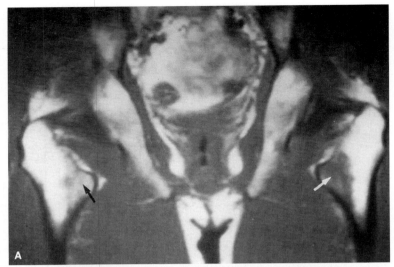

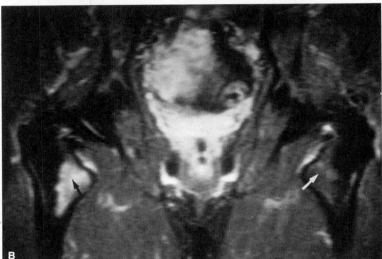

FIGURE 15-49. Non-Hodgkin's lymphoma in a 36-year-old man after monoclonal antibody therapy. **(A)** On a T1-weighted coronal image, a low signal intensity area within the left trochanter simulating tumor (*white arrow*) can be identified. A mild decrease in signal intensity in the right lesser trochanter (*black arrow*) appears less ominous. **(B)** On the corresponding coronal STIR image, a markedly hyperintense tumor is present in the right lesser trochanter (*black arrow*) and a mildly hyperintense normal red marrow signal intensity is seen in the left lesser trochanter (*white arrow*).

lymphoma by the significantly increased signal intensity in lymphomatous infiltration.

In long term fatty replacement of bone marrow after radiation therapy for Hodgkin's disease, studied by Kauczor and colleagues,[66] there is an increase in relative fat signal in the thoracic and lumbar spines, without signs of marrow degeneration, 15 to 126 months after radiation therapy. Nonirradiated pelvic and femoral marrow, however, demonstrates a relative decrease in fat signal intensity, indicating marrow reconversion. In patients receiving radiation therapy for cervical carcinoma, signal intensity changes in pelvic marrow can be detected as early as 8 days after the initiation of radiation therapy. A complete fatty marrow pattern is observed 6 to 8 weeks after radiation therapy.[67] Adjacent nonirradiated marrow demonstrates lesser degrees of similar signal intensity changes on T1-weighted and STIR images.

Histiocytic Proliferative Disorders

HISTIOCYTOSIS X. Three related diseases—eosinophilic granuloma, Letterer-Siwe disease, and Hand-Schüller-Christian disease—are included under the designation histiocytosis X. Although all three represent neoplasia of a special form of histiocyte, known as the Langerhans cell, they differ with respect to the extent of organ involvement and prognosis.

Eosinophilic granuloma, a unifocal bone lesion, is a benign disorder that typically occurs in children and young adults.[68] In some cases, spontaneous healing and fibrosis occur within a year or two of presentation. Other cases require curettage or local irradiation. MR findings in these nonaggressive lesions are characterized by areas of low signal intensity on T1-weighted images and increased signal intensity on T2-weighted images (Fig. 15-50). Long-bone involvement, typically diaphyseal, may affect the metaphysis

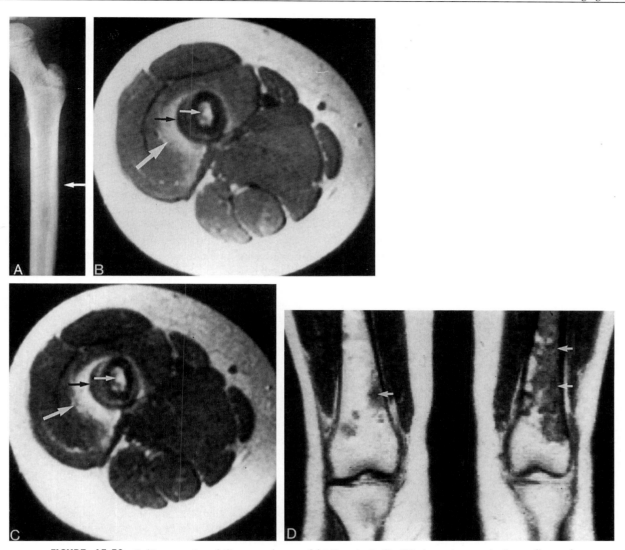

FIGURE 15-50. Solitary eosinophilic granuloma of histiocytosis X. (**A**) An anteroposterior radiograph shows thickened periosteal reaction (*arrow*) along the lateral femoral cortex. Bright signal intensity perilesional edema (*large white arrow*) and marrow involvement (*small white arrow*), and low signal intensity thickened medial femoral cortex (*black arrow*) are seen on (**B**) intermediate weighted and (**C**) T2-weighted images (TR, 2000 msec; TE, 20,60 msec). (**D**) On a T1-weighted coronal image, eosinophilic granuloma of histiocytosis X can be seen involving the femoral diaphysis and metaphysis with patchy areas of low signal intensity histiocytic infiltration (*arrows*) (TR, 600 msec; TE, 20 msec).

or extend to the physeal plate. There may also be localized bone expansion, indicated by a low signal intensity sclerotic peripheral border. Eosinophilic granulomas may be associated with perilesional or peritumoral edema. In the vertebral body, eosinophilic granuloma may present as a vertebral plana with diffuse infiltration of the vertebral body. Typical characteristics on T1- and T2-weighted images, however, are nonspecific for the diagnosis of eosinophilic granuloma. Age, in addition to location and morphology of signal intensity changes, are important in determining a differential diagnosis.

The multifocal form of the disease, known as Hand-Schüller-Christian disease, usually presents in patients younger than 5 years of age. Systemic symptomatology is common; the classic triad of calvarial bone lesions, exophthalmos, and diabetes insipidus (caused by posterior pituitary or hypothalamic involvement) are diagnostic for Hand-Schüller-Christian disease.

The most aggressive form of histiocytosis X is Letterer-Siwe disease, which classically affects infants and young children. It involves virtually all of the organs of the body, including bone marrow. Current chemotherapy has improved the prognosis for this disease; a 40% to 50% 5-year survival rate has been attained.[69]

Myeloma

Multiple myeloma, the most common primary neoplasm of bone, is caused by the uncontrolled proliferation of malignant plasma cells within the marrow.[70] The neoplastic plasma cells secrete nonfunctional monoclonal immunoglobulins, and these immunoglobulins can be measured in the serum or urine to aid in the diagnosis. The plasma cells also produce an osteoclastic stimulating factor, responsible for the skeletal destruction (punched-out osteolytic lesions and diffuse osteopenia) seen in multiple myeloma.[70,71] The peak incidence of multiple myeloma is between 50 and 60 years of age, and the disease is extremely rare in patients younger than 40 years of age. Amyloidosis may occasionally complicate myeloma.

There are two variants of myeloma: the solitary bone plasmocytoma and extramedullary plasmocytoma. Solitary lesions, or plasmacytomas, are more common in young or middle-aged adults, and may be accompanied by back pain and cord compression. The sclerotic presentation of multiple myeloma is rare, and has been termed the *POEMS syndrome* (P for progressive sensorimotor polyneuropathy; O for osteosclerotic bone lesions; E for endocrine abnormalities including diabetic mellitus, adrenal insufficiency and hypothyroidism; M for an increase in serum M protein; and S for skin thickening with increased pigmentation).[72,73]

MAGNETIC RESONANCE APPEARANCE. Imaging is important in the diagnosis of multiple myeloma. However, nuclear scintigraphy using technetium is limited, and there must be significant medullary bone involvement before osteoporosis or lytic lesions can be detected on plain film radiography. Involvement of the marrow is characteristically multifocal—a finding clearly demonstrated on MR scans[74] (Figs. 15-51 and 15-52). The patchy asymmetric process of focal deposits is distinguishable from metastases by signal intensity characteristics and morphology. Multiple myeloma may also present as a complete marrow replacement, simulating leukemia (Fig. 15-53). MR imaging of the spine in early myeloma may show involvement in both symptomatic and asymptomatic patients[68] (Fig. 15-54). Areas of involvement demonstrate low signal intensity on T1-weighted images and bright signal intensity on T2-weighted, STIR, and Gd-DTPA enhanced images.[75] Short TI inversion recovery images demonstrate greater lesion contrast than that seen on corresponding conventional T2-weighted images. The percentage of bone marrow involvement may not correlate with the MR appearance, however.[76]

MR findings in multiple myeloma patients who have responded to chemotherapy include resolution of the abnormal marrow or a persistent marrow abnormality without associated contrast enhancement.[77,78] A pattern of peripheral rim enhancement may also be seen, and it, too, correlates with a positive response to chemotherapy. A partial response to treatment is characterized by conversion from a diffuse to a variegated or focal marrow pattern, with decreased signal intensity in areas of marrow previously showing persistent contrast enhancement with intravenous gadolinium.

Metastatic Disease of the Marrow

In adults, marrow metastases usually result from carcinoma of the prostate (Fig. 15-55), breast (Fig. 15-56), lung (Figs. 15-57 and 15-58), kidney (Fig. 15-59), gastrointestinal tract (Fig. 15-60), and melanoma of the skin (Fig. 15-61). In pediatric patients, the most common primaries that metastasize to the marrow are neuroblastoma, rhabdomyosarcoma, and Ewing's sarcoma (Fig. 15-62). Marrow invasion occurs by hematogenous dissemination, and the high frequency of metastases to pelvic bones and vertebrae is attributed to the abundant vascular supply afforded by the vertebral venous plexus, which serves as a major venous pathway.[79] Metastatic tumor deposits in the marrow can be accompanied by necrosis, fibrosis, bone destruction (osteolytic activity) or bone production (osteoblastic activity)[80] (Fig. 15-63).

MAGNETIC RESONANCE APPEARANCE. The potential contrast between metastatic tumor and normal adult marrow is high, because almost all metastatic tumors are characterized by long T1 and variably long T2 relaxation times. T1-weighted SE sequences are very useful in this situation. Short TI inversion recovery images have even higher contrast between metastatic tumor and normal or irradiated marrow. The latter has a characteristic appearance on MR scans.

text continues on page 1211

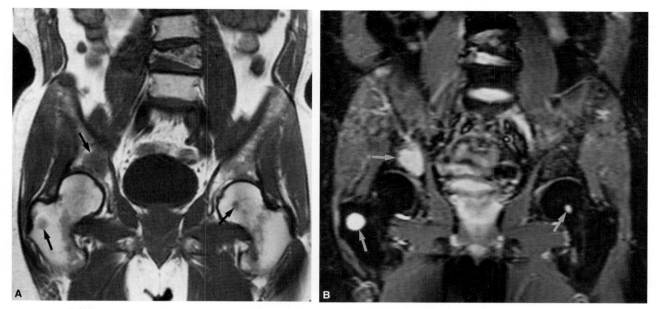

FIGURE 15-51. Myeloma (*arrows*) showing discrete multifocal presentation with normal marrow interspersed on a T1-weighted coronal image (**A**). In these patients, marrow biopsy specimens may not be representative of marrow elsewhere. This patient has been treated with chemotherapy and demonstrates a generalized low signal intensity background on STIR images, indicating fatty marrow transformation. The persistent lesions (*arrows*) are hyperintense on STIR coronal image (**B**).

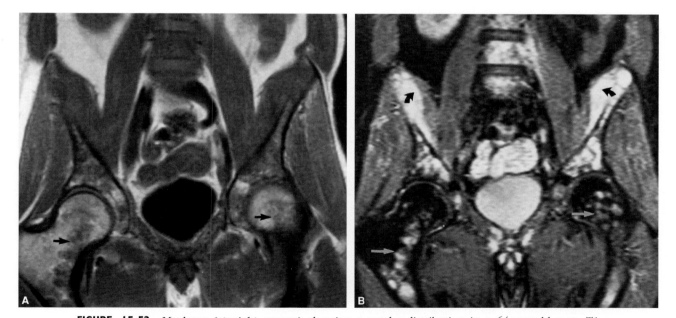

FIGURE 15-52. Myeloma (*straight arrows*) showing a patchy distribution in a 64-year-old man. T1-weighted (**A**) and STIR (**B**) coronal images demonstrate the extramedullary extent of the tumor violating the iliac crests (*curved arrows*) bilaterally and medially.

continued

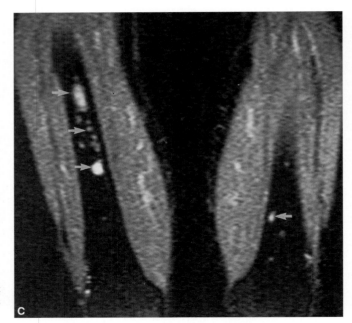

FIGURE 15-52. *Continued.* Hyperintense focal femoral involvement (*straight arrows*) is shown on a STIR coronal image through the femurs (**C**).

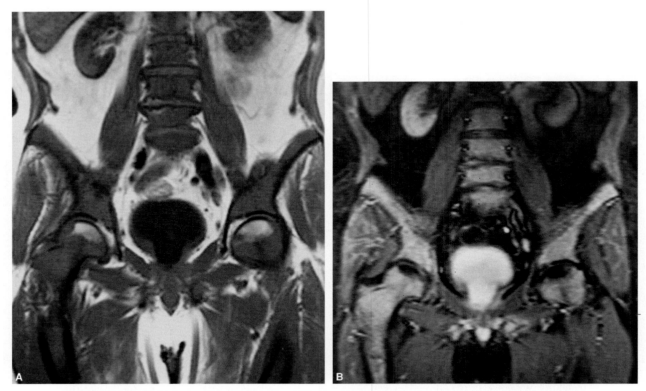

FIGURE 15-53. Multiple myeloma. There is a diffuse pattern of involvement of the red marrow and most of the yellow (fatty) marrow of the pelvis (**A, B**) and femur (**C**). Myeloma is hypointense on T1-weighted coronal images (**A**) and hyperintense on STIR coronal images (**B, C**). *continued*

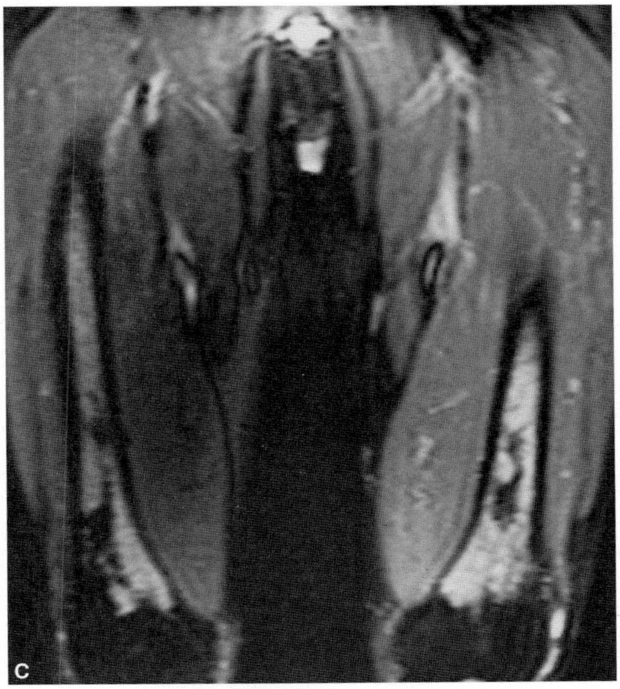

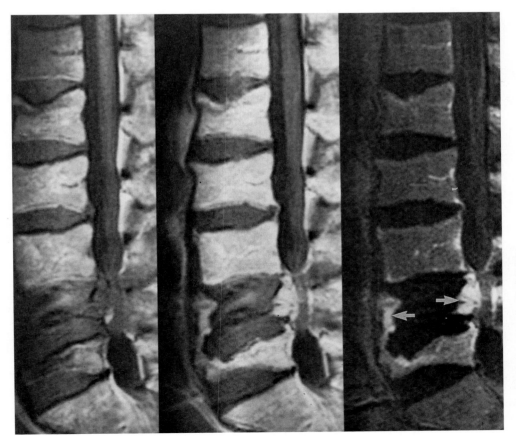

FIGURE 15-53. *Continued*

FIGURE 15-54. Lumbar plasmacytoma and myeloma in a patient with elevated urinary light chains and low back pain. An image subtraction technique was used to subtract the precontrast T1-weighted sagittal image (*far left*) from the postcontrast enhanced image (*middle*) to yield a substraction image (*far right*) more sensitive to changes of enhancement (*arrows*) and relative hyperperfusion. The L4 vertebral body is destroyed by myeloma/plasmacytoma. Epidural extension is present.

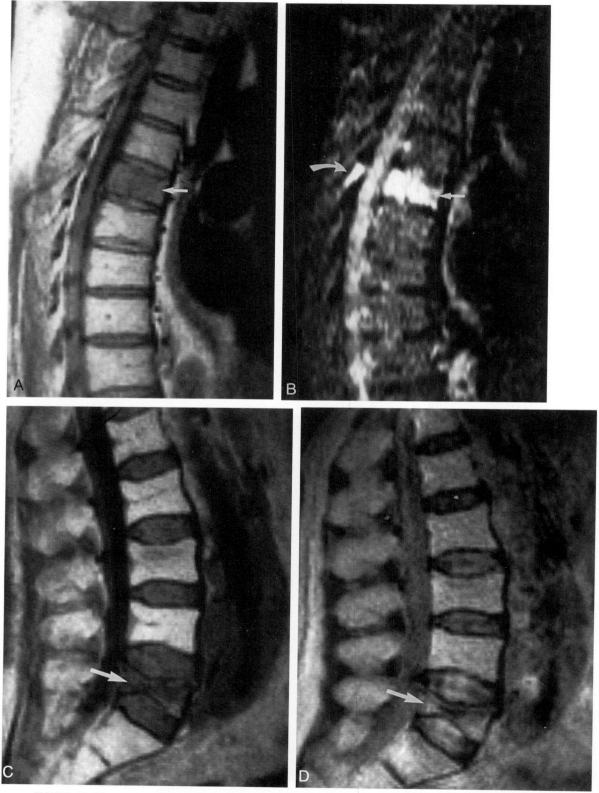

FIGURE 15-55. Prostate carcinoma that has metastasized to the spine (*straight arrows*) demonstrates (**A**) low signal intensity on a T1-weighted sagittal image and (**B**) high signal intensity on a STIR sequence. In addition, posterior element involvement (*curved arrow*) is uniquely demonstrated on the STIR image. In a different patient, the affected L5 vertebral body demonstrates (**C**) low signal intensity on a T1-weighted image, and (**D**) high signal intensity on a Gd-DTPA–enhanced image. Gadolinium contrast administration allows enhancement of the tumor while the cerebrospinal fluid remains low in signal intensity.

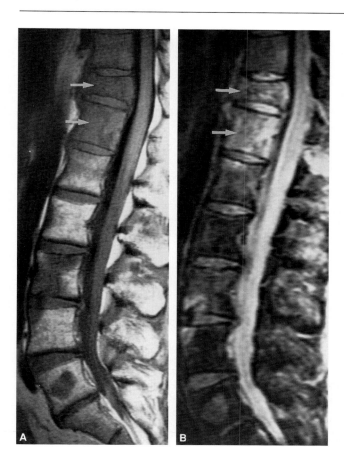

FIGURE 15-56. Metastatic breast carcinoma. This patient received lumbar spine irradiation and has evidence of multiple metastatic lesions (*arrows*), which are hypointense on a T1-weighted sagittal image (**A**) and hyperintense on a STIR sagittal image (**B**). The greatest degree of hyperintensity is seen in the more active lesions (*arrows*).

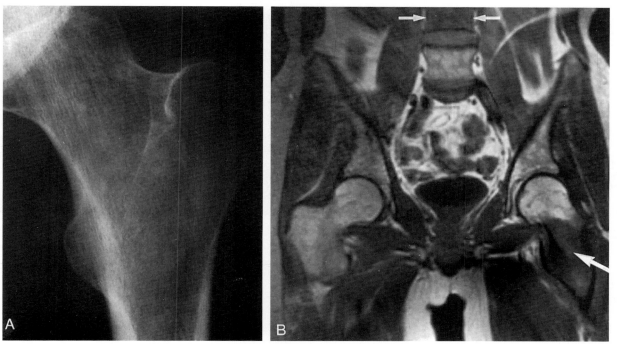

FIGURE 15-57. *Continued*

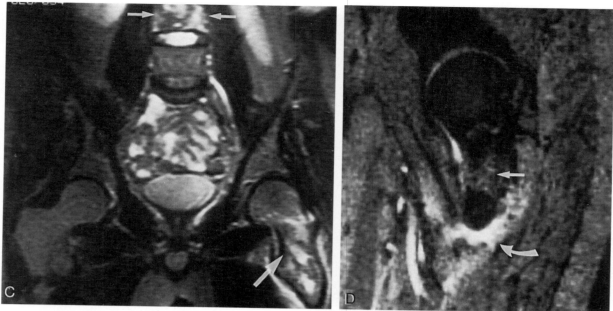

FIGURE 15-57. *Continued.* (**A**) An anteroposterior radiograph is negative for metastatic lung carcinoma. (**B**) T1-weighted and (**C**) T2-weighted images show low and high signal intensity, respectively, in L4 (*small arrows*) and the proximal femur (*large arrow*) (**B**: TR, 800 msec; TE, 20 msec; **C**: TR, 2000 msec; TE, 60 msec). (**D**) A sagittal T2*-weighted image shows a high signal intensity metastatic deposit (*straight arrow*) and peritumoral edema (*curved arrow*) (TR, 400 msec; TE, 30 msec; flip angle, 30°).

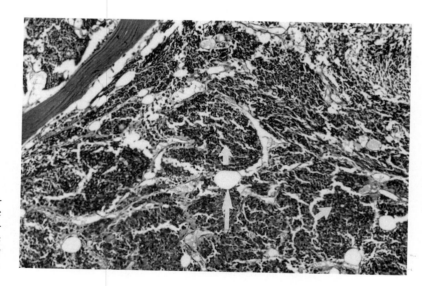

FIGURE 15-58. Extensive bone marrow replacement secondary to metastatic small cell carcinoma of the lung. The marrow is hypercellular and composed of small hyperchromatic cells (*short arrow*), which have replaced the normal hematopoietic elements. Few fat cells (*long arrow*) are present (H & E; original magnification ×120).

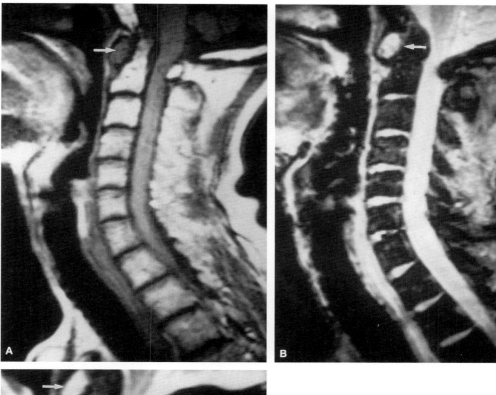

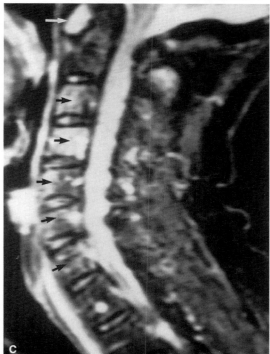

FIGURE 15-59. (A) A T1-weighted sagittal image of the cervical spine in a patient with metastatic renal cell carcinoma shows low signal intensity tumor replacement of fatty marrow in the anterior arch of the atlas (*white arrow*). Subtle, mild signal intensity inhomogeneity of C3 through C7 is present (TR, 500 msec; TE, 20 msec). (B) A T2*-weighted image shows increased signal intensity in C1 (*white arrow*) with a limited increase in metastatic tumor in C3 through C7 (TR, 400 msec; TE, 15 msec; flip angle, 20°). (C) A STIR image shows hyperintense marrow tumor in C1 (*white arrow*) and C2 through C7 (*black arrows*) (TR, 2000 msec; TI, 160 msec; TE, 43 msec).

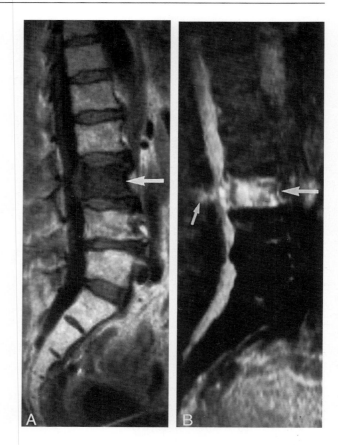

FIGURE 15-60. Colon carcinoma metastatic to L4 (*large arrows*) demonstrates (**A**) low signal intensity on a T1-weighted sagittal image and (**B**) high signal intensity on a STIR sequence. The STIR image displays spinous process involvement as well (*small arrow*).

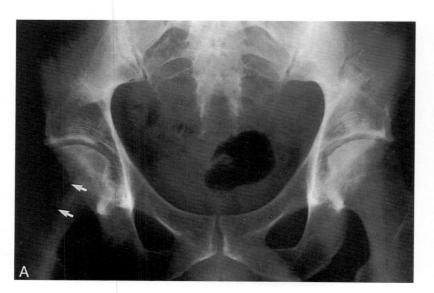

FIGURE 15-61. (**A**) On an anteroposterior radiograph, a metastatic melanoma lesion is seen as a lytic area in the lateral femoral neck (*arrows*). *continued*

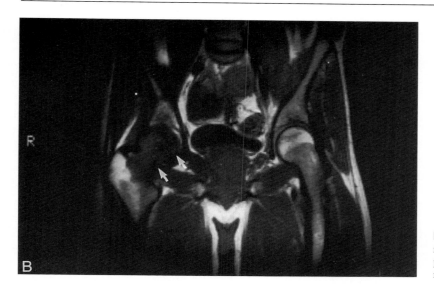

FIGURE 15-61. *Continued.* (**B**) On a T1-weighted coronal image, nonspecific low signal intensity marrow replacement (*arrows*) is evident (TR, 500 msec; TE, 30 msec).

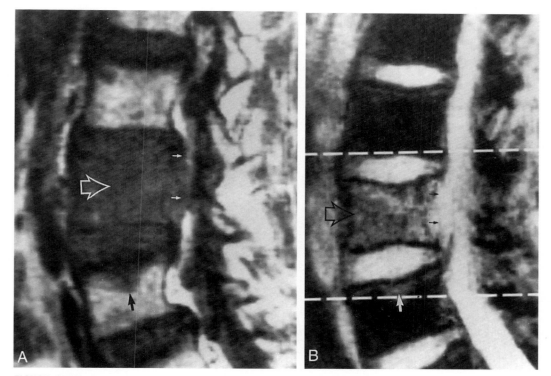

FIGURE 15-62. Ewing's sarcoma metastatic to L3 (*open arrows*) with epidural involvement (*small solid arrows*) demonstrates (**A**) low signal intensity on a T1-weighted image and (**B**) high signal intensity on a T2*-weighted image. Schmorl's node of the L5 endplate (*large solid arrows*) should not be mistaken for tumor (**A**: TR, 600 msec; TE, 30 msec; **B**: TR, 400 msec; TE, 25 msec; flip angle, 30°).

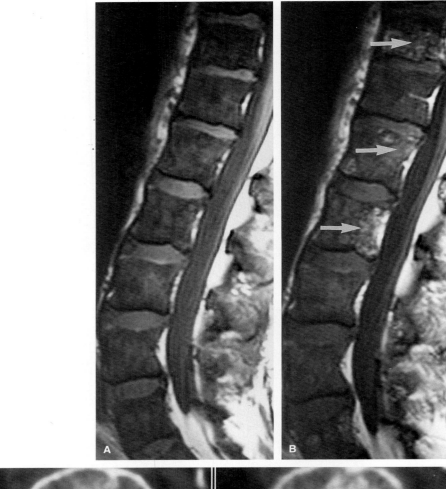

FIGURE 15-63. Metastatic breast carcinoma with diffuse blastic marrow involvement. (**A**) Hypointense vertebral bodies are shown on a T1-weighted sagittal image. (**B**) Postcontrast T1-weighted sagittal image demonstrates patchy enhancement (*arrows*) correlating with lesions that remained active after treatment. (**C**) CT scan shows residual dense osteosclerotic changes.

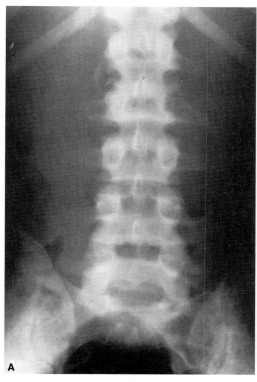
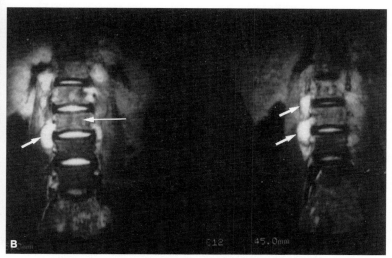

FIGURE 15-64. Coccidioidomycosis. Biopsy-proven coccidioidomycosis with marrow hyperemia and adenopathy. The findings (ie, vertebral body and pedicle erosion) simulate lymphoma on a plain film radiograph (**A**) and adenopathy (*short arrows*) and marrow lesions (*long arrow*) on a coronal STIR image (**B**) (**B**: TR, 1400 msec; TI, 140 msec; TE, 40 msec).

The T2 relaxation time of metastatic deposits is often unpredictably variable, and lesions may be difficult to separate from normal fatty marrow. Depending on the degree of T2 prolongation versus the amount of blastic bone, the net signal is often variable, heterogeneous, and may even be decreased due to decreased proton density.

Short TI inversion recovery and short TR/TE sequences have replaced the more time-consuming T2-weighted pulse sequences in most cases. If spinal cord or thecal sac impingement is suspected, however, T2-weighted scans are useful, because increased signal in the cerebrospinal fluid improves the detection of sac compression. Although STIR sequences also result in bright cerebrospinal fluid, spatial resolution is not as good. Since the tumor is also of high signal intensity, it may be difficult to distinguish between the tumor and cerebrospinal fluid.

Short TI inversion recovery scans are used to screen the axial skeleton for metastatic disease. If this sequence shows no focal areas of high signal intensity, the likelihood of microscopic marrow tumor involvement is low. Symptomatic individuals, however, occasionally have an inhomogeneous distribution of red marrow that may simulate metastatic disease, particularly in the proximal femurs. Osteomyelitis or infection may have to be excluded on clinical grounds (Fig. 15-64). Adenopathy or extension across the disc space indicates infection.

Metastatic disease has been successfully detected on MR T1-weighted and STIR images, even when bone scans are negative or equivocal (Fig. 15-65). MR imaging provides an excellent means of assessing soft-tissue involvement, including adenopathy (Fig. 15-66), and Gd-DTPA enhancement is useful in the assessment of pathologic fractures and epidural spread (Fig. 15-67). Metastatic lesions may show isointensity with adjacent vertebral body marrow on non–fat-suppressed contrast enhanced images (Fig. 15-68). The morphology of the posterior vertebral body cortex should be evaluated for convexity, a sign associated with metastatic tumor extension. A chronic, benign compression fracture frequently demonstrates fat marrow signal intensity (ie, bright on T1-weighted images, dark on STIR images). In more acute compression fractures, subchondral reaction often parallels the endplate without the more central or heterogeneous involvement seen in metastatic disease. Disease progression and peritumoral reaction can be monitored on baseline or serial MR studies (Fig. 15-69).

Schweitzer and coworkers[81] have described the ''bull's-eye sign'' (a focus of high signal intensity in the center of a lower signal intensity osseous marrow abnormality, seen on T1-weighted images) as a specific indicator of normal hematopoietic marrow and not metastatic disease.[81] However, both the halo sign (a peripheral rim

text continues on page 1215

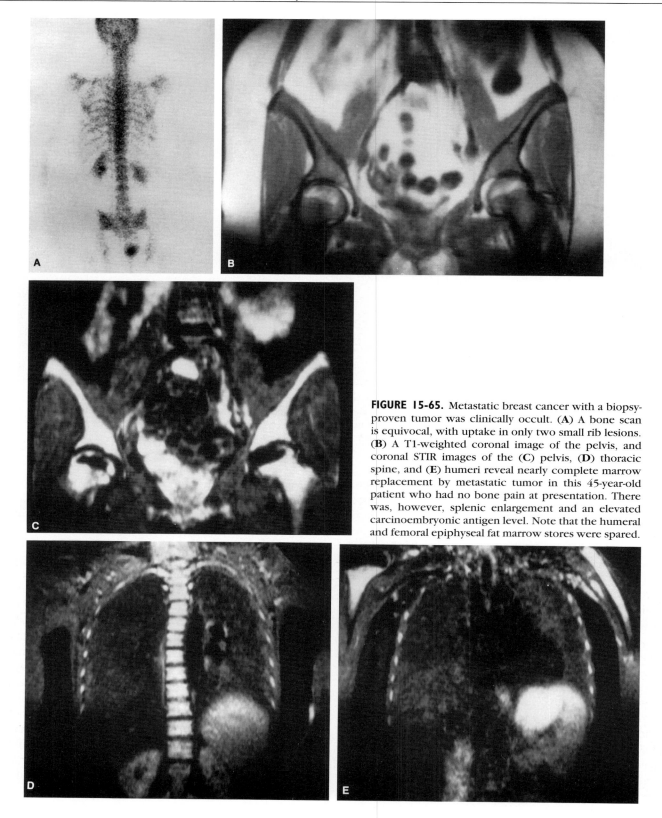

FIGURE 15-65. Metastatic breast cancer with a biopsy-proven tumor was clinically occult. (**A**) A bone scan is equivocal, with uptake in only two small rib lesions. (**B**) A T1-weighted coronal image of the pelvis, and coronal STIR images of the (**C**) pelvis, (**D**) thoracic spine, and (**E**) humeri reveal nearly complete marrow replacement by metastatic tumor in this 45-year-old patient who had no bone pain at presentation. There was, however, splenic enlargement and an elevated carcinoembryonic antigen level. Note that the humeral and femoral epiphyseal fat marrow stores were spared.

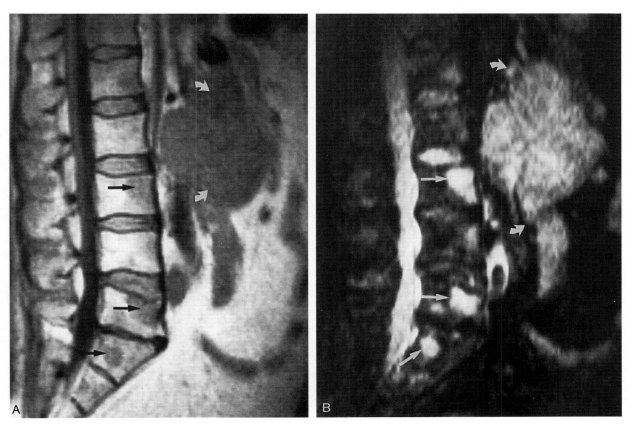

FIGURE 15-66. Metastatic carcinoma of the testis involving the lumbar spine (*straight arrows*) and peri-aortic lymph nodes (*curved arrows*) demonstrates low signal intensity on a T1-weighted image (**A**) and high signal intensity on a STIR sequence (**B**).

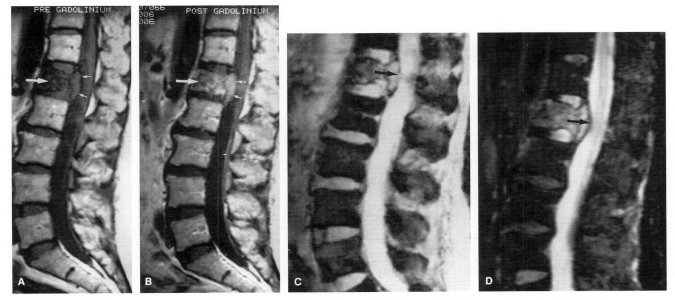

FIGURE 15-67. Metastatic lung carcinoma. T1-weighted sagittal images (**A**) before and (**B**) after Gd-DTPA administration show metastatic tumor infiltration (*large arrows*) and aggressive extension through the posterior vertebral cortex (*small arrows*). The tumor is enhanced on the post–Gd-DTPA image (TR, 500 msec; TE, 20 msec). A comparison of (**C**) sagittal T2*-weighted and (**D**) STIR images reveals posterior convexity of the L1 vertebral body, a sign characteristic of aggressive metastatic marrow replacement (**C**: TR, 400 msec; TE, 15 msec; flip angle, 20°; **D**: TR, 2000 msec; TI, 140 msec; TE, 40 msec).

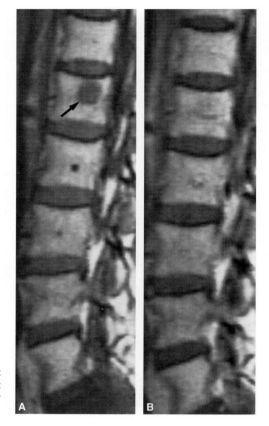

FIGURE 15-68. 42-year-old woman with breast cancer. A metastatic focus (*arrow*) that is hypointense on a T1-weighted sagittal image (**A**) displays isointensity on a postcontrast enhanced image (**B**). If only postgadolinium images are obtained, the isointense marrow lesions are very difficult to detect.

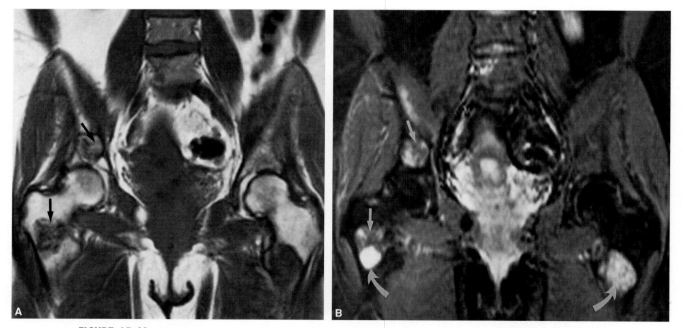

FIGURE 15-69. Partial response to therapy for breast cancer in a 62-year-old woman. There is partial fatty replacement (*straight arrows*) of right proximal femur and supraacetabular metastasis on T1-weighted coronal image (**A**) and corresponding diminution of hyperintensity on STIR image (**B**). Viable tumor (*curved arrows*) is seen as areas of greatest hyperintensity on STIR sequence (**B**). With complete response to therapy, the STIR signal intensity resolves and may be even lower than surrounding marrow, reflecting either bony or fatty transformation. Sclerotic margins are well seen in right supraacetabular lesion on T1-weighted scan (**A**).

of increased signal intensity around an osseous lesion seen on T2-weighted images) and diffuse signal hyperintensity on T2-weighted images have been found to correlate with metastatic disease. The halo sign, most commonly seen in osteoblastic metastases from prostate cancer, is thought to occur secondary to trabecular destruction with a resultant fluid-filled gap. Mucinous or cellular tissue could contribute to hyperintense signal intensity on T2-weighted sequences.

The term *healing flare response* has been used to describe treated skeletal metastases from breast cancer. Healing flare is characterized by increased radiotracer uptake and radiographic (including CT) demonstration of sclerotic changes in previously documented osteolytic or mixed skeletal metastases.[82] MR imaging can also be used to demonstrate healing flare and interval sclerosis (Fig. 15-70). Healing flare in skeletal metastases does not correlate with survival rate (patients with stable metastases after hormonal treatment or chemotherapy live as long), and the increased uptake on bone scans may give the false appearance of more extensive metastasis. Therefore, in monitoring therapy to determine the success of treatment, it is important to correlate bone scans, which show increased uptake with conventional radiographs, CT, or MR imaging.

Lipid Storage Diseases

Gaucher's Disease

Gaucher's disease is a metabolic storage disorder caused by deficient activity of glucocerebrosidase, a lysosomal enzyme. There are three phenotypic forms of Gaucher's disease. Type 1, the common adult form, spares the central nervous system but progressively involves the osseous system and viscera. Types II and III are much rarer childhood forms that have neurological manifestations. The progressive histiocytic proliferation secondary to accumulation of undegraded glycolipids results in displacement of normal hematopoietic cells in the marrow, eventually resulting in peripheral blood cytopenia. Bone erosion may result and precipitate fractures. Necrosis of bone marrow (ie, osteonecrosis) may be associated with this disorder.[83]

MAGNETIC RESONANCE APPEARANCE. Glucocerebroside-laden cells produce patchy, coarse, decreased signal intensity on T1- and T2-weighted images,[68,83] which does not increase on STIR images (there is shortening of the T2 relaxation time in the glucocerebroside component of the Gaucher cell) (Fig. 15-71). Marrow changes in Gaucher's disease have a

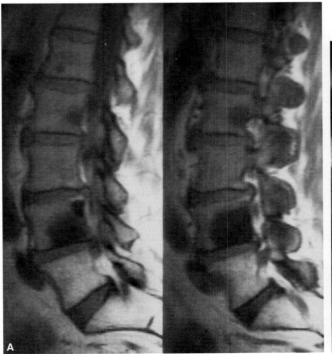

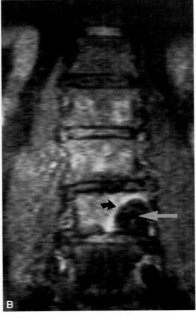

FIGURE 15-70. MR appearance of flare phenomenon. Two weeks after orchiectomy, interval bone scans showed increased uptake (more than prior to surgery). **(A)** T1-weighted sagittal images display hypointense osteoblastic metastases from a prostate primary. **(B)** The corresponding STIR coronal image demonstrates a hypointense osteoblastic lesion (*straight arrow*) with a hyperintense rim (*curved arrow*) due to increased osteoblast activity and hyperemia.

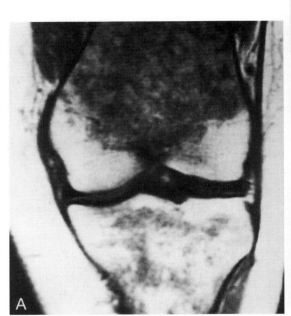
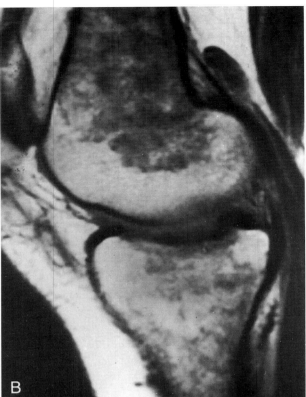

FIGURE 15-71. Accumulation of lipid in reticuloendothelial cells in Gaucher's disease. Low signal intensity marrow infiltration can be seen extending into the epiphysis on (**A**) T1-weighted coronal and (**B**) sagittal images. There may be relative sparing of the epiphyses and apophyses until later stages of disease (TR, 800 msec; TE, 30 msec).

predilection for the hematopoietic marrow stores in the axial skeleton, pelvis, and metaphyses of long bones. When the appendicular skeletal is affected, the disease progresses from proximal-to-distal epiphyseal involvement. In extensive marrow disease, there is generalized distal involvement. Preferential involvement of the distal femurs causes the characteristic Erlenmeyer flask deformity. The mucopolysaccharidoses, which are an unrelated group of hereditary disorders characterized by dwarfism and a specific enzyme deficiency, demonstrate relative hyperintensity on STIR images (Fig. 15-72).

Marrow infarction, a complication of Gaucher's disease, is seen on T1-weighted images as sharply demarcated lesions of low signal intensity. The bright signal intensity described by Rosenthal and colleagues represents unaffected fatty marrow.[68] Short TI inversion recovery and fat-suppressed T2-weighted FSE images depict increased signal intensity in subacute and acute infarcts. With marrow fibrosis, decreased marrow signal intensity is seen on T1-weighted images with no increase in signal intensity on STIR sequences. Although red marrow signal characteristics may be seen in Gaucher's disease, they are less noticeable than in other marrow infiltrative disorders such as lymphoma. Increased splenic vol-

ume and decreased spinal fat fractions correlate with the severity of the disease.[84] Displacement of normal marrow fat with Gaucher's cells results in bulk T1 increases due to the higher T1 value of water compared with fat.[85]

Avascular necrosis in patients with type I Gaucher's disease has been correlated with liver size and marrow signal intensity changes (ie, decreased signal intensity on T1-weighted images and increased signal intensity on T2*-weighted sequences).[86] Blooming or magnetic susceptibility in splenic nodules are thought to represent iron deposits. Symptomatic management of avascular necrosis (bed rest, analgesics, and non–weight-bearing of the involved extremity) is recommended during this stage of bone crisis.[87]

Iron Storage Assessment

To assess iron stores directly, it is usually necessary to sample one of the two iron-storing organs, the liver or the bone marrow. Marrow iron stores are normal or mildly increased in anemias caused by chronic disease and thalassemia minor, and in homozygous hemoglobinopathies such as sickle cell disease. Iron stores are greatly increased in chronic condi-

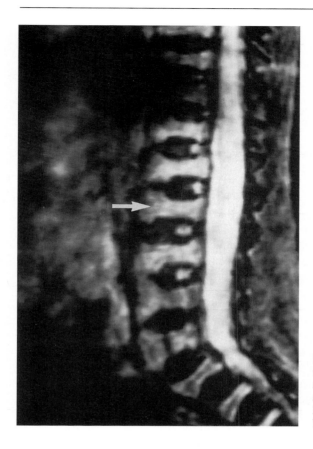

FIGURE 15-72. A sagittal STIR image in a child with mucopolysaccharidosis type IV (also known as Morquio-Brailsford disease or Morquio's syndrome). The accumulation of mucopolysaccharides, secondary to deficiency of galactosamine-6-sulfate sulfatase, produces hyperintensity on STIR contrast (*arrow*). Note the platyspondyly (ie, flattening) and slight rounding of the vertebral bodies.

tions requiring repeated blood transfusions, such as thalassemia major and myeloproliferative myelodysplastic syndrome, as well as in long-standing aplastic anemia. In hemochromatosis, intestinal iron absorption and deposition is increased (Fig. 15-73). Errors of iron quantification are common due to the small amount of the biopsy sample and the chelation effect of the decalcified marrow biopsy specimen.[88]

Stored iron can also be assessed by evaluating urinary excretion of iron after the administration of a chelating agent, usually deferoxamine. This test is useful in detecting iron overload, but is less accurate in assessment of iron deficiency states.[89]

Another method of estimating iron stores, an in vivo method based on the magnetic susceptibility of ferritin in hemosiderin, was studied in rats.[90] MR imaging can also be used to assess iron stores. Iron stores of ferritin and hemosiderin cause decreased fatty marrow signal intensity on T1-

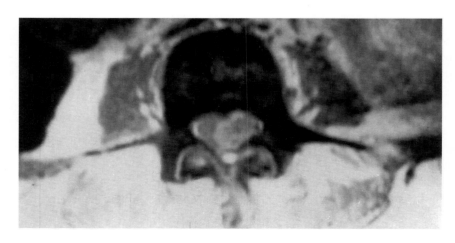

FIGURE 15-73. Iron deposition in hemochromatosis demonstrates diffuse low signal intensity on a T1-weighted axial image. This simulates the appearance of a gradient refocused or STIR sequence (TR, 1000 msec; TE, 20 msec).

and T2-weighted images. As yet, there are no studies that correlate the amount of iron deposition with the degree of decrease in marrow signal intensity.

Bone Marrow Changes in Females, Athletes, and Smokers

As mentioned, signal intensity changes representing reconversion of fatty marrow to hematopoietic marrow can be depicted on T1-weighted and STIR images. During pregnancy, accelerated erythropoiesis, representing an actual increase of approximately 25% in the red cell mass, takes place, as does an increase in circulating erythropoietin in the last two trimesters. Human placental lactogen has been shown to stimulate erythropoiesis in the mouse. Additionally, deficiencies of iron during pregnancy may result in anemia, making the finding of marrow reconversion during pregnancy not surprising.[91]

A common observation in the mature skeleton of women is red marrow inhomogeneity in metaphyseal and diaphyseal sites (Fig. 15-74). The cause has not been fully elucidated,[92] but one theory implicates a latent iron deficient state as the stimulus for marrow reconversion. In latent iron deficiency, the patient may be asymptomatic and blood hemoglobin levels may be normal. More sophisticated testing, however, shows elevated erythrocyte protoporphyrin levels and absence of stainable iron in the marrow.[93] Delayed (ie, incomplete) conversion of red to yellow marrow also produces inhomogeneity. Red marrow stores, of low signal intensity on T1-weighted images, demonstrate isointensity on T2*-weighted images, minimal hyperintensity on T2-weighted images, and varying degrees of increased signal intensity on STIR images (Fig. 15-75). Mild to moderate obesity in women is also associated with this pattern of marrow inhomogeneity.

Hematopoietic bone marrow hyperplasia has been identified in marathon runners and is thought to be a normal variant representing a response to sports-induced anemia.[94] In this population group, there is relative sparing of both the epiphysis (distal femur) and proximal tibia. Poulton and coworkers[95] also found bone marrow reconversion in the knee in heavy smokers, younger adult patients, and obese women who are heavy smokers.[95] This pattern of reconversion, also a normal variant, may involve the metaphysis of both the femur and tibia.

Patients with anorexia nervosa, commonly accompanied by anemia and leukopenia, also develop marrow changes that have been studied in the spine, pelvis, and proximal femurs. Two histologic patterns of marrow change are seen. In one there is decreased marrow cellularity with an increase in fat, and in the other there is a reduction in both fat and hematopoietic cells with an increase in extracellular material rich in hyaluronic acid (serous atrophy). Serous atrophy is characterized by water-like signal intensity on MR images

(ie, decreased signal intensity on T1-weighted images and hyperintensity on T2-weighted images).[96] Early fat conversion produces increased signal intensity on T1-weighted images.

Aplastic Anemia

In aplastic anemia, the marrow is extremely hypoplastic (ie, yellow) and exhibits less than 30% residual hematopoietic elements microscopically (Fig. 15-76). Aplastic anemia is believed to be caused by injury or failure of a common pluripotential stem cell affecting all hematopoietic cell lines. It sometimes presents as an acute disorder, or it may have a more prolonged chronic course, with signs and symptoms related to the pancytopenia.[97]

The etiology is unknown in approximately 50% of patients, in which case the anemia is diagnosed as idiopathic aplastic anemia. The remainder of cases are attributed to exposure to drugs, chemicals, toxins, radiation, and severe viral infections. Uncommonly, congenital disorders such as Fanconi's anemia may be accompanied by a genetic predisposition to aplastic anemia. Although a mild form of aplastic anemia may be successfully treated with marrow-stimulating drugs such as androgens, the mainstay of therapy is bone marrow transplantation.[98] Iatrogenically induced aplastic marrows are encountered in the course of aggressive chemotherapy in the treatment of acute leukemia or in preparation for bone marrow transplantation. Radiotherapy may result in focal aplastic marrow.

MAGNETIC RESONANCE APPEARANCE. Aplastic marrow is characterized by increased signal intensity on T1-weighted images and intermediate signal intensity on T2-weighted images. These signal intensity changes are attributed to replacement of hematopoietic marrow by fatty marrow.[99,100] On T1-weighted images, focal low signal intensity heterogeneity is seen during treatment for aplastic anemia. This heterogeneity may represent hematopoiesis recovery or fibrosis. Although MR imaging demonstrates primarily high signal intensity fatty marrow in aplastic anemia, islands of hematopoiesis may produce a patchy appearance of lower signal intensity areas surrounded by bright signal intensity fat on T1-weighted images. Aplastic anemia may be difficult to discriminate from normal bone marrow in adult patients because of conversion to fatty marrow signal intensity. Diagnosis and monitoring of aplastic anemia may be improved with chemical-shift imaging techniques.

Hemoglobinopathies

Sickle Cell Anemia

Approximately 0.15% of black children in the United States are homozygous for hemoglobin S (HbS) and have full-blown sickle cell disease. This disorder is caused by a

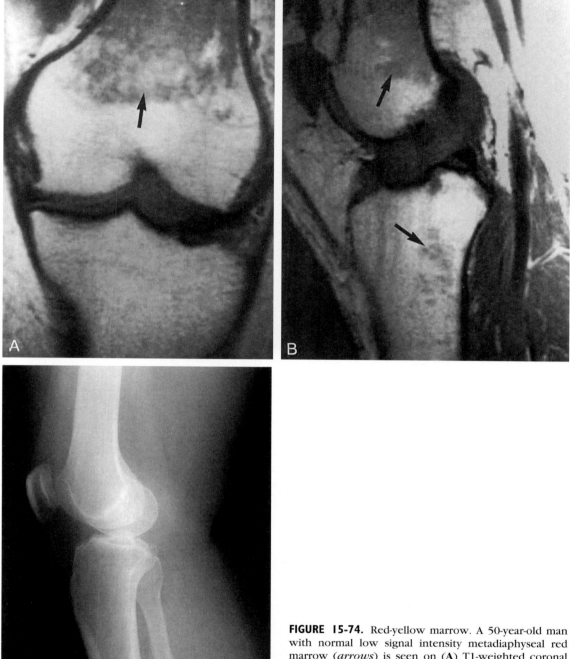

FIGURE 15-74. Red-yellow marrow. A 50-year-old man with normal low signal intensity metadiaphyseal red marrow (*arrows*) is seen on (**A**) T1-weighted coronal and (**B**) sagittal images. The epiphyseal regions demonstrate uniform yellow marrow signal intensity. This finding of marrow inhomogeneity is considered a normal variant. (**C**) A conventional lateral radiograph is shown for comparison.

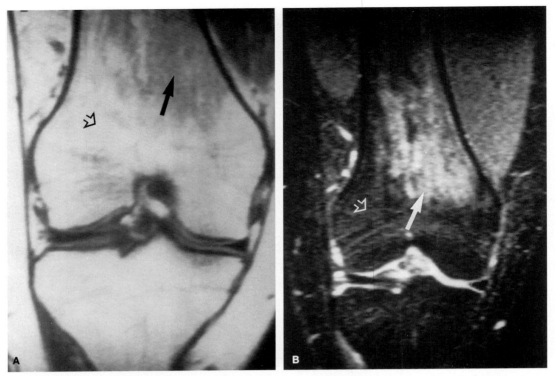

FIGURE 15-75. Normal red marrow and yellow marrow inhomogeneity in metaphyseal diaphyses in a 40-year-old woman. **(A)** A T1-weighted coronal image displays bright signal intensity fatty marrow (*open arrow*) and lower signal intensity hematopoietic or red marrow (solid arrow). **(B)** A corresponding coronal STIR image shows dark fat marrow (*open arrow*) and increased signal intensity red marrow (*solid arrow*).

specific molecular lesion: the substitution of valine for glutamic acid at the beta chain of hemoglobin.[101] When oxygen tension is reduced, erythrocytes containing HbS become sickle shaped. These rigid, nondeformable sickle cells cause occlusion of small vessels, and their abnormal shape subjects them to premature pitting by the spleen, resulting in accelerated red blood cell destruction (ie, hemolytic anemia). These two features, small vessel occlusion and hemolytic anemia,

account for the various clinical manifestations in sickle cell disease. Like other patients with congenital hemolytic anemia, sickle cell patients demonstrate radiographic abnormalities due to expansion of the red marrow. Vascular occlusion leads to a development of bony infarctions.

MAGNETIC RESONANCE APPEARANCE. Sickle cell anemia is characterized by yellow to red marrow reconversion with

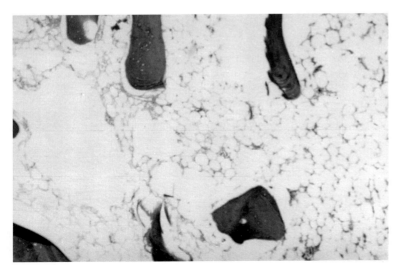

FIGURE 15-76. Bone marrow exhibits marked hypocellularity and is essentially 100% fat in aplastic anemia (H & E; original magnification ×100).

low to intermediate signal intensity hematopoietic marrow identified on T1-weighted images, and hematopoietic or red marrow characteristics on STIR images (Fig. 15-77). Marrow conversion can involve the diaphysis, metaphysis, and epiphysis.[102,103] Patients with marrow ischemia may present with bone marrow infarction, depicted on MR images (Fig. 15-78). Acute infarcts may demonstrate increased signal intensity on T2-weighted images.

Thalassemia

The thalassemias are a diverse group of congenital disorders in which there is a defect in the synthesis of one or more of the subunits of hemoglobin. As a result of the decreased production of hemoglobin, red blood cells are microcytic and hypochromic. Thalassemias are quantitative abnormalities of synthesis of either the beta or alpha hemoglobin subunit. As a result of the imbalance in the subunit synthesis, patients exhibit varying degrees of ineffective erythropoiesis and hemolytic anemia. The severity of the resultant anemia is related to the number of the deficient subunit chains, which, in turn, is related to whether gene expression is homozygous, intermediate, or heterozygous.[104]

MAGNETIC RESONANCE APPEARANCE. As in sickle cell anemia, MR scans in thalassemia major demonstrate low to intermediate signal intensity within hematopoietic marrow, involving both fatty and red marrow stores (ie, epiphyseal extension). In thalassemia minor, MR imaging demonstrates increased red marrow stores and delayed development of ossification centers.[13]

Miscellaneous Marrow Lesions

Paget's Disease

Paget's disease is characterized by initial uncontrolled osteoclastic activity (ie, bone resorption), followed by vascular fibrous connective tissue production, and finally osteo-blastic activity (ie, bone production). In the final stages, bone is composed of dense trabecular bone organized in a haphazard fashion, resulting in irregular, mosaic cement lines. The composition of this altered bone is disorganized and, although dense, it is structurally weak and prone to fracture.

Paget's disease is most likely to affect individuals older than 40 years of age who are primarily of European extraction. Serum alkaline phosphatase levels are markedly increased in this disorder. Various electron-microscopic studies have implicated viral agents related to measles or respiratory syncytial viruses as possible etiologic agents. This disorder may involve a limited portion of the skeleton or may be more generalized. Pelvic bones are most commonly involved, followed in incidence by the femur, skull, tibia, lumbosacral spine, dorsal spine, clavicles, and ribs. Secondary malignant sarcomatous transformation arises in preexisting Paget's disease in less than 1% of cases.[105]

MAGNETIC RESONANCE APPEARANCE. In the lytic, mixed, and sclerotic presentations of Paget's disease, a coarsened appearance of the marrow is identified on T1-weighted images[106] (Fig. 15-79). Although no increase in signal intensity is observed on T2-weighted or T2*-weighted images, bright signal intensity may be identified on STIR images. The sclerotic pattern of Paget's may resemble diffuse osteonecrosis with widespread low signal intensity marrow replacement on T1-, T2-, or T2*-weighted images (Fig. 15-80).

Localized Osteoporosis

Reflex sympathetic dystrophy, or Sudeck's atrophy, is a painful neurovascular disorder.[107] Dystrophic soft-tissue changes, swelling, distal extremity predilection, and periarticular as well as diffuse osteoporosis are characteristic. Reflex dystrophy syndrome is mediated by the sympathetic

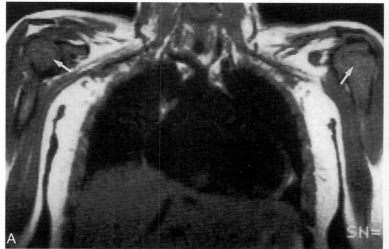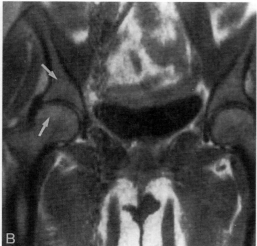

FIGURE 15-77. T1-weighted coronal images show diffuse low signal intensity (*arrows*) in (**A**) the humeri and (**B**) the pelvis in two patients with sickle cell anemia and persistent red marrow hypercellularity (TR, 800 msec; TE, 20 msec).

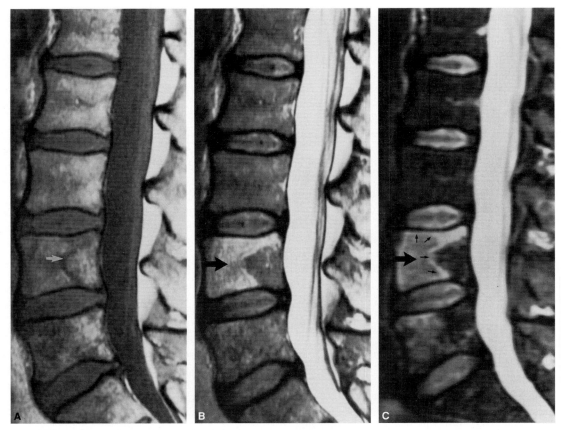

FIGURE 15-78. Sickle cell anemia with acute vertebral body marrow infarction. Ischemic marrow is isointense on T1-weighted sagittal image (**A**) although a well-demarcated hypointense interface (*arrow*) is present between the anterior two thirds and posterior one third of the vertebral body. Marrow infarction (*large arrow*) is hyperintense on corresponding T2-weighted fast spin-echo (**B**) and fast spin-echo STIR (**C**) images. Note the hyperintensity is greatest peripherally (*small arrows*) on the STIR sequence (**C**). In contrast to acute ischemia, chronic infarction maintains hypointensity on both T1- and T2-weighted images.

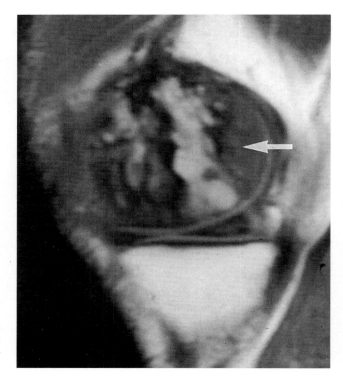

FIGURE 15-79. On a T1-weighted sagittal image, coarse-fibered bone in Paget's disease is seen as areas of low signal intensity intermixed with high signal intensity yellow marrow, creating an inhomogeneous appearance in the medial femoral condyle (*arrow*) (TR, 800 msec; TE, 20 msec).

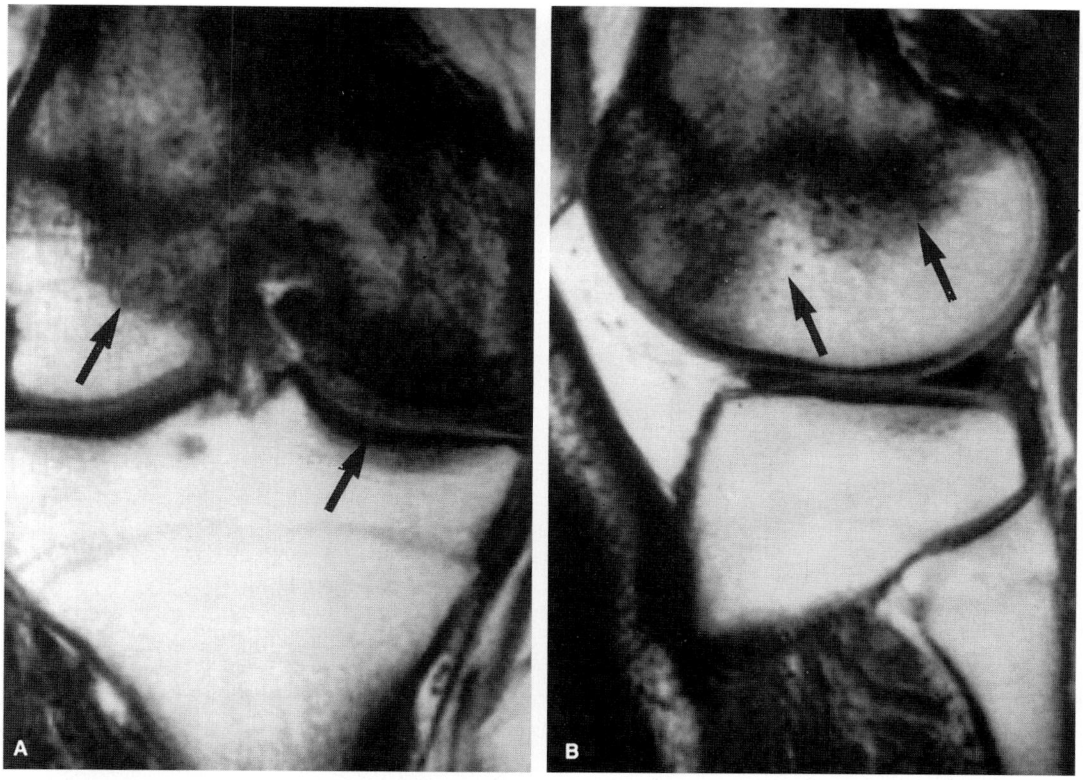

FIGURE 15-80. T1-weighted (**A**) coronal and (**B**) sagittal images in a patient with Paget's disease show geographically well-defined lysis and low signal intensity sclerosis (*arrows*) extending into the subarticular region of the distal femur. Initial tibial involvement is frequently diaphyseal (TR, 600 msec; TE, 20 msec).

nervous system and may be initiated by minimal trauma or fracture. T1-weighted and STIR images are more sensitive than T2*-weighted or conventional T2-weighted images in identifying hyperemic marrow (Fig. 15-81). Periarticular low signal intensity regions are displayed on T1-weighted images, whereas corresponding STIR images demonstrate a diffusely hyperintense signal intensity.

Transient regional osteoporosis is a self-limited condition characterized by localized osteoporosis and pain. The etiology is unknown. The joint space and articular cartilage are preserved, in contrast to septic arthritis. Transient regional osteoporosis is subdivided into regional migratory osteoporosis and transient osteoporosis of the hip. Regional migratory osteoporosis involves the joints of the lower extremity (the knee, ankle, and foot), is most likely to occur in middle-aged patients, and is symptomatic for 6 months to 1 year. Unlike reflex sympathetic dystrophy, there is frequent clinical recurrence in other joints. Transient osteoporosis of the hip typically affects middle-aged men, although it was initially described in women in the third trimester of pregnancy. Either hip may be involved, with a self-limited course of demineralization and pain.

MAGNETIC RESONANCE APPEARANCE.   On T1-weighted images, femoral head and neck hyperemia demonstrates low signal intensity on T1-weighted images and increased signal intensity on T2-weighted and STIR images (Fig. 15-82). The acetabulum is not usually involved, although joint effusions are common. Since early avascular necrosis may present with similar MR findings (in fact, transient osteoporosis of the hip may represent an early reversible stage of avascular necrosis), an osteonecrotic focus should be excluded on follow-up examination.

Acquired Immunodeficiency Syndrome

Patients with AIDS exhibit a multitude of disorders that may be reflected in various bone marrow changes.[108] Infectious disorders, particularly disseminated *Mycobacterium* (Fig. 15-83), *Cryptococcus*, or *Histoplasma* infections, may extensively involve the marrow. Histopathologically, discrete granulomas are not typically formed in immunodeficient patients. Instead, the causative organisms are detected within histiocytic aggregates and sheets. A diffuse histiocytic proliferation related to viral infection (virus-associated hemophagocytic syndrome) has been observed in patients with AIDS.

High-grade lymphomas are frequently observed in AIDS patients and may involve the bone marrow in apatchy or diffuse manner. Occasionally, lymphoma presents

text continues on page 1227

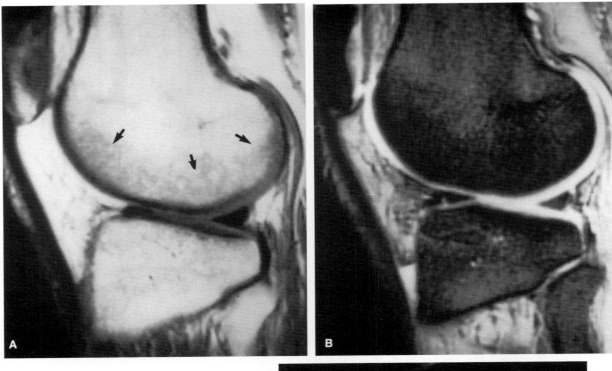

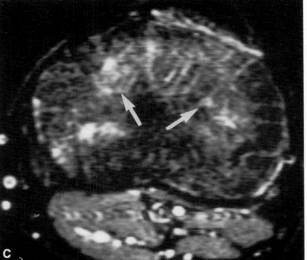

FIGURE 15-81. Reflex sympathetic dystrophy (Sudeck's atrophy). **(A)** A T1-weighted sagittal image shows subarticular low signal intensity marrow (*arrows*) (TR, 600 msec; TE, 20 msec). **(B)** The corresponding T2*-weighted sagittal image is unremarkable (TR, 600 msec; TE, 15 msec; flip angle, 20°). **(C)** An axial STIR image through the proximal tibia shows marrow edema (*arrows*) with hyperintense signal intensity (TR, 2000 msec; TI, 160 msec; TE, 43 msec).

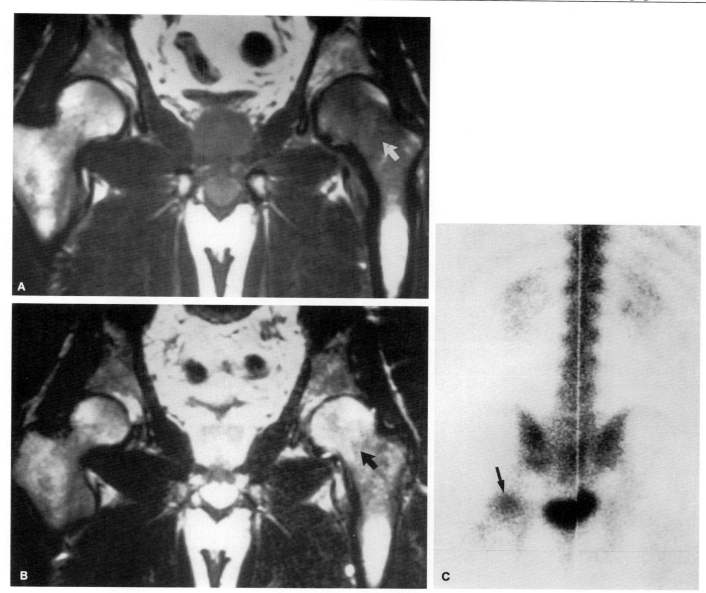

FIGURE 15-82. Transient osteoporosis of the hip. **(A)** A T1-weighted coronal image shows low signal intensity in the left femoral head and neck (*arrow*) without an osteonecrotic focus (TR, 600 msec; TE, 20 msec). **(B)** On the corresponding T2-weighted coronal image, there is increased signal intensity in the left femoral head and neck (*arrow*) (TR, 2000 msec; TE, 80 msec). **(C)** A posterior view technetium bone scan shows uptake in the left femoral head (*arrow*).

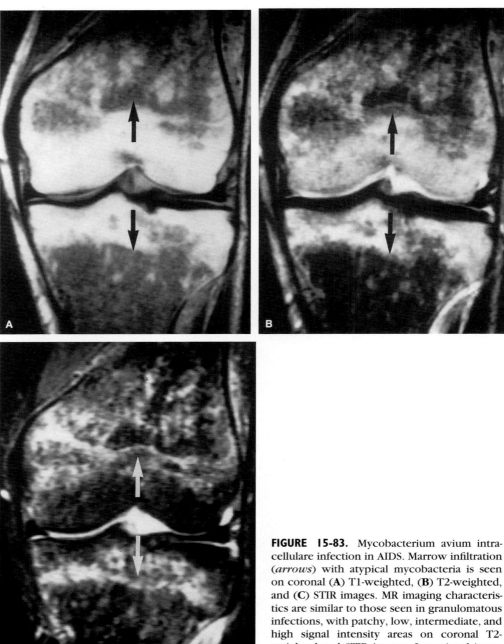

FIGURE 15-83. Mycobacterium avium intracellulare infection in AIDS. Marrow infiltration (*arrows*) with atypical mycobacteria is seen on coronal (**A**) T1-weighted, (**B**) T2-weighted, and (**C**) STIR images. MR imaging characteristics are similar to those seen in granulomatous infections, with patchy, low, intermediate, and high signal intensity areas on coronal T2-weighted and STIR images. Low signal intensity areas on T1-weighted images tend to remain dark on T2-weighted and STIR images.

as extensive marrow necrosis associated with severe bone pain.

Some nonspecific changes reported in the bone marrow of AIDS patients include serous atrophy of fat with hypocellular marrow and accumulation of hyaluronic acid, hypocellularity, and decreased storage iron.[109,110]

References

1. Kricun ME. Red-yellow marrow conversion: its effect on the location of some solitary bone lesions. Skeletal Radiol 1985;14:1019.
2. Moore SG, Dawson KL. Magnetic resonance appearance of red and yellow marrow in the femur: spectrum with age. Radiology 1990;175:219.
3. Vogler JB III, Murphy WA. Bone marrow imaging. Radiology 1988;168:679.
4. Dooms GC, et al. Bone marrow imaging: magnetic resonance studies related to age and sex. Radiology 1985;155:429.
5. Weiss L. Histopathology of the bone marrow. In: Gordon AS, ed. Regulation of hematopoiesis. New York: Appleton-Century-Crofts, 1970.
6. Quesenberry P, Levitt L. Hematopoietic stem cells. N Engl J Med 1979;301:755.
7. Ogawa M, Porter PN, Naleabata T. Renewal and commitment to differentiation of hematopoietic stem cells. Blood 1983;61;823.
8. Vogler JB, Murphy WA. Bone marrow imaging. Radiology 1988;168:679.
9. Custer RP, Ahlfeldt FE. Studies on the structure and function of the bone marrow. J Lab Clin Med 1932;17:960.
10. Le Bruyn PPH, Breen PC, Thomas TB. The microcirculation of the bone marrow. Anat Rec 1970;168:55.
11. Piney A. The anatomy of the bone marrow. Br Med J 1922;2:792.
12. Maniatus A, Vavassoli M, Crosby WH. Factors affecting the conversion of yellow to red marrow. Blood 1971;37:581.
13. Moore SG, Sebag GH. Primary disorders of bone marrow. In: Cohen MD, Edwards MK, eds. Magnetic resonance imaging of children. Philadelphia: Decker, 1990:765.
14. Wehrli FW, et al. Mechanisms of contrast in NMR imaging. J Comput Tomogr 1984;8:369.
15. Mitchell DG, et al. The biophysical basis of tissue contrast in extracranial MR imaging. AJR 1987;149:831.
16. Mirowitz SA, Apicella P, Reinus WR, Hammerman AM. MR imaging of bone marrow lesions: relative conspicuousness on T1-weighted, fat-suppressed T2-weighted, and STIR images. AJR 1994;162:215.
17. Olson DL, et al. Magnetic resonance imaging of the bone marrow in patients with leukemia, aplastic marrow and lymphoma. Invest Radiol 1986;21:540.
18. Waitches G, Zawin JK, Poznanski AK. Sequence and rate of bone marrow conversion in the femora of children as seen on MR imaging: are accepted standards accurate? AJR 1994;162:1399.
19. Zawin K, Jaramillo D. Conversion of bone marrow in the humerus, sternum and clavicle: changes with age on MR images. Radiology 1993;188:159.
20. Dawson KL, Moore SG, Rowland JM. Age-related marrow changes in the pelvis: MR and anatomic findings. Radiology 1992;183:47.
21. Duda SH, Laniado M, Schick F, et al. Normal bone marrow in the sacrum of young adults: differences between the sexes seen on chemical-shift MR imaging. AJR 1995;164:935.
22. Mirowitz SA. Hematopoietic bone marrow within the proximal humeral epiphysis in normal adults: investigation with MR imaging. Radiology 1993;188:689.
23. Custer RP. Studies on the structure and function of bone marrow. I. Variability of the hemopoietic pattern and consideration of method for examination. J Lab Clin Med 1932;17:951.
24. Arndt WF III, Truax AL, Barnett FM, et al. MR diagnosis of bone contusions of the knee: comparison of coronal T2-weighted fast spin-echo with fat saturation and fast spin-echo STIR images with conventional STIR images. AJR 1996;166:119.
25. Sebag GH, Moore SG. Effect of trabecular bone on the appearance of marrow in gradient echo imaging of the appendicular skeleton. Radiology 1990;174:855.
26. Brateman L. Chemical shift imaging: a review. AJR 1987;146:971.
27. Foon KA, Casciato DA. Acute leukemia. In: Casciato DA, Lowitz BB, eds. Manual of clinical oncology, 2nd ed. Boston: Little, Brown, 1990:386.
28. Foon KA, Todd RF. Immunologic classification of leukemia and lymphoma. Blood 1986;68:1.
29. Moore SG, et al. Bone marrow in children with acute lymphocytic leukemia: MR relaxation times. Radiology 1986;160:237.
30. Rosen BR, et al. Hematologic bone marrow disorders: quantitative chemical shift MR imaging. Radiology 1988;169:799.
31. Thomsen C, et al. Prolonged bone marrow T1-relaxation in acute leukemia: in vivo tissue characterization by magnetic resonance imaging. Magn Reson Imaging 1987;5:251.
32. Sugmura K, et al. Bone marrow diseases of the spine: differentiation with T1 and T2 relaxation times in MR imaging. Radiology 1987;165:541.
33. Jensen KE, et al. Changes in T1 relaxation process in the bone marrow following treatment in children with acute lymphoblastic leukemia: a magnetic resonance imaging study. Pediatr Radiol 1990;20:464.
34. McKinstry CS, et al. Bone marrow in leukemia and aplastic anemia: MR imaging before, during and after treatment. Radiology 1987;162:701.
35. Wittels B. Bone marrow biopsy changes following chemotherapy for acute leukemia. Am J Surg Pathol 1980;4:135.
36. Islam A, Catovsky D, Galton DA. Histological study of bone marrow regeneration following chemotherapy for acute myeloid leukemia and chronic granulocytic leukemia in blast transformation. Br J Haematol 1980;45:535.
37. Gerard EL, Ferry JA, Amrein PC, et al. Compositional changes in vertebral bone marrow during treatment for acute leukemia: assessment with quantitative chemical shift imaging. Radiology 1992;183:39.
38. Vande Berg BC, Schmitz PJ, Scheiff JM, et al. Acute myeloid leukemia: lack of predictive value of sequential quantitative MR imaging during treatment. Radiology 1995;197:301.
39. Foon KA, Casciato DA. Chronic leukemias. In: Casciato DA, Lowitz BB, eds. Manual of clinical oncology, 2nd ed. Boston: Little, Brown, 1990:360.
40. Adamson JW, Fialkow PJ. Pathogenesis of the myeloproliferative syndromes. Br J Haematol 1978;38:299.
41. Wiernik PH. The chronic leukemias. In: Kelley WN, ed. Textbook of internal medicine, vol 1. Philadelphia: JB Lippincott, 1989:1177.
42. Deisseroth AL, Wallerstein RO. Bone marrow failure. In: Kelley WN, ed. Textbook of internal medicine, vol 1. Philadelphia: JB Lippincott, 1989:1202.
43. Moore MAS. Pathogenesis in myelofibrosis. In: Hoffman AV, ed. Recent advances in hematology. Edinburgh: Churchill Livingstone, 1982:132.
44. Burke JS. The value of the bone marrow biopsy in the diagnosis of hairy cell leukemia. Am J Clin Pathol 1978;70:876.
45. Golomb HM. Hairy cell leukemia. In: Williams WJ, et al, eds. Hematology. New York: McGraw-Hill, 1983:999.
46. Thompson JA, et al. MRI of bone marrow in hairy cell leukemia: correlation with clinical response to alpha-interferon. Leukemia 1987;1:315.

47. Fletcher BD, Wall JE, Hanna SL. Effect on hematopoietic growth factors on MR images of bone marrow in children undergoing chemotherapy. Radiology 1993;189:745.

48. Ryan SP, Weinberger E, White KS, et al. MR imaging of bone marrow in children with osteosarcoma: effect of granulocyte colony-stimulating factor. AJR 1995;165:915.

49. Morstyn G, Souza L, Keech J, et al. Effects of granulocyte colony stimulating factor on neutropenia induced by cytotoxic chemotherapy. Lancer 1988;1:667.

50. Jabubowski AA, Souza L, Kelly F, et al. Effects of human granulocyte colony stimulating factor in a patient with idiopathic neutropenia. N Engl J Med 1989;320:38.

51. Gale RP, Champlin RE. Bone marrow transplantation in acute leukemia. Clin Haematol 1986;15:851.

52. Nadler BW. Malignant lymphoma. In: Harrison TR, ed. Principles of internal medicine, 12th ed. New York: McGraw-Hill, 1991:1608.

53. Chau NJ, Blume KG. Bone marrow transplantation. Part II. Autologous. West J Med 1990;152:46.

54. O'Reilly RG. Allogenic bone marrow transplantation: current state and future directions. Blood 1983;62:941.

55. Horowitz MM, Gale RP, Sandel PM, et al. Graft versus leukemia reaction after bone marrow transplantation. Blood 1990;75:55.

56. Stevens SK, et al. Repopulation of marrow affer transplantation: MR imaging with pathologic correlation. Radiology 1990;175:213.

57. Fletcher BD, Crom DB, Krance RA, Kun LE. Radiation-induced bone abnormalities after bone marrow transplantation for childhood leukemia. Radiology 1994;191:231.

58. McKenna RW, Hernandez JA. Bone marrow in malignant lymphoma. Hematol Oncol Clin North Am 1988;2:617.

59. O'Caroll DL, McKenna RW, Brunning RD. Bone marrow histology in Hodgkin's disease. Cancer 1976;38:1717.

60. Coller BS, Chabner BA, et al. Frequencies and patterns of bone marrow involvement in non-Hodgkin's lymphomas. Am J Hematol 1977;3:105.

61. Shields AF, et al. The detection of bone marrow involvement by lymphoma using magnetic resonance imaging. J Clin Oncol 1987;5:225.

62. Linden A, et al. Malignant lymphoma: bone marrow imaging versus biopsy. Radiology 1989;173:335.

63. Richard MA, et al. Low field strength magnetic resonance imaging of bone marrow in patients with malignant lymphoma. Br J Cancer 1988;57:412.

64. Stevens SK, et al. Early and late bone marrow changes after irradiation: MR evaluation. Am J Roentgenol 1990;154:745.

65. Casamassima F, et al. Hematopoietic bone marrow recovery after radiation therapy: MRI evaluation. Blood 1989;73:1677.

66. Kauczor HU, Dietl B, Brix G, et al. Fatty replacement of bone marrow after radiation therapy for Hodgkin disease: quantification with chemical shift imaging. J Magn Reson Imaging 1993;3:575.

67. Blomlie V, Rofstad EK, Skjonsberg A, et al. Female pelvic bone marrow: serial MR imaging before, during, and after radiation therapy. Radiology 1995;194:537.

68. Rosenthal DI, et al. Evaluation of Gaucher disease using magnetic resonance imaging. J Bone Joint Surg [Am] 1986;68:802.

69. Murra JM. Histiocytoses in bone tumors: clinical, radiologic and pathologic correlations. Philadelphia: Lea & Febiger, 1989:1021.

70. Bergsagel DE. Plasma cell myeloma. In: Williams WJ, et al, eds. Hematology. New York: McGraw-Hill, 1983:1078.

71. Mundy GR, et al. Evidence for the accretion of an osteoclast stimulating factor in myeloma. N Engl J Med 1976;291:1041.

72. Goldman AB. Multiple myeloma. In: Tavera SJM, Ferucci JT, eds. Radiology diagnosis, imaging, intervention. Philadelphia: JB Lippincott, 1994.

73. Resnick D, Greenway CD, Bardwick P, et al. Plasma cell dyscrasia with polyneuropathy, organomegaly, endocrinopathy, and skin changes: the POEMS syndrome. Radiology 1981;140:17.

74. Moulopoulos LA, Varma DGK, Dimopoulos MA, et al. Multiple myeloma: spinal MR imaging in patients with untreated newly diagnosed disease. Radiology 1992;185:833.

75. Rahmouni A, Divine M, Mathieu D, et al. Detection of multiple myeloma involving the spine: efficacy of fat-suppression and contrast-enhanced MR imaging. AJR 1993;160:1049.

76. Libshitz, HI, Malthouse SR, Cunningham D, MacVicar AD. Multiple myeloma: appearance at MR imaging. Radiology 1992;182:833.

77. Moulopoulos LA, Dimopoulos MA, Alexanian R, Leeds NE. Multiple myeloma: MR patterns of response to treatment. Radiology 1994;193:441.

78. Rahmouni A, Divine M, Mathieu D, et al. MR appearance of multiple myeloma of the spine before and after treatment. AJR 1993;160:1053.

79. Jaffe HL. Tumors and tumorous conditions of the bones and joints. Philadelphia: Lea & Febiger, 1961:589.

80. Anner RM, et al. Frequency and significance of bone marrow involvement by metastatic solid tumors. Cancer 1977;39:1337.

81. Schweitzer ME, Levine C, Mitchell DG, et al. Bull's-eyes and halos: useful MR discriminators of osseous metastases. Radiology 1993;188:249.

82. Janicek MJ, Hayes DF, Kaplan WD. Healing flare in skeletal metastases from breast cancer. Radiology 1994;192:201.

83. Lanir A, et al. Gaucher disease: assessment with MR imaging. Radiology 1986;161:239.

84. Rosenthal DI, Barton NW, McKusick KA, et al. Quantitative imaging of Gaucher's disease. Radiology 1992;185:841.

85. Johnson LA, Hoppel BE, Gerard EL, et al. Quantitative chemical shift imaging of vertebral bone marrow in patients with Gaucher's disease. Radiology 1992;182:451.

86. Terk MR, Esplin J, Lee K, et al. MR imaging of patients with Type 1 Gaucher's disease: relationship between bone and visceral changes. AJR 1995;165:599.

87. Katz K, Horev G, Grunebaum M, Yosipovitch Z. The natural history of osteonecrosis of the femoral head in children and adolescents who have Gaucher's disease. J Bone Joint Surg 1996;78:14.

88. Fong TP, et al. Stainable iron in aspirated and needle biopsy specimens of marrow: a source of error. Am J Hematol 1977;2:47.

89. Harker LA. Evaluation of storage iron by chelates. Am J Med 1968;45:105.

90. Bauman JH. Estimation of hepatic iron stores by in vivo measurement of magnetic susceptibility. J Lab Clin Med 1967;70:246

91. Jepson JH, et al. Erythropoietin in plasma of pregnant mice and rays. Com J Physiol Pharmacol 1968;45:573.

92. Deutsch AL, et al. Incidental detection of hematopoietic hyperplasia on routine knee MR imaging, AJR 1989;153:655

93. Wintrobe M. Iron deficient and iron deficiency anemia. In: Wintrobe M, ed. Clinical hematology, 8th ed. Philadelphia: Lea & Febiger, 1981:618.

94. Shellock FG, Morris E, Deutsch AL, et al. Hematopoietic bone marrow hyperplasia: high prevalence on MR images of the knee in asymptomatic marathon runners. AJR 1992;158:335.

95. Poulton TB, Murphy WD, Duerk JL, et al. Bone marrow reconversion in adults who are smokers: MR imaging findings. AJR 1993;161:1217.

96. VandeBerg BC, Malghem J, Devuyst O, et al. Anorexia nervosa correlation between MR appearance of bone marrow and severity of disease. Radiology 1994;193:859.

97. Gale RP, et al. Aplastic anemia: biology and treatment. Ann Intern Med 1981;95:477.

98. Camitta BM, et al. Aplastic anemia: pathogenesis, diagnosis, treatment and prognosis. N Engl J Med 1982;306:645.

99. McKinstry CS, Steiner TR, et al. Bone marrow in leukemia and aplastic anemia: MR imaging before, during, and after treatment. Radiology 1987;162:701.

100. Kaplan PA. Bone marrow patterns in aplastic anemia: observations with 1.5-T MR imaging. Radiology 1987;164:441.

101. Benz ED. The hemoglobinopathies. In: Kelley WN, ed. Textbook of internal medicine. Philadelphia: JB Lippincott, 1989:1423.

102. Sebes JI, et al. Diagnostic imaging of bone and joint abnormalities associated with sickle cell hemoglobinopathies. AJR 1989;152:1153.

103. Van Zanten TEG, et al. Imaging of bone marrow with magnetic resonance during a crisis and in chronic forms of sickle cell disease. Clin Radiol 1989;40:486.

104. Henry J. Clinical diagnosis and management. Philadelphia: WB Saunders, 1984:679.

105. Cotran RS, Robbins SL. The musculoskeletal system. In: Pathologic basis of disease, 4th ed. Philadelphia: WB Saunders, 1989:1328.

106. Roberts MC, et al. Paget disease: MR imaging findings. Radiology 1989;173:341.

107. Malkin LH. Reflex sympathetic dystrophy syndrome following trauma to the foot. Orthopaedics 1990;13:851.

108. Steinbach LS, Tehranzadeh J, Fleckenstein JL, et al. Human immunodeficiency virus infection: musculoskeletal manifestations. Radiology 1993;186:833.

109. Osborne BM, Guarda LA, Bertler JJ. Bone marrow biopsies in patients with the acquired immunodeficiency syndrome. Hum Pathol 1984;15:1048.

110. Seaman JP, Kjeldsberg CR, Linhur A. Gelatinous transformation of the bone marrow. Hum Pathol 1978;9:685.

Magnetic Resonance Imaging in Orthopaedics & Sports Medicine, Second Edition,
edited by David W. Stoller. Lippincott-Raven Publishers, Philadelphia, © 1997.

Chapter 16

Bone and Soft-Tissue Tumors

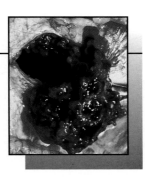

David W. Stoller
James O. Johnston
Terri M. Steinkirchner

The superior contrast discrimination provided by magnetic resonance (MR) imaging has proved extremely valuable in the assessment of bone and soft-tissue tumors.[1–17] T1 and T2 relaxation times are prolonged in a variety of malignant tissue types; therefore, malignant change tends to demonstrate low to intermediate signal intensity on T1-weighted images, and bright signal intensity on T2-weighted images. Although computed tomography (CT) may provide superior cortical detail, MR imaging is much more sensitive to marrow involvement by edema or tumor and provides soft-tissue definition of the surrounding musculature, fascial planes, and neurovascular bundles without artifact from cortical bone.

IMAGING TECHNIQUES

In the evaluation of tumors, a combination of both T1 and conventional T2 weighting, fat-suppressed T2-weighted fast spin-echo, or gradient-echo techniques is essential. With short TI inversion recovery (STIR) imaging sequences, T1 and T2 contrast are additive.[18,19] T1-weighted images provide excellent contrast for identification of marrow, cortical, and soft-tissue involvement. In particular, T1-weighted images allow differentiation between fat and tumor, as well as definition of muscle planes and separate anatomic compartments.

Gadolinium has been used to enhance contrast on T1-weighted images to better characterize osseous and soft-tissue tumor involvement.[10,14,16,20–22] On gadolinium-enhanced images, regions of low signal intensity are thought to represent areas of nonviable tumor or necrosis (Fig. 16-1). Gadolinium-enhanced images may also be useful for differentiating peritumoral edema from underlying tumor and recurrent tumor from scar or fibrosis.[23]

T2-weighted images are valuable in distinguishing muscle from tumor and can increase diagnostic specificity in evaluating marrow infiltration, seen as areas of low signal intensity on T1-weighted images.

Magnetic resonance may not be as sensitive as CT to cortical disruption, fine periosteal reactions, and small calcifications, although the sensitivity of MR imaging versus CT needs further documentation. With proper imaging planes and resolution, we have been able to distinguish early endosteal and cortical erosions, as well as periosteal changes on MR images (Fig. 16-2). Although each MR examination must be tailored to the patient and pathology in question, certain general guidelines can be followed. The longitudinal extent of tumors can be seen on T1-weighted coronal or sagittal images. If a lesion is difficult to differentiate from (ie, is isointense with) adjacent tissues, either a conventional T2, fat-suppressed T2-weighted fast spin-echo, T2*, or STIR sequence should be obtained. T1- and T2-weighted images (including fat-suppressed T2-weighted fast spin-echo or STIR sequences) in the axial plane provide the most important images in delineating the relationship of a tumor to adjacent neurovascular structures and compartments— essential information in preoperative limb salvage planning. In addition, the proximal and distal extent of tumor involvement can be assessed by evaluating multiple axial sections. The region of abnormality should be positioned as close to

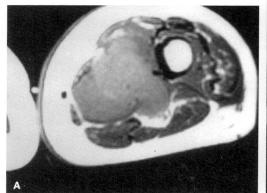

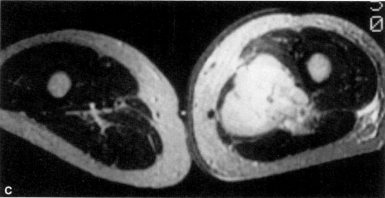

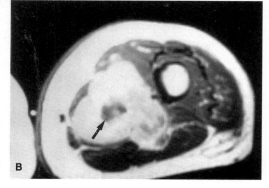

FIGURE 16-1. T1-weighted images (**A**) before and (**B**) after Gd-DTPA administration show malignant fibrous histiocytoma. The tumor is enhanced after intravenous injection of gadolinium. Central tumor necrosis remains unenhanced (*arrow*) (TR, 500 msec; TE, 20 msec). (**C**) On the corresponding T2-weighted axial image, the tumor demonstrates increased signal intensity, but central necrosis is not seen (TR, 2000 msec; TE, 80 msec).

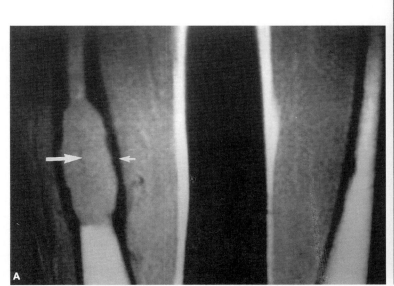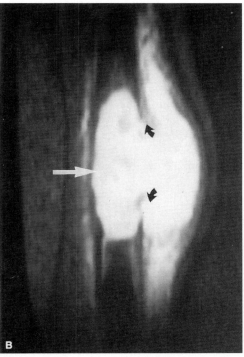

FIGURE 16-2. Ewing's sarcoma (*large straight arrows*) of the right femoral shaft is seen on (**A**) coronal T1-weighted and (**B**) sagittal short TI inversion recovery (STIR) images. Cortical thickening (*small straight arrow*) demonstrates low signal intensity on the coronal T1-weighted image. Histologically confirmed hyperintense subcortical tumor infiltration (*curved arrows*) is identified with STIR contrast (**A:** TR, 600 msec; TE, 30 msec; **B:** TR, 1400 msec; TI = 100 msec; TE, 40 msec).

the center of the coil as possible. The patient's position—prone or supine—is determined by the area of abnormality. Prior to imaging the particular region of interest, a large field-of-view localizer using an increased diameter surface coil or body coil may be necessary to exclude skin lesions or to accurately determine the proximal and distal extension of a large mass.

GENERAL MAGNETIC RESONANCE APPEARANCE

Direct multiplanar imaging facilitates improved preoperative and pretherapy evaluation of the exact extent of a lesion. In addition, since there is minimal artifact from nonferromagnetic implants with MR imaging, it is often possible to identify postoperative and posttreatment fibrous tissues not seen on CT. A tumor bed with postoperative scarring demonstrates low signal intensity on both T1- and T2- (including fat-suppressed T2-weighted fast spin-echo) weighted images. If, however, T1- and T2-weighted images show intermediate and high signal intensity, respectively, the possibility of recurrent tumor is more likely. This distinction often cannot be made on CT scans.

It is often not possible to distinguish benign from malignant lesions of bone and soft tissue on the basis of MR signal characteristics alone. Both benign and malignant lesions may demonstrate areas of low signal intensity on T1-weighted images and increased signal intensity on T2-weighted images. Malignant lesions tend to be more extensive, involving marrow, cortical bone, and soft tissues; but these criteria do not always distinguish benign from malignant lesions. No correlations have been shown matching T1 and T2 relaxation times with corresponding histopathology.[24] If the neurovascular bundle is involved, the lesion is likely to be malignant. A fluid-fluid level is a nonspecific finding in bone and soft-tissue lesions. Tumors with fluid-fluid levels include fibrous dysplasia, simple bone cysts, malignant fibrous histiocytoma (MFH), osteosarcoma, aneurysmal bone cysts, hemangioma, and synovial sarcoma.[25]

Infectious processes (eg, osteomyelitis) and benign neoplasms have been found to have a low signal intensity peripheral margin in 33% of patients.[26] This margin is rarely seen in malignant lesions because a well-defined sclerotic interface is not present. It is important to perform MR studies prior to biopsy, to avoid postsurgical inflammation and edema that may prolong T2 values of uninvolved tissues. Muscle edema is nonspecific and may be associated with trauma, infection, and vascular insults. On T1-weighted images, high signal intensity in the surrounding musculature can be seen in atrophy with fatty infiltration or neuromuscular disorders, and should not be mistaken for tumor. Venous varicosities may scallop subcutaneous tissue and demon-

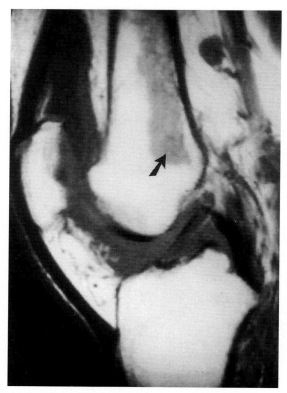

FIGURE 16-3. Red marrow inhomogeneity (*arrow*) without extension across the physeal scar can be seen in the diaphysis and metaphysis of the femur on a T1-weighted sagittal image (TR, 600 msec; TE, 20 msec).

strate low signal intensity on T1-weighted images. This appearance is characteristic, and can be distinguished from neoplastic soft-tissue extension or tumor vascularity.

Red-to-yellow marrow conversion in middle-aged women (marrow inhomogeneity is especially common in obese women with a history of smoking) is seen in metaphyseal or diaphyseal areas of low signal intensity (ie, red marrow) without extension into the epiphysis (Fig. 16-3). These lesions become isointense with adjacent marrow on heavily T2-weighted images and demonstrate increased signal intensity on STIR images. Inhomogeneity of metaphyseal red and yellow marrow may also be observed in the immature skeleton.

BONE TUMORS

Benign Lesions

Benign Osteoblastic Lesions

OSTEOID OSTEOMA. Osteoid osteomas are small, benign, osteoblastic lesions characteristically seen in younger patients (between 7 and 25 years of age).[27] They are composed of osteoid and trabeculae of newly formed osseous tissue embedded in a substriated, highly vascularized osteogenic connective tissue with a surrounding peripheral zone of dense sclerotic bone. They rarely exceed 1 cm in diameter and are usually located in either the spongiosa or the cortex of the bone. Most commonly, they affect long tubular bones; the femur is the most common site of involvement. The

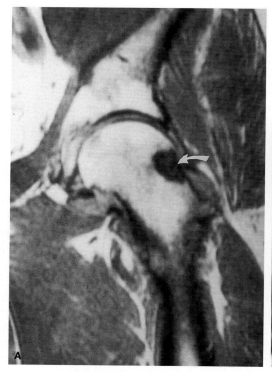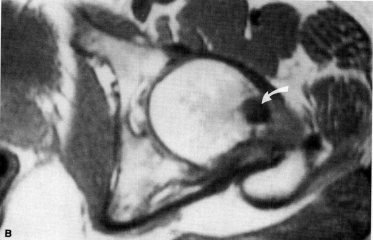

FIGURE 16-4. On T1-weighted (**A**) coronal and (**B**) axial images, subcortical osteoid osteoma is seen as a low signal intensity nidus (*curved arrows*) in the left femoral neck (TR, 600 msec; TE, 20 msec).

clinical hallmark of this lesion is pain that is most prominent at night and can be relieved with salicylates (ie, aspirin).[27-29]

Magnetic Resonance Appearance. On T1-weighted images, the nidus of the lesion demonstrates low to intermediate signal intensity (Figs. 16-4 through 16-6). On T2-weighted images, the central nidus demonstrates moderate to increased signal intensity.[30,31] Intracapsular osteoid osteomas of the hip usually cause a synovial inflammatory response and are associated with joint effusions and variable reactive marrow edema.[32,33] Reactive sclerosis demonstrates low signal intensity on T1- and T2-weighted images. There may be extensive marrow edema associated with osteoid osteomas, and STIR or fat-suppressed T2-weighted fast spin-echo sequences can be used to screen for this reactive edema. Occasionally, increased vascularity directed toward the nidus can be seen on MR images (Fig. 16-7). Thin section CT may be necessary to identify the nidus in intracortical lesions, however.[34] Enhancement with gadolinium in the presence of a reactive soft-tissue mass with myxomatous change may be mistaken for a malignant tumor or osteomyelitis.[15] CT-guided percutaneous excision and percutaneous radiofrequency ablation techniques have been used for treatment.[35-38]

OSTEOBLASTOMA. Initially known as giant osteoid osteoma, osteoblastoma commonly presents in patients between 10 and 20 years of age.[15,29,39] Local pain is inconsistently relieved with salicylates. Osteoblastoma most frequently involves the flat bones or posterior osseous elements of the vertebrae. Histologically, osteoblastomas present a more variable picture than osteoid osteomas. There is well-vascularized connective tissue containing osteoid and primitive woven bone rimmed by osteoblasts. In contrast to osteoid osteoma, trabecular maturation, degree of calcification, and overall architectural patterns vary greatly in osteoblastoma.[29] A diffuse inflammatory response involving bone and adjacent soft tissue was reported in one MR study of a case of vertebral osteoblastoma.[40] Signal intensity may be heterogeneous or homogeneous on T2-weighted images. CT may be more accurate for the identification of small foci of matrix calcification. Local excision involves marginal or intralesional resection with curettage.[15]

Benign Chondroblastic Lesions

ENCHONDROMA. Enchondromas are benign intramedullary lesions composed of circumscribed lobules of hyaline cartilage that occasionally exhibit flecks of calcification. Cellularity may be increased in tumors in children and adolescents, but these histologic features do not imply chondrosarcoma. Radiologic findings are critical for accurate diagnosis.[41] Approximately 40% to 65% of solitary enchondromas occur in the hands, and approximately 25% occur in the long tubular bones.[29,41] Multiple enchondromatosis (Ollier's disease) was originally described in 1899. This rare, nonhereditary disorder is characterized by multiple asymmetric chondromatous lesions. In childhood, these lesions predispose the bone to fracture; in adulthood, there is an increased risk of malignant transformation.[42] Lesions that continue to grow after the cessation of normal body growth should raise the suspicion of malignant transformation. Treatment of atypical or symptomatic enchondromas include marginal or intralesional resection.[15] Autologous or allograft bone grafting is required in defects in large and weight-bearing bones.

Magnetic Resonance Appearance. Magnetic resonance imaging is useful in identifying enchondromas, which are well defined and demonstrate low signal intensity on T1-weighted images. Satellite cartilaginous foci are often seen in association with enchondromas. Chondroid elements demonstrate hyperintensity on T2-weighted, T2*-weighted, or STIR images (Figs. 16-8 and 16-9). In the multiple enchondromas of Ollier's disease, the foci of cartilaginous tissue or matrix are seen as areas of low to intermediate signal intensity on T1-weighted images and high signal intensity on T2-weighted images (Figs. 16-10

text continues on page 1242

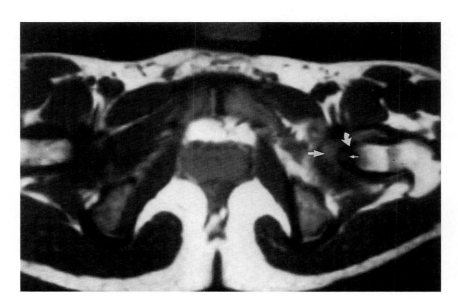

FIGURE 16-5. T1-weighted axial image of intracortical osteoid osteoma of the left femoral neck. A circular nidus of intermediate signal intensity (*small straight arrow*), low signal intensity cortical thickening (*curved arrow*), and intermediate signal intensity effusion (*large straight arrow*) can be seen (TR, 600 msec; TE, 20 msec).

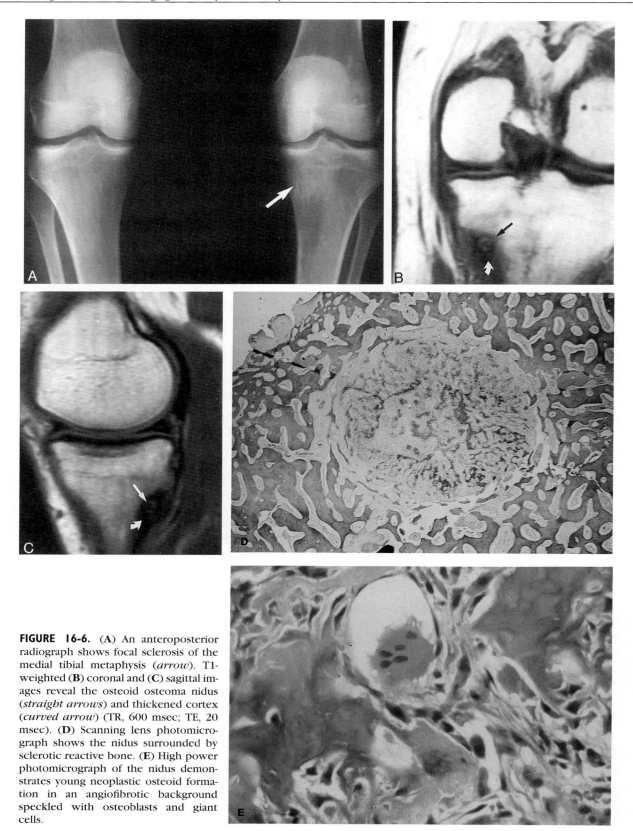

FIGURE 16-6. (A) An anteroposterior radiograph shows focal sclerosis of the medial tibial metaphysis (*arrow*). T1-weighted (**B**) coronal and (**C**) sagittal images reveal the osteoid osteoma nidus (*straight arrows*) and thickened cortex (*curved arrow*) (TR, 600 msec; TE, 20 msec). (**D**) Scanning lens photomicrograph shows the nidus surrounded by sclerotic reactive bone. (**E**) High power photomicrograph of the nidus demonstrates young neoplastic osteoid formation in an angiofibrotic background speckled with osteoblasts and giant cells.

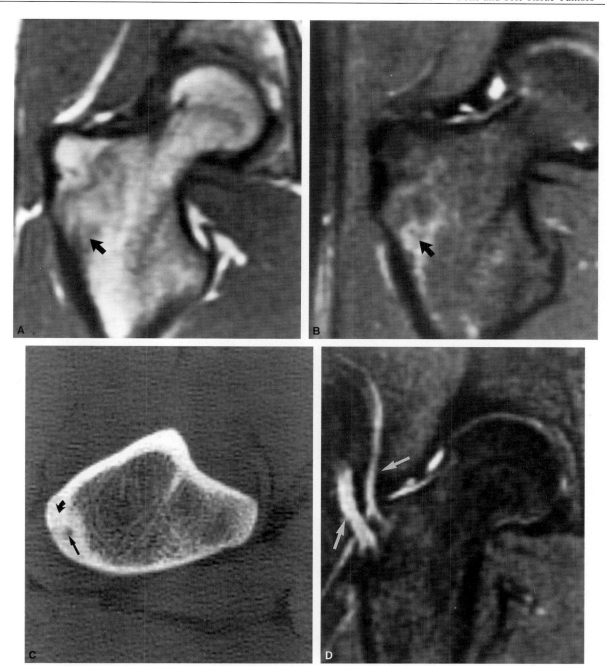

FIGURE 16-7. Cortex-based osteoid osteoma adjacent to the greater trochanter. Mild reactive subchondral marrow edema (*arrow*) is hypointense on T1-weighted (**A**) and hyperintense on fat-suppressed T2-weighted fast spin-echo (**B**) coronal images. (**C**) Localized cortical thickening (*curved arrow*) and nidus (*straight arrow*) are best appreciated on corresponding axial CT image. (**D**) Hypervascularity with feeding vessels (*arrows*) to the nidus are present on fat-suppressed T2-weighted fast spin-echo coronal image. Feeding vessels originate from surrounding soft tissues.

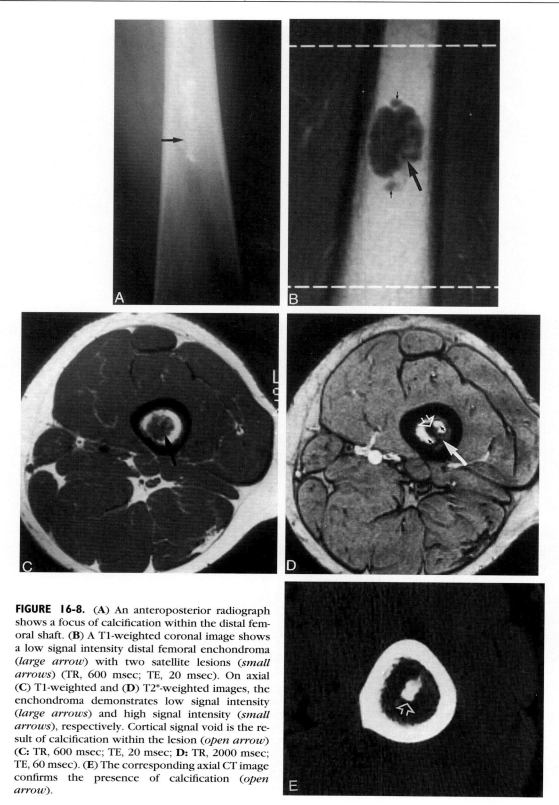

FIGURE 16-8. (**A**) An anteroposterior radiograph shows a focus of calcification within the distal femoral shaft. (**B**) A T1-weighted coronal image shows a low signal intensity distal femoral enchondroma (*large arrow*) with two satellite lesions (*small arrows*) (TR, 600 msec; TE, 20 msec). On axial (**C**) T1-weighted and (**D**) T2*-weighted images, the enchondroma demonstrates low signal intensity (*large arrows*) and high signal intensity (*small arrows*), respectively. Cortical signal void is the result of calcification within the lesion (*open arrow*) (**C:** TR, 600 msec; TE, 20 msec; **D:** TR, 2000 msec; TE, 60 msec). (**E**) The corresponding axial CT image confirms the presence of calcification (*open arrow*).

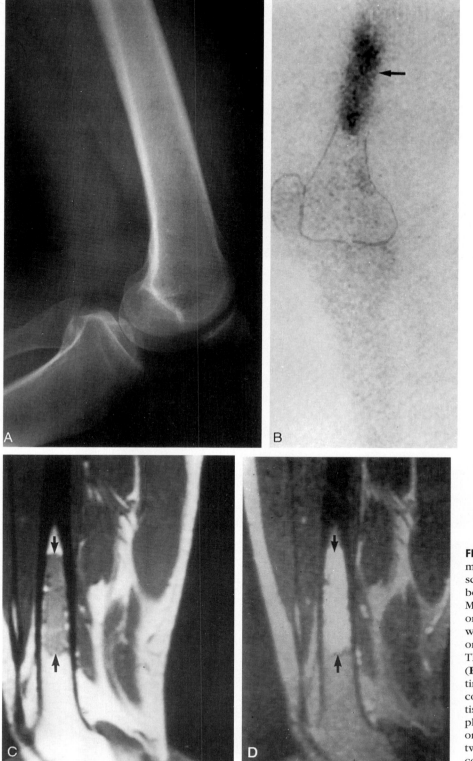

FIGURE 16-9. (**A**) A lateral radiograph is unremarkable for enchondroma. (**B**) On nuclear scintigraphy, there is uptake of ^{99m}TC-MDP bone tracer in the distal femur (*arrow*). On MR scans, benign enchondroma (*arrows*) demonstrates (**C**) low signal intensity on a T1-weighted image and (**D**) high signal intensity on a T2-weighted image (**C:** TR, 1000 msec; TE, 20 msec; **D:** TR, 2000 msec; TE, 60 msec). (**E**) Gross appearance of chondroid tissue at time of surgery prior to curettement. (**F**) Popcorn-like appearance of friable chondroid tissue during curettement. (**G**) Low power photomicrograph at outer edge of tumor demonstrating a benign noninvasive interface between chondroid matrix and surrounding cortical-cancellous bone.   *continued*

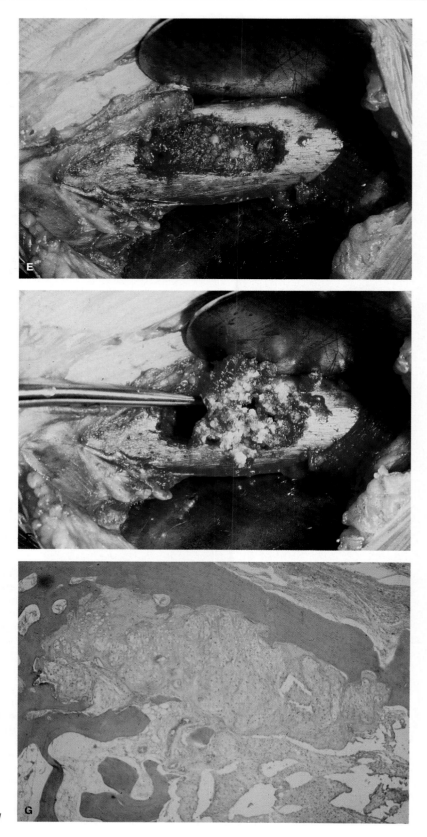

FIGURE 16-9. *Continued*

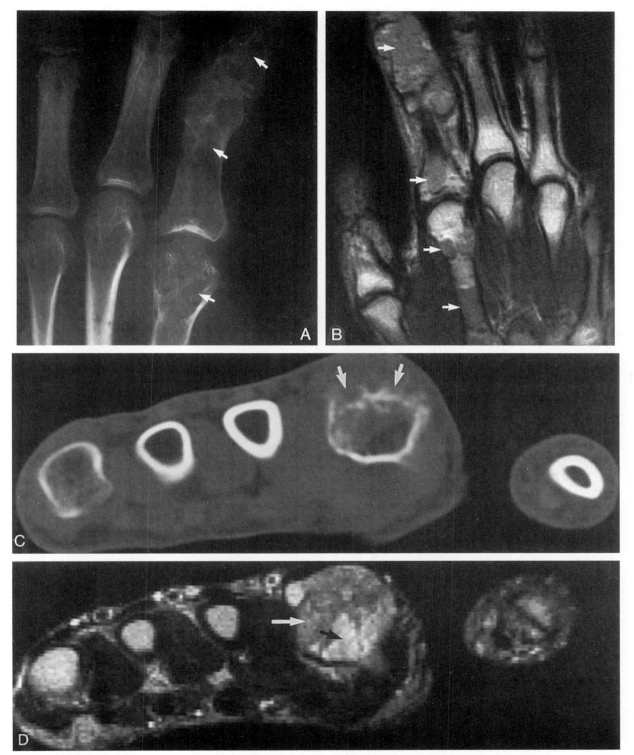

FIGURE 16-10. Ollier's disease. **(A)** An anteroposterior radiograph and **(B)** a T1-weighted coronal image show multiple enchondromatous foci (*arrows*) in the second ray. **(B:** TR, 1000 msec; TE, 40 msec). **(C)** Corresponding axial CT image shows cortical irregularity (*arrows*). **(D)** On an axial spin-echo T2-weighted sequence, increased signal intensity is seen in cartilaginous foci (*black arrow*) within the affected digit (*white arrow*) (TR, 2000 msec; TE, 80 msec).

and 16-11). This appearance is secondary to the long T1 and T2 relaxation times of chondroid tissue. Enchondromas in Ollier's disease may show aggressive features such as cortical irregularities, without malignant degeneration (see Fig. 16-10). Enchondromas are common in the tubular bones of the hands and feet (Fig. 16-12).

Enchondromas can be differentiated from bone infarcts by the following features[43,44]:

- Lack of central fat signal intensity on T1-weighted images
- Peripheral borders that are not as serpiginous as those seen in infected tissue
- Central areas of increased signal intensity on T2-weighted images.

Central calcifications are best seen on T2*-weighted images (Fig. 16-13). However, it is difficult to differentiate enchondroma from low grade chondrosarcoma on the basis of signal intensity alone. The presence of a positive bone scan in the absence of pain cannot be used as a criteria for malignant conversion of enchondromas. Nonaggressive features include the absence of a soft-tissue mass and absence of interval growth on serial MR studies.

In juxtacortical or periosteal chondroma, soft-tissue calcification may mimic myositis ossificans (Figs. 16-14 and 16-15). Localized increases in signal intensity on T2-weighted images may occur without underlying involvement of the adjacent bone.[45]

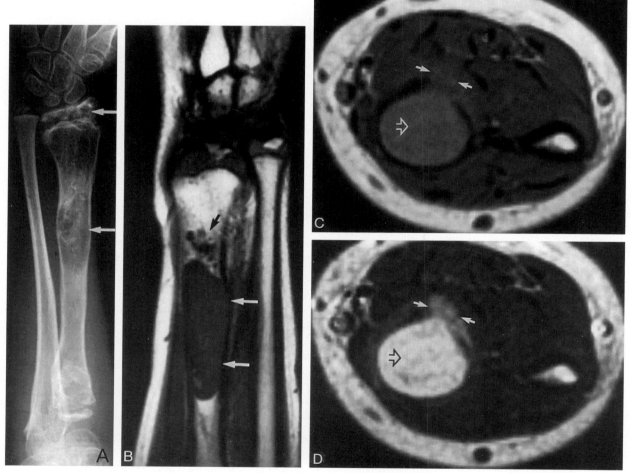

FIGURE 16-11. Ollier's disease. (A) An anteroposterior forearm radiograph demonstrates proximal and distal radius lesions (*arrows*). (B) A T1-weighted coronal image of distal radius lesions shows satellite enchondromas (*black arrow*) and a larger low signal intensity focus of enchondroma (*white arrows*) (TR, 600 msec; TE, 20 msec). Enchondroma (*open arrows*) on axial (C) T1-weighted and (D) T2-weighted images demonstrates low and high signal intensity, respectively, with disruption of cortical bone (*solid arrows*). Enchondromas in Ollier's disease may exhibit aggressive features in the absence of malignant transformation (C: TR, 600 msec; TE, 20 msec; D: TR, 2000 msec; TE, 60 msec).

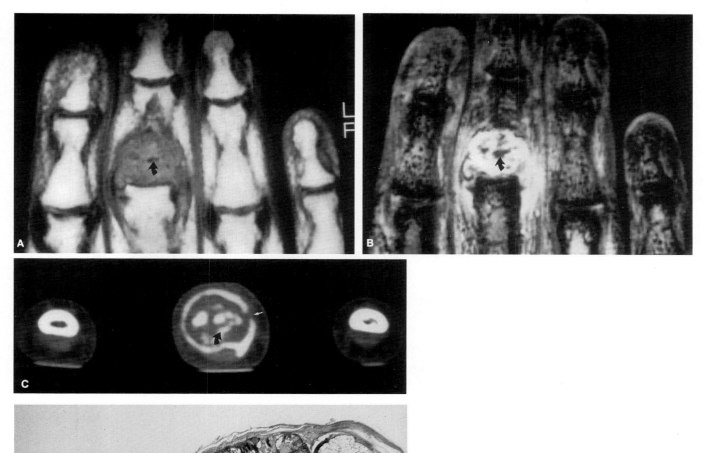

FIGURE 16-12. Expansile enchondroma of the base of the middle phalanx is seen on coronal (**A**) T1-weighted and (**B**) T2*-weighted images. Central calcification can be seen (*arrows*). (**C**) The corresponding CT image shows central stippled chondroid tumor calcification (*black arrow*) and cortical interruption (*white arrow*). (**D**) Gross macrosection of a similar enchondroma in the proximal phalanx of another patient demonstrates extensive thinning and dilation of the cortical structures and extension to the proximal articular cartilage.

OSTEOCHONDROMA. Osteocartilaginous exostosis (osteochondroma) is one of the most common bone tumors in children. Solitary osteochondroma is a frequent lesion, and opinions differ as to whether it represents a true neoplasm or a developmental physeal growth defect.[41] The vast majority of these lesions present in patients younger than 20 years of age. With the exception of a proliferative cartilage cap, the spongiosa and cortex in exostosis are continuous with the adjacent shaft. The thickness of the cartilaginous cap correlates with the age of the patient.[41] In children or adolescents, the cap may be as thick as 3 cm. In adults, however, the cap is thinner, presumably secondary to wear and tear.

Findings of a cartilage cap thicker than 1 cm, an irregular cartilaginous cap, renewed growth with pain in an adult, or a combination of these raises the possibility of chondrosarcomatous transformation.[29,41,46,47] Such malignant transformation is rare (less than 1%) in solitary osteochondroma, but has been reported with increased frequency in cases of multiple osteocartilaginous exostoses.

Magnetic Resonance Appearance. Osteochondromas are metaphyseal-based tumors that usually involve the long bones (Fig. 16-16). When the flat bones are involved, the
text continues on page 1248

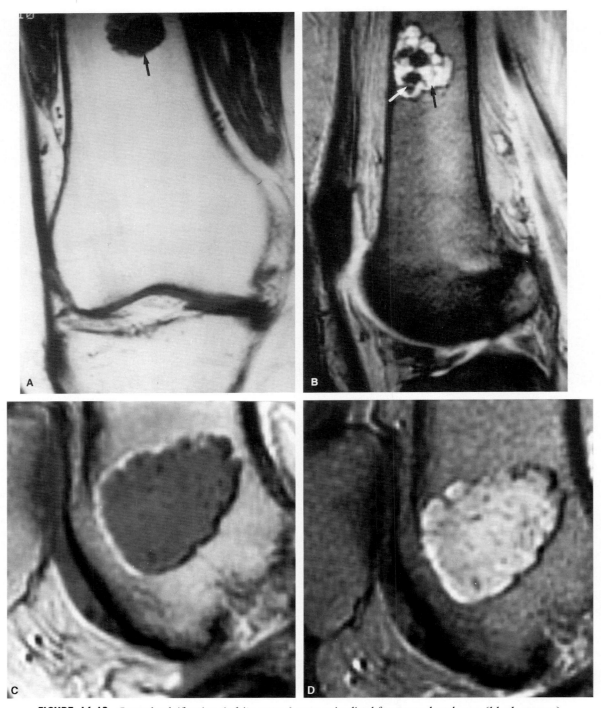

FIGURE 16-13. Central calcification (*white arrow*) occurs in distal femur enchondroma (*black arrows*). (**A**) Compared with a T1-weighted coronal image, the chondroid tissue is (**B**) hyperintense on a T2*-weighted sagittal image (**A:** TR, 600 msec; TE, 20 msec; **B:** TR, 400 msec; TE, 15 msec; flip angle, 20°). Central calcifications are less conspicuous when using conventional T2-weighted sequences as shown in another patient on intermediate (**C**) and T2-weighted (**D**) images.

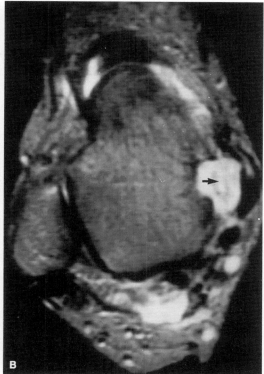

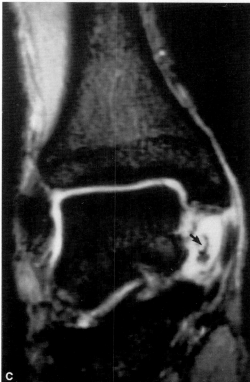

FIGURE 16-14. Periosteal (ie, juxtacortical) chondroma located inferior to the medial malleolus is seen on axial (**A**) intermediate weighted and (**B**) T2-weighted images and on (**C**) a coronal T2*-weighted image. Central cartilage and osseous tissue is low in signal intensity on all pulse sequences (*arrows*). Periosteal chondromas often occur adjacent to tendon or ligament insertions (**A, B:** TR, 2000 msec; TE, 20, 80 msec; **C:** TR, 400 msec; TE, 20 msec; flip angle, 25°).

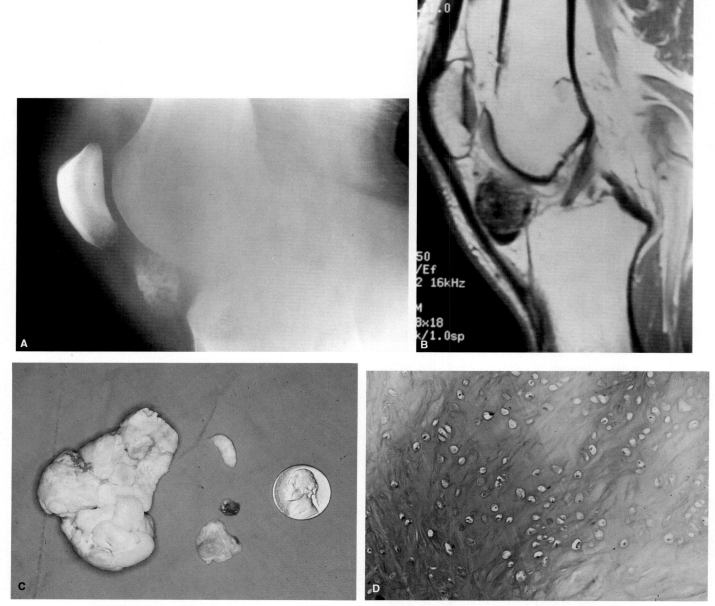

FIGURE 16-15. (A) Radiograph of the knee of a young adult male with a heavily calcified juxtaarticular chondroma in the infrapatellar fat pad. (B) T1-weighted sagittal image demonstrates the low signal character of this heavily calcified chondroid lesion just beneath the patellar ligament. (C) Gross appearance of the resected specimen with the upper faceted surface representing its prior articulation with the femoral condyle. (D) Low power photomicrograph of benign-appearing chondrocytes in a heavily calcified chondroid matrix.

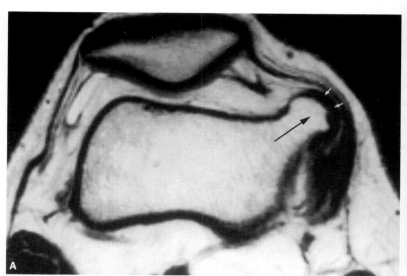

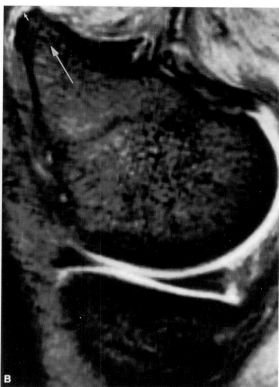

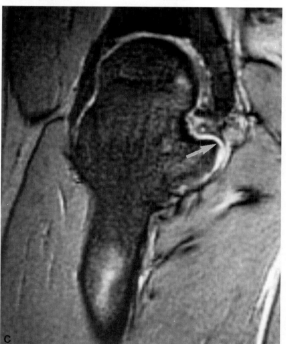

FIGURE 16-16. Osteochondroma. Metaphyseal exostosis with continuity of marrow and cortex (*long arrows*) is present. The cartilage cap (*short arrows*) demonstrates (**A**) low to intermediate signal intensity on a T1-weighted image and (**B**) high signal intensity on a T2*-weighted image (**A:** TR, 600 msec; TE, 20 msec; **B:** TR, 400 msec; TE, 15 msec; flip angle, 20°). (**C**) In another patient an osteochondroma arising from the region of the lesser trochanter demonstrates a thin, uniform hyperintense cartilage cap (*arrow*) as seen on a T2*-weighted coronal image of the right hip.

lesion may present with a more cauliflower or expansile configuration (Figs. 16-17 and 16-18). On MR examination, benign osteochondromas are isointense with normal marrow. The intact cartilage cap demonstrates intermediate signal intensity on T1-weighted images and high signal intensity on T2-weighted images. With malignant degeneration, the signal intensity of the exostosis decreases on T1-weighted images and increases on T2-weighted images. Disruption of the high signal intensity cartilaginous cap may also be observed with aggressive tumor invasion. T2*-weighted and fat-suppressed T2-weighted fast spin-echo sequences are useful in defining the thickness of the cartilaginous cap (as mentioned earlier, it may be as thick as 3 cm in adolescents and less than 1 cm in adults). Dispersed calcifications in the cartilaginous cap, as well as increased thickness of the cap, are features of malignant transformation that can be identified on MR scans (Fig. 16-19). MR imaging is superior to CT in demonstrating inflammatory changes that accompany

enlargement of the bursa exostotica covering the cartilaginous cap (Fig. 16-20). This bursa is hypointense on T1-weighted images and hyperintense on T2, fat-suppressed T2-weighted fast spin-echo, or STIR sequences. Gadolinium administration causes enhancement of the periphery of the bursa exostotica only. Growth deformity is associated with multiple exostoses[48] (Fig. 16-21).

Geirnaerdt and colleagues have described a pattern of septal enhancement with gadolinium-enhanced MR imaging, which is helpful in identifying transformation of osteochondromas to low-grade chondrosarcomas.[14] The enhancing curvilinear septa are thought to correlate histologically with fibrovascular septa around and between lobules of paucicellular cartilage and cystic mucoid tissue. Osteochondromas without signs of malignant transformation show a peripheral enhancement of fibrovascular tissue covering the nonenhanced hyaline cartilage cap without evidence of fibrovascular septa. Despite the presence of septa in low-grade chon-

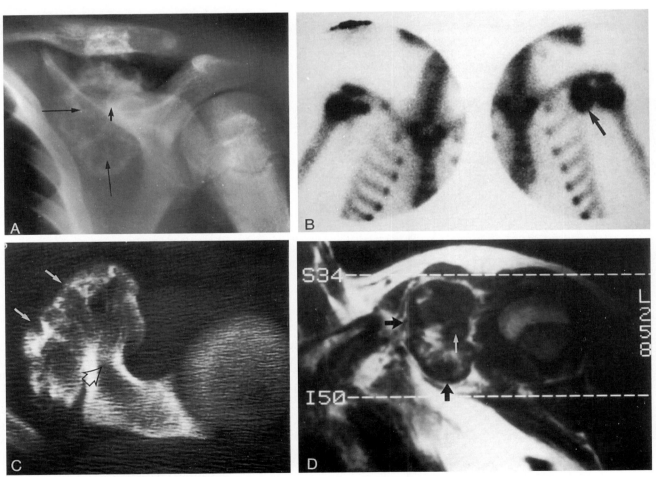

FIGURE 16-17. Benign osteochondroma. **(A)** An anteroposterior radiograph shows a cauliflower-like bony excrescence (*long arrows*) arising from the coracoid process (*short arrow*). **(B)** Nuclear scintigraphy shows increased uptake of bone tracer in region of left coracoid. **(C)** On an axial CT image, the enlarged cartilage cap (*white arrows*) can be seen continuous with cortex and spongiosa of adjacent bone (*open arrow*). **(D)** On a T1-weighted coronal image, a low signal intensity mass can been seen emanating from the low spin density coracoid (*white arrow*). The cartilage cap is difficult to distinguish from the cortex without a T2-weighted pulse sequence (TR, 600 msec; TE, 20 msec).

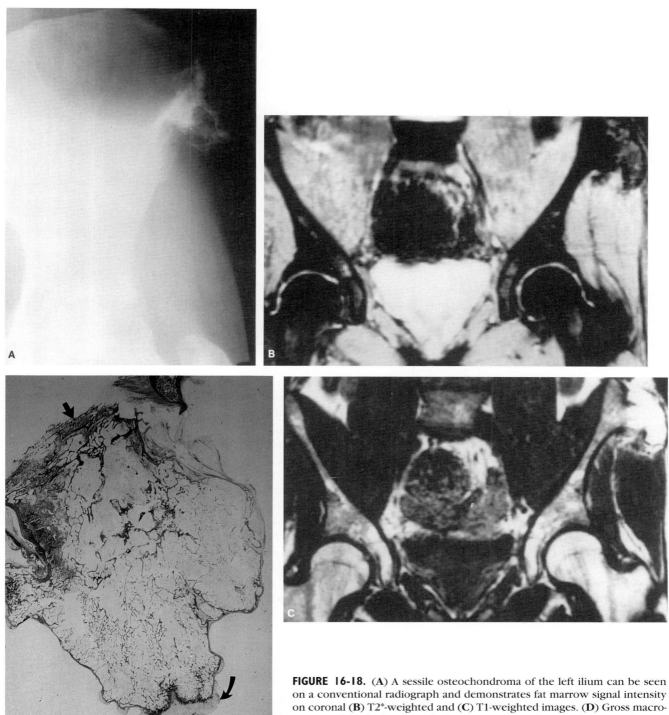

FIGURE 16-18. (A) A sessile osteochondroma of the left ilium can be seen on a conventional radiograph and demonstrates fat marrow signal intensity on coronal (B) T2*-weighted and (C) T1-weighted images. (D) Gross macrosection of similar lesion with the short arrow indicating the cortical origin and the curved arrow pointing to the small cartilaginous cap with friable atrophic fatty cancellous bone between.

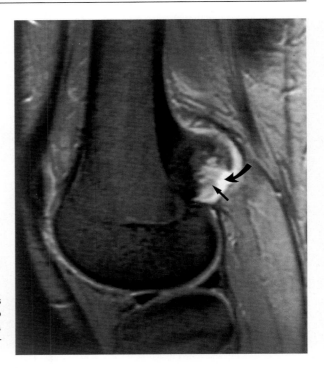

FIGURE 16-19. Osteochondroma of the knee with a change in MR findings including the development of dispersed calcifications in the cartilaginous cap (*straight arrow*), increased thickness of the cartilaginous cap (*curved arrow*), and enlargement of the lesion—features suggesting initial malignant transformation. T2*-weighted sagittal image.

drosarcoma, these patterns of enhancement are not observed in high-grade chondrosarcomas. Crim and Seeger point out that these findings have not been validated in a sufficient number of patients to conclude that septal enhancement is a specific sign for low-grade chondrosarcoma.[49] In fact, fibrovascular septa are uncommon in grade 1 chondrosarcoma. Additional studies need to be performed to more precisely determine the benefit of gadolinium enhancement in the diagnosis of grade 1 chondrosarcomas.

Symptomatic osteochondromas can be treated with simple resection of the base and cartilaginous tissue, including the perichondrium surrounding the cap.

CHONDROBLASTOMA. The benign chondroblastoma is an epiphyseal cartilage tumor that generally arises in a long tubular bone and occurs most frequently in the second decade of life.[50] Joint effusion may accompany periarticular

bone involvement. Histologic findings include a cellular proliferation of chondroblasts with irregularly dispersed multinucleated osteoclast giant cells.[50] In 50% of cases, benign peripheral sclerosis, intralesional punctate lace-like calcifications, and chondroid are present. Older lesions may exhibit necrosis, resorption, or reparative fibrosis with metaplastic osseous areas. These features all contribute to the variability seen in this lesion. Treatment involves biopsy followed by curettage. Intralesional curettage may be combined with freezing with liquid nitrogen or application of phenol. Bony defects require autogenous or allogenic local graft, and, depending on the degree of subchondral erosions, reconstruction of joint surfaces.[15]

Magnetic Resonance Appearance. Benign chondroblastomas demonstrate a well-defined area of low to intermediate signal intensity on T1-weighted images and heterogeneity

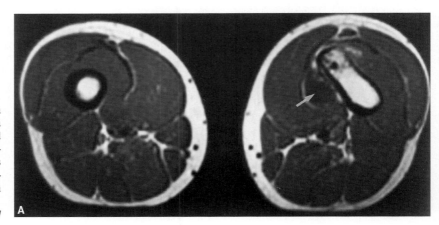

FIGURE 16-20. Bursa exostotica associated with a femoral osteochondroma. The bursa exostotica (*straight arrow*) is hypointense on a T1-weighted axial image (**A**), hyperintense on a fat-suppressed T2-weighted fast spin-echo image (**B**), and demonstrates peripheral enhancement (*curved arrow*) after administration of intravenous gadolinium contrast as seen on a fat-suppressed T1-weighted axial image (**C**).

continued

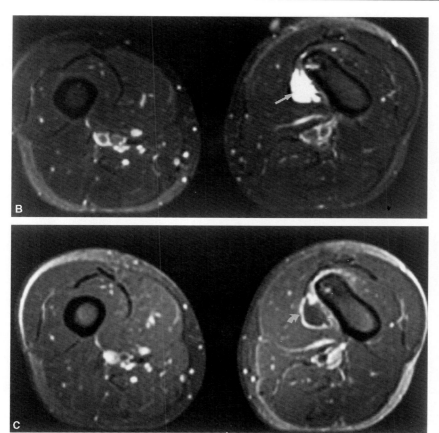

FIGURE 16-20. *Continued*

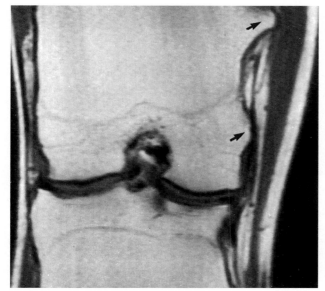

FIGURE 16-21. Undertubulation of the knee and exostosis (*arrows*) are seen on a T1-weighted coronal image of multiple hereditary exostosis (TR, 600 msec; TE, 20 msec).

with increased signal intensity in a noncalcified chondroid matrix on T2-weighted images (Figs. 16-22 and 16-23). Typically, the long-bone epiphyses of the humerus, tibia, or femur are affected. MR imaging can be used to identify eccentric locations and the associated sclerotic border.[51] Epiphyseal and metaphyseal marrow edema associated with a diametaphyseal periosteal reaction is a frequent finding, seen in up to 57% of cases of long-bone involvement.[52] MR imaging is sensitive to this extensive reactive marrow edema, which demonstrates decreased signal intensity on T1-weighted images and increased signal intensity on T2-weighted or STIR images (Fig. 16-24). T2-weighted images are useful in demonstrating the lobular internal architecture and fine lobular margins of the lesion.[53]

Benign Fibrous and Related Lesions

FIBROUS CORTICAL DEFECT. Fibrous cortical defects, histologically identical to large nonossifying fibromas (see later), demonstrate low to intermediate signal intensity on T1-weighted images and intermediate to increased signal intensity on T2*-weighted and fat-suppressed T2-weighted fast spin-echo images. The increased signal intensity ob-

text continues on page 1254

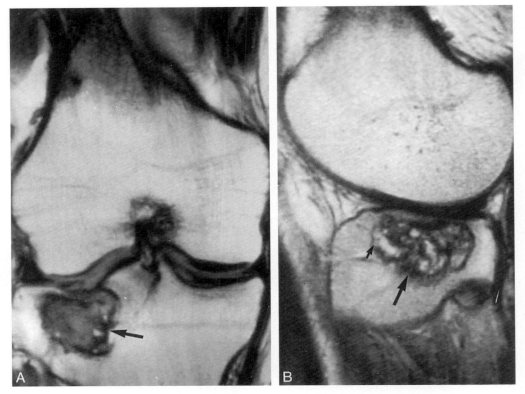

FIGURE 16-22. (A) On a T1-weighted coronal image, chondroblastoma of the tibial epiphysis (*arrow*) demonstrates intermediate signal intensity (TR, 600 msec; TE, 20 msec). (B) On a T2-weighted sagittal image, the chondroblastoma (*large arrow*) demonstrates nonuniform increased signal intensity (*small arrow*) (TR, 2000 msec; TE, 60 msec).

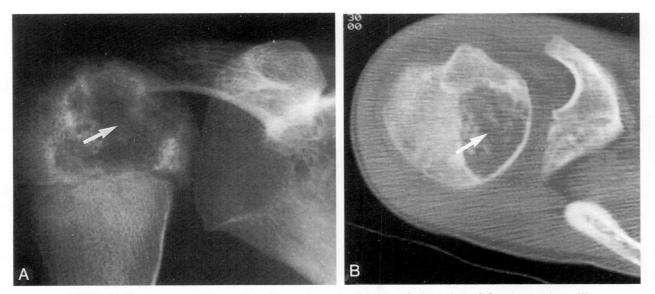

FIGURE 16-23. Chondroblastoma of the humeral epiphysis is identified as a lytic defect (*arrows*) on (A) an anteroposterior radiograph and (B) an axial CT scan. On a T2-weighted sequence, a cartilage tumor (*straight black arrows*) of the humeral head (*curved white arrows*) (C) demonstrates low to intermediate signal intensity on the first echo and (D) is an inhomogeneous area of mixed signal intensity on the second echo (TR, 1500 msec; TE, 20, 60 msec). (E) Gross macrosection of a similar case with chondroblastic nidus (*curved arrow*) and the transitional reactive bone interface (*straight arrow*) seen also in osteoblastomas. (F) High power photomicrograph of the nidus with typical polyhedral-shaped chondroblasts scattered in a "chicken wire" chondroid matrix.

continued

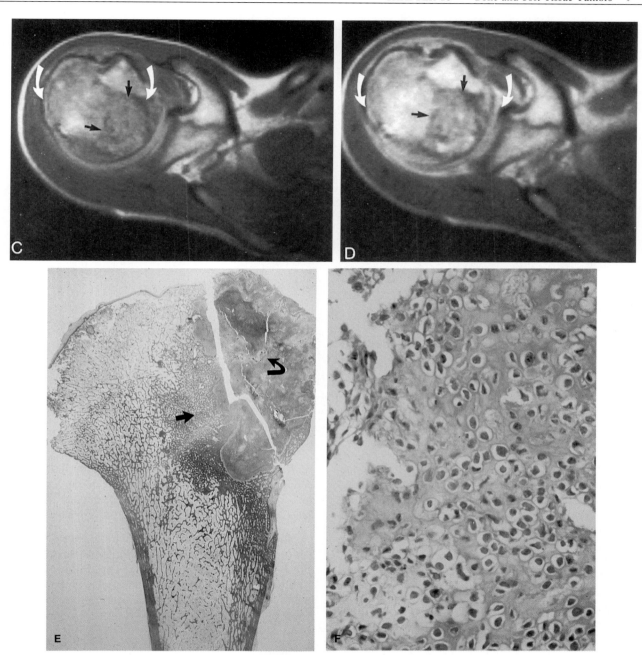

FIGURE16-23. *Continued*

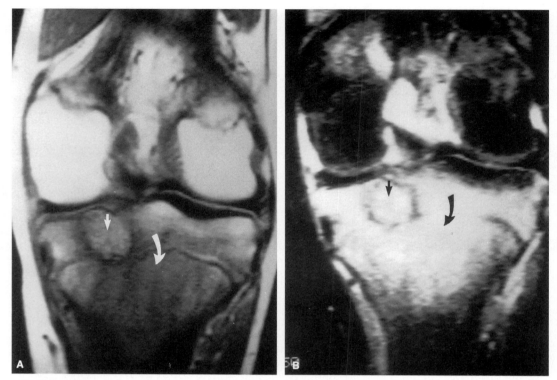

FIGURE 16-24. Extensive marrow edema (*curved arrows*) in reaction to epiphyseal-based chondroblastoma (*straight arrows*) demonstrates low signal intensity on a T1-weighted image (**A**) and hyperintensity on a short TI inversion recovery image (**B**).

served on T2-weighted images is secondary to T2 prolongation in the varied cellular constituents (eg, fibrous stroma, multinucleated giant cells, foam cells, cholesterol crystals, stromal red blood cells in hemorrhage)[29] (Fig. 16-25). Fibrous cortical defects have a predilection for the diaphyses of long bones.[15]

NONOSSIFYING FIBROMA. Nonossifying fibromas are frequently found in the long bones of children and are thought to represent one end of the spectrum of benign cortical defects with encroachment on the medullary cavity. Histologically, both nonossifying fibromas and fibrous cortical defects are composed of spindle-shaped fibroblasts arranged in an interlacing pattern. Unlike the fibrous cortical defect, nonossifying fibromas are more commonly found in the metaphyseal area.[15] On T1-weighted images, these lesions are usually low in signal intensity and have a lobulated contour with an eccentric epicenter (Figs. 16-26 and 16-27). T2, fat-suppressed T2-weighted fast spin-echo, or STIR images may demonstrate areas of hyperintensity. Nonossifying fibromas may also display a central area of fat signal intensity isointense to adjacent marrow, especially during healing or involution (Fig. 16-28).

Gadolinium has been used to enhance the peripheral border in fibrous metaphyseal defects.[54] Benign fibrous histiocytomas, also histologically similar to nonossifying fibromas, is present in an older population group and may be associated with symptoms of bone pain and local recurrence after treatment.[51] Nonsymptomatic fibrous cortical defects and nonossifying fibromas do not require treatment.[15] A pathologic fracture may occur through a nonossifying fibroma.

OSSIFYING FIBROMA. Ossifying fibromas are benign fibro-osseous lesions that most commonly arise in the facial bones of young female patients.[29] These lesions, as opposed to fibrous dysplasia, are well demarcated and therefore amenable to surgical curettage and enucleation. The histologic features of this lesion consist of random trabecular woven bone or dystrophic calcification set in a fibrous stroma.

PERIOSTEAL DESMOID. The periosteal desmoid is a fibrous proliferation of the periosteum involving the posteromedial cortex of the medial femoral condyle. The sclerotic saucer-shaped lesion is usually hypointense on T1- and T2-weighted images. A distal femoral cortical irregularity, called a linea aspera, is seen in a similar age group (10 to 20 years) and may be related to traction of the adductor magnus aponeurosis. This lesion may, in fact, represent a variant of the periosteal desmoid (Fig. 16-29). Biopsy should not be performed on periosteal desmoids, and they require no treatment.

Hyman and colleagues used MR imaging to identify an excavation of the distal femoral metaphysis corresponding to the origin of the medial head of the gastrocnemius muscle.[55]

text continues on page 1258

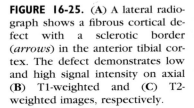

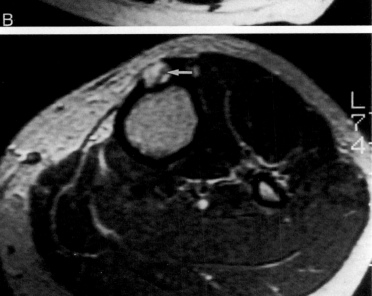

FIGURE 16-25. (**A**) A lateral radiograph shows a fibrous cortical defect with a sclerotic border (*arrows*) in the anterior tibial cortex. The defect demonstrates low and high signal intensity on axial (**B**) T1-weighted and (**C**) T2-weighted images, respectively.

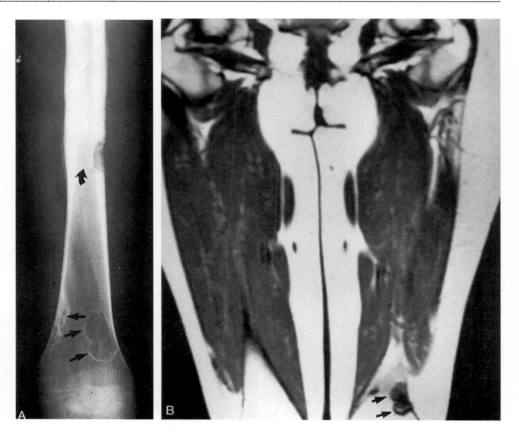

FIGURE 16-26. **(A)** An anteroposterior radiograph shows the sclerotic border (*straight arrows*) of a nonossifying fibroma. An incidental biopsy site for Ewing's sarcoma can also be seen (*curved arrow*). **(B)** T1-weighted image shows lobulated low signal intensity in the distal femoral metaphysis (*arrows*) (TR, 600 msec; TE, 20 msec).

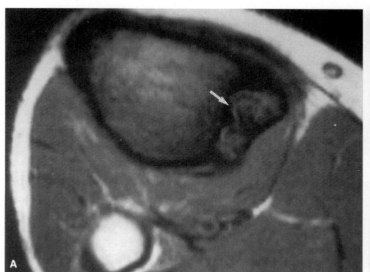

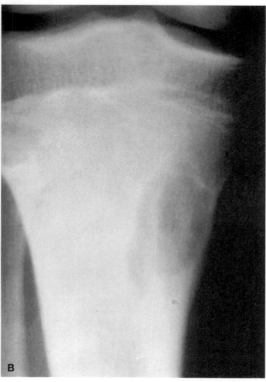

FIGURE 16-27. **(A)** A T1-weighted axial image shows nonossifying fibroma (*arrow*) with a pathologic fracture (TR, 500 msec; TE, 20 msec). **(B)** Corresponding anteroposterior radiograph displays the eccentric location of the lesion.

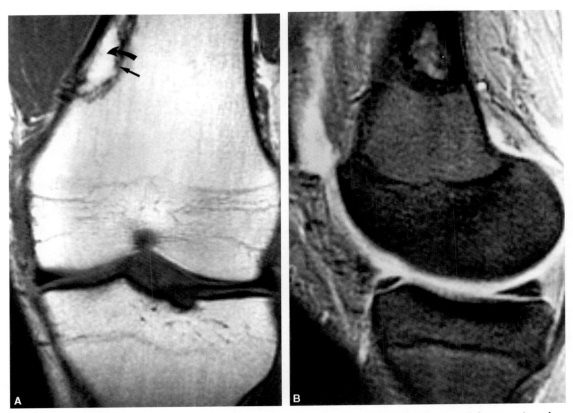

FIGURE 16-28. Nonossifying fibroma with low signal intensity sclerotic border (*straight arrow*) and marrow fat central signal intensity (*curved arrow*). T1-weighted coronal (**A**) and T2*-weighted sagittal (**B**) images.

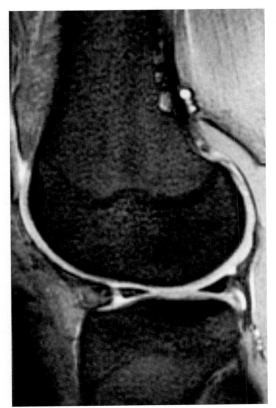

FIGURE 16-29. Femoral cortical irregularity distal to the linea aspera (*arrow*). This area of cortical roughening is usually located more medially, along the posterior femoral cortex than shown on this T2*-weighted image. Both the periosteal desmoid and distal femoral cortical irregularity may resemble a fibrous cortical defect. There is mild hyperintensity identified in the base of this lesion.

Stress-induced remodeling was inferred by the presence of inflammation along the floor of the excavation. The high signal intensity edema associated with the inflammation could be mistaken for a malignant bone tumor on T2-weighted images.

FIBROUS DYSPLASIA AND OSTEOFIBROUS DYSPLASIA. Monostotic fibrous dysplasia and osteofibrous dysplasia demonstrate low signal intensity on T1-weighted images and isointensity to increased signal intensity on T2-weighted images (Fig. 16-30). The lesions are bordered by a thick, low signal intensity sclerotic border, and the homogeneous increased signal intensity seen on T2-weighted images is less than that of fluid (Fig. 16-31). The femoral neck is a common location for monostotic fibrous dysplasia. The lesions in polyostotic fibrous dysplasia (Fig. 16-32) are similar, but polyostotic fibrous dysplasia is a more aggressive condition. The shepherd's crook deformity is caused by a pathologic fracture at the femoral neck. Treatment of fibrous dysplasia involves cortical grafting or implant fixation to stabilize the long bone.[15]

The intracortical cystic lesions of osteofibrous dysplasia (Kempson-Campanacci lesion) may mimic adamantinoma and demonstrate heterogeneity on T2-weighted images (Fig. 16-33). Osteofibrous dysplasia is a benign lesion with a predilection for the tibia in children, affecting the proximal to mid-segment of the anterior tibial cortex. Anterior bowing, cortical disruption and medullary cavity involvement may occur. Anterior tibial cortical disruption may be associated with reactive muscle edema and present with anterior compartment-like symptoms (Fig. 16-34). Fat-suppressed T2-weighted fast spin-echo or STIR sequences are sensitive to these soft-tissue changes.

Benign Tumors and Non-Neoplastic Lesions

UNICAMERAL BONE CYST. A solitary unicameral bone cyst enters into the differential diagnosis of benign bone lesions. In patients younger than 16 years of age, unicameral bone cysts may occur in the proximal humerus or femur, in close proximity to the cartilaginous growth plate, and they may recur following surgical removal. Malignancy in a solitary unicameral bone cyst has been reported, but it is extremely rare. Treatment includes steroid injection or curettage and bone grafting.[15]

Magnetic Resonance Appearance. The unicameral bone cyst has a characteristic MR appearance. On T1-weighted images, it is well defined and demonstrates low signal intensity secondary to simple fluid within the cyst. On T2-weighted images, the fluid contents demonstrate uniformly increased signal intensity. Internal hemorrhage may alter T1 and T2 signal characteristics. A low signal intensity peripheral border representing reactive sclerosis often demarcates this lesion.[51] Although fracture may occur as a complication, there should be no associated soft-tissue mass (Fig. 16-35).

text continues on page 1263

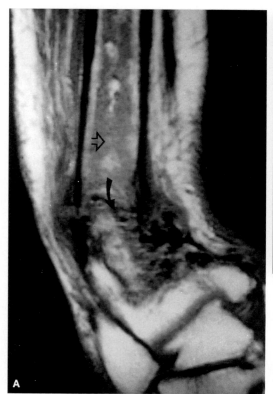

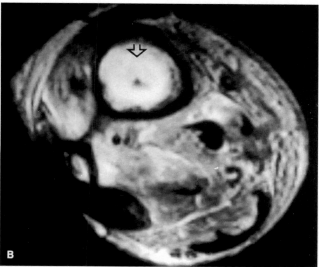

FIGURE 16-30. Fibrous dysplasia (*open arrows*) with pathologic fracture (*curved arrow*) involving the distal tibial diaphysis and metaphysis. Fibrous tissue expansion of the medullary cavity is low to intermediate in signal intensity on a coronal T1-weighted image (**A**) and bright in signal intensity on an axial T2-weighted image (**B**).

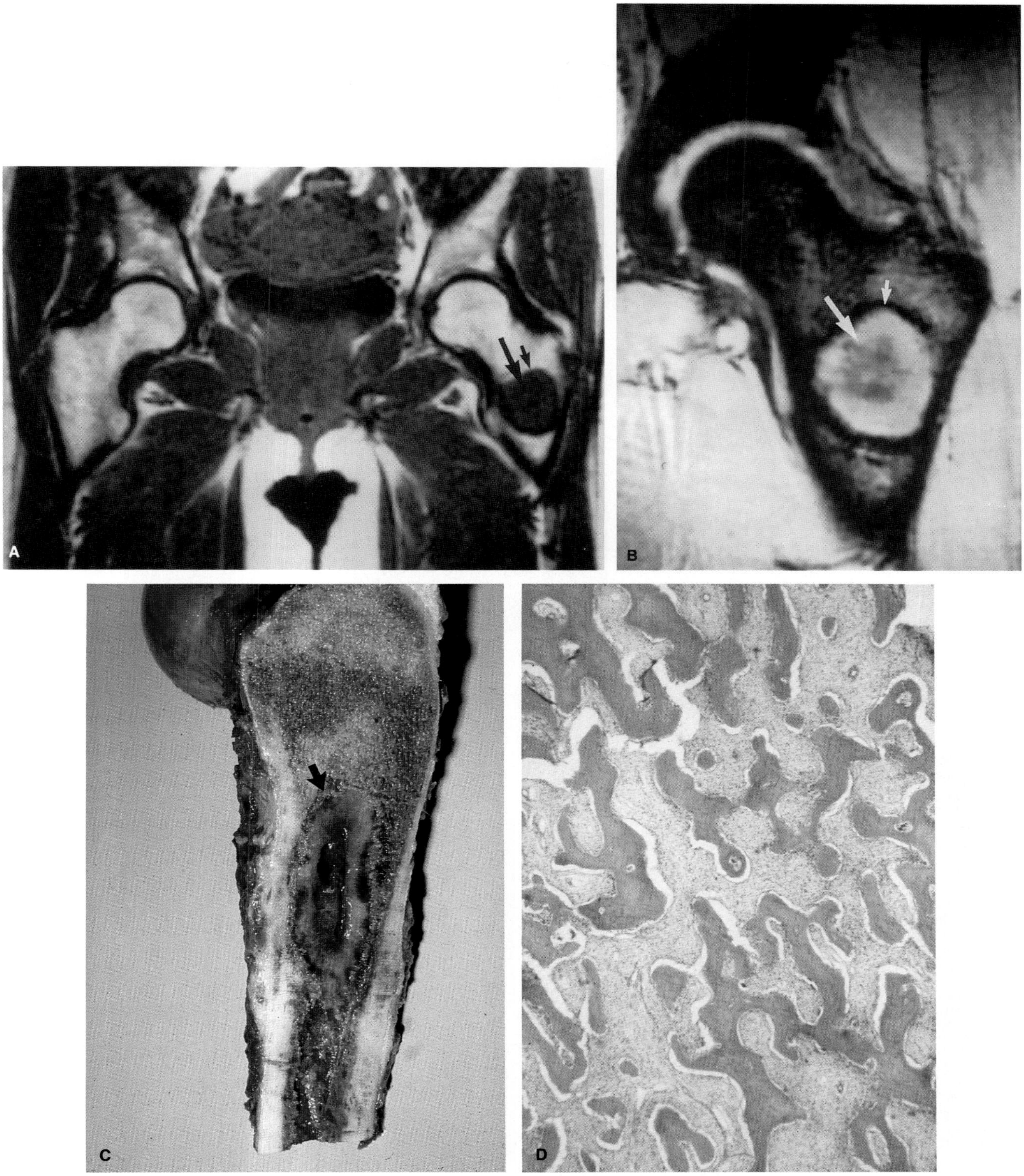

FIGURE 16-31. Monostotic fibrous dysplasia (*large arrows*) of the left femoral neck — a common location — demonstrates low signal intensity on a coronal T1-weighted image (**A**) and increased signal intensity on a coronal T2*-weighted image (**B**). Note the central area of lower signal intensity on the T2*-weighted image and the thick cortical low signal intensity sclerotic rind (*small arrows*). (**C**) Sagittal section of a gross specimen with the arrow indicating the sclerotic rind at the periphery of the monostotic lesion. (**D**) Low power photomicrograph demonstrating the alphabet soup configuration of the metaplastic trabecular bone in a background of dysplastic fibrous tissue.

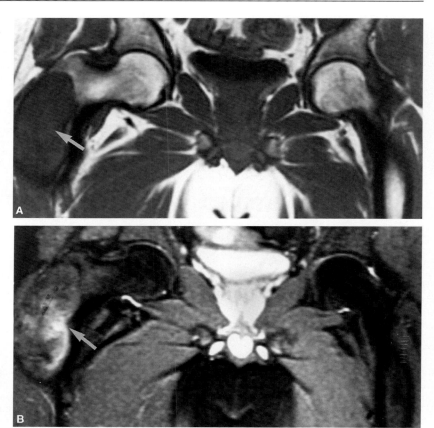

FIGURE 16-32. A large lesion of fibrous dysplasia (*arrow*) in the femoral neck in a patient with polyostotic fibrous dysplasia. T1 (**A**) and T2* (**B**) coronal images. The lesion demonstrates central inhomogeneity on the T2*-weighted coronal image.

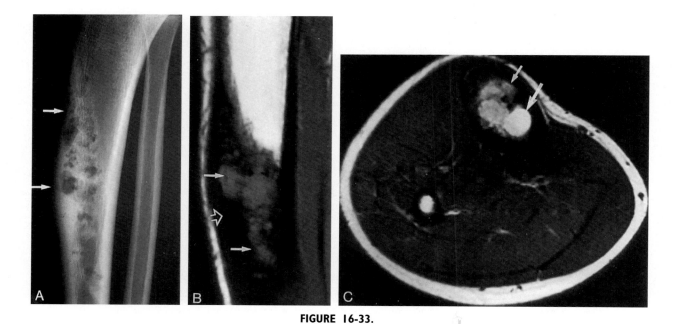

FIGURE 16-33.

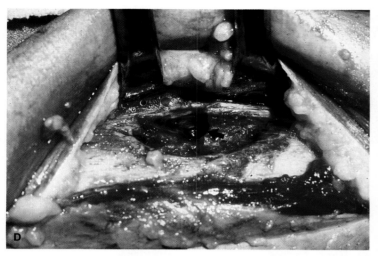

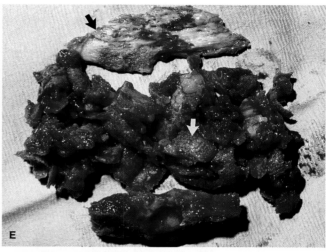

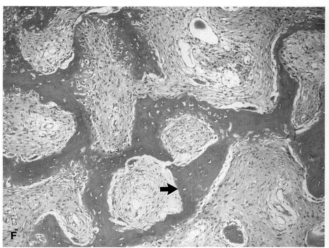

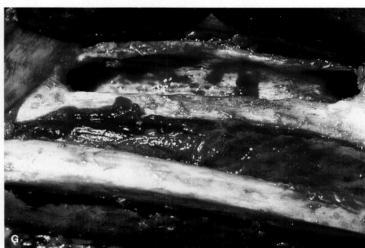

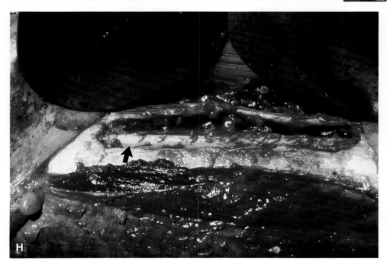

FIGURE 16-33. *Continued.* (**A**) Lateral radiograph shows a sclerotic, bubbly lesion in the anterior tibial shaft (*arrows*). (**B**) T1-weighted sagittal image shows intermediate signal intensity osteofibrous dysplasia (*solid arrows*) and low signal intensity thickened cortical tissue (*open arrow*) (TR, 600 msec; TE, 20 msec). (**C**) A T2-weighted axial image shows increased signal intensity within fibrous dysplasia (*small arrow*), separate from the tibial shaft (*large arrow*) (TR, 2000 msec; TE, 60 msec). (**D**) Gross appearance of lesion after unroofing the thin overlying cortex. The arrow is pointing down to a macrocyst in the fibrous matrix. (**E**) Reactive undersurface of cortical window (*black arrow*) and gritty-appearing fibrous tissue (*white arrow*) after surgical curettement. (**F**) Low power photomicrograph indicating alphabet soup metaplastic bone (*arrow*) in fibrous stroma. (**G**) Surgical appearance of cortical shell following complete debulking of fibrous tissue. (**H**) Surgical photomicrograph after placement of adjacent fibular strut into the cortical shell (*arrow*).

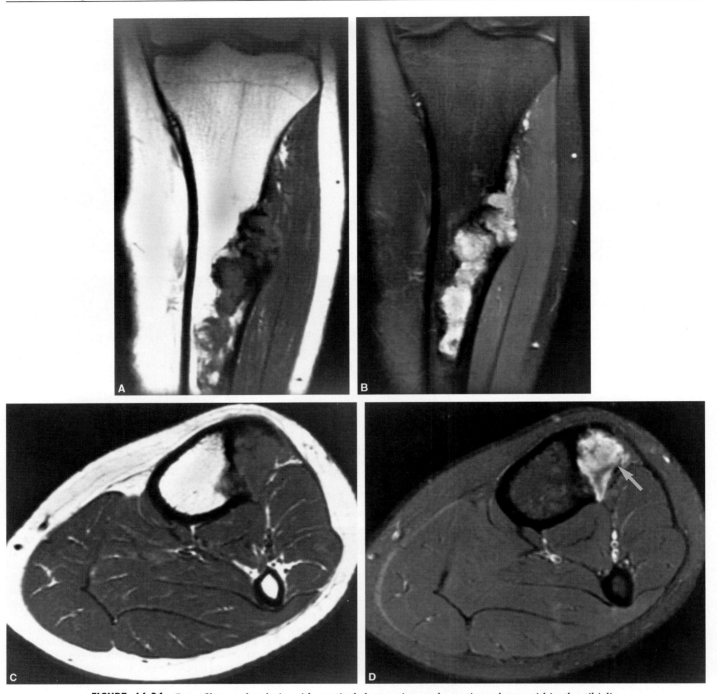

FIGURE 16-34. Osteofibrous dysplasia with cortical destruction and reactive edema within the tibialis anterior muscle group (*arrow*). This lesions presented with symptoms of anterior compartment syndrome. (**A**) T1 and (**B**) fat-suppressed T2-weighted fast spin-echo coronal images. (**C**) T1, (**D**) fat-suppressed T2-weighted fast spin-echo, and (**E**) fast spin-echo STIR axial images.

continued

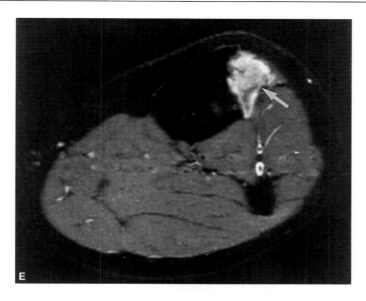

FIGURE 16-34. *Continued*

ANEURYSMAL BONE CYST.   The aneurysmal bone cyst is an expansile, blood-filled lesion that is osteolytic on conventional radiographs. In the hip or pelvis, aggressive cortical expansion and soft-tissue extension may simulate a malignant process or pseudotumor. Aneurysmal bone cysts, which occur in children and young adults (approximately 80% occur in patients younger than 20 years of age), are most commonly found in the posterior osseous elements of the vertebrae and the shafts of the long bones.[56] They are reported to involve the femur in 13% of cases and the innominate bone in 9% of cases. Aneurysmal bone cysts contain varying amounts of blood, fluid, and fibrous tissue. In many cases, they arise from preexisting bone lesions such as a giant cell tumor, osteoblastoma, chondroblastoma, fibrous dysplasia, or chondromyxoid fibroma.[56] Histologic features include blood-filled channels supported by a fibrous septum, which contains multinucleated giant cells and osteoid. Careful microscopic assessment is required to rule out the elusive telangiectatic variant of osteosarcoma, which may mimic an aneurysmal bone cyst both clinically and radiographically.[56–58]

The favored theory regarding the pathogenesis of aneurysmal bone cysts suggests an altered vascular flow resulting in local circulatory failure.[56] The Armed Forces Institute of Pathology (AFIP) endorses the theory that the aneurysmal bone cyst occurs secondary to hemorrhagic ''blow-out'' in a preexisting lesion.[59] In the AFIP classification, juxtacortical lesions are grouped with cystic subperiosteal giant cell tumors or subperiosteal myositis ossificans. Central lesions, attributed to secondary changes in preexisting lesions, are identified by the predominant lesion or tumor histology present. Intramedullary lesions without any associated preexisting lesion are thought to represent giant cell tumors of bone. Curettage

and bone grafting are used for treatment.[15] Local adjuvants include freezing with liquid nitrogen and application of phenol.

Magnetic Resonance Appearance.   On MR examination, aneurysmal bone cysts tend to be well circumscribed but heterogeneous, with areas of both low and high signal intensity.[60] The expansile lesion may have internal septations, fluid-fluid levels, and areas of bright signal intensity on both T1- and T2-weighted images, depending on the chronicity of the associated hemorrhage[61] (Figs. 16-36 and 16-37). The fluid-fluid level probably represents layering of uncoagulated blood within the lesion.[62] On T1-weighted images, increased signal intensity in the gravity-dependent layer represents methemoglobin. It may be difficult to exclude the possibility of malignancy when severe inhomogeneity of signal intensity is observed. Cortical bowing and septation (ie, trabeculation) may be seen in a low signal intensity contour of cortical bone.

HEMANGIOMA.   Hemangiomas are benign bone lesions classified as capillary, cavernous, or venous vascular proliferations. Those hemangiomas that are highly cellular may be confused with a malignant vascular neoplasm.[63] Hemangiomas may occur in patients from 20 to 60 years of age, but the incidence increases after middle age. The spine and flat bones of the skull and mandible are most frequently involved. When there is vertebral involvement, standard radiographs demonstrate coarse vertical trabeculations with a corduroy-cloth appearance.

Magnetic Resonance Appearance.   Hemangiomas are variable in MR appearance and may demonstrate low, intermediate, or high signal intensity on T1-weighted images (Fig. 16-38). There is usually some increase in signal intensity on

text continues on page 1269

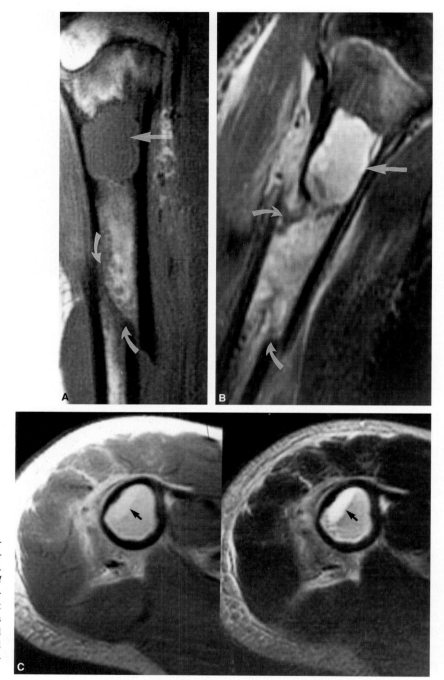

FIGURE 16-35. Centrally located and well-circumscribed unicameral or simple bone cyst of the proximal diaphysis of the humerus (*straight arrow*). A complication of a pathologic fracture (*curved arrows*) is identified on intermediate weighted sagittal image (**A**) and fat-suppressed T2-weighted fast spin-echo coronal image (**B**). The cystic contents are hyperintense on the fat-suppressed T2-weighted fast spin-echo image (**B**). A hemorrhagic fluid-fluid level (*arrow*) is shown on conventional T2-weighted spin-echo axial images (**C**).

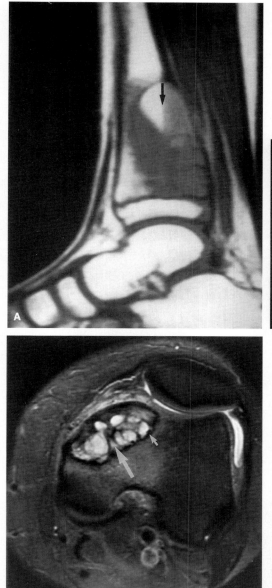

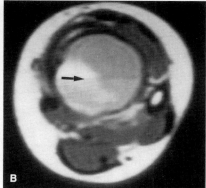

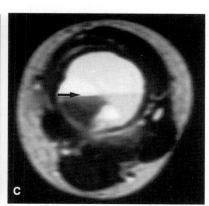

FIGURE 16-36. A metaphyseal-based aneurysmal bone cyst is eccentric and expansile, with a hemorrhagic fluid-fluid level (*arrows*) as seen on sagittal T1-weighted images (**A**) and intermediate weighted images (**B**), and on axial T2-weighted image (**C**). (**D**) Fat-suppressed T2-weighted fast spin-echo axial image in a separate case demonstrates multiple cysts (cystic loculations) with different signal intensities (*large arrow*) within an aneurysmal bone cyst of the distal femur. The low signal intensity rim is indicated (*small arrow*).

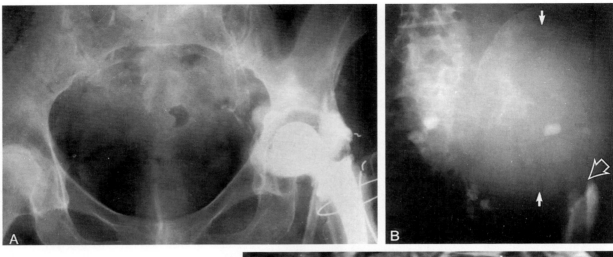

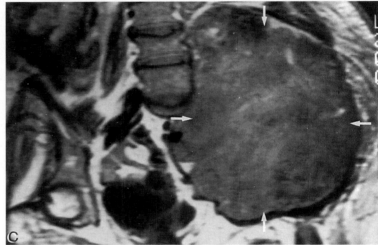

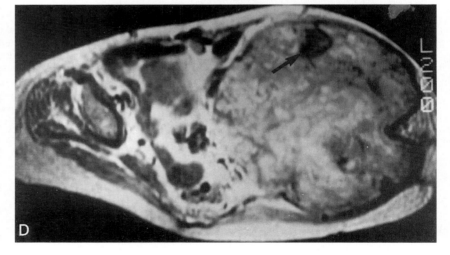

FIGURE 16-37. Aneurysmal bone cyst. (A) The initial anteroposterior radiograph shows a left total-hip prosthesis. (B) A later anteroposterior radiograph shows the progression of aggressive lytic destruction of the left hemipelvis (*solid arrows*) and proximal femur (*open arrow*) by a soft tissue density mass. (C) A T1-weighted coronal image defines the extent (*arrows*) of this well-marginated mass (TR, 500 msec; TE, 20 msec). Axial (D) intermediate weighted and (E) T2-weighted images show characteristic low signal intensity hemosiderin deposits (*solid arrows*) mixed with high signal intensity hemorrhagic elements (*open arrow*) (D, E: TR, 2000 msec; TE, 20, 60 msec). (F) Corresponding axial CT image of the lesion (*arrows*) is nonspecific for hemorrhagic constituents. (G) Gross specimen showing undersurface of outer shell of reactive bone with spongy hemorrhagic granulation tissue (*white arrow*). (H) Low power photomicrograph of the mossy outer lining of cyst with reactive giant cell (*black arrow*). continued

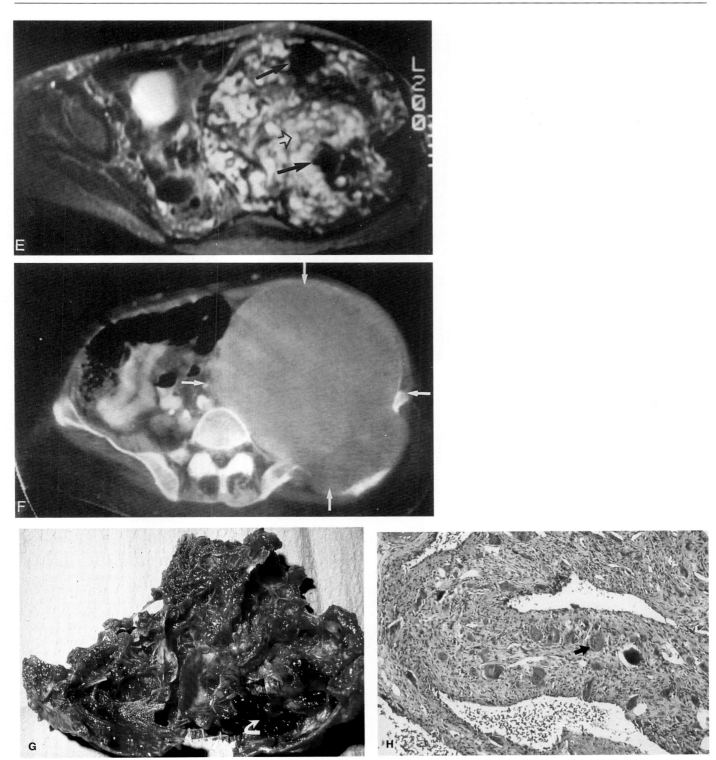

FIGURE 16-37. *Continued*

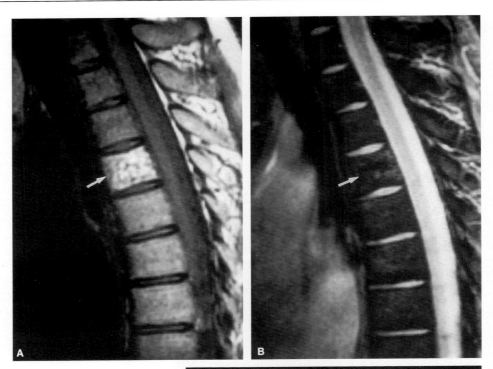

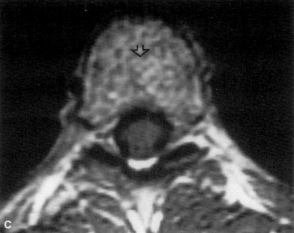

FIGURE 16-38. (A) T1-weighted sagittal image shows thoracic vertebral body involvement with a bright signal intensity hemangioma (*arrow*) (TR, 600 msec; TE, 20 msec). (B) Corresponding T2*-weighted sagittal image does not show significant increased signal intensity (*arrow*) (TR, 400 msec; TE, 15 msec; flip angle, 20°). Hemangiomas, however, frequently display increased signal intensity on T2-weighted or short TI inversion recovery images. (C) The hemangioma (*arrow*) has a corduroy appearance on a T1-weighted axial image (TR, 600 msec; TE, 20 msec).

T2-weighted or STIR sequences. Reinforced trabeculae are more difficult to appreciate on MR images than CT scans.

INTRAOSSEOUS LIPOMA. Intraosseous lipomas are rare, constituting approximately 0.1% of bone tumors.[26] Approximately 10% of these are discovered within the calcaneus.[26] Both simple bone cysts and lipomas exhibit a pyramidal shape and are situated in the center of the trigonum calcis, which raises the question of some form of relationship between the two entities. However, the precise explanation remains uncertain.[26]

The staging classification for intraosseous lipomas has three categories based on the degree of histologic involvement.[26,64] In stage 1 tumors, viable fat cells can be demon-strated; in stage 2 tumors, there are both viable fat cells and mixed areas of fat necrosis and calcification; and in stage 3 tumors, necrotic fat, calcification, cyst formation, and reactive woven bone are present.

Magnetic Resonance Appearance. An intraosseous lipoma can be differentiated from a simple cyst in the calcaneus by diffuse fat signal intensity or a thick rind of adipose tissue. This tissue demonstrates bright signal intensity on T1-weighted images and circumscribes a central hemorrhagic component, which demonstrates low signal intensity on T1-weighted images and bright signal intensity on T2-weighted images (Fig. 16-39). In addition to their appearance in the calcaneus, intraosseous lipomas are known to affect the long tubular bones, including the fibula, tibia, and femur (Fig. 16-40). Intraosseous

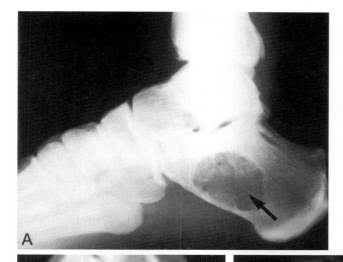

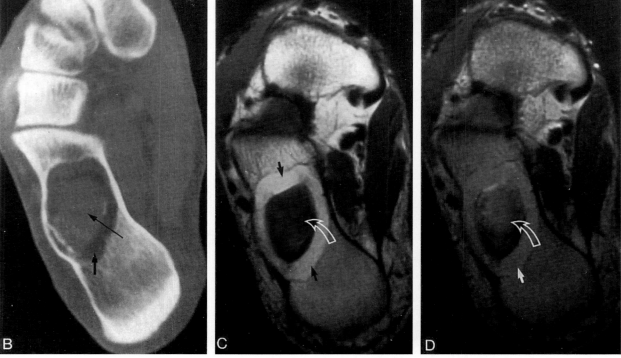

FIGURE 16-39. (**A**) Lateral radiograph shows an intraosseous lipoma as a lytic area in the calcaneus (*arrow*). (**B**) The corresponding axial CT image delineates the low-attenuation periphery (*short arrow*) and higher-attenuation central component (*long arrow*). (**C**) On a T1-weighted image, the high signal intensity fat (*solid arrows*) surrounds the low signal intensity hemorrhagic fluid contents (*curved arrow*) (TR, 600 msec; TE, 20 msec). (**D**) On a T2-weighted axial image, the fat periphery demonstrates decreased signal intensity (*solid arrow*), whereas central fluid contents (*curved arrow*) generate increased signal intensity (TR, 2000 msec; TE, 60 msec).

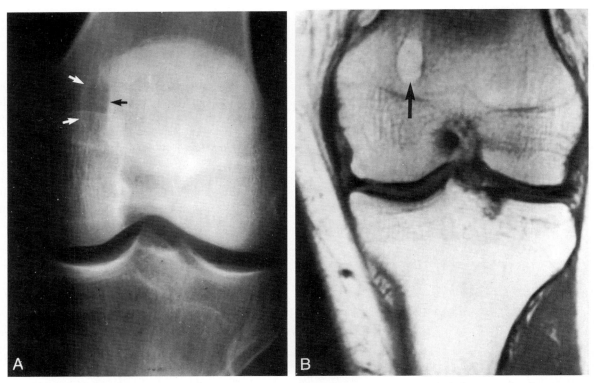

FIGURE 16-40. Intraosseous lipoma (*arrows*) of the distal femur is seen as (**A**) a lytic lesion with sclerotic borders on a conventional radiograph and as (**B**) a high signal intensity focus on a T1-weighted coronal image.

lipomas demonstrate the same signal intensity as that of fat (ie, bright on T1-weighted images and intermediate on T2-weighted images), and therefore appear black on STIR images, for which fat signal intensity is nulled.

BONE INFARCT. Bone infarcts, usually metaphyseal based, are circumscribed by a serpiginous low signal intensity border that corresponds to the rim of reactive sclerosis that is often detected in plain radiographs[65] (Fig. 16-41). In the acute and subacute stages, signal from the central island of the infarct is isointense with fatty marrow signal. With T2 weighting there may be linear bright signal parallel with the outline of the lesions. Except for location, the imaging characteristics of subarticular degeneration and sclerosis may be similar to those seen in bone infarcts. Bone infarcts can be differentiated from subarticular degeneration and sclerosis when they occur in subchondral bone.

EOSINOPHILIC GRANULOMA. The solitary and diffuse lesions of eosinophilic granuloma may be confused with osteo-

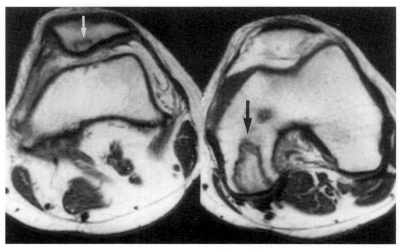

FIGURE 16-41. Low signal intensity circumscribed bone infarcts are present in the patella (*white arrow*) and medial femoral condyle (*black arrow*), as seen on a T1-weighted axial image. Central fat marrow signal intensity is characteristic of bone infarction. The location of an infarct in the medial femoral condyle should be viewed as having the same significance as osteochondritis or an osteonecrotic lesion (TR, 500 msec; TE, 20 msec).

myelitis or Ewing's sarcoma on MR images. Subperiosteal new bone and high signal intensity peritumoral edema have been identified on both T1- and T2-weighted images[66,67] (Fig. 16-42). The site of histiocytic proliferation demonstrates increased signal intensity on T2-weighted images. Treatment involves biopsy and curettage with or without grafting.[15]

Benign/Malignant Lesions

Giant Cell Tumor

Giant cell tumors exhibit unpredictable biologic behavior. They can be aggressive and are usually treated by surgical removal. Forty percent recur locally, and approximately 10%

to 20% have potential for malignant transformation.[68] Others exhibit local soft-tissue extension or systemic tumor implantation. The majority of these tumors are seen in patients 20 to 40 years of age.[68,69] The long tubular bones are most commonly affected, and giant cell tumors often present around the knee (eg, distal femur, proximal tibia) and abut the subchondral bone.[70] When spinal bones are involved, there is a predilection for anterior elements (ie, vertebral bodies). Giant cell tumors of bone originate in the distal metaphysis of the long bones and abut the physeal plate.[71] They do not occur in or cross the physis prior to fusion of the epiphysis and metaphysis, at which time the tumor occupies a subchondral position.

Histologically, these tumors exhibit a uniform distribution of giant cells against a cellular background of ovoid

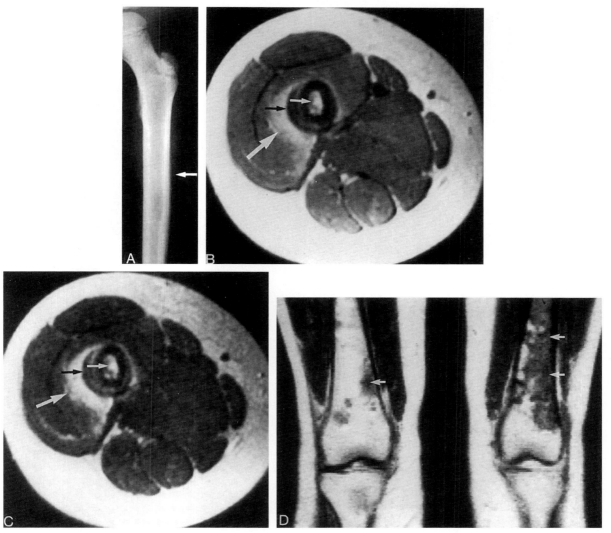

FIGURE 16-42. Solitary eosinophilic granuloma of histiocytosis X. (**A**) An anteroposterior radiograph shows thickening periosteal reaction (*arrow*) along the lateral femoral cortex. Bright signal intensity perilesional edema (*large white arrow*) and marrow involvement (*small white arrow*) and low signal intensity thickened medial femoral cortex (*black arrow*) are seen on (**B**) intermediate weighted and (**C**) T2-weighted images (TR, 2000 msec; TE 20, 60 msec). (**D**) A T1-weighted coronal image of eosinophilic granuloma of histiocytosis X involving the femoral diaphysis and metaphysis shows patchy areas of low signal intensity histiocytic infiltration (*arrows*) (TR, 600 msec; TE, 20 msec).

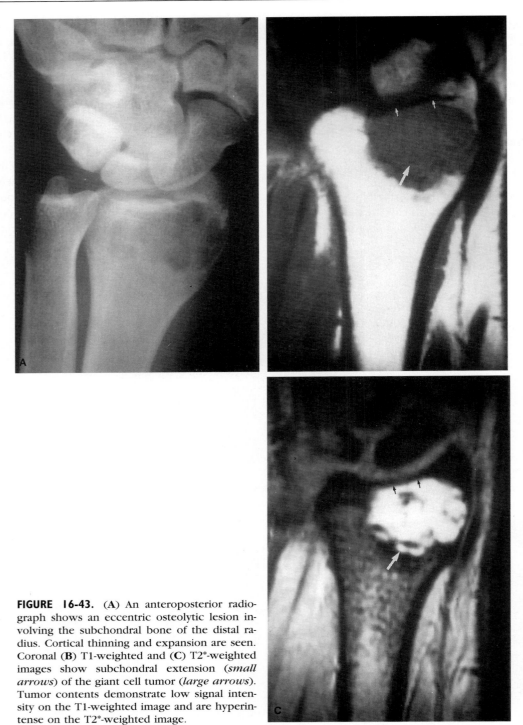

FIGURE 16-43. **(A)** An anteroposterior radiograph shows an eccentric osteolytic lesion involving the subchondral bone of the distal radius. Cortical thinning and expansion are seen. Coronal **(B)** T1-weighted and **(C)** T2*-weighted images show subchondral extension (*small arrows*) of the giant cell tumor (*large arrows*). Tumor contents demonstrate low signal intensity on the T1-weighted image and are hyperintense on the T2*-weighted image.

spindle stromal cells that exhibit mitotic activity. Osteoid foci can be seen within these lesions and are usually associated with areas of hemorrhage or within a fracture callus.[68] A histologic grading system was instituted in an attempt to predict the biologic aggressiveness of these lesions, but it has fallen out of favor in light of unpredictable behavior in the presence of histologically benign features. Tumor implantation at distant sites, typically the lungs, in patients with histologically benign giant cell tumors occurs in approximately 1% to 3% of cases.[68] These implants are regarded as passive vascular transports related to surgical curettage. If these pulmonary lesions are identical histologically to the primary giant cell tumor, they generally do not lead to the demise of the patient.

Malignant transformation, which can occur in a previously benign-appearing giant cell tumor, usually follows irradiation of the original tumor.[19,21,24,25]

MAGNETIC RESONANCE APPEARANCE.

The MR appearance of giant cell tumors of the long bones is generally well defined. They demonstrate low to intermediate signal intensity on T1-weighted images and high signal intensity on T2-weighted images[71] (Figs. 16-43 and 16-44). Heterogeneity in T2-weighted images may represent central areas of liquefaction, hemorrhage, or necrosis (Fig. 16-45). Aoki and colleagues reported MR detection of hemosiderin in 63% of giant cell tumors.[72] The low signal intensity hemosiderin is

attributed to extravasated erythrocytes in the tumor and the phagocytic function of the tumor cells. Areas of hemosiderin were most evident on gradient-echo sequences.

T2, STIR, or gradient refocused images may help to identify areas of tumor recurrence after excision and packing with methylmethacrylate (Fig. 16-46). Recurrent tumors have been identified on MR scans with low to intermediate signal intensity on T1-weighted sequences and high signal intensity on T2-weighted sequences. Fluid-fluid levels can sometimes be seen on MR scans, but are not revealed on corresponding CT sections.[73] Areas of necrosis (ie, signal inhomogeneity), cortical erosion, and associated effusions may also be identified on MR images. Intratumoral hemorrhage may produce bright signal intensity on T1- and T2-weighted images, although the tumor generally demonstrates low signal intensity on T1-weighted images and increased signal intensity on T2-weighted images.

Soft-tissue involvement and rare joint invasion can be evaluated with pretherapeutic MR staging.[74] A thin rim of sclerotic bone may be identified at the tumor interface with uninvolved fatty marrow in less aggressive lesions. Contrast inhomogeneity and multilobular configuration was seen in one case of giant cell tumor involving the flat pubic bone of the pelvis.

Because of the high rate of recurrence with curettage or intralesional resection, a more extensive approach, with an en bloc resection, has been attempted.[15] This technique is not without its own complications, however, including infection, resorption, collapse, and fracture. More extensive local excision (with wide decortication of bone overlying the tumor), combined with the use of polymethylmethacrylate cement, has been used in an attempt to remove adequate tissue without destabilizing the surgical area.

Malignant Lesions

Since the primary component of most malignant bone tumors has prolonged T1 and T2 tissue relaxation times, these tumors demonstrate low signal intensity on T1-weighted images and bright signal intensity on T2-weighted images.[1] Nonuniformity of signal intensity is most evident on T2-weighted images, in areas of necrosis or hemorrhage. Neurovascular bundle encasement, peritumoral edema, and irregular margins are secondary evidence of the malignant nature of these lesions.

Except in cases of postradiation marrow edema, extensive marrow involvement by edema or tumor is highly suggestive of either a malignancy or an infection. When there is marrow involvement in neoplastic or inflammatory disease, the MR signal characteristics depend on whether the marrow in the affected limb is yellow or red. On T1-weighted images, neoplastic or inflammatory involvement of yellow marrow demonstrates low signal intensity within or adjacent to bright marrow fat, and increased signal intensity with progressive T2 weighting. When the affected limb

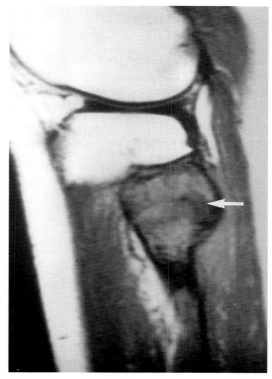

FIGURE 16-44. Expansile giant cell tumor (*arrow*) of the proximal fibula demonstrates low signal intensity on a T1-weighted sagittal image (TR, 600 msec; TE, 20 msec).

text continues on page 1276

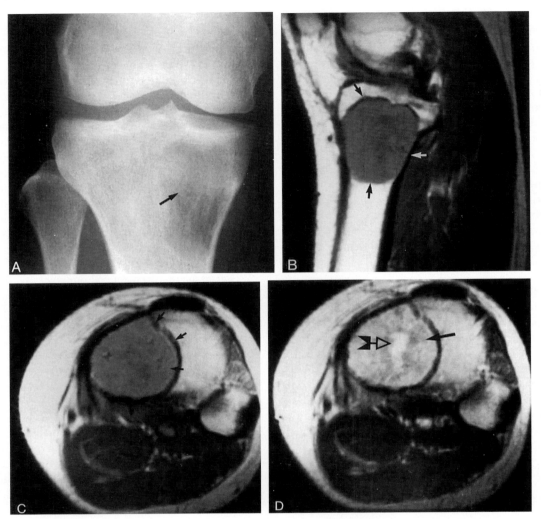

FIGURE 16-45. Giant cell tumor. **(A)** Radiograph shows a lytic focus on the medial tibial metaphysis and epiphysis (*arrow*). T1-weighted **(B)** sagittal and **(C)** axial images demonstrate an eccentric, well-circumscribed low signal intensity tumor (*black arrows*) with intact overlying cortex (*white arrow*) (TR, 600 msec; TE, 20 msec). **(D)** T2-weighted image shows central necrosis (*flagged arrow*) within the high signal intensity lesion (*straight arrow*) (TR, 2000 msec; TE, 60 msec). **(E)** Surgical photograph of the friable hemorrhagic reddish brown solid fleshy tumor tissue being curetted through a large cortical window. **(F)** High power photomicrograph with polyhedral stromal cells (*short arrow*) with a nuclear pattern similar to that seen in reactive giant cells (*long arrow*). **(G)** Surgical photograph of the cleaned out inner wall of tumor cloaca ready for reconstruction with either a bone graft or bone cement. **(H)** Anteroposterior radiograph 2 years after surgery with reinforcement Steinmann pins in the cement to reduce risk of fracture.

continued

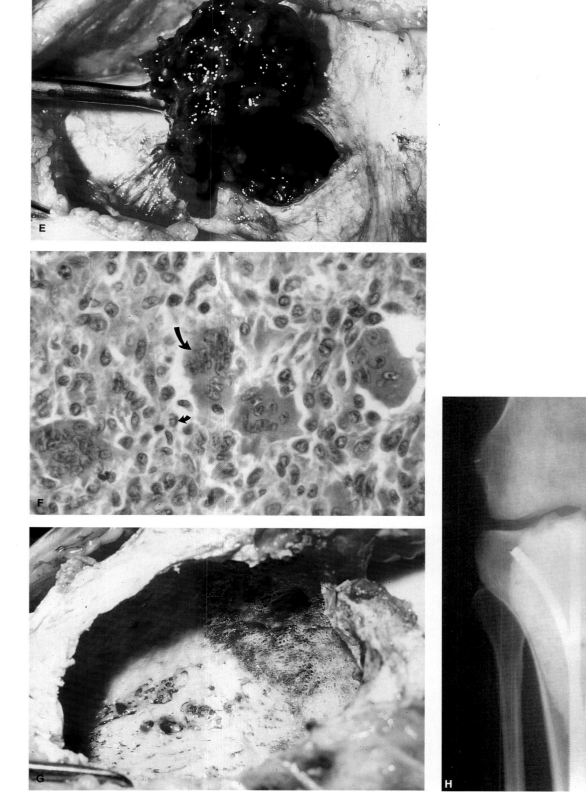

FIGURE 16-45. *Continued*

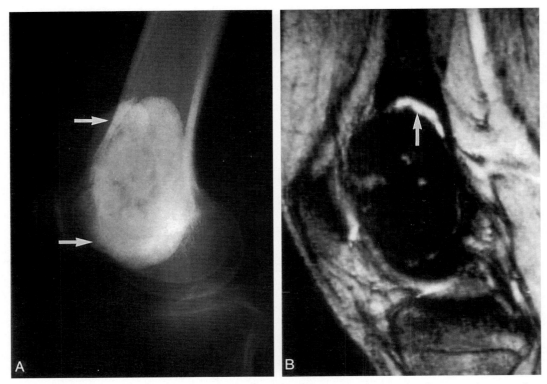

FIGURE 16-46. (**A**) Lateral radiograph shows a methylmethacrylate packed cavity after operative resection of giant cell tumor (*arrows*). (**B**) Corresponding T2*-weighted sagittal image reveals a recurrent giant cell tumor, which demonstrates bright signal intensity (*arrow*). Methylmethacrylate generates dark signal intensity (TR, 400 msec; TE, 30 msec; flip angle, 30°).

is primarily red marrow, however, lesions often appear isointense with normal hematopoietic marrow on T1-weighted images and bright on T2-weighted images.

In the postoperative evaluation of malignant neoplasms, initial edema and inflammatory changes demonstrate low signal intensity on T1-weighted images and bright signal intensity on T2-weighted images. This bright signal intensity on T2-weighted images is feathery, infiltrative, and conforms to the contour of the muscle. With increased time, the surgical field is replaced with fibrous tissue that demonstrates low to intermediate signal intensity on T1- and T2-weighted scans. Postoperative hematomas and seromas are well marginated, confined to the region of surgery, and demonstrate uniform increased signal intensity with long TR and TE settings. Chronic hemorrhage with hemosiderin deposits remains dark on T1- and T2-weighted images because of the paramagnetic effect of iron.

Certain MR changes, including the following, strongly suggest tumor recurrence:

- The reappearance of edema, characterized by low signal intensity on T1-weighted images and bright signal on T2-weighted images
- A new area of increased signal intensity on T2-weighted images with a corresponding area of intermediate signal intensity on T1-weighted images
- A change in the contour of a muscle or postoperative surgical field, such that the margins are convex instead of concave.

Osteosarcoma

Osteosarcoma is the most common primary malignant bone tumor in childhood. Except for multiple myeloma, osteosarcomas are the most common primary malignancy of bone and are considered one of the most aggressive and histologically varied neoplasms. The identifying feature of all osteosarcomas is the presence of malignant stromal cells that produce osteoid. From a clinical viewpoint, there are two main categories of osteosarcoma, primary (de novo) and secondary.[42,75]

PRIMARY OSTEOSARCOMA. Primary (de novo) conventional osteosarcomas most often affect individuals younger than 20 years of age. There is a slight predominance in male patients. In 96% of cases, the tumor develops in the long bones and limbs. The lesion is usually metaphyseal, destroys trabecular and cortical bone, invades the soft tissues, and may extend into the epiphysis.[75]

The role of genetic factors in the pathogenesis of osteosarcoma is of particular interest in children. Patients with genetic retinoblastoma who have a point mutation at chromosome 13q14 band demonstrate a 500-fold increased risk of developing osteosarcoma.[47] Cytogenic and molecular techniques have uncovered the Rb gene, a tumor suppressor gene that plays a role in the pathogenesis of osteosarcoma.[47]

Suppression of the p53 gene appears to be common in osteosarcoma.[76]

SECONDARY OSTEOSARCOMA.
Osteosarcoma in older individuals (secondary osteosarcoma) arises in a setting of preexisting bone disease (eg, Paget's disease, bone infarcts) or after exposure to a mutagenic event such as irradiation (Fig. 16-47). In osteosarcoma associated with Paget's disease, bones other than the long bones (eg, the pelvis, skull, facial bones, and scapula) are involved. Osteosarcomas arising in Paget's disease have a poorer prognosis than more conventional de novo osteosarcomas.[47]

CLASSIFICATION.
Several pathologic patterns of osteosarcomas have been identified. Histologic assessment of telangiectatic osteosarcomas is especially difficult, because the viable cells and anaplastic cells are obscured by hemorrhage and necrosis or camouflaged within benign reactive cells of the walls, which simulates an aneurysmal bone cyst.[56,57] Some hold that telangiectatic osteosarcomas have a more aggressive clinical course. On conventional radiographs, the telangiectatic variant appears lytic because of the lack of demonstrable bone production. Magnetic resonance scans show an aggressive, destructive lesion, usually accompanied by an associated soft-tissue mass. The inhomogeneity of signal intensity, with both low and high signal intensity areas on T1- and T2-weighted images, reflects the high degree of vascularity and the presence of large hemorrhagic cystic spaces (Fig. 16-48).

Approximately 10% of primary osteosarcomas are tremendously rich in bone production (ie, sclerosing or osteo- blastic osteosarcoma).[75] At times, the bone and osteoid are deposited in massive solid amounts. Frequently, the mineralization extends into the soft tissues.[77] Blastic components remain low in signal intensity on T1- and T2-weighted images, but associated peritumoral edema or nonsclerotic areas generate increased signal intensity on heavily T2-weighted or STIR images.

Chondroblastic osteosarcoma is seen in approximately 5% of cases.[75] The generation of chondroid elements, whether benign or malignant, contributes to increased signal intensity on T2-weighted images.

Osteosarcomas that produce large amounts of spindly fibroblasts are classified as fibroblastic osteosarcoma, seen in approximately 4% of cases.[75] There is no convincing evidence that chondroblastic or fibroblastic subtypes of osteosarcoma have different prognoses.[75]

Central, low-grade osteosarcoma, a rare type of osteosarcoma arising in medullary bone, is so well differentiated that it is frequently mistaken for a benign condition both radiologically and histopathologically. Patients are usually young adults and may have had symptoms for years at the time of presentation. Much of the lesion appears well circumscribed, simulating fibrous dysplasia. A search for small foci of cortical destruction may be essential for accurate diagnosis. The prognosis in low-grade osteosarcoma is excellent. Metastasis occurs late, if ever; but local recurrences may be a serious problem if surgery is inadequate.[75] On MR scans, the low-grade central osteosarcoma may be difficult to distinguish from a conventional osteosarcoma, which has an identical radiographic appearance.

There are three additional subtypes of osteosarcomas,

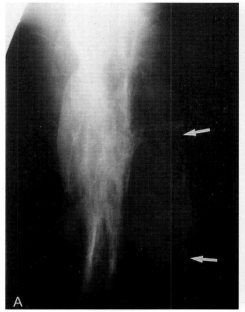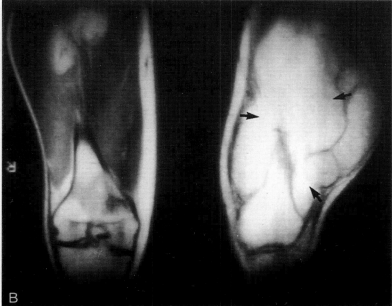

FIGURE 16-47. Tumoral callus (*arrows*) in osteogenesis imperfecta of the femur is seen on (**A**) an anteroposterior radiograph and (**B**) a T1-weighted coronal image. Exuberant osteoid tissue demonstrates normal yellow marrow signal intensity. No malignant degeneration to osteosarcoma is seen.

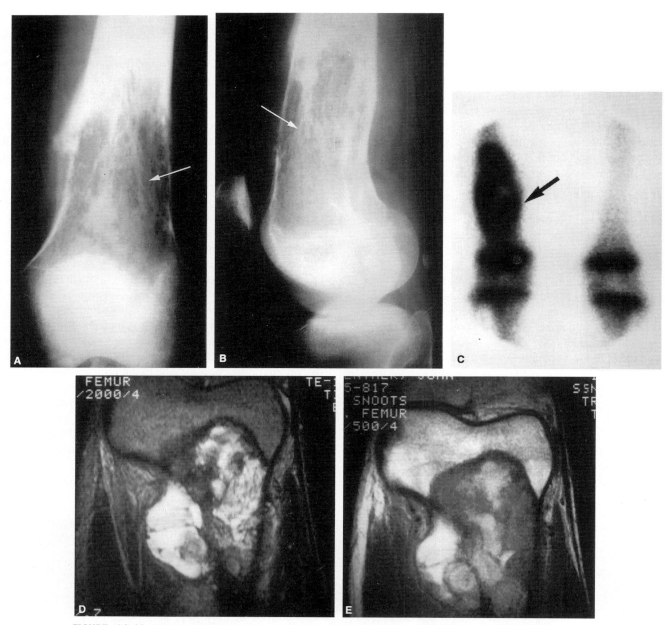

FIGURE 16-48. Telangiectatic osteosarcoma. (**A**) Anteroposterior and (**B**) lateral radiographs show an osteolytic tumor (*arrows*) with trabecular and cortical destruction. (**C**) Bone scintigraphy shows uptake of tracer in the distal femur (*arrow*). Uptake is present beyond the confines of the femur (ie, the convex margins). Coronal (**D**) T1-weighted and (**E**) T2-weighted images show intraosseous and extraosseous tumor extension with heterogeneous cystic hemorrhagic components (**D**: TR 500 msec; TE 30 msec; **E**: TR 2000 msec; TE 120 msec).

referred to as juxtacortical osteosarcomas. They account for 7% of all osteosarcomas and arise on the surface of the bone rather than within the medulla. These juxtacortical subtypes are periosteal osteosarcoma, parosteal osteosarcoma, and high-grade surface osteosarcoma.

Periosteal osteosarcoma, which accounts for 0.3% of all osteosarcomas, favors the diaphyseal surface of long tubular bones and forms an irregular thickened cortex. Histologically, hyaline chondrosarcomatous elements are a prominent feature.[78] Parosteal osteosarcoma, another rare form of osteo-

sarcoma (0.8%) occurs most frequently on the metaphyseal surface of long tubular bones within the parosteal soft tissue, and forms a lobulated mass. Histologically it is characterized by a fibrous proliferation surrounding parallel lamellar bony spicules. The fibrous component can appear externally bland, mimicking a fibrous dysplasia. Unlike periosteal osteosarcomas, chondrosarcomatous elements are minimal or absent in parosteal osteosarcomas.[79,80]

MR imaging performed in the early stages of developing myositis ossificans may display changes, which can be mistaken for a more aggressive process, such as parosteal or periosteal osteosarcoma.[81] Rim enhancement with intravenous contrast injection and hyperintensity on T2-weighted images mimics the appearance of an abscess or necrotic tumor.

TREATMENT OF OSTEOSARCOMA. The management of patients with conventional osteogenic sarcoma has changed dramatically since the early 1970s for two reasons. First is the introduction of adjuvant multidrug chemotherapy, which has changed the prognosis for survival from 25% at 5 years to the present figure of 75%. The effectiveness of preoperative chemotherapy is assessed by evaluating the clinical picture of reduced pain and tumor size. Imaging studies are also helpful in monitoring the effectiveness of chemotherapy by quantifying the amount of tumor necrosis taking place after the first or second cycle of chemotherapy. The degree of chemotherapy tumor necrosis is further quantified by the pathologist, who gives a percentile determination to the surgical specimen taken at the time of amputation or limb salvage resection. If this percentage is greater than 90%, the survival prognosis climbs to an 85% to 90% 5-year survival, compared with only 50% to 60% for the nonresponder group.[76]

The second major event that took place in the 1970s was the advent of total joint replacement surgery, which was rapidly applied to the local management of osteosarcoma by means of limb salvage reconstruction instead of ablative amputation. Presently, limb salvage reconstructive procedures are used in 90% of cases, with a local recurrence rate

of 6% and a prosthetic survival rate of 83% at 5 years and 67% at 10 years.[82,83] A modular titanium system with a rotating hinge device for the knee joint has been used in the United States since 1982 with a high degree of success (see Fig. 16-54F). The major cause for failure is stress shielding secondary to stem loosening. This is avoided in newer systems with more compliant, stress-sharing fixation devices.

MAGNETIC RESONANCE APPEARANCE. Magnetic resonance imaging affords superior marrow and soft-tissue discrimination in the evaluation of osteosarcoma. Osteosarcoma, chondrosarcoma, giant cell tumors, and Ewing's sarcoma are statistically the primary bone neoplasms that are likely to involve the lower extremities. The distal femur, proximal tibia, and humerus are common sites of involvement in conventional osteosarcoma (Fig. 16-49). With MR imaging, intramedullary marrow involvement, soft-tissue extension, skip-lesion metastases, and postoperative recurrence can be accurately assessed (Figs. 16-50 and 16-51). Marrow infiltration can be mapped on MR scans, even when standard radiographic results are negative or when conventional radiographic findings are misleading.[84] In addition to occurring as a primary extremity neoplasm, osteosarcoma is a known complication of osteogenesis imperfecta, and tumoral callus may mimic osteosarcoma (see Fig. 16-47). MR imaging can be used to differentiate exuberant bone, which is isointense with yellow marrow, from osteosarcoma, which causes both T1 and T2 prolongation. In addition, MR scans of aggressive, dedifferentiated osteosarcomas may demonstrate a necrotic, hemorrhagic fluid-fluid level within the more distal marrow

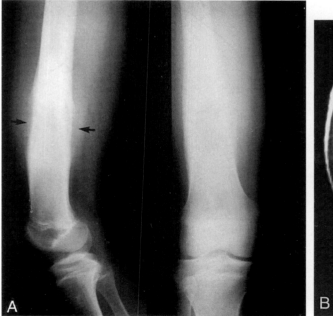
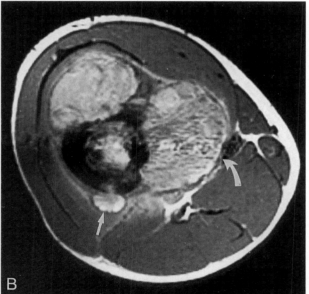

FIGURE 16-49. Osteosarcoma. (**A**) Anteroposterior (*left*) and lateral (*right*) radiographs show aggressive cortical destruction with periosteal reaction (*arrow*). Axial (**B**) intermediate weighted and (**C**) T2-weighted images show a high signal intensity tumor with cortical transgression (*curved arrows*) and soft-tissue extension (*straight arrows*).

continued

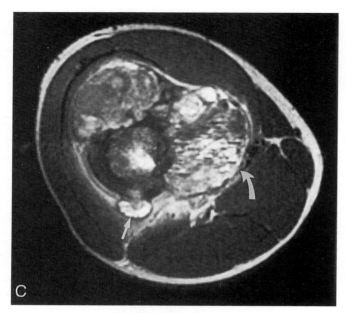

FIGURE 16-49. *Continued*

cavity, a unique feature not seen on corresponding CT (Fig. 16-52).

In many cases, there is MR evidence of tumor crossing the physis, although this extension is not evident on conventional radiographs (Fig. 16-53). In general, osteosarcomas tend to demonstrate low signal intensity on T1-weighted sequences and high signal intensity on T2-weighted sequences. Specific cellular constituents (eg, fibrous, chondroid, blastic, or telangiectatic components), however, can modify signal characteristics.[77]

There is excellent correlation between the MR appearance of the extent of marrow, cortical bone, and soft-tissue involvement and the gross pathologic specimen[85] (Fig. 16-54). Lesions that are primarily blastic, and therefore sclerotic on plain film radiographs, demonstrate low signal intensity on both T1- and T2-weighted sequences (Fig. 16-55). However, even in lesions with extensive sclerosis, areas of increased signal intensity may be identified on T2-weighted images. Hemorrhagic components within telangiectatic osteosarcoma demonstrate focal areas of high signal intensity on T1- and T2-weighted images. Skip lesions and multiple sites of involvement are common in multicentric osteosarcoma, which affects a younger age group[86] (Fig. 16-56).

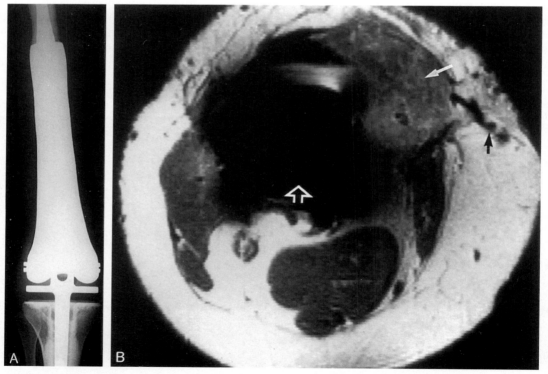

FIGURE 16-50. Postoperative osteosarcoma. **(A)** An anteroposterior radiograph shows limb salvage with a total knee prosthesis. **(B)** The corresponding intermediate weighted axial image shows postoperative fibrous tissue (*solid white arrows*), the surgical incision site (*solid black arrows*), and a prosthesis signal artifact (*open arrow*) (TR, 1500 msec; TE, 40 msec).

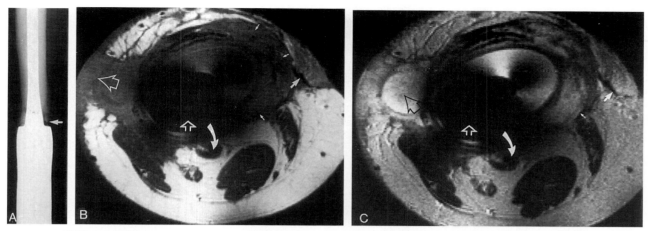

FIGURE 16-51. Interval postoperative osteosarcoma with infection. **(A)** An anteroposterior radiograph shows cortical irregularity at the prosthesis-bone interface (*arrow*). An abscess formation in lateral soft tissues (*large open arrows*) demonstrates low signal intensity on an axial T1-weighted image **(B)** and high signal intensity on an axial T2-weighted image **(C)**. A metallic artifact (*small open arrows*), fibrous tissue (*small solid arrows*), the surgical incision site (*large solid arrows*), and the popliteal vessels (*curved arrows*) are shown (**B:** TR, 600 msec; TE, 20 msec; **C:** TR, 2000 msec; TE, 60 msec).

In cases of parosteal osteosarcoma, the precise involvement of cortex and marrow can be assessed using sagittal plane images (Fig. 16-57). Both edema and tumor extension may encase vessels, and multiple axial images are usually necessary to distinguish edema that conforms and tracks along specific muscle groups.

MR imaging is superior to CT in determining the exact extent of marrow involvement by tumor and edema, particularly important in limb salvage procedures (Fig. 16-58). MR imaging is also sensitive in identifying joint invasion by osteosarcoma; however, false-positive interpretations may result in overstaging of the tumor.[87] Contrast enhancement is helpful in identifying joint involvement. The effectiveness of preoperative chemotherapy is determined by evaluation

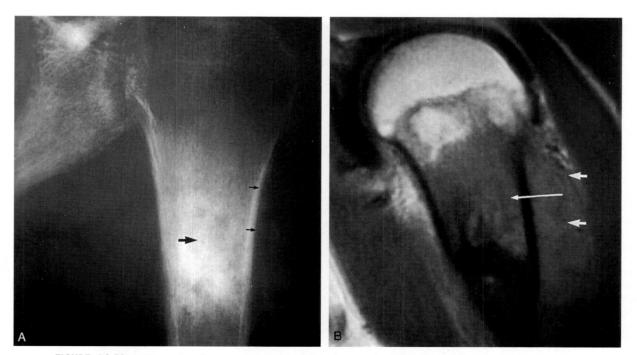

FIGURE 16-52. Differentiated osteosarcoma involving the proximal humerus. **(A)** An anteroposterior radiograph shows sclerosis (*large arrow*) and aggressive periosteal reaction (*small arrows*). **(B)** The corresponding T1-weighted coronal image demonstrates a soft-tissue mass (*short arrows*) and marrow involvement (*long arrow*) (TR, 600 msec; TE, 20 msec).

continued

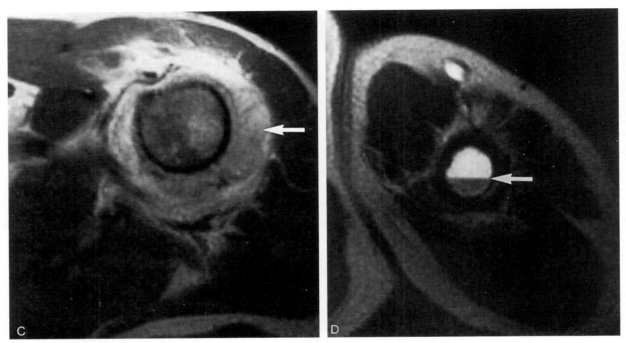

FIGURE 16-52. *Continued.* T2-weighted axial images display increased intensity proximally in the circumferential soft-tissue component (*arrow*) (**C**) and a fluid-fluid level (*arrow*) in area of marrow necrosis distally (**D**) (**C, D:** TR, 2000 msec; TE, 60 msec).

of the sensitivity of the tumor to chemotherapy. Although this can be approximated on a clinical and radiologic basis, histopathologic assessment of the amount of tumor necrosis in the postresection specimen remains the best way to evaluate response.[76] Direct coronal or sagittal MR images of the tumor are also helpful in planning preoperative or postoperative therapeutic regimens. Prior to surgery, interval responses of both tumor and edema to chemotherapy can be monitored by serial MR scans, including contrast-enhanced MR images[88–92] (Fig. 16-59). Fast dynamic contrast-enhanced sequences are especially useful for identifying re-

text continues on page 1288

FIGURE 16-53. (**A**) An anteroposterior radiograph shows lytic metaphyseal-based osteosarcoma with aggressive cortical destruction (*white arrow*). No extension of tumor is seen proximal to the physeal line (*black arrow*). (**B**) The corresponding T1-weighted coronal image shows low signal intensity marrow infiltration involving the epiphysis, metaphysis, and proximal diaphysis (*solid straight arrow*). A soft-tissue mass with cortical breakthrough involves the medial tibial metaphysis (*open arrow*). The biopsy site, which is packed with gelfoam, is shown as a dark focus of low signal intensity (*curved arrow*) (TR, 800 msec; TE, 25 msec).

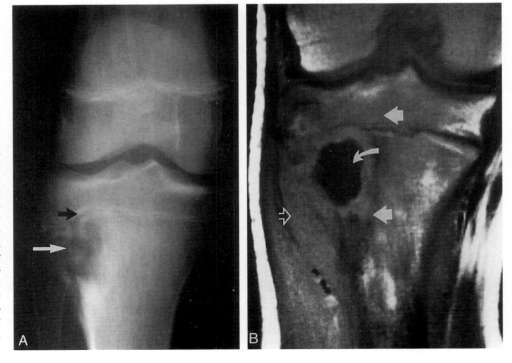

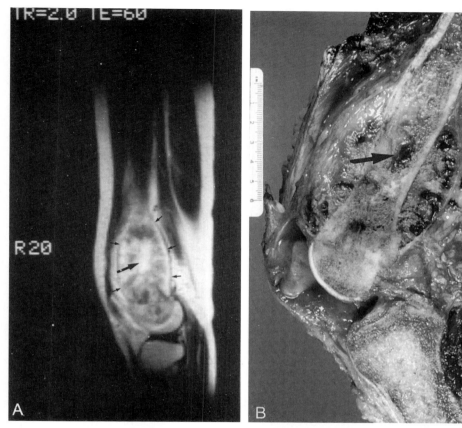

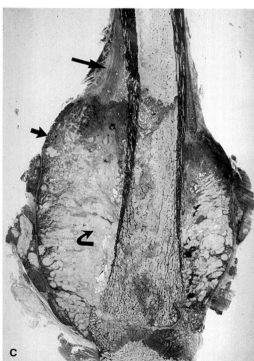

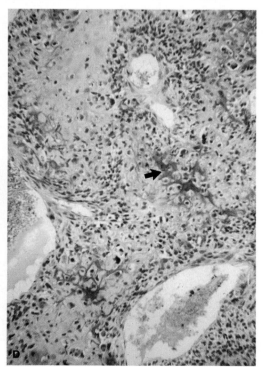

FIGURE 16-54. (**A**) A T2-weighted sagittal image shows osteosarcoma involving the femoral metaphysis (*small arrows*). Bright contrast portions of the high signal intensity tumor represent necrosis with hemorrhage (*large arrow*) (TR, 2000 msec; TE, 60 msec). (**B**) The corresponding gross specimen shows central tumor necrosis (*arrow*). (**C**) Macrosection of amputated specimen cut in the coronal plane displaying a large extracortical tumor mass with various tissue types, including young tumor osteoid at the outer edge (*short arrow*) contrasting to malignant chondroid tissue (*curved arrow*) that would be higher signal on T2-weighted images. Long arrow indicates Codman's reactive triangle. (Reprinted with permission from Skinner HB, ed. Current diagnosis and treatment in orthopaedics. Norwalk, CT: Appleton & Lange, 1995.) (**D**) Low power photomicrograph of malignant tumor osteoid indicated by arrow.   *continued*

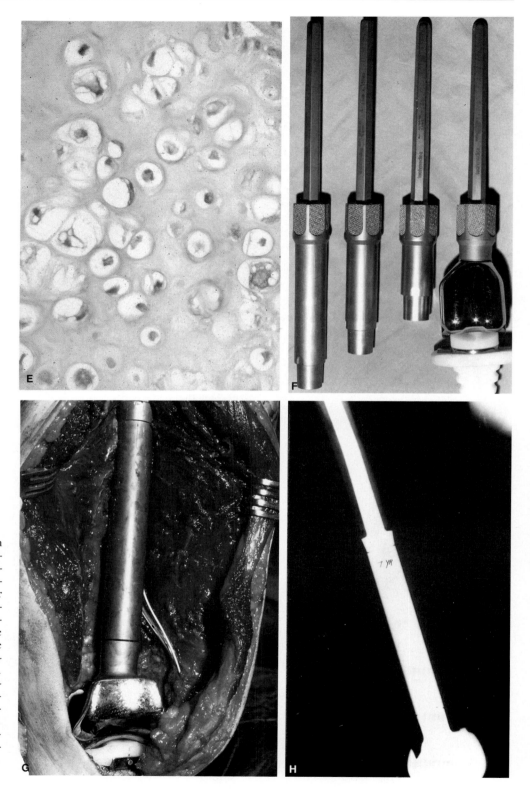

FIGURE 16-54. *Continued.* (**E**) High power photomicrograph of the malignant chondroid portion of heterogeneous tumor tissue. (**F**) Photograph of the titanium modular rotating hinge prosthesis used in reconstructive limb salvage surgery following wide surgical resection of the distal femur. (**G**) Photograph of the implant at the time of surgical reconstruction prior to wound closure. (**H**) Radiographic appearance in lateral projection 7 years following surgery. (**F** and **H** reprinted with permission from Meyer JL, Vaeth JM, eds. Frontiers in radiation therapy and oncology: organ conservation in curative cancer treatment, vol 27. Basel: S Karger AG, 1993.)

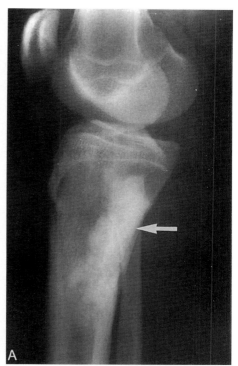

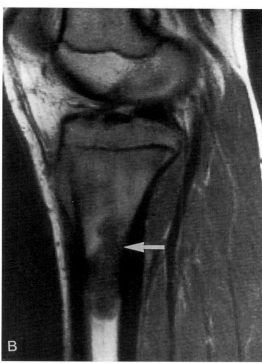

FIGURE 16-55. (A) A lateral radiograph shows a sclerotic response (*arrow*) to osteoblastic osteosarcoma. (B) The corresponding T1-weighted sagittal image shows a low signal intensity blastic tumor (*arrow*) (TR, 600 msec; TE, 20 msec).

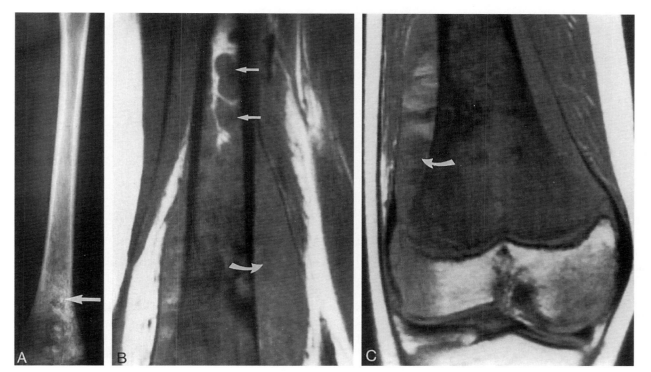

FIGURE 16-56. (A) An anteroposterior radiograph shows distal femoral lytic sclerotic reaction (*arrow*) to multicentric osteosarcoma. (B) Skip lesions (*straight arrows*) are seen on a T1-weighted sagittal image. (C) These lesions are located proximal to the primary tumor focus on T1-weighted coronal image. A soft-tissue mass is identified on both the sagittal and coronal views (*curved arrows*) (B, C: TR, 600 msec; TE, 20 msec). (D) Intermediate weighted and (E) T2-weighted axial images show increased signal intensity in the marrow and surrounding soft tissue (D, E: TR, 2000 msec; TE, 20, 60 msec). *continued*

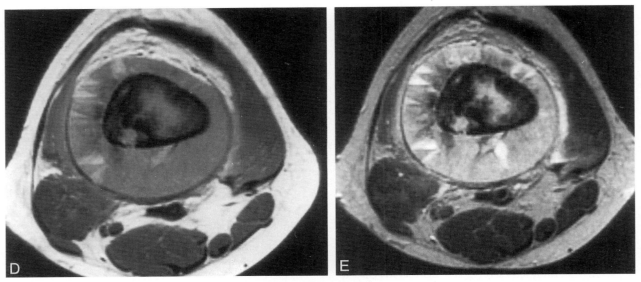

FIGURE 16-56. *Continued*

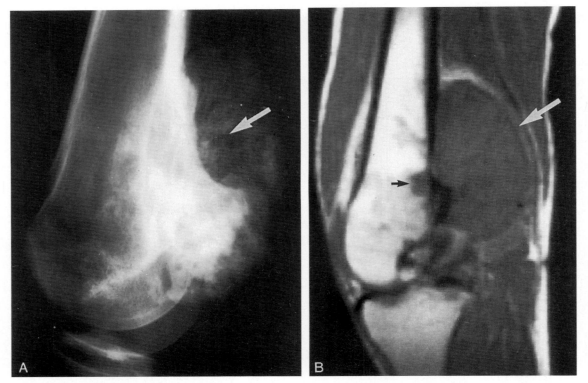

FIGURE 16-57. (**A**) A lateral radiograph shows posterior sclerosis and a soft-tissue osteoid (*arrow*). (**B**) On a T1-weighted sagittal image, soft-tissue parosteal osteosarcoma demonstrates low signal intensity (*white arrow*). The focus of marrow involvement (*black arrow*) was not revealed on plain film radiographs (TR, 600 msec; TE, 20 msec). (**C**) Gross appearance of resected specimen with an osseous tumor nodule (*arrow*) projecting posteriorly between the femoral condyles. (**D**) Surgical specimen cut in the coronal plane demonstrating the surface characteristics of the parosteal osteosarcoma. (**E**) Low power photomicrograph showing the low-grade histology of this osteoid-forming sarcoma. *continued*

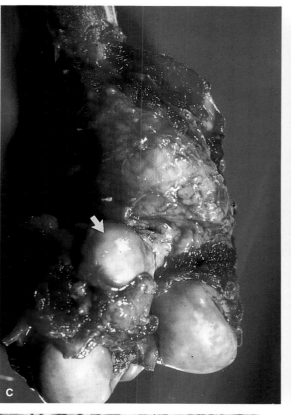

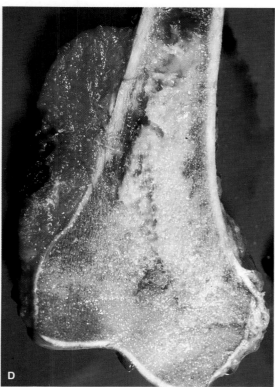

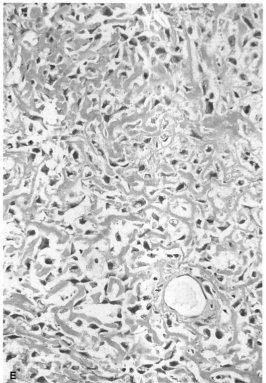

FIGURE 16-57. *Continued*

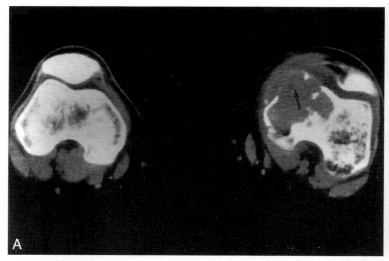
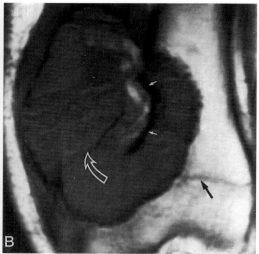

FIGURE 16-58. (**A**) An axial CT scan shows cortical breakthrough and a soft-tissue mass (*arrow*), which are characteristic of osteosarcoma. (**B**) A coronal T1-weighted image defines the proximal and distal extent of the tumor across the physis (*black arrow*), the degree of soft-tissue involvement (*curved open arrow*), and the degree of cortical destruction (*white arrows*) on a single section (TR, 600 msec; TE, 20 msec).

sidual tumor prior to surgery.[92] Viable tumor is correlated with a short (less than 6 second) time interval between arterial enhancement and tumoral enhancement. Pan and colleagues reported on four MR patterns found in postchemotherapy osteosarcoma[89]:

1. A dark pattern of low to intermediate signal intensity areas on T1- and T2-weighted images, corresponding to calcified osteoid or cartilage matrix, dense granulation tissue, and hemosiderin

2. A mottled or speckled pattern of intermediate signal intensity on T1-weighted images and high signal intensity on T2-weighted images, best appreciated on T2-weighted images, corresponding to tumor matrix, edematous granulation tissue, and hemosiderin deposits

3. A distinct multicystic or bubbly appearance in the cystic pattern, of intermediate to high signal intensity on T1-weighted images and high signal intensity on T2-weighted images, thought to correspond to either blood-filled cysts with viable tumor cells or tumor matrix mixed with edematous granulation

FIGURE 16-59. (**A**) On an anteroposterior radiograph, blastic osteosarcoma appears as a sclerotic metaphyseal focus. (**B**) On a T1-weighted coronal image, the lesion is seen as a low signal intensity area of marrow replacement (*arrows*) (TR, 1000 msec; TE, 40 msec). The interval response to monthly chemotherapy in the first (**C**), second (**D**), and third (**E**) months of treatment is seen on T2-weighted images. Although the blastic foci of the tumor (*black arrows*) remain unchanged, popliteus muscle edema (*white arrows*) decreases with continued chemotherapy. The unfused tibial apophysis is demarcated (*open arrow*). (**F**) An anatomic gross section shows blastic tumor (*white arrows*) and tibial apophysis (*open arrow*) (**C** through **E**: TR, 2000 msec; TE, 60 msec).

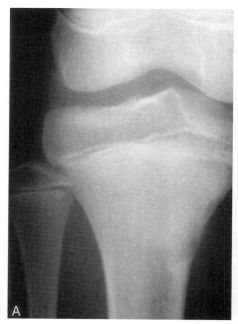
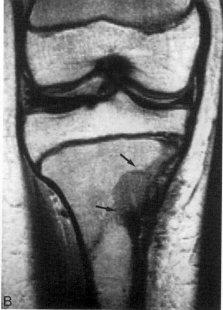

continued

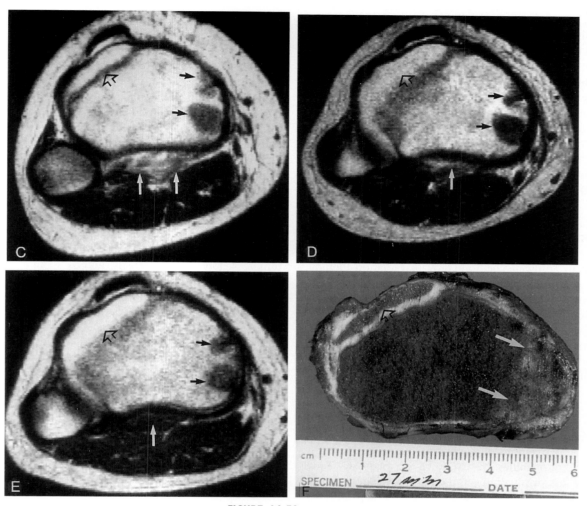

FIGURE 16-59. *Continued*

tissue; however, foci of residual viable tumor cannot be specifically diagnosed

4. Skip metastases, a reduction in peritumoral edema, the development of a dark rim of collagenous capsule continuous with the periosteum, bone infarcts, and intramedullary vascular channels can all be identified.

Holscher and colleagues have reported a correlation between a positive response to chemotherapy and signal intensity changes on T2-weighted images in the extraosseous tumor component and changes in overall tumor volume.[88] No correlation was observed between chemotherapy and intraosseous tumor signal intensity or volume and histology. Sanchez and colleagues have studied patients receiving intraarterial chemotherapy and reported similar signal intensities in viable tumor, necrosis, edema, and hemorrhage, which demonstrated the limitations of unenhanced spin-echo images in the accurate assessment of the percentage of tumor necrosis.[93]

Chondrosarcoma

Chondrosarcomas occur about one half as often as osteogenic sarcomas. They are malignant cartilage-producing neoplasms, which arise primarily in adulthood and old age. The peak incidence is in the fourth, fifth, and sixth decades of life. Chondrosarcomas most commonly arise in the central skeleton (the pelvis and ribs) and within the metadiaphysis of the femur and humerus. More than in other primary bone malignancies, their clinical and biologic behavior depends on their histologic grade, which is proportional to the level of anaplasia. Grade 1 (ie, well-differentiated) chondrosarcomas consist of pure hyaline cartilage exhibiting mild anaplasia and mild increased cellularity. Cellularity and anaplasia are greatest in poorly differentiated or grade 3 variants. The 5-year survival rates of patients with grades 1, 2, and 3 disease are approximately 90%, 81%, and 43%, respectively.[47] Grades 1 and 2 neoplasms (ie, the majority of chondrosarcomas) do not usually metastasize, whereas grade 3 neoplasms demonstrate a tendency to form hematogenous metastases. The majority of chondrosarcomas, approximately 75%, arise de novo and are considered primary chondrosarcomas. The remainder, secondary chondrosarcomas, arise by malignant transformation of preexisting cartilaginous lesions such as multiple enchondromatosis (eg, Ollier's disease or Maffucci's syndrome) and exostosis, especially multiple osteochondromatosis.[47] These neoplasms, whether situated peripherally or centrally, are composed of characteristic lobules of gray-white translucent tissue with spotty calcification.[47] The adjacent cortex may be thickened or eroded, with extension of the neoplasm into the surrounding soft tissues (Fig. 16-60).

TREATMENT OF CHONDROSARCOMA.

Unlike osteosarcoma and Ewing's sarcoma, low-grade chondrosarcomas are not responsive to adjuvant chemotherapy or radiation therapy. Instead, these tumors are considered surgical problems and must be removed with clean margins—if at all possible—in which case the 5-year survival rate is approximately 81%.[94] Figure 16-61 shows a typical primary central chondrosarcoma of the proximal humerus that has been treated by a wide resection of the proximal 15 cm (6 inches) of the humerus and reconstructed with a combination of a metallic Neer prosthesis and a cadaver allograft. Tendinous tags have been left intact for reattachment to the original structures, allowing for excellent limb function for many years to come. Preoperative MR imaging is extremely helpful in planning these reconstructive procedures by providing accurate evaluation the extent of tumor growth down the medullary canal and out into the surrounding soft tissue. These same preoper-

ative imaging studies assist the prosthesis manufacturers in the design of the prosthetic implant.

MAGNETIC RESONANCE APPEARANCE.

The epicenter of a primary, central chondrosarcoma can be located in the metaphysis or diaphysis of a long bone.[95] The cortex is irregularly thinned, and a circumferential periosteal reaction may appear to contain the lesion. Dedifferentiated chondrosarcomas are more aggressive and show rapid growth, cortical destruction, and the frequent association of an extraosseous component. MR imaging can be used to characterize changes of marrow involvement prior to medullary expansion (Fig. 16-62). T2*-weighted images are sensitive to matrix calcifications and associated soft-tissue masses (see Fig. 16-61). On T2- and T2*-weighted images, calcifications are identified as low signal intensity foci that contrast with the bright signal intensity tumor. A low signal intensity fibrous septum may also be seen, separating homogeneous high signal intensity lobules of hyaline cartilage.[62] Heterogeneity of signal intensity correlates with higher grade, more cellular lesions.[96] Gadolinium administration may produce enhancement in a ring and arc septal pattern. However, the clinical application of contrast-enhanced imaging needs further evaluation.[14,49]

Secondary chondrosarcoma develops in a preexisting enchondroma or osteochondroma (Fig. 16-63). Although extremely rare in childhood, chondrosarcoma has been known to arise from malignant transformation of an enchondroma in Ollier's disease. On T2-weighted images, these areas demonstrate greater signal intensity than adjacent enchondromas. Malignant degeneration or transformation can be inferred by the presence of frank cortical disruption, soft-tissue exten-

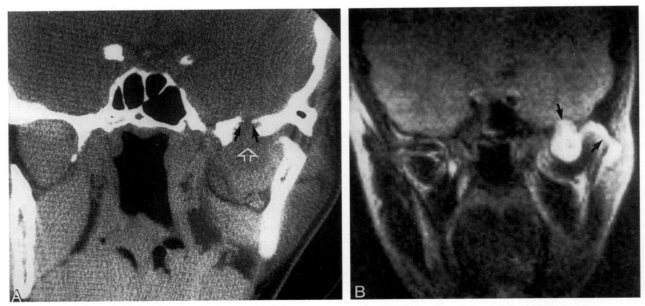

FIGURE 16-60. Chondrosarcoma of the temporomandibular joint. (**A**) Direct coronal CT shows a vague low attenuation mass (*open arrow*) and cortical destruction (*solid arrows*) extending to the middle cranial fossa. (**B**) The corresponding T2-weighted coronal image shows the exact location and boundaries of the bright signal intensity tumor (*arrows*).

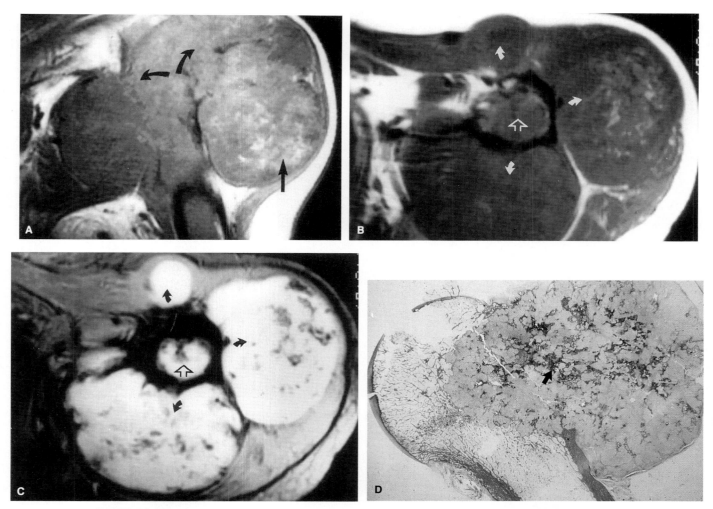

FIGURE 16-61. (**A**) A coronal T1-weighted image shows aggressive destruction of the proximal humerus (*curved arrows*) with a large soft-tissue component (*straight arrow*). This is characteristic of chondrosarcoma. Axial (**B**) T1-weighted and (**C**) T2*-weighted images show the degree of anterior, posterior, and lateral tumor extension (*curved arrows*), as well as the degree of marrow expansion (*open arrows*) (**A, B:** TR 600 msec; TE, 20 msec; **C:** TR 400 msec; TE, 20 msec; flip angle 25°). (**D**) Macrosection of tumor breaking out of the humoral head beneath the deltoid muscle with benign enchondral ossification (*white arrow*), which is seen as signal void on T2-weighted images. (Reprinted with permission from Henderson C, Wilson C, Phillips T, Debas H, Northfelt D, eds. Current cancer diagnosis and treatment. Norwalk, CT: Appleton & Lange, in press.) (**E**) High power photomicrograph demonstrating numerous dividing chondroblasts (*arrow*) typical of chondrosarcoma. (**F**) Surgical photograph of allograft used in limb salvage reconstruction following wide resection with rotator cuff tendon (*arrow*). (**G**) Long-stem metallic Neer prosthesis with pectoralis tendon allograft (*arrow*). (**H**) Photograph of completed alloprosthetic reconstruction with reattachment of the rotator cuff (*curved arrow*) and pectoralis and latissimus dorsi tendons (*straight arrow*). (**I**) Postoperative anteroposterior radiograph with Neer stem cemented into the distal humerus. (**G** through **I** reprinted with permission from Meyer JM, Vaeth JM, eds. Frontiers of radiation therapy and oncology: organ conservation in curative cancer treatment, vol 27. Basel, S Karger AG, 1993.)

continued

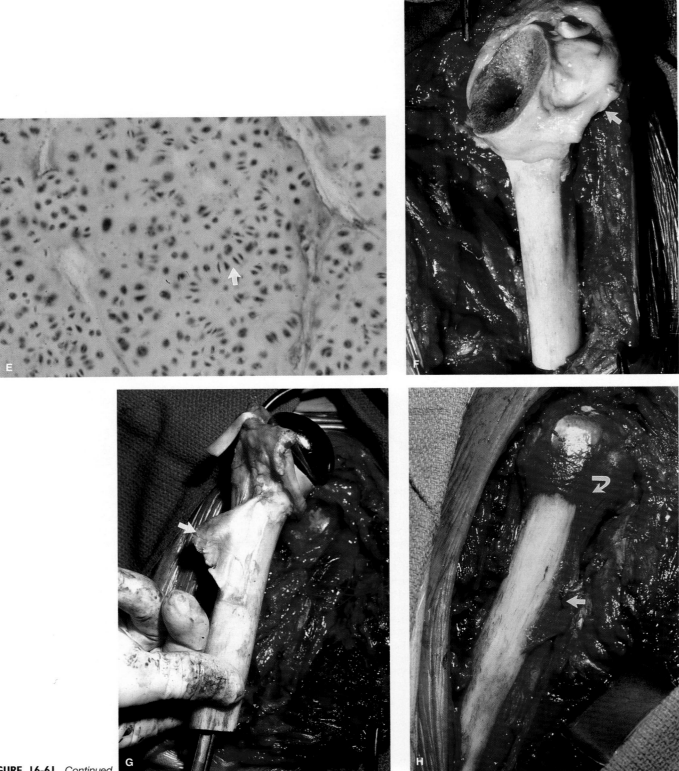

FIGURE 16-61. *Continued*

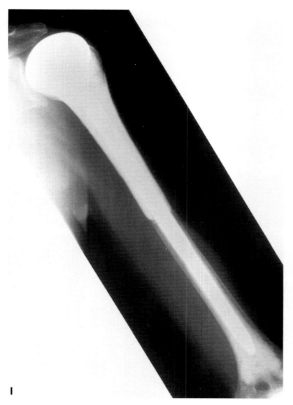

I

FIGURE 16-61. *Continued*

sion, periosteal reaction, and disproportionate size of lesion relative to satellite enchondromas. Although these findings have been confirmed by pathologic evaluation, reliable MR criteria have not been developed to characterize these aggressive cartilage lesions.

MR imaging is useful in the evaluation of aggressive extraskeletal mesenchymal chondrosarcoma, where soft-tissue origin is common.[97] In these extraskeletal lesions, MR imaging demonstrates enhancement, lobulation, and extent of disease; whereas CT is more accurate in characterizing calcifications.

Ewing's Sarcoma

Ewing's sarcoma is seen primarily during the last part of the first decade and the first one half of the second decade of life. It is the second most common malignant bone tumor in childhood, and although any bone in the body may be affected, the femur, ilium, humerus, and tibia are the most common sites. Ewing's sarcoma is one of the malignant round cell tumors involving bone. Although its histogenesis remains uncertain, evidence suggests a neuroectodermal origin.[98] Translocation of the long arms of chromosomes 11 and 22 have been found in Ewing's sarcoma.[99]

TREATMENT OF EWING'S SARCOMA.   Just as with osteosarcoma, the prognosis for Ewing's sarcoma has changed dramatically since the early 1970s with the advent of multi-

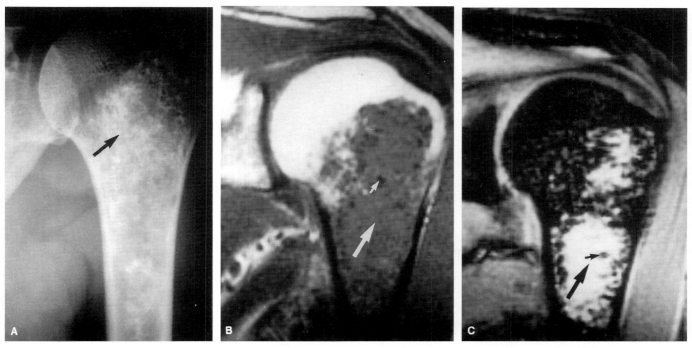

FIGURE 16-62. (A) An anteroposterior radiograph of the left shoulder shows characteristic annular and comma-shaped calcifications within central or medullary chondrosarcoma (*arrow*). Coronal (B) T1-weighted and (C) T2*-weighted images more accurately depict proximal marrow involvement (*large arrows*). Calcifications are seen as dark signal intensity foci (*small arrows*). The chondroid matrix is hyperintense on the T2*-weighted image.

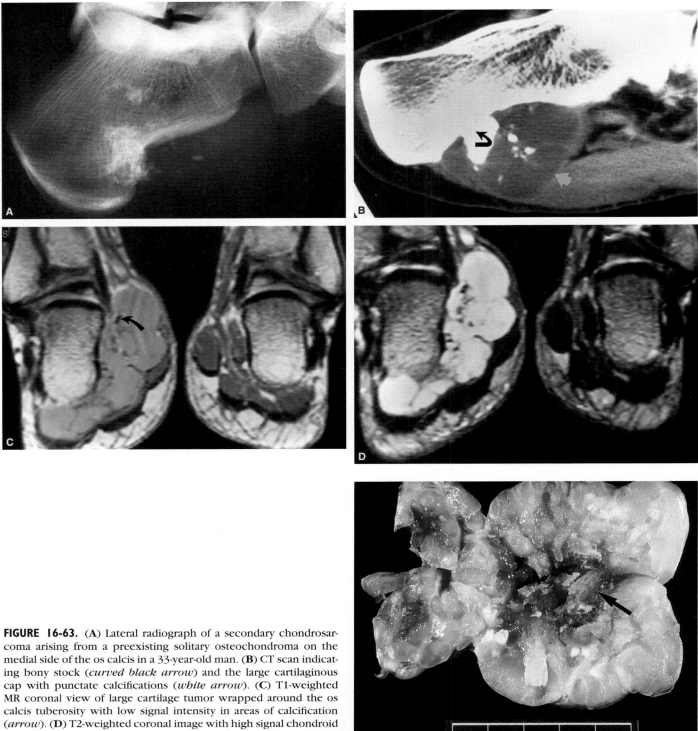

FIGURE 16-63. (A) Lateral radiograph of a secondary chondrosarcoma arising from a preexisting solitary osteochondroma on the medial side of the os calcis in a 33-year-old man. (B) CT scan indicating bony stock (*curved black arrow*) and the large cartilaginous cap with punctate calcifications (*white arrow*). (C) T1-weighted MR coronal view of large cartilage tumor wrapped around the os calcis tuberosity with low signal intensity in areas of calcification (*arrow*). (D) T2-weighted coronal image with high signal chondroid tissue. (E) Photograph of surgical specimen with arrow indicating bony base surrounded by a large cartilaginous cap.

drug adjuvant chemotherapy (including cyclophosphamide, ifosfamide, doxorubicin [Adriamycin], methotrexate, and vincristine). The 10-year survival rate is now 55% to 70%.[100] The effectiveness of chemotherapy can be monitored with MR imaging (see Figs. 16-69A and 16-69B), and these same imaging studies can assist the surgeon in planning surgical resection of the tumor and limb salvage reconstruction. If the tumor can be successfully removed with safe margins, there is no need for postoperative radiation therapy, and the prognosis for survival is increased to 74%.[101] For nonresectable tumors—such as large tumors of the pelvis, femur, or spine—adjuvant radiation therapy rather than surgery is used in conjunction with chemotherapy. In these cases, the prognosis is less favorable.

MAGNETIC RESONANCE APPEARANCE. Ewing's sarcoma demonstrates low signal intensity on T1-weighted sequences and bright signal intensity on T2, T2*-weighted, and STIR sequences[102,103] (Fig. 16-64). Marrow involvement and peritumoral edema are clearly delineated (Fig. 16-65).

Because the soft-tissue component of Ewing's sarcoma is usually substantial, MR evaluation is superior to CT or to plain film radiography, especially in the distal extremities (Fig. 16-66). Since MR imaging provides excellent delineation of soft tissues, the extent of muscular and neurovascular involvement in extraosseous Ewing's sarcoma can also be

assessed (Fig. 16-67). In addition, Ewing's sarcoma originating in bone marrow can be identified in the early stages, before cortical erosion and periostitis have developed (Fig. 16-68). Multilamellar periosteal reactions and an atypical pattern of cortical thickening and saucerization in Ewing's sarcoma have also been identified on MR scans.[104] The rare periosteal Ewing's sarcoma can be distinguished from the more common medullary and soft-tissue Ewing's sarcoma because of its location, predominance in males, lack of presenting metastases.[105] MR imaging has been used after chemotherapy to more accurately define tumor margins and assess the interval decrease in adjacent peritumoral edema (Fig. 16-69).

Plasmacytoma

Plasmacytoma is a solitary neoplasm of plasma cells that sometimes converts into multiple myeloma.[106] Solitary plasmacytomas affect the middle age group (50 years) and frequently target the spine and pelvis. A solitary lytic or expansile lesion is common, although an ivory vertebral pattern has been reported in the spine. Magnetic resonance characteristics of plasmacytoma are nonspecific low to intermediate signal intensity on T1-weighted images and high signal intensity on T2-weighted images (Fig. 16-70). Aggressive cortical disruption and infiltration into soft tissue and adjacent

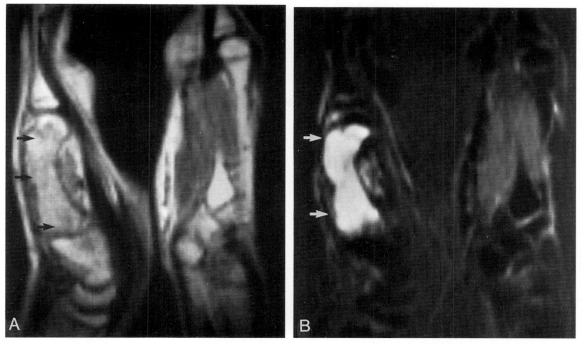

FIGURE 16-64. (**A**) Ewing's sarcoma (*arrows*) of the metacarpal in a patient undergoing radiation therapy is seen on a conventional T1-weighted sagittal image (TR, 900 msec; TE, 40 msec). (**B**) A short TI inversion recovery image shows high signal intensity contrast (*arrows*) in the infiltrated bone. The normal marrow appears black (TR, 400 msec; TI, 125 msec; TE, 40 msec).

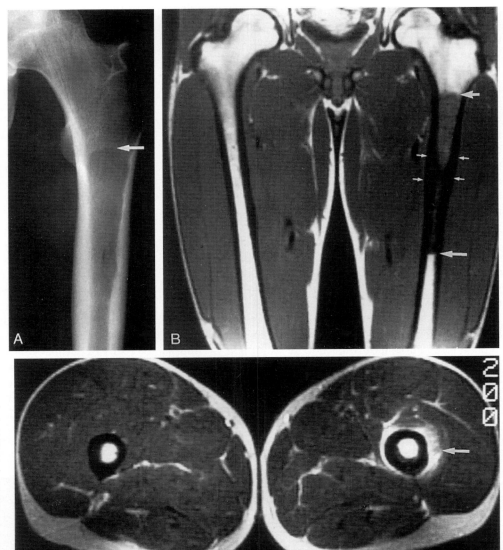

FIGURE 16-65. (A) An anteroposterior radiograph demarcates the proximal extent of medullary involvement (*arrow*) in Ewing's sarcoma. (B) The corresponding T1-weighted coronal MR image reveals both proximal (*medium arrow*) and distal (*large arrow*) marrow extension and periosteal thickening (*small arrows*) (TR, 500 msec; TE, 20 msec). (C) A T2-weighted axial image shows high signal intensity peritumoral edema (*arrow*) without an associated soft-tissue mass (TR, 2000 msec; TE, 60 msec).

structures, with discontinuity of adjacent low signal intensity cortical bone, can be identified on MR examination.

Adamantinoma

Adamantinoma of bone is a rare neoplasm with an uncertain histogenesis. The tibia is the site of involvement in 90% of cases. Immunohistochemical data indicate an epithelial nature. Histologically, there is a spectrum of patterns ranging from spindled to squamoid, with characteristic basaloid cells. The peak incidence is in the third to fourth decades of life. Although these tumors are slow growing and appear histologically bland, approximately 20% metastasize.[107]

The MR imaging characteristics of adamantinoma may be similar to lesions of osteofibrous dysplasia, with low signal intensity sclerosis identified on T1- and T2-weighted images (Fig. 16-71). Peritumoral edema or small focal areas of hyperintensity may be identified within the tibial cortex. These areas of increased signal intensity may correspond to osteolytic defects adjacent to sclerotic bone. Adamantinomas are characteristically located in the middle one third of the tibia and have a cortical or eccentric epicenter.

Metastatic Disease

Magnetic resonance is very sensitive in evaluating metastatic disease.[108–111] Skeletal metastases of known origin usually involve the breast or prostate, whereas metastases of unknown origin often originate in the lung or kidney.[112] In

text continues on page 1304

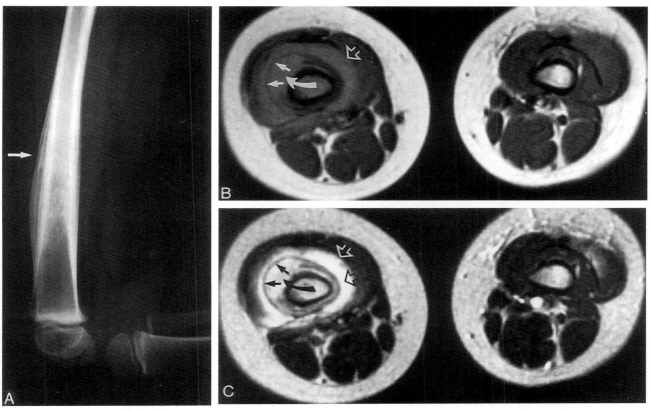

FIGURE 16-66. (**A**) A lateral radiograph shows an "onion skin" periosteal reaction in Ewing's sarcoma of the femur (*arrow*). Axial (**B**) T1-weighted and (**C**) T2-weighted images show a low signal intensity periosteal reaction (*solid arrows*), peritumoral edema (*open arrows*), and marrow and soft-tissue components (*curved arrows*). Edema, marrow, and soft-tissue components demonstrate low signal intensity on the T1-weighted image and bright signal intensity on the T2-weighted image (**B:** TR, 600 msec; TE, 20 msec; **C:** TR, 2000 msec; TE, 60 msec).

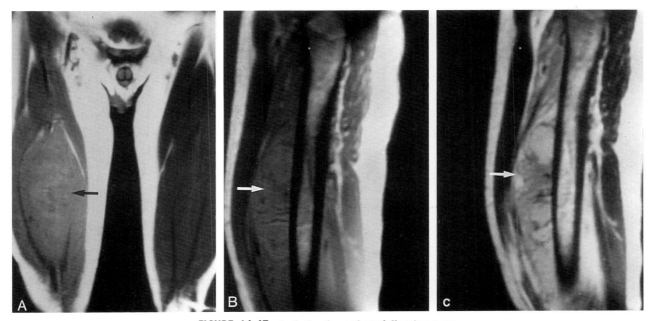

FIGURE 16-67. **A–C.** *See legend on following page.*

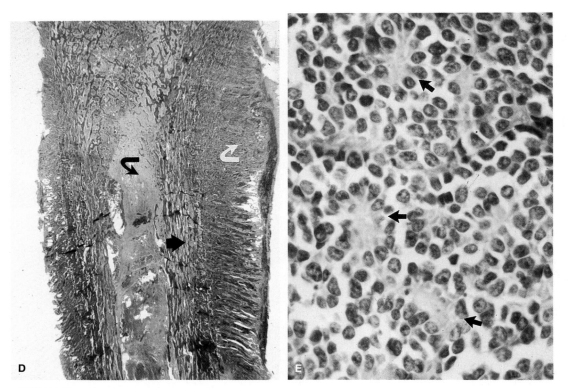

FIGURE 16-67. (A) On a balanced (intermediate weighted) image, extraosseous Ewing's sarcoma demonstrates intermediate signal intensity (*arrow*) (TR, 1500 msec; TE, 40 msec). On a T1-weighted image (**B**), signal intensity of the sarcoma (*arrows*) is low and on a T2-weighted image (**C**) is high (**B**: TR, 600 msec; TE 20 msec; **C**: TR, 2000 msec; TE, 60 msec). In a separate case, pathologic specimen shows both osseous and soft-tissue involvement. (**D**) Macrosection of resected femur with necrotic tumor in marrow canal (*curved black arrow*), tumor permeation through cortical bone (*straight black arrow*), and large viable extracortical tumor mass (*curved white arrow*). (**E**) High power photomicrograph with solid sheet of blue cells organized in colonies or pseudorosettes.

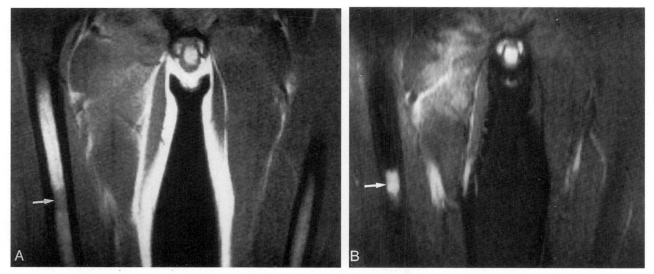

FIGURE 16-68. (**A**) On a T1-weighted image, early marrow involvement (*arrow*) of Ewing's sarcoma is seen as a focus of decreased signal intensity (TR, 600 msec; TE, 20 msec). (**B**) On a short TI inversion recovery image, the focus of involved marrow (*arrow*) shows increased signal intensity (TR, 1400 msec; TI, 125 msec; TE, 40 msec).

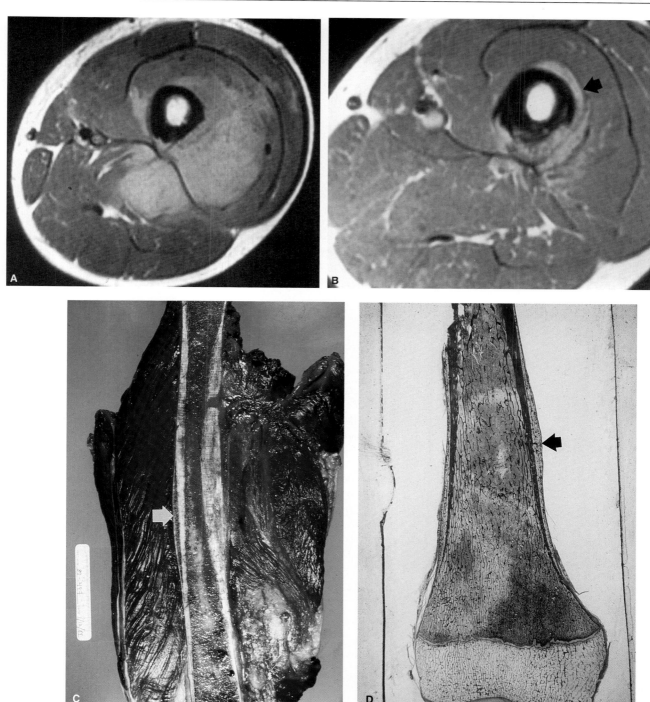

FIGURE 16-69. (A) Proton density axial image of a 12-year-old boy with extensive intermediate signal, soft-tissue abnormality representing a Ewing's sarcoma arising from the femur as the result of extensive round cell infiltrate and edema into the surrounding muscle compartments. (B) Same proton density study after two cycles of chemotherapy with dramatic shrinkage of the tumor margins (*arrow*). (C) Photograph of the amputated specimen with arrow indicating same tumor margin seen in **B**. (D) Gross macrosection of same specimen with extracortical tumor margin indicated by arrow.

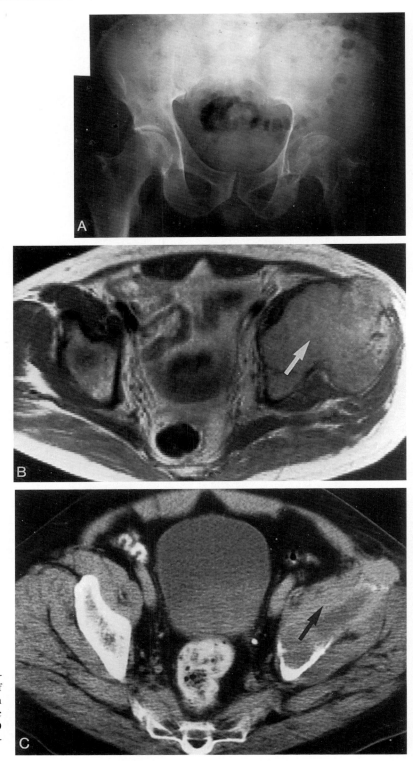

FIGURE 16-70. Plasmacytoma of the ilium. (**A**) An antero-posterior radiograph of the pelvis shows destruction of the left ilium. (**B**) A T1-weighted axial MR image reveals an intermediate signal intensity mass (*arrow*) with aggressive cortical transgression and soft-tissue extension (TR, 600 msec; TE, 20 msec). (**C**) An axial CT image shows disrupted cortical bone (*arrows*).

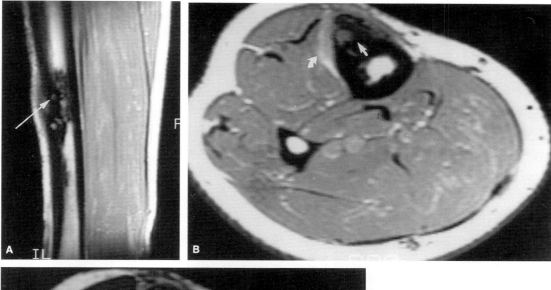

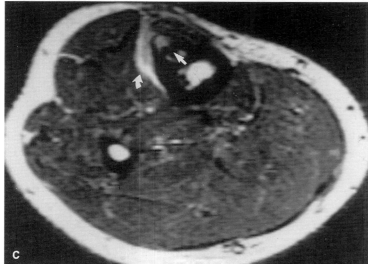

FIGURE 16-71. (A) A T1-weighted sagittal image shows an eccentric, sclerotic, low signal intensity adamantinoma in the anterior tibial diaphysis (*arrow*). Axial intermediate weighted images (**B**) and T2-weighted images (**C**) show a focal area of cortical hyperintensity (*straight arrows*) and peritumoral edema (*curved arrows*).

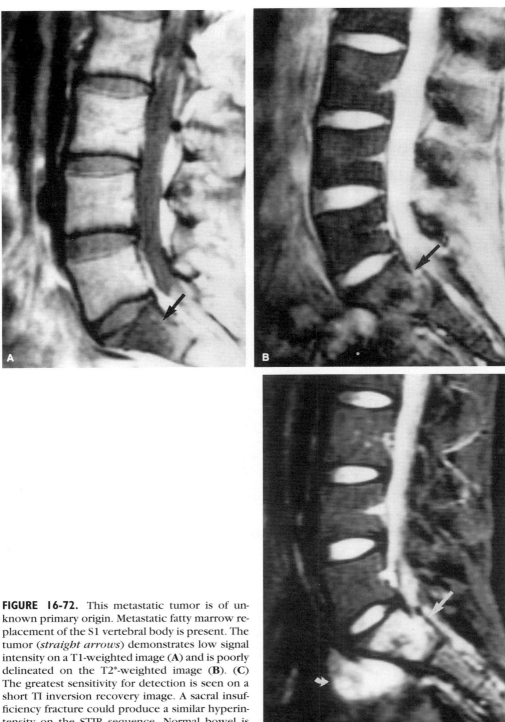

FIGURE 16-72. This metastatic tumor is of unknown primary origin. Metastatic fatty marrow replacement of the S1 vertebral body is present. The tumor (*straight arrows*) demonstrates low signal intensity on a T1-weighted image (**A**) and is poorly delineated on the T2*-weighted image (**B**). (**C**) The greatest sensitivity for detection is seen on a short TI inversion recovery image. A sacral insufficiency fracture could produce a similar hyperintensity on the STIR sequence. Normal bowel is identified anterior to S1 (*curved arrow*).

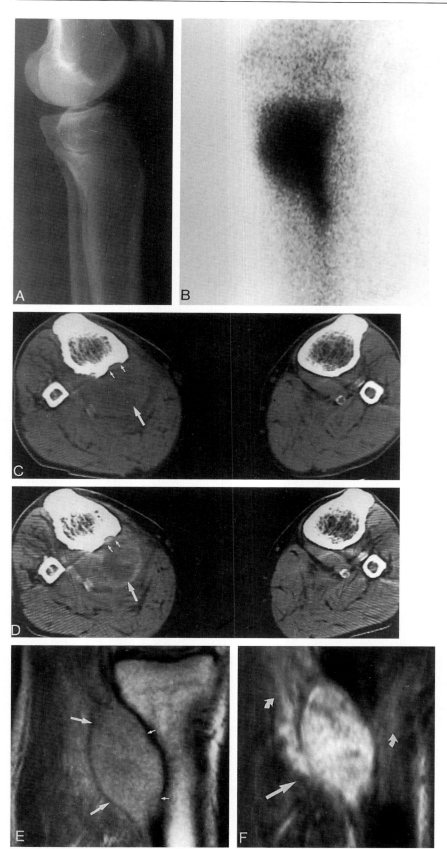

FIGURE 16-73. (A) A lateral radiograph shows subtle cortical irregularity, indicative of metastatic melanoma, along the proximal posterior tibial cortex. (B) Technetium bone scintigraphy reveals an uptake of tracer in the posterior tibia and soft tissues. Axial CT scans (C) before and (D) after contrast enhancement show hypervascularity of the soft-tissue mass (*large arrows*). Posteromedial cortical erosion is also shown (*small arrows*). (E) On a T1-weighted sagittal image, the intermediate signal intensity metastatic melanoma is an elliptical mass (*large arrow*) invading the low signal intensity posterior tibial cortex (*small arrows*). (F) On the corresponding short TI inversion recovery image, the metastatic melanoma (*straight arrow*) demonstrates high signal intensity, as well as reactive marrow and soft-tissue edema (*curved arrows*).

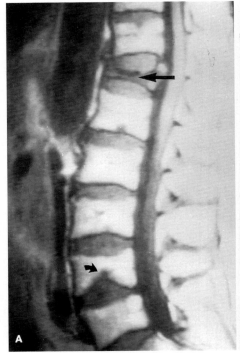
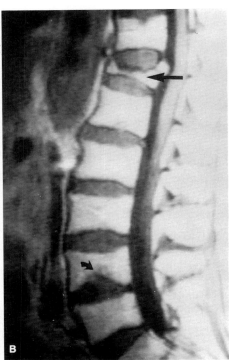

FIGURE 16-74. In metastatic lung cancer, T1-weighted sagittal images (**A**) before and (**B**) after Gd-DTPA enhancement show a pathologic fracture at T12 (*straight arrows*). A nonenhanced benign compression fracture at L4 is also indicated (*curved arrows*) (TR, 500 msec; TE, 30 msec).

general, metastatic bone disease appears as focal lesions that involve both cortical bone and marrow and demonstrate low signal intensity on T1-weighted sequences and bright signal intensity on T2-weighted sequences. T1-weighted and STIR sequences are more sensitive than T2*-weighted scans in identifying increased signal intensity in metastatic deposits or surrounding edema (Figs. 16-72 and 16-73). Gadolinium has been used to enhance

osseous and soft-tissue metastases on T1-weighted images (Figs. 16-74 and 16-75). Neuroblastomas frequently metastasize to both bone and soft tissue (eg, paraspinal lesions) (Fig. 16-76). Nuclear scintigraphy may produce false-positive scan results or may be negative even with very aggressive lesions (Fig. 16-77). Metastatic deposits can be identified on MR scans in patients with negative findings on conventional radiographs (Fig. 16-78). Vascu-

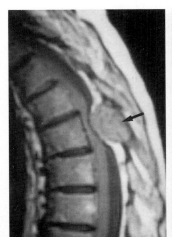
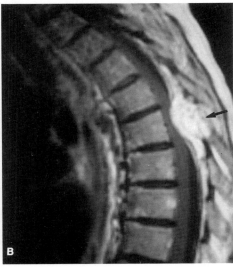

FIGURE 16-75. This metastatic adenocarcinoma (*arrows*) is from an unknown primary source. Sagittal T1-weighted images (**A**) before and (**B**) after Gd-DTPA enhancement show the tumor epicenter in the posterior elements of the thoracic spine, resulting in extradural cord compression (TR, 500 msec; TE, 20 msec).

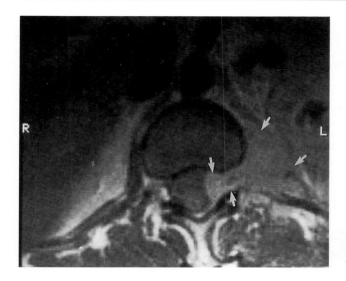

FIGURE 16-76. Metastatic neuroblastoma has infiltrated the left neural foramina (*arrows*) on this intermediate weighted image (TR, 2000 msec; TE, 28 msec).

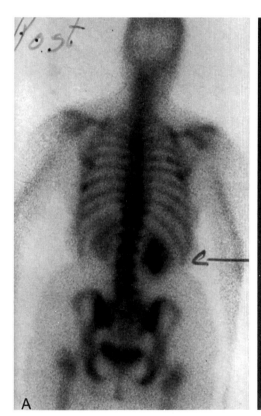

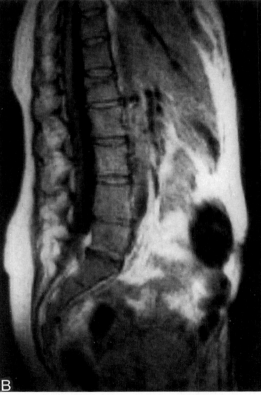

FIGURE 16-77. (**A**) Technetium bone scan is unremarkable in a patient with aggressive metastatic breast carcinoma. (**B**) T1-weighted and (**C**) short TI inversion recovery images show low and high signal intensity, respectively, in diffuse marrow involvement of the entire thoracic and lumbar spines. (**D**) The corresponding axial CT scan confirms lytic destruction of cancellous cortical bone. *continued*

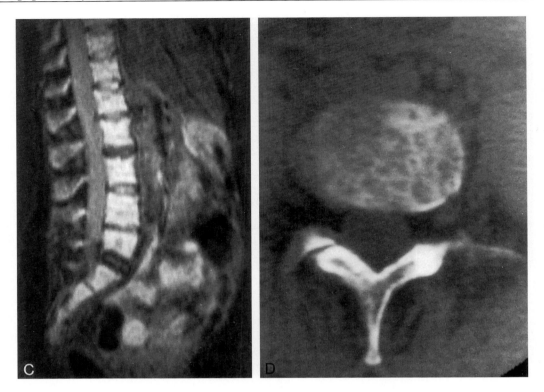

FIGURE 16-77. *Continued*

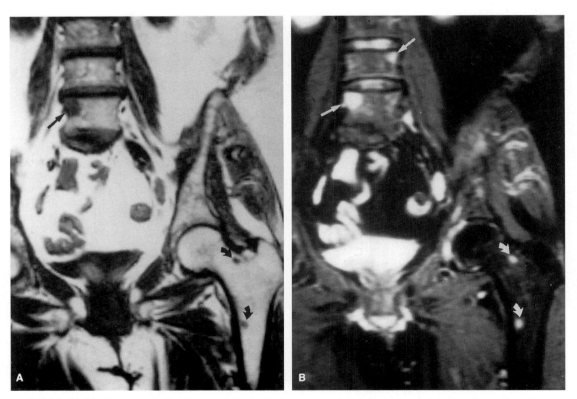

FIGURE 16-78. Unsuspected metastatic breast carcinoma was not detected on routine radiographs of the spine or hip. Coronal T1-weighted images (**A**) and short TI inversion recovery (STIR) images (**B**) reveal metastatic foci in the L4 and L5 vertebral bodies (*straight arrows*) and left proximal femur (*curved arrows*). Note the greater sensitivity (ie, contrast) on the STIR image, which highlights the L4 metastatic tumor that is not seen on the T1-weighted image (**A:** TR, 500 msec; TE, 20 msec; **B:** TR, 2000 msec; TI, 160 msec; TE, 40 msec).

larity may assist in determining the site of tumor origin (eg, renal cell carcinoma with low signal intensity vessels; Fig. 16-79). High bone detail in cortical or trabecular destruction may require correlation with corresponding CT scans (Fig. 16-80).

The MR appearance of metastatic lesions is nonspecific for the site of origin.[21] Peritumoral soft-tissue edema may be observed in the absence of a soft-tissue mass. Sequential postcontrast MR images can help to differentiate tumor from perineoplastic edema.[23] Osteolytic metastatic lesions, commonly from carcinoma of the lung or breast, often demonstrate a more uniform signal intensity on T1- and T2-weighted images than do mixed sclerotic or osteoblastic deposits from carcinoma of the prostate or medulloblastoma (Fig. 16-81). Lesions of enostosis or osteopoikilosis may mimic blastic metastatic deposits; however, no aggressive features are associated with enostosis or osteopoikilosis (Figs. 16-82 and 16-83).

Primary Lymphoma of Bone

Originally designated "reticulum cell sarcoma of bone," this clinicopathologic disorder is now defined as a malignant lymphoma that arises within the medullary cavity of a single bone and occurs without concurrent regional lymph node or visceral involvement within a 6-month period[113,114] (Fig. 16-84). This rare disorder represents approximately 2% to 3% of malignant bone tumors and 5% of all extranodal lymphomas. Although all pathohistologic types of non-Hodgkin's lymphoma have been reported to occur in bone, large cell (ie, reticulum cell) lymphoma is the most common.

Primary lymphoma of bone carries a better prognosis than disseminated non-Hodgkin's lymphoma with secondary involvement of bone.[115] Mulligan and Kransdorf have reported sequestration in 11% of cases of primary lymphoma.[116] Sequestra also occur in osteomyelitis, eosinophilic granuloma, fibrosarcoma, MFH, and desmoplastic fibroma.

SOFT-TISSUE NEOPLASMS

In the evaluation of soft-tissue tumors, MR imaging offers the following advantages over CT[4,5,117–121]:

- Both cortical and marrow involvement can be evaluated
- Improved depiction of the tissue planes surrounding the lesion and muscle textural patterns
- Assessment of neurovascular involvement.

Gadolinium enhancement may be used to further characterize the extent, degree of necrosis, and recurrence of soft-tissue tumors.[122–124]

MR demonstrates changes of radiation therapy and chemotherapy in the treatment of soft-tissue sarcomas.[125] These changes include irradiation effects on the epiphyseal plates (which are widened) and metaphysis, and suppression of myeloid elements. Chemotherapy-related myeloid suppression may lead to anemia, neutropenia, and subsequent stimulation of hematopoietic marrow. Pretherapy MR imaging and spectroscopy have been used by Sostman and colleagues

text continues on page 1312

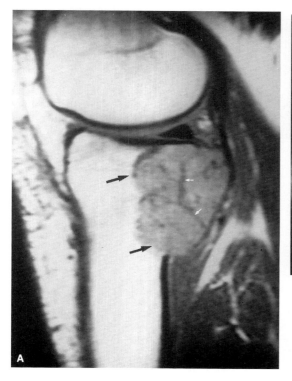

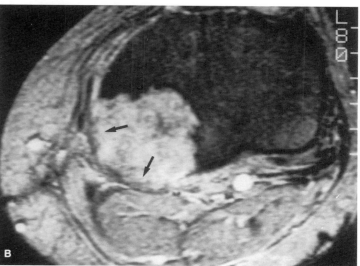

FIGURE 16-79. (**A**) A T1-weighted sagittal image shows expansile destruction of the posterior tibial cortex (*black arrows*) caused by metastatic renal cell carcinoma. Tumor vascularity is seen in low signal intensity linear segments (*white arrows*) (TR, 600 msec; TE, 200 msec). (**B**) The corresponding axial T2*-weighted image shows hyperintense metastasis violating the posterior tibial cortex (*arrows*) (TR, 500 msec; TE, 20 msec; flip angle, 25°).

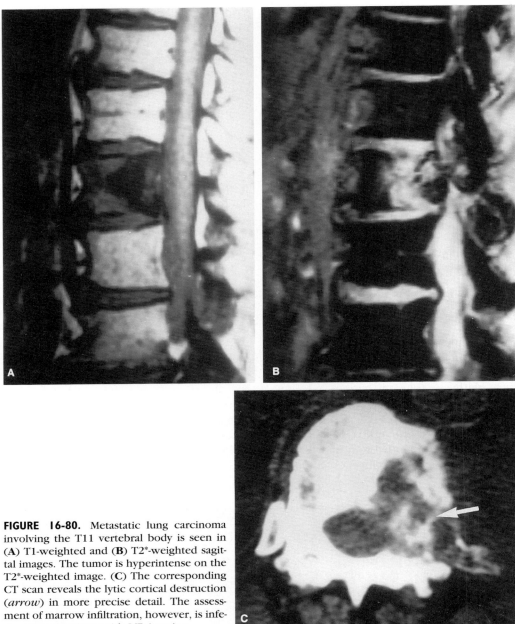

FIGURE 16-80. Metastatic lung carcinoma involving the T11 vertebral body is seen in (**A**) T1-weighted and (**B**) T2*-weighted sagittal images. The tumor is hyperintense on the T2*-weighted image. (**C**) The corresponding CT scan reveals the lytic cortical destruction (*arrow*) in more precise detail. The assessment of marrow infiltration, however, is inferior in comparison with MR imaging.

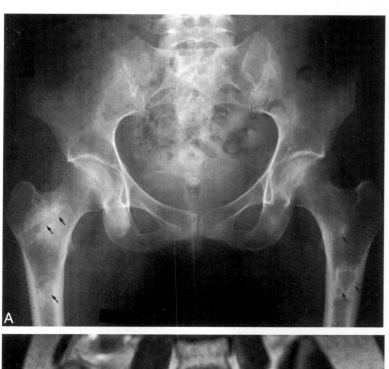

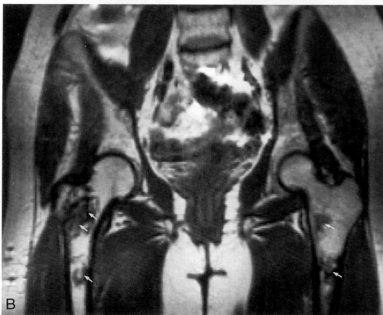

FIGURE 16-81. (A) An anteroposterior radiograph of the pelvis shows mixed lytic and sclerotic femoral lesions (*arrows*). (B) On the corresponding T1-weighted coronal image, metastatic deposits of medulloblastoma (*arrows*) demonstrate nonuniform low to intermediate signal intensity (TR, 500 msec; TE, 40 msec).

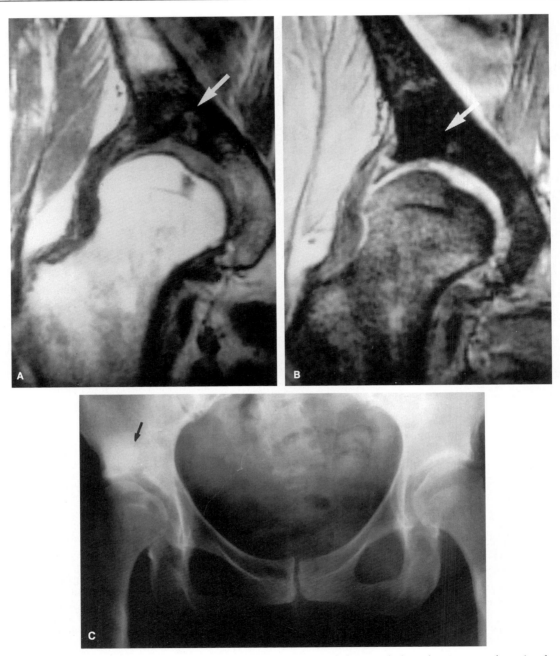

FIGURE 16-82. A large enostosis (ie, bone island; *arrows*) of the acetabulum demonstrates low signal intensity on coronal T1-weighted images (**A**) and T2*-weighted images (**B**). Without the aggressive features of soft-tissue mass or marrow hyperemia, this lesion should not be diagnosed as a sclerotic metastasis (**A:** TR, 500 msec; TE, 20 msec; **B:** TR, 400 msec; TE, 20 msec; flip angle, 25°). (**C**) The corresponding anteroposterior radiograph shows a superior acetabular sclerotic focus (*arrow*).

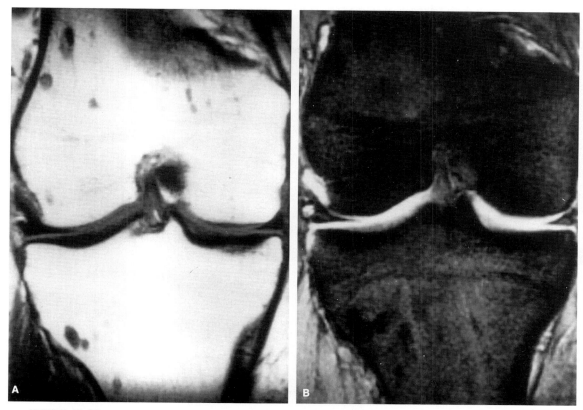

FIGURE 16-83. Asymptomatic low signal intensity multiple bone islands are seen on coronal T1-weighted images (**A**) and T2*-weighted knee images (**B**). The morphology and distribution of these islands are characteristic of osteopoikilosis (**A:** TR, 600 msec; TE, 20 msec; **B:** TR, 400 msec; TE, 15 msec; flip angle, 20°).

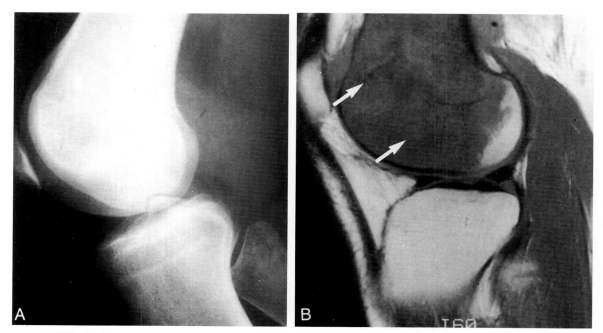

FIGURE 16-84. (**A**) A lateral radiograph is negative in a patient with osseous lymphoma. (**B**) On a T1-weighted sagittal image, low signal intensity lymphomatous marrow replacement is seen crossing the physeal scar and involving the subchondral bone (*arrows*) (TR, 800 msec; TE, 20 msec).

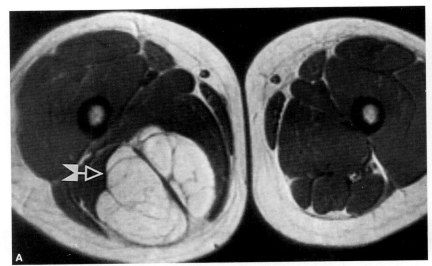
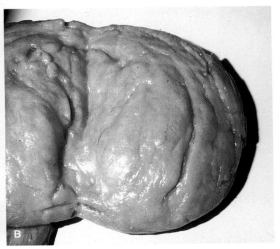
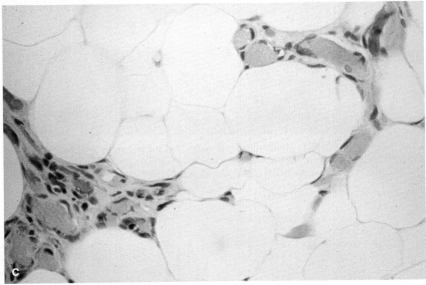

FIGURE 16-85. **(A)** A lipoma (*arrow*) located between the semimembranosus and semitendinosus muscles demonstrates subcutaneous fat signal intensity on a T1-weighted axial image (TR, 600 msec; TE, 20 msec). **(B)** Photograph of resected specimen. **(C)** High power photomicrograph shows benign lipocytes.

in predicting the prognosis of patients with soft-tissue sarcomas.[126] By monitoring the relationship between pretherapy pH and T2 with tumor necrosis, they determined that higher values were associated with increased tumor necrosis.

Benign Soft-Tissue Neoplasms

Benign soft-tissue tumors are usually homogeneous and clearly marginated, and do not involve neurovascular structures. Malignant soft-tissue lesions tend to be inhomogeneous, with irregular margins and surrounding muscle edema. With long TR/TE sequences (TR, 2500 msec; TE, 80 msec), a tumor may demonstrate higher signal intensity than associated edema.

Fibromatosis

Axial and sagittal planar images may be used to assess the fibrous lesions of plantar fibromatosis. These fibrous nodules, which involve the plantar aponeurosis, demonstrate low signal intensity on T1- and T2-weighted sequences. Xanthofibromas may also demonstrate low signal intensity on T1- and T2-weighted images. In one series of 26 patients, the MR appearance of soft-tissue fibromatosis was variable, with hyperintense, isointense, hypointense, or mixed signal intensity relative to adjacent skeletal muscle.[127] Increased signal intensity on T1-weighted images was attributed to fat, protein, or both. Lesions of fibromatosis may also show varying degrees of increased signal intensity on T2, T2*, and STIR protocols.

Lipoma

Soft-tissue lipomas are homogeneous and clearly marginated, with or without internal fibrous separations. Lipomas are the most frequent of the soft-tissue tumors, and they usually appear in the fifth or sixth decades of life. Most commonly, these soft-tissue neoplasms are found in the subcutaneous regions of the back and shoulder, but they can be found in any subcutaneous location. Less frequently, they occur in deeper locations such as within the thigh, anterior mediastinum, retroperitoneum, or gastrointestinal wall. Deep-seated intramuscular lipomas, especially in the paraspinal region, are rarely encapsulated; these frequently recur.[128]

MAGNETIC RESONANCE APPEARANCE. Lipomas demonstrate bright signal intensity on T1-weighted images and do not increase in signal intensity on T2 or fat-suppressed T2-weighted fast spin-echo weighted sequences[4] (Figs. 16-85 and 16-86). On STIR images, the fat signal in these lesions is nulled (Fig. 16-87). Low signal intensity septations may be seen within these lesions on T1- and T2-weighted images. Lipomas do not show contrast enhancement after intravenous injection of a paramagnetic material.

Deep lipomas occurring in the extremities commonly involve either the shoulder or thigh. Although intramuscular lipomas are almost always well-defined lesions, on occasion they may have ill-defined borders and may demonstrate infiltration into adjacent muscle tissue (Fig. 16-88). MR imaging is useful for presurgical evaluation of parosteal lipomas, clearly identifying associated muscle atrophy and nerve involvement.[129]

Hemangioma

Hemangiomas can occur in bone or soft tissues, and may vary widely in appearance. Histopathologically, they range from the cavernous type, with very large vascular spaces separated by fibrous tissue, to the capillary type—very cellular and lacking fibrous septa (Figs. 16-89 through 16-91).

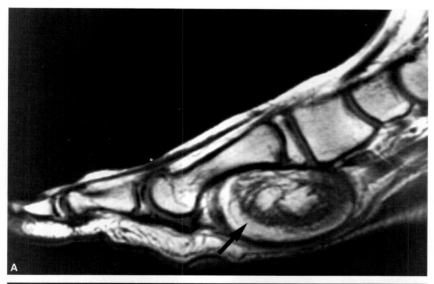

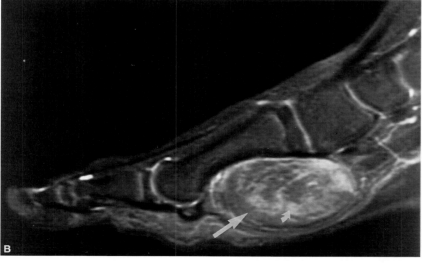

FIGURE 16-86. Plantar lipoma (*straight arrow*) of the foot showing fat signal intensity on T1-weighted sagittal image (**A**), which suppresses on fat-suppressed T2-weighted fast spin-echo sagittal image (**B**). This lipoma was in a weight-bearing location and demonstrated atypical features of inflammation (*curved arrow*), as characterized by poorly defined hyperintense areas on the fat-suppressed T2-weighted fast spin-echo sequence (image **B**).

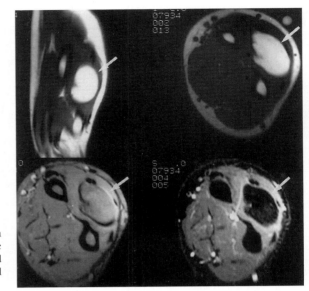

FIGURE 16-87. Lipoma (*arrows*) demonstrates bright fat signal intensity on T1-weighted sagittal (*top left*) and axial (*top right*) images. Lipomatous tissue is isointense with surrounding musculature and soft tissue on a T2*-weighted axial image (*bottom left*), and demonstrates dark signal intensity on an axial short TI inversion recovery image (*bottom right*).

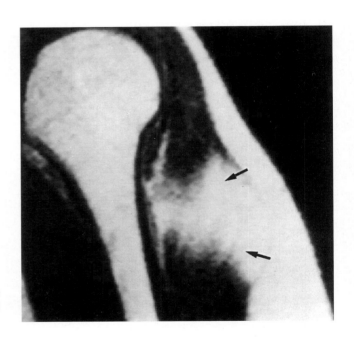

FIGURE 16-88. A high signal intensity lipoma (*arrows*) is infiltrating the deltoid muscle laterally on a T1-weighted coronal image (TR, 500 msec; TE, 31 msec).

Intramuscular hemangiomas (Figs. 16-92 and 16-93) are noncircumscribed tumors with a predilection for the thigh muscles of young adults.[130] Pain is frequently the presenting symptom. The intramuscular type of hemangioma is associated with variable amounts of fat, smooth muscle, myxoid stroma, and hemosiderin. Although clearly benign histologically, these intramuscular hemangiomas may recur.[128]

MAGNETIC RESONANCE APPEARANCE. Hemangiomas demonstrate low to intermediate signal intensity on T1-weighted images and bright signal intensity on T2-weighted images[131] (see Fig. 16-92). Because of paramagnetic effects, central hemorrhage with hemosiderin deposits or peripheral hemosiderin-laden macrophages demonstrate low signal intensity on T1- and T2-weighted images. In selected cases, feeding vessels can be identified on STIR images (see Fig. 16-93). There may be secondary involvement of cortical bone (Fig. 16-94).

Hemangiopericytoma

Hemangiopericytomas are hypervascular soft-tissue tumors thought to originate from the capillary cell wall.[29] Pericytes (ie, cells present in the walls of capillaries and venules) can be demonstrated with electron microscopy and identified

as the exact cell of origin. Most of these neoplasms are small, but, on rare occasions, they may achieve diameters of 8 cm or more. Despite a benign histopathologic pattern, hemangiopericytomas can recur, and as many as 50% metastasize to lungs, bone, and liver. Their biologic behavior, therefore, cannot always be predicted from histology. Hemangiopericytomas usually present as a deep, soft-tissue mass of the thigh.[128]

MAGNETIC RESONANCE APPEARANCE. The peripheral arterial branching seen in angiograms is depicted on T2-weighted MR images as an intricately packed network of vessels demonstrating signal void. It is in contrast to the adjacent tumor, which is bright (Fig. 16-95).

Ganglion Cyst

Ganglion cysts, thin-walled cysts filled with clear mucinous fluid, occur in soft tissues near joints. They are most commonly found around the hands and feet, especially the wrist, and are believed to represent either synovial herniations or mucinous degenerations of dense fibrous connective

text continues on page 1318

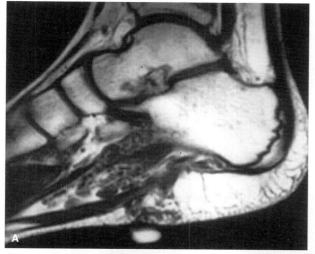

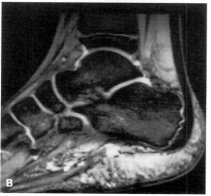

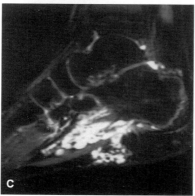

FIGURE 16-89. Hemangioma with dilated, serpiginous vessels in the plantar aspect of the foot demonstrates low signal intensity on a T1-weighted sagittal image (**A**), and bright signal intensity on T2*-weighted (**B**) and short TI inversion recovery (STIR) (**C**) images. Characteristic extension to the skin and subcutaneous tissues is most accurately defined on T1-weighted and STIR images (**A:** TR, 600 msec; TE, 20 msec; **B:** TR, 400 msec; TE, 20 msec; flip angle, 25°; **C:** TR, 2000 msec; TI, 160 msec; TE, 43 msec).

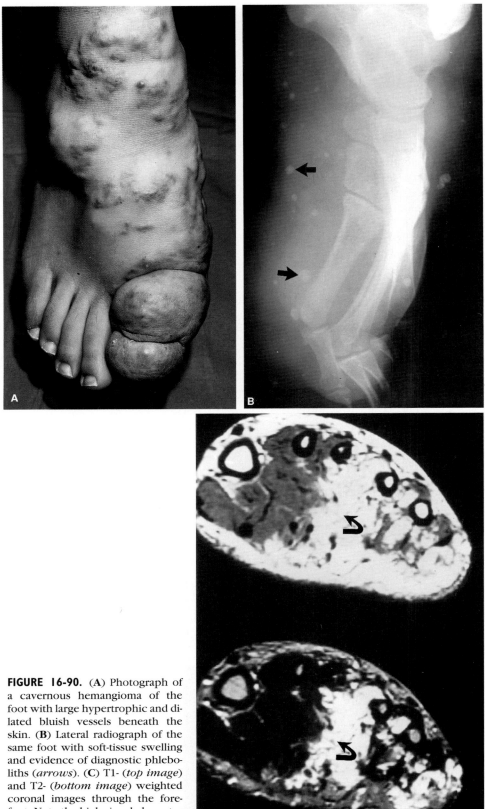

FIGURE 16-90. (A) Photograph of a cavernous hemangioma of the foot with large hypertrophic and dilated bluish vessels beneath the skin. (B) Lateral radiograph of the same foot with soft-tissue swelling and evidence of diagnostic phleboliths (*arrows*). (C) T1- (*top image*) and T2- (*bottom image*) weighted coronal images through the forefoot. Note the high signal character of the hemangioma (*arrows*).

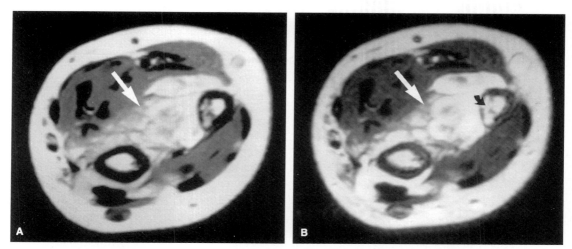

FIGURE 16-91. Axial intermediate weighted (**A**) and T2-weighted (**B**) images show hyperintense hemangioma with lobulated, sinusoidal, blood-filled spaces (*straight arrows*). Marrow and cortex hemangiomatous tissue is shown (*curved arrow*).

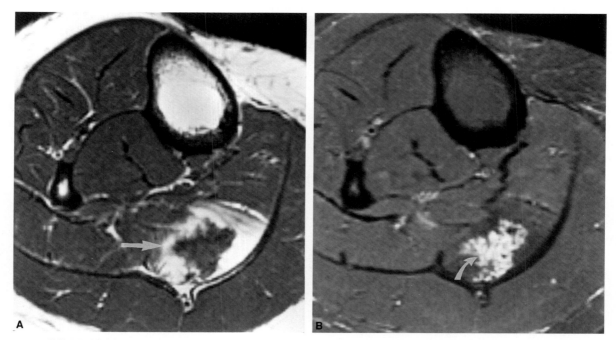

FIGURE 16-92. Intramuscular hemangioma of the soleus muscle group on T1-weighted axial image (**A**) and fat-suppressed T2-weighted fast spin-echo image (**B**). Fat content within the hemangioma (*straight arrow*) is bright on the T1-weighted scan (**A**) and suppresses on fat-suppressed T2-weighted fast spin-echo scan (**B**). The vascular component demonstrates the reverse pattern, demonstrating low signal on the T1-weighted scan (**A**) and lobulated hyperintensity (*curved arrow*) on fat-suppressed T2-weighted fast spin-echo (image **B**).

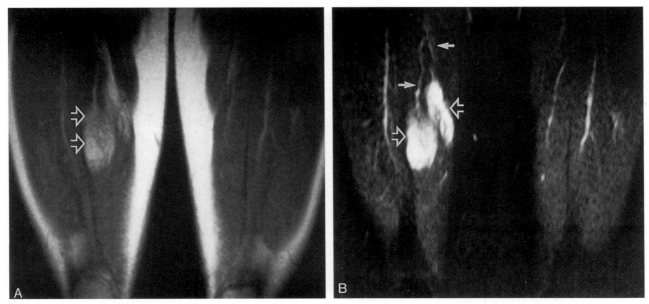

FIGURE 16-93. High signal intensity hemangioma (*open arrows*) of the vastus medialis muscle is seen on both T1-weighted (**A**) and short TI inversion recovery (STIR) (**B**) coronal images. The supplying vessels demonstrate high signal intensity contrast in the STIR sequence (*solid arrows*). The symmetry of vessel size with adjacent vasculature excludes arteriovenous fistula from the differential diagnosis (**A:** TR, 600 msec; TE, 20 msec; **B:** TR, 1400 msec; TI, 125 msec; TE, 40 msec).

tissue, possibly related to trauma. Occasionally, these lesions may erode adjacent bone (periosteal ganglia) and become totally intraosseous.[132,133] The most common site of intraosseous ganglion cysts is the medial malleolus of the tibia. Synovial ganglion cysts project into the soft tissues, are well defined, and demonstrate low signal intensity on T1 weighted images and high signal intensity on T2-weighted images (Fig. 16-96). Septations, when present, are best seen on T2-weighted images, where they are outlined by the bright signal intensity of fluid.

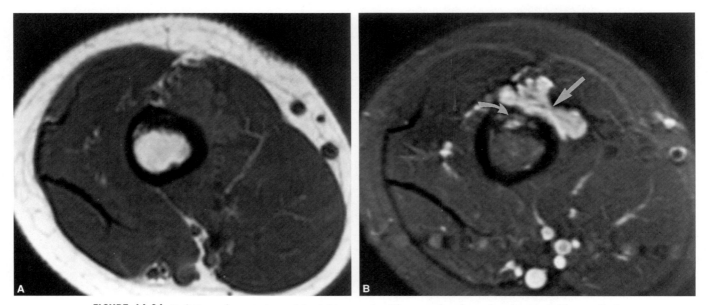

FIGURE 16-94. Soft-tissue hemangioma (*straight arrow*) with secondary bone involvement. The cortical hyperintensity (*curved arrow*) could be mistaken for an infectious tract. The hemangioma is hypointense on the T1-weighted axial image (**A**), hyperintense on the fat-suppressed T2-wieghted fast spin-echo image (**B**), and enhances with intravenous gadolinium on a fat-suppressed T1-weighted image (**C**). The site of cortical extension (*arrow*) is displayed on 3D CT images (**D**). *continued*

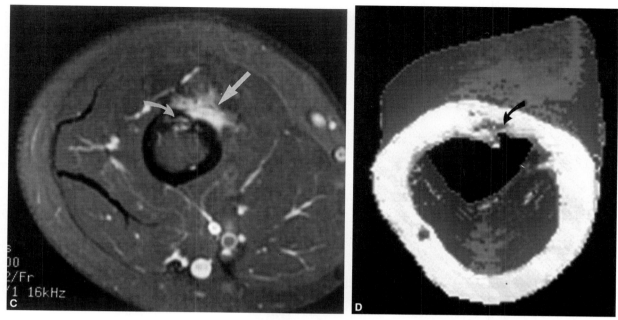

FIGURE 16-94. *Continued*

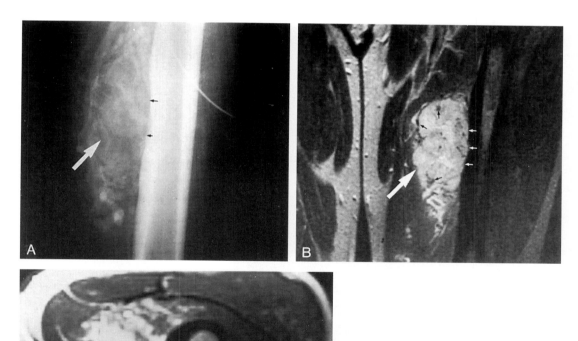

FIGURE 16-95. (**A**) Hemangiopericytoma of the vastus medialis and intermedius muscles shows hypervascularity (*large arrow*) and erosion of the adjacent cortex (*small arrows*) on a plain film radiograph. T2-weighted coronal images (**B**) and axial images (**C**) show low signal intensity hypervascularity (*small black arrows*), cortical erosion (*small white arrows*), and bright signal intensity (*large arrow*). (**D**) The corresponding axial CT scan shows a vague soft-tissue mass (**B, C:** TR, 2000 msec; TE, 60 msec). *continued*

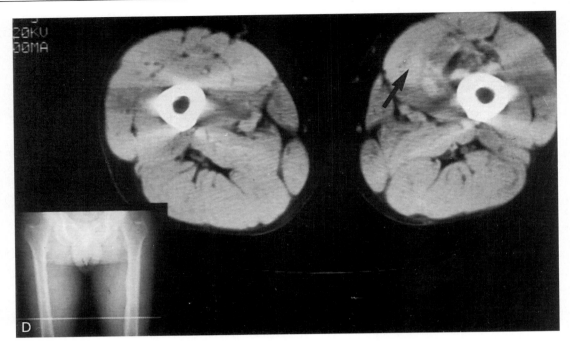

FIGURE 16-95. *Continued*

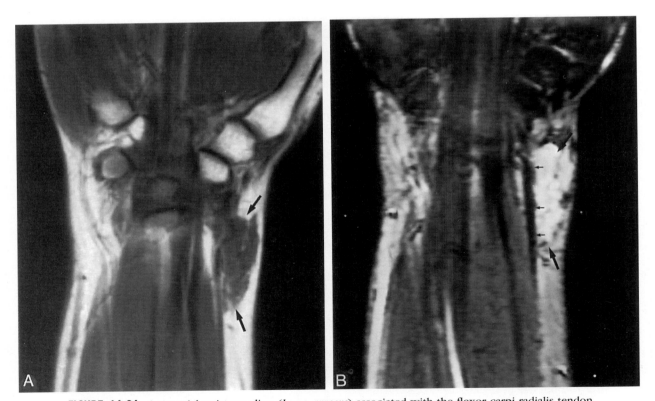

FIGURE 16-96. A synovial wrist ganglion (*large arrows*) associated with the flexor carpi radialis tendon (*small arrows*) is seen on both coronal T1-weighted (**A**) and T2*-weighted (**B**) images, and on axial T1-weighted (**C**) and T2-weighted (**D**) images. The relationship of the cyst (*curved arrow*) to the flexor tendon (*medium arrow*) is evident on the axial images. Mucinous synovial contents demonstrate low signal intensity on the T1-weighted scans and high signal intensity on the T2-weighted scans (**A, C:** TR, 600 msec; TE, 20 msec; **B:** TR, 400 msec; TE, 30 msec; flip angle, 30°; **D:** TR, 2000 msec; TE, 60 msec).

continued

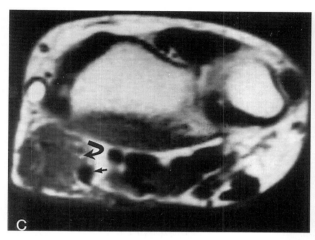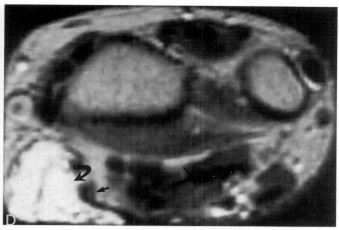

FIGURE 16-96. *Continued*

Hemorrhage

Intramuscular hemorrhage and venous or arterial thrombosis may present with pain and can simulate a soft-tissue mass (Figs. 16-97 and 16-98).

Arteriovenous Malformation

Arteriovenous malformations of the soft tissues are seen as an irregular tangle of vessels that demonstrate low signal intensity on T1- and T2-weighted images in areas of rapidly flowing blood. Arteriovenous malformations in Klippel-Weber-Trenaunay syndrome (unilateral cutaneous capillary hemangiomas, varicose veins, and local soft-tissue and osseous hypertrophy) are associated with bone lesions and are hyperintense on T2, fat-suppressed T2-weighted fast spin-echo, and STIR sequences (Fig. 16-99). The high signal intensity lesion has a serpiginous morphology or pattern of tangled vessels. Low signal intensity foci of hemosiderin or vessels can also be seen.

Desmoid Tumor

Desmoid tumors (ie, aggressive fibromatosis) exhibit biologic aggressiveness that lies somewhere between a reactive fibrous proliferation and a low-grade fibrosarcoma.[128] These lesions appear most frequently in the second to fourth decades, although they may occur at any age. They are usually large, infiltrative, poorly demarcated fibrous masses that tend to recur if incompletely surgically excised. They do not, however, exhibit the ability to metastasize. The desmoid tumor of soft tissue may present in the popliteal fossa and infiltrate surrounding musculature.[128,134]

MAGNETIC RESONANCE APPEARANCE. Desmoid tumors are characterized by low signal intensity fibrous bands traversing the tumor, which demonstrates low to intermediate signal intensity on T1-weighted images and high signal intensity on T2- and T2*-weighted images (Fig. 16-100). In contrast, juvenile fibromatosis demonstrates uniformly low signal intensity on T1-

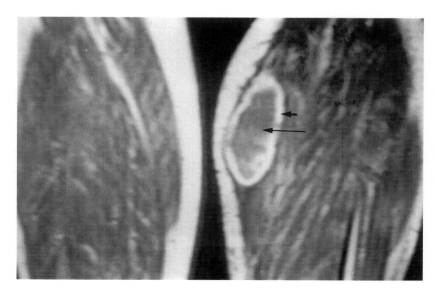

FIGURE 16-97. Subacute soleus muscle hemorrhage (*long arrow*) demonstrates a high signal intensity periphery (*short arrow*) on T1-weighted coronal image (TR, 800 msec; TE, 20 msec).

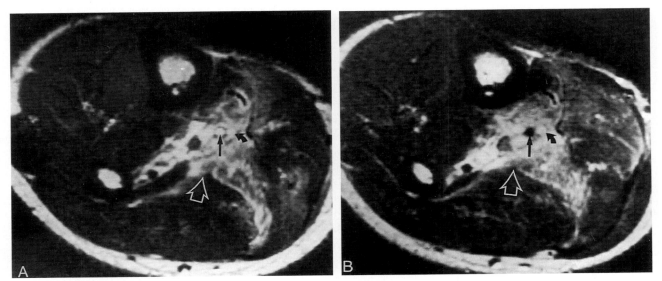

FIGURE 16-98. Arterial embolus. (**A**) Slow flow in the posterior tibial artery (*solid straight arrow*) and vein (*curved arrow*) demonstrates high signal intensity on T2-weighted axial image. Surrounding muscle edema (*open arrow*) also demonstrates high signal intensity (TR, 2000 msec; TE, 80 msec). (**B**) Lack of flow in the posterior tibial artery on an inferior axial image is seen as a signal void (*solid straight arrow*), whereas the adjacent vein maintains high signal intensity (*curved arrow*). Edema (*open arrow*) conforms to the regional arterial supply (TR, 2000 msec; TE, 80 msec).

and T2-weighted images. An association between multicentric fibromatosis and metaphyseal dysplasia (widening and flaring of the metaphysis and cortical thinning) has been reported.[135]

Juvenile Fibromatosis

Juvenile fibromatosis is a locally invasive tumor that demonstrates low signal intensity on T1- and T2-weighted images (Fig. 16-101). It resembles fibrous desmoid tumors and may recur after initial excision.

Cystic Hygroma

Cystic hygromas, usually found in the neck, exhibit the same signal intensity as fluid on T1- and T2-weighted im-

text continues on page 1327

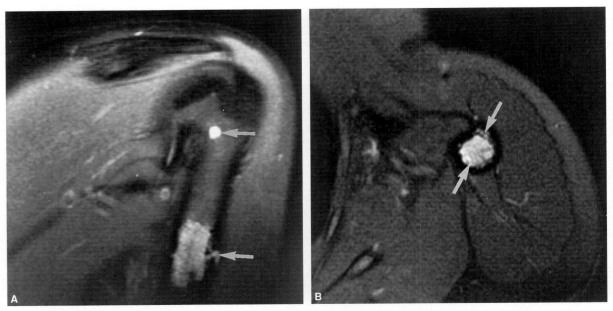

FIGURE 16-99. Osseous lesions of arteriovenous malformations (*arrows*) in Klippel-Weber-Trenaunay disease. Vascular lesions are hyperintense on coronal (**A**) and axial (**B**) fat-suppressed T2-weighted fast spin-echo images.

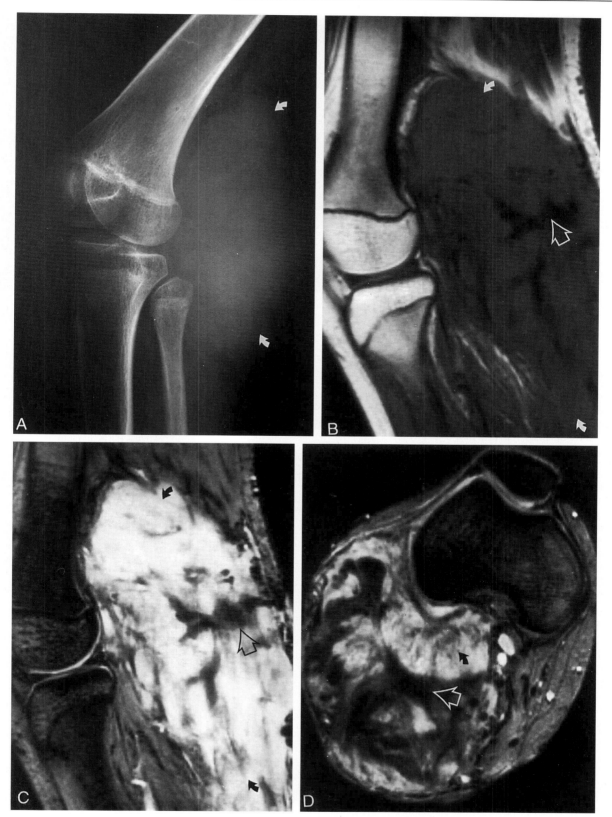

FIGURE 16-100. A–D. *See legend on following page.*

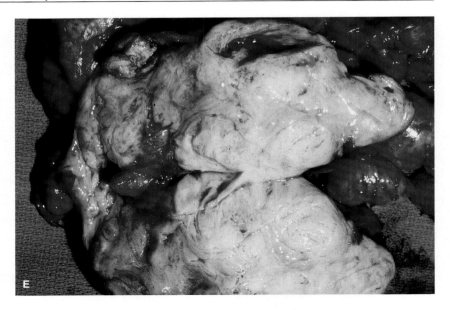

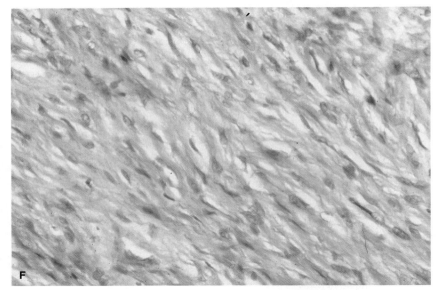

FIGURE 16-100. (**A**) A lateral radiograph shows a popliteal soft-tissue mass (*curved arrows*). (**B**) A T1-weighted sagittal image shows an intermediate signal intensity desmoid tumor (*curved arrows*) and dark signal intensity fibrous bands (*open arrow*) (TR, 600 msec; TE 20 msec). (**C**) Sagittal and (**D**) axial T2*-weighted images show a high signal intensity tumor (*curved arrows*) with low signal intensity fibrous stroma (*open arrows*) (TR, 400 msec; TE 30 msec; flip angle, 30°). (**E**) Photograph of gross specimen showing the white appearance of the heavily collagenized tissue. (**F**) High power photomicrograph of benign but aggressive collagen-producing fibroblastic tissue.

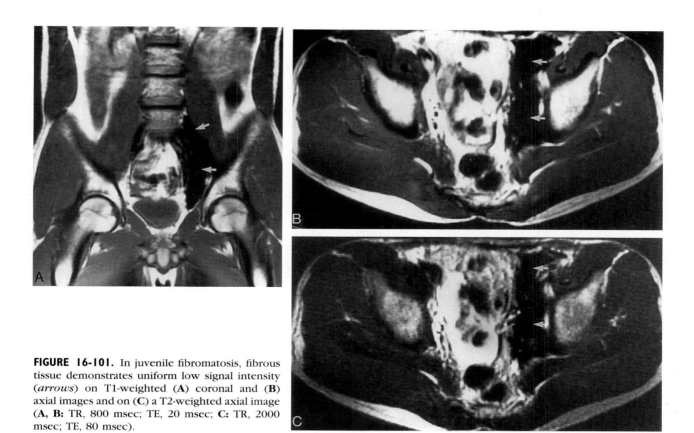

FIGURE 16-101. In juvenile fibromatosis, fibrous tissue demonstrates uniform low signal intensity (*arrows*) on T1-weighted (**A**) coronal and (**B**) axial images and on (**C**) a T2-weighted axial image (**A, B:** TR, 800 msec; TE, 20 msec; **C:** TR, 2000 msec; TE, 80 msec).

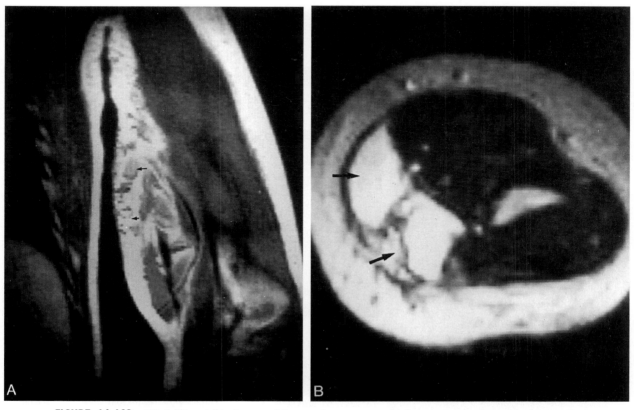

FIGURE 16-102. (**A**) A T1-weighted coronal image shows areas of inhomogeneous low signal intensity (*arrows*) in the axillary subcutaneous fat; these are indicative of cystic hygroma (TR, 500 msec; TE, 40 msec). (**B**) On a T2-weighted axial image through the upper arm, the fluid-filled cystic structures (*arrows*) demonstrate high signal intensity (TR, 2000 msec; TE, 60 msec).

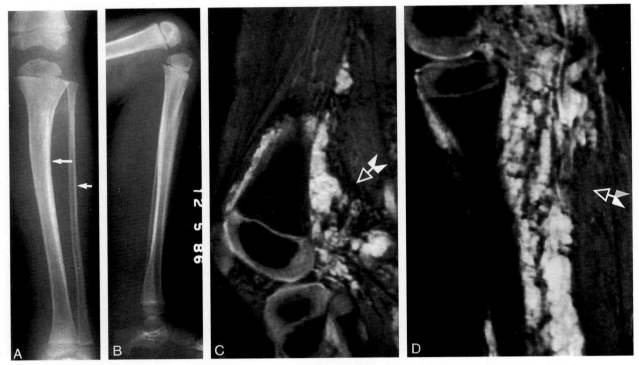

FIGURE 16-103. Neurofibromatosis in a 5-year-old child. Tibial dysplasia-bowing (*long arrow*) and a gracile fibula (*short arrow*) are seen on (**A**) anteroposterior and (**B**) lateral radiographs. On T2*-weighted images, high signal intensity plexiform neurofibromas (*flagged arrows*) can be seen from the popliteal fossa (**C**) to the soft tissue posterior to the tibia (**D**) (**C, D:** TR, 400 msec; TE, 30 msec; flip angle, 30°).

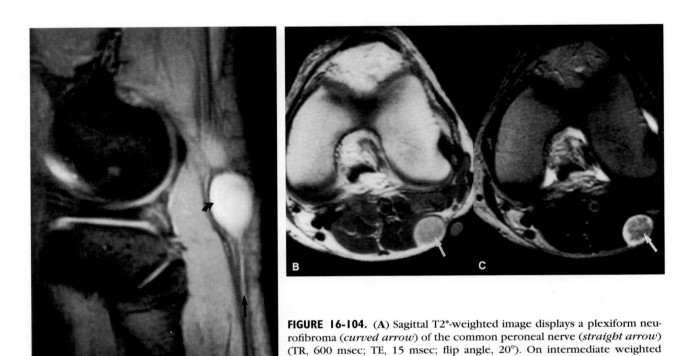

FIGURE 16-104. (**A**) Sagittal T2*-weighted image displays a plexiform neurofibroma (*curved arrow*) of the common peroneal nerve (*straight arrow*) (TR, 600 msec; TE, 15 msec; flip angle, 20°). On intermediate weighted images (**B**) and T2-weighted images (**C**), individual distended fascicles (*arrows*) can be seen (**B, C:** TR, 2000 msec; TE, 20, 80 msec).

ages[136] (Fig. 16-102). In one case involving the axilla, recurrence, after initial resection, was identified in MR examination.

Neurofibromatosis

Neurofibromatosis is a hereditary, autosomal dominant, hamartomatous disorder that involves the neuroectoderm, mesoderm, and endoderm. Neurofibromas represent an unencapsulated nerve sheath lesion, which occurs in three forms:

1. Solitary localized nodules
2. Diffuse thickening of skin and subcutaneous tissues
3. "Plexiform" tumor representing worm-like multinodular growths that expand to contiguous major or minor nerves. The plexiform pattern is characteristic of neurofibromatosis.[128]

MAGNETIC RESONANCE APPEARANCE. In neurofibromatosis, MR imaging is used not only to evaluate the soft-tissue extent of disease, but also to assess spinal canal, adjacent cortical bone, and marrow involvement.[137] Neurofibromas demonstrate low to intermediate signal intensity on T1-weighted sequences and uniform bright signal intensity on T2-weighted images. They also demonstrate increased signal intensity on T2*-weighted images (Fig. 16-103) and on gadolinium-enhanced T1-weighted images.

Plexiform neurofibromas may be distinguished from nonplexiform types by the presence of longitudinal tracking along neural fascicles in a lobulated fashion (see Figs.

16-103 and 16-104). A malignant schwannoma may originate from a peripheral nerve or a neurofibroma (Fig. 16-105). These tumors also demonstrate hyperintensity on T2*-weighted images. Heterogeneity may be appreciated on T2-weighted axial images. The nonplexiform lesions that do not involve multiple fascicles are more likely to infiltrate into adjacent tissue and are visualized with greater signal inhomogeneity (Fig. 16-106).

Malignant Soft-Tissue Neoplasms

Liposarcoma

Arising from primitive mesenchymal cells rather than adult fat cells, liposarcomas appear anywhere in the body without regard to adipose tissue. They are frequently found in the extremities, and the myxoid type commonly involves the thigh and popliteal region.[138] Peak incidence is in the fifth to seventh decades. These neoplasms arise in deep structures, and, although they appear deceptively well circumscribed, they are commonly multilobular, with projections that creep between tissue planes. Areas of hemorrhage, necrosis, and cystic softening may be present. Four histopathologic variants have been characterized: (1) well differentiated, (2) round cell, (3) myxoid, and (4) pleomorphic.

text continues on page 1331

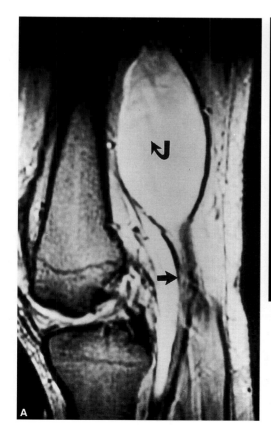

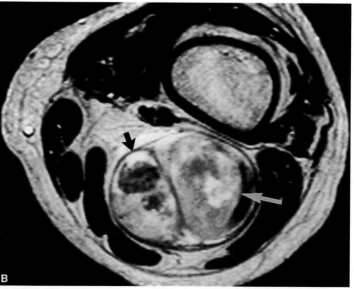

FIGURE 16-105. (A) T2*-weighted sagittal image of a malignant schwannoma with high signal mass of tumor (*curved arrow*) in sciatic nerve posterior to distal femur and posterior tibial and common peroneal branches (*black arrow*). (B) Axial T2-weighted images through the distal portion of the tumor just before the sciatic nerve divides into the posterior tibial nerve (*black arrow*) and the common peroneal nerve (*white arrow*). (C) Intraoperative photograph of the tumor before resection. The main tumor mass (*curved arrow*) and distal branches (*straight arrows*) can be seen.

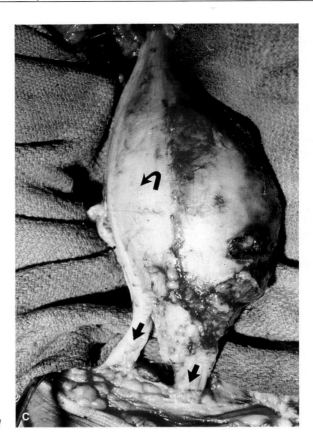

FIGURE 16-105. *Continued*

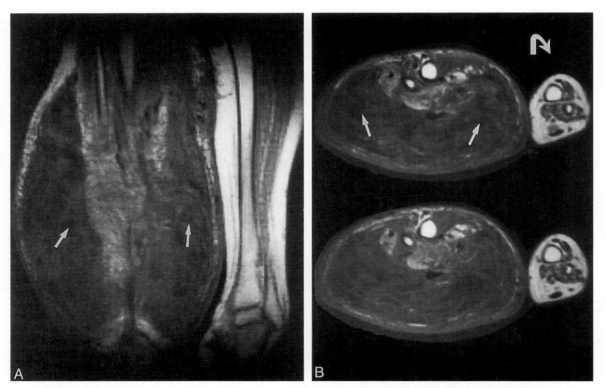

FIGURE 16-106. T1-weighted **(A)** coronal and **(B)** axial images show a large, infiltrating, neoplexiform neurofibroma invading and replacing soft-tissue elements in the leg. Lower signal intensity areas of inhomogeneity represent fibrous components (*straight arrows*). The opposite leg is shown for comparison (*curved arrow*) (TR, 500 msec; TE, 40 msec).

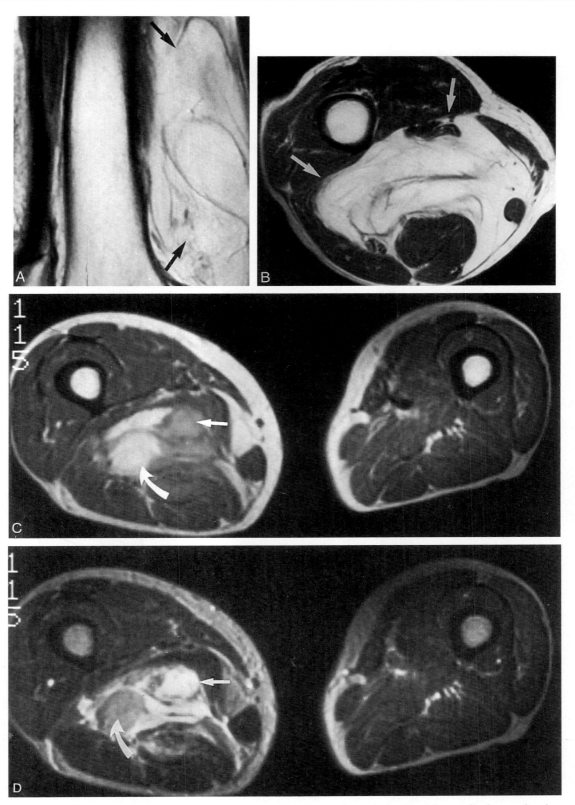

FIGURE 16-107. T1-weighted (**A**) sagittal and (**B**) axial images through the distal femur display popliteal high signal intensity lipomatous tissue (*arrows*) in the popliteal fossa (TR, 500 msec; TE, 20 msec). (**C**) An intermediate weighted axial image shows sarcomatous change at a lower signal intensity (*straight arrow*) than adjacent lipomatous tissue (*curved arrow*) (TR, 2000 msec; TE, 20 msec). (**D**) Flip-flop of signal intensity occurs on a T2-weighted axial image. On this scan, the liposarcoma demonstrates high signal intensity (*straight arrow*), whereas the adjacent lipoma is isointense with subcutaneous fat (*curved arrow*) (TR, 2000 msec; TE, 60 msec).

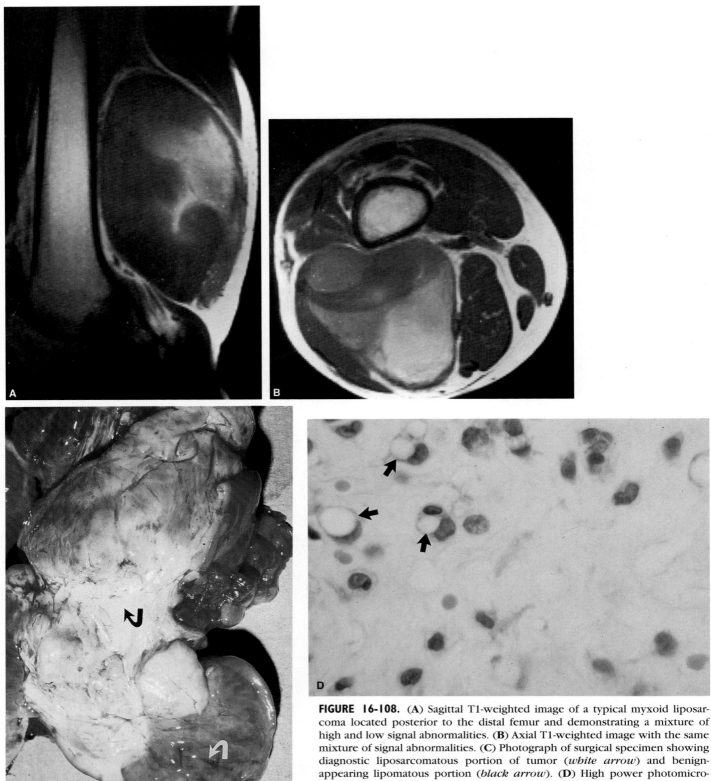

FIGURE 16-108. (**A**) Sagittal T1-weighted image of a typical myxoid liposarcoma located posterior to the distal femur and demonstrating a mixture of high and low signal abnormalities. (**B**) Axial T1-weighted image with the same mixture of signal abnormalities. (**C**) Photograph of surgical specimen showing diagnostic liposarcomatous portion of tumor (*white arrow*) and benign-appearing lipomatous portion (*black arrow*). (**D**) High power photomicrograph of liposarcoma showing signal ring lipoblasts (*arrows*) in a myxoid stroma obtained from the reddish tan portion of the gross specimen which correlates with the low signal portion of the MR image.

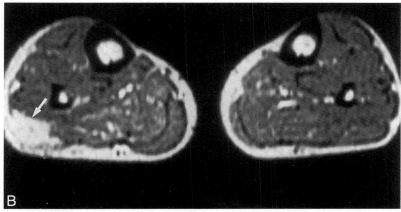

FIGURE 16-109. (A) A T1-weighted coronal image shows a posterolateral soft-tissue mass that is isointense with muscle (*arrow*) (TR, 600 msec; TE, 20 msec). (B) The leiomyosarcoma (*arrow*) shows a uniform increase in signal intensity on the T2-weighted axial image (TR, 2000 msec; TE, 60 msec).

Myxoid liposarcomas are the most commonly observed variant. Biologic aggressiveness and a tendency for distant metastases are expressed primarily in the round cell and pleomorphic variants.

MAGNETIC RESONANCE APPEARANCE. Liposarcomas are more inhomogeneous than lipomas[128,139] (Fig. 16-107). On T1-weighted images, lesions with a greater cellular component may demonstrate lower signal intensity relative to fatty elements. Focal areas of malignant change within a lipomatous matrix demonstrate low to intermediate signal intensity on T1-weighted sequences and high signal intensity on T2-weighted sequences.[140] Well-differentiated liposarcomas demonstrate fat composition with thick septa, which are hyperintense on T2-weighted images.[135] Myxoid tumors are mildly heterogeneous, and the more aggressive round-cell and pleomorphic subtypes are more heterogeneous. Heterogeneity is associated with high-grade liposarcomas. Although well-differentiated subtypes contain fat, other histopathologic types may not demonstrate fat signal intensity. Myxoid liposarcomas have a more cystic appearance on MR images (Fig. 16-108). Gadolinium enhancement may help to demonstrate central myxoid degeneration, not always seen on unenhanced T2-weighted images.

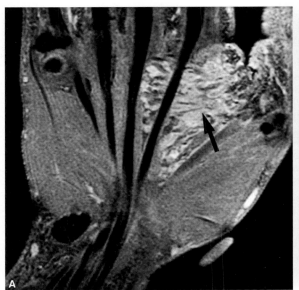

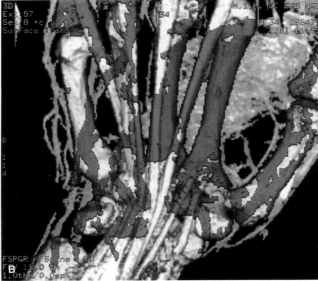

FIGURE 16-110. Neurofibrosarcoma (*arrow*) of the hand is hyperintense on spoiled grass coronal image (A) and displayed in blue on 3D MR rendering (B).

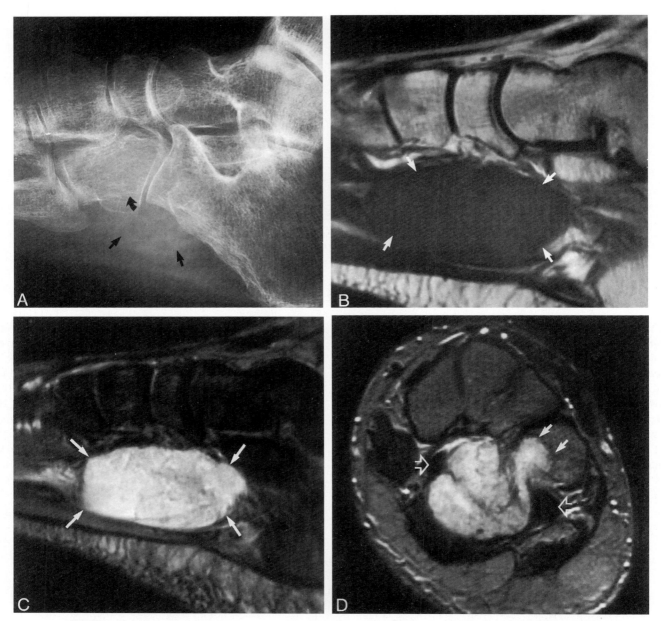

FIGURE 16-111. Synovial sarcoma. (**A**) A lateral radiograph shows a subtle plantar soft-tissue mass (*straight arrows*). Localized osteoporosis and distortion of normal trabecular lawn are seen in the adjacent cuboid (*curved arrow*). The corresponding sagittal (**B**) T1-weighted and (**C**) T2*-weighted images show a large, primary, soft-tissue synovial sarcoma (*arrows*) that demonstrates low and high signal intensity, respectively (**B:** TR, 600 msec; TE, 20 msec; **C:** TR, 400 msec; TE, 30 msec; flip angle, 30°). (**D**) An axial T2-weighted image shows cuboid bone invasion (*solid arrows*) and the proximity of the sarcoma to the flexor and peroneal tendons (*open arrows*) (TR, 2000 msec; TE, 60 msec). (**E**) Gross surgical specimen taken from the foot. (**F**) High power photomicrograph demonstrating the typical biphasic pattern of the synovial sarcoma with epithelioid cells (*black arrow*) and fibroblastic spindle cells (*white arrow*).

continued

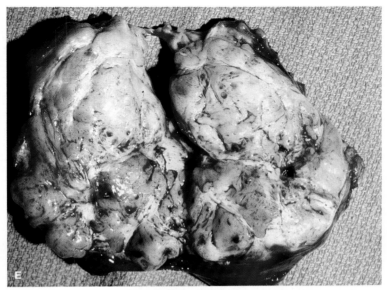

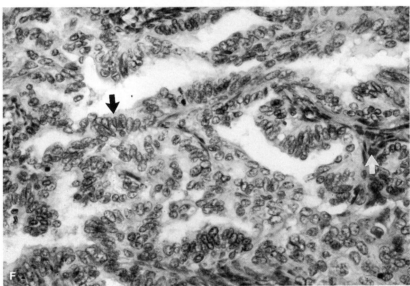

FIGURE 16-111. *Continued*

Leiomyosarcoma

Leiomyosarcoma demonstrates isointensity with muscle tissue on T1-weighted images and a uniform increase in signal intensity on T2-weighted images (Fig. 16-109).

Neurofibrosarcoma

The development of neurofibrosarcoma may be characterized by irregular areas of necrosis and heterogeneity on T1- and T2-weighted images. Areas of hyperintensity can be appreciated on gradient-echo images (Fig. 16-110).

Synovial Sarcoma

The term synovial sarcoma is considered a misnomer, because studies do not support the synovial cell as the cell of origin for these tumors. Instead, a multipotential mesen-chymal cell has been identified as the likely source.[128,141] Synovial sarcomas tend to occur in younger patients, 15 to 35 years of age, in close proximity to joints. They commonly involve the lower extremities in an extraarticular location. Less than 10% of these tumors arise within the joint cavity. In one patient with recurrent intraarticular synovial sarcoma, a nodule of malignant tissue was detected adjacent to the anterior horn of the lateral meniscus.

Spotty calcification is present in 15% of cases, and the histopathologic pattern is biphasic with epithelial and spindled areas.[128] Synovial sarcomas have a propensity to metastasize to lymph nodes.

MAGNETIC RESONANCE APPEARANCE.   MR imaging is useful for staging the intraarticular and extraarticular involve-

text continues on page 1336

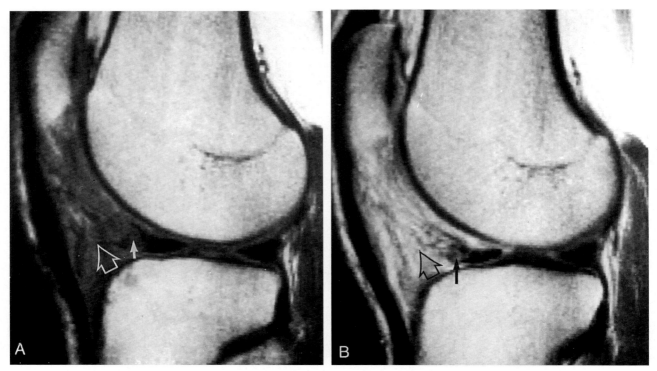

FIGURE 16-112. A recurrent intraarticular synovial sarcoma nodule is seen adjacent to the anterior horn of the lateral meniscus on sagittal (**A**) T1-weighted and (**B**) T2-weighted images. Infrapatellar fat pad edema (*open arrows*) and sarcoma (*solid arrows*) demonstrate low signal intensity on the T1-weighted image and high signal intensity on the T2-weighted image.

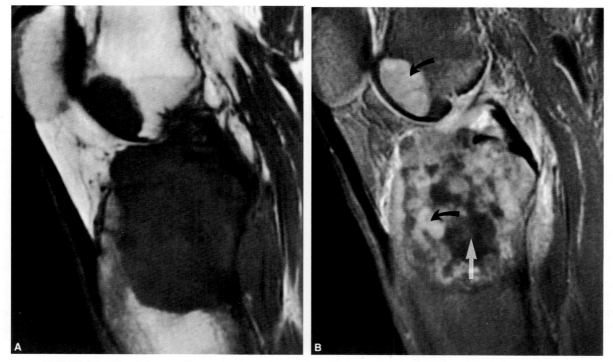

FIGURE 16-113. Malignant fibrous histiocytoma in the proximal tibia crosses the joint and presents as a second lesion in the distal femur on T1-weighted (**A**) and fat-suppressed intravenous gadolinium-enhanced T1-weighted (**B**) sagittal images. Tumor necrosis is hypointense (*straight arrow*), whereas viable tumor enhances (*curved arrows*) on fat-suppressed sequence (image **B**).

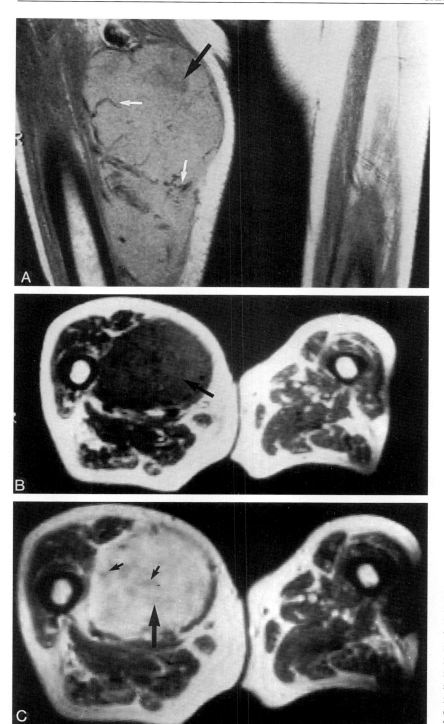

FIGURE 16-114. (A) Malignant fibrous histiocytoma is seen as a large tumor mass (*black arrow*) involving the medial thigh compartment on an intermediate weighted coronal image. Tumor hypervascularity is indicated (*white arrows*) (TR, 1800 msec; TE, 40 msec). On axial (**B**) T1-weighted and (**C**) T2-weighted images, the lesion (*large arrows*) demonstrates low and high signal intensity, respectively. Areas of tumor inhomogeneity are apparent on T2-weighted image (*small arrows*) (**B:** TR, 600 msec; TE, 20 msec; **C:** TR, 2000 msec; TE, 60 msec).

ment of synovial sarcomas (Fig. 16-111). We used it to evaluate a series involving the ankle and foot, and found that the propensity of synovial sarcoma to track along tendon sheaths and to invade adjacent bone allowed prospective MR diagnosis in five of six cases. The lesions demonstrate low to intermediate signal intensity on T1-weighted images and are homogeneously bright on T2-weighted images. It is important to note that the increased signal intensity on T2 or fat-suppressed T2-weighted fast spin-echo sequences is less than that of fluid, and should not be mistaken for a cystic fluid collection or ganglion if intermediate signal intensity areas are present. Small areas of central necrosis can be seen as regions of higher signal intensity. Focal calcifications, although detected on MR images, are better delineated on CT scans. A heterogeneous, multilocular mass with internal septation may be the characteristic feature on MR images. Extensive loculations with multiple fluid-fluid levels secondary to hemorrhage have also been observed.[142] Infrapatellar fat-pad edema, as well as recurrent tumor, display increased signal intensity on T2-weighted images (Fig. 16-112).

Malignant Fibrous Histiocytoma

Malignant fibrous histiocytoma of both bone and soft tissue has been characterized on MR images[143] (Figs. 16-113 and 16-114). MFH is a soft-tissue sarcoma that occurs most frequently in patients 50 to 70 years of age. Areas of hemorrhage and necrosis are commonly seen within this often large, multinodular, hypervascular tumor. Magnetic resonance features of MFH are nonspecific. Signal inhomogeneity with low to intermediate intensity on T1-weighted images and high intensity on T2-weighted images reflects the distribution of hemorrhage, necrosis, and calcification. Low signal intensity vessels correspond to hypervascular regions of the tumor. This lesion may be mistaken for a traumatic fluid collection (ie, hemorrhage) when the signal intensity is homogeneous and no aggressive features are seen. Intravenous gadolinium enhancement is useful in this situation, since fluid will not enhance. MFH of bone may cross the joint space (see Fig. 16-113). This is best appreciated on fat-suppressed intravenous-enhanced MR images.

Fibrosarcoma

Fibrosarcoma is a rare malignant tumor with a fibrous, proliferative matrix devoid of any cartilage, osteoid, or bone. Fibrosarcoma of bone has a poorer prognosis than primary soft-tissue fibrosarcoma.[143] Magnetic resonance characteristics of fibrosarcoma include low signal intensity on T1-weighted images, reflecting histologic differentiation; hyperintensity on T2-weighted images; and areas of enhancement with intravenous gadolinium[144] (Fig. 16-115). Soft-tissue fibrosarcoma may be identified with or without evidence of secondary cortical erosion or destruction. Fibrosarcomas that occur in children are different from those seen in adults. In

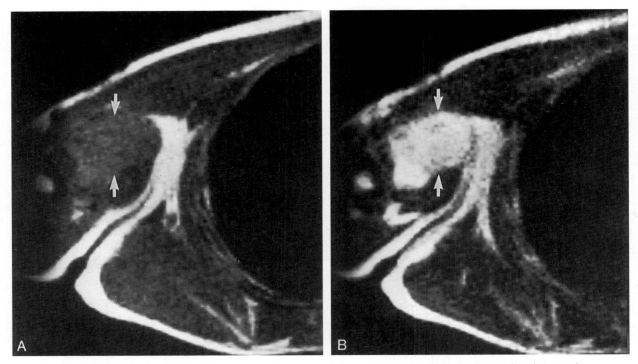

FIGURE 16-115. A soft-tissue fibrosarcoma (*arrows*) of the upper arm involves the biceps brachii muscle group medially. The tumor demonstrates (**A**) low signal intensity on a T1-weighted axial image and (**B**) high signal intensity on a T2-weighted axial image (**A:** TR, 500 msec; TE, 28 msec; **B:** TR, 1500 msec; TE, 56 msec).

children, the tumor usually occurs within the first 2 years of life, and the prognosis is more favorable than in adults.

References

1. Zimmer WD, et al. Magnetic resonance imaging of bone tumors: comparison with CT. Radiology 1985;155:709.
2. Bloem JL, et al. Magnetic resonance imaging of primary malignant bone tumors. RadioGraphics 1987;7:425.
3. Wetzel LH, et al. A comparison of MR imaging and CT in the evaluation of musculoskeletal masses. RadioGraphics 1987;7:851.
4. Petasnick JP, et al. Soft-tissue masses of the locomotor system: comparison of MR imaging with CT. Radiology 1986;160:125.
5. Totty WG, et al. Soft tissue tumors: MR imaging. Radiology 1986;160:135.
6. Tehranzadeh J, et al. Comparison of CT and MR imaging in musculoskeletal neoplasms. J Comput Assist Tomogr 1989;13:466.
7. Dalinka NK, et al. Use of magnetic resonance imaging in the evaluation of bone and soft-tissue tumors. Radiol Clin North Am 1990;28:461.
8. Lenkinski RE, et al. Combined MR imaging and spectroscopy of bone and soft tissue tumors. J Comput Assist Tomogr 1990;14:1.
9. Sundaram M, et al. MR imaging of tumor and tumorlike lesions of bone and soft tissue. AJR 1990;155:817.
10. Benedikt RA, Jelinek JS, Kransdorf MJ, et al. MR imaging of soft-tissue masses: role of gadopentetate dimeglumine. JMRI 1994;4:485-490.
11. Frassica FJ, Thompson RC. Evaluation, diagnosis, and classification of benign soft-tissue tumors. J Bone Joint Surg [Am] 1996;78A:126.
12. Moulton JS, Blebea JS, Dunco DM, et al. MR imaging of soft-tissue masses: diagnostic efficacy and value of distinguishing between benign and malignant lesions. AJR 1995;164:1191.
13. Crim JR, Seeger LL, Yao L, et al. Diagnosis of soft-tissue masses with MR imaging: can benign masses be differentiated from malignant ones? Radiology 1992;185:581.
14. Geirnaerdt MJA, Bloem JL, Eulderink F, et al. Cartilaginous tumors: correlation of gadolinium-enhanced MR imaging and histopathologic findings. Radiology 1993;186:813.
15. Gitelis S, Wilkins R, Conrad EV. Benign bone tumors. J Bone Joint Surg [Am] 1995;77A;1756.
16. Verstraete KL, DeDeene Y, Roels H, et al. Benign and malignant musculoskeletal lesions: dynamic contrast-enhanced MR imaging-parametric "first-pass" images depict tissue vascularization and perfusion. Radiology 1994;192:835.
17. Lang P, Grampp S, Vahlensieck M, et al. Primary bone tumors: value of MR angiography for preoperative planning and monitoring response to chemotherapy. AJR 1995;165:135.
18. Porter B, et al. Magnetic resonance imaging of bone marrow disorders. Radiol Clin North Am 1986;24:269.
19. Golfieri R, et al. Role of the STIR sequence in magnetic resonance imaging examination of bone tumours. Br J Radiol 1990;63:251.
20. Erlemann R. Musculoskeletal neoplasms: dynamic Gd-DTPA enhanced MR imaging: reply. Radiology 1990;177:288.
21. Erlemann R, et al. Musculoskeletal neoplasms: fast low-angle shot MR imaging with and without Gd-DTPA. Radiology 1990;176:489.
22. Erlemann R, et al. Musculoskeletal neoplasms: static and dynamic Gd-DTPA-enhanced MR imaging. Radiology 1989;171:767.
23. Lang P, Honda G, Roberts T, et al. Musculoskeletal neoplasm: perineoplastic edema versus tumor on dynamic postcontrast MR images with spatial mapping of instantaneous enhancement rates. Radiology 1995;197:831.
24. Pettersson H, et al. Musculoskeletal tumors: T1 and T2 relaxation times. Radiology 1988;167:783.
25. Tsai JC, et al. Fluid-fluid level: a nonspecific finding in tumors of bone and soft tissue. Radiology 1990;175:779.
26. Mirra JM, Picci P. Tumors of fat. In: Mirra J, ed. Bone tumors: clinical, radiologic, and pathologic correlations. Philadelphia: Lea & Febiger, 1989:1480.
27. Lichentenstein L. Osteoid osteoma. In: Lichentenstein L, ed. Bone tumors, 5th ed. St Louis: CV Mosby, 1977:89.
28. Cohen MD, Herrington TM, et al. Osteoid osteoma: 95 cases and a review of the literature. Semin Arthritis Rheum 1983;12:265
29. Resnick D, Kyriakos M, Greenway G. Tumors and tumor-like lesions of bone: imaging and pathology of specific lesions. In: Resnick D, Niwayama G, eds. Diagnosis of bone and joint disorders, 2nd ed. Philadelphia: WB Saunders, 1988:3621.
30. Harms SE, et al. MRI of the Musculoskeletal system. In: Scott WW, et al, eds. CT of the musculoskeletal system. New York: Churchill Livingstone, 1987:171.
31. Glass RBG, et al. MR imaging of osteoid osteoma. J Comput Assist Tomogr 1986;10:1065.
32. Schlesigner AK, et al. Intracapsular osteoid osteoma of the proximal femur: findings on plain films and CT. AJR 1990;154:1241.
33. Goldman AB, Schneider R, Pavlov H. Osteoid osteomas of the femoral neck: report of four cases evaluated with isotopic bone scanning, CT and MR imaging. Radiology 1993:186:227.
34. Assoun J, Richardi G, Railhac JJ, et al. Osteoid osteoma: MR imaging versus CT. Radiology 1994;191:217.
35. Towbin R, Kaye R, Meza MP, et al. Osteoid osteoma: percutaneous excision using a CT-guided coaxial technique. AJR 1994;164:945.
36. Assoun J, Railhac JJ, Bonnevialle P, et al. Osteoid osteoma: Percutaneous resection with CT guidance. Radiology 1993;188:541.
37. Rosenthal DI, Alexander A, Rosenberg AE, Springfield D. Ablation of osteoid osteomas with a percutaneously placed electrode: a new procedure. Radiology 1992;183:29.
38. Rosenthal DI, Springfield DS, Gebhardt MC, et al. Osteoid osteoma: percutaneous radio-frequency ablation. Radiology 1995;197:451.
39. Kroon HM, et al. Osteoblastoma: clinical and radiologic findings in 98 new cases. Radiology 1990;175:783.
40. Crim JR, et al. Widespread inflammatory response to osteoblastoma: the flare phenomenon. Radiology 1990;177:835.
41. Milgram JW. The origin of osteochondromas and enchondromas: a histopathologic study. Clin Orthop 1983;174:264.
42. Liu J, et al. Bone sarcomas associated with Ollier's disease. Cancer 1987;59:1376.
43. Crim JR, et al. Enchondroma protuberans: report of a case and its distinction from chondrosarcoma and osteochondroma adjacent to an enchondroma. Skeletal Radiol 1980;19:431.
44. Unger EC, et al. MR imaging of Maffucci syndrome. AJR 1988;150:351.
45. Vives M, Dormans JP, Conard K. Periosteal chondroma: orthopaedic implications. Contemp Orthop 1995;30:217.
46. Evans HL, et al. Prognostic factors in chondrosarcoma of bone: a clinicopathologic analysis with emphasis on histologic grading. Cancer 1977;40:818.
47. Cotran R, et al. The Musculoskeletal system. In: Cotran R, et al, eds. Robbins' pathologic basis of disease. Philadelphia: WB Saunders, 1989:1336.
48. Schmale GA, Conrad EV, Raskind WH. The natural history of hereditary multiple exostoses. J Bone Joint Surg 1994;986.
49. Crim JR, Seeger LL. Diagnosis of low-grade chondrosarcoma. Radiology 1993;189:503.
50. Springfield DS, et al. Chondroblastoma: a review of 70 cases. J Bone Joint Surg [Am] 1985;67:748.
51. Greenspan A. Orthopaedic radiology: a practical approach. New York: Gower Medical Publications, 1988:15.2.
52. Brower AC, et al. Frequency and diagnostic significance of periostitis in chondroblastoma. AJR 1990;154:309.
53. Weatherall PT, Maale GE, Mendelsohn DB, et al. Chondroblastoma: classic and confusing appearance at MR imaging. Radiology 1994;190:467.

54. Fletscher BD, et al. Musculoskeletal neoplasms: dynamic Gd-DTPA–enhanced MR imaging. Radiology 1990;177:287.

55. Hyman AA, Heiser WJ, Kim SIE, et al. An excavation of the distal femoral metaphysis: a magnetic resonance imaging study. J Bone Joint Surg [Am] 1995;77A:1897.

56. Ruiter DJ, von Rijssel TG, VanderVelde EA. Aneurysmal bone cysts: a clinicopathological study of 105 cases. Cancer 1977;39:2231.

57. Kaufman RA, Towbin RB. Telangiectatic osteosarcoma simulating the appearance of an aneurysmal bone cyst. Pediatr Radiol 1982;11:102.

58. Huvos AG, Rosen G, Bretsky SS, Butler A. Telangiectatic osteogenic sarcoma: a clinicopathologic study of 124 patients. Cancer 1982;49:1679

59. Kransdorf MJ, Sweet DE. Aneurysmal bone cyst: concept, controversy, clinical presentation, and imaging. AJR 1995;164:573.

60. Munk PL, et al. MR imaging of aneurysmal bone cysts. AJR 1989;153:99.

61. Beltran J, et al. Aneurysmal bone cysts: MR imaging at 1.5T. Radiology 1985;158:689.

62. Moore SG. Tumors of the musculoskeletal system. In: Cohen MD, ed. Magnetic resonance imaging of children. Philadelphia: BC Decker, 1990.

63. Mirra JM. Vascular tumors. In: Mirra J, ed. Bone tumors: clinical, radiologic, and pathologic correlations. Philadelphia: Lea & Febiger, 1989:1335.

64. Milgram JW. Intraosseous lipomas: radiologic and pathologic manifestations. Radiology 1988;167:155.

65. Munk PL, et al. Immature bone infarcts: findings on plain radiographs and MR scans. AJR 1989;152:547.

66. Haggstrom JA, et al. Eosinophilic granuloma of the spine: MR demonstration. J Comput Assist Tomogr 1988;12:344.

67. Hayes CW, Conway WF, Sundaram M. Misleading aggressive MR imaging appearance of some benign musculoskeletal lesions. Radiographics 1992;12:1119.

68. Mirra J. Giant cell tumors. In: Mirra J, ed. Bone tumors: clinical, radiologic, and pathologic correlations. Philadelphia: Lea & Febiger, 1989:941.

69. Eckardt JJ, Grogan TJ. Giant cell tumors of bone. Clin Orthop 1986;204:45.

70. Brandy TJ, et al. NMR imaging of forearms in healthy volunteers and patients with giant-cell tumors of bone. Radiology 1982;144:549.

71. Mosrer RP, et al. Giant cell tumor of the upper extremity. Radiographics 1990;10:83.

72. Aoki J, Tanikawa H, Ishii K, et al. MR findings indicative of hemosiderin in giant cell tumor of bone: frequency, cause and diagnostic significance. AJR 1996;166:145.

73. Stark DD, Bradley WG, eds. Magnetic resonance imaging. St Louis: CV Mosby, 1988:1323.

74. Herman SD, et al. The role of magnetic resonance imaging in giant cell tumor of bone. Skeletal Radiol 1987;16:635.

75. Mirra J, Gold R, Picci P. Osseous tumors of intramedullary origin. In: Mirra J, ed. Bone tumors: clinical, radiologic, and pathologic correlations. Philadelphia: Lea & Febiger, 1989:303.

76. Picci P, Bacci G, Companacci M, et al. Histologic evaluation of necrosis in osteosarcoma induced by chemotherapy: regional mapping of viable and nonviable tumor. Cancer 1985;56:1515.

77. Seeger LL, et al. Cross-sectional imaging in the evaluation of osteogenic sarcoma. Semin Roentgenol 1989;24:174.

78. Farr G, Huvos A. Juxtacortical osteogenic sarcoma: an analysis of 14 cases. J Bone Joint Surg [Am] 1972;54:1205.

79. Companacci M, Picci P, et al. Parosteal osteosarcoma. J Bone Joint Surg [Am] 1984;66:313.

80. Mirra J, ed. Bone tumors: clinical, radiologic, and pathologic correlations. Philadelphia: Lea & Febiger, 1989:1743.

81. Shirkhoda A, Armin A, Bis KG, et al. MR imaging of myositis ossificans: variable patterns at different stages. JMRI 1995;5:287.

82. Malawer MM, et al. Prosthetic survival and clinical results with use of large segment replacements in the treatment of high grade bone sarcomas. J Bone Joint Surg 1995;771:1154.

83. McDonald DJ. Limb-salvage surgery for treatment of sarcomas of the extremities. AJR 1994;163:509.

84. Rosenberg ZS, Lev S, Schmahmann S, Steiner GC. Osteosarcoma: subtle, rare and misleading plain film features. AJR 1995;165:1209.

85. Gillespy T III, et al. Staging of intraosseous extent of osteosarcoma: correlation of preoperative CT and MR imaging with pathologic macroslides. Radiology 1988;167:765.

86. Hopper KD, et al. Osteosarcomatosis. Radiology 1990;175:233.

87. Schima W, Amann G, Stiglbauer R, et al. Preoperative staging of osteosarcoma: efficacy of MR imaging in detecting joint involvement. AJR 1994;163:1171.

88. Holscher HC, et al. Value of MR imaging in monitoring the effect of chemotherapy in bone sarcomas. AJR 1990;154:763.

89. Pan G, et al. Osteosarcoma: MR imaging after preoperative chemotherapy. Radiology 1990;174:517.

90. Hanna SL, Reddick WE, Parham DM, et al. Automated pixel-by-pixel mapping of dynamic contrast-enhanced MR images for evaluation of osteosarcoma response to chemotherapy: preliminary results. JMRI 1993;3:849.

91. Holscher HC, Bloem JL, Vanel D, et al. Osteosarcoma: chemotherapy-induced changes at MR imaging. Radiology 1992;182:839.

92. Vanderwoude HJ, Bloem JL, Verstraete KL, et al. Osteosarcoma and Ewing's sarcoma after neoadjuvant chemotherapy: value of dynamic MR imaging in detecting viable tumor before surgery. AJR 1995;165:593.

93. Sanchez RB, et al. Musculoskeletal neoplasms after intraarterial chemotherapy: correlation of MR images with pathologic specimens. Radiology 1990;175:237.

94. Huvos AG. Bone tumors. Philadelphia: WB Saunders 1991:343.

95. Springfield DS, Gebhardt MC, McGuire MH. Chondrosarcoma: a review. J Bone Joint Surg [Am] 1996;78A:141.

96. Cohen EK, et al. Hyaline cartilage-origin bone and soft tissue neoplasms: MR appearance and histologic correlation. Radiology 1988;167:477.

97. Shapeero LG, Vanel D, Covanet D, et al. Extraskeletal mesenchymal chondrosarcoma. Radiology 1993;186:819.

98. Yunis EJ. Ewing's sarcoma and related small round cell neoplasms in children. Am J Surg Pathol 1986;10(Suppl):54.

99. Turc-Carel C, Phillip T, Berger MP, et al. Chromosome study of Ewing's sarcoma (ES) cell lines: consistency of a reciprocal translocation (11:22) (q24:ql2). Cancer Genet Cytogenet 1984;12:1.

100. Rosen G, et al. Ewing's sarcoma: ten-year experience with adjuvant chemotherapy. Cancer 1981;47:2204.

101. Wilkins RM, et al. Ewing's sarcoma of bone: experience with 140 patients. Cancer 1986;58:2552.

102. Boyko OB, et al. MR imaging of osteogenic and Ewing's sarcoma. AJR 1987;148:317.

103. Frouge C, et al. Role of magnetic resonance imaging in the evaluation of Ewing's sarcoma: a report of 27 cases. Skeletal Radiol 1988;17:387.

104. Mueller DL, Grant RM, Riding MD, Coppes MJ. Cortical saucerization: an unusual imaging finding of Ewing's sarcoma. AJR 1994;163:401.

105. Shapeero LG, Vanel D, Sundaram M, et al. Periosteal Ewing's sarcoma. Radiology 1994;191:825.

106. Frassica DA, et al. Solitary plasmacytoma of bone: Mayo Clinic experience. Int J Radiat Oncol Biol Phys 1989;16:43.

107. Huvos AG. Adamantinoma of long bones: a clinicopathologic study of 14 cases with vascular origin suggested. J Bone Joint Surg [Am] 1975;57:148.

108. Gold RH, et al. integrated approach to the evaluation of metastatic bone disease. Radiol Clin North Am 1990;28:471.

109. Avrahami E, et al. Early MR demonstration of spinal metastases in patients with normal radiographs and CT and radionuclide bone scans. J Comput Assist Tomogr 1989;13:598.

110. Colman LK, et al. Early diagnosis of spinal metastases by CT and MR studies. J Comput Assist Tomogr 1988;12:423.

111. Smoker WRK, et al. The role of MR imaging in evaluating metastatic spinal disease. AJR 1987;149:1241.

112. Rougraff BT, Kneisl JS, Simon MA. Skeletal metastases of unknown origin. J Bone Joint Surg [Am] 1993;75A:1276.

113. Boston H, et al. Malignant lymphoma (so-called reticulum cell sarcoma) of bone. Cancer 1974;34: 1131.

114. Ostrowski M, et al. Malignant lymphoma of bone. Cancer 1986;12:2646.

115. Demas BE, et al. Soft-tissue sarcomas of the extremities: comparison of MR and CT in determining the extent of disease. AJR 1988;150:615.

116. Mulligan ME, Kransdorf MJ. Sequestra in primary lymphoma of bone: prevalence and radiologic features. AJR 1993;160:1245.

117. Kransdorf MJ, et al. Soft-tissue masses: diagnosis using MR imaging. AJR 1989;153:541.

118. Sundaram M, et al. Magnetic resonance imaging of soft tissue masses: an evaluation of 53 histologically proven tumors. Magn Reson Imaging 1988;6:237.

119. Berquist TH, et al. Value of MR imaging in differentiating benign from malignant soft-tissue masses: study of 95 lesions. AJR 1990;155:1251.

120. Sundaram M, et al. Soft-tissue masses: histologic basis for decreased signal (short T2) on T2-weighted MR images. AJR 1987;148:1247.

121. Biondetti PR, Ehman RL. Soft tissue sarcomas: use of textural patterns in skeletal muscle as a diagnostic feature in postoperative MR imaging. Radiology 1992;183:845.

122. Herrlin K, et al. Gadolinium-DTPA enhancement of soft tissue tumors in magnetic resonance imaging. Acta Radiol 1990;31:233.

123. Fletscher BD, et al. Musculoskeletal neoplasms: dynamic Gd-DTPA−enhanced MR imaging. Radiology 1990;177:287.

124. Vanel D, Shapeero LG, DeBaere T, et al. MR imaging in the follow-up of malignant and aggressive soft-tissue tumors: results of 511 examinations. Radiology 1994;190:263.

125. Mullen LA, Berdon WE, Ruzal-Shapiro C, Levin TL. Soft tissue sarcomas: MR imaging findings after treatment in three pediatric patients. Radiology 1995;195:413.

126. Sostman HD, Prescott DM, Dewhirst MW, et al. MR imaging and spectroscopy for prognostic evaluation in soft tissue sarcomas. Radiology 1994;190:269.

127. Quinn SF, et al. MR imaging in fibromatosis: results in 26 patients with pathologic correlation. AJR 1991;156:539.

128. Braaks J. Disorders of soft tissue. In: Sternberg S, ed. Diagnostic surgical pathology, vol 1. New York: Raven Press, 1989:161.

129. Murphey MD, Johnson DL, Bhatia PS, et al. Parosteal lipoma: MR imaging characteristics. AJR 1994;162:105.

130. Buetow, PC, et al. Radiologic appearance of intramuscular hemangioma with emphasis on MR imaging. AJR 1990;154:563.

131. Hawnaur JM, et al. Musculoskeletal hemangiomas: comparison of MRI with CT. Skeletal Radiol 1990;19:251.

132. Bullough P. Joint diseases. In: Sternberg S, ed. Diagnostic surgical pathology, vol 1. New York: Raven Press, 1989:214.

133. Abdelwahab IF, Kenan S, Hermann G, et al. Periosteal ganglia: CT and MR imaging features. Radiology 1993;188:245.

134. Sundaram M, et al. Synchronous multicentric desmoid tumors (aggressive fibromatosis) of the extremities. Skeletal Radiol 1988;17:16.

135. Disler DG, Alexander AA, Mankin HJ, et al. Multicentric fibromatosis with metaphyseal dysplasia. Radiology 1993;187:489.

136. McCarthy SM, et al. Magnetic resonance imaging of fetal anomalies in utero: early experience. AJR 1985;145:677.

137. Levine E, et al. Malignant nerve-sheath neoplasms in neurofibromatosis: distinction from benign tumors by using imaging techniques. AJR 1987;149:1059.

138. Sundaram M, et al. Myxoid liposarcoma: magnetic resonance imaging appearances with clinical and histological correlation. Skeletal Radiol 1990;19:359.

139. Dooms GC, et al. Lipomatous tumors and tumors with fatty component: MR imaging potential and comparison of MR and CT results. Radiology 1985;157:479.

140. London J, et al. MR imaging of liposarcomas: correlation of MR features and histology. J Comput Assist Tomogr 1989;13:832.

141. Tsumyoshi M. Synovial sarcoma: a clinicopathologic and ultrastructural study of 42 cases. Acta Pathol 1983;33:23.

142. Morton MJ, et al. MR imaging of synovial sarcoma. AJR 1991;156:337.

143. Petasnick JP, et al. Soft-tissue masses of the locomotor system: comparison of MR imaging with CT. Radiology 1986;160:125.

144. Beltran J, et al. Gadopentetate dimeglumine-enhanced MR imaging of the musculoskeletal system. AJR 1991;156:457.

Magnetic Resonance Imaging in Orthopaedics & Sports Medicine, Second Edition,
edited by David W. Stoller. Lippincott-Raven Publishers, Philadelphia, © 1997.

Chapter 17

Magnetic Resonance Imaging of Muscle Injuries

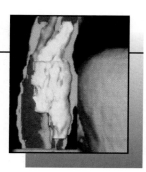

Frank G. Shellock
James L. Fleckenstein

Magnetic resonance (MR) imaging is a valuable tool in the study of skeletal muscle anatomy, exercise physiology, and traumatized tissue.[1-42] Compared with other diagnostic imaging techniques, MR imaging offers several important advantages over and above its exquisite sensitivity for the identification of compositional changes that occur in association with muscle damage. The transient, physiologic phenomenon of exercise-induced enhancement observed on MR images of active muscles can be used to evaluate recruitment patterns and to assess the effect of rehabilitation techniques.[10-12,18,26,32,34,35,37,38,41] Cross-sectional area, architecture, and three-dimensional volumetric renderings of skeletal muscle may also be accurately determined using MR imaging.[18-28] These MR imaging applications can contribute to the further assessment or treatment of muscle injuries and their sequelae.

MR imaging also circumvents traditional obstacles in the clinical evaluation of muscle injuries. The high sensitivity of MR imaging in the detection of muscle damage allows improved delineation and classification of the various types of exertional muscle injuries. This sensitivity can also be used to substantiate muscle as the source of pain in a broad range of patients with musculoskeletal complaints, and does so on the basis of a positive finding rather than by excluding

the vast variety of other lesions that may mimic muscle injuries. MR imaging complements the clinical grading of strains by spatially localizing which muscles are involved and determining whether there are associated complications, including hematoma, fascial tear, fibrosis, ossification, and muscle herniation.

Fundamental mechanisms underlying the adverse sequelae of injuries, such as myositis ossificans and fatty replacement of necrotic muscle, can be monitored noninvasively with the use of MR imaging. In addition, measurements of injured muscle mass and correlation with strength decrement may prove useful in physical rehabilitation and in athletic strength training. Finally, the fact that MR imaging appears to be a safe imaging modality and can be used to monitor the natural course of exertional muscle injury suggests that insight into the possible relationships between acute and chronic injuries will be forthcoming in the near future.

MR IMAGING TECHNIQUE

Magnetic resonance imaging is sensitive to both acute and chronic alterations in water content, including those associated with total water as well as with the extracellu-

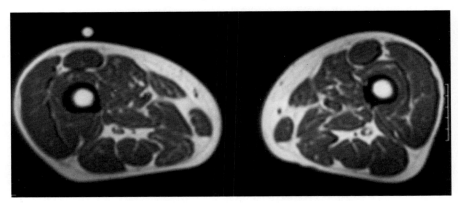

FIGURE 17-1. T1-weighted axial image of bilateral thighs obtained to evaluate muscle anatomy (TR/TE, 600/20 msec).

lar and intracellular compartments.[9–11,43] Increased water content, a hallmark sign of muscle necrosis and bleeding that occurs in conjunction with muscle injuries, correlates with increases in both T1 and T2 proton relaxation times.[9–11,43] Increased water content is also associated with acute exercise-induced changes in muscle.[18,38,39,41] It important to understand the various mechanisms responsible for the specific types of water content alterations that may be observed on MR images of muscle (as discussed later in this chapter) and to utilize the appropriate imaging parameters and techniques for a optimum evaluation of the affected area.

T1-weighted (short repetition time [TR]/short echo time [TE]) spin-echo pulse sequences are relatively insensitive to the fluid changes that occur in association with muscle injuries as well as those that occur with exercise.[1,18,38,39,41] Using this imaging technique, the signal intensity may be either slightly increased or decreased, depending on the exact T1, T2, and spin-density changes and the repetition time and echo time used for imaging.[18,38,39,41] T1-weighted spin-echo pulse sequences are helpful, however, in detecting of the presence of certain processes that have short T1 relaxation times, such as subacute hematoma and fatty infiltration of muscles. In addition, T1-weighted spin-echo pulse sequences are useful for showing normal and abnormal muscle morphology[18,38,39,41] (Fig. 17-1). Morphologic changes are commonly observed with severe muscle injuries.

Gradient-echo pulse sequences have been used to study muscle injuries, muscle anatomy, and exercise-induced enhancement of muscle, with relatively high temporal resolution.[18,38,41] This is usually accomplished using gradient-echo techniques with T2* contrast, using a flip angle selected to minimize the effects of T1 differences on the image. Gradient-echo pulse sequences with T1-weighted contrast (eg, radiofrequency spoiled gradient-echo) may be used for anatomic depiction of muscle anatomy because they produce an outlining or ''India ink'' effect at the interface between the muscle and fascia[18,38] (Fig. 17-2). This facilitates the determination of individual muscle groups and is especially useful when examining complex anatomy.

Increased relaxation times, as well as increases in spin density, are generally additive to signal intensity using a short tau (inversion time) inversion recovery (STIR) sequence.[44,45] Therefore, STIR images are preferable for identifying the water content changes seen in muscle injuries and due to exercise.[18,38,39,41,45] Suppression of signal from fat, which may be mistaken for muscle edema on spin-echo pulse sequences, is also achieved with the STIR sequence. It should be noted that the signal suppression of fat using STIR is not specific, and that the MR signal from subacute hematoma may also be suppressed when its T1 relaxation time is similar to that of fat. Despite this important caveat, STIR pulse sequences are considered to be nearly ideal for identifying and evaluating muscle injuries.[18,38,39,41]

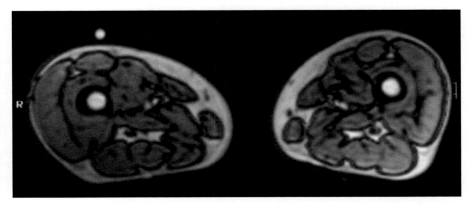

FIGURE 17-2. The same axial plane section location as seen in Figure 17-1, obtained using a spoiled gradient-echo pulse sequence with ''T1-weighted–like'' contrast. This sequence produces an outlining or ''India ink'' effect at the interface between the muscle and fascia, improving the depiction of muscle anatomy. This greatly facilitates the determination of individual muscle groups and is especially useful when examining complex anatomy (TR/TE, 51/3.6 msec, flip angle, 20°).

Conventional STIR imaging is somewhat limited by the relatively long acquisition time required. Acquisition time can be minimized by decreasing the repetition time, the number of excitations, and the number of phase encoding steps.[45] Inversion recovery fast spin-echo (IR-FSE) or "turbo" pulse sequences also permit a substantial reduction in image acquisition time, with tissue contrast characteristics that are only slightly different than those obtained using conventional STIR parameters[46] (Fig. 17-3).

T2-weighted (long TR/long TE) spin-echo pulse sequences can be used to detect water content changes that occur in muscle as a result of injury or exercise, but this technique is usually less sensitive than STIR pulse sequences.[18,38,41] Chemical shift selective suppression technique (ie, fat saturation) used in conjunction with T2-weighted spin-echo imaging improves the ability to detect alterations in the water content of tissue. T2 contrast can also be achieved with very short image acquisition times using fast spin-echo or turbo pulse sequences.

An obvious advantage to using MR imaging for the assessment of muscle is that multiple imaging planes can be used to maximize the information obtained. Typically, axial plane images allow simultaneous visualization of the muscles in a cross section of an extremity and they are usually the most informative. Comparison of muscle

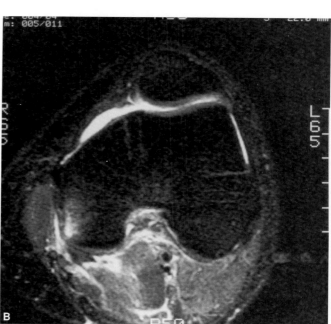

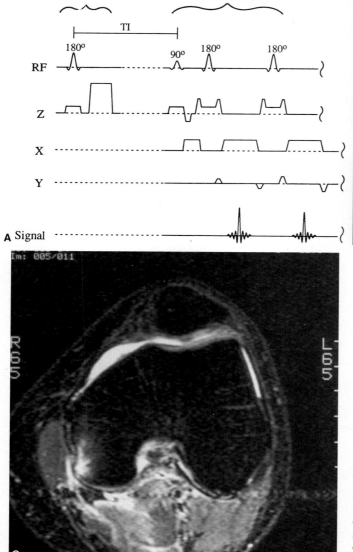

FIGURE 17-3. (A) Schematic of inversion recovery, fast spin-echo pulse sequence. *(B) Axial plane standard STIR image of the knee at the level of the femoral condyle showing bone contusion and soft tissue edema secondary to an impact injury (TR/TI/TE, 2000/130/35 msec). (C) Same section location as seen in image **B**, obtained using an IR-FSE pulse sequence (TR/TI/TE, 3600/150/35 msec). Note the similar anatomic and pathologic features shown on the STIR image compared with the image obtained with the IR-FSE pulse sequence.

signal intensity between groups is also facilitated on axial plane images. Longitudinal plane images are used to localize bony landmarks and to evaluate the extent of any signal intensity changes that may be present.

EXERCISE-INDUCED CHANGES

Transient, exercise-induced changes in MR imaging characteristics of skeletal muscle result from a complex combination of several different processes that produce increases in spin density and T1 and T2 relaxation times.[18,30,31,38,39,47–49] The increased signal intensity seen in muscle due to exercise must be differentiated from signal intensity changes related to muscle injuries. Therefore, a thorough discussion of MR imaging and exercise-induced changes is warranted.

Effects of Changes in Muscle Water Content

Low-intensity, submaximal exercise causes an increase in muscle water content that is primarily due to changes in the extracellular compartment. Maximal-intensity exercise also causes an increase in muscle water, which is relatively greater in intracellular than extracellular water content.[50] These water content changes are caused by the production of lactate and other substrates associated with a shift of water out of the vascular compartment and into the interstitial and intracellular spaces.[38,50] As a result of these alterations in muscle water content, there is a short-term (ie, 10 minutes or less, depending on pulse sequence and other factors) increase in signal intensity that is seen during or immediately after exercise[38,41,50] (Fig. 17-4).

Effects of Perfusion and Glycogenolysis

Multiple studies have demonstrated that perfusion is not required for the exercise-induced increase in MR signal intensity to occur in skeletal muscle. For example, Archer and colleagues[48] used the ischemic clamp model of exercise to determine the potential role of tissue perfusion on the signal changes seen on MR images of exercised muscle. Proton relaxation times were serially estimated in healthy volunteers before exercise, after exercise in the presence of vascular occlusion, during vascular reocclusion after 1 minute of reperfusion, and after reinstitution of continuous flow. This investigation corroborated earlier work that showed blood flow was not required for signal increases associated with exercise.[10,31,48] Furthermore, the study demonstrated that reperfusion caused an additional increase in relaxation time, whereas continuous flow after exercise was associated with a decrease in T2.[48] These different phases of the MR imaging response to exercise represent the dynamic aspects of water shifts during and after exercise.

Morvan and coworkers[36] performed MR imaging, phos-

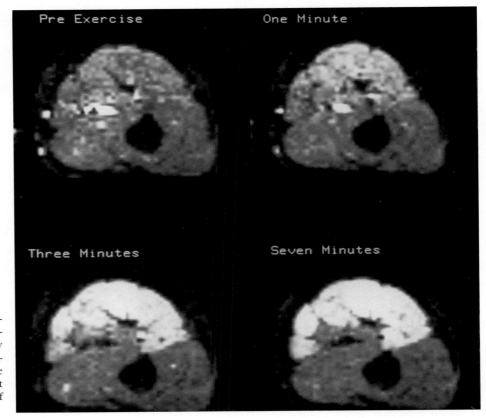

FIGURE 17-4. MR imaging of skeletal muscle during exercise. Axial echo planar images obtained during hamstring curl activity show exercise-induced enhancement of involved muscles. Images shown are before exercise, at 1 minute, at 3 minutes, and at 7 minutes. Note recruitment pattern of muscles related to duration of activity.

phorus 31 MR spectroscopy, and duplex Doppler ultrasound during exercise to examine the relationship between blood flow and MR imaging signal changes and the intracellular pH of muscle. The results support the view that, although circulatory conditions may play a role in the maximum T2 variation during exercise, they do not directly explain the T2 changes. In addition, the correlations involving intracellular pH support the concept that metabolic events in exercising muscle play a role in mediating transcapillary fluid movement.[36]

One theory is that osmotically induced water shifts, secondary to lactate production, contribute to the signal intensity changes observed in exercising skeletal muscle.[30,31,38] This hypothesis is supported by MR imaging studies performed in patients with myophosphorylase deficiency, which causes impaired glycolysis and absent lactate production after exercise. According to this theory, without lactate production the diffusion of water from blood to active muscle should be impaired. The observation that exercise-induced changes in T2 relaxation times are negligible in patients with myophosphorylase deficiency is consistent with impaired transudation of water.[30,31,38] Exertional hyperemia is normal or exaggerated in these patients, further supporting the observation that blood flow is not primarily responsible for the signal intensity changes seen on MR images.[30,31,38]

Effects of Temperature

Tissue proton relaxation characteristics are dependent on a variety of factors, including the static magnetic field strength of the MR system and the temperature of the tissue.[51] A simple linear relationship has been observed between T1 relaxation times and temperatures over the range of 20° and 50°C.[51]

Several biological factors influence tissue temperature, including metabolic state and blood flow. Increases in temperature are known to have a greater effect on T1 than on T2. However, it does not appear that the temperature change that occurs in muscles during exercise (which may on the order of 2° to 3°C) is sufficient to account for the increase in T1 values associated with muscular activity.[48,51]

Effects of Exercise "Intensity"

The exercise-induced contrast enhancement of muscles seen on T2-weighted images has been reported to be dependent on the generated force or severity of work associated with the activity.[38,52,53] In other words, the greater the effort required for the exercise regimen, the larger the increase in signal intensity and T2 values that are observed. However, the degree of the change in signal intensity may have a nonlinear dependence associated with the "intensity" of exercise.[41]

The relationship between muscle activity and signal in-

tensity changes observed on MR imaging is apparently a function of the type of exercise performed, the fiber composition of the involved muscles, the physical training level of the subject, as well as a variety of other factors.[26,35,38,49,52,53] Therefore, any direct correlation between exercise levels and T2 changes should not be assumed unless documented in multiple subjects using MR imaging criteria.

Effects of Eccentric Versus Concentric Actions

The increased signal intensity detected immediately after exercise is much greater in muscles involved in concentric (shortening) actions than in those used in eccentric (lengthening) actions[12] (Fig. 17-5). When subjected to the same relative work load, muscles performing concentric actions expend more energy than do those performing eccentric actions.[54-75] Concentric work is associated with increased oxygen consumption, more activated motor units, and more lactate production for the same power output.[54-57] Because increases in T2 values and signal intensity are related to exercise intensity, and eccentric actions require less energy expenditure than do concentric actions, it is not surprising that muscles performing concentric actions have a greater increase in signal intensity than do muscles performing eccentric actions.[12]

MR IMAGING OF MUSCLE INJURIES

Muscle injuries—including strain-related injuries, delayed onset muscle soreness (DOMS), chronic overuse syndromes, and various other forms of muscle pathology—are easily identified using MR imaging techniques.[1,18,38,39,41] In addition, certain myopathies are optimally evaluated by identifying underlying morphologic alterations, functional response to exercise, and by monitoring response to therapy.[1,18,38,39,41]

Muscle Injury and Pain

Pain occurs as part of a continuum in acute and chronic muscle injuries.[58] The inability to determine objectively the presence of a pathologic abnormality has long hampered the clinical and scientific evaluation of traumatized muscle. Thus, it is not surprising that categorization and nomenclature of exertion-related muscle injuries varies among authors.[58-62]

Clinical factors that may vary in muscle injuries include whether the related pain occurs acutely during the exercise (acute strain) or whether it only develops following a time delay (DOMS).[55] In addition, there apparently is a distinct group of patients who engage in chronic, repetitive muscular activity, including both recreational activities (eg, runners, baseball pitchers) and occupational activities (eg, typists,

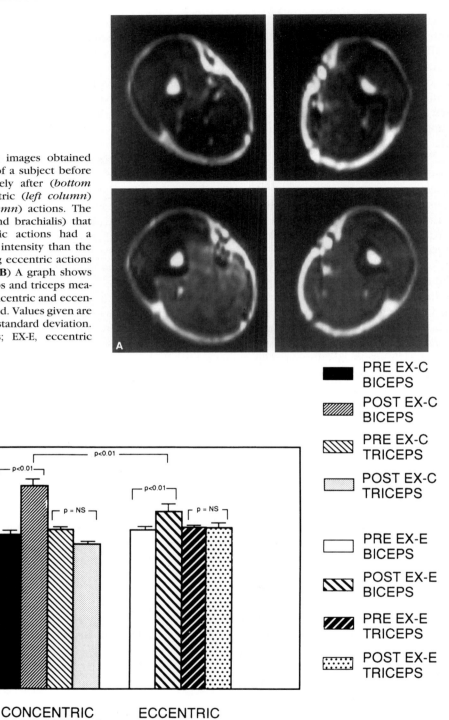

FIGURE 17-5. (**A**) Axial images obtained through the upper arms of a subject before (*top row*) and immediately after (*bottom row*) performing concentric (*left column*) and eccentric (*right column*) actions. The active muscles (biceps and brachialis) that performed the concentric actions had a greater increase in signal intensity than the active muscles performing eccentric actions (TR/TE, 2000/80 msec). (**B**) A graph shows the T2 values of the biceps and triceps measured before and after concentric and eccentric actions were performed. Values given are means plus or minus the standard deviation. EX-C, concentric actions; EX-E, eccentric actions.

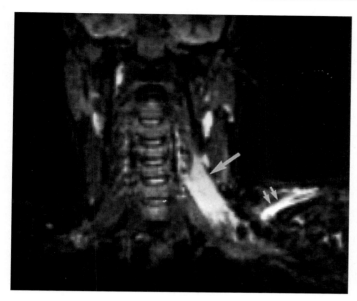

FIGURE 17-6. Cervical strain. Coronal STIR image of the neck and shoulders of a woman following a motorcycle accident. Diffusely abnormal signal intensity is obvious in the left scalenus anterior muscle (*arrow*) as well as the left supraspinatus (*double arrows*). Other areas of bright signal intensity in the neck are due to the normal STIR appearance of blood flowing slowly in veins. (Reprinted with permission from Fleckenstein JL, et al. Locomotor system assessment by muscle magnetic resonance imaging. Magn Reson Q 1991;7:79.)

musicians) who experience pain associated with specific movements. This condition has a variety of names, including chronic overuse syndrome, chronic injury,[58] chronic strain,[60] chronic myalgia,[63] repetition strain injury,[64,65] overuse injury,[66] and cumulative trauma disorder.[67] Admittedly, repetition strain injury is a controversial entity,[64] but the National Institute of Occupational Safety and Health has estimated that for certain occupations, 15% to 20% of employees are at risk for developing this condition.[67]

To appreciate the importance of accurately grading traumatized muscle, one need only consider the high frequency with which lumbar or cervical strain is diagnosed in emergency rooms without objective evidence to support the diagnosis.[67] It is not surprising that this lack of evidence contributes to the enormous expense of low back pain and "whiplash" injuries, since a battery of negative test results frequently follows these presentations. With MR imaging,

it is possible to obtain objective information about muscle pathology in paraspinal strains and other work-related muscle problems (Figs. 17-6 and 17-7), information that might not only modify medical management of such patients but also aid in appropriate legal judgments and decisions about worker's compensation.

Muscle Strain

Muscle strain has been defined as an indirect injury to muscle caused by excessive stretch.[68] Muscle strains appear to occur in areas with the highest proportion of fast-twitch, type II muscle fibers (eg, rectus femoris, biceps femoris, and medial gastrocnemius muscles).[68,69] In addition, muscles that are moved in an eccentric manner appear to be predisposed to strain.[68,69] Early reports indicated that the midsubstance loca-

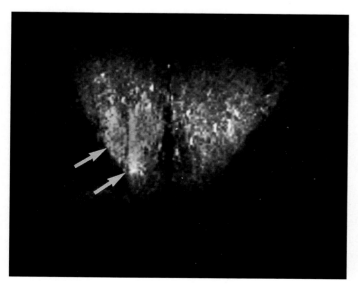

FIGURE 17-7. Lumbar strain. A construction worker had severe paraspinous muscle spasm while lifting at work. Coronal STIR image shows abnormal signal intensity in the latissimus dorsi muscles, which is worse on the right side (*arrows*). The routine lumbar spine MR examination was entirely normal. (Reprinted with permission from Fleckenstein JL, et al. Locomotor system assessment by muscle magnetic resonance imaging. Magn Reson Q 1991;7:79.)

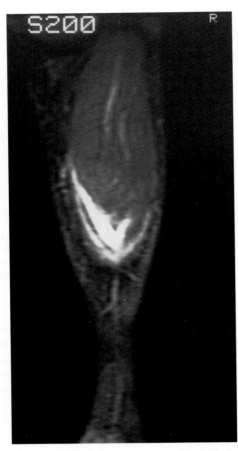

FIGURE 17-8. Coronal STIR image shows grade 1 strain of the gastrocnemius (TR/TE/TI, 2200/35/160 msec).

tion was the most common site of muscle strain,[70] and a grading system for this type of strain was developed.[59,60]

More recently, research reports based on work with animal models has verified the clinical observation that the muscle-tendon unit (MTU) is the weakest link in the locomotor system.[68,69] A simple grading system of MTU strains has been advanced in which injuries are characterized as mild, moderate, or severe.[68,69] According to this scheme, if weakness is absent, the strain is mild, or first degree, and is believed to represent injury in the absence of myofascial disruption (Fig. 17-8). In order to be categorized as a mild strain, pathologic findings must be restricted to mild inflammatory cell infiltration, edema, and swelling. In moderate, or second degree, strains, weakness is associated with a variable degree of separation of muscle from tendon or fascia (Fig. 17-9). In severe, or third degree strains, myofascial separation is complete and there is an associated lack of muscle function (Fig. 17-10).

Although initially appealing, such a grading system for characterizing muscle injuries may be deceptively simplistic. In fact, the clinical evaluation of muscle strains is admitted to be very difficult,[58,60-62] even more so than injuries of tendons or bones.[60] Only when the muscle bunches up on contraction is complete muscle rupture a straightforward clinical diagnosis. However, associated edema or hematoma may prevent palpation of the fascial defect.[68,71] In addition, the fact that synergists are recruited when a single muscle is disrupted hinders the detection of muscle strains and limits the accuracy of clinical assessment. It may also be difficult to detect a muscle strain when the affected muscle is located in a deep site relative to intact, normal muscles. Furthermore, the apparent degree of weakness is dependent upon the presence of spasm, pain, guarding, and hematoma, all of which can occur in the absence of a fascial tear. Further complicating the clinical picture is the fact that on the one hand large fascial tears may be associated with relatively little muscle abnormality, and on the other the MTU may be functionally impaired because of muscle spasm, even when it is structurally intact.[60] Fluid collections also frequently accompany strains, making the assessment of the injured muscle even more problematic.[69] Fluid collections themselves may be a cause of swelling and weakness in the absence of fascial tear.

By providing objective morphologic data, MR imaging allows accurate assessment of the integrity of strained muscles, the MTU, the tendon, and the tendo-osseous unit. Edema, within or around the muscles, depending on the stage

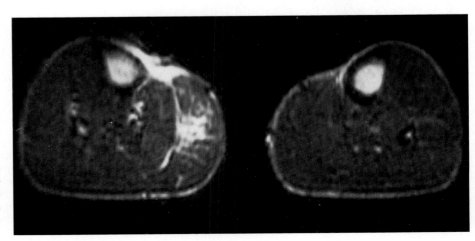

FIGURE 17-9. Axial image of grade 2 strain of the gastrocnemius. There is focal disruption of the muscle architecture as well as increased signal intensity associated with edema and interstitial hemorrhage (TR/TE, 2000/80 msec).

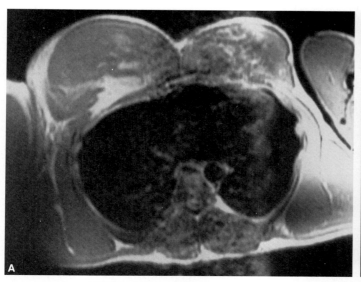
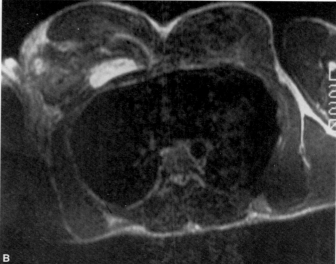

FIGURE 17-10. Grade 3 strain of the pectoralis. Rupture and retraction of the right pectoralis in a weight lifter that occurred during maximum weight bench pressing. Note the marked distortion of the anatomy as well as the localized edema. A focal hematoma shows high signal intensity on (**A**) T1-weighted and (**B**) T2-weighted images (**A**: TR/TE, 600/20 msec; **B**: TR/TE, 2000/80 msec).

of healing, is also identified on MR images.[2,3] The MTU is frequently found to be the point of rupture, the extent of associated tendinous injury can be evaluated (Fig. 17-11), and appropriate therapy needs can then be addressed.

When an associated fascial or tendinous tear is small,

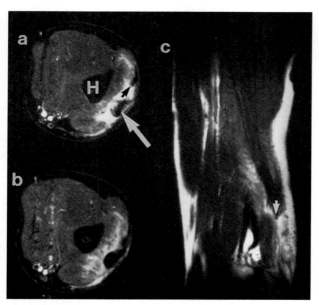

FIGURE 17-11. Triceps rupture. (**A, B**) Contiguous axial STIR and (**C**) coronal T2-weighted images obtained at the level of the distal triceps show extensive areas of high signal intensity intervening between the retracted tendon (*white arrow*) and the humerus (H). Discontinuity is evident (**C**) between the remaining intact tendon (*black arrow*) and the retracted portion (*arrow*). The longitudinal image shows retraction of the MTU portion superiorly (**A, B**: TR/TI/TE, 1500/30/100 msec; **C**: TR/TE, 2000/80 msec).

the injury can safely be managed conservatively. However, when a muscle is completely or nearly completely ruptured, early surgery is indicated. Fibrosis and retraction of the muscle may cause an inferior functional result, even after only a short delay.[60] The use of MR imaging to distinguish focal hematomas from swollen, edematous muscles may also guide clinical management (Fig. 17-12). The former may be treated by drainage, whereas the latter are often treated with wrapping procedures for compression and support of the injured area.[72]

Because weakness from muscle strains can devastate an athlete's performance or cause disability in laborers, and because these injuries may be recurrent, precise definition of the injured muscles is important for optimal management.[68] Regardless of which of the various classification schemes may be used, it is most important for the radiologist to localize the lesion, estimate the volume and severity of muscle involvement, and determine the presence or absence of clinically important associated abnormalities.

Delayed Onset Muscle Soreness

Pathophysiology

Muscle pain that occurs several hours to days after the activity is referred to as DOMS (as opposed to a muscle strain, which usually has corresponding pain that occurs during or immediately following a muscle contraction).[55–57] The painful symptoms associated with DOMS typically increase in intensity during the first 24 hours after exertion, peak from 24 to 72 hours after the activity, and then subside. The degree of soreness is related to both the intensity of the

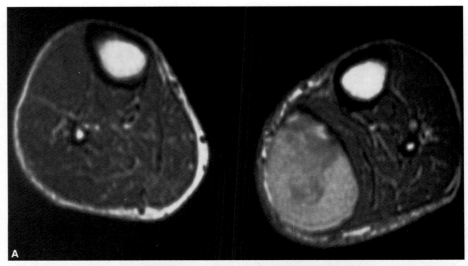

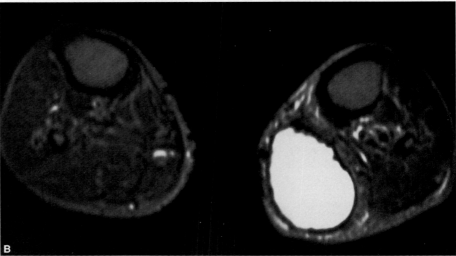

FIGURE 17-12. Hematoma complicating calf strain. (**A**) Focal hematoma can be diagnosed when T1 shortening, due to methemoglobin, causes high signal intensity on this axial T1-weighted image (TR/TE, 600/20 msec). (**B**) Hemosiderin causes T2 shortening, seen as decreased signal intensity in the rim of the hematoma on this axial T2-weighted image (TR/TE, 2000/80 msec).

muscular contraction and the duration of exercise, with intensity appearing to be the most important factor.[55–57,74–76]

A number of clinical correlates are associated with DOMS, including increases in intramuscular fluid pressure, elevations in plasma enzymes, myoglobinemia, and abnormal muscle histology and ultrastructure.[74–77] Biopsy of involved muscles may reveal free erythrocytes and mitochondria in the extracellular spaces, myofibrillar disorganization, and Z-band alterations, including misregistrations, bisections, and extensions.[74–76] Disruption of sarcomeres may be seen at 24 to 48 hours, with regeneration beginning within 3 days after exertion.[74–76] Exercise-induced muscle pain associated with DOMS may be related to disruption of the connective tissue elements in the muscles or their attachments and to the increase in intramuscular fluid pressure.[55–57,74–77] Exertional rhabdomyolysis appears to be an extreme form of DOMS.[18,41]

The pathophysiology of DOMS is incompletely understood. As with muscle strains, one of the major difficulties in the investigation of DOMS is the inability to localize precisely the involved muscle and to characterize the extent of injury. With MR imaging studies, however, it is possible to obtain information to better characterize the muscle abnormalities associated with DOMS.

All physical activity involves some combination of concentric (shortening), isometric (no change in length), and eccentric (lengthening) muscle actions.[55,57,77] Eccentric actions are most likely to produce muscle damage, and, therefore, exercise involving isolated eccentric actions is typically used to produce experimental muscle damage that takes the form of DOMS[57,59,74–77] (Fig. 17-13). In studies on MR imaging of muscle injuries related to DOMS, eccentric actions were typically used to induce the damage.

MR Appearance

In DOMS, as in muscle strains, muscle T1 and T2 proton relaxation times increase, consistent with the presence of edema.[1,18,41,42] The overall MR imaging appearance of DOMS is quite similar to that of muscle strains. In both conditions, perifascial fluid-like collections can sometimes be seen in the early phase of injury[41,42] (Fig. 17-14). These

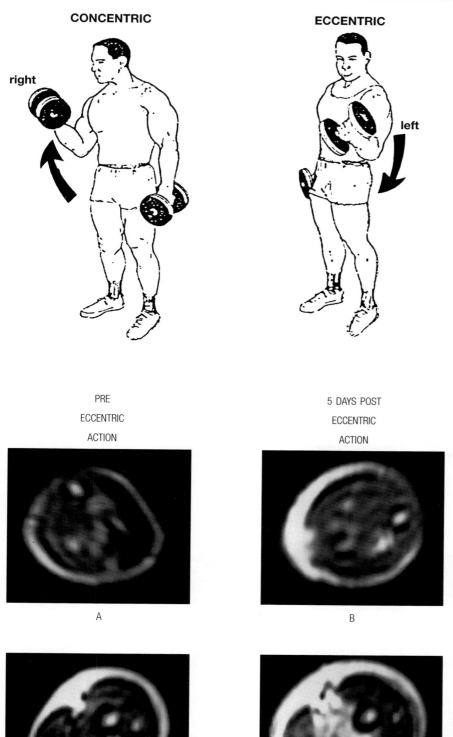

CONCENTRIC

right

ECCENTRIC

left

FIGURE 17-13. Concentric and eccentric muscle actions. This diagram shows the two types of muscle action. The right extremity is performing a concentric action (shortening), as the weight is raised during performance of a biceps curl. The left extremity is performing an eccentric action (lengthening) as the weight is lowered during the biceps curl. Eccentric actions are typically involved in the development of delayed onset muscle soreness (DOMS).

PRE
ECCENTRIC
ACTION

5 DAYS POST
ECCENTRIC
ACTION

A

B

C

D

FIGURE 17-14. T2-weighted axial images obtained from the middle upper arm and middle forearm of a subject before (**A, C**) and on day 5 after (**B, D**) exercise involving eccentric actions. There is increased signal intensity of the brachialis and deep biceps muscles (**D**) as well as increased signal intensity localized to the subcutaneous tissue of the forearm (**B**) that is distal to the site of the muscle injury (TR/TE, 2000/80 msec).

recede concurrent with resolution of symptoms and normalization of creatine kinase and other enzyme levels.[41,42] Unfortunately, the similarity in MR imaging appearances of strains and DOMS makes it difficult to distinguish between the two clinical syndromes on the basis of MR imaging changes alone.

In one study of the MR imaging appearance of calf muscles immediately following ankle plantarflexion,[2] it was found that although both gastrocnemius heads and the soleus were acutely stressed by the exercise (by MR imaging criteria), this did not accurately predict which muscles subsequently became injured. When pain and rhabdomyolysis developed 24 to 72 hours after the activity (ie, in DOMS), MR imaging showed marked alterations in the appearance of the medial head of the gastrocnemius, a finding consistent with necrosis.[2]

In a subsequent study,[4] it was found that eccentric (ie, lengthening) muscle actions produced DOMS and attendant MR imaging abnormalities, whereas concentric (ie, shortening) muscle actions produced neither.[4] This study supports the important role of eccentric actions in the development of DOMS, as well as the ability of MR imaging to confirm this impression and to study the natural history of this condition (Figs. 17-15 and 17-16). For muscles injured performing eccentric actions, there was a correlation between the peak T2 increases and the decreases in muscle function[6] (see Fig. 17-16). There was also a direct relationship between the volume of muscle damaged and the decrease in muscle strength.[6,18] MR imaging signs of muscle injury persisted for a prolonged period of time, despite a resolution of symptoms and return of muscle function to baseline values within a period of 10 to 12 days.[6] Additionally, there were alterations in a cross-sectional muscle area that corresponded with the accumulation of edema, which is known to occur as a result of performing eccentric actions.[4]

The accumulation of interstitial fluid seen with DOMS is probably a response to the myofibrillar disintegration that follows eccentric actions, which require extreme tension.[4] On T2-weighted images, signal intensity gradually increases for a few days after the initial exercise, peaks after several

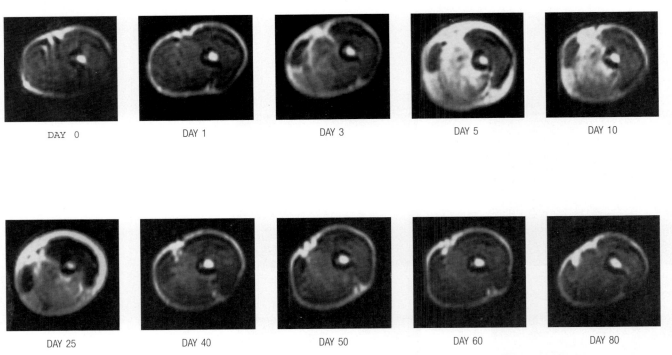

DAY 0   DAY 1   DAY 3   DAY 5   DAY 10

DAY 25   DAY 40   DAY 50   DAY 60   DAY 80

FIGURE 17-15. T2-weighted axial images obtained from the middle upper arm of the subject before (day 0) and serially after performance of eccentric muscle actions. The slight peripheral shading of the image obtained on day 0 was caused by contact of the subject's arm with the bore of the magnet during MR imaging. Anatomy is best depicted on the day 1 image, which shows a subtle increase in signal intensity in the biceps and brachialis muscles. The day 3 image shows a more diffuse pattern and a greater increase in signal intensity in the brachialis and almost the entire biceps muscle. The lateral aspect of the biceps, however, appears to have been unaffected throughout the time of the MR evaluation. The peak increased signal intensity is seen on day 5, along with the greatest distortion in the anatomy of the affected muscles. On days 10 and 25, the increased signal intensity is diminished compared with day 5, and it is further reduced on days 40, 50, and 60. Note also the marked increase in the circumference of the affected muscles, which is most apparent on images obtained on days 3, 5, 10, and 25. The image obtained on day 80 shows a return to baseline with regard to signal intensity as well as the size of the affected muscles. This subject had severe symptoms of pain, soreness, and joint stiffness associated with eccentric muscular actions (TR/TE, 2000/80 msec).

ECCENTRIC MUSCLE ACTION T2 VALUES

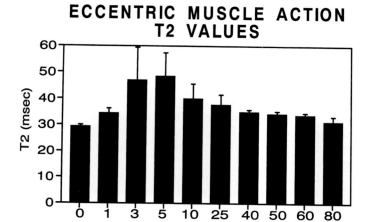

FIGURE 17-16. A graph of the T2 relaxation times of the muscles before (day 0) and after (days 1, 3, 5, 10, 25, 40, 50, 60, and 80) exercise involving eccentric actions. A statistically significant ($P < 0.05$) increase in T2 relaxation times existed for each subsequent postexercise imaging interval compared with T2 relaxation times before exercise (day 0). Values given are means plus or minus the standard deviation. The "T" lines at the top of each bar represent the plus range of the standard deviation.

days, and slowly decreases toward normal over a period as long as 80 days[4] (see Fig. 17-15).

Interestingly, studies on DOMS show that there is a delay between the onset of severe symptoms and the peak signal abnormalities seen on MR imaging, and clinical symptoms are not, therefore, a reliable means of assessing the severity or extent of muscle injury associated with DOMS.[2,42] MR imaging may be used to detect subclinical muscle injuries and to monitor the course of DOMS, as well as other mechanisms of muscle damage.[2,18,41,42]

Different patterns of affected muscles, demonstrated by increased signal intensity, have been described in DOMS[2,4] (Fig. 17-17). These different patterns may be related to the specific muscle group involved, the type of fiber composition of the muscles, the level of training of the individual, the type of activity that caused the DOMS, and various biomechanical factors. There may also be collections or "streaks"

of increased signal intensity seen in subcutaneous sites distal to the affected muscle in DOMS[2] (see Fig. 17-14). These have been ascribed to myoglobin.

Nurenberg and colleagues[42] conducted another study of DOMS to determine if there was a correlation between the degree of the delayed increase in MR signal intensity of muscle after exertional injury and the amount of ultrastructural damage present. The highest correlations are found when T1-weighted and proton density pulse sequences are used to evaluate signal intensity. These results differ those of previous studies, which indicated that more prominent delayed signal intensity increases are found on T2-weighted images. The discrepancy in these findings can be explained by differences in the level of exertion, the severity of pain, and the extent of muscle involvement. More sustained exercise causes more severe muscle damage and edema (free water), resulting in greater increased signal intensity on T2-weighted images.[42] Correlation between the graded amount of DOMS and the degree of ultrastructural injury is poor.[42] However, the good correlation observed between signal intensity changes and degree of ultrastructural injury suggests that assessment of signal intensity associated with muscle injury may be used to determine the severity of damage.[42]

Chronic Overuse Syndrome

As mentioned earlier, chronic overuse syndrome refers to a broad group of disorders characterized by pain or stiffness that develops as a result of repetitive movements used in certain occupations or recreational activities (Figs. 17-18 through 17-20). The pathophysiology of overuse syndromes is largely unknown, despite the considerable attention paid to it in the literature and in the work place. Tenosynovitis, tendinitis, and muscle pathophysiology have each been implicated. In sum, it seems fair to identify the musculotendinous unit as the primary site of involvement, as it is in other muscle injuries. In this context, MR imaging allows not only objective substantiation of a patient's complaint, but the relative degree of tendinous and muscular involvement at the MTU can also be specified. It is hoped that such

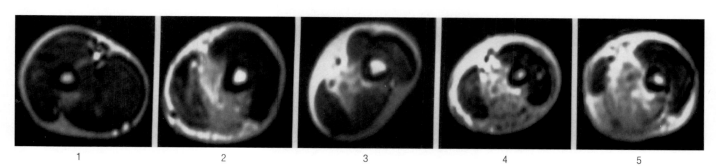

FIGURE 17-17. Delayed onset muscle soreness (DOMS). T2-weighted axial images obtained from the middle upper arms of five different subjects on day 5 after performing biceps curl exercise involving eccentric actions. Note the variability in the pattern of increased signal intensity affecting the biceps and brachialis muscles (TR/TE, 2000/80 msec).

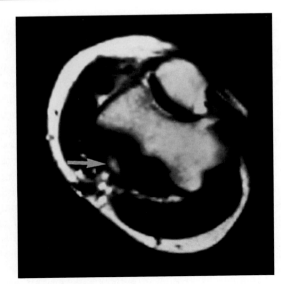

FIGURE 17-18. Occupational overuse syndrome, "waitress elbow." MR imaging in a waitress who complained of several days of progressive pain near her elbow. Pain was exacerbated by holding her cocktail tray, ultimately forcing her to stop work. Axial plane images obtained with a TR/TE of 1000/80 msec demonstrate a focus of high signal intensity (*arrow*) at the site of pain. Both the MRI abnormality and symptoms resolved during 1 week off work, and symptoms did not recur.

identification will aid in directing other studies of chronic overuse syndromes. Perhaps then, appropriate preventative measures and rehabilitation programs will be optimally directed at the specific pathology responsible.

Chronic overuse syndrome has various presentations. For example, there may be irritation at the muscle-tendon junction or tenosynovitis may occur along with an inflammatory reaction caused by adhesions between the tendon and surrounding synovium. If the strain at this site is not eliminated, chronic inflammatory reaction results in further pain, swelling, and edema.

Like other categories of exertional injury, chronic overuse syndrome is in part poorly understood because of the traditional lack of objective tests to confirm the presence of tissue abnormality.[2,18] For example, it has been stated that traditional diagnostic radiological tests tend to be normal in such cases. MR imaging appears to fill this void in the diagnostic approach to chronic overuse syndrome, as seen in cases of recurrent "waitress elbow," "tennis elbow," and "Achilles tendinitis" (see Figs. 17-18 through 17-20). These cases demonstrate that MR images display objective confirmation of the presence of tissue abnormality and suggest that the degree of muscle abnormality may often be underestimated in these conditions. The occurrence of abnormalities similar to those seen in chronic overuse syndrome in top marathon runners raises the question of whether this injury is best categorized as DOMS, acute strain, or chronic overuse.

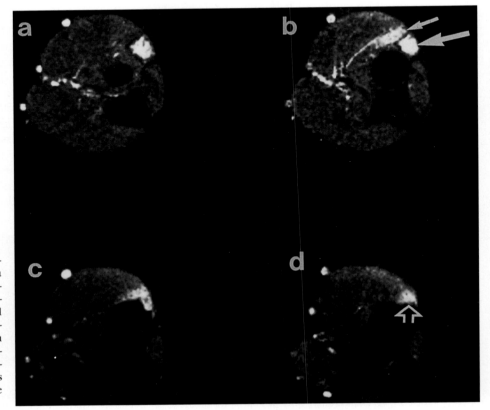

FIGURE 17-19. Recreational overuse syndrome, "tennis elbow." MR imaging in a patient who curtailed his frequency of playing tennis because of progressively increasing exertional pain over the lateral humeral epicondyle. Contiguous 1 cm axial STIR images, proceeding from (**A**) distal through (**D**) proximal show focal signal intensity increases in the extensor digitorum communis (*long arrow*) and extensor carpi radialis brevis (*short arrow*), where they originate from the lateral epicondyle (*arrowhead*).

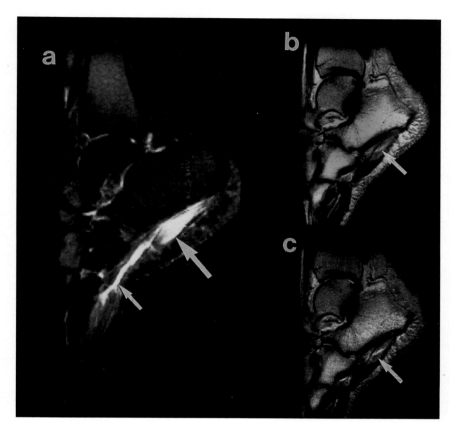

FIGURE 17-20. Recreational overuse syndrome, "plantar fasciitis." MR imaging in a patient who stopped aerobic workouts because of progressive heel pain during exercise. **(A)** Sagittal STIR image shows extensive edema in the flexor digitorum brevis (*large arrow*). A prominent vein is also evident (*small arrow*). On comparable images obtained with a TR/TE of 2000/40 msec **(B)** and a TR/TE of 2000/80 msec **(C)**, the high signal intensity associated with muscle edema is less conspicuous (*arrows*).

The appropriate role of MR imaging in the evaluation of chronic overuse syndrome has yet to be defined. However, MR imaging of the apparent injury may be used to determine the muscle or muscles involved, to localize and grade the edema-like process within affected muscle, and to assess associated soft tissue abnormalities.[2,18] This information may contribute to understanding the pathogenesis of chronic overuse syndrome.

Interstitial Hemorrhage and Hematoma

Both interstitial hemorrhage and hematoma are commonly found in association with muscle injuries.[1,2,18,39] Interstitial hemorrhage is bleeding that occurs between the damaged connective tissues, whereas a hematoma is a discrete collection of blood confined to a restricted location.[1,18,39] An increase in the size of the affected muscle may be seen in both of these entities.[1,39]

The MR appearance varies, depending on the static magnetic field strength of the MR system, the "timing" of the evaluation of the blood-containing tissue, and the relative degree of edema at the injury site.[17,39] If MR imaging is conducted within 48 hours of injury, interstitial hemorrhage and hematoma have a signal intensity similar to muscle on T1-weighted pulse sequences and hyperintense on STIR pulse sequences.[17,39] During the subacute or chronic stage

(ie, seven to 300 days after injury), the water content decreases and the protein content increases, and the hematoma has moderately decreased T1 and T2 relaxation times (see Fig. 17-12). This produces a signal intensity similar to that of fat on a T1-weighted pulse sequence. In addition, the tissues are affected by the presence of oxyhemoglobin, deoxyhemoglobin, and red blood cells.[17,39,78] This results in T1 shortening due to oxidative denaturation of hemoglobin and the production of methemoglobin. The concentration of methemoglobin increases over an 80 to 90 hour period following the injury, and the shortening of the T1 relaxation time of the blood-containing tissue follows the time course of methemoglobin production.[17,39,78]

In hematoma, the overall effect on T1-weighted images is a pattern of heterogeneous signal intensity during the subacute stages. With T2-weighted pulse sequences acquired on an MR system with a high static magnetic field strength, there is a focal area of low signal intensity, corresponding to the preferential T2 shortening secondary to deoxyhemoglobin within intact red cells.[17,39,78] In long-standing hematoma, T1-weighted images demonstrate low signal intensity.

In comparison, the signal characteristics of interstitial hemorrhage (ie, low signal intensity on T1-weighted images and high signal intensity on T2-weighted images during the acute stage,[17,39,78]) may be due primarily to the concomitant presence of edema, but this is poorly documented. The high signal intensity associated with interstitial hemorrhage does not appear to change considerably over time, probably because of the high free water content relative to soft tissue due to the presence of inflammation in the later stages following muscle injury[17,39,78] (see Fig. 17-9). Additional investigations are needed to clarify the MR appearance of interstitial hemorrhage.

MUSCLE CONTUSION

A muscle contusion is differentiated from strain-related damage by the mechanism of injury.[18,39,79] A contusion of muscle is any compressive or concussive form of direct trauma to the tissue and is typically caused by a blunt object.[39] Muscle contusions are often experienced by athletes who engage in contact sports in which a body part or object strikes the muscle, causing the injury.[39] Clinically, bruising of the superficial tissue is present.

Jackson and Feagin[79] suggested the following grading system for the severity of contusions based on the relative restriction of the range of motion of the adjacent joint. In addition, they correlated prognosis with the grade of injury.

- *Mild contusion*: Active or passive range of motion is limited by less than one third of normal. Patients have an average of 6 days of disability.
- *Moderate contusion*: Active motion is limited to one third to two thirds of the normal range of motion, usually due to the presence of muscle spasms. Patients have an average of 56 days of disability.
- *Severe contusion*: Active motion is limited by greater than two thirds of the normal range of motion. Patients have longer than 60 days of disability.

The proposed criteria for muscle contusion include superficial capillary rupture, interstitial hemorrhage, edema, and an inflammatory reaction.[18,39] Although the MR imaging appearance of muscle contusion is a direct reflection of the combination of the factors just mentioned,[18,39] it is highly variable and oftentimes cannot be distinguished from a grade 1 or grade 2 muscle strain (Fig. 17-21). Therefore, close clinical correlation is extremely helpful, especially since there has been no peer-reviewed investigation published that describes the expected appearance of contusion on MR imaging. A known complication of muscle contusion is the development of myositis ossificans,[18,39] which is the localized formation of nonneoplastic heterotopic bone and cartilage in soft tissues.[39,80]

MUSCLE CONTRACTURE AND RHABDOMYOLYSIS

Muscle contracture refers to muscle shortening occurring without repetitive action potentials. Indeed, this electrical difference between cramp, with its high-frequency action potentials, and contracture is basic[18,41] (Figs. 17-22 and 17-23). Muscle contracture occurs most often in metabolic

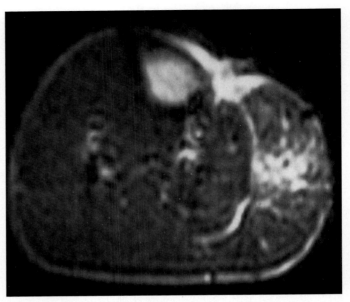

FIGURE 17-21. Contusion. MR images of the gastrocnemius in a soccer player who sustained a contusion injury. The MR appearance on this axial image in contusion is similar to that seen in grade 1 or grade 2 muscle strains (TR/TE, 2000/80 msec).

disorders, such as in patients with inherited defects of glycolytic enzymes (eg, myophosphorylase deficiency or McArdle's disease).[5,18,41]

After the contracture, patients typically develop elevated serum creatine kinase levels and, when severe, pigmenturia and acute renal failure. During the contracture, there typically is intense pain. In some diseases, such as phosphofructokinase deficiency, patients may have few or no symptoms and yet have marked rhabdomyolysis. In these patients, MR imaging may show extensive zones of myonecrosis and fatty infiltration.[5,18,41] Although not specific, the coexistence of muscle edema, atrophy, and fatty infiltration is a very significant finding and should suggest a myopathic or neurogenic disorder.[18,41]

Rhabdomyolysis may occur in patients who do not have any metabolic disorder. Indeed, there are myriad predisposing causes for the development of rhabdomyolysis.[7,18] However, the MR imaging appearance is typical and not different from the pattern of muscle edema seen in most other muscle injuries, including metabolic myopathies.[7,18,41]

SEQUELAE OF MUSCLE INJURIES

One of the sequelae of muscle injury is further injury. For example, an incomplete muscle rupture may predispose to a complete rupture.[13] In this context, it is interesting to note that MR alterations seen in both strains and DOMS persist for much longer than any other clinical evidence of injury.[2,4] Clinical and scientific implications of this fact are currently being investigated. Obviously, it would be of great importance to known whether or not

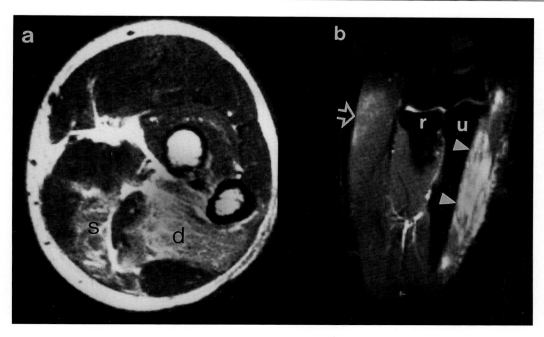

FIGURE 17-22. Muscle contracture in lactate dehydrogenase deficiency. (**A**) T2-weighted axial image of the proximal forearm obtained 24 hours after handgrip-induced contracture. Note that edema is present in the deep (d) and superficial (s) finger flexors (TR/TE, 2000/80 msec). (**B**) A coronal STIR image shows the relationship between the injured flexor digitorum profundus (*arrowheads*) to the ulna (u). Lateral to the radial head (r), a smaller region of necrosis is evident in the extensor carpi radialis (*open arrowhead*).

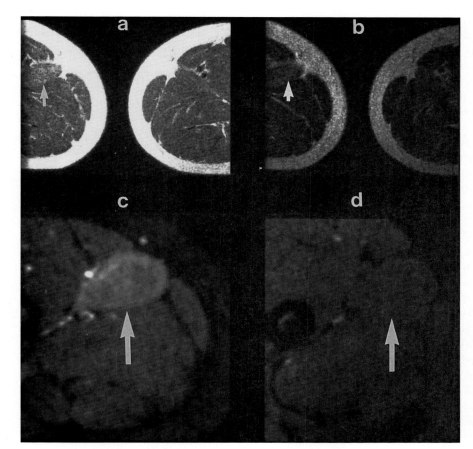

FIGURE 17-23. Thigh muscle contracture in McArdle's disease. (**A, B**) Spin-echo images of the thighs show questionably increased signal intensity in the right adductor longus (*arrows*) (**A**: TR/TE, 1500/30 msec; **B**: TR/TE, 1500/60 msec). (**C**) The abnormality was unequivocal using the STIR sequence (*arrow*). (**D**) STIR image 3 months later documents complete healing, without sequelae.

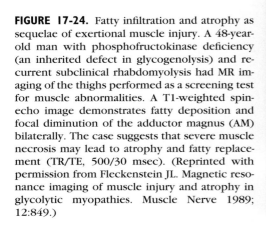

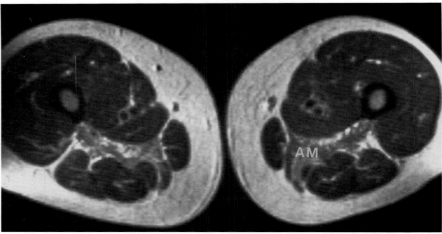

FIGURE 17-24. Fatty infiltration and atrophy as sequelae of exertional muscle injury. A 48-year-old man with phosphofructokinase deficiency (an inherited defect in glycogenolysis) and recurrent subclinical rhabdomyolysis had MR imaging of the thighs performed as a screening test for muscle abnormalities. A T1-weighted spin-echo image demonstrates fatty deposition and focal diminution of the adductor magnus (AM) bilaterally. The case suggests that severe muscle necrosis may lead to atrophy and fatty replacement (TR/TE, 500/30 msec). (Reprinted with permission from Fleckenstein JL. Magnetic resonance imaging of muscle injury and atrophy in glycolytic myopathies. Muscle Nerve 1989; 12:849.)

a persisting abnormality within the previously strained muscle of an athlete predicts that the strain will recur with resumption of intense exercise. Although the significance of the marked prolongation of MR abnormalities in muscle injuries is unclear, it remains a new opportunity for the noninvasive study of muscle healing.

One practical implication of the delayed disappearance of edema from muscle after excessive exercise is the MR detection of evidence of previous muscle injury beyond the patient's memory of such an event. This implies a potential source of serendipitously observed MR abnormalities. On the other hand, this radiographic finding may be the only clue to the true origin of the patient's musculoskeletal complaints.

Other sequelae of muscle injuries (including fibrosis, fatty replacement, and muscle ossification), although infrequent, are also detectable and differentiable using MR imaging. Fibrosis contributes to difficulties during surgery when treatment is delayed.[60] As discussed earlier, fatty replacement of traumatized muscle is rare, but occurs with regularity in patients with specific myopathies[5] (Fig. 17-24). Ossification of muscle is not uncommon in muscle contusion, and can be detected by MR imaging (Fig. 17-25). This presents an exciting prospect for future investigations, because MR imaging also detects adjacent muscle edema that is undetectable by other means. Thus, the potential exists for detecting myositis before the occurrence of ossification. In this way, it is hoped, an intervention might be optimally applied to the precise muscle at risk, so that ossification can be prevented.

Another complication of muscle injuries detectable by MR imaging is compartment syndrome.[13] In this condition, edema or hemorrhage occur within intact fascial boundaries, creating a closed compartment in which increases in muscle pressure impair blood and oxygen delivery. This may be an indication for immediate surgical decompression. Because lower extremity deep venous thrombosis and compartment syndrome may both present with painful swollen legs, the correct diagnosis is occa-

sionally unclear. Used for this purpose, MR imaging simultaneously evaluates the status of vessels, subcutaneous tissues, and bone marrow in addition to the muscles. MR monitoring of exertion-induced changes in muscle relaxation times has been used to improve assessment of chronic compartment syndrome, the diagnostic criterion for which is said to be abnormal, progressive elevation of the muscle proton T1 relaxation time during recovery after exercise.[13]

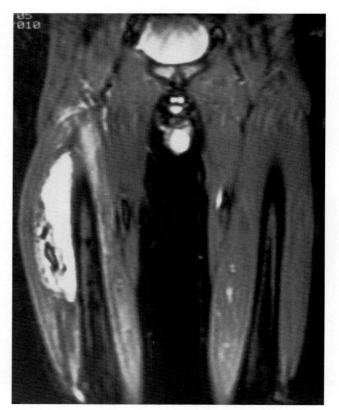

FIGURE 17-25. Sequelae of exertional muscle injury, myositis ossificans. This coronal STIR image shows extensive increased signal intensity in the right quadriceps. A focal area of bone is evident in the soft tissue of the vastus lateralis.

ASSESSMENT OF MUSCLE INJURIES AND REHABILITATION TECHNIQUES

Muscle recruitment patterns can be determined for specific movements by comparing MR images obtained before exercise with those obtained either during or immediately after the activity is performed[2,18,38,41] (Fig. 17-26). In this way, MR imaging may be used to identify and characterize the muscles involved in specific movements in order to determine the affected area secondary to a muscle injury and to evaluate the effectiveness of a physical rehabilitation technique. For example, MR imaging has been used to examine recruitment patterns of the lumber muscles in normal subjects, in patients with chronic low back pain without surgery, and in patients with chronic low back pain with surgery, as they performed the Roman chair extension exercise,[26] a commonly performed rehabilitation activity. In this study, the Roman chair extension exercise produced increased signal intensity on MR images of the lumbar paraspinal extensor muscles within a few repetitions. At peak exercise levels, the signal intensity of the multifidus and the longissimus/iliocostalis were different for the different subject groups, suggesting a preferential utilization of the multifidus.[26]

Furthermore, MR imaging demonstrated static and dynamic differences in lumbar paraspinal musculature. Compared with normal subjects, patients with chronic low back pain who had had prior surgery demonstrated increased MR signal intensity of the multifidus and longissimus/iliocostalis at rest, and an attenuated signal intensity response after exercise.[26] The increased signal intensity of the paraspinal mus-

cles in the patients with chronic back pain has been attributed to either residual injury or denervation, and the attenuated exercise enhancement may be related to changes in muscle composition following surgery and/or related deconditioning of the muscles.[26]

DETERMINATION OF MUSCLE MASS

Assessment of muscle mass using MR imaging is useful for a precise determination of the extent and distribution of muscle injuries, evaluating responses to physical rehabilitation programs, and for monitoring the progression of muscle degeneration associated with certain locomotor disorders.[18,41] Because of its superior soft tissue contrast and the lack of ionizing radiation, MR imaging is considered to be a suitable method for quantifying muscle cross-sectional area for intraindividual and interindividual analysis of muscle size.[19,22-25,27] In addition, MR imaging has been shown to provide accurate information regarding in vivo muscle architecture, as described by Fukunaga and colleagues[19] and Narici and colleagues[22-24] This information is critical for a complete evaluation of muscle function, because the maximum force exerted by a muscle is related to the total cross-sectional area of all of the fibers in a group, and the maximum rate of shortening is related to the length of the longest fibers within the muscle.

The assessment of muscle function secondary to injury is often of added value when characterizing the extent and ultimate effect of the damaged tissue.[6] For example, MR

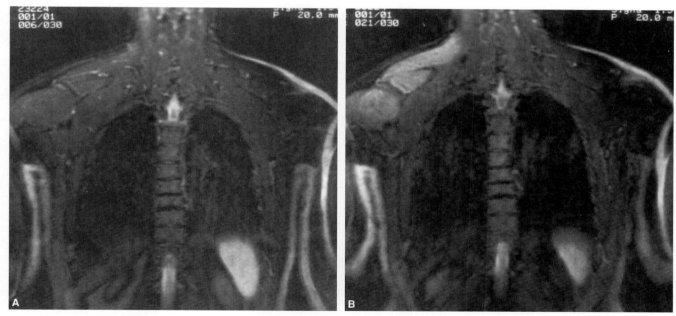

FIGURE 17-26. MR imaging showing exercise-induced changes in signal intensity. Coronal plane IR-FSE images obtained immediately before (**A**) and after (**B**) the subject performed unilateral, side-lateral dumb bell raise exercise. Note the high signal intensity changes seen in the muscles of the rotator cuff. This information is often useful for evaluation of rehabilitation programs designed for training specific muscle groups (TR/TI/TE, 3600/35/160 msec).

imaging has been used to determine the correlation between the volume of muscle damage with a reduction in strength.[6] MR images can be reformatted using commercially available, three-dimensional computer software in order to provide a more realistic depiction of muscle anatomy, volume, and morphology on a single image, as opposed to viewing muscle on multiple consecutive two-dimensional images.[18]

A three-dimensional reconstruction of MR images of muscle can easily delineate normal and injured muscles, as well as demonstrate muscle pathology related to morphologic alterations[4,26,27] (Fig. 17-27). A three-dimensional reconstruction also permits spatial correlation of the affected muscle in one image instead of having to rely on multiple sections.[18]

PITFALLS OF MR IMAGING OF MUSCLE INJURIES

Magnetic resonance imaging pitfalls or "look-alikes" of exertional muscle injury span all categories of disease. For example, the MR signal changes seen with muscle damage may be very similar to changes caused by other forms of trauma or pathology, including neoplasm, radiation, denervation, bacterial infection, polymyositis, hemorrhage, and even

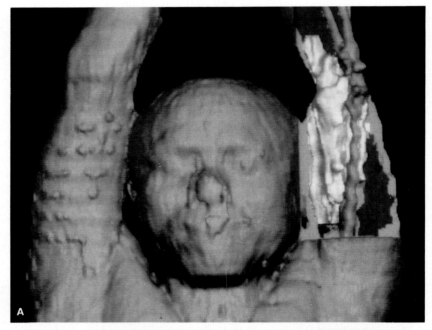

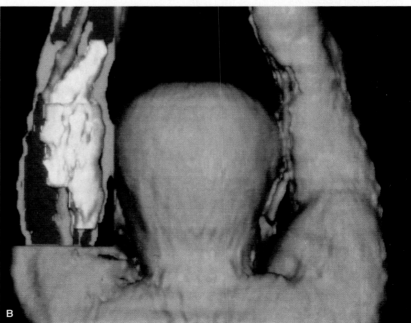

FIGURE 17-27. Three-dimensional reconstructions of exertional muscle injury. T2-weighted axial images (TR/TE, 2000/80 msec) superimposed on high-resolution (TR/TE, 600/20 msec) images shown in (**A**) anterior and (**B**) posterior projections reveal high signal intensity primarily localized in the muscle-tendon junction of the biceps and brachialis muscles.

acute exercise.[1,2,18,39,41] As discussed earlier, the sequelae of muscle damage may also mimic the precipitating injuries. Therefore, it is advisable to obtain a thorough clinical history and to correlate the findings with MR imaging results.

References

1. Ehman RL, Berquist TH. Magnetic resonance imaging of musculoskeletal trauma. Radiol Clin North Am 1986;24:291.
2. Fleckenstein JL, Weatherall PT, Parkey RW, Payne JA, Peshock RM. Sports-related muscle injuries: evaluation with MR imaging. Radiology 1988;172:793.
3. De Smet AA, Fisher DR, Heiner JP, Keene JS. Magnetic resonance imaging of muscle tears. Skeletal Radiol 1990;19:283.
4. Shellock FG, Fukunaga T, Mink JH, Edgerton VR. Serial MRI evaluation of exertional muscle injury: concentric vs. eccentric actions. Radiology 1991;179:659.
5. Fleckenstein JL, Peshock RM, Lewis SF, Haller RG. Magnetic resonance imaging of muscle injury and atrophy in glycolytic myopathies. Muscle Nerve 1989;12:849.
6. Shellock FG, Fukunaga T, Day K, Mink JH, Edgerton VR. Serial MRI and Cybex testing evaluations of exertional muscle injury: concentric vs. eccentric actions [abstr]. Med Sci Sports Exer 1991;23:110.
7. Lamminen AE, Hekali PE, Tiula E, Suramo I, Korhola OA. Acute rhabdomyolysis: evaluation with magnetic resonance imaging compared with computed tomography and ultrasonography. Br J Radiol 1989;62:326.
8. Polak JF, Jolesz FA, Adams DE. Magnetic resonance imaging of skeletal muscle prolongation of T1 and T2 subsequent to denervation. Invest Radiol 1988;23:365.
9. Jolesz FA, Schwartz LH, Sreter E, et al. Proton NMR of fast and slow twitch muscles and the effects of stimulation. Proc Soc Magn Reson Med 1986;2:444.
10. Fleckenstein JL, Canby RC, Parkey RW, Peshock RM. Acute effects of exercise on MR imaging of skeletal muscle in normal volunteers. AJR 1988;15:231.
11. Fleckenstein JL, Bertocci LA, Nunnally RL, Parkey RW, Peshock RM. Exercised-enhanced MR imaging of variations in forearm muscle anatomy and use: importance in MR spectroscopy. AJR 1989;153:693.
12. Shellock FG, Fukunaga T, Mink JH, Edgerton VR. Acute effects of exercise on skeletal muscle: concentric vs eccentric actions. AJR 1991;156:765.
13. Amendola A, Rorabeck CH, Vellett D, Vezina W, Rutt B, Nott L. The use of magnetic resonance imaging on exertional compartment syndromes. Am J Sports Med 1990;18:29.
14. Fisher MR, Dooms GC, Hricak H, Reinhold C, Higgins CB. Magnetic resonance imaging of the normal and pathologic muscular system. Magn Reson Imaging 1986;4:491.
15. Fleckenstein JL, Burns D, Murphy K, Jayson H, Bonte F. Differential diagnosis of bacterial myositis in AIDS: MRI evaluation. Radiology 1991;179:653.
16. Murphy WA, Totty WG, Carroll JE. MRI of normal and pathologic skeletal muscle. AJR 1986;146:565.
17. Dooms GC, Fisher MR, Hricak H, Higgins CB. MR imaging of intramuscular hemorrhage. J Comput Assist Tomogr 1985;9:908.
18. Fleckenstein JL, Shellock FG. Exertional muscle injuries: magnetic resonance imaging evaluation. Top Magn Reson Imaging 1991;3:50.
19. Fukunaga T, Roy RR, Shellock FG, et al. Physiological cross-sectional area of human leg muscles based on magnetic resonance imaging. J Orthop Res 1992;10:926.
20. LeBlanc A, Gogia P, Schneider V, Krebs J, Schonfeld E, Evans H. Calf muscle area and strength changes after five weeks of horizontal bed rest. Am J Sports Med 1988;16:624.

21. Beneke R, Neuerbug J, Bohndorf K. Muscle cross-section measurement by magnetic resonance imaging. Eur J Physiol 1991;63:424.
22. Narici MV, Roi GS, Landoni L. Force of knee extensor and flexor muscles and cross-sectional area determined by nuclear magnetic resonance imaging. Eur J Appl Physiol 1988;57:39.
23. Narici MV, Roi GS, Landoni L, Minetti AE, Cerretelli P. Changes in force, cross-sectional area and neural activation during strength training and detraining of the human quadriceps. Eur J Appl Physiol 1989;59:310.
24. Narici MV, Landoni L, Minnetti AE. Assessment of human knee extensor muscle stress from in vivo physiological cross-sectional area and strength measurements. Eur J Appl Physiol 1992;65:438.
25. McColl RW, Fleckenstein JL, Bowers J, Theriault G, Peshock RM. Three-dimensional reconstruction of skeletal muscle from MRI. Comput Med Imaging Graph 1992;16:363.
26. Flicker PL, Fleckenstein JL, Ferry K, et al. Lumbar muscle usage in chronic low back pain: MRI evaluation 1993.
27. Bowers J, Theriault G, Fleckenstein J, et al. Three-dimensional reconstruction of skeletal muscle in health and disease. J Magn Reson Imaging 1991;1:235.
28. Engstrom CM, Loeb GE, Reid JG, Forrest WJ, Avruch L. Morphometry of the human thigh muscles: a comparison between anatomical sections and computer tomographic and magnetic resonance images. J Anat 1991;176:139.
29. Shellock FG, Mink JH, Deutsch AL. MR imaging of muscle injuries. Appl Radiol 1994;23:11.
30. Fleckenstein JL, Haller RG, Lewis SF, et al. Absence of exercise-induced MRI enhancement of skeletal muscle in McArdle's disease. J Appl Physiol 1991;71:961.
31. Fleckenstein JL, Haller RG, Bertocci LA, Parkey RW, Peshock RM. Glycogenolysis, not perfusion, is the critical mediator or exercise-induced muscle modifications on MR images. Radiology 1992;183:25.
32. Peshock R, Fleckenstein J, Payne J, Lewis S, Mitchell J, Haller R. Muscle usage patterns during cycling: MRI evaluation. Med Sci Sports Exerc 1990;22:S91.
33. McCully K, Shellock FG, Bank W, Posner J. The use of nuclear magnetic resonance to evaluate muscle injury. Med Sci Sports Exerc 1992;24:537.
34. Fleckenstein JL, Watumull D, Bertocci LA, et al. Finger-specific flexor recruitment in humans: depiction by exercise-enhanced MRI. J Appl Physiol 1992;72:1974.
35. Jeneson JAL, Taylor JS, Vigneron DB, et al. 1H MR imaging of anatomical compartments with the finger flexor muscles of the human forearm. Magn Reson Med 1990;15:491.
36. Morvan D, Vilgrain V, Arrive L, Nahum H. Correlation of MR changes with doppler US measurements of blood flow in exercising normal muscle. J Magn Reson Imaging 1992;2:645.
37. Shellock FG, Horrigan J, Mink JH, Deutsch A. MRI of muscle recruitment patterns associated with different shoulder exercises. J Magn Reson Imaging 1994;WIP:S25.
38. Shellock FG, Fleckenstein J, Tyson L. MR Imaging of skeletal muscle exercise physiology and pathophysiology. In: Fleckenstein J, ed. Diagnostic imaging of skeletal muscle. New York: Springer-Verlag, 1996.
39. Mink JH. Muscle injuries. In: Mink JH, Reicher MA, Crues JV, Deutsch AL, eds. MRI of the knee. New York: Raven Press, 1995:401.
40. LeBlanc A, Evans H, Schonfeld E, et al. Changes in nuclear magnetic resonance (T2) relaxation of limb tissue with bed rest. Magn Reson Med 1987;4:487.
41. Fleckenstein JL, Weatherall PT, Bertocci LA, et al. Locomotor system assessment by muscle magnetic resonance imaging. Magn Reson Q 1991;7:79.
42. Nurenberg P, Giddings C, Stray-Gundersen J, Fleckenstein JL, Gonyea WJ, Peshock RM. MR imaging-guided muscle biopsy for correlation of increased signal intensity with ultrastructural change and delayed-onset muscle soreness after exercise. Radiology 1992;184:865.
43. Herfkens RJ, Sievers R, Kaufman L, et al. Nuclear magnetic resonance imaging of the infarcted muscle: a rat model. Radiology 1983;147:761.

44. Dwyer AJ, Frank JA, Sank VJ, Reinig JW, Hickey AM, Doppman JL. Short-TI inversion recovery pulse sequence: analysis and initial experience in cancer imaging. Radiology 1988;168:827.

45. Fleckenstein JL, Archer B, Barker B, Vaughn T, Parkey RW, Peshock RM. Fast, short tau inversion recovery imaging. Radiology 1991;179:499.

46. Shellock FG, Schatz CJ, Hahn P. MRI evaluation of traumatic TMJ abnormalities: comparison between T2 weighted and STIR pulse sequences. J Magn Reson Imaging 1994;WIP:S25.

47. Fischer MJ, Meyer RA, Adams GR, Foley JM, Potchen EJ. Direct relationship between proton T2 and exercise intensity in skeletal muscle MR images. Invest Radiol 1990;25:480.

48. Archer BT, Fleckenstein JL, Bertocci LA, et al. Effect of perfusion on exercised muscle: MR imaging evaluation. J Magn Reson Imaging 1992;2:407.

49. Cohen MS, Shellock FG, Nadeau KA, et al. Acute muscle T2 changes during exercise [book of abstracts]. Soc Magn Reson Med 1991;107.

50. Sjorgaard G, Saltin B. Extra- and intracellular water spaces in muscles of man at rest and with dynamic exercise. Am J Physiol 1982;12:R271.

51. Nelson TR, Tung SM. Temperature dependence of proton relaxation times in vitro. Magn Reson Imaging 1987;5:189.

52. Weidman ER, Charles HC, Negro-Vilar R, Sullivan MJ, MacFall JR. Muscle activity localization with 31P spectroscopy and calculated T2 weighted 1H images. Invest Radiol 1991;26:309.

53. Charles HC, Covington TD, Cobb FR, Kennedy JE, Negro-Vilar R, Sullivan MJ. Heterogeneous patterns of skeletal muscle metabolism after bicycle ergometry as assessed with T2 weighted H-1 MR imaging mapping [book of abstracts]. Soc Magn Reson Med 1991;107.

54. Adams GR, Duvoisin MR, Dudley GA. Magnetic resonance imaging and electromyography as indexes of muscle function. J Appl Physiol 1992;73:1578.

55. Armstrong RB. Mechanisms of exercise-induced delayed onset muscular soreness: a brief review. Med Sci Sports Exerc 1984;16:529.

56. Evans WJ, Cannon JG. The metabolic effects of exercise-induced muscle damage. In: Holloszy JO, ed. Exercise and sport sciences reviews. Baltimore: Williams & Wilkins, 1991:99.

57. Abraham WM. Factors in delayed muscle soreness. Med Sci Sports 1977;9:11.

58. Kibler WB. Clinical aspects of muscle injury. Med Sci Sports Med 1990;22:450.

59. Glick JM. Muscle strains: prevention and treatment. Physician Sports Med 1980;8:73.

60. O'Donoghue DH. Principals in the management of specific injuries. In: Treatment of injuries to athletes, 4th ed. Philadelphia: WB Saunders, 1984:51.

61. Ryan AJ. Quadriceps strain: rupture and charley horse. Med Sci Sports 1969;1:106.

62. Oakes BW. Hamstring muscle injuries. Aust Fam Physician 1984;13:587.

63. Larsson SE, Bengtsson A, Bodegard L, Henricksson KG, Larsson J. Muscle changes in work-related chronic myalgia. Acta Orthop Scand 1988;59:552.

64. Repetition strain injury [editorial]. Lancet 1987;ii(8554):316.

65. Ireland DC. Repetitive strain injury. Aust Fam Physician 1986;15:415.

66. Lockwood AH. Medical problems of musicians. N Engl J Med 1989;320:221.

67. Frymoyer JW, Mooney V. Occupational orthopaedics. J Bone Joint Surg 1986;68:469.

68. Garrett WE. Injuries to the muscle-tendon unit. Instr Course Lect 1988;37:275.

69. Garrett WE. Muscle strain injuries: clinical and basic aspects. Med Sci Sports Exerc 1990;22:436.

70. Gilcreest EL. Rupture of muscles and tendon, particularly subcutaneous rupture of biceps flexor cubiti. JAMA 1925;84:1819.

71. Tarsney FF. Rupture and avulsion of the triceps. Clin Orthop 1972;83:177.

72. Herring SA. Rehabilitation of muscle injuries. Med Sci Sports Exerc 1990;22:453.

73. Bobbert MF, Hollander AP, Huining PA. Factors in delayed onset muscular onset soreness of man. Med Sci Sports Exerc 1986;18:75.

74. Jones DA, Newham DJ, Round JM, Tolfree SEJ. Experimental human muscle damage: morphological changes in relation to other indices of damage. J Physiol 1986;375:435.

75. Newham DJ, McPhail G, Mills KR, Edwards RHT. Ultrastructural changes after concentric and eccentric contractions of human muscle. J Neurol Sci 1983;61:109.

76. Clarkson PM, Tremblay I. Exercise-induced muscle damage, repair, and adaptation in humans. J Appl Physiol 1988;65:1.

77. Friden J, Sfakianos PN, Hargens AR. Muscle soreness and intramuscular fluid pressure: comparison between eccentric and concentric load. J Appl Physiol 1986;61:2175.

78. Swensen SJ, Keller PL, Berquist TH, et al. Magnetic resonance of hemorrhage. AJR 1985;145:921.

79. Jackson DW, Feagin JA. Quadriceps contusions in young adults: relationship of severity of injury to treatment and prognosis. J Bone Joint Surg [Am] 1973;55:95.

80. Amendola M, Glazer GM, Agha Z, et al. Myositis ossificans circumscripta: computed tomographic diagnosis. Radiology 1983;149:775.

Index

Page numbers followed by *f* indicate figures; page numbers followed by *t* indicate tabular material.